Diseases of the Veins

Diseases of the Veins

SECOND EDITION

NORMAN L BROWSE Kt, MD, FRCS, FRCP

Emeritus Professor of Surgery, United Medical and Dental Schools of Guy's and
St Thomas's Hospitals.
Hon. Consulting Surgeon, St Thomas's Hospital, London, UK

KEVIN G BURNAND MS, FRCS

Professor of Surgery, United Medical and Dental Schools of Guy's and St Thomas's Hospitals.
Consultant Surgeon, St Thomas's Hospital, London, UK

ALLAN T IRVINE MRCP, FRCR

Honorary Senior Lecturer, St Thomas's Hospital.
Consultant Radiologist, Department of Radiology, United Medical and Dental Schools of
Guy's and St Thomas's Hospitals, London, UK

NICHOLAS M WILSON BSc, MS, FRCS

Consultant Vascular Surgeon, Department of Surgery, Royal Hampshire County Hospital,
Winchester, Hampshire, UK

A member of the Hodder Headline Group
LONDON • SYDNEY • AUCKLAND
Co-published in the USA by Oxford University Press, Inc., New York

First published in Great Britain in 1988
Second edition published in Great Britain in 1999
by Arnold, a member of the Hodder Headline Group,
338 Euston Road, London NW1 3BH
http://www.arnoldpublishers.com

Co-published in the United States of America by
Oxford University Press, Inc.,
198 Madison Avenue, New York, NY 10016
Oxford is a registered trademark of Oxford University Press

Whilst the advice and information in this book is believed to be true and
accurate at the date of going to press, neither the authors nor the publisher
can accept any legal responsibility or liability for any errors or omissions
that may be made. In particular (but without limiting the generality of the
preceding disclaimer) every effort has been made to check drug dosages;
however, it is still possible that errors have been missed. Furthermore,
dosage schedules are constantly being revised and new side-effects
recognized. For these reasons the reader is strongly urged to consult the
drug companies' printed instructions before administering any of the drugs
recommended in this book.

British Library Cataloguing in Publication Data
A catalogue record for this book is available from the British Library

Library of Congress Cataloging-in-Publication Data
A catalog record for this book is available from the Library of Congress

ISBN 0 340 58894 2

Publisher: Annalisa Page
Project Editor: Melissa Morton
Production Editor: James Rabson
Production Controller: Helen Whitehorn
Cover designer: Terry Griffiths

Typeset in 10/11 Times
Composition by Scribe Design, Gillingham, Kent
Printed and bound in Great Britain by The Bath Press, Avon

Dedication

To the memory of Dr Michael Lea Thomas,
radiologist, pioneer phlebographer, colleague, friend
and co-author of the first edition of this book

Contents

Preface to the second edition — xi
Acknowledgements to the second edition — xii
Preface to the first edition — xiii
Acknowledgements to the first edition — xiv

1 **Milestones, pebbles and grains of sand** — **1**
References — 21

2 **Embryology and radiographic anatomy** — **23**
Development and congenital
   anomalies — 23
Anatomy of the lower limb veins — 30
Anatomy of the upper limb veins — 44
References — 47

3 **Physiology and functional anatomy** — **49**
Physiology — 49
The functional anatomy of the calf
   pump — 55
The physiology of the calf pump — 57
The causes of calf pump failure — 59
The arm veins — 62
References — 62

4 **Techniques of investigation** — **67**
Clinical examination — 69
Investigations that provide images of the
   veins and/or thrombus — 72
Investigations that provide images of
   thrombus in the lungs — 108
Investigations of venous function — 112
Commentary — 130
References — 132

5 **Varicose veins: pathology** — **145**
Epidemiology — 145
Aetiology — 147
Pathology — 156
References — 158

6 **Varicose veins: diagnosis** — **163**
The symptoms caused by varicose veins — 163
History — 169
Physical signs of varicose veins — 169
Summary — 177
Special investigations of the superficial
   veins — 178
Definition of the extent and connections
   of varicosities — 182
Special investigations of the deep veins — 183
Suggested diagnostic pathways — 185
References — 187

7 **Varicose veins: natural history and
   treatment** — **191**
The natural history of untreated and
   uncomplicated varicose veins — 191
Treatment: general — 193
Surgical treatment of varicose veins — 195
Injection sclerotherapy — 231
Alternative treatments of varicose veins — 237
Results of treatment — 237
Varicose veins of pregnancy and vulval
   varicosities — 239
Treatment of dilated intradermal venules — 241
Treatment of the complications of
   varicose veins — 241
References — 241

8   Deep vein thrombosis: pathology   **249**
Prevalence and incidence of deep vein
  thrombosis   249
Aetiology of deep vein thrombosis   254
Temporal changes in a deep vein
  thrombus   273
References   276

9   Deep vein thrombosis: diagnosis   **291**
Practical significance of the symptoms
  and signs   299
Investigations   301
Clinical application of tests for deep
  vein thrombosis   308
Conclusions   310
References   311

10   Deep vein thrombosis: treatment   **319**
Thrombolysis   320
Thrombectomy   329
Anticoagulation   340
Defibrinogenation   351
Summary   352
References   353

11   Deep vein thrombosis: prevention   **359**
Pharmacological methods of
  prevention   360
Mechanical methods of prevention   368
Commentary   371
References   373

12   Chronic deep vein incompetence   **385**
Normal valves   385
Pathology   387
Pathophysiology   389
Diagnosis   389
Treatment   394
Commentary   404
References   405

13   Chronic deep vein obstruction   **409**
Pathology   409
Clinical presentation   415
Investigations   416
Treatment   419
References   425

**14   Acquired obstruction of the inferior
     vena cava (IVC)**   **429**
Pathology   429
Clinical presentation   430
Investigations   431
Treatment   437
Prognosis   440
References   441

**15   The calf pump failure syndrome:
     pathology**   **443**
The effect of deep vein thrombosis
  on vein function   444
The effect of thrombosis on calf pump
  function   454
The effect of calf pump failure on the
  microcirculation of the lower limb   458
Prevalence   466
References   467

**16   The calf pump failure syndrome:
     diagnosis**   **473**
Diagnosis   473
Investigations   479
References   483

**17   The calf pump failure syndrome:
     treatment**   **485**
Natural history   485
Treatment   486
References   500

18   Venous ulceration: pathology   **505**
Prevalence and incidence of venous
  ulceration   505
Aetiology of venous ulceration   508
The pathology of a venous ulcer   521
References   525

19   Venous ulceration: diagnosis   **531**
The clinical features of venous ulceration   531
Investigations   537
Differential diagnosis of leg ulcers   539
Investigation of a venous ulcer   562
References   566

**20   Venous ulceration: natural history and
     treatment**   **571**
Natural history   571
Treatment   573
Prevention of ulcer recurrence   591
References   598

21   Pulmonary embolism   **605**
Pulmonary thromboembolic disease   605
Investigations   610
Diagnosis   616
Differential diagnosis   616
Natural history and prognosis   616
Treatment   617
Prophylaxis of pulmonary embolism   622
Some other special situations in
  pulmonary embolic disease   623
Other forms of pulmonary
  embolism which may mimic
  thromboembolism   624
References   625

22 Prevention of pulmonary embolism 631
Primary prevention (through the
prevention of deep vein thrombosis) 632
Secondary prevention (prevention of
embolism from established
thrombosis) 636
References 651

23 Superficial thrombophlebitis 657
Pathology 657
Diagnosis 659
Treatment 660
References 662

24 Congenital venous abnormalities 665
Pathology 665
Congenital vena caval obstruction 670
Klippel–Trenaunay syndrome 671
Popliteal vein entrapment 686
References 686

**25 Occlusion of the veins of the upper
arm and neck 689**
Axillary/subclavian vein thrombosis 689
Superior vena caval occlusion and
thrombosis 702
References 707

26 Venous injury 711
Incidence 711
Classification 714
Clinical presentation 717
Investigation 717
Treatment: general considerations 717
References 726

27 Venous tumours 731
Cystic degeneration of the vein wall 731
Venous (cavernous) haemangioma 732
Leiomyoma and leiomyosarcoma of
the vein wall 742
References 745

Index 747

Preface to the second edition

It is ten years since the first edition of *Diseases of the Veins* was published. In those years three developments have encouraged the growth of research into the problems of venous pathophysiology. First, the refinement of duplex ultrasound scanning has allowed many clinicians to become directly involved in the study of the physiology and pathology of venous disease. Secondly, an increased understanding of the role of, and interactions between, the circulating blood cells and the vascular endothelium has stimulated research into the changes in the microcirculation precipitated by an inadequate venous return, especially those that lead to venous ulceration. Thirdly, this new knowledge, combined with the accessibility of the new methods of investigation, has stimulated the formation of many Societies and Associations, particularly in the USA, dedicated to the promotion of research and the promulgation of our understanding of venous problems.

These developments have influenced the contents of this second edition of *Diseases of the Veins*. The most obvious change is a considerable increase in the number of references at the end of each chapter. The other changes are less obvious and consist mainly of a reappraisal, but sometimes abandonment, of some theories and treatments based on a better, though still incomplete, understanding of the physiology, diagnosis and treatment of venous disease derived from the published research studies and clinical trials of the past ten years.

Although many small pieces of new knowledge have increased our overall understanding of venous disease, major problems remain unsolved. We still do not know why 'primary' varicose veins develop. We still do not know which aspects of calf pump dysfunction are the important precursors of venous ulceration. We still do not know how calf pump failure causes the tissue necrosis that we see as venous ulceration. We know how we can reduce the incidence of postoperative deep vein thrombosis and probably pulmonary embolism but cannot abolish either and when thrombosis has occurred we cannot restore the affected veins and their valves to normal.

This edition summarizes the position in 1997–98. We hope that future editions will contain the answers that diligent clinical and laboratory research will provide to the many questions that this edition leaves unanswered.

London 1998
NLB
KGB
ATI
NMW

Acknowledgements to the second edition

Dr Michael Lea Thomas – our first edition co-author and expert phlebographist – died in 1991. We are most grateful that Dr Alan Irvine, his successor at St Thomas's, agreed to take over the authorship of the radiographic and ultrasonic aspects of this book. We are also fortunate that Mr Nicholas Wilson, vascular surgeon, friend and former Resident, agreed to take on the revision of a number of chapters. The individual contribution of these two new co-authors is not itemized within the book because the whole is a joint effort with a common style. Their contributions have nevertheless been considerable and significant.

Two chapters required a level of expert experience and knowledge that the four main authors could not provide. Professor Roger Hall, Professor of Clinical Cardiology, RPGMS, kindly revised the chapter on Pulmonary Embolism previously written by Dr Graham Miller. Dr Beverley Hunt, Consultant Haematologist at St Thomas's Hospital, helped to revise and update the chapter on the aetiology of venous thrombosis, especially the section on thrombophilia. We are most grateful for their help.

Dr Jarosz, Senior Registrar in Dr Irvine's department, gave valuable help with the sections on CT and MRI scanning.

Even in this modern world of computers, word processors and hard disks, someone has to transfer authors' thoughts into words on disks and manuscripts. Mrs Julia Hague has given us invaluable secretarial support aided by Mrs Carole Goodall, Mrs Liz Paine and Miss Janine Lawrence.

This revision has taken longer and been a far greater task than originally anticipated. We thank all the staff of Arnold for their patience and encouragement.

We wanted all the clinical photographs in this edition to be in colour. We are extremely grateful that Mr GJ Collyer, Research Director of Seton–Scholl Ltd, agreed to provide the financial sponsorship that has enabled us to achieve this ambition. Seton Healthcare's support of this book is but a small part of its overall support and sponsorship of clinical research into the problems of venous disease for which we are especially grateful.

Preface to the first edition

Interest in the physiology and pathology of the veins has waxed and waned over the centuries. The development of methods of measuring blood pressure and blood flow gave an enormous impetus to the study of the circulation but the new methods were mainly applied to the heart and arteries. For the first forty years of this century the veins could truly be thought of as the Cinderella of the circulation, neglected, and almost forgotten.

The past forty years has seen a steady change in this attitude brought about by the efforts of a relatively small number of physiologists, surgeons and radiologists such as Kenneth Franklin, Edwin Wood, John Shepherd, John Ludbrook, Robert Linton, Harold Dodd, Frank Cockett, Robert May, Carl Arnoldi, JC dos Santos, Gunnar Bauer, T Greitz, A Gullmo and Orsen Almen.

The scientific study of venous disease began when JC dos Santos introduced phlebography. By chance the beginning of our own interest in venous thrombosis, pulmonary embolism, venous ulceration, the post-thrombotic syndrome and varicose veins coincided with the invention and acceptance of the X-ray contrast media that made phlebography safe – a technical 'breakthrough' that enabled our inquisitiveness to flourish, produce over 300 publications and to write this book.

A book describing and criticizing every publication about the veins would extend into many volumes. We therefore chose to write a book which analyses and discusses what we consider to be the important publications on venous disease but which also presents our own views and attitudes to venous problems, with ample references for the reader who wishes to seek out the sources on which our opinions are based.

We hope that the result is a practical, readable book containing something for medical students, residents and consultants, which quotes facts but which questions current views and stimulates the reader to begin his own enquires.

We are particularly indebted to Dr Graham Miller for his excellent chapter on Pulmonary Embolism. All the other chapters have been written by ourselves.

Two areas have been intentionally omitted, the intracerebral veins and the portal venous system, because disorders for these veins are usually fully discussed in textbooks of neurosurgery and gastroenterology as they tend to present to specialists in these fields rather then to generalists or phlebologists.

Many of the views presented in this book have developed from our association with the physiologists, radiologists and surgeons already mentioned, our former research associates and residents, J Ackroyd, MR Andress, P Baskerville, R Beard, JN Bowles, GM Briggs, A Chilvers, EW Fletcher, L Gray, P Jarrett, G Layer, R Leach, D Negus, T O'Donnell, A Pimm, J Waters, S Whitehead, and our excellent Technical Staff, D Rutt, D Sizeland, Marian Morland and Gill Clemenson. This book is the fruit of all our labours. We hope it is a worthwhile contribution to the dissemination of knowledge about diseases of the veins.

London, 1988
NLB
KGB
MLT

Acknowledgements to the first edition

All three of us owe much to the stimulation of our colleagues and teachers. Many have been mentioned in the preface but three deserve special mention, John Shepherd, John Kinmonth and Frank Cockett. Our interest in the veins and the peripheral circulation would never have begun if we had not met and worked with these men.

Our research has depended upon the devoted support of the technical staff of the Department of Surgery and Radiology of St Thomas' Hospital, London, guided by Mr DL Rutt, Senior Chief Medical Laboratory Scientific Officer and Miss DA Hannigan, Senior Radiographer.

The illustrations have been produced by Mr TW Brandon and his colleagues in the Department of Photography.

We are most grateful to Sterling Research Laboratories for defraying the cost of coloured illustrations.

The burden of typing the manuscript has fallen on our secretaries, Julia Hague, Solveig Joannides, Barbara Neal and Linda Lewis. In addition to working on the manuscript, Vivienne Beckett and David Sizeland have catalogued and checked all the references.

We are greatly indebted to all those mentioned and many others for their support and encouragement and particularly to our Publishers, Edward Arnold, who encouraged us to write the book yet accepted the delays that are inevitable when busy clinicians try to write.

CHAPTER 1

Milestones, pebbles and grains of sand

Time, and the judgement of our successors, will decide which of the papers on venous disease published in this century have made a major contribution to the advancement of our knowledge and understanding. Even the smallest paper helps to expand our knowledge. The greatest house needs grains of sand in its cement to hold the bricks and the keystones in place.

This chapter presents the publications, in chronological order, which we think have advanced contemporary understanding. They show that man has had a considerable empirical understanding of the treatment of venous problems for at least 2000 years but that a real appreciation of the physiological and pathological processes involved had to await the greatest advance of all, William Harvey's description of the circulation of the blood.

The story begins in Ancient Egypt.

1550 BC

The first 'venous' publication?

The Ebers papyrus was written in 1550 BC. One section contains a description of three types of lump, together with the advice that two types can be treated surgically but 'certain serpentine windings are not to be operated upon because that would be "head on the ground"'.

Majno and others[16,20,23] have suggested that the term 'serpentine windings' means varicose veins which should not be incised lest a fatal ('head on the ground') haemorrhage occur. If this interpretation is correct, this is the first known publication about the treatment of varicose veins.

Ebers Papyrus, 1550 BC.

4TH CENTURY BC

The first illustration of a varicose vein?

Figure 1.1 is a votive tablet found at the foot of the Acropolis in Athens. It shows the medial side of a massive leg with a long serpentine swelling which has all the characteristics of a varicose vein. Is the small mortal performing a Trendelenburg test on his God, or does the God have gross hypertrophy of the limb with congenitally abnormal veins? This is the oldest known illustration of a varicose vein. Perhaps Doctor Amynos, to whom the tablet is dedicated, was one of the world's first phlebologists.

6TH CENTURY BC

The first description of a function for the veins?

In his description of the life and works of Alcmaeon of Croton, Codellas states that Alcmaeon believed that 'sleep was the retreat of blood to the veins and awakening its forth pouring' and that death was caused by 'the total retreat of blood to the veins'.[9]

The Works of Alcmaeon of Croton, 6th century BC.

460–377 BC

Hippocrates and the veins

There are many references to the vascular system and to ulcers in the works of Hippocrates. [1,8,18]

In *De Carnibus* he states that 'two vessels arise from the heart, the one called an artery the other

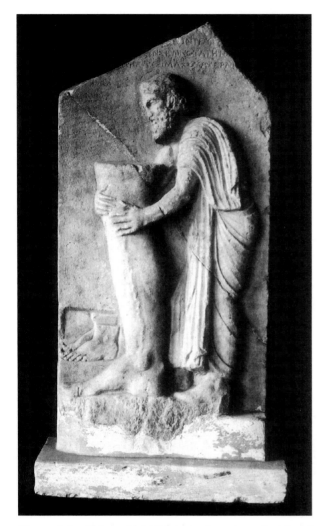

Figure 1.1 This votive tablet was found on the site of the sanctuary (temple) of the hero, Doctor Amynos, at the base of the west side of the Acropolis in Athens. According to the inscription, it was offered and dedicated to Doctor Amynos by Lysimachidis of Acharnes, son of Lysimachos. It is estimated to date from the end of the 4th century BC. It is the earliest known depiction of varicose veins. (We are grateful to the National Archeological Museum of Greece for permission to reproduce this illustration and for the historical information.)

called a vein'. When discussing wounds he describes the fact that a loose tourniquet will cause excessive bleeding whereas a tight tourniquet may cause gangrene.

In *De Ulceribus* he states that 'in the case of an ulcer it is not expedient to stand, more especially if the ulcer be situated in the leg' and then describes the causes of ulcers including, possibly, venous thrombosis. He also says, 'We must avoid wetting ulcers except with wine, unless the ulcer be situated near a joint, for the dry is nearer to the sound and the wet to the unsound'.

A little later he warns, 'When a varix is on the fore part of the leg and is superficial, or below the flesh, and the leg is black and seems to stand in need of having the blood evacuated from it, such swellings are not by any means to be cut open, for generally large ulcers are the consequences of the incisions'. Is this a warning against the treatment of superficial thrombophlebitis in the gaiter area of the leg by incision and evacuation of the thrombosis?

Majno[21] has compiled a description of how Hippocrates would have treated a fat woman with varicose veins and a venous ulcer based on the many references to ulcers found throughout the Hippocratic texts. He suggests that Hippocrates would have given the following advice:

- Wash the ulcer, only puncture it once in a while lest a large sore follow.
- If necessary, cut out the ulcer and then compress it to squeeze out the blood and humours.

Perhaps this is the first reference to compression dressings for venous ulceration even though the main objective was to keep the ulcer open to let out the 'evil humours'.

Hippocrates. *De Ulceribus* and *De Carnibus*, 460–377 BC.

479–300 BC

Did the Chinese recognize venous ulceration?

The Yellow Emperor's Classic of Internal Medicine was written by Huang Ti Nei Ching Su Wen. Although the Yellow Emperor lived in 2600 BC, the book was probably written between 479 and 300 BC, making it contemporary with Hippocrates. It certainly describes the treatment of ulcers but whether it refers to varicose veins depends entirely upon the translator's interpretation of the ancient text.[30] This interpretation varies considerably in different translations, making it difficult to decide whether the Chinese physicians recognized a connection between venous abnormalities and ulceration.

Huang Ti Nei Ching Su Wen. *The Yellow Emperor's Classic of Internal Medicine*, 400 BC.

335 BC

Veins are different from arteries

Praxagoras of Cos was probably the first physician to differentiate between arteries and veins when, on postmortem evidence, he mistakenly stated that the veins contained blood whereas the arteries contained air.[17,27]

The Writings of Praxagoras, 335 BC.

270 BC

The ligation of blood vessels. The beginning of vascular surgery

The foundation of the Alexandrian School of Medicine in Egypt and the innovations of its two greatest physicians, Herophilos and Erasistratos, were the progenitors of vascular surgery. These physicians invented artery forceps and were the first to ligate blood vessels, thus controlling bleeding and making surgery possible.[22] They noticed that the valves of the heart stopped retrograde blood flow[19] and, although they thought that the arteries contained air, Erasistratos knew that a tourniquet caused congestion of the venous blood in a limb but did not know how this occurred because he did not appreciate that the blood circulated.[6,24] Burggraeve states that Herophilos discovered the lacteals.[5]

The works of these remarkable men were lost when the great library at Alexandria was destroyed in AD 391, a tragic event that delayed the advance of medicine for 1000 years.

200 BC

Indian ulcers

The practice of medicine developed in India at the same time and just as swiftly as in the Mediterranean. The main textbook of Indian surgery was *The Sushruta Samhita* which describes the treatment of ulcers with maggots to clear away necrotic material, curettage, and dressings using leaves. It also describes the use of Chinese cloth bandage for the treatment of ulcers. The inelastic material would have acted in the same way as a modern impregnated bandage.

The Sushruta Samhita, 200 BC. Translated by KL Bhishogratna. Chowkhamba Sanskrit Series Office. India, Varanasi 1907–1911.

AD 14–37

Roman ulcers

Celsus was the great Roman physician. He lived during the Emperorship of Tiberius. In many of the Hippocratic texts it is not clear whether the term ulcer is used in its modern sense or as a collective noun that includes all forms of wounds. Celsus distinguished between wounds and ulcers[7] and advised the use of plasters and linen bandages to pull ulcers together. He described the ligation of veins that were bleeding, the double clamping and division of veins between ligatures, and treated varicose veins by avulsion and cauterization. He used antiseptics on wounds and described the four cardinal physical signs of inflammation.

Celsus AC. *De Medicina*, AD 25.

AD 130–200

Galen: the beginning of varicose vein surgery

Galen of Pergamum described the treatment of ulcers and varicose veins by venesection. He noticed that the walls of the veins were always much thinner than the walls of the arteries and that veins contained dark blood. He described the use of silk ligatures and advised that varicose veins should be treated by incision and tearing out with a blunt hook.[15,31]

The Works of Claudius Galen, AD 130–200

AD 502–575

According to Anning, Aetius of Amida redescribed the ligation of varicose veins in the 6th century AD.[2]

AD 900

Keep the ulcer open!

In AD 900 Avicenna was still supporting the Hippocratic view that ulcers should not be allowed to heal because they were a site from which 'evil humours' could escape. If an ulcer did heal, he advised that it should be deliberately broken down again.[29]

Avicenna. *De Ulceribus*, Lib IV, 10th century.

1306

Wrong reasons, right result

Although Maitre Henri de Mondeville described the use of bandages on the limbs to drive out the 'evil humours' from ulcers, he correctly realized that compression bandaging helped the ulcer to heal.[25] He would probably have explained ulcer healing by claiming that it was no longer needed once the bandages had expelled all the bad humours.

Chirurgie de Maitre Henri de Mondeville, 1302–1320.

1452

The anatomy of the veins as seen by a great artist

The masterly anatomical drawings of Leonardo da Vinci (Figures 1.2–1.4) show how clearly he

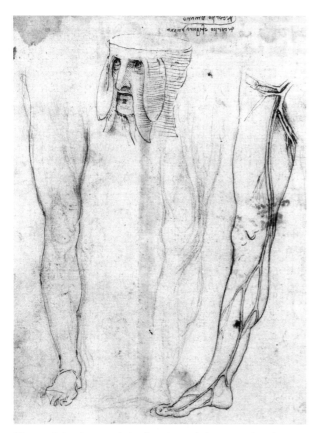

Figure 1.2 Leonardo's drawing of the superficial veins of the lower limb. This leg did not have a posterior arch vein, often called Leonardo's vein, nor are any communicating veins visible. (Royal Library, Windsor Castle. R.L. 1 2624R [QV3r] Copyright reserved. Reproduced by gracious permission of Her Majesty The Queen.)

observed the venous system. Interestingly, the leg in Figure 1.2 does not have a posterior arch vein, which is often called Leonardo's vein, and no communicating veins are shown.

1510–1590

A local compression dressing

Ambroise Paré described the ligation of varicose veins and the long saphenous vein in the thigh.[26] While he was employed as a surgeon to Henri II in 1553, he cured the ulcer of his captor, Lord Vandeville, by regular bandaging. His method was to 'roule the leg beginning at the foote and finishing

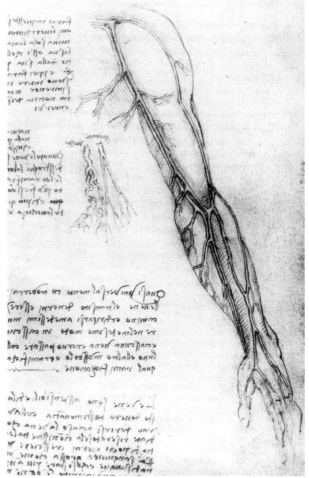

Figure 1.3 Leonardo's drawing of the superficial veins of the arm. (Royal Library, Windsor Castle. R.L. 1 9027R [formerly ANBIOr] Copyright reserved. Reproduced by gracious permission of Her Majesty The Queen.)

at the knee, not forgetting a little bolster upon the varicose veine'.

The Works of Ambroise Paré, c. 1560–1580.

1547–1580

Venous valves

In 1562 Fallopius stated that Amatus Lusitanus testified to him that Gian Battista Canano had described the valvular fold in the azygos vein to him (Amatus) in 1547. It is possible that this was the first description of a venous valve. In 1551 Amatus Lusitanus stated that the veins contained valves and

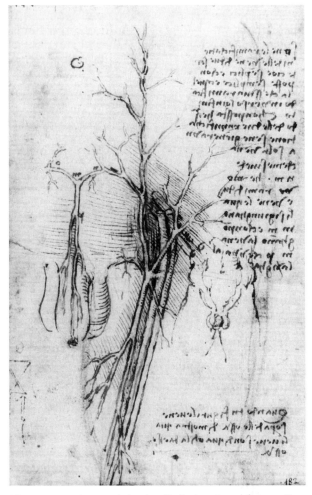

Figure 1.4 Leonardo's detailed drawing of the tributaries of the long saphenous vein in the groin. (Royal Library, Windsor Castle. R.L. 191 13R [Q1V8r] Copyright reserved. Reproduced by gracious permission of Her Majesty The Queen.)

that it was he who had given proof of this a thousand times since 1547. Whether Gian Canano or Amatus Lusitanus was the first to demonstrate the valves will never be known. Franklin[12] and Friedenwald[13] reviewed the arguments over the historical precedence but came to no conclusion. Withington[32] and Friedenwald[13] concluded that Lusitanus showed the valves to Canano, Friedenwald believing that Fallopius misunderstood the description of the dissections in Ferrara in 1547, which were conducted by Canano and Lusitanus together.

Lusitanus A. *Centuriae 1*, Curat. 52, 1551; *Centuriae V*, Curat. 70, 1560.

1514–1564

The first complete anatomical description of the veins (but no valves!)

Vesalius described the venous system in detail. It seems certain that he was told about the valves by Canano in 1546, when visiting Ratisborn. He then looked for them himself, could not find them and subsequently denied their existence.[14]

Vesalius Fabrica, 1555.

1585

A drawing of a valve, at last

Figure 1.5 is believed to be the first recorded drawing of a valve in a vein. It was published by Saloman Alberti in 1585.

Alberti, S. *De Valvatis Membraneis Quorundam Vasorum*. Tres orations. Norimb, 1585.

1593–1603

A full description of the valves

Hieronymus Fabricius of Aquapendente redescribed the valves in his work entitled *De Venarum Ostiolis* after he had demonstrated them at public dissections in 1579. He noticed that they stopped retrograde flow but thought that they participated in the control of the ebb and flow of blood described by Galen.

Fabricius may have described the relationship between gangrene and venous thrombosis in his book *Gangraena et Sphacelo*, and he definitely

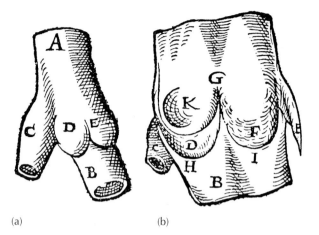

(a)   (b)

Figure 1.5 These illustrations, published by Saloman Alberti in 1585, are the first known drawings of a venous valve. (a) This shows the outside of a leg vein (AB) with muscle tributary (C). D and E are the bulging valve sinuses. (b) This shows the opened veins with the mouth of the tributary (K), the valve cusp (E) cut away to reveal the sinus (F), the agger of each cusp (H and I) and the cornua of the cusps (G).

described the double ligature and division between the ligatures of varicose veins in the book *Opera Chirurgica*.

It is significant that William Harvey worked with Fabricius between 1599 and 1603 and that Fabricius was a pupil of Fallopius who was in turn a pupil of Vesalius.

Fabricius H. *De Venarum Ostiolis*, 1603.
Fabricius H. *De Gangraena et Sphacelo*. Cologne, 1593.
Fabricius H. *Opera Chirurgica*, 1593.

1597

Gangrene associated with 'stopped' veins and arteries

Peter Lowe described two forms of gangrene. One was painful, pale, soft and black and 'in pressing on it with thy fingers, it falleth downe and riseth not', i.e. was oedematous. The other was extremely painful, very cold and associated with loss of movement and feeling. He noticed that the former, which he believed followed unresolved 'inflammation', was associated with venous and arterial occlusions, and great quantities of blood in the limb. He did not know that the blood circulated but seems to be describing two distinct forms of gangrene – venous gangrene and arterial gangrene.

Lowe P. *The Whole Course of Chirurgie*. 1597; Chapter 5.

1620

A connection between varicose veins and ulcers

In 1620 Fallopio stated that 'varices carry faeculent humours which cause ulceration'.[11]

Fallopio G. *La Chirurgica*. Venice, 1620.

1628

The great revolution: the blood circulates

William Harvey published *De Motu Cordis* in 1628. This work produced the greatest revolution of physiological thought since medicine began and was the foundation of our present understanding of the circulation. Figure 1.6 illustrates the fundamental observation made by Harvey that the valves in the veins are there to ensure undirectional blood flow.

Harvey W. *Exercitatio Anatomica de Motu Cordis et Sanguini in Animalibus*. Frankfurt: W Fitzer, 1628.

1644

Venous occlusion observed

Schenck described an occlusion of the inferior vena cava.

Schenck. *Observationum Medicum Rariorum*. 1644. Lugduni. Lib3; 339.

1669

The first use of the term 'venous tone' and the first description of the calf muscle pump

Richard Lower used the words 'relaxato venarum tono' in his book *De Corde*. This is the first description of 'venous tone'. In his next book, *Tractatus de Corde Item de Motu et Colore Sanguinis et Chyli in eum Transitu*, Lower clearly appreciated the effect of the limb muscles on blood flow, so giving the first description of the peripheral muscle venous pump.

Lower R. *De Corde*. 1669.
Lower R. *Tractatus de Corde Item de Motu et Colore Sanguinis et Chyli in eum Transitu*. London: Allestry, 1670.

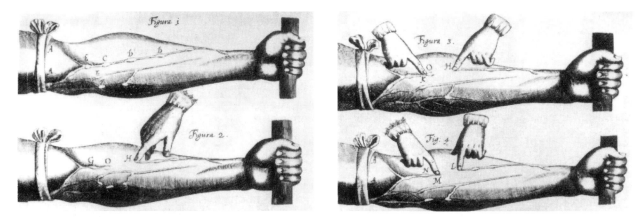

Figure 1.6   The illustration from *De Motu Cordis* that depicts the simple but incontrovertible experiment that convinced William Harvey that the blood circulates.

In *Figure 1* the text states: 'Let an arm be ligated above the elbow in a living human subject as if for blood letting. [AA] At intervals there will appear, especially in country folk and those with varicosis, certain so to speak nodes and swellings [BCDEF] not only where there is a point of diversion [EF] but even where none exists [CD] and those nodes are produced by valves, which show up in this way in the outer part of the hand or of the elbow. If by milking the vein downwards with the thumb or a finger [*Figure 2*, O to H] you try to draw blood away from the node or valve [*Figure 2*, O], you will see that none can follow your lead because of the complete obstacle provided by the valve; you will also see that the portion of vein [*Figure 2*, O H] between the swelling and the drawn-back finger has been blotted out, though the portion above the swelling or valve is fairly distended [*Figure 2*, O G]. If you keep the blood thus withdrawn [back to H] and the vein thus emptied, and with your other hand exert a pressure downward towards the distended upper part of the valves [*Figure 3*, K], you will see the blood completely resistant to being forcibly driven beyond the valve [*Figure 3*, O]. And the greater the effort you put into your performance, the greater will be the swelling and distension of the vein which you will see at the valve or swelling [*Figure 3*, O], though below that the vessel is empty [*Figure 3*, H O].

Moreover, if, with the arm ligated as before [AA] and the veins swelling up, you press on one of them some distance [*Figure 4*, L] below a selected swelling or valve, and thereafter with a finger [M] stroke the blood upwards to the region above the valve [N], you will see that part of the vein remaining empty and the blood to pass back through the valve [as in *Figure 2*, H O]. When, however, you take your finger [*Figure 2*, H] away, you will see the stretch of vein fill up again from the parts below, and become as in *Figure 1*, D C. *Whence it is clearly established that the blood moves the veins from parts below to those above and to the heart, and not in the opposite way.*' (Authors' italics.)

(Based on KJ Franklin's translation of *De Motu Cordis*. Springfield, IL: CC Thomas, 1957.)

1676

'Varicose' ulcers and a compression stocking

Richard Wiseman, Sergeant Surgeon to Charles II and a neighbour of Richard Lower, redescribed the association between varicose veins and ulceration. He appreciated the effect that venous dilatation had on the valves and used the term 'varicose ulcer'. He invented a leather lace-up stocking for the treatment of venous disease of the lower limb which was the forerunner of the modern elastic stocking (see Figure 20.2) and also described a case of postpartum white leg.

In 1652 Wiseman was an assistant to Edward Molins, Surgeon to St Thomas's Hospital, and so would have worked at St Thomas's, a privilege enjoyed by the authors who have often considered reintroducing his lace-up stocking to their own practice.

Figure 1.7(a-d) shows four abstracts from Wiseman's book which describes the treatment of varicose veins and varicose ulcers and reveals his deep understanding of the problems.

Wiseman R. *Severall Chirurgicall Treatises*. London: Royston and Took, 1676.

(a)

and suffers the rest of the stream to pass by it. This most commonly happens in-cutaneous Vessels, where the Veins have no assistance from muscular Flesh which by frequent pressure would otherwise be apt to squeeze it forwards. To which it may be added, that the Valves of the Vein so swelled, whether naturally or accidentally, are weakened, and do not sufficiently support the Blood in its ascent; so that, falling down upon the sides of the Vessel, the weight of it is too great to be driven forward by the venal motion of the Blood.

(b)

The *Varices* ought not to be cured, unless they be painful, or that they be Cure. extended into a large Tumour, or ulcerate and bleed much: for, as I have said, they preserve Health. But if there be a necessity of curing them, it ought to begin with Purging and Bleeding, not once or twice, but often repeated; and if the *Viscera* be in fault, they ought to be strengthned and amended; after which the Cure may be endeavoured by astringent and exsiccant Medicaments, and those to be applied with convenient Bandage, to press back the Blood coagulating in the Vessel, and moderately resist the Current. If these suffice not, then, according to the ancient practice, you are to proceed by Section, dividing the Skin, and separating the Teguments; and having raised the varicous Vein, you are to pass a Ligature above and another beneath it, making a deligation of them; then-slit the Vein, cast out the gross Blood, and afterwards digest and heal it, as is after said in an *Aneurisma*. With what success this hath been done, you may read in the Works of *Fabricius Hildanus:* and whether the Pain be

(c)

2. Observat. of a Simple Ulcer. Such another was commended to my hands by Doctor *Weatherly*. The Ulcer was in the Leg, and had been very vexatious to the Patient: it was accompanied with some little Fluxion, enough to relax the Parts, and keep the Ulcer from digesting, and consequently from healing. I dressed it as in the former Observation hath been said; only instead of a Rowler I put on a laced Stocking: by the wearing of which the Humours were restrained, and the Patient cured himself in a few days by the Unguents fore-mentioned.

(d)

which it swelled, and became more humid. After some while, when I saw the temper of the Member alter, I ordered a laced Stocking to be put on, for that I could not with a Rowler make such a Compression so near the Ancle as I would, without causing a swelling in his Foot. I dressed it with Pled-

Figure 1.7 Excepts from Richard Wiseman's book *Several Chirurgicall Treatises*, 4th edition. London: Benjamin Tooke, 1705.

(a) Book I Chapter XIV 'Of a Varix', page 64, lines 10–16. This refers to superficial thrombophlebitis which Wiseman considered occurred in cutaneous vessels because there is no 'assistance to blood flow from the muscles', a clear reference to the calf muscle pump, and also states that 'the valves of dilated veins are weakened and cannot support the blood'.

(b) Book I Chapter XIV 'Of a Varix', page 65, lines 12–15. A description by Wiseman of the surgical method for curing varicose veins. After describing the surgical cure he says 'I have never met one patient that cared to hear of the Cure by ligature nor indeed have I seen any great reason for it. For if the unsightliness and pain be in the legs it may be helped by the wearing of a laced stocking'.

(c) Book II Chapter II 'Of a Simple Ulcer', page 166, lines 25–31. This describes the use of the laced stocking instead of a bandage (Rowler) followed by ulcer healing in a few days.

(d) Book II Chapter III 'Of Ulcers with Intemperies', page 171, lines 14–17. This describes the application of local compression with the laced stocking. Wiseman observes that tight compression with a bandage caused swelling of the foot.

1688

Tumours spread inside veins

Blancardus observed the spread of a tumour within the lumen of a vein when he described an inferior vena cava 'filled with neoplastic "steatomatous" matter'.

Blancardus. *Anatomica Practica Rationalis.* 1688; Obs. XVI: 38.

1733

Measurement of venous pressure

The Reverend Stephen Hale measured arterial and venous pressures in conscious animals.

Hale S. *Statistical Essays Containing Haemastatics or an Account of Some Hydraulic and Hydrostatical Experiments made on the Blood and Blood-vessels of Animals.* Vol. 2. London: W Innys and R Manby, 1733.

1758

Gravity

Sharp, in his book *A Treatise on the Operations of Surgery*, stated that 'the indisposition of these sores (leg ulcers) is in some measure owing to the gravitation of the humours downward', thus showing an appreciation that gravity affects the blood and interstitial fluid within the lower limb. Newton had described his Laws of Gravity 71 years earlier in 1687.

Sharp. *A Treatise on the Operations of Surgery.* London: Touson, 1758.

1759–1768

Milk oedema

Pusoz, Levrat and Astrud all thought that post-puerperal white leg was caused by excess milk in the legs.

Pusoz N. *Traites des Accouchemens.* Paris: Deslandes, 1759.
Levret. *L'art des Accouchmens,* 3rd edition. Paris: Didot, 1766.
Astrud J. *Traite de Maladies des Femmes.* Paris: Cavelier, 1761–1765.

1769

A system opposed to coagulation

Morgagni noticed that the blood failed to clot after a sudden death.

Morgagni GB. *De Sedibus et Causis Morborum per Anatomen Indigatis.* Venice, 1769.

1784

Lymphoedema

White suggested that the postpuerperal white leg was caused by rupture of the lymphatics.

White C. *An Enquiry into the Nature and Cause of the Swelling in One or Both Legs which Sometimes Happens to Lying Women.* Warrington, 1784.

1786

Venous oedema

Haller described the oedema that follows the ligation or obstruction of a major vein.

Haller A. *First Lines of Physiology,* 1786.

1793

Stasis causes thrombosis

Baillie gave the first British description of inferior vena cava obstruction and stated that a reduction in the rate of blood flow leads to thrombosis. This was perhaps the first reference to 'stasis' as a cause of thrombosis.

Ballie M. *Transactions of a Society for the Improvement of Medical and Chirurgical Knowledge* I, 1793; 119.

1794

Fright keeps the blood liquid

John Hunter noticed that the blood of a stag hunted to death had not coagulated.

Hunter J. *A Treatise on the Blood, Inflammation and Gunshot Wounds.* London, 1794; 26.

1797

Hydrostatic forces matter

Home stated that the patient's height and weight affected the pressure in the veins and the development of ulcers. He also said that the symptoms of venous disease varied with the weather.

Home E. *Practical Observations on the Treatment of Ulcers on the Legs Considered as a Branch of Military Surgery*. London: Nichol, 1797.

1799

A paste bandage

In a book on the management of all forms of leg ulcer, Baynton reported that ulcers were situated on the distal part of the limb because they were remote from 'the foundation of life and heat' and were at a disadvantage for the return of blood and lymph from the legs. He introduced a primitive form of paste bandage.

Baynton T. *A New Method of Treating Old Ulcers of the Legs*. Bristol: Emery and Adams, 1799.

1810

White leg is not exclusively a complication of pregnancy

Ferriar described a case of phlegmasia alba dolens associated with typhus and, though he still thought this was caused by a lymphatic abnormality, this is probably the first description of deep vein thrombosis other than in childbirth.

Ferriar J. An affectation of the lymphatic vessels hitherto misunderstood. *Medical Histories and Reflections* 1810; Vol. 3: 129.

1822

The relationship between phelgmasia alba and thrombosis finally established

Davis described how deep vein thrombosis caused phlegmasia alba dolens and re-emphasized its relationship to childbirth.

Davis DD. The proximate cause of phlegmasia dolens. *Med Chir Trans* 1822; 12.

1824

A thesis on venous disease

In 1824 Briquet wrote a detailed thesis on venous disease. He pointed out that phlebectasy was most pronounced in the superficial veins near large communications with deep veins. He understood that the calf muscles acted as a pump but thought that all the blood flowed out of the lower limb through the superficial veins, having passed from the deep to the superficial veins through the communicating veins.

Briquet. *Thèse de Paris*, 1824.

Physiological explanations of therapy

Astley Cooper stated that compression of varicose veins restored the competence of the valves. He also reiterated the importance of varicose veins in the genesis of leg ulcers.

Cooper A. *The Lectures of Sir Astley Cooper Bart. on the Principles and Practice of Surgery*. London: Thomas, 1824.

1845

An invention that revolutionized medical science

Francis Rynd invented the hypodermic needle in 1845. This ultimately led to the development of sclerotherapy, the measurement of intravascular pressures and the analysis of blood samples.

1846

A clinical test of saphenous vein incompetence

Brodie described reflux down the long saphenous vein and its prevention by direct digital pressure. This was the first description of a clinical test of venous incompetence. He used plaster and bandages to heal ulcers and recognized that some dressings caused skin sensitivity reactions.

Brodie B. *Lectures on Pathology and Surgery*, 1846.

1852

Intimal injury causes thrombosis

Rokitansky reported that venous thrombosis occurred in a vein at the site of an injury or where the vein was adjacent to an area of inflammation. He came very close to describing Virchow's well-known triad, which was published 8 years later.

Rokitansky C. Venous thrombosis due to vein injury, neighbouring inflammation, or blood changes. In: *Pathological Anatomy, 4.* London: Sydenham Society, 1852; 336.

1854

The medicated compressing bandage

Unna described the use of a non-compliant plaster dressing for the treatment of ulcers, which became known as the 'Unna boot'.

Unna PG. Veber Paraplaste eine neue form medikaneutoser Pflaster. 1854. *WienMed Wochenschr* 1896; **46:** 1854.

1855

A connection between deep and superficial vein incompetence

Verneuil, in his book on varicose veins, described the anatomy of the veins of the leg in detail and stated that varicose veins were caused by incompetence of the deep veins.

He observed that the valves in the communicating veins, which he also described, stopped blood flowing from the deep to the superficial system.

Verneuil A. Du siège réel et primitif des varices des membres inférieurs. *Gazette Medicale Paris* 1855; **10:** 524.

1859

The source of pulmonary emboli, the causes of thrombosis, and a hint of fibrinolysis

Virchow described the association between thrombosis in the legs and emboli in the lung in 1846 and, later in other publications, and his seminal book *De Cellular Pathologie*, he described the three predisposing causes of thrombosis – changes in the vessel wall, the blood flow and the blood. He also recorded that blood remained fluid in the capillaries after death.

Propagating thrombus and pulmonary emboli were clearly depicted in Virchow's great book (Figures 1.8–1.10).

Virchow R. Die Verstopfung den Lungenarteries und ihre Folgen. *Beitr Exp Pathol Physiol* 1846; 21.
Virchow R. Neuer Fall von todlicher Emboli der Lungerarteries. *Arch Pathol Anat* 1856; **10:** 225.
Virchow R. *Die Cellular Pathologie.* Berlin: Verlag von August Hirschwald, 1859.

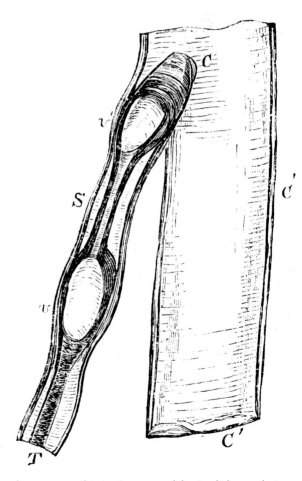

Figure 1.8 This is Figure 69 of the English translation of *Virchow's Cellular Pathology* (1860). It shows 'thrombosis of the saphenous vein(s), thrombi seated on the valves (v,v') in the process of softening and connected by more recent and thinner portions of coagulum: Prolongation of the plug (C) projecting beyond the mouth of the saphenous vein into the femoral vein'.

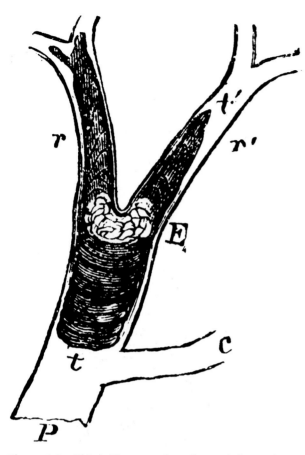

Figure 1.9 This is Figure 72 from the English translation of Virchow's *Cellular Pathology* (1860). It illustrates the features of a pulmonary embolus. 'The embolus (E) is astride the angle formed by the division of the pulmonary artery (P). The capsulating (secondary) thrombus (t and t') reaches in front of the embolus (t) to the next highest collateral vessel, behind the embolus (t') it fills in great measure the diverging branches (r and r') ultimately terminating in the form of a cone.'

1863

Bed rest and elevation

In his book *Rest and Pain,* Hilton observed that venous ulcers were frequently above the medial malleolus, that ulcers can be healed by rest and that incompetent communicating veins are probably ulcerogenic.

Hilton J. *Rest and Pain.* London: Bell and Daldy Lecture IX, 1863.

1864

The beginning of sclerotherapy

In his book on varicose veins, Chapman reported that a Frenchman, Monsieur Pravaz, 'has tried to sclerose varicose veins by injecting perchloride of iron'.

Chapman HT. *Varicose Veins, their Nature, Consequence and Treatment.* London: Churchill, 1864.

1866

Thrombosis damages the valves – a classic example of clinical and autopsy observation

In 1866 John Gay published a book based on a series of Lettsomian lectures. The illustrations in this book are obviously hand drawn by Gay from autopsy dissections and are rather crude, but they clearly show the communicating veins and the posterior arch vein (Figures 1.11–1.14).

Gay appreciated that leg ulcers were more difficult to heal if varicose veins were present, commenting

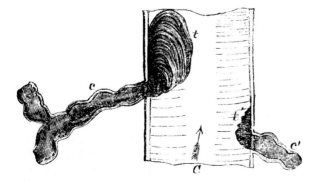

Figure 1.10 This is Figure 71 of the English translation of Virchow's *Cellular Pathology* (1860). It shows 'two small varicose circumflex veins of the thigh filled with autochthonous (original) thrombus projecting beyond the orifices into the trunk of the femoral vein. The prolonged thrombus (t) is produced by concentrically opposed deposits from the blood. The prolonged thrombus (t') is irregular because fragments (emboli) have become detached from it'. This figure clearly shows that Virchow had seen and recorded how thrombus is formed by successive layers of thrombus deposition producing what are now called the 'Lines of Zahn', 15 years before the mechanism was described by Zahn.[33]

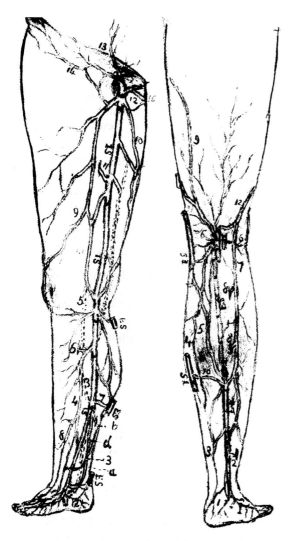

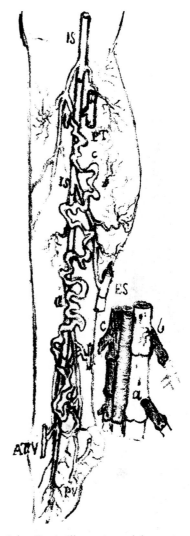

Figure 1.11   This drawing from John Gay's lecture on 'Varicose Disease of the Lower Extremities' shows the anatomy of the long and short saphenous vein. It depicts and labels the posterior arch vein (which he calls the loop vein) (3) and the medial communicating veins (b, d and 6).

Figure 1.12   John Gay's illustration of the varicose veins in the right leg of a 56-year-old woman who died of erysipelas of the left leg. The inset shows the tributaries of the posterior tibial veins filled with old thrombus (6). The text states that 'the posterior tibial artery was so encrusted that its cavity was almost entirely obliterated'. An example of combined venous and arterial insufficiency.

that 'when the varicose veins are relieved the ulcers are as readily cured as ulcers in general'. His drawings clearly show post-thrombotic deep vein damage and even old thrombi in the deep veins, the significance of which he fully appreciated and recognized.

Gay J. *On Varicose Disease of the Lower Extremities*. Lettsomian Lecture. London: Churchill, 1866.

1868

Venous not varicose ulcers

Spender published his book on ulcers and venous disease 2 years after Gay's book, and similarly recorded the fact that ulcers could occur in the absence of varicose veins if there had been

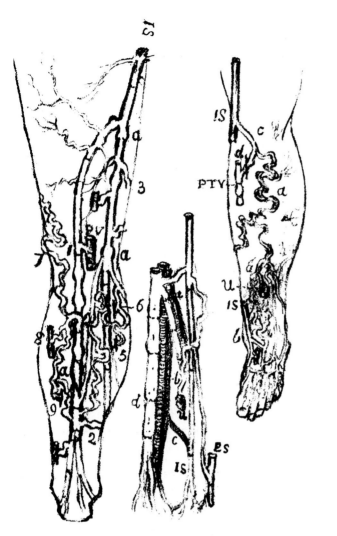

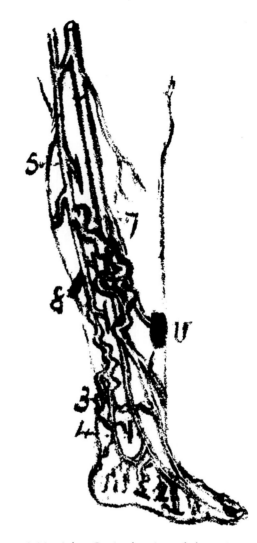

Figure 1.13 John Gay's dissection of the left leg of a 55-year-old man with ulcers on both legs. The anterior view shows the long saphenous vein connecting with the posterior tibial vein (PTV), and in the inset a vein from beneath the ulcer (u) connecting with the saphenous vein and a deep vein (b). The text states: 'The peroneal and the outer posterior tibial venae comitantes were narrowed throughout, and their channels obstructed by an old blood clot which pervaded their tributaries to the first valves as well as a large branch (inset, c) by which the latter of these veins was connected with the internal saphena.'

Figure 1.14 John Gay's drawing of the veins on the medial side of the leg of a 56-year-old man with a venous ulcer. It clearly shows the posterior arch vein and the text describes three communicating veins at sites 3, 5 and 8.

post-thrombotic damage to the deep veins, the first indication that the term varicose was misleading. Both Gay and Spender referred to venous rather than varicose ulcers.

Spender JK. *A Manual of the Pathology and Treatment of Ulcers and Subcutaneous Diseases of the Lower Limbs*. London: Churchill, 1866.

1870

The long saphenous vein is often normal when its tributaries are varicose

In Holmes' *Surgery*, Callender pointed out that superficial varices mainly occur in the tributaries of the long saphenous vein, not in the long saphenous vein itself.

Callender, in Holmes' *Surgery*, 1870.

1871

Primary venous tumours

Perl described a primary vein wall tumour.

Perl L. Ein Fall von Sarkom der Vena Cava Inferior. *Virchows Arch Pathol Anat* 1871; **53:** 378.

1878

Elastic compression bandages

In 1878 Martin wrote a long letter to the *British Medical Journal* describing the use of India-rubber bandages for the treatment of leg ulcers. He gave a detailed description of their method of application and the way in which they produced compression.

Martin HA. The India-rubber bandage for ulcers and other diseases of the legs. *Br Med J* 1878; **2:** 624–6.

1891

The logical surgical treatment of long saphenous incompetence

Trendelenburg described the ligation of the long saphenous vein in the upper third of the thigh to prevent long saphenous vein reflux. He did not advocate a flush ligation of the long saphenous vein at the sapheno-femoral junction.

Trendelenburg F. Uber die Unterbindung der Vena Saphena magna bie unterschenkel varicen. *Beitr Clin Chir* 1891; **7:** 195.

1894

The first operation for deep venous insufficiency

Parona (cited by Turner Warwick[28]) described ligation of the popliteal vein for venous problems because he believed that superficial varicose veins were secondary to deep varicose veins.

Parona. Poloclinico. *Chirurgie* 1894; **8:** 9.

1894

The connection between surgery and deep vein thrombosis

Von Strauch observed and recorded the occurrence of deep vein thrombosis after a surgical operation.

Von Strauch M. Uber venen Thrombose der unteren Extremitaten nach Koliotomien bei Bechenhock Largering und Athernarkose. *Zentrac Gynak* 1894; **18:** 304.

1895

A test of deep vein obstruction

Perthes described his walking test for detecting obstruction of the deep veins.

Perthes G. Uber die Operation der Unterschenkel-varicen nach Trendelenburg. *Dtsch Med Wochenschr* 1895; **21:** 253.

1896

The principles underlying the production of tissue fluid

Starling measured the osmotic pressure of plasma proteins and explained how it counterbalanced the intracapillary hydrostatic pressure, thus ending the long dispute between those who believed interstitial fluid was a filtrate and those who believed it was a secretion and explaining how venous hypertension caused oedema.

Starling EH. On the absorption of fluids from the connective tissue spaces. *J Physiol (Lond)* 1896; **19:** 312–26.

1899

Silent and symptomatic thrombosis

Welch described 'bland' and 'infective' thrombus. He noticed that pulmonary emboli could come from latent as well as from overt deep vein thrombosis. This was the beginning of the notion that there were two types of thrombosis – thrombophlebitis and phlebothrombosis – a concept which has now been abandoned.

Welch WH. In: Albutt C. *A System of Medicine*. London: Macmillan, 1899; **6:** 155.

1905 AND 1906

Stripping

Keller and Mayo described techniques for stripping out the long saphenous vein.

Keller. A new method of extirpating the internal saphenous and similar veins in varicose conditions. *N Y J Med* 1905; **82**: 385.
Mayo CH. Treatment of varicose veins. *Surg Gynecol Obstet* 1906; **2**: 385.

1906

The advent of reconstructive venous surgery

Carrel and Guthrie, in their Nobel prize winning work on vascular anastomosis, made the first attempts at vein transplantation.

Carrel A, Guthrie CC. Uniterminal and biterminal venous transplantation. *Surg Gynecol Obstet* 1906; **2**: 266.

1911

The beginning of physiological measurements on peripheral veins

Hooker noticed that exercise affected the pressure in the veins of the lower limb but he did not measure it precisely.

Hooker DR. The effect of exercise upon the venous blood pressure. *Am J Physiol* 1911; **28**: 235.

1916 AND 1917

Primary and secondary varicose veins

Homans described the treatment of varicose veins and classified them as primary if the deep veins were normal, and as secondary if the deep veins showed evidence of post-thrombotic damage. He suggested that leg ulcers were caused by post-thrombotic deep vein damage and introduced the concept that venous stasis was the ultimate cause of venous ulceration.

Homans J. The operative treatment of varicose veins and ulcers, based upon a classification of these lesions. *Surg Gynecol Obstet* 1916; **22**: 143.
Homans J. The aetiology and treatment of varicose ulcers of the leg. *Surg Gynecol Obstet* 1917; **24**: 300.

1923

Phlebography

Berberich and Hirsch described their first attempt at venography using strontium bromide.

Berberich J, Hirsch S. Die roentgenographische Dorstellung der Arterien und Venen am Lebenden Menschen. *Klin Wochenschr* 1923; **2**: 2226.

1924

The pathology of the thrombus

Aschoff, in his lectures on pathology, argued that iliofemoral thrombus began at the groin and propagated downwards. He also described the pathological features of thrombus formation and growth, which Virchow had drawn 65 years earlier (see Figure 1.10).

Aschoff L. *Lecture Notes on Pathology*. New York: Hoeber, 1924.

1926

Venous thrombectomy

Basy described a case of thrombosis of the right axillary vein treated by phlebotomy, removal of the thrombus and suture of the vein. This is probably the first description of venous thrombectomy.

Basy L. Thrombose de la veine axillaire droite (thrombophlebite par effort). Phlebotomie, ablation de caillots, suture de la veine. *Meme Acad Chir* 1926; **52**: 529.

1928

Anatomy of venous valves

Franklin's historical survey of the discovery of the valves of the veins signalled a resurgence of interest in venous physiology and pathology.

Franklin KJ. Valves in veins. An historical survey. *Proc R Soc Med Sect Hist Med* 1928; **21**: 1.

1930

'Gravitational' ulcers and safer phlebography

Dickson Wright described the use of local dressings and adhesive bandages (Elastoplast) for the treatment of venous ulcers and introduced the term 'gravitational' ulcer. Ratschow introduced the first water-soluble X-ray contrast material, a di-iodinated pyridine derivative, for phlebography.

Ratschow M. Uroselektan in der Vasographie unter spezieller Berucksichtigung der Varkographie. *FortschrRontgenstr* 1930; **42:** 37.

Wright D. Treatment of varicose ulcers. *Br Med J* 1930; **2:** 996.

1931

An early 'gold standard'

In 1931 Turner Warwick published an important monograph on varicose veins which stimulated interest in the surgical treatment of venous disease. Much of his thoughts were based on the work of Gay, Spender, Briquet and Verneuil. In this book he described the 'bleed-back' test which is still used at operation to test the competence of the valves in the communicating veins.

Turner Warwick W. *The Rational Treatment of Varicose Veins and Varicocele.* London: Faber, 1931.

1933

Fibrinolysis

Tillett and Garner observed that the haemolytic streptococcus produced a substance which broke down fibrin.

Tillett WS, Garner RL. The fibrinolytic activity of haemolytic streptococci. *J Exp Med* 1933; **58:** 485.

1934

The measurement of venular capillary pressure

Landis made direct measurement of the pressure at the arterial and venous end of capillary loops and explained how the pressure gradient between these sites (32 to 12 mmHg) affected the movement of water and solutes from the blood into the tissue spaces. Sixty years were to elapse before the relationship between the disturbance of this mechanism caused by an inadequate calf muscle pump and venous ulceration was re-examined.[3,4,10]

Landis EM. Capillary pressure and capillary permeability. *Physiol Rev* 1934; **14:** 404–81.

1936

Plasmin

Schmitz described the nature of plasmin.

Schmitz A. Uber die Proteinase des fibrins. *Z Physiol Chem* 1936; **224:** 89.

1937

The destructive effect of thrombosis

Edwards and Edwards showed that a venous thrombosis destroyed the valves but was frequently followed by recanalization.

This year also saw the publication of Franklin's important monograph on the physiology of the veins, the first book of our era solely concerned with this topic.

Edwards FA, Edwards JE. The effect of thrombophlebitis on the venous valve. *Surg Gynecol Obstet* 1937; **65:** 320.

Franklin KJ. *A Monograph on Veins.* Springfield, IL: Thomas, 1937.

Heparin

After many years of basic research, Murray and his co-workers described the use of heparin in animals as a form of preventing thrombosis after vascular injury. This was followed by Crafoord's description of the use of heparin in man.

Murray DWG, Jaques LB, Perrett TS, Best CH. Heparin and the thrombosis of veins following injury. *Surgery* 1937; **2:** 163.

Crafoord CC. Preliminary report on post-operative treatment with heparin as a preventative of thrombosis. *Acta Chir Scand* 1937; **79:** 407.

Natural fibrinolysis

In 1937 MacFarlane described postoperative hyperfibrinolysis.

MacFarlane RG. Fibrinolysis following operation. *Lancet* 1937; **1:** 10.

1938

Thrombectomy and the mechanism of venous gangrene

Gregoire established that gangrene can be caused by deep vein thrombosis, and Lawen described the removal of a thrombus from a leg vein.

Gregoire M. La phlébite bleu (phlegmatia caerulea dolens). *Presse Med* 1938; **46:** 1313.

Lawen A. Weitere erfahrungen uber operative Thrombanentfernung bei venethrombose. *Arch Klin Chir* 1938; **193:** 723.

Clinical phlebography

Dos Santos described a clinically applicable technique of phlebography.

Dos Santos JC. La phlébographie directe. Conception, technique, premier résultats. *J Int Chir* 1938; **3:** 625.

Communicating vein ligation

In 1938 Linton described the operation of subfascial ligation of the medial lower leg communicating veins.

Linton RR. The communicating veins of the lower leg and the operative technique for their ligation. *Ann Surg* 1938; **107:** 582.

1939

Heparin and deep vein thrombosis

Crafoord described the use of heparin for the treatment of postoperative deep vein thrombosis.

Crafoord C. Heparin and post-operative thrombosis. *Acta Chir Scand* 1939; **82:** 319.

Thrombectomy accepted

Leriche described a technique of thrombectomy for deep vein thrombosis.

Leriche R, Geisendorf W. Résultats d'une thrombectomie précoce avec resection veineuse dans une phlébite grave des deux membres inférieurs. *Presse Med* 1939; **47:** 1239.

'osis or 'tis

Oschner and DeBakey established (temporarily) the use of the terms 'phlebothrombosis' and 'thrombophlebitis' in an extensive review of the current knowledge of venous thrombosis.

Oschner A, DeBakey M. Therapy of phlebothrombosis and thrombophlebitis. *Southern Surgeon* 1939; **8:** 269.

1940

The clinical application of phlebography

Bauer applied phlebography to define the state of the deep veins in patients with deep vein thrombosis. This important publication set the scene for our present understanding of the post-thrombotic syndrome and the value of anticoagulant therapy.

Bauer G. A venographic study of thromboembolic patients. *Acta Chir Scand* 1940; **84:** Suppl 61.

1941

The prevention of postoperative thrombosis with heparin

Crafoord and Jorpes attempted to prevent postoperative deep vein thrombosis by fully anticoagulating their patients with heparin. These patients had no pulmonary emboli, and surprisingly few bleeding complications in spite of the fact that they were given doses of 30 000–40 000 units daily.

Crafoord C, Jorpes E. Heparin as a prophylactic against thrombosis. *JAMA* 1941; **116:** 2831.

The effect of heparin on established deep vein thrombosis

Bauer continued his studies with phlebography and showed that the exhibition of anticoagulants early in the course of a deep vein thrombosis stopped its progression.

Bauer G. Venous thrombosis. Early diagnosis with aid of phlebography and abortive treatment with heparin. *Arch Surg* 1941; **43:** 463.

1942

The post-thrombotic syndrome

By performing further phlebograms on the patients he had studied 5 or more years earlier, Bauer was able to describe the sequelae of deep vein thrombosis. He showed that a large proportion of patients who had had a major deep vein thrombosis developed post-thrombotic sequelae.

Bauer G. A roentgenological and clinical study of the sequels of thrombosis. *Acta Chir Scand* 1942; **86:** Suppl 74.

1946

Physiological fibrinolysis

MacFarlane and Biggs, having observed that blood, taken after an operation which had clotted, later dissolved spontaneously, developed the concept that trauma, fear and anaesthesia stimulate fibrinolytic activity.

MacFarlane also developed the concept of the coagulation cascade.

MacFarlane RG, Biggs R. Observations on fibrinolysis, spontaneous activity associated with surgical operations and trauma. *Lancet* 1946; **2:** 862.

1947

Tissue plasminogen activator

In 1947 Astrup and Permin described tissue plasminogen activator, the initiator of fibrinolysis.

Astrup T, Permin PM. Fibrinolysis in the animal organism. *Nature* 1947; **159:** 681.

1948

The Bisgaard regimen

Bisgaard described his method of massage and bandaging for the treatment of venous ulceration.

Bisgaard H. *Ulcers and Eczema of the Leg. Sequels of Phlebitis.* Copenhagen: Munksgaard, 1948.

Fibrinolysis balances coagulation

MacFarlane and Biggs described the presence of intrinsic fibrinolysis within the blood and postulated that it acted as a counterbalance to the coagulation system.

MacFarlane RG, Biggs R. Fibrinolysis: its mechanism and significance. *Blood* 1948; **3:** 1167.

1949

A test of venous function

Pollack and Wood measured the pressure in the saphenous vein at the ankle while the subject was standing and lying down and observed that the venous pressure fell during exercise.

Pollack AA, Taylor BE, Myers TT, Wood EH. The effect of exercise and body position on the venous pressure at the ankle in patients having venous valvular defects. *J Clin Invest* 1949; **28:** 559.
Pollack AA, Wood EH. Venous pressure in the saphenous vein at the ankle in man during exercise and changes in posture. *J Appl Physiol* 1949; **1:** 649.

1950

Low-dose heparin for the prevention of deep vein thrombosis

De Takats suggested that the injection of a low dose of heparin would prevent deep vein thrombosis after operation.

De Takats G. Anticoagulant therapy in surgery. *JAMA* 1950; **142:** 527.

1951–1954

Therapeutic thrombolysis

Astrup described the isolation of a substance, derived from tissues, which was capable of activating the proteolytic enzymes in the blood. This was the beginning of the era of thrombolysis.

Innerfield, Schwarz and Angrist showed that trypsin dissolved thrombi; and Johnson and Tillett showed that intravascular thrombi could be dissolved by streptokinase.

Clifton and Sherry showed that plasmin could dissolve artificially induced femoral vein thrombi and arterial thrombi.

Mullertz showed that there is always a degree of fibrinolytic activity in human blood.

Astrup T. The activation of a proteolytic enzyme in the blood by animal tissue. *Biochem J* 1951; **50:** 5.
Astrup T. Stage A. Isolation of a soluble fibrinolytic activator from animal tissue. *Nature* 1952; **170:** 929.
Clifton EE, Grossi CE, Connamela DA. Lysis of thrombi produced by sodium morrhuate in the femoral vein of dogs by human plasmin (fibrinolysin). *Ann Surg* 1954; **139:** 52.
Innerfield I, Schwarz A, Angrist A. Intravenous trypsin. The anticoagulant fibrinolytic and thrombolytic effects. *J Clin Invest* 1952; **31:** 1049.
Johnson AJ, Tillett WS. The lysis in rabbits of intravascular blood clots by streptococcal fibrinolytic system (streptokinase). *J Exp Med* 1952; **95:** 449.
Mullertz S. A plasminogen activator in spontaneously active human blood. *Proc Soc Exp Biol Med* 1953; **82:** 291.
Sherry S. Titchner A, Gottesman L, Wasserman P, Troll W. The enzymatic dissolution of experimental arterial thrombi in the dog by trypsin, chromotrypsin and plasminogen activators. *J Clin Invest* 1954; **33:** 1303.

1953

'Blow-out veins'

In 1953 Cockett described the 'ankle blow-out syndrome' and its treatment by the extrafascial ligation of incompetent communicating veins. This paper revived European interest in the surgical treatment of venous ulceration.

Cockett FB, Jones DE. The ankle blow-out syndrome. A new approach to the varicose ulcer problem. *Lancet* 1953; **1:** 17.

1954

Phlebography for all

In 1954 sodium diatrozoate (a tri-iodinated contract material) was introduced, heralding the widespread use of contrast phlebography. These agents are no longer in use, having been replaced by the much safer, virtually non-thrombogenic, low osmolality, non-ionic media.

Almen T. Contrast agent design: some aspects of the synthesis of water soluble contrast agents of low osmolality. *J Theor Biol* 1969; **24:** 216.

A deep vein bypass operation

Warren and Thayer published the first description of the use of the saphenous vein for bypassing a post-thrombotic occlusion of the superficial femoral vein.

Warren R, Thayer T. Transplantation of the saphenous vein for postphlebitic stasis. *Surgery* 1954; **35:** 867.

1956

Education

In 1956 Dodd and Cockett published their book on the treatment of venous disease of the lower limb. This book became the standard textbook on the treatment of venous disease and stimulated many surgeons throughout the world to develop an interest in this field of surgery.

Dodd H, Cockett FB. *The Pathology and Surgery of the Veins of the Lower Limb.* Edinburgh: Livingstone, 1956.

1957

Bed rest and thrombosis

Gibbs published a detailed description, based on autopsy studies, of the site of venous thrombosis and its relation to rest in bed.

Fontaine discussed the value of venous thrombectomy and reported that Leriche had performed a venous thrombectomy in the 1920s.

Gibbs NM. Venous thrombosis of the lower limb with particular reference to bed rest. *Br J Surg* 1957; **45:** 209.

Fontaine R. Remarks concerning venous thrombosis and its sequelae. *Surgery* 1957; **41:** 6.

1958

A source of fibrinolytic activator

Todd described the production of a fibrinolytic activator from the wall of the veins. This was the beginning of our understanding of the role the endothelium and other cells in the production of fibrinolytic activator.

Todd AS. Fibrinolysis autographs. *Nature* 1958; **181:** 495.

Femoro-femoral vein bypass

In 1958 Palma described his femoro-femoral bypass operation for the relief of iliac vein obstruction.

Palma EC, Risi F, De Campo F. Tratamiento de los trastornos postflebiticos mediante anastomosis venosa safeno-femoral contro-lateral. *Bull Soc Surg Uruguay* 1958; **29:** 135.

1959

The first proof that pulmonary embolism can be prevented

In 1959 Sevitt and Gallagher published a study which showed that oral anticoagulants significantly reduced the mortality and the incidence of fatal pulmonary embolism following hip fractures.

Sevitt S, Gallagher NG. Prevention of venous thrombosis and pulmonary embolism in injured patients. A trial of anticoagulant prophylaxis with phenindione in middle aged and elderly patients with fractured necks of femur. *Lancet* 1959; **2:** 981.

Streptokinase will lyse venous thrombi

In 1955 Tillett, Johnson and McCarty demonstrated that streptokinase can be given safely to humans, and then showed that it could lyse artificially induced human venous thrombi *in vivo*.

Tillett WS, Johnson AJ, McCarty WR. The intravenous infusion of the streptococcal fibrinolytic principle (streptokinase) into patients. *J Clin Invest* 1955; **34:** 169.

Johnson AJ, McCarty WR. The lysis of artificially induced intravascular clots in man by intravenous infusion of streptokinase. *J Clin Invest* 1959; **38:** 1627.

1960

The detection of venous thrombi with radioisotopes

Hobbs and Davies described a series of animal experiments which showed that labelled fibrinogen could be used to detect the presence of venous thrombosis. This study led to the development of the Fibrinogen Uptake Test, a method of diagnosis that has greatly enlarged our understanding of the aetiology and natural history of venous thrombosis in all types of patient.

Hobbs JT, Davies JWL. Detection of venous thrombosis with ^{131}I labelled fibrinogen in the rabbit. *Lancet* 1960; **2:** 134.

1960–1995

From the 1960s onwards there has been a vast expansion in the number of publications concerning venous disease. It would be invidious to pick out the contributions of any of our many friends and colleagues from around the world for special mention because only time will tell whether contemporary contributions will be considered to be significant by our successors. The life expectancy of many of our current methods of investigation and treatment is unpredictable. The fibrinogen uptake test has already been abandoned following the appearance of the AIDS virus. The development of diagnostic ultrasound has taken 20 years but has now replaced many established methods of anatomical and physiological investigation and is probably the greatest advance of the past 10 years. Consequently, the remainder of this book refers solely to the factual content of the many hundreds of recent publications, the contents of which indicate how much thought and development have gone into the investigation and treatment of venous disease. You, the reader, must decide whether they are milestones, pebbles or grains of sand.

References

1. Adams EF. *The Genuine Works of Hippocrates.* London: Sydenham Press, 1949.
2. Anning ST. Historical aspects. In: Dodd H, Cockett FB, eds. *The Pathology and Surgery of Veins of the Lower Limb.* Edinburgh: Livingstone, 1956.
3. Browse NL, Burnand KG. The postphlebitic syndrome: a new look. In: Bergan JJ, Yao JST, eds. *Venous Problems.* Chicago: Year Book Publishers, 1978; 395–404.
4. Browse NL, Burnand KG. The cause of venous ulceration. *Lancet* 1982; **2:** 243–5.
5. Burggraeve A. *Etudes sur Andre Vésale Gaud.* Annott-Braeckman, 1841.
6. Caelius Aurelianus. *De Morbis Chronicis.* II. 186/Amman; 416.
7. Celsus AC. *Of Medicine in Eight Books.* Trans by J Grieve. London: Wilson & Durham, 1756.
8. Chadwick J, Mann WN. *The Medical Works of Hippocrates.* Oxford: Blackwell, 1950.
9. Cocellas PS. Alcmaeon of Groton, his life, work and fragments. *Proc R Soc Med* 1932; **25:** 1041.
10. Fagrell B. Microcirculatory disturbances: the final cause for venous leg ulcers. *Vasa* 1982; **11:** 101–3.
11. Fallopio G. *La Chirurgica di Cabriel Fallopio.* Trans by Cio Petro Maffei. Venice, 1620.
12. Franklin KJ. Valves in veins, an historical review. *Proc R Soc Med (Sect Hist Med)* 1927; **21:** 1.
13. Friedenwald H. Amatus Lusitanus. *Bull Inst Hist Med* 1937; **5:** 603.
14. Friedenwald H. Amatus Lusitanus. *Bull Inst Hist Med* 1937; **5:** 644.
15. Galen C. *Glaudi Galeni Opera Omnia.* CG Kühn, ed. Lipsiae. Off Libr C Cnobochii 1821–1833. 22 vols.
16. Ghalioungni P. *The House of Life (PerAnAh).* Amsterdam/Israel, 1973; 81 and 83.
17. Harris CRS. *The Heart and Vascular System in Ancient Greek Medicine from Alcmaeon to Galen.* Oxford: Clarendon, 1973; 108.
18. Littré E. *Oeuvres Complètes d'Hippocrate: Traduction Nouvelle avec le Texte Grec en Regard.* Paris: Baillière, 1839–1861 (10 vols).
19. Lonie IM. The paradoxical text 'On the Heart'. *Medical History* 1973; **17:** Part 11, p. 137.
20. Majno G. *The Healing Hand.* Cambridge, MA: Harvard University Press, 1975; 90.
21. Majno G. *The Healing Hand.* Cambridge, MA: Harvard University Press, 1975; 153.
22. Majno G. *The Healing Hand.* Cambridge, MA: Harvard University Press, 1975; 328.
23. Major RH. *A History of Medicine.* Oxford: Blackwell, 1954; Vol. 1.
24. Michler M. *Die Alexandrinschen Chirurugen. Eine Sammlung und Answertung ihre Gragmente.* Wiesbaden: Steiner, 1968; 13.
25. Mondeville H de. *Chirurgie de Maitre Henri Mondeville composée de 1306 à 1320.* Trans by E Nicaise. Paris: Alcan, 1893.
26. Paré A. *The Works of that Famous Surgeon Ambrose Paré.* Trans by T Johnson. London: Cotes and du Gard, 1649.
27. Soury J. *Le Système Nerveux Central. Structure et Fonctions. Histoire Critique de Théories et des Doctrines.* Paris: Carré et Naud, 1899.
28. Turner Warwick W. *The Rational Treatment of Varicose Veins and Varicocele.* London: Faber & Faber, 1931.
29. Underwood M. *A Treatise upon Ulcers of the Legs.* London: Mathews, 1783.

30. Veith I. *Huang Ti Nei Ching Su Wen. The Yellow Emperor's Classic of Internal Medicine.* Berkeley, CA: University of California Press, 1966.
31. Walsh J. Galen's writings and influences inspiring them. *Am Med Hist* 1934; **Part I:** 14.

32. Withington J. *Medical History from the Earliest Times.* London, 1894; 276.
33. Zahn W. Untersuchungen über Thrombose. Bildung der Thromben. *Virchows Arch Pathol Anat* 1875; **62:** 81.

CHAPTER 2

Embryology and radiographic anatomy

Development and congenital anomalies	23	Anatomy of the upper limb veins	44
Anatomy of the lower limb veins	30	References	47

A knowledge of the normal anatomy of the venous system and its many variations is essential for a full understanding of venous disease. As much of living anatomical knowledge is derived from contrast phlebography, this chapter is deliberately presented as radiological anatomy with surgically important features emphasized where appropriate.

Development and congenital anomalies

Initially, the cardinal veins form the main venous drainage system of the embryo. They consist of the anterior cardinal veins, which drain the cephalic part of the embryo, and the posterior cardinal veins, which drain the remaining part of the body of the embryo. The anterior and posterior cardinal veins join before entering the sinus horn to form the short common cardinal veins. During the fourth week the cardinal veins form a symmetrical system.

During the fifth to the seventh week of embryonic life a number of additional veins are formed: the subcardinal veins, which mainly drain the kidneys; the sacrocardinal veins which drain the lower extremities; and the supracardinal veins which drain the body wall by way of the intercostal veins, thereby taking over the function of the posterior cardinal veins (Figure 2.1a).

Characteristic of the formation of the vena caval system is the appearance of anastomoses between left and right so that blood from the left is channelled to the right side.

The anastomosis between the anterior cardinal veins develops into the left brachio-cephalic (innominate) vein. Most of the blood from the left side of the head and the upper extremities is then channelled to the right. The terminal portion of the left posterior cardinal vein entering the left brachio-cephalic vein is retained as a small vessel, the left superior intercostal vein. This vessel receives blood from the second and third intercostal spaces. The superior vena cava is formed by the right common cardinal vein and the proximal portion of the right anterior cardinal vein.

The anastomosis between the subcardinal veins is formed by the left renal vein. When this communication has been established, the left subcardinal vein disappears and only its distal portion remains as the left gonadal vein. Hence the right subcardinal vein becomes the main drainage channel and develops into the renal segment of the inferior vena cava.

The anastomosis between the sacrocardinal veins is formed by the left common iliac vein. The right sacrocardinal vein finally becomes the sacrocardinal segment of the inferior vena cava. When the renal segment of the inferior vena cava connects with the hepatic segment, which is derived from the right vitelline vein, the inferior vena cava is complete. It consists then of a hepatic segment, a renal segment and a sacrocardinal segment.

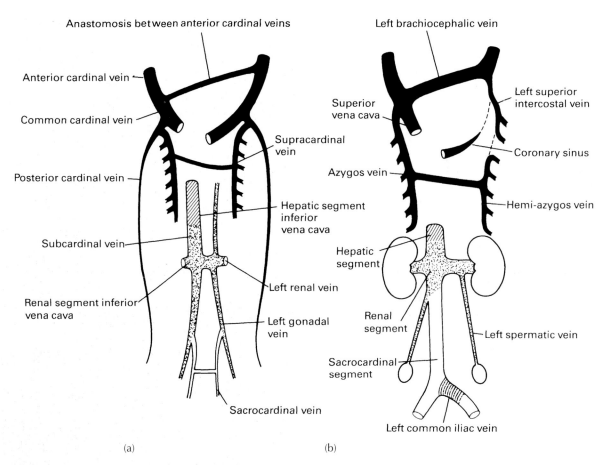

Figure 2.1 Diagrams showing the development of the inferior vena cava, the azygos veins and the superior vena cava. (a) In the seventh week. Note the anastomoses which have formed between the subcardinal, the supracardinal, the sacrocardinal and the anterior cardinal veins. (b) The venous system at birth. Note the three components of the inferior vena cava. (After Langman.[25])

With the obliteration of the major portion of the posterior cardinal veins, the supracardinal veins gain in importance. The fourth to eleventh right intercostal veins empty into the right subcardinal vein, which, together with a portion of the posterior cardinal vein, form the azygos vein. On the left the fourth to seventh intercostal veins enter the left supracardinal vein. After development of a communicating vessel between the two supracardinal veins the left supracardinal vein enters into the azygos vein and this is then known as the hemi-azygos vein (Figure 2.1b).[25]

This complex development, coupled with the persistence of parts of the embryological trunks, gives rise to a number of anomalies.[29] It has been estimated that 1% of otherwise normal subjects have anomalies of the inferior vena cava or its tributaries.[36]

Two anomalies of the inferior vena cava are of particular clinical interest, a double inferior vena cava below the renal veins, and hypoplasia or complete absence of the inferior vena cava.

A double inferior vena cava exists if the left sacrocardinal vein fails to lose its connection with the left subcardinal vein. The incidence of this anomaly is between 0.2 and 3%.[21] The two cavae may be of equal size but the right cava is usually larger. The left inferior vena cava drains into the right inferior vena cava via the left renal vein (Figure 2.2a and b).

Absence of the inferior vena cava occurs when the right subcardinal vein fails to connect with the liver. Blood from the lower half of the body returns to the heart by the azygos vein and the superior vena cava. The hepatic veins enter the right atrium directly from below. This anomaly is usually associated with other cardiac malformations (Figure 2.3a and b).[25]

A persistent left sacrocardinal vein resulting in a left-sided inferior vena cava has an incidence of

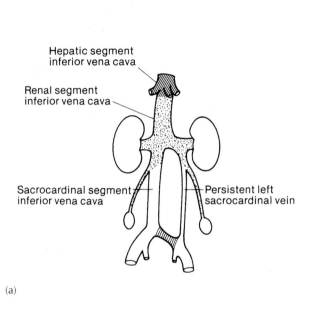

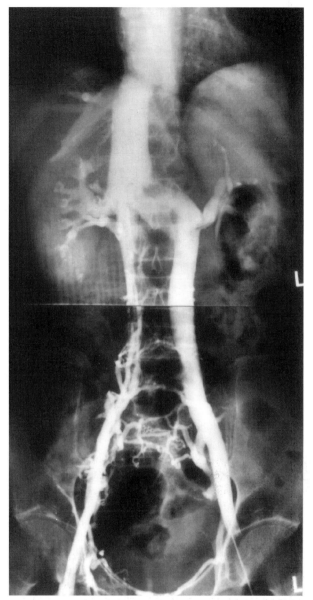

Figure 2.2 (a) Diagram of a double inferior vena cava at lumbar level caused by persistence of the left sacro-cardinal vein. (After Langman.[25]) (b) Duplication of the inferior vena cava shown by phlebography. The plexus of vessels to the right of the spine are remnants of a full sized right-sided vessel which has become thrombosed following plication for pulmonary embolism. A phlebogram was not carried out preoperatively and the patient had a pulmonary embolus through the left vena cava.

(a)

(b)

0.2–0.5%.[15,20,42] The left inferior vena cava drains into the left renal vein, crosses the spine and continues cranially as a normal right-sided inferior vena cava (Figure 2.4).

Persistence of the right posterior cardinal vein results in a retrocaval or retroiliac ureter. The distal ureter lies dorsal to the inferior vena cava. This anomaly is recognized on an excretion urogram or retrograde ureterogram by the medial displacement of the ureter. When a ureter is obstructed by this abnormality of the inferior vena cava the pelvi-calyceal system and proximal third of the ureter is dilated (Figure 2.5). Failure of the anastomosis between the two sacrocardinal veins leads to agenesis of the left common iliac vein (see Chapter 23).[26]

The most common congenital anomaly of the superior vena cava is a persistent left superior vena cava. This occurs in 0.3% of the population but more frequently (4.3%) in patients with congenital heart disease.[6,7] Although a left superior vena cava may occur in isolation, it is more often found in association with a separate right superior vena cava. The left superior vena cava drains into the coronary sinus (Figure 2.6a). Another anomaly is a double

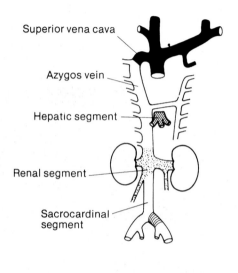

(a)

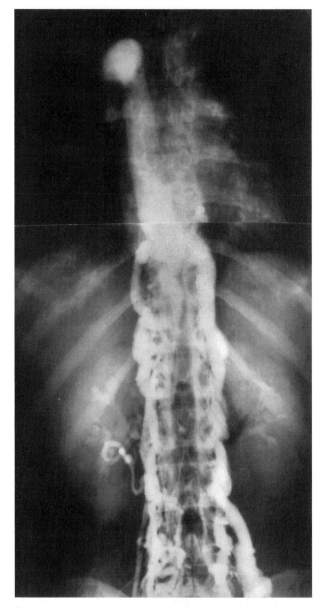

(b)

Figure 2.3   (a) Diagram of an absent inferior vena cava. The lower half of the body is drained by the azygos vein which enters the superior vena cava. The hepatic vein enters the heart at the site of the inferior vena cava. (After Langman.[25]) (b) A phlebogram showing absence of the inferior vena cava. The venous return is through both ascending lumbar veins and the azygos and hemi-azygos veins. This was thought to be congenital in origin because it was noted early in life and there was no history to suggest venous thrombosis.

superior vena cava caused by persistence of the left anterior cardinal vein and failure of the left brachio-cephalic (innominate) vein to develop (Figure 2.6b).

Development of the limb veins

The primitive capillary plexus of the flattened limb buds organizes to form a peripheral border vein which serves as the primitive outflow tract for blood brought in by the axial arteries. Along the cranial border of the limb bud this vein is small and largely disappears, but on the caudal margin it transforms into a permanent vessel. The border vein appears in the arm and leg between the sixth and eighth weeks, the adult venous anatomy being outlined during the next 2 weeks.

In the arm the radial extension of the border vein atrophies, the ulnar portion of the vein persists to form, at different levels, the subclavian, axillary and basilic veins. The border vein originally opens into the posterior cardinal vein but as the heart descends, the subclavian vein ultimately opens into the precardinal (internal jugular) vein. The cephalic

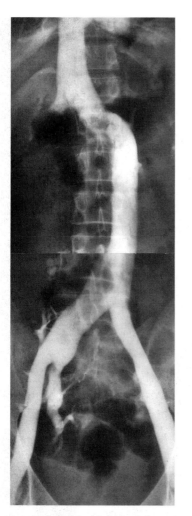

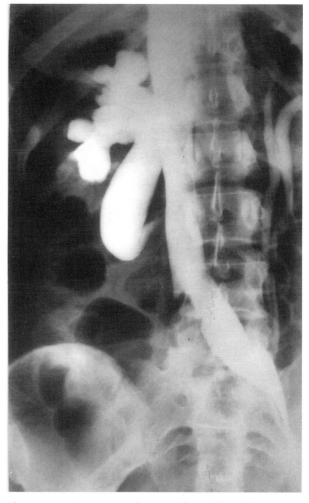

Figure 2.4 A pure left-sided inferior vena cava. The vein crosses to the right to continue cranially as an otherwise normal inferior vena cava.

Figure 2.5 A retrocaval ureter shown by inferior vena cavography. The calyces and upper ureter on the right are dilated due to obstruction by the abnormal inferior vena cava. Below the obstruction the ureter is displaced towards the midline. The excretion urogram resulted from the contrast injection for the phlebogram. The vena cava is not distorted by the position of the ureter.

vein develops secondarily in association with the radial border vein. At first the cephalic vein anastomoses with the external jugular vein but finally it opens into the axillary vein. The external jugular veins and the subclavian veins develop independently and attach later.

In the leg the tibial continuation of the primitive border vein disappears while the fibular segment largely persists. The long saphenous vein arises separately from the posterior cardinal vein, gives off the femoral and posterior tibial veins, and then incorporates the tibial border vein at the level of the knee. Distally, the border vein develops into the anterior tibial and short saphenous veins.[2]

Abnormal development of these systems gives rise to some of the congenital venous anomalies which are discussed in Chapter 23.

STRUCTURE OF VEINS

The walls

The walls of the veins, like those of the arteries, are composed of three coats, the tunica intima, the tunica media and the tunica adventitia. The main difference between the walls of the arteries and those of the veins is that, in the latter, there is a comparative weakness of the muscular layer and a much smaller proportion of elastic tissue. In small veins these coats are difficult to distinguish.

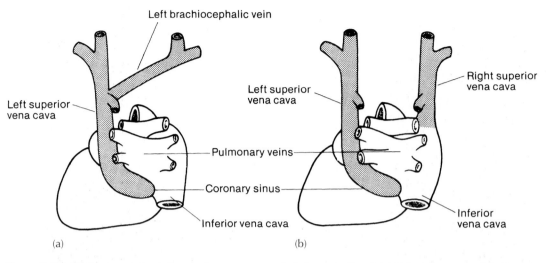

Figure 2.6 (a) Diagram of a left superior vena cava draining into the right atrium by way of the coronary sinus (dorsal view). (b) A double superior vena cava. The communicating (brachio-cephalic) vein between the two anterior cardinal veins has failed to develop. (After Langman.[25])

The media varies considerably between veins of different calibre. In the venules it is thin and composed almost exclusively of muscle. In the medium sized veins it consists of a thick layer of connective tissue with elastic fibres and some smooth muscle fibres, usually arranged circumferentially. The larger veins such as the femoral, iliac, axillary, subclavian and innominate veins have much less smooth muscle in the tunica media, and in the inferior and superior venae cavae smooth muscle is almost entirely absent. The saphenous veins contain large amounts of smooth muscle in their walls.

Valves

Unlike arteries, veins possess valves which direct the blood flow towards the heart. The valves have two leaflets consisting of folds of intima reinforced with an intervening layer of connective tissue.

There are no valves in the superior and inferior venae cavae but there are valves in the tributaries from both the upper and lower limbs, the number of valves increasing towards the periphery of each limb. Valves do not appear to play an important part in controlling the circulation within the upper limbs and there is no equivalent of the calf and thigh muscle pumps in the arm. Venous return is largely the result of 'vis a tergo' in the upper limbs.[35] Consequently, although thrombosis in upper limb veins damages the valves as severely as it does in the lower limb, it rarely produces serious late sequelae.

The valves in the lower limb play an important role in controlling the direction of blood flow (see Chapter 3).

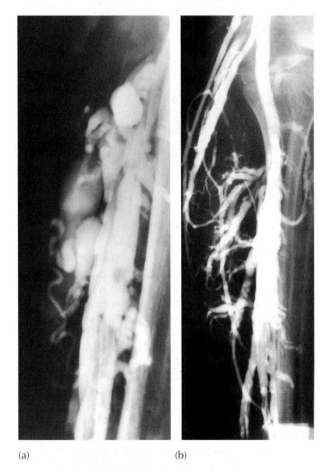

(a)   (b)

Figure 2.7 (a) Soleal muscle veins which are baggy and valveless. (b) Normal calf veins. There are numerous valves in the gastrocnemius veins, and in the paired stem veins.

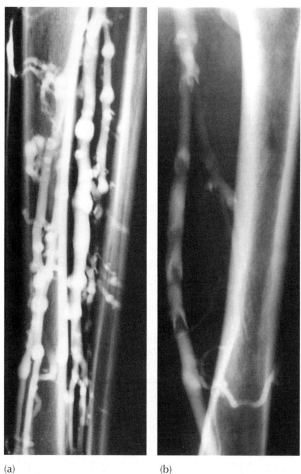

(a) (b)

Figure 2.8 (a) Valves in the stem veins of the calf causing a 'string of beads' appearance. (b) Valves in the superficial and deep femoral veins and the popliteal vein. There are fewer valves in these more proximal veins. In this phlebograph the clearly defined bicuspid valves are clearly shown because a Valsalva manoeuvre is being performed.

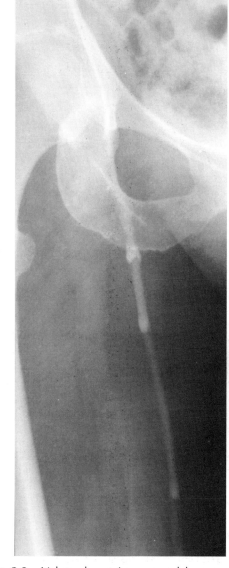

Figure 2.9 Valves shown in a normal long saphenous vein by a Valsalva manoeuvre.

There are no valves in the sinusoidal veins of the soleal muscles (Figure 2.7a) but the venous arcades which drain the soleal and gastrocnemius muscles have numerous valves (Figure 2.7b). All the deep veins of the calf are densely valved with valves occurring at approximately 2 cm intervals (Figure 2.8a). The popliteal vein usually has two valves in the region of the knee joint; damage to these valves may have serious consequences on the calf muscle pump.[3] There is a valve in the femoral vein just distal to its junction with the deep femoral vein in 90% of all legs and a valve in the upper third of the popliteal vein just distal to the adductor canal in 96% of legs. The other valves in the deep veins of the thigh are inconstant in number and position and not only vary from person to person but also vary between the right and left legs (Figure 2.8b).[13,40] There are eight to ten valves in the long and short saphenous veins. There is invariably a valve at the proximal end of the long saphenous vein which is thought to be important in preventing reflux down the long saphenous vein (Figure 2.9).

The valves in the communicating veins between the superficial and deep venous systems of the leg are arranged so that blood flows from the superficial to the deep veins, and the high pressure in the deep venous system is prevented from reaching the superficial veins. The valves in the communicating veins are both superficial and deep to the deep fascia (Figure 2.10).

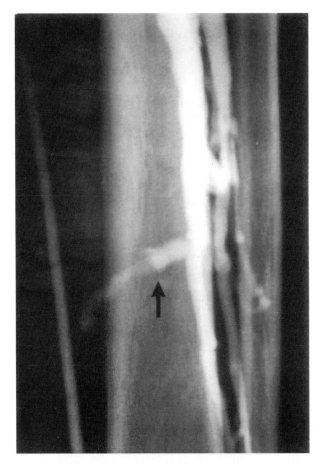

Figure 2.10 A phlebograph showing a valve in a normal communicating vein 10 cm above the ankle joint (arrowed). Venous valves are frequently shown to be slightly incompetent on phlebography.

There is some doubt about the significance of the valves in the communicating veins of the feet; it seems likely that these veins are only partly valved so that blood can flow from the feet into both the deep and superficial venous systems.[17,23] As a consequence of this bidirectional flow in the foot, in contrast to the situation in the rest of the leg, the foot veins have no major haemodynamic importance.

Anatomy of the lower limb veins

The foot veins

The venous drainage of the foot consists of the following systems:

- The superficial dorsal venous arch (i.e. the long and short saphenous vein, joined together by the arch and its tributaries)
- The plantar cutaneous arch joining the medial and lateral marginal veins
- The deep venous system of the sole (i.e. the lateral and medial plantar veins, which become the posterior tibial veins)
- The communicating veins, which connect the deep and superficial networks (Figure 2.11a and b).[37]

The deep veins of the leg

The deep veins of the lower leg consist of three paired stem veins which are venae commitantes accompanying the arteries: the anterior tibial veins, the posterior tibial veins and the peroneal veins. Each vein may divide into several trunks which surround the artery and anastomose freely with each other. The anterior tibial veins drain the blood from the dorsum of the foot and run in the deep part of the anterior (extensor) compartment close to the interosseous membrane. The posterior tibial veins are formed by the confluence of the superficial and deep plantar veins behind the ankle joint beneath the flexor retinaculum. The peroneal veins lie directly behind and medial to the fibula.

In a phlebograph taken in an antero-posterior or postero-anterior projection with the foot internally rotated, the peroneal veins lie between the images of the tibia and fibula, the anterior tibial veins lie more laterally, often overlying the fibula, and the posterior tibial veins lie medially, running obliquely upwards to cross the lower third of the shaft of the tibia. Individual veins are easier to identify in a lateral projection (Figure 2.12a and b). Collectively, these veins are referred to as the stem veins of the calf. The main deep veins of the lower limb are shown diagrammatically in Figure 2.13.

The veins of the calf muscles are either large, baggy and valveless, the so-called sinusoidal veins which are dilated segments of the venous arcades joining the posterior tibial and peroneal veins (see Figure 2.7), or thin and straight with valves (Figure 2.14). The former predominate in the soleal muscle and the latter in the gastrocnemius muscles.

In the upper part of the calf the paired stem veins merge to form single trunks and then unite at different levels to form the popliteal vein. If they unite above the knee joint they produce an apparently duplicated popliteal vein (Figure 2.15). The veins from the soleus muscle drain into the stem veins or the lower part of the popliteal vein. The

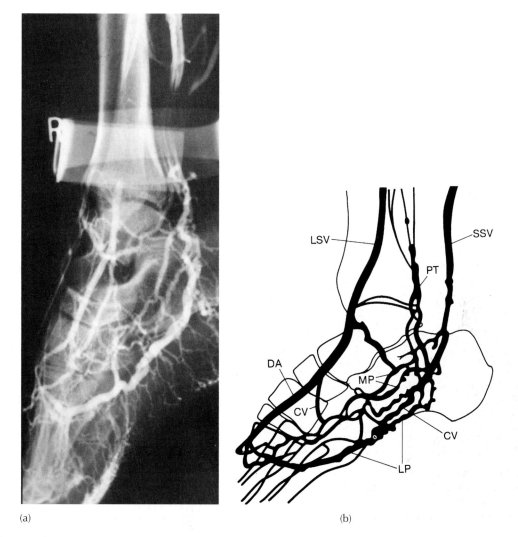

(a) (b)

Figure 2.11 (a) A normal foot phlebograph. (b) Schematic drawing of the foot veins. LSV, long saphenous vein; SSV, short saphenous vein; PT, posterior tibial veins; DA, dorsal venous arch (medial limb); MP, medial plantar vein; LP, lateral plantar vein; CV, communicating veins connecting the medial plantar veins with the medial limb of the dorsal venous arch and the lateral plantar veins with the lateral marginal vein. (After Pegum and Fegan.[37])

veins from the gastrocnemius muscles drain into the lower and upper parts of the popliteal vein (see Figure 2.14).

The deep veins of the thigh

The superficial femoral vein is the continuation of the popliteal vein and on a phlebograph passes obliquely upwards and medially across the lower third of the femur. Approximately 9 cm below the inguinal ligament it receives the deep femoral vein which is only demonstrated fully in about a third of phlebographs when there is a direct connection between the lower part of the superficial femoral vein and a tributary of the deep femoral vein (Figure 2.16). Mavor and Galloway[30] found the deep femoral vein connecting directly to the popliteal vein in 38% of limbs and with a tributary to the popliteal vein in 48%. These findings suggest that ligation of the femoral vein below the entrance of the deep femoral vein may often be ineffective in preventing thrombus from propagating up from the popliteal vein into the femoral vein.[30]

There are frequent and considerable variations in the anatomy of the popliteal vein, the superficial femoral vein and the deep femoral vein. Duplication occurs in 2% of legs. It has been suggested that the classical anatomical pattern is present in only 16% of legs.[8]

The common femoral and external iliac veins

The common femoral vein is formed by the confluence of the superficial femoral and deep femoral veins and becomes the external iliac vein as it passes beneath the inguinal ligament. As the inguinal ligament is not visible on a radiograph, its level must be inferred from a knowledge of its anatomical position. The distinction between the common femoral vein and external iliac vein is somewhat artificial, and tributaries commonly ascribed to one often drain into the other. The external iliac vein is the continuation of the common femoral vein. It runs from the inguinal ligament to the sacroiliac joint where it is joined inferomedially by the internal iliac vein emerging from the true pelvis (Figure 2.17). The main

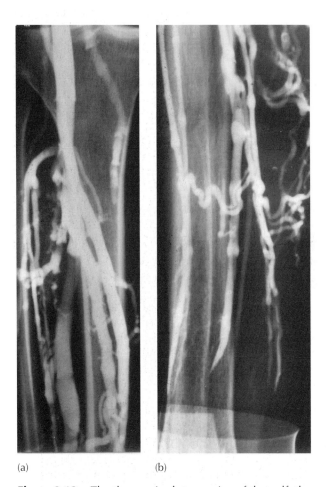

(a)   (b)

Figure 2.12 The three paired stem veins of the calf: the anterior tibial, peroneal and posterior tibial veins. In the upper part of the calf the veins merge into single trunks and then unite to form the popliteal vein. (a) Anterior projection with the foot internally rotated. (b) Lateral projection. The lateral phlebograph gives a better demonstration of the individual stem and muscle veins of the calf. The veins which lie behind the tibia and pass upwards towards it are always the posterior tibial veins. Interconnections between the deep veins are common.

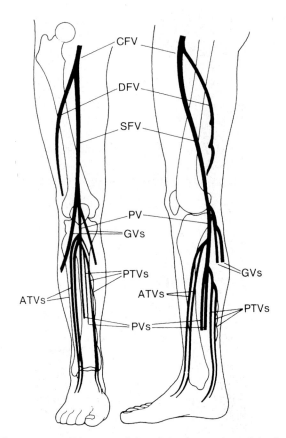

Figure 2.13 Diagram of the main deep veins of the leg. PVs, peroneal veins; ATVs, anterior tibial veins; PTVs, posterior tibial veins; GVs, gastrocnemius veins; PV, popliteal vein; CFV, common femoral vein; SFV, superficial femoral vein; DFV, deep femoral vein. (After May and Nissl.[32]) The terms common femoral, superficial femoral and deep femoral vein are frequently used clinically and throughout this book even though they are not absolutely accurate anatomical terms.

tributaries of the external iliac vein anastomose with each other across the floor of the pelvis to form important collaterals in iliac vein obstruction (Figure 2.18a and b).[31]

The common iliac veins

The common iliac veins are short wide vessels which ascend from the level of the sacroiliac joints to unite on the right side of the fifth lumbar vertebra to form the inferior vena cava. The right common iliac vein and the inferior vena cava run upwards in an almost straight line whereas the left common iliac vein runs transversely to join the left common iliac vein at a right angle. At this level the left common iliac vein is pushed forwards by the convexity of the lumbosacral spine and crossed by the right common iliac artery. This

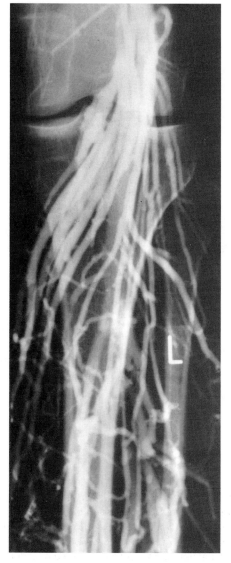

Figure 2.14 The gastrocnemius veins. These veins which drain the gastrocnemius muscles are straight and valved and join the upper popliteal vein. They tend to be multiple with up to seven medial and lateral tributaries.

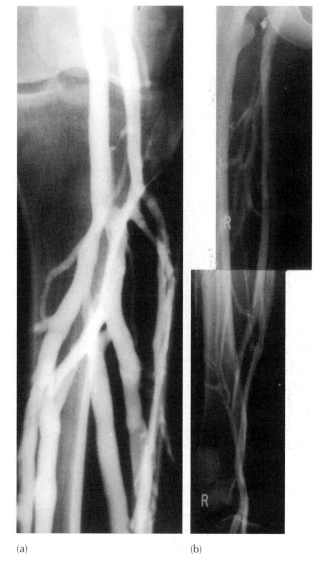

(a) (b)

Figure 2.15 (a) A phlebograph of a double popliteal vein caused by a high termination of the stem veins of the calf. (b) A phlebograph showing double popliteal, superficial and deep femoral veins.

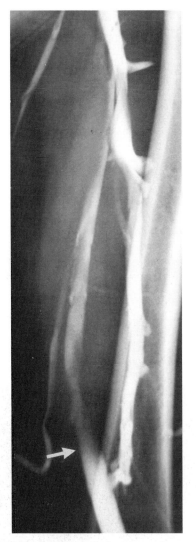

Figure 2.16 A phlebograph showing a direct connection between the superficial (white arrow) and deep femoral veins so that both fill completely. This direct communication occurs in about one-third of all legs and has surgical implications for ligation to prevent propagation of popliteal vein thrombosis.

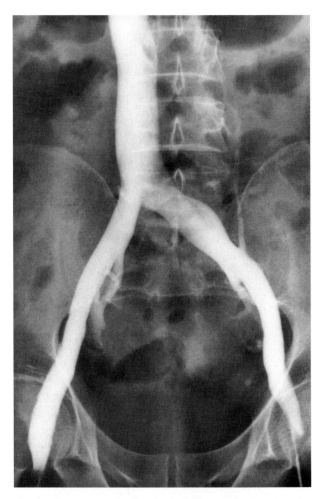

Figure 2.17 A normal pelvic phlebograph showing the external iliac veins, the common iliac veins and the lower inferior vena cava. The internal iliac veins are shown with a Valsalva manoeuvre as far as competent valves permit. There is a slight translucency at the termination of the left common iliac vein due to compression by the right common iliac artery. This is a normal appearance found in about half of all iliac phlebographs.

causes a variable degree of antero-posterior compression at the termination of the left common iliac vein which appears as a radiological filling defect in approximately 50% of pelvic phlebograms (see Figure 2.17). Excessive compression at this site may predispose to thrombosis and is discussed in detail in Chapter 9. The only tributary of the common iliac vein is the ascending lumbar vein which is larger on the left side than on the right side. The vein forms one of the main collateral pathways around a common iliac vein or lower inferior vena caval obstruction. Its iliac tributaries, draining the muscles of the false pelvis, form collaterals in external iliac vein obstruction (Figure 2.19).

The internal iliac veins

The internal iliac veins are formed on the floor of the true pelvis by the gluteal, internal pudendal and

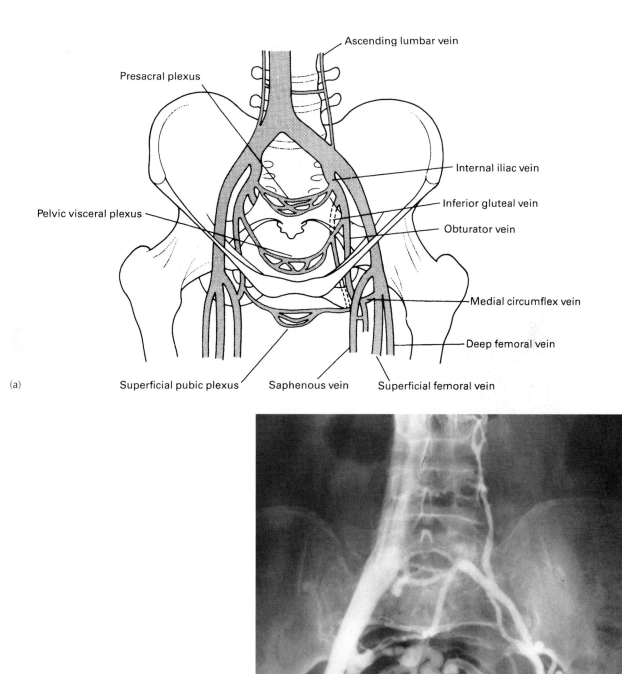

Ascending lumbar vein

Presacral plexus

Internal iliac vein

Pelvic visceral plexus

Inferior gluteal vein

Obturator vein

Medial circumflex vein

Deep femoral vein

(a)

Superficial pubic plexus   Saphenous vein   Superficial femoral vein

Figure 2.18 (a) Diagram of the potential collateral pathways in pelvic vein obstruction. (After Mavor and Galloway.[32]) (b) A pelvic phlebograph with left common iliac vein occlusion and replacement of the left external iliac vein by a collateral representing a vena commitans of the adjacent artery. Note the extensive collateral circulation from left to right through the pubic veins and the visceral and presacral plexuses.

(b)

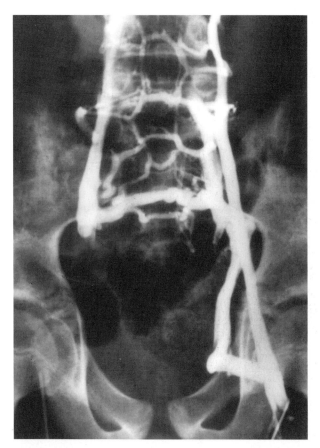

Figure 2.19 A left femoral vein injection phlebograph showing localized occlusion of the left common iliac vein, probably congenital in origin. There are collaterals from the presacral plexus, both ascending lumbar veins, and the vertebral plexuses. An enlarged obturator vein joining the left internal iliac vein is also a collateral.

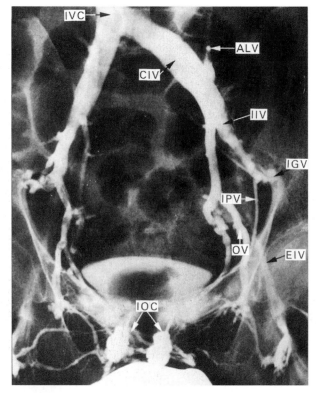

Figure 2.20 The internal iliac veins shown by bilateral intraosseous injections into the pubic bones in the supine position. This technique allows complete visualization of all the tributaries but is rarely required. IOC, intraosseous cannulae; IIV, internal iliac vein; EIV, external iliac vein; CIV, common iliac vein; IVC, inferior vena cava; ALV, ascending lumbar vein; OV, obturator vein; IPV, internal pudendal vein; IGV, inferior gluteal vein.

obturator veins together with the veins of the sacral and visceral pelvic plexuses. These plexuses may form valuable collaterals across the pelvis in unilateral common iliac vein obstruction (Figure 2.18a and b). The internal iliac veins can only be fully demonstrated radiologically by the intraosseous technique (Figure 2.20).

The inferior vena cava

The inferior vena cava is formed by the confluence of the common iliac veins at the level of the fifth lumbar vertebra and terminates at the right atrium (Figure 2.21a and b). It lies to the right of the vertebral bodies and receives a variable number of short, wide lumbar veins which connect with the vertebral venous plexuses, the left gonadal vein, the right renal vein, the right adrenal vein, the phrenic veins and the hepatic

veins. Many of these tributaries can only be shown by selective phlebography.

Potential routes for collaterals in inferior vena caval obstruction are almost limitless and the most complete analysis of these is that of Pleasants[39] but this was before the advent of vena cavography.[12] Ferris *et al.* have described the channels most often demonstrated by phlebography,[14,15] and even these may require special techniques such as balloon occlusion cavography, selective catheterization or intraosseous studies to show them fully. Ferris and his colleagues, for convenience, divided the collaterals into central, intermediate, portal and superficial groups. The central channels comprise the lumbo-azygos system, the vertebral plexuses and the cava above the occlusion; the intermediate channels comprise the gonadal veins, the ureteric veins and the left renal-azygos system; the portal collaterals are via the rectal plexus; and the

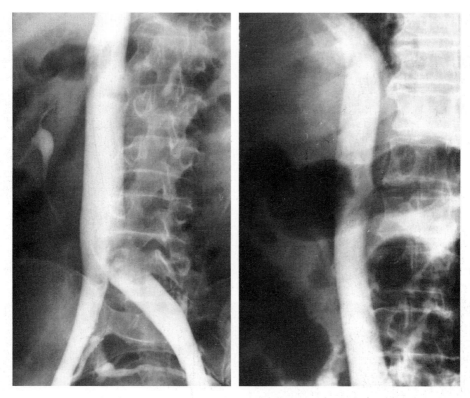

Figure 2.21 A normal inferior vena cavagraph. (a) Antero-posterior projection. (b) 20 degree left anterior oblique projection. The cava lies to the right of the vertebral column. Non-opacified blood can be seen entering from the renal veins and hepatic veins.

extensive superficial routes include the superficial epigastric, the circumflex iliac veins, the thoraco-abdominal, the lateral thoracic and the axillary veins together with the superior vena cava (Figure 2.22a, b and c).[16,27]

THE SUPERFICIAL VEINS OF THE LOWER LIMB

The superficial venous system of the leg consists of two main veins, the long and short saphenous veins (both of which are valved) and their tributaries (Figure 2.23).

The long saphenous vein

The long saphenous vein is formed by the union of the veins from the medial side of the sole of the foot with the medial dorsal veins. It runs upwards in front of the medial malleolus along the length of the antero-medial aspect of the limb, gradually inclining posteriorly to pass behind the medial condyles of the tibia and femur. It is accompanied by the saphenous branch of the femoral nerve which may

be avulsed if the vein is stripped below the knee. In the thigh the long saphenous vein runs in a slight curve towards its junction with the femoral vein, the breadth of two fingers (3 cm) below and lateral to the pubic tubercle, at the fossa ovalis. Just before it enters the fossa, it is joined by the superficial circumflex iliac, the superficial inferior epigastric and the superficial external pudendal veins (and occasionally by the deep internal pudendal vein, although this usually drains directly into the common femoral vein) together with as many as seven other superficial unnamed veins (Figure 2.24).[18] The long saphenous vein receives several tributaries in its course along the lower leg. The medial superficial veins from the sole join it near its anatomical origin and the posterior arch vein joints its posterior aspect in the upper leg. The posterior arch vein is important because it is connected to the deep venous system by at least two or three major medial ankle communicating veins. It should be noted that stripping the long saphenous vein from the ankle upwards does not avulse these communicating veins. The anterior superficial tibial vein joins the long saphenous vein at about the same level as the posterior arch vein (see Figure 2.23).

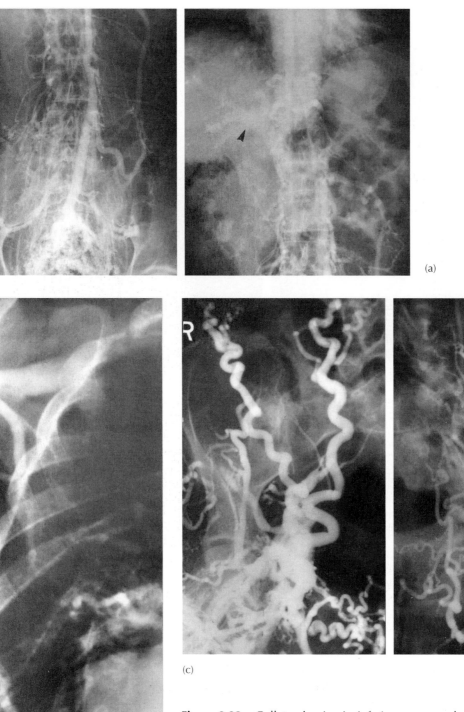

(a)

(c)

(b)

Figure 2.22   Collateral veins in inferior vena caval obstruction. (a) Deep collaterals from the rectal venous plexus joining the portal vein (arrow) via the inferior mesenteric vein. (b) Lateral thoracic veins joining the axillary vein demonstrated by intraosseous pertrochanteric phlebography. (c) The lower inferior vena cava and the external and common iliac veins are occluded. The superficial collateral veins bypassing the obstruction are the superficial epigastric veins medially and the superficial circumflex iliac veins laterally. These collaterals should be clinically obvious.

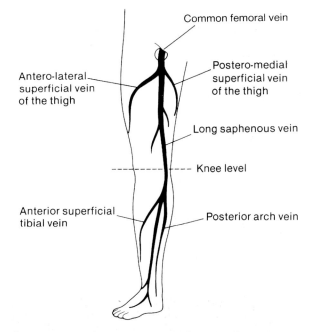

Figure 2.23 shows labels: Common femoral vein, Antero-lateral superficial vein of the thigh, Postero-medial superficial vein of the thigh, Long saphenous vein, Knee level, Anterior superficial tibial vein, Posterior arch vein.

Figure 2.23 The anatomy of the superficial venous system of the lower extremity. (After Haeger.[18])

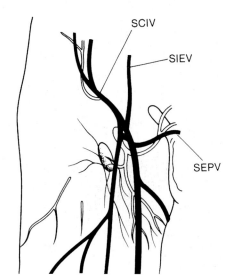

Figure 2.24 shows labels: SCIV, SIEV, SEPV.

Figure 2.24 The most constant tributaries of the saphenous vein in the fossa ovalis. SIEV, superficial inferior epigastric vein; SEPV, superficial external pudendal vein; SCIV, superficial circumflex iliac vein.

Two large tributaries join the long saphenous vein in the thigh. They are probably best referred to as the postero-medial and antero-lateral superficial veins of the thigh. The postero-medial vein usually originates from a confluence of veins on the postero-medial border and the posterior aspect of

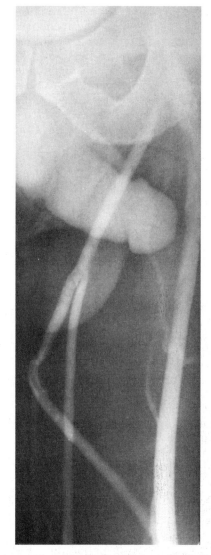

Figure 2.25 The postero-medial superficial vein of the thigh shown by saphenography. This vein and the antero-lateral superficial vein of the thigh may be quite large and mistaken for the main long saphenous vein at surgery.

the thigh. It often connects with the upper part of the short saphenous vein just before that vein pierces the deep fascia. It runs around the medial aspect of the thigh as it ascends and ends by joining the upper part of the long saphenous vein. The antero-lateral superficial vein of the thigh runs from the lateral aspect of the knee obliquely across the anterior aspect of the thigh to join the long saphenous vein usually just below its termination but sometimes as low as 15 cm below the fossa ovalis. Both medial and lateral superficial thigh veins may be quite large and can be mistaken at operation for the main long saphenous vein (Figures 2.23, 2.25).

There are many variations of anatomy in the region of the fossa ovalis where the long saphenous vein joins the common femoral vein, mainly consisting of the direct entry of one or more of the tributaries of the long saphenous vein into the common femoral vein.[10] These variations will be recognized at the time of surgery if the sapheno-femoral junction is adequately displayed. Varicography or saphenography can give preoperative information about these anatomical variations (see Chapters 4 and 6).

In approximately 15–20% of legs the superficial external pudendal artery crosses in front of the long saphenous vein. This can be safely divided to expose the deep structures of the sapheno-femoral junction. The reported frequency of duplication or reduplication of the long saphenous vein varies between 1% and 27%.[19,33] In the authors' experience, based on saphenography in patients without previous surgery for varicose veins, the frequency of duplication is approximately 5%. There are two rare, but clinically important, variations of the termination of the long saphenous vein; a low termination in which the saphenous vein joins the femoral vein 3–5 cm below the inguinal ligament with the external pudendal and superficial epigastric veins joining at the usual higher site,[4] and a high termination in which the long saphenous vein terminates in a vein in the subcutaneous tissues of the abdominal wall.[43]

The short saphenous vein

The short saphenous vein begins at the outer border of the foot behind the lateral malleolus as a continuation of the dorsal venous arch.[22] It is joined above the malleolus by a communicating vein which may be important when ulcers are present in this area. It enters the popliteal vein between the heads of the gastrocnemius muscle. The short saphenous vein is best seen in the lateral projection of a phlebograph where it can be seen lying superficially and following the curve of the calf muscles (Figure 2.26). There are a number of variable connections between the long and short saphenous vein in the region of the knee and these may cause confusion when trying to decide whether varices are connected to dorsal tributaries of the long saphenous vein or to tributaries of the short saphenous vein. The short saphenous vein usually joins the posterior aspect of the popliteal vein lateral to the tibial nerve producing a characteristic 'S'-shaped loop on a saphenogram. Duplication of the short saphenous vein, in contrast to that of the long saphenous vein, is extremely rare – 0.25%.[24] The close proximity of a lateral gastrocnemius vein which may be indistinguishable from the short saphenous vein is often

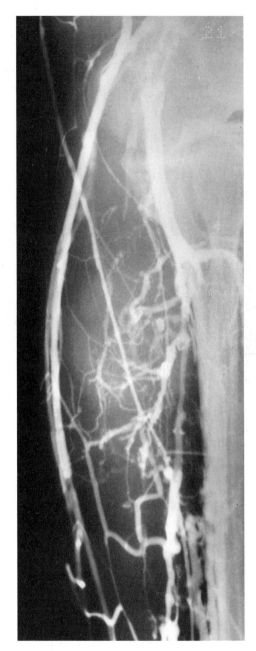

Figure 2.26 The short saphenous vein shown by short saphenography. The vein can be recognized in a lateral projection lying superficially in the subcutaneous tissues following the curve of the calf muscles.

mistaken for duplication (Figure 2.27). Approximately 60% of all short saphenous veins join the popliteal vein in the popliteal fossa within 8 cm of the knee joint; 20% join the long saphenous vein via the postero-medial or antero-lateral superficial thigh veins at varying levels in the thigh; and the remainder join the superficial femoral vein, the

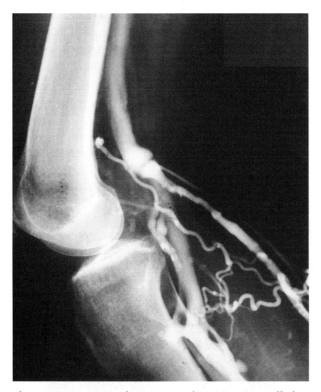

Figure 2.27 A saphenogram showing a small but entirely normal short saphenous vein joining the popliteal vein in the popliteal fossa. Deep to this is a lateral gastrocnemius vein which is often mistaken for a duplication.

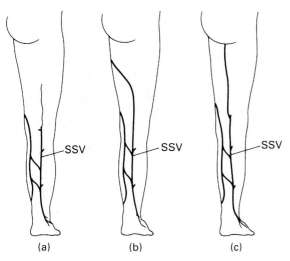

(a) (b) (c)

Figure 2.28 Diagrams of the variations in termination of the short saphenous vein (SSV). (a) A small tributary extending superficially onto the back of the thigh. (b) The short saphenous vein joining the superficial postero-medial vein of the thigh which drains into the long saphenous vein. (c) The short saphenous vein passing deeply to join a gluteal vein draining into the internal iliac vein. (After Kosinski.[24])

deep femoral vein, or even tributaries of the internal iliac veins (Figure 2.28a, b and c).[25,35] Wherever the principal termination, and however high, there is usually a small vestigial connection with the popliteal vein. As the precise termination of the short saphenous vein is difficult to find by clinical examination, the site of its termination by saphenography, varicography, can be very useful as a preoperative investigation (Figure 2.29).

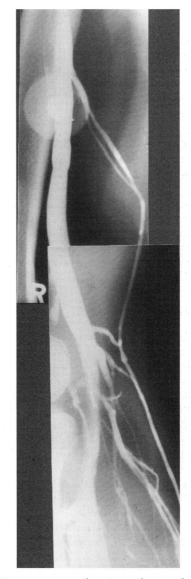

Figure 2.29 A montage showing a short saphenous vein with a high termination into the superficial femoral vein in the thigh. Note that there is a tributary joining the popliteal vein at the usual site in the popliteal fossa. The ball-bearings are of known size and enable correction for magnification to be made when assessing the diameter of the vein for use for bypass surgery.

The communicating veins

The deep and superficial venous system of the lower extremity are separated by fascia and joined by communicating veins with valves which direct the blood from the superficial to the deep venous system. These communicating veins are sometimes called perforating veins because they pierce the deep fascia (see Chapter 3). The communicating veins have been further divided into direct (i.e. connecting a superficial vein directly with a deep vein) or indirect, when the connection is through one or more sinusoids in the muscles.[28] This distinction is somewhat artificial but the direct communicating veins are generally more constant in position, larger and haemodynamically more important than the indirect veins.

The largest communicating veins are the terminations of the long and short saphenous veins where they join the deep venous system but they are only part of a system of more than 100 veins in each leg which connect the superficial to the deep veins. The communicating veins of the foot allow the blood to pass in either direction and are of little physiological importance.

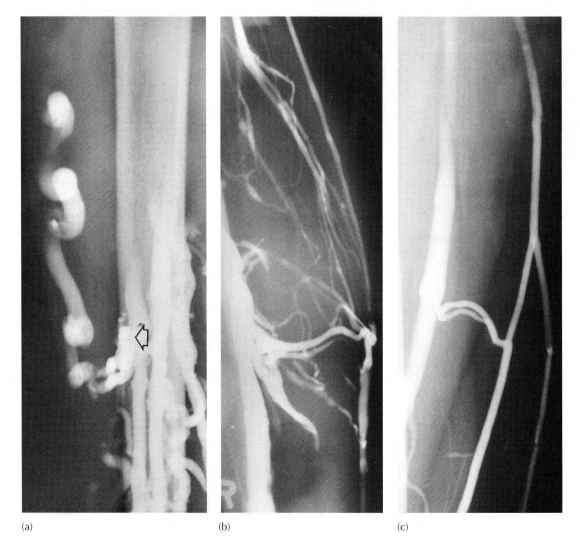

(a)   (b)   (c)

Figure 2.30   Examples of communicating veins shown by ascending phlebography. (a) A medial ankle communicating vein of Cockett. The vein demonstrated here is incompetent because it fills from the posterior tibial (i.e. a deep vein), it is dilated and joins a varicose vein. (b) The soleus 'point'. This communicating vein connects veins in the soleal muscle with the short saphenous vein or its tributaries. The gastrocnemius point (not illustrated, see Figure 2.31) connects veins in the gastrocnemius muscle with the superficial veins. (c) Mid-thigh communicating veins (Dodd's group). These veins in Hunter's canal are frequently multiple. The two veins shown here are almost certainly competent, being less than 3 mm in diameter.

In the lower leg there are medial and lateral communicating veins. On the medial side there is one communicating vein just below the medial malleolus and three or four above the malleolus behind the tibia. The medial lower leg communicating veins, often called Cockett's veins, connect the posterior arch vein with the posterior tibial veins but do not drain directly into the long saphenous vein (Figure 2.30a).[9] The lowest medial communicating vein is usually found at approximately 7 cm, the middle vein at 12 cm and the upper vein 18 cm above the tip of the medial malleolus. A further communicating vein may be present above these.[34] Another communicating vein which may become incompetent is situated on the medial aspect of the calf 10 cm below the knee joint. It joins the main trunk of the long saphenous vein to the posterior tibial veins and is sometimes called Boyd's vein.[5]

The most important communicating vein on the lateral side of the lower leg is not constant in position. It connects the short saphenous vein with the peroneal veins anywhere from just above the lateral malleolus to the junction of the lower and middle thirds of the calf. Two more constant communicating veins also joining the short saphenous vein with the peroneal veins are situated posteriorly approximately 5 cm and 12 cm above the os calcis. These are the two posterior mid-calf communicating veins

which sometimes cause recurrent varicose veins. They join the short saphenous vein or its tributaries to the soleal or gastrocnemius muscle veins near the midline (Figure 2.30b) and are referred to as the soleal and gastrocnemius points.

In the thigh there are several connections between the long saphenous vein and the femoral vein. The most important group, sometimes called Dodd's veins[11] consist of one or more veins which pass through the subsartorial (Hunter's) canal to join the long saphenous vein with the superficial femoral vein (Figure 2.30c). These veins are usually, but not invariably, destroyed when the long saphenous vein is stripped out and so are an important cause of recurrent varicose veins. After saphenous ligation, without stripping, an incompetent mid-thigh communicating vein may be responsible for an early recurrence of varicose veins on the medial aspect of the leg in the region of the knee.

The most important communicating veins of the legs are shown diagrammatically in Figure 2.31.

Whilst the communicating veins which have been described are relatively constant and surgically important, other communicating veins may be the cause of primary or secondary varicose veins or ulceration at unusual sites. For this reason their accurate localization by ascending phlebography or varicography is often required as discussed in Chapter 4.

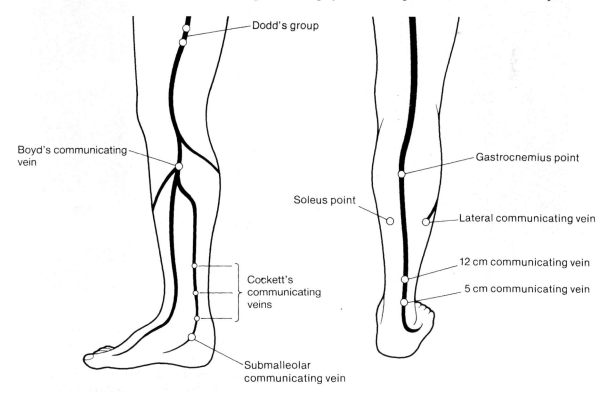

Figure 2.31 Diagram of the clinically important communicating veins of the leg. (a) Medial view. (b) Postero-lateral view. (After May and Nissl.[34])

Anatomy of the upper limb veins

The upper limb has a superficial and a deep system of veins, both of which drain into a single outflow tract, the axillary vein. The superficial veins drain the dorsal aspect of the hand laterally through the cephalic vein, and medially through the basilic vein. At the elbow these veins are joined by the median cubital vein and the blood is carried proximally by both the cephalic and basilic veins which join the deep veins at different levels near the shoulder. The basilic vein pierces the fascia of the upper arm to join the deep brachial vein and become the axillary vein. The cephalic vein pierces the clavipectoral fascia to join the axillary vein (Figure 2.32a). The deep veins draining the palmar surface of the hand continue as paired venae commitantes of the radial and ulnar arteries. A third group of veins, the interosseous veins, join with the radial and ulnar veins to form a pair of brachial veins which become in turn the axillary, subclavian and brachio-cephalic (innominate) veins.

The right and left brachio-cephalic veins unite to form the superior vena cava which descends on the right of the ascending aorta to enter the right atrium at the level of the third costar cartilage (Figure 2.33). In its upper half the superior vena cava is covered on its anterior, posterior and right side by the pleura. In its lower half it lies within the pericardium. Before it enters the pericardium it is joined posteriorly by the azygos vein.

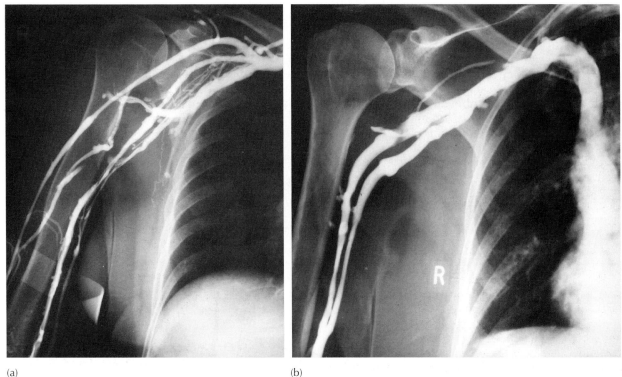

(a)   (b)

Figure 2.32 (a) A phlebograph showing the superficial veins of the arm. The cephalic vein is often paired, as in this example. Both cephalic veins can be seen on the lateral aspect of the upper arm entering the axillary vein just below the medial part of the clavicle. The basilic vein can be seen on the medial aspect of the arm. It passes deeply to join the usually paired brachial veins to become the axillary vein at the outer border of the scapula. The phlebograph is not taken in the true anatomical position of the arm which is why the cephalic and basilic veins are not as clearly separated as they are in life or when shown diagrammatically. (b) The deep veins of the arm. The paired brachial veins become the axillary vein at the outer border of the scapula. At the outer border of the first rib the axillary vein continues as the subclavian vein. The brachio-cephalic (innominate) vein is formed behind the sterno-clavicular joint by the junction of the subclavian and the internal jugular vein. The innominate vein can be seen in this phlebograph passing downwards to enter the superior vena cava. Before doing so it is joined by the right innominate vein and both veins drain into the right atrium.

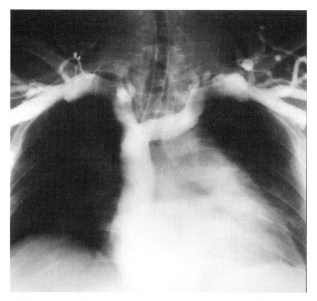

Figure 2.33 A normal superior vena cava, formed by the confluence of the brachio-cephalic (innominate) veins, entering the right atrium.

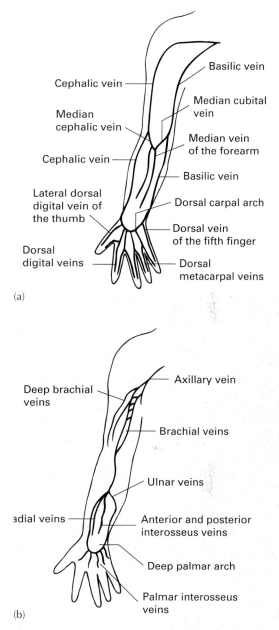

Figure 2.34 (a) Diagram of the superficial veins of the upper limb. (b) Diagram of the deep veins of the upper limb.

The axillary vein begins, by definition, at the lower border of the subscapularis muscle but as this cannot be seen on radiographs it is usually considered to begin at the outer border of the scapula. It ends at the outer border of the first rib where it becomes the subclavian vein which in turn ends just medial to the midpoint of the clavicle. The brachio-cephalic veins are formed by the junction of the subclavian and internal jugular veins behind the sterno-clavicular joints and end where they unite to form the superior vena cava behind the lower border of the fifth right costal cartilage (see Figure 2.32b).

The usual arrangement of the superficial and deep veins of the upper limb are shown diagrammatically in Figure 2.34a and b.

Variations in the anatomy of the veins of the upper limb occur frequently but as primary varicose veins are absent in the upper limb, venous surgery is rarely required and the variations are therefore much less significant than those of the lower limb. Sometimes the median cubital vein is large and carries all or most of the blood from the cephalic into the basilic vein, the proximal part of the cephalic vein being either absent or proportionally diminished. The accessory cephalic vein arises from small tributaries on the back of the forearm and from the ulnar side of the dorsal venous network and joins the cephalic vein below the elbow. In some arms it arises from the cephalic vein above the wrist and joins it higher up. A large oblique tributary frequently joins the cephalic vein on the back

of the forearm. Sometimes the brachio-cephalic veins open independently into the right atrium, the right vein taking the course of the normal superior vena cava and the left vein becoming a persistent left superior vena cava (see Figure 2.6a).

The superficial and deep veins of the arm are linked by a few valved communicating veins, one of the largest being in the cubital fossa. The venous drainage of the upper limb is largely the result of cardiac function, and as there is no muscle pump the valves have little physiological importance. These differences between the upper and lower limbs, which presumably evolved in parallel with man's erect posture, may explain why pathological conditions of the upper limb of venous origin are so uncommon. Only a few patent veins are required for adequate venous drainage and most venous occlusions are rapidly compensated by collaterals. Few, if any, symptoms occur if thrombosis in the upper limb veins damages the valves.[38] Valvular incompetence does not produce symptoms in the upper limb.

The azygos and vertebral venous systems

Venous blood enters the heart via the superior and inferior vena cava. If either or both of these veins is obstructed, drainage is maintained by collaterals formed mainly by the azygos and vertebral venous systems.[1,44]

The origin of the azygos vein is inconstant but it can generally be regarded as the continuation of the ascending lumbar vein into the thorax.

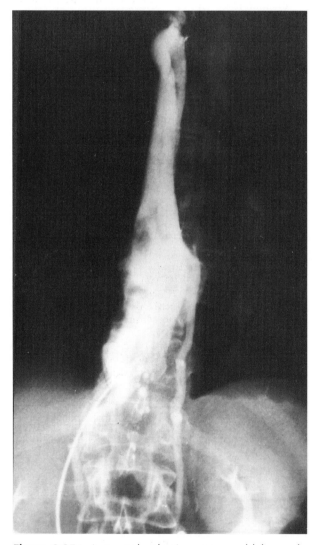

Figure 2.35 A normal selective azygos phlebograph. The right ascending lumbar vein becomes the azygos vein as it enters the thorax. On the left of this phlebograph the ascending lumbar vein can be seen passing upwards becoming the hemi-azygos vein and crossing the midline at D9 to enter the azygos vein.

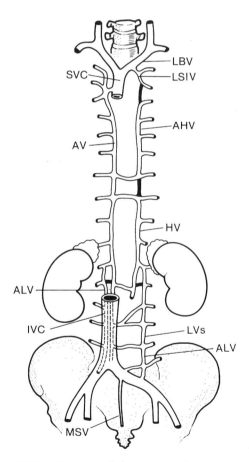

Figure 2.36 Diagram of the azygos, hemi-azygos and ascending lumbar veins. Shaded segments indicate variable communications. IVC, inferior vena cava; ALV, ascending lumbar veins; SVC, superior vena cava; LBV, left brachio-cephalic vein; LSIV, left superior intercostal vein; AHV, accessory hemi-azygos vein; HV, hemi-azygos vein; AV, azygos vein; LVs, lumbar veins; MSV, median sacral vein. All these veins, together with the vertebral plexuses, are potential collaterals in superior vena cava obstruction. (After Hemingway.[20])

Similarly, the hemi-azygos vein is the continuation of the left ascending lumbar vein. In approximately 60% of people the left renal vein communicates with the hemi-azygos system. The hemi-azygos vein crosses the vertebral column at the level of the ninth lumbar vertebra to join the azygos vein. The azygos vein ascends into the thorax to the level of the fourth thoracic vertebra where it passes anteriorly to join the superior vena cava (Figure 2.35).

In approximately 0.5% of the population the azygos vein continues upwards in a more lateral position before entering the superior vena cava at a higher level, giving rise to an azygos lobe of the right lung.[20] The azygos and hemi-azygos veins have a few imperfect valves but their tributaries have functioning venous valves. The veins of the vertebral column form an intricate plexus extending along its entire length, divisible into the external and internal plexuses, outside and inside the vertebral canal. These veins are devoid of valves, anastomose freely with each other, and drain into the intercostal veins, and into the ascending lumbar veins through the intervertebral veins.

In aplasia or hypoplasia or obstruction to either the superior or inferior vena cava, the azygos systems and the vertebral plexuses provide the main channels for venous drainage (Figure 2.36).[11,20] Apart from these circumstances the detailed anatomy of this complex and inconstant venous network is of little practical importance.

References

1. Abrams HL. The vertebral and azygos veins. In: Abrams HL, ed. *Angiography*, 3rd edition. Boston: Little Brown, 1983; 895.
2. Arey LB. *Development Anatomy*. Philadelphia and London: WB Saunders, 1974.
3. Basmajian JV. The distribution of valves in the femoral, external, iliac and common iliac veins and their relationship to varicose veins. *Surg Gynecol Obstet* 1952; **95:** 537.
4. Bevan PE, Green SH, Stammers FAR. Low termination of the internal saphenous vein. *Br Med J* 1956; **1:** 610.
5. Boyd AM. Discussion on primary treatment of varicose veins. *Proc R Soc Med* 1948; **41:** 633.
6. Campbell M, Deuchar DC. Left sided superior vena cava. *Br Heart J* 1954; **16:** 423.
7. Cha ME, Khoury GH. Persistent left superior vena cava: radiologic and clinical significance. *Radiology* 1972; **103:** 375.
8. Cockett FB. Abnormalities of the deep veins of the leg. *Postgrad Med J* 1954; **30:** 512.
9. Cockett FB. The pathology and treatment of venous ulcers of the leg. *Br J Surg* 1955; **43:** 260.
10. Daseler EH, Anson BJ, Reimann AF, Beaton LE. The saphenous venous tributaries and related structures in relation to the technique of high ligation. *Surg Gynecol Obstet* 1946; **82:** 53.
11. Dodd H. The varicose tributaries of the superficial femoral vein passing into Hunter's canal. *Postgrad Med J* 1959; **35:** 18.
12. dos Santos R. Phlébographie d'une veine cava inférieure suture. *J Urol Med Chir* 1935; **39:** 586.
13. Eger SA, Casper SL. Etiology of varicose veins from the anatomic aspect based on dissections of 38 adult cadavers. *JAMA* 1943; **123:** 148.
14. Ferris EJ. The inferior vena cava. In: Abrams HL, ed. *Angiography*, 3rd edition. Boston: Little Brown, 1983.
15. Ferris EJ, Hipona FA, Kahn PC, Phillips E, Shapiro JH. *Venography of the Inferior Vena Cava and its Branches*. Baltimore: Williams & Wilkins, 1969.
16. Fletcher EWL, Lea Thomas M. Chronic postthrombotic obstruction of the inferior vena cava investigation by cavography. A report of two cases. *Am J Roentgenol* 1968; **102:** 363.
17. Hach W. *Phlebographie der Bein – und Beckenvenen*. Konstantz: Schnetztor Verlag, 1976.
18. Haeger K. Practical anatomy. In: Haeger K, ed. *Venous and Lymphatic Disorders of the Leg*. Lund: Scandinavian University Books, 1966.
19. Haeger K. The anatomy of the veins of the leg. In: Hobbs JT, ed. *The Treatment of Venous Disorders*. Lancaster: MTP Press, 1977.
20. Hemingway AP. Venography. In: Grainger RG, Allison DJ, eds. *Diagnostic Radiology*. Edinburgh: Churchill Livingstone, 1986.
21. Hirsch DM, Chan K. Bilateral inferior vena cava. *JAMA* 1963; **18S:** 729.
22. Holinshead WH. *Anatomy for Surgeons*. Volume 3. Philadelphia: Harper and Row, 1982; 603.
23. Jacobsen B. The venous drainage of the foot. *Surg Gynecol Obstet* 1970; **131:** 22.
24. Kosinski G. Observations on the superficial venous system of the lower extremity. *J Anat* 1926; **60:** 131.
25. Langman J. *Medical Embryology*, 4th edition. Baltimore/London: Williams & Wilkins, 1981; 191.
26. Lea Thomas M, Posniak HV. Agenesis of the iliac veins. *J Cardiovasc Surg* 1984; **25:** 64.
27. Lea Thomas M, Fletcher EWL, Cockett FB, Negus D. Venous collaterals in external and common iliac vein obstruction. *Clin Radiol* 1967; **18:** 403.
28. Le Deutu A. *Recherches Anatomiques et Considerations Physiologiques sur la Circulation Vein use du Pied et de la Jambe*. Thesis, Paris: 1967.
29. McClure EF, Butler EG. The development of the vena cava inferior in man. *Am J Anat* 1925; **35:** 331.
30. Mavor GE, Galloway JMD. The iliofemoral venous segment as a source of pulmonary emboli. *Lancet* 1967; **1:** 871.
31. Mavor GE, Galloway JMD. Collaterals of the deep venous circulation of the lower limb. *Surg Gynecol Obstet* 1967; **125:** 561.

32. May R, Nissl R. *Die Phlebographie der Unteren Extremitat.* Stuttgart: Thieme, 1959.

33. May R, Nissl R. Surgery of the veins of the leg and pelvis. In: May R, ed. *Anatomy.* Stuttgart: Georg Thieme, 1979.

34. May R, Nissl R. Nomenclature of the surgically most important connecting veins. In: May R, Patsch H, Staubesand J, eds. *Perforating Veins.* Munich: Urban & Schwarzenberg, 1981.

35. Mullarky RE. *The Anatomy of Varicose Veins.* Springfield, IL: Thomas, 1965.

36. Negus D. The surgical anatomy of the veins of the lower limb. In: Dodd H, Cockett FB, eds. *The Pathology and Surgery of the Veins of the Lower Limb.* Edinburgh: Churchill Livingstone, 1976.

37. Pegum JM, Fegan WG. Physiology of venous return from the foot. *Cardiovasc Res* 1967; **1:** 249.

38. Picard JD. *La Phlebographie des Membres Inférieurs et Supérieurs.* Paris: Expansion Scientifique Francaise, 1975.

39. Pleasants JH. Obstruction of inferior vena cava with a report of 18 cases. *Johns Hopkins Hosp Rep* 1911; **16:** 363.

40. Powell T, Lynn RB. The valves of the external, iliac, femoral and upper third of the popliteal veins. *Surg Gynecol Obstet* 1951; **92:** 453.

41. Raivio E. Untersuchungen uber die Venen der unteren Extremitaten mit besonderer Berucksichtigung der gegenseitigen Verbindungen zwischen den oberflachigen und tiefen Venen. *Ann Med Exp Fenn* 1948; **26:** 1.

42. Seib GA. The azygos system of veins in American whites and American negroes, including observations on the inferior caval venous system. *Am J Phys Anthropol* 1934; **19:** 39.

43. Sieglbauer F. *Lehrbuch der Normalen. Anatomie des Menschen.* Wien: Urban & Schwarzenberg, 1944.

44. Yao JST, Neiman HL. Upper extremity venography. In: Neiman HL, Yao ST, eds. *Angiography of Vascular Disease.* New York: Churchill Livingstone, 1985.

CHAPTER 3

Physiology and functional anatomy

Physiology	49	The causes of calf pump failure	59
The functional anatomy of the calf pump	55	The arm veins	62
The physiology of the calf pump	57	References	62

Although the veins form almost one-half of the circulatory system and contain two-thirds of the blood, our understanding of venous physiology has lagged behind our understanding of arterial physiology.

There are two reasons why the physiology of the veins has been neglected. First, there are no obvious fatal venous diseases. Consequently, there has not been the stimulus from the physician to the physiologist to explore venous physiology in the way that there has been the stimulus from physicians to investigate the kidney, bowel, heart and arteries. Secondly, veins are extremely difficult to study. Their variable anatomy, ever changing pressure and flow characteristics and susceptibility to so many local external influences makes measurement of their physiological properties difficult to achieve and interpret. Fortunately, the last 40 years have witnessed a tremendous improvement in measurement techniques and many of these methods have been applied to the veins. There are now numerous books on venous physiology, the subject is vast.[4,34,84] The purpose of this chapter is to introduce some of the important aspects of venous physiology which are relevant to the study of abnormalities of the peripheral veins and, in particular, the function of the calf muscle pump.

Physiology

Venous pressure

The pressure in a foot vein which is measured *when the subject is supine* represents the increment of pressure that remains after the dissipation of the kinetic energy generated from the heart by the resistance of the arterioles and capillaries. It is approximately 15 mmHg (2.0 kPa). The right atrial pressure is normally between 0 and 2 mmHg so the venous return to the heart when the subject is supine is generated by a pressure gradient of 13–15 mmHg.

When the body is erect, the column of blood between the heart and the foot exerts a gravitational force – the hydrostatic pressure. Provided this column of blood is not interrupted at any point, the foot vein pressure is then 15 mmHg plus the pressure exerted by the column of blood between the foot and the point used as the zero reference for the pressure measurement – usually the level of the manubrium sterni. This hydrostatic pressure is exerted equally by the blood in the arteries and the veins, so the perfusion pressure, the pressure difference between the arteries and veins, is unchanged. In a man who is 180 cm (6 ft) tall the

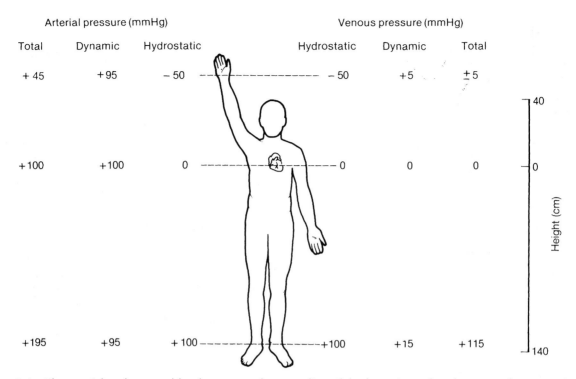

Arterial pressure (mmHg)   Venous pressure (mmHg)

Total	Dynamic	Hydrostatic		Hydrostatic	Dynamic	Total
+ 45	+ 95	− 50		− 50	+ 5	± 5
+ 100	+ 100	0		0	0	0
+ 195	+ 95	+ 100		+ 100	+ 15	+ 115

Height (cm): 40 / 0 / 140

Figure 3.1   The arterial and venous blood pressure when standing. If the heart is used as the zero reference point for pressure measurements, the pressure at any point in the circulation is the sum of the dynamic pressure generated by the heart and the hydrostatic pressure exerted by the column of blood between the site of measurement and the zero reference point.

hydrostatic pressure (the gravitational potential energy) is approximately 100 mmHg. This means that the measured foot vein pressure will be 100 + 15 mmHg and the mean foot arterial pressure will be 100 + 90 mmHg, the pressure gradient across the capillaries remaining unchanged (Figure 3.1).

If only the pressure measurements are considered, it may seem that arterial blood is flowing from the heart to the foot against the pressure gradient. It is, but the gravitational energy (not the pressure) is 0 mmHg at the foot and 100 mmHg at heart level because the energy resides at the top of the column of blood. Thus the total energy at heart level is 200 mmHg (the 100 mmHg of kinetic pressure energy generated by the heart plus the gravitational energy of 100 mmHg) whereas the total energy at the ankle is 90 mmHg (the 90 mmHg kinetic pressure energy produced by the heart plus no gravitational energy). The blood is flowing down to the foot against the pressure gradient but with the energy gradient.

The vein wall contains the same mixture of muscle fibres, elastin and collagen arranged in the tunica adventitia, media and interna as other blood vessels. The collagen and muscle fibres are arranged in a spiral. The smooth muscle supplies the active tone, and the elastin and collagen supply the passive elasticity.

When a vein relaxes, it collapses flat. As it distends it passes through an eliptical form to become circular (Figure 3.2). The resistance to blood flow becomes less as the cross-section changes from an elipse to a circle. Until the cross-section becomes circular, the vein can accommodate an increasing volume of blood without a significant increase in distending pressure. The distending pressure is the transmural pressure (i.e. the intraluminal pressure

Cross-section of vein lumen

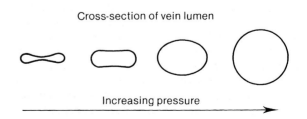

Increasing pressure

Figure 3.2   When a vein is collapsed its transverse section is 'dumb-bell'-shaped. As it distends it becomes elliptical before becoming circular. The resistance to flow becomes slightly less as it changes from an elipse to a circle.

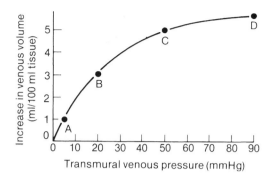

Figure 3.3 The pressure–volume curve of the veins of the lower limb. Between points A and B an increase in volume of 0.5 ml/100 ml tissue causes an increase in pressure of 4 mmHg. Between points C and D the same volume change increases the pressure by 50 mmHg.

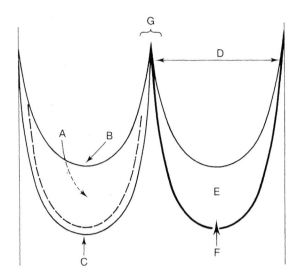

Figure 3.4 The nomenclature of the valve. A, sinus; B, free border of cusp; C, attached border of cusp; D, cornua; E, cusp; F, agger; G, commissure. (Redrawn after Franklin.[34])

minus the extraluminal [tissue] pressure). Once the cross-section is circular, further increases in volume are associated with a disproportionate increase in pressure (i.e. the pressure–volume curve has reached its plateau) (Figure 3.3).

The shape of the pressure–volume curve is particularly relevant to venous disease in the lower limb. The erect posture or venous obstruction distends the distal superficial limb veins so that when the body is upright they are always full and circular in cross-section. In these circumstances the addition of even a small volume of blood by a disordered pump leaking through incompetent communicating veins will cause a significant increase in superficial venous pressure. This is illustrated in the pressure–volume curve in Figure 3.3; a 0.5 ml/100 ml change of volume anywhere between A and B causes only a small (4 mmHg) change in pressure whereas the same change in volume between C and D increases the pressure by 50 mmHg. For similar reasons, the rate at which the pressure rises during venous refilling in veins whose compliance has been damaged by thrombosis will also be greater.[75]

The veins contain two-thirds of the total blood volume. Blood volume is generally controlled by the kidney responding to alterations of its blood flow and through hormonal control of tubular function. Rapid changes in the volume of blood in different parts of the circulation are usually controlled by reflex changes of venous tone in response to changes in central venous pressure, which is in turn regulated by arteriolar and venular resistance.

The valves

The direction of venous blood flow is controlled by the valves.[41]

Vein valves are bicuspid. The cusps of the valves of the superficial veins lie with their free edges parallel to the skin surface.[29]

The distribution of the valves in the veins of the lower limb is shown in Figure 5.3, page 148.[57,74] The inferior vena cava and common iliac veins have no valves and 75% of external iliac veins have no valves, but only 25% of common femoral veins are valveless. It has been suggested that the lack of valves in the iliac and common femoral veins is the starting point for the development of a progressive descending valvular incompetence that causes varicose veins (see Chapter 5).[58] Below the inguinal ligament the number of valves in each segment steadily increases so that the calf veins have valves which are 5 cm apart. Valves are present in veins of 1 mm diameter, but not in smaller veins or the venules.[86]

The terms given to each part of a valve are shown in Figure 3.4. The valve sinus is always wider than the vein above and below the cusps,[23] and so it has been postulated that the valve cusps do not lie flat against the wall of the vein when the valve is open but float in the bloodstream parallel to the longitudinal axis of the vein. There are three reasons for believing that this is correct:

1. The valves are often seen in this position on phlebographs and during B mode ultrasound imaging.
2. This is the ideal position to ensure that the cusps close when retrograde flow occurs

because, if they lie flat against the vein wall, they will not fill and balloon out into the bloodstream as reflux begins, whereas, if they lie in the bloodstream away from the vein wall, some refluxing blood must flow into the sinus and push the valve towards the midline.

3. Thrombosis frequently starts in a valve sinus which suggests that they always contain some blood.[38]

The valves in the axial veins stop the blood flowing away from the heart. The valves in the communicating veins of the calf stop blood flowing from the deep to the superficial veins but the valves in the communicating veins of the foot point in the opposite direction and tend to prevent blood flowing from the superficial veins on the dorsum of the foot to the deep veins in the muscles of the sole of the foot.[37,70]

Valves are extremely strong even though they are just a thin sheet of collagen fibres covered with endothelium.[3]

The mechanical properties of strips of normal human femoral vein valve cusp cut parallel to the free edge of the cusp, and longitudinal and circumferential strips of the vein wall are shown in Figure 3.5. The valve cusps are stronger and more elastic than the vein wall. Although calculations of tensile strength have to be related to the thickness of the tissue being studied, this only partly explains the difference in tensiometer measured tensile strength and breaking strain between the valves and the vein wall. There is no doubt that the valves are extremely strong structures.

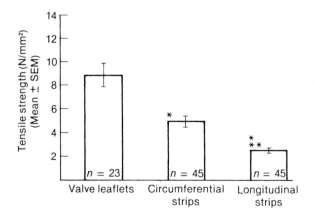

Figure 3.5 The tensile strength of valve cusps and circumferential and longitudinal strips of human femoral vein.[3] * Strength significantly different from valve leaflet. $P < 0.001$. ** Strength significantly different from circumferential strip. $P < 0.001$.

Circumferential strips of vein are slightly less elastic than longitudinal strips (possibly because of the disposition of the spiral fibres) but circumferential strips from the sinus are more elastic – a property which may help the sinus to 'balloon out' more easily and turn the combined cavities of the two valve sinuses into a sphere.

It is customary to think of valve function as solely the result of cusp movement. In fact it is a complex change involving cusp movement and valve sinus distension which tightens the edges of the cusps by separating the commissures. If this does not happen and the valve edge remains loose, because of lack of vein distensibility or because the free edges of the cusps elongate, the edge of the cusp may evert (prolapse) and the valve become incompetent (see Figure 12.9, page 395).

Venous blood flow

Venous blood flow in the lower limb is produced by the 'vis a tergo', the calf pump and the changes of intra-abdominal and intrathoracic pressure. These factors are discussed later in the section describing the physiology of the calf pump (page 57). Venous tone has an effect on the rate of blood flow but is more involved in the distribution of the blood throughout the body.

Venous tone

Active and variable tone is provided by the smooth muscle in the tunica media. The passive tone is provided by the elastic properties of the vein wall; this cannot be changed and, in the resting state, is probably the major source of tone. Deep vein thrombosis and ageing both affect the elastic properties of the vein wall.[81] Most veins have little active tone when the body is at rest, especially the large collecting deep veins of the limbs and trunk.

Changes in tone are mediated through the sympathetic nerves, by circulating vasoactive substances and local metabolites. Changes of venous tone are part of a number of cardiovascular reflexes which jointly control body temperature, blood volume and blood pressure (Figure 3.6).

The smooth muscle of the vein wall constricts when stimulated by noradrenaline.[40,62,106] Acetylcholine can cause both constriction and relaxation.[2,50,76,95] Most prostaglandins dilate the veins but some cause venoconstriction.[39,60] Many other putative transmitter substances may affect venous tone.[20]

All veins have an adrenergic innervation,[26,46] through nerve endings which terminate in the tunica media.[22] The density of the nerve endings varies from vein to vein.[10] The splanchnic and cuta-

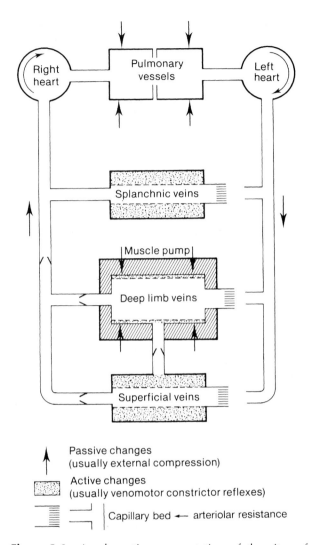

Passive changes
(usually external compression)

Active changes
(usually venomotor constrictor reflexes)

Capillary bed ← arteriolar resistance

Figure 3.6 A schematic representation of the sites of passive (usually external compression) and active (usually venomotor constrictor reflexes) changes of venous volume. (Adapted from Shepherd.[84])

neous veins have a rich innervation whereas the veins of skeletal muscles have few endings and so show a minimal response to sympathetic nerve stimulation.[54]

Sympathetic adrenergic stimulation causes venoconstriction.[17] Some parasympathetic nerves (e.g. the vagus) have an acetylcholine mediated constrictor effect.[19] Venodilatation is normally achieved through a reduction in adrenergic tone, provided this is present. Active neurogenic vasodilatation mediated through the autonomic nervous system remains unproven.

Sympathetic venous tone is controlled from the brain stem[8] in which there are pressor and depressor

areas which cause venoconstriction and venodilatation, respectively, by modifying the sympathetic discharge. A few venous reflexes are spinal,[16] but the majority pass through the brain stem. There is also an important thermoregulatory area in the preoptic region of the hypothalamus which controls the tone of the subcutaneous veins.[98]

Tone in the subcutaneous veins is affected by the following:

- emotion and pain, which cause venoconstriction[28,61]
- Sleep, which causes venorelaxation[97]
- An increased body-core temperature (pyrexia), which causes venorelaxation[77]
- A deep breath, which causes venoconstriction[16,24,78]
- Exercise, which causes venoconstriction[11,12]
- Standing upright, which causes a transient venoconstriction.[79]

Overall, the most important reflex role of the subcutaneous veins is in thermoregulation. The only other potent causes of reflex venoconstriction are emotional stress and changes in ventilation.

The apparent venoconstriction and dilatation seen in response to local cooling and heating is mainly a passive effect secondary to changes in arteriolar resistance and blood flow. Local temperature changes have only a small direct effect on the vein wall but do modify the response of the veins to thermoregulatory reflexes.[1,98,105] Thus the veins of a hand placed in hot water are dilated by two mechanisms, a small direct reflex reduction in the tone of the veins and an increased blood flow and consequently an increased venous filling secondary to reflex arteriolar dilatation.

There is a local vasoconstricting 'venoarteriolar reflex' that originates in the veins. Venular pressures above 25 mmHg initiate a noradrenergic axon reflex that causes local arteriolar vasoconstriction. This reduces arteriolar blood flow and consequently venular distension.[42] This reflex may be damaged in patients with long-standing venous hypertension and its loss may be involved in the pathogenesis of venous ulceration.

Changes in blood pressure have little or no effect on the subcutaneous veins.[30] Orthostatic hypotension is an arteriolar, not a venous, failure.

A reduced partial pressure of oxygen in the inhaled air causes venoconstriction, probably via a chemoreceptor reflex.[44]

The veins also respond to local stimuli. A direct injury usually causes venospasm but, conversely, venospasm can be overcome by repeated gentle blunt trauma (e.g. tapping with the finger).[35]

There are myelinated nerve fibres in the vein wall,[103] some of which are involved in the perception

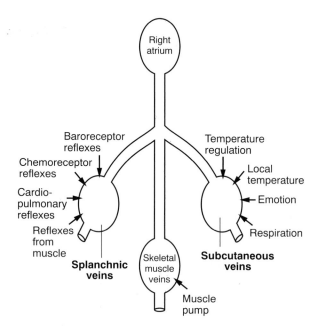

Figure 3.7 The reflexes that control the tone, resistance and capacity of the three main categories of veins. (Adapted after Shepherd, *Phlebologie* 1984, **1:** 25.)

of pain, some in detecting changes of temperature and some in the pressure/stretch reflexes.[89]

The many cardiovascular reflexes which affect the veins and help control the circulation are summarized in Figure 3.7.

The endothelium

The endothelium of the blood vessels not only provides an antithrombotic lining but also manufactures and secretes a number of substances which affect the tone of the underlying smooth muscle cells, the condition of the blood, and the interstitial fluid. Vascular endothelium is a secretory organ.

Endothelial cells produce prostacyclin which is a vasodilator, endothelium-derived relaxing factor,[36] and another vasodilator and endothelium-derived hyperpolarizing factor, probably nitric oxide,[51] which produces a brief vasodilation.

At the same time endothelial cells produce at least three contracting factors, endothelin,[104] cyclo-oxygenase[49] and angiotensin II. Most of the studies of these factors have been made on arterial endothelium and arterioles. How important these substances are in the control of venular tone is not clear, for in addition, and particularly in veins, arachidonic acid, adenosine triphosphate (ATP), adenosine diphosphate (ADP) and thrombin also produce endothelium-dependent vasoconstriction.[25,63]

Endothelial cells also produce coagulation factor VIII, and activators of fibrinolysis. The precise role of the endothelium in factor VIII production is not clear.[48] Insufficient factor VIII causes a bleeding diathesis – haemophilia – but the endothelium is not the sole source of this factor and haemophilia is mainly caused by a loss of hepatic production of factor VIII. Nevertheless, vascular endothelium does participate in the control of the levels of circulating coagulation factors.

The prostacyclins produced by the endothelium have antiplatelet aggregating as well as vasodilator properties.[99] Whether they play a role in preventing the adherence of platelets to the endothelium itself or to any uncovered collagen is uncertain but it is believed that the antithrombotic effect of endothelium is related to the balance between platelet thromboxane and endothelium prostacyclin production.

The endothelial cells of the veins are a major source of fibrinolytic activator. Whereas coagulation factors and prostacyclin are produced by all vascular endothelium, much more fibrinolytic activator is produced by the endothelium of the major veins and their vasa venora than by the endothelium of arteries.

The existence of a system opposed to coagulation has been known for many years.[59,64] Its site of production was established when Todd showed that slices of veins incubated on fibrin plates produced areas of fibrinolysis.[92–94] The effect of this endothelial activity on the blood can be demonstrated by measuring the increased fibrinolytic activity which follows venous congestion.[52,68,83,91]

The presence of a small but natural and varying blood fibrinolytic activity derived from the venous endothelium led Fearnley to propose the concept of 'natural fibrinolysis'.[31,32,80]

Many workers have since sought a connection between thrombotic disease and reduced fibrinolytic activity.[21,33,47] Nilsson[67] and the authors[15] have shown such a relationship between recurrent thrombosis and vein wall fibrinolytic activity; we also found a reduced fibrinolytic activity in patients with severe chronic venous insufficiency.[18]

The inability of normal lower leg veins to produce as much fibrinolytic activator as arm veins and the relationship between venous pressure and activator release[53,69,102] (Figure 3.8) mean that venous pressure changes and venomotor reflexes cannot be considered to have only a haemodynamic effect. Changes in vein wall configuration, tension and pressure will all affect the productive capacity of the endothelium, adding another dimension to our difficulties in understanding the effects of calf pump malfunction on the microcirculation.

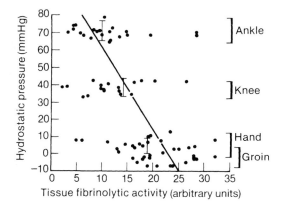

Figure 3.8 The relationship between vein wall fibrinolytic activity and resting (hydrostatic) venous pressure in 20 patients. The lower the hydrostatic pressure the greater the activator activity.[53]

The functional anatomy of the calf pump

The deep and superficial veins of the lower limb occupy two distinct compartments, separated by the deep fascia. Although there are many different types of vein in each compartment, they can, for physiological purposes, be regarded collectively as two entities, a deep chamber and a superficial chamber (Figure 3.9).[14]

The deep compartment (the pump chamber)

The deep compartment below the knee forms the chamber of the calf pump. The soleal sinuses and gastrocnemius veins actually lie within the muscles. The posterior, anterior tibial, and peroneal veins lie between the muscles. The intermuscular veins are not compressed by muscular contraction as forcefully as the intramuscular veins, and they also act as the outflow tract for the foot. All the deep veins of the calf join to form the popliteal vein which is the calf pump outflow tract. As this vein continues up the limb it passes through the 'thigh' pump but in a position, the subsartorial canal, that protects it from much of the compressive forces generated by thigh muscle contraction. The outflow tract continues through the abdomen and the thorax where it is subject to the intermittent positive and negative pressures associated with respiration. The influence of these extramural pressures is discussed later.

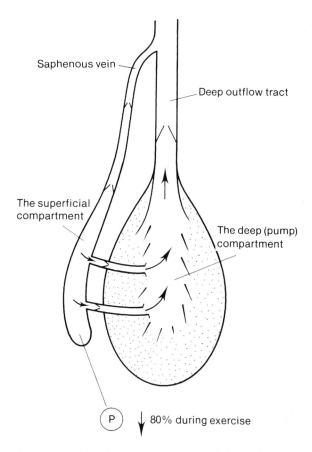

Figure 3.9 The functional anatomy of the veins of the lower limb. The arrows indicate the normal direction of blood flow. During exercise the superficial vein pressure falls by 80%.

The superficial compartment

The superficial compartment comprises a network of venules and veins in the skin and subcutaneous tissues that empty into both the deep (pump) chamber and the pump outflow tract. The two main superficial veins, the long and short saphenous veins, drain directly into the outflow tract, but there are many other connections between the superficial veins and the veins of the deep compartment.

The superficial tributaries of the saphenous systems collect blood from the skin and subpapillary dermal plexus and then progressively unite to form the two main veins. The saphenous veins themselves lie in a deeper layer of the subcutaneous tissues underneath a thin but quite strong layer of connective tissue. The veins in the dermal plexus and the subcutaneous fat are well situated for their role in thermoregulation but are poorly supported against distending forces.

The valves ensure that blood flows into the pump and towards the heart. Blood leaves the superficial compartment by flowing up the saphenous veins into the femoral or popliteal veins or directly into the pump through the many communicating veins.[13,90]

Communications between the superficial and deep compartments

The superficial compartment has two large constant connections with the outflow tract, the sapheno-femoral and the sapheno-popliteal junctions (see Figures 2.23 and 2.28, pages 39 and 41). They are protected by valves that normally prevent reflux from the deep to the superficial compartments. The common femoral and popliteal veins are not inside the muscle pumps. They lie relatively unsupported in the loose fatty connective tissue which surrounds the femoral and popliteal neurovascular bundles.

In addition to these two main communications between the deep outflow tract and the superficial compartment there are many other veins that drain into veins beneath the deep fascia which are within the pump, though not always actually within the muscles.

The named communicating veins on the medial aspect of the lower leg (see Figures 2.30 and 2.31a, pages 42 and 43) connect the superficial veins with the posterior tibial veins. These veins do not connect the long saphenous vein directly to the deep compartment but drain the whole superficial system, including the long saphenous vein, into the pump indirectly through their connections with the posterior arch vein.

There are also a number of communicating veins on the lateral and posterior aspects of the limb that connect the superficial veins with the peroneal vein and veins within the soleus and gastrocnemius muscles (see Figure 2.31b, page 43).

In addition to the named communicating veins, there are between 50 and 100 small unnamed veins which connect the deep and superficial systems. Anatomically, they are similar in muscle and collagen content to superficial veins. They are usually accompanied by a small artery and are primarily venae comitantes of the artery. They do not play a significant part in the normal physiology of the calf pump.

The valves in the communicating veins are arranged so that they prevent flow from the deep to the superficial compartments. There may be one, two or three valves depending upon the length and course of the vein. The valves are invariably in that part of the vein beneath the deep fascia (Figure 3.10).[53,54,71,72]

The course of the communicating veins beneath the deep fascia varies according to their destination.

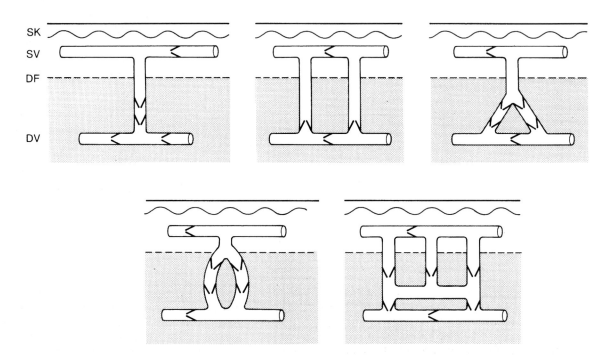

Figure 3.10 The position of the valves and some common variations of the communicating veins. (Redrawn after Pirner.[71]) SK, skin; SV, superficial vein; DF, deep fascia; DV, deep vein. Shaded area = muscle pump.

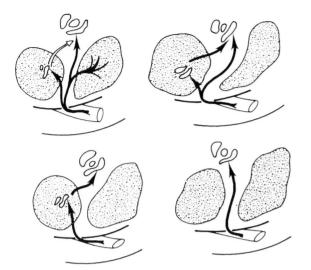

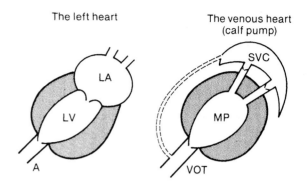

Figure 3.12 A comparison between the left side of the heart and the calf pump. LA, left atrium; LV, left ventricle; A, aorta; SVC, superficial venous compartment; MP, deep venous compartment (the muscle pump); VOT, venous outflow tract. Continuing the analogy: mitral incompetence = communicating vein incompetence; myocardial failure = calf muscle weakness; aortic incompetence = deep vein valve incompetence in the outflow tract; aortic stenosis = deep vein obstruction in the outflow tract.

Figure 3.11 Variations in the pathways taken by veins connecting the superficial to the deep veins. (Adapted from Stolic.[87])

Some are short and direct, others run between or into muscles before connecting with the intermuscular veins.[19] It is not known whether these variations have any pathophysiological significance (Figure 3.11).

Phlebologists argue about the generic name of these veins. Many like to call them perforating rather than communicating veins because they pierce the deep fascia, and some anatomists think the term 'communicating vein' should be reserved for veins that connect vessels within the same compartment.

Nevertheless, the important physiological role of these veins is the connection that they make between the deep and superficial compartments. We therefore prefer the term communicating vein on physiological grounds and do not call them 'perforators' or 'blow outs'. Others have also expressed a preference for this term.[55,57,87]

The physiology of the calf pump

The action of the calf pump is best understood if the many superficial and deep veins are considered as two compartments with a few interconnections and a single outflow tract. It is, however, important to remember that the superficial compartment communicates with both parts of the deep compartment, the pump chamber and the outflow tract.

The calf pump has been called the peripheral heart. We have found it helpful to develop this comparison because the left side of the heart is also a two chamber system. Figure 3.12 compares our compartmentalized concept of the calf pump with that of the left side of the heart. The calf pump is the equivalent of the left ventricle. The venous outflow tract is the equivalent of the aorta and its valve. The superficial compartment is the equivalent of the left atrium, and the communicating veins are comparable to the mitral valve. The difference between the leg and the heart is that there is a direct connection between the superficial compartment and the pump outflow tract which, if it was present in the heart and not protected by a valve, would be equivalent to a large arteriovenous fistula and add a considerable load to the heart. This is exactly what happens when saphenous vein incompetence refills the superficial chamber with regurgitating blood and subsequently overloads the pump.

The pump

Systole

When the calf muscles and the muscles in the deep posterior compartment of the lower leg contract, they raise the pressure in and around all the structures contained within the deep fascia. All the intramuscular veins are completely compressed because the muscles generate pressures of 200–300 mmHg.[7,57,100] The pressure in tissues which are deep to the fascia but outside the muscles does not rise as high but reaches levels of 100–150 mmHg.[45,56,88]

These pressures squeeze the blood out of the veins, the valves ensuring that the blood flows only towards the heart. Flow from the deep to the superficial compartment is prevented by the valves in the communicating veins.[5]

The large veins within the gastrocnemius and soleus muscles form the main chamber of the pump but all the other deep veins participate.

The average volume of the calf is 1500–2000 ml, and its contained calf blood volume is 60–70 ml.[101] Continuous exercise reduces the calf blood volume by 1.5–2.0 ml/100 ml. Most of this reduction is from compression of the veins in the pump chamber. The average expelled volume is therefore approximately 30–40 ml, only 50% of all the blood within the pump. The pump will normally expel this volume in four to five contractions, though one single sustained contraction can expel almost as much. When the rate of exercise increases, the muscle blood flow may increase to 20–30 ml/100 ml/min. This places an additional load of 600 ml/min on the calf pump. The calf must contract at least 20 times every minute to expel this increased blood flow. Normal walking at 80 steps/min contracts each calf 40 times/min so the pump can easily deal with the high blood flow of exercise hyperaemia.

The outflow tract from the pump, the popliteal vein, is a very large bore vein which offers virtually no resistance to flow. As the gradient of 10–15 mmHg between the small veins and the heart is sufficient to ensure venous blood flow when the subject is supine, the increase in gradient of 100–200 mmHg produced by the pump[6] is more than enough to ensure an adequate rapid venous return to the heart during vigorous erect muscle exercise. An obstruction to flow within the popliteal vein seriously impedes calf pump function.

Diastole

The pump chamber is refilled by the arterial inflow and the flow from the superficial compartment during diastole. Just as blood flows from the left atrium to the left ventricle during ventricular diastole, so blood flows from the superficial to the deep compartment when the calf muscles relax.[13]

At the moment when the calf muscles relax their contained veins are empty, at zero pressure and as yet unfilled by arterial inflow. As the veins are collapsed they are also unaffected by hydrostatic pressure. Conversely, the superficial veins are full and subjected to hydrostatic pressure plus the remnant of cardiac generated pressure, the

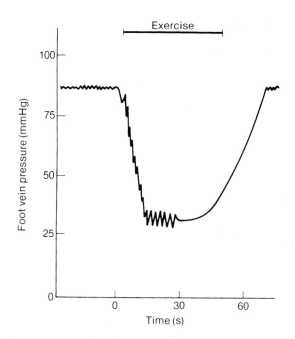

Figure 3.13 The changes in foot vein pressure during heel raising exercise. In a normal limb the pressure drops by 60–80% and, after exercise, takes 15–25 seconds to return to resting levels.

'vis a tergo'. The pressure gradient between the two compartments is therefore 100–110 mmHg. Blood immediately flows from the superficial to the deep compartment through the many communicating veins.[13] This empties the superficial compartment and reduces its pressure.[9,43,45,73,82,85,96] Measurements of foot vein pressure during exercise show it to fall by 60–80% (Figure 3.13). This reduction in pressure is essential for the preservation of healthy skin and subcutaneous tissues. The exposure of the subcutaneous veins to a persistent high pressure may eventually cause cell death (see Chapter 15).

Thus calf pump activity performs two vital functions:

1. It ensures venous return from the lower limbs during exercise.
2. It reduces superficial vein pressure thus removing the damaging effect of the hydrostatic pressure that is inseparable from man's upright posture.

It is therefore normal to have a low pressure in the subcutaneous veins during exercise and when supine. Superficial vein pressure only rises when standing still and when the calf pump fails. The absence of venous hypotension during exercise is the ultimate cause of almost all 'venous' pathology.

Respiration

Movements of the diaphragm affect the resistance of the outflow tract because they change intra-abdominal and intrathoracic pressure. During inspiration the abdominal pressure increases and obstructs venous return. At the same time the intrathoracic pressure falls so that the pressure gradient between the abdomen and thorax increases, encouraging venous blood flow from the abdominal to the thoracic veins.[65,66] Thus during inspiration blood flow from the limbs to the abdomen is impeded but blood flow from the abdomen to the thorax is accelerated.[27]

As soon as each inspiration stops, the abdominal pressure falls and venous blood flow recommences from the lower limbs to the abdomen. There is still a positive but smaller gradient between the abdomen and the chest so blood flow from the abdomen to the chest continues.

Flow from the upper limbs into the chest is directly related to the positive and negative intrathoracic pressures of respiration.

The causes of calf pump failure

The pump

Four abnormalities may reduce the efficiency of the pump itself.

Muscle weakness

Weakness of the calf pump is the equivalent of heart failure. The calf muscles rapidly waste and weaken with disuse. Disuse accompanies major injuries, neurological disease, vascular insufficiency, debilitating diseases, myositis, and bone and joint pain. If the veins and their valves are normal, a weak calf muscle alone rarely causes symptoms of venous insufficiency but, if there is a pre-existing venous abnormality and the muscle becomes weak, symptoms are exacerbated.

Sometimes venous disease itself causes calf muscle wasting. A painful venous ulcer or fibrous ankylosis of the ankle joint caused by chronic venous insufficiency may cause the patient to limp to avoid painful ankle movements. The absence of calf contractions exacerbates the venous hypertension and its complications and causes calf muscle disuse atrophy. A vicious circle develops as valve damage causes skin complications, which cause pain and walking difficulties, which diminish pump function, which causes further deterioration of the skin.

Pump chamber contraction (reduced end-diastolic volume)

Extensive deep vein thrombosis may leave many of the deep veins of the calf, within and between the muscles, permanently occluded or thick, stiff and narrow with incompetent valves. They cannot hold all the blood delivered to them during pump diastole, so that pump vein pressure between calf contractions rises rapidly. The undamaged patent veins dilate and their valves become incompetent. These secondary changes, added to the damage caused by the deep vein thrombosis, cause the pump to fail.

The volume of blood that can be squeezed from the calf by external compression is reduced in patients with old deep vein damage.[101]

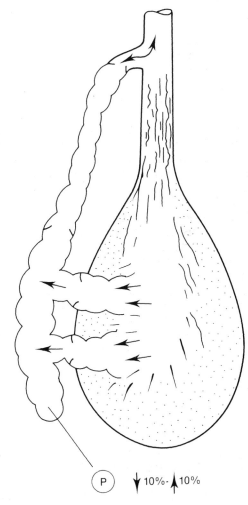

Figure 3.14 Outflow tract obstruction. Deep vein obstruction causes upstream dilatation of the veins in the pump chamber and secondary incompetence of the communicating veins because these veins become part of the collateral outflow tract. During exercise the foot vein pressure will fall slightly or even rise.

Pump chamber dilatation (increased end-diastolic volume)

Obstruction to the outflow of blood from the pump caused by occlusion of veins within the pump or in the main outflow tract causes the veins within the pump to dilate and their valves to become secondarily incompetent. Valvular incompetence of the intramuscular veins alone may not be particularly important but, if the communicating veins become incompetent, calf pump efficiency is seriously reduced. A major degree of outflow obstruction is usually caused by axial vein thrombosis.

Pump vein valve incompetence

All veins lying along the axis of the limb need valves to prevent retrograde flow. Not all the veins within the calf muscles have valves (e.g. the soleal sinuses), but these particular vessels are U-shaped with both ends emptying towards the heart.

An absence of valves in the deep veins puts additional strain on the valves in the communicating veins.

Isolated segments of deep veins with damaged valves rarely cause symptoms, presumably because the potential volume of reflux into them is small. Extensive destruction of the valves can, however, cause venous claudication as well as communicating vein incompetence.

Outflow tract obstruction (Figure 3.14)

Anything that blocks the outflow of blood from the pump will cause secondary dilatation of the veins within the pump and the communicating veins.

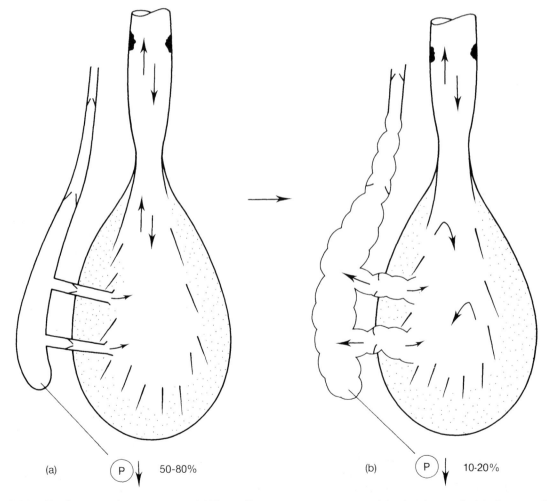

(a) P 50-80%   (b) P 10-20%

Figure 3.15 Outflow tract incompetence. (a) The calf pump can compensate for pure deep vein (outflow tract) incompetence by increasing its output. (b) If the dilatation of the veins within the pump affects the communicating veins the pump begins to fail and foot vein pressure is only reduced by 10–20% during exercise.

Collateral vessels are rarely adequate and therefore obstruction usually causes a slow but progressive deterioration of calf pump efficiency, just as aortic stenosis affects cardiac function.

Once the communicating veins dilate and become incompetent, they become collateral vessels by carrying blood out into the superficial system during calf pump systole to bypass the deep obstruction.

Outflow tract incompetence (Figure 3.15)

Pure deep vein incompetence without obstruction is uncommon. The pump refills rapidly during diastole and has to eject more blood during systole. The pump develops a high end-diastolic volume. Provided the muscle is strong and the communicating veins remain competent, this abnormality rarely causes symptoms. Ultimately, the veins within the pump and the communicating veins dilate and become incompetent and the symptoms of venous insufficiency begin to appear.

Communicating vein incompetence (Figure 3.16)

Communicating veins have been mentioned repeatedly throughout this discussion on calf pump insufficiency. Their valves form an essential protection between the high pressures that develop within the pump and the low pressures produced by the pump in the subcutaneous compartment. If their valves fail, the pump pushes blood into the superficial veins as well as into the outflow tract during systole. The situation is analogous to mitral valve incompetence. The clinical effect depends upon the balance between forward normal outflow tract blood flow, retrograde communicating vein flow and superficial compartment distension, the latter determines the effect of the retrograde flow on superficial pressure.

The two causes of communicating vein valve incompetence are:

- valve cusp destruction by thrombosis and/or valve ring dilatation secondary to a downstream post-thrombotic venous obstruction or
- the result of the progressive vein dilatation of the primary varicose vein diathesis.

Superficial vein incompetence (Figure 3.17)

A segment of a superficial vein with incompetent valves may become dilated and tortuous but will not damage the local tissues provided there is a competent valve between it and the deep veins and the cutaneous venules. Superficial vein incompetence is mainly a cosmetic problem. Its only effect

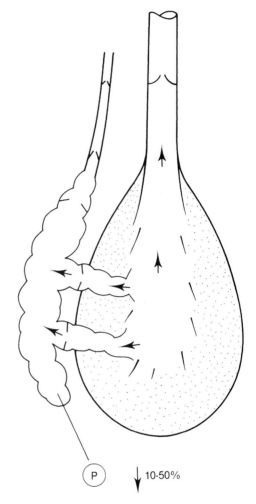

Figure 3.16 Communicating vein incompetence. Incompetence of the veins within the pump usually following deep vein thrombosis, sometimes in the communicating veins themselves, leads to dilatation and incompetence of the communicating veins, so allowing reflux of blood into the superficial compartment during calf muscle contraction. Communicating vein dilatation and valvular incompetence may also occur as part of the varicose vein diathesis. The arrows indicate the direction of blood flow. During exercise the foot vein pressure falls by 10–50%.

on calf pump function is to increase the volume of blood that has to be pumped out of the lower leg. Incompetent superficial veins (varicose veins) only contain 5–10% of the total blood in the lower limb, but the volume of blood refluxing through them may be considerable. Eventually, usually after very many years, this added load can impair calf pump function and cause skin damage. Long-standing primary varicose veins can cause venous ulceration.

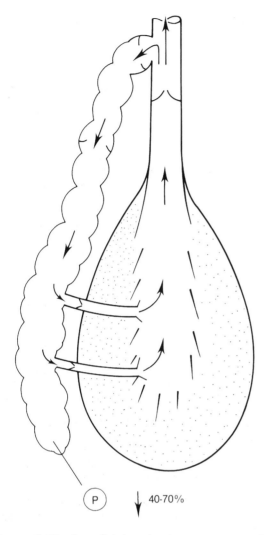

Figure 3.17 Superficial vein incompetence allows blood to reflux down the superficial veins but, providing the communicating veins are competent, the calf pump can usually cope with the additional load and reduce the foot vein pressure during exercise by 40–70%. This is why simple superficial varicose veins are an uncommon cause of venous ulceration.

The arm veins

The anatomy of the arm veins is described in Chapter 2. The arm muscles exert a pumping effect which is similar to that of the calf muscles but the superficial veins form a greater part of the outflow tract than the superficial veins in the leg and the valves in the communicating veins point in the opposite direction. As the hydrostatic pressure in the arms is so low, venous malfunction never causes the skin changes and ulceration which are seen in the lower limb.

References

1. Abdel-Sayed WA, Abboud FM, Calvelo MG. Effect of local cooling on responsiveness of muscular cutaneous arteries and veins. *Am J Physiol* 1970; **219:** 1772.
2. Ablad B, Mellander S. Comparative effects of hydralazine, sodium nitrate and acetylcholine on resistance and capacitance vessels and capillary filtration in skeletal muscle in the cat. *Acta Physiol Scand* 1963; **58:** 319.
3. Ackroyd JS, Pattison M, Browse NL. A study of the mechanical properties of fresh and preserved human femoral vein wall and valve cusps. *Br J Surg* 1985; **72:** 117–19.
4. Alexander RS. The peripheral venous system. In: Hamilton WF, Dow P, eds. *Handbook of Physiology. Section 2. Circulation.* Bethesda, MD: American Physiological Society, 1963; 1075.
5. Almen T, Nylander G. Serial phlebography of the normal lower limb during muscular contraction and relaxation. *Acta Radiol Scand* 1962; **57:** 264.
6. Barcroft H, Dornhorst AC. Demonstration of the muscle pump in the human leg. *J Physiol (Lond)* 1949; **108:** 39.
7. Barcroft H, Dornhorst AC. The blood flow through the human calf during rhythmic exercise. *J Physiol (Lond)* 1949; **109:** 402–11.
8. Baum T, Hosko MJ. Response of resistance and capacitance vessels to central nervous stimulation. *Am J Physiol* 1965; **209:** 236.
9. Beecher HK, Field ME, Krogh A. The effect of walking on the venous pressure at the ankle. *Scand Arch Physiol* 1936; **73:** 133.
10. Bevan JA, Hosmer DW, Ljung B, Pegram BL, Su C. Innervation pattern and neurogenic response of rabbit veins. *Blood Vessels* 1974; **11:** 172.
11. Bevegard BS, Shepherd JT. Changes in tone of limb veins during supine exercise. *J Appl Physiol* 1965; **20:** 1.
12. Bevegard BS, Shepherd JT. Effect of local exercise of forearm muscles on forearm capacitance vessels. *J Appl Physiol* 1965; **20:** 968.
13. Bjordal R. Simultaneous pressure and flow recordings in varicose veins of the lower extremity. *Acta Chir Scand* 1970; **136:** 309–26.
14. Browse NL. The treatment of venous insufficiency of the lower limb. *Vasc Diagn Ther* 1982; **3:** 27–34.
15. Browse NL, Gray L, Jarrett PEM, Morland M. Blood and vein wall fibrinolytic activity in health and vascular disease. *Br Med J* 1977; **1:** 478–81.
16. Browse NL, Hardwick PJ. The deep breath venoconstriction reflex. *Clin Sci* 1969; **37:** 125–35.
17. Browse NL, Lorenz RR, Shepherd J. Response of capacity and resistance vessels of dog's limb to sympathetic nerve stimulation. *Am J Physiol* 1966; **210:** 95.
18. Burnand KG, Browse NL. The postphlebitic leg and venous ulceration. In: Russell RCG, ed. *Recent Advances in Surgery 11.* Edinburgh: Churchill Livingstone, 1982; 225.

19. Burnstock G. Evolution of the autonomic innervation of visceral and cardiovascular systems in vertebrates. *Pharmacol Rev* 1969; **21:** 247.

20. Burnstock G. Local mechanisms of blood-flow control by perivascular nerves and endothelium. *J Hypertens* 1990; **8 (Suppl 7):** 95–106.

21. Chakrabarti R, Birks PM, Fearnley GR. Origin of blood fibrinolytic activity from veins and its bearing on the fate of venous thrombi. *Lancet* 1963; **1:** 1288.

22. Coimbra A, Ribeiro-Silva A, Osswald W. Fine structural and autoradiographic study of the adrenergic innervation of the dog lateral saphenous vein. *Blood Vessels* 1974; **11:** 128.

23. Cotton LT. Varicose veins. Gross anatomy and development. *Br J Surg* 1961; **48:** 589.

24. Deluis W, Kellerova E. Reaction of arterial and venous vessels in the human forearm and hand to deep breath or mental strain. *Clin Sci* 1971; **40:** 271.

25. DeMay JG, Vanhoutte PM. Heterogenous behaviour of the canine arterial and venous wall, importance of the endothelium. *Circ Res* 1982; **51:** 439–47.

26. Donegan JF. The physiology of the veins. *J Physiol (Lond)* 1921; **55:** 226.

27. Duamarco JL, Rimini R. Energy and hydraulic gradients along systemic veins. *Am J Physiol* 1954; **178:** 215.

28. Duggan JJ, Love VL, Lyons RH. A study of reflex venomotor reactions in man. *Circulation* 1953; **7:** 869.

29. Edwards EA. The orientation of venous valves in relation to body surfaces. *Anat Rec* 1936; **64:** 369.

30. Epstein SE, Beiser GD, Stampfer M, Braunwald E. Role of the venous system in baroreceptor mediated reflexes in man. *J Clin Invest* 1968; **47:** 139.

31. Fearnley GR. A concept of natural fibrinolysis. *Lancet* 1961; **1:** 992.

32. Fearnley GR. *Fibrinolysis*. Baltimore, MD: Williams & Wilkins, 1965.

33. Fearnley GR, Banfort GU, Fearnley E. Evidence of diurnal fibrinolytic rhythm with a simple method of measuring natural fibrinolysis. *Clin Sci* 1957; **16:** 645–50.

34. Franklin KJ. *A Monograph on Veins*. Springfield, IL: Thomas, 1937.

35. Franklin KJ, McLachlin AD. Dilatation of veins in response to tapping in man and in certain other mammals. *J Physiol* 1936; **88:** 257–60.

36. Furchgott RF, Zawadski JU. The obligatory role of endothelial cells in the relaxation of arterial smooth muscle by acetylcholine. *Nature* 1980; **288:** 373–6.

37. Gardner AMN, Fox RH. The venous pump of the human foot. *Bristol Med Chir J* 1983; **109:** 112.

38. Gibbs NM. Venous thrombosis of the lower limbs with particular reference to bedrest. *Br J Surg* 1957; **45:** 209.

39. Greenberg RA, Sparks HV. Prostaglandins and consecutive vascular segments of the canine hind limb. *Am J Physiol* 1969; **216:** 567.

40. Haddy FJ, Fleishman M, Emanuel D. Effect of epinephrine, norepinephrine and serotonin upon systemic small and large vessel resistances. *Circ Res* 1957; **5:** 247.

41. Harvey W. *Exercitatio Anatomica de Motu Cordis et Sanguinis in Animalibus*. Francofurti: Sumptibus Gulielusi Fizeri, 1628.

42. Henrikson O, Skagen K. Local and central sympathetic vasoconstrictor reflexes in human limbs during orthostatic stress. In: Christensen NJ, Henriksen O, Lassen NA, eds. *The Symphatho-adrenal System. Alfred Benzou Symposium 23.* Copenhagen: Munksgaard, 1988.

43. Henry JP. The influence of temperature and exercise on venous pressure in the foot when in the erect posture. *Am J Med* 1948; **4:** 619.

44. Hintze A, Throh HL. Das ferhalten der menschlichen handvenen bei akuter arterieller hypoxie. *Pflügers Arch Ges Physiol* 1961; **274:** 227.

45. Hojensgard IC, Stürup H. Static and dynamic pressures in superficial and deep veins of the lower extremity in man. *Acta Physiol Scand* 1953; **27:** 49–67.

46. Hooker DR. The veno-pressor mechanism. *Am J Physiol* 1918; **46:** 591.

47. Isacson S. Low fibrinolytic activity of blood and vein walls in venous thrombosis. *Scand J Haematol* 1971; **Suppl 16**.

48. Jaff EA, Hoyer LW, Nachman RL. Synthesis of antihaemophilic factor antigen by cultured human endothelial cells. *J Clin Invest* 1973; **52:** 2757.

49. Katusic ZS, Vanhoutte PM. Superoxide anion and endothelial regulation of arterial tone. *Semin Perinatol* 1991; **15:** 30–3.

50. Kjellmer I, Odelram M. The effect of some physiological vasodilators on the vascular bed of skeletal muscle. *Acta Physiol Scand* 1965; **63:** 94.

51. Komori K, Vanhoutte PM. Endothelium-derived hyperpolarising factor. *Blood Vessels* 1990; **27:** 238–45.

52. Kwaan HC, Lo R, McFadzean AJS. Production of plasma fibrinolytic activity within veins. *Clin Sci* 1957; **16:** 241.

53. Leach RD, Clemenson G, Morland M, Browse NL. The relationship between venous pressure and vein wall fibrinolytic activity. *J Cardiovasc Surg* 1982; **23:** 505–8.

54. Lesh TA, Rothe CF. Sympathetic and haemodynamic effects on capacitance vessels in dog skeletal muscles. *Am J Physiol* 1969; **217:** 819.

55. Linton RR. John Homan's impact on diseases of the veins of the lower extremity with special reference to deep thrombophlebitis and the post-thrombotic syndrome with ulceration. *Surgery* 1977; **81:** 1–11.

56. Ludbrook J. The musculo-venous pumps of the human lower limb. *Am Heart J* 1966; **71:** 635–41.

57. Ludbrook J. *Aspects of Venous Function in the Lower Limbs*. Springfield, IL: Thomas, 1966.

58. Ludbrook J, Beales G. Femoral venous valves in relation to varicose veins. *Lancet* 1962; **1:** 79.

59. Macfarlane RK. Fibrinolysis following operation. *Lancet* 1937; **1:** 10–12.

60. Mark AL, Schmid PG, Eckstein JW, Wendling MG. Venous responses to prostaglandin F2~. *Am J Physiol* 1971; **220:** 222.

61. Marshall RJ, Shepherd JT. *Cardiac Function in Health and Disease*. Philadelphia: WB Saunders, 1966.

62. Mellander S. Comparative studies on the adrenergic neuro-hormonal control of resistance and capacitance blood vessels in the cat. *Acta Physiol Scand* 1960; **50: Suppl 176**.

63. Miller VM, Vanhoutte PM. Nitric oxide may not be the only endothelium-derived relaxing factor in canine femoral veins. *Am J Physiol* 1989; **257:** 1910–16.

64. Mole RH. Fibrinolysis and the fluidity of the blood postmortem. *J Pathol Bacteriol* 1948; **60:** 413.

65. Moreno AH, Burchell AR, Vanderwonde R, Burke J H. Respiratory regulation of splanchnic and systemic venous return. *Am J Physiol* 1967; **213:** 455.

66. Moreno AH, Katz AI, Gold LD. An integrated approach to the study of the venous system with steps toward a detailed model of the dynamics of venous return to the right heart. *IEEE Trans Biomed Eng* 1969; **16:** 308.

67. Nilsson IM, Isacson S. New aspects of the pathogenesis of thromboembolism. In: Allgower M, ed. *Progress in Surgery 11*. Basel: Karger, 1973; 46.

68. Nilsson IM, Robertson B. Effect of venous occlusion on coagulation and fibrinolytic components in normal subjects. *Thromb Diath Haemorrh* 1968; **20:** 397–408.

69. Pandolfi M, Nilsson IM, Robertson B, Isacson S. Fibrinolytic activity of human veins. *Lancet* 1967; **2:** 127–8.

70. Pegum JM, Fegan WG. Physiology of venous return from the foot. *Cardiovasc Res* 1967; **1:** 249.

71. Pirner F. Uber die Bedentung Form und Art der Klappen in den V communicates der unteren Extremitat. *Anat Anz* 1956; **103:** 450–60.

72. Pirner F. Die Bedentung der insuff V.perforans fur die Kramfaderoperation. *Chir Praxis* 1963; **7:** 112–19.

73. Pollack AA, Wood EH. Venous pressure in the saphenous vein at the ankle in man during exercise and changes in posture. *J Appl Physiol* 1949; **1:** 649.

74. Powell T, Lynn RB. The valves of the external iliac, femoral and upper third of the popliteal vein. *Surg Gynecol Obstet* 1951; **92:** 453–5.

75. Raju S, Fredericks R, Lishman P, Neglen P, Morano J. Observations on the calf pump mechanism. Determinates of post exercise pressure. *J Vasc Surg* 1993; **17:** 459–69.

76. Rice AJ, Long JP. An unusual venoconstriction induced by acetylcholine. *J Pharmacol Exp Ther* 1966; **151:** 423.

77. Rowell LB. Human cardiovascular adjustments to exercise and thermal stress. *Physiol Rev* 1974; **54:** 75.

78. Samueloff SL, Bevegard BS, Shepherd JT. Temporary arrest of circulation to a limb for the study of venomotor reactions in man. *J Appl Physiol* 1966; **21:** 341.

79. Sammueloff SL, Browse NL, Shepherd JT. Response of capacity vessels in human limbs to head-up tilt and suction on the lower body. *J Appl Physiol* 1966; **21:** 47.

80. Samuels PB, Webster DR. The role of venous endothelium in the inception of thrombosis. *Ann Surg* 1962; **136:** 422.

81. Schina MJ, Neumyer MM, Healy DA, Atnip RG, Thiele BL. Influence of age on venous physiologic parameters. *J Vasc Surg* 1993; **18:** 749-52.

82. Seiro V. Uber Blutdruck und Blulkreislauf in den Krampfadern der unteren Extremitaten. *Acta Chir Scand* 1938; **80:** 41.

83. Shaper AG, Marsh NA, Patel I, Kater F. Response of fibrinolytic activity to venous occlusion. *Br Med J* 1975; **3:** 571–3.

84. Shepherd JT, Vanhoutte PM. *Veins and their Control*. Philadelphia: WB Saunders, 1975.

85. Smirk RH. Observations on the causes of oedema in congestive heart failure. *Clin Sci* 1936; **2:** 317.

86. Stanbesand J, Rulffs W. Die klappen kleiner venen. *Z Anat Entwickl Gesch* 1958; **120:** 392.

87. Stolic E. Terminology, division and systematic anatomy of the communicating veins of the lower limb. In: May R, Partsch H, Straubesand J, eds. *Perforating Veins*. Wien: Urban & Schwarzenberg, 1981; 19–34.

88. Stürup H, Hojensgard IC. Venous pressure in the deep veins of the lower extremity of patients with primary and post thrombotic varicose veins. *Acta Chir Scand* 1950; **99:** 526–36.

89. Thompson FJ, Barnes CD. Evidence for thermosensitive elements in the femoral vein. *Life Sci I* 1970; **90:** 309.

90. Tibbs DJ, Fletcher EWL. Direction of flow in superficial veins as a guide to venous disorders in lower limbs. *Surgery* 1983; **93:** 758–67.

91. Tighe JR, Swan UT. Fibrinolysis in venous obstruction. *Clin Sci* 1963; **25:** 219–22.

92. Todd AS. Fibrinolysis autographs. *Nature* 1958; **181:** 495–6.

93. Todd AS. Histological localization of fibrinolysis activator. *J Pathol Bacteriol* 1959; **78:** 281–3.

94. Todd AS. Localisation of fibrinolytic activity in tissues. *Br Med Bull* 1964; **20:** 200.

95. Vanhoutte PM, Shepherd JT. Venous relaxation caused by acetylcholine acting on the sympathetic nerves. *Circ Res* 1973; **32:** 259.

96. Walker AJ, Longland CJ. Venous pressure measurement in the foot in exercise as an aid to investigation of venous disease in the leg. *Clin Sci* 1950; **9:** 101.

97. Watson WE. Distensibility of the capacity blood vessels of the human hand during sleep. *J Physiol (Lond)* 1962; **161:** 392.

98. Webb Peploe MM, Shepherd JT. Response of superficial limb veins of the dog to changes in temperature. *Circ Res* 1968; **22:** 737.

99. Weksler BB, Marcus AJ, Jaff EA. Synthesis of prostaglandin I_2 by cultured human and bovine endothelial cells. *Proc Natl Acad Sci USA* 1977; **74:** 3922.

100. Wells HS, Youmans JB, Miller DG. Tissue pressure, intracutaneous, subcutaneous and intramuscular, as related to venous pressure, capillary filtration and other factors. *J Clin Invest* 1938; **17:** 489–99.

101. Whitehead S, Clemenson G, Browse N L. The assessment of calf pump function by isotope plethysmography. *Br J Surg* 1983; **70:** 675–9.
102. Wolfe JHN, Morland M, Browse NL. The fibrinolytic activity of varicose veins. *Br J Surg* 1979; **66:** 185–7.
103. Woollard HH. The innervation of blood vessels. *Heart* 1926; **13:** 319.
104. Yanagisawa M, Kurichara H, Kimura S. A novel potent vasoconstrictor peptide produced by vascular endothelial cells. *Nature* 1988; **332:** 411–15.
105. Zitnik RS, Ambrosioni E, Shepherd JT. Effect of temperature on cutaneous venomotor reflexes in man. *J Appl Physiol* 1971; **31:** 507–12.
106. Zsoter T, Tom H. Adrenoreceptive sites in the veins. *Br J Pharmacol Chemother* 1967; **31:** 407.

CHAPTER 4

Techniques of investigation

Clinical examination	69	Investigations of venous function	112
Investigations that provide images of the veins and/or thrombus	72	Commentary	130
		References	132
Investigations that provide images of thrombus in the lungs	108		

There are many different methods available for the investigation of the venous system. None provides complete information on either the anatomy or the function of the veins. They vary from simple clinical examination to methods using modern sophisticated electronic apparatus. Each method has its own particular advantages, and disadvantages, and sometimes three or four different methods actually measure the same thing. There are, for example, four methods of calf plethysmography, all of which measure the change in blood volume within the calf, and these, together with foot volumetry and photoplethysmography, make six techniques that measure calf pump function.

It is essential to understand which aspect of venous anatomy or function a test measures and how accurately it does this. Knowledge of the methodology of the tests, though secondary to this understanding, is also very important when interpreting the results. Furthermore, this chapter not only describes all the tests in common use but also describes some that have, for a variety of reasons, become obsolete because the latter give insight into how our understanding of the veins and venous pathology has developed. Each section concentrates upon the principle of each test, the method and the reasons for inaccuracies. The place of each test in the investigation of specific conditions is discussed in the relevant chapter.

It has become customary to express the value of a test, not only in terms of accuracy, but also in terms of sensitivity, specificity and predictive value.

These are mathematical forms of assessment which are undoubtedly useful when evaluating a new test, but they should also be used to evaluate any test, however old, when you introduce it into your own regimen of investigation as a way of comparing your own ability to perform the test against the published results of other workers.

These mathematical expressions of validity depend upon a comparison between the test being evaluated and an established test of the same function whose accuracy is known. The key word in the preceding sentence is 'accurate'. The most accurate test available is commonly referred to as *the gold standard*. Unfortunately, there are few gold standards in venous investigation. Phlebography almost comes up to the 100% accuracy level required of a gold standard for anatomical delineation but there are no perfect tests of venous physiological function. When talking about the specificity or sensitivity of a test, therefore, always remember to specify or enquire about the gold standard against which the new test is being compared. More often than not you will find that the gold standard is not totally reliable (a base metal, often gold lacquer covering lead). After such a discovery you will properly appreciate the value of the calculated expressions of sensitivity and specificity.

Accuracy, sensitivity and specificity

Accuracy is a word we all understand. It is the simple expression of the number of correct diagnoses obtained by the test, whether they be positive or negative, as a proportion of the total number of tests performed ($\times$ 100 to make it a percentage).

$$\text{Accuracy} = \frac{\text{Number of correct tests}}{\text{Total number of tests}} \times 100$$

The numerator, which is the total number of correct tests, both positive and negative, is based upon a comparison with the gold standard.

The *sensitivity* of a test tells you how often a positive test actually indicates real disease. It is therefore the ratio between the number of correctly positive tests and the true incidence of the disease.

$$\text{Sensitivity} = \frac{\begin{array}{c}\text{Number of correct}\\\text{positive tests}\end{array}}{\text{Number with disease}} \times 100$$

The numerator is determined by the gold standard, the denominator is the sum of the correct positive tests and the incorrect negative tests (true positives plus false negatives) again determined by comparison against the gold standard.

The *specificity* of a test tells you how often a negative test actually indicates no disease.

$$\text{Specificity} = \frac{\begin{array}{c}\text{Number of correct}\\\text{negative tests}\end{array}}{\text{Number without disease}} \times 100$$

The denominator is the sum of the correct negative tests and the incorrect positive tests (true negative plus false positive).

We find the terms sensitivity and specificity confusing. They are words whose literal meanings bear no relation to what they are trying to tell us – the ability to detect disease and the ability to identify the absence of disease, respectively. Unfortunately, they have become firmly established amongst those workers who have developed and who perform many of these non-invasive vascular laboratory tests and therefore we all have to remember their definitions.

The question that the clinician is more likely to ask, apart from overall accuracy, is 'How often is a positive (or a negative) test likely to be correct?' This question implies that a test may be better at detecting disease than detecting normality, or *vice versa*. This question can be easily answered by calculating what has become known as the positive (or negative) predictive value – another cumbersome expression which would be much simpler and easier to comprehend if it was changed to positive (or negative) test accuracy.

Positive test accuracy

$$\begin{array}{l}\text{Positive test}\\\text{accuracy (positive} =\\\text{predictive value)}\end{array} \frac{\begin{array}{c}\text{Number of correct}\\\text{positive tests}\end{array}}{\begin{array}{c}\text{Number of}\\\text{positive tests}\end{array}} \times 100$$

The numerator is derived from a comparison against the gold standard. The denominator is all the positive tests, that is the sum of the correct (true) and the incorrect (false) positive tests.

Negative test accuracy

This is similar to positive test accuracy.

$$\begin{array}{l}\text{Negative test}\\\text{accuracy (negative} =\\\text{predictive value)}\end{array} \frac{\begin{array}{c}\text{Number of correct}\\\text{negative tests}\end{array}}{\begin{array}{c}\text{Number of}\\\text{negative tests}\end{array}} \times 100$$

The denominator is the sum of the correct and the incorrect negative tests (true negatives and false negatives).

Example
Suppose you have developed a new test of venous thrombosis which you have performed on 300 limbs and compared against phlebograms performed on the same limbs, the phlebogram being accepted as the gold standard, even though we know that it is not quite 100% accurate.

Two hundred of the new tests are positive, 100 tests are negative. When, however, the tests are compared against the phlebograms:

- 180 of the new test's positive results are correct (true positives)
- 20 of the new test's positive results are incorrect (false positives)
- 70 of the new test's negative results are correct (true negatives)
- 30 of the new test's negative results are incorrect (false negatives).

Overall accuracy of the test is

$$\frac{180 + 70}{300} \times 100 = 83\%$$

Positive test accuracy (positive predictive value) of the test is

$$\frac{180}{200} \times 100 = 90\%$$

Negative test accuracy (negative predictive value) of the test is

$$\frac{70}{100} \times 100 = 70\%$$

Sensitivity of the test is

$$\frac{180}{180 + 30} \times 100 = 86\%$$

Specificity of the test is

$$\frac{70}{70 + 20} \times 100 = 77\%$$

These calculations suggest that our new test is moderately good. Overall it gets the answer right in four of five cases (accuracy 83%). It is, however, better when a thrombosis is present (nine out of ten positive test accuracy) than when the leg is normal (seven out of ten negative test accuracy). Overall its ability to detect disease is 86% (sensitivity) and its ability to exclude disease is almost as good – 77% (specificity).

Think about these ways of expressing the value of a test and decide which you most readily understand and prefer.

Clinical examination

The many and varied symptoms and signs of venous disease are described and discussed in those chapters dealing with specific venous abnormalities. The majority of symptoms and signs are non-specific.[160, 280]

History

Venous disease affects all age groups, though varicose veins in children are likely to be associated with a congenital rather than an acquired abnormality, and deep vein thrombosis is rare in children.

Pain, swelling and unsightliness are the dominant symptoms.

Superficial venous insufficiency causes a dull aching pain which is relieved by rest; deep vein thrombosis causes a persistent, more severe pain. Venous outflow obstruction, whether acute (following a deep vein thrombosis) or chronic, causes a bursting pain during muscle exercise. A patient with an acute thrombosis is unlikely to try to walk because the muscles are also painful at rest.

Night cramps are common.

Swelling of the leg may be localized, or general. General swelling may vary from a little oedema around the ankle to gross swelling of the whole limb. There is no difference between the swelling of deep vein thrombosis and that of chronic venous insufficiency; it is a low protein oedema caused by the venous obstruction.

Unsightliness is related to the size and extent of the varicose veins, intradermal venules, pigmentation, scarring and swelling.

A carefully taken clinical history is an essential part of the investigation of venous disease and often helps exclude or pinpoint other differential diagnoses. Chest symptoms in a patient with deep vein thrombosis should always be assumed to be caused by pulmonary embolism until proved otherwise.

Examination

Always examine the legs twice, first when the patient is standing and then when the patient is lying down, except when muscle pain and discomfort are severe.

Inspection

Three abnormalities may be visible on inspection: dilated superficial veins, changes in the skin and swelling.

Dilated veins may be large incompetent tortuous subcutaneous veins (i.e. varicose veins) or fine intradermal venules ('venous stars'). The position of the dilated veins may indicate their anatomical origin and connections. Veins on the medial side of the thigh are most likely to be connected to the long saphenous system but below the knee the position of a varicose vein does not allow its attribution to any particular system. A varicose vein on the medial side of the calf may be connected to the long saphenous system but it could be connected to the short saphenous system or it could be independent of both.

Skin changes range from mild eczema and pigmentation through thickening and hardening of the skin and fat (lipodermatosclerosis) to weeping eczema and frank ulceration. Although the majority of these skin changes are found on the lower medial third of the lower leg, they can occur anywhere. Conversely, other forms of ulceration more common on other parts of the leg can occur in the 'gaiter' area and so it should never be assumed that skin changes are venous in origin just because of their site. The clinical features of venous ulcers are discussed in Chapter 19. The presence of skin changes indicates a severe disturbance of calf pump function, whereas quite large varicose veins may exist with little or no functional abnormality.

The extent of diffuse swelling caused by venous disease usually correlates with the site and severity of the venous outflow obstruction. Localized swelling is usually caused by local inflammatory changes (e.g. superficial thrombophlebitis).

Palpation

The size and tension of the veins can easily be assessed with the finger tips. The presence of an *expansile cough impulse* indicates the absence of functioning valves between the palpating finger and the thorax. Always examine for this impulse at the sapheno-femoral junction, whether there be a palpable vein or not, and over any other visible veins. Veins that cannot be seen can often be felt, especially in the thigh.

A calf that is the site of a deep vein thrombosis will be warmer than the normal calf.[331] Recently thrombosed veins are firm, incompressible and tender. The tenderness fades with the inflammation but the vein gets harder and the overlying skin often becomes pigmented.

Skin changes are not usually tender to palpation except when there is acute lipodermatosclerosis when the skin, which is red–brown, and the fat, which is thickened with a palpable edge between it and the normal tissues, are both tender.

The surface of an ulcer is painful if it is infected or necrotic. Clean, healing chronic venous ulcers are usually neither painful nor very tender.

The oedema of venous obstruction is soft and 'pits' easily with firm pressure.

The thickening of lipodermatosclerosis sometimes looks like oedema but is hard and incompressible and can even become calcified. Veins amongst thickened hard tissues feel like hollow pits when the patient is lying flat and the venous pressure is low. It is easy to be misguided by this appearance into thinking that these pits are fascial defects corresponding to the site of superficial-to-deep communicating veins.[47]

Deep tenderness within the muscles, particularly the calf, is a physical sign of deep vein thrombosis but also of a multitude of other abnormalities within the muscle such as local trauma, myositis, arteritis, ischaemia and malignant change. Varicose veins rarely cause muscle tenderness. Even in conditions where deep vein thrombosis is the most likely diagnosis (e.g. postoperation) calf tenderness has a positive test accuracy of only 50% (using the fibrinogen uptake test as the gold standard).[220] Nevertheless, it is important to palpate the deep tissues of the leg as well as the skin, subcutaneous tissues and veins. Attempts to quantify tenderness by applying known pressures with a pneumatic cuff have not been helpful.[31,262,264]

Careful palpation may reveal tender defects in the deep fascia on the medial side of the lower leg which sometimes correspond to the site of dilated communicating veins.[47]

Percussion

A dilated blood-filled vein will conduct a percussion impulse in the direction of normal blood flow and retrogradely if the valves are incompetent. Thus tapping on a vein and feeling downstream should be used as a method for detecting the course and connections of a dilated vein, whereas tapping and feeling upstream should be used as a way of testing for incompetent valves in the segment of vein between the two hands.[84]

Auscultation

Do not forget to place a stethoscope over large bunches of varicosities, especially if they are in an abnormal position. On rare occasions there will be a 'machinery murmur', indicating the presence of an arteriovenous fistula.

Elevation

If the veins in a limb are distended when the patient is lying down, slowly raise the limb until the veins collapse. The height to which the limb has to be raised corresponds to the pressure in the veins and indicates the severity of the venous obstruction.

Clinical classification

The American Vascular Societies have proposed the following classification of the clinical severity of the symptoms and signs of chronic venous insufficiency:[337]

- Class 0 – asymptomatic
- Class 1 – mild insufficiency causing mild discomfort (heaviness, painful varicosities), mild ankle swelling, local or generalized dilatation of subcutaneous veins
- Class 2 – moderate insufficiency causing hyperpigmentation in the gaiter area, moderate oedema, subcutaneous fibrosis (without ulceration, prominent local or regional dilatation of subcutaneous veins)
- Class 3 – severe insufficiency causing chronic pain, ulceration or preulcer changes (atrophie blanche, painful lipodermatosclerosis, and/or severe oedema).

This classification has now been extended and broadened by the American Venous Forum by the addition of anatomical, aetiological and pathological data. This new classification is known as the

Table 4.1 The CEAP classification*

C	For **C**linical signs (grade$_{0-6}$), supplemented by ($_A$) for asymptomatic and ($_S$) for symptomatic presentation
E	For **E**tiologic classification (**C**ongenital, **P**rimary, **S**econdary)
A	For **A**natomical distribution (**S**uperficial, **D**eep, or **P**erforator, alone or in combination)
P	For **P**athophysiological dysfunction (**R**eflux or **O**bstruction, alone or in combination)

C: Clinical signs

Class 0	No visible or palpable signs of venous disease
Class 1	Telangiectases or reticular veins
Class 2	Varicose veins
Class 3	Edema
Class 4	Skin changes ascribed to venous disease (e.g. pigmentation, venous eczema, lipodermatosclerosis)
Class 5	Skin changes as defined above with healed ulceration
Class 6	Skin changes as defined above with active ulceration

E: Aetiology

Congenital (E_C)
Primary (E_P) – with undetermined cause
Secondary (E_S) – with known cause
* Postthrombotic
* Posttraumatic
* Other

P: Pathophysiology

Reflux (P_R)
Obstruction (P_O)
Reflux and obstruction ($P_{R,O}$)

A: Anatomy

Segment no.

Segment no.	Superficial veins (A_S)
1	Telangiectases/reticular veins
2	Greater (long) saphenous (GSV) – above knee
3	Greater (long) saphenous (GSV) – below knee
4	Lesser (short) saphenous (LSV)
5	Nonsaphenous
	Deep veins (A_D)
6	Inferior vena cava
7	Common iliac
8	Internal iliac
9	External iliac
10	Pelvic – gonadal, broad ligament, other
11	Common femoral
12	Deep femoral
13	Superficial femoral
14	Popliteal
15	Crural – anterior tibial, posterior tibial, peroneal (all paired)
16	Muscular – gastrocnemial, soleal, other
	Perforating veins (A_P)
17	Thigh
18	Calf

*A consensus statement. *Vasc Surg* 1996; **30**: 5–11.

CEAP classification and is set out in Table 4.1. The Forum also produced a clinical scoring system but, as the different symptoms and signs are not weighted against each other, it has doubtful clinical or research value.

General examination

No patient complaining solely about a venous problem should have just their veins examined. It is essential to examine all the systems of the limb, particularly the arteries and nerves, and the whole patient. Varicose veins can be caused by abdominal tumours. Deep vein thrombosis and superficial thrombophlebitis can be secondary to occult carcinoma, especially of the lung, stomach, pancreas and kidney. Failure to examine the whole patient even though he/she presents with only a few varicose veins is negligent.

The tourniquet tests

The tourniquet tests are simple bedside tests which help to assess the direction of blood flow and the source of refilling of the superficial veins.[62,66,120,406] They are therefore very simple function tests but are described here because they should always be part of the routine of clinical examination. They are tests whose accuracy very much depends on the operator (i.e. they get more accurate as the experience and understanding of the clinician performing the test grows).

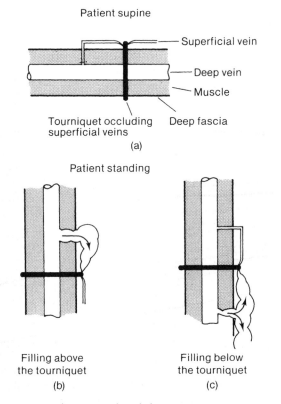

Patient supine

Superficial vein

Deep vein

Muscle

Tourniquet occluding
superficial veins

Deep fascia

(a)

Patient standing

Filling above
the tourniquet

Filling below
the tourniquet

(b)

(c)

Figure 4.1 The principle of the tourniquet test. (a) A tourniquet is placed around the leg to occlude the superficial veins when the patient is supine and the superficial veins empty. The patient is then asked to stand. (b) Filling of the veins above the tourniquet indicates an incompetent deep-to-superficial communication above the tourniquet. (c) Filling of the veins below the tourniquet indicates an incompetent connection below the tourniquet.

If the subcutaneous veins of the lower limb are occluded by a narrow tourniquet placed around the limb when the patient is lying down, filling of the veins below the tourniquet when the patient stands up indicates that there is an incompetent connection between the deep and superficial veins below the tourniquet (Figure 4.1).

The level of this incompetent connection can be determined by repeating the test with the tourniquet at different levels or by using multiple tourniquets. Venous filling can be accelerated by mild exercise, such as repeated heel raising.

If the tourniquet is placed around the limb when the patient is standing and the superficial veins are distended, exercise should reduce the pressure and volume of blood in the veins below the tourniquet if the deep veins are functioning normally, and increase their pressure and volume if the deep veins are

obstructed. This test, usually called Perthes' test,[327] is more difficult to perform than the simpler reflux test, which is loosely called Trendelenburg's test.[62]

Tourniquet tests are useful in patients with chronic venous insufficiency and especially in those with superficial varicosities (see Chapter 6). In conjunction with clinical examination they provide a sufficient understanding of the venous abnormality for management decisions in 80–90% of patients with simple varicose veins (see Chapter 7), but it must always be remembered that tourniquets do not always occlude the superficial veins[265,281] and reflux can be more accurately detected with a hand-held Doppler flow detector (see page 121).

Investigations that provide images of the veins and/or thrombus

PHOTOGRAPHY

Colour photographs can be used to record the size and extent of superficial varicosities and ulcers. There are many examples of the value of colour photography throughout this book.

Photographs are the only way in which changes in the appearance of the skin may be recorded over a period of time but they are only useful if the photographic technique is carefully controlled and kept constant for each photograph. Widmer used photography effectively as part of his prevalence study of venous disease in Basle.[432] The important aspects of his technique are given below.

Position

The patient must stand in a standardized reproducible position with legs apart and feet externally rotated as much as possible to ensure that the whole of the inner side of both legs is visible on the anterior view, and the lateral sides are visible on the posterior view. Oedema is best shown in an anterior view with the long axis of the foot in the sagittal plane.

Views

Anterior, posterior and oblique views (at a standard angle) should be taken.

Lighting

Although oblique lighting gives shadows which reveal large varicosities, it does not illuminate the skin sufficiently to reveal fine intradermal veins. A direct light does not give many shadows but demonstrates minor colour differences in the skin much more clearly. The intensity and colour of the light used must be kept constant. A flash is not necessary if optimum lighting and a good camera are used.

Colour

Colour film reveals minor variations of skin pigmentation but intradermal venules show up better on black and white film. The type and brand of film must not be altered as different brands have different colour sensitivities.

Camera

Any good camera will suffice provided the focal distance, aperture and exposure are kept constant.

The changes in ulcers may also be recorded with serial photographs provided the same constraints about constant position, lighting, film and camera are applied. Serial close-up views are most informative provided a centimetre scale is placed on the skin to enable measurements from the photograph to be calibrated.

INFRA-RED PHOTOGRAPHY

The blood in the superficial veins heats the overlying skin. This temperature difference can be detected by infra-red photography, a method which is less sensitive but similar to thermography. Large veins appear as dark areas, even intradermal venules show up, but the technique is not very valuable except when the clinician suspects that there are many varices that he cannot see or feel (Figure 4.2).

THERMOGRAPHY

A thermographic system detects differences in skin temperature by measuring the infra-red emissions from the skin with an infra-red detector – usually indium–antimonide or cadmium–mercury–telluride cooled with liquid nitrogen. The object under study is scanned by a scanning camera which focuses the infra-red emissions onto the detector. The electrical impulses from the detector are converted into a video signal so that a visual television image is produced which can be examined directly or photographed with a polaroid camera.[95]

If the patient is lying in bed, the legs can be scanned from the foot of the bed by viewing them through a mirror held over them at an angle of 45°.

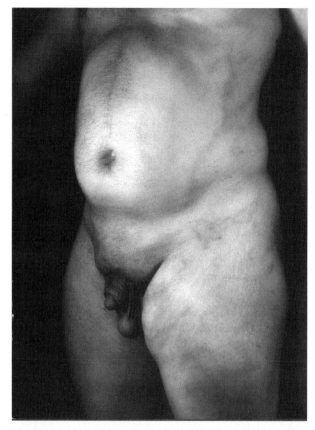

Figure 4.2 An infra-red photograph of a patient with an occlusion of the inferior vena cava. There were no visible veins on the abdominal wall but the infra-red photograph revealed dilated subcutaneous collateral veins on the lateral side of the abdomen.

To examine the deep veins, the legs must be elevated to eliminate superficial venous pooling.[97]

It is important for the limbs to be exposed for 10 minutes in an ambient temperature of 18–20°C and in a room without any draughts. Any movement of air will affect the thermogram. The common convention is to display the hot areas as white and the cold areas as black. It is, however, best to focus the image so that there is the maximum number of grey tones. Some systems have a colour coded presentation.

The normal image of the leg reveals an even temperature throughout with a slightly colder area over the tibia and patella anteriorly and a warmer area over the popliteal fossa posteriorly (Figure 4.3a and b). Sometimes the image has a mottled appearance caused by irregular warm and cool spots. The mechanism and reason for these local variations in skin blood flow is not known.

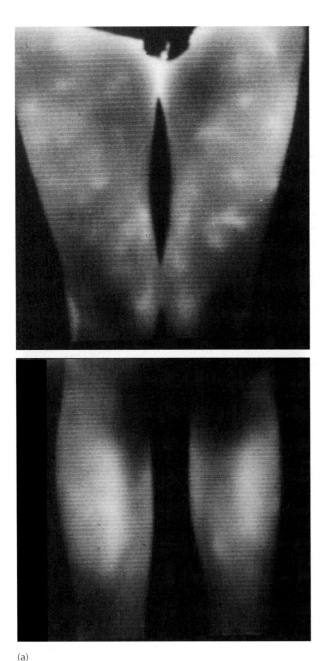

(a)

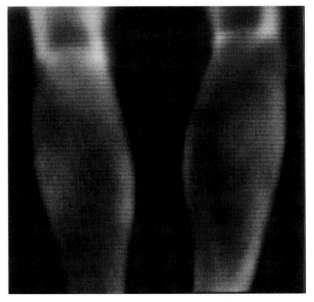

(b)

Figure 4.3 Normal thermograms. (a) The anterior view of the thighs and lower legs. White areas are hot; black areas are cold. The legs are symmetrical; the skin over the patellae and subcutaneous borders of the tibiae is cooler (blacker) than the skin over the muscles in the adjacent anterior compartment. (b) The posterior view of the calves. (We are indebted to Dr ED Cooke for providing these thermograms.)

Deep vein thrombosis

This causes an increase in the temperature of the overlying skin. This was first recorded as a clinical observation in 1939[331] and was confirmed with thermography in the early 1970s.[97] Examples of positive thermograms are shown in Figure 4.4. Other conditions which may cause a temperature increase and be confused with deep vein thrombosis are: superficial thrombophlebitis, acute infection, acute arthritis, trauma, ruptured Baker's cysts, Paget's disease of bone, osteomyelitis and bone tumours. The first four of these conditions also give false-positive results with the fibrinogen uptake test.

Cooke compared thermography against phlebography for the diagnosis of deep vein thrombosis in 164 patients.[95] Thermography had a positive test accuracy of 92%, and a negative test accuracy of 93%. The overall accuracy was 93%. Other investigators[347,351] have obtained similar results but it must

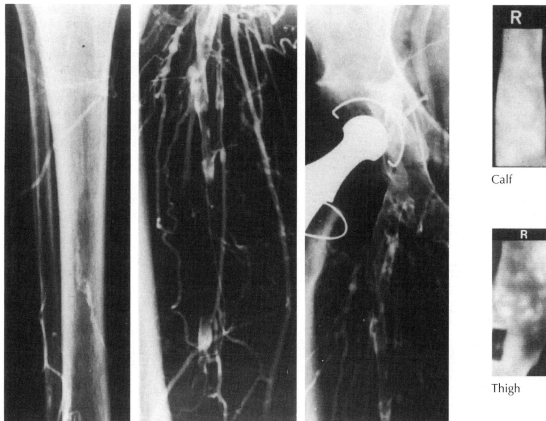
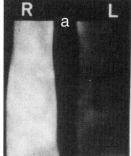
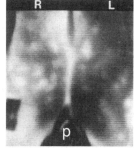

Calf

Thigh

Figure 4.4 A thermogram and phlebograph of a patient with a complete right calf, femoral and iliac vein thrombosis following a hip replacement operation. The right calf and thigh show an increased temperature with loss of the normal cool area over the patella and tibia. These images are obtained through a mirror and are therefore reversed and upside down. p, pubis; a, ankle. (We are indebted to Dr ED Cooke for providing these illustrations.)

be remembered that the clinicians managing these patients had excluded patients with clinical evidence of conditions expected to cause false positives before proceeding to thermography. The published studies of thermography show that it is accurate but it has not been widely adopted because the equipment is expensive and the setting up of the test and the control of the environment is cumbersome and time consuming.

Varicose veins

Varicose veins do not show up on the thermogram if the patient is supine. If the patient stands, the veins appear as irregular lines over the leg; these lines are similar to those seen on an infra-red photograph.

Incompetent communicating veins

If the leg is emptied of blood, a superficial vein occluding tourniquet placed below the knee, and the leg then put in a dependent position, the sites at which any blood flows from the deep to the superficial system, through incompetent communicating veins, become hot and can be seen on a thermogram. This effect has been used to detect and pinpoint the position of incompetent communicating veins. The accuracy of the method can be increased by cooling the skin of the leg with cold towels before performing the test. This technique has been compared with phlebography and the Turner Warwick 'bleed-back test' at operation.[322,356,436] Compared with operation, thermography has a positive test accuracy of 87% and a negative test accuracy of 84%.

Chronic deep vein insufficiency

It has been claimed that in 20% of all patients with chronic venous insufficiency the calf is warmer than a normal calf; this abnormality is detectable by thermography.[96] The increased temperature is patchy and uneven and can therefore be distinguished from the uniform temperature rise of deep vein thrombosis. It is increased by exercise.[158,169] The significance of this observation and its mechanism needs further investigation but it has been suggested that patients with this abnormality have a ninefold increase in the incidence of postoperative deep vein thrombosis.

LIQUID CRYSTAL THERMOGRAPHY

The introduction of liquid crystal thermography has provided a simpler and cheaper detector.

The heat sensitive cholesteric crystals are incorporated into a latex sheet which is stretched across a plastic frame. These crystals, which are brown when cool, become yellow, green and ultimately blue as they become warmer. Different sheets are provided to cover different ranges of temperature. The frame is incorporated into a rig which holds a Polaroid camera and flash gun. The patient lies prone with the calves exposed to room air for 10 minutes. The frame is then placed over the calves and the colour changes recorded, visually or photographically 30 seconds later. The same process is repeated over the thighs and lower legs with the patient lying supine. Any area, not over visible varicose veins in one of the limbs with a temperature greater by 0.7°C than an adjacent area, is likely to be overlying a site of deep vein thrombosis. Bilateral symmetrical warm areas do not indicate underlying deep vein thrombosis. This inability to detect bilateral disease is a serious deficiency of the technique. Because this test is simple and easy to perform, it has been used as a way of excluding deep vein thrombosis,[351] but published studies[176,362] have reported specificities (correct identification as normal) of 83% and 53% as against sensitivities (correct identification of thrombosis) of 100% and 97%. These results imply that it should not be used as a way of excluding thrombosis but as a way of confirming a clinical diagnosis and indicating further investigation. However, even when used in this manner, known causes of false positives such as local cellulitis, local trauma, superficial thrombophlebitis and local collections of dilated veins should be looked for and considered as contraindications to the test. It is not surprising, therefore, that this test has not been widely adopted for the diagnosis of deep vein thrombosis.

THE FIBRINOGEN UPTAKE TEST (FUT)

Sadly, this test can no longer be used because it is not possible to prepare fibrinogen that can be guaranteed free of either the acquired immune deficiency syndrome (AIDS) virus, or the hepatitis viruses. This test undoubtedly facilitated a tremendous expansion of our understanding of the prevalence and aetiology of deep vein thrombosis, especially postoperative thrombosis, and if a safe fibrinogen could be manufactured would again be used in many clinical trials. Alternatives using other isotope-labelled substances that participate in the coagulation mechanism are available but have not proved as simple and effective as the fibrinogen uptake test. Because of the important contribution that this test has made to our understanding of venous thrombosis and in the hope that it will be possible to revive it, we have retained in this edition a full description of its methodology, application and accuracy.

The possibility that venous thrombi would incorporate radioactive fibrinogen as they formed was first tested in the rabbit by Hobbs and Davies in 1960,[177] but studies with different isotopes were necessary before the test used today became fully validated.[25,46,154,300,319]

All thrombi are metabolically active, they are not 'silent backwaters' of the circulation. Fibrinogen is not only taken from the circulation and converted into fibrin as a thrombus forms but fibrinogen diffuses in and out of the thrombus throughout its early life. As the fibrin in the thrombus polymerizes and the thrombus ages, the exchange of molecules between it and the blood become less.

The fibrinogen uptake test (FUT) depends upon the incorporation of injected radioactive fibrinogen by thrombus and the detection of the localized radioactivity by external scintillation counting.[138,305] Fibrinogen cannot be autoclaved and the introduction of small pools of donors and testing them for hepatitis B antigen (Australia antigen) and HIV (human immunodeficiency viruses) cannot eliminate the risk of giving a patient a serum-transmitted disease; consequently, this test can no longer be used.

Method

The patient is given 100 mg of potassium iodide on the day before the labelled fibrinogen is given and daily thereafter for 14 days to block the uptake of radioactive iodine by the thyroid gland. In emergency situations the potassium iodide and the fibrinogen can be given together because the quantity of free iodine released during the first 24 hours is extremely small and most unlikely to damage the cells of the thyroid gland.

The patient should lie comfortably on a bed or couch with the legs elevated (30°) above the heart, to eliminate pooling of blood in the legs.

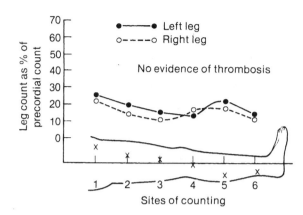

Figure 4.5 The fibrinogen uptake test of two normal legs. The count rates over the points marked 1–6 are recorded as a percentage of the precordial count. The slight variations in radioactivity are caused by the varying quantities of blood in the tissues beneath the scintillation counter. This study was performed with a 4 inch collimator.

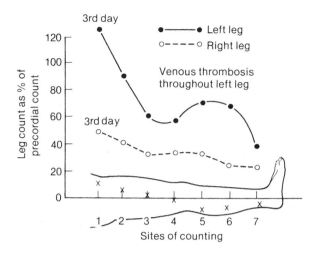

Figure 4.6 A patient with a raised fibrinogen uptake test (4 in collimator) throughout the left leg 3 days after an abdominal operation. The difference between the legs at points 1, 2, 5 and 6 were greater than 15 percentage points and persisted for 24 hours. This patient had a calf and femoral vein thrombosis.

The legs are examined with a hand-held scintillation counter and ratemeter[203] along the line of the femoral vein in the thigh, over the popliteal fossa, and down the centre or either side of each calf.

A standard sodium iodide crystal and 7.5 cm collimator will view an area of tissue 10 cm in diameter to a depth of 5 cm. With such a counter the points for counting should be 10 cm apart. The smaller crystal and collimator of the common portable ratemeter views an area 5 cm in diameter to a depth of 10 cm, so counting points should be 5 cm apart.

In the early days of the test the radioactivity was measured in counts/min using a scaler and a timer; the development of small portable ratemeters replaced this rather cumbersome apparatus.

The counts emitted from the precordium (the fourth left interspace adjacent to the sternum) are adjusted on the ratemeter to read 100%. The counts from each point along both legs are then recorded as percentages of the precordial count (Figures 4.5 and 4.6).

The initial studies comparing ^{125}I-fibrinogen uptake with phlebography used a scaler and timer and showed that a difference of 15 percentage points developing between adjacent sites on the same leg or between identical sites on the opposite leg was diagnostic of a thrombosis. Comparisons between the scaler/timer system and the portable ratemeter showed that a difference of 20 percentage points was necessary to make a positive diagnosis with the ratemeter. The increased count rate

must persist for more than 24 hours to be significant. Daily investigations are performed to detect changes in the configuration of the thrombus.

The information is kept on a sheet or displayed graphically (Figure 4.6). A graph makes comparisons easier and shows the day-to-day changes occurring in the thrombus.

Application

This test is best used for the detection of thrombus in circumstances when it is expected that thrombosis will occur (e.g. after operation or during a severe medical illness) so that the radioactive fibrinogen is given before the event.

The FUT has been the main research tool used for the study of the prevalence of venous thrombosis and for testing methods of prophylaxis, and in some centres for screening high risk patients.

It can be used to confirm the diagnosis of established thrombosis but as thrombus ages so the accuracy of the test diminishes and different diagnostic criteria are required.[71]

Accuracy

Any condition that causes a deposition of fibrin, intravascular or extravascular, will give a positive test.[69,202] Inflammation, bruises, haematomata, arthritis and fresh wounds will all give false-positive results (Figure 4.7); it must be remembered that in all the studies comparing this test with phlebography,

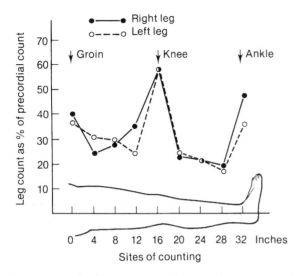

Figure 4.7   The fibrinogen uptake test of a patient with acute rheumatoid arthritis of the knees and ankles. This was initially interpreted as a positive test until the joints were examined. A phlebograph was normal.

most of these conditions have been diagnosed clinically and excluded from the study. The FUT is only accurate when limbs with disorders that would cause false-positive scans are excluded.

False negatives occur when ageing thrombus does not take up fibrinogen[71] and when there are fresh thrombi in the upper half of the thigh or pelvic veins[138,305] where the background radioactivity from blood and urine masks the relatively small increase of radioactivity present in a thrombus. These are serious disadvantages and mean that the FUT can only be used to study or detect calf and lower thigh thrombosis.

The positive and negative test accuracy for thrombi developing after the injection of the radioactive fibrinogen, below the mid-thigh, having excluded obvious causes of false positives by clinical examination and confirmed that the abnormality is persistent (24 hours), is over 95%, when compared with phlebography. Some investigators considered that this test should have been used as the gold standard of calf thrombosis, and it has been suggested that it could replace phlebography for the diagnosis of deep vein thrombosis if it was combined with impedance plethysmography.[190,191]

The positive test accuracy for established thrombus when compared with phlebography is 75% for thrombi less than 7 days old and 65% for thrombi more than 14 days old. These tests may take 48 hours to become positive. Thus, the FUT is not of practical value in the diagnosis of established thrombosis, except when combined with other

screening tests which exclude major vein thrombi and indicate that a 48-hour delay in waiting for the test result is safe.

THE RADIOACTIVE PLASMIN UPTAKE TEST

This is an example of one of the other labelled clotting factor tests that have been developed but which have not been found to be as good or convenient as the fibrinogen uptake test.

The slow entry of fibrinogen into established thrombus stimulated a search for a substance that would enter thrombi faster and more easily and so be suitable for the diagnosis of established thrombi. Labelled porcine plasmin was found to do this and it has been used as a clinical test.[4,46,116,311]

This test can detect established unilateral thrombi within 30 minutes of the injection of the labelled plasmin but because of the method of expressing the level of radioactivity, bilateral symmetrical thrombi are often missed. The advantage of this technique is the rapidity of the result and the absence of radiation of the thyroid gland. Its disadvantage, apart from its failure to detect bilateral disease, is the short half-life of the isotope (6 hours) which means that the plasmin must be labelled for each test and cannot be stored on the shelf.

This test has not been generally adopted because of the difficulties mentioned above together with a low specificity of 40% (i.e. a poor ability to detect the absence of disease).

DUPLEX ULTRASOUND

Physics and instrumentation

A sound wave can be produced in a medium by placing a vibrating source in contact with it, causing particles in the medium to vibrate. The resulting disturbance propagates away from the source and is attenuated, scattered and reflected by the medium. In medical ultrasound a piezoelectric transducer serves as the source and detector of sound waves.

Speed of sound

The propagation speed for sound waves is dependent on the medium through which it is travelling; for soft tissues it is 1540 m/s.

Frequency and wavelength

The frequency of the sound wave is determined by number of oscillations per second of the source.

Diagnostic ultrasound uses frequencies in the 1–15 MHz range. The wavelength is the distance over which the acoustic disturbance repeats itself.

Attenuation

As the sound wave propagates through tissue its density diminishes with the distance travelled. The main sources of attenuation are absorption, reflection and scattering. The rate of attenuation is not constant through soft tissues, with attenuation higher for muscle and lower for fluid-filled structures, such as veins. For most soft tissues the attenuation is proportional to the frequency. This means that higher frequency sound waves are more severely attenuated than lower frequency waves. Thus the higher the frequency of the ultrasound beam the shorter it can penetrate through soft tissue. Consequently, higher frequency ultrasound beams are used to access superficial structures.

Reflection

When an ultrasound beam strikes an interface between two tissues having different acoustic properties, part of the beam is reflected and part transmitted. If the reflected wave travels back to the ultrasound source it is detected as an echo. The strength of the reflected wave is proportional to the acoustic impedance of the material. Acoustic impedance (Z) is defined as the speed of ultrasound in a material multiplied by its density.

Scattering

This occurs at acoustic interfaces whose dimensions are small. The energy is scattered in all directions.

The Doppler effect

This is the change of frequency that occurs whenever there is relative motion between the sound source and the reflector.

Ultrasonic Doppler equipment is commonly used for detecting and evaluating blood flow in veins. The sources of echo signals are the red blood cells flowing in the vessel.

Pulse-echo ultrasound

Ultrasound can be used to image interfaces. An ultrasonic transducer is placed in direct contact with the skin. The transducer emits brief pulses of sound. The transducer also serves as a receiver for echoes transmitted back from interfaces from the original sound pulse. There are four types of real time transducers:

- Mechanical scanners – single or multiple transducers are oscillated within a single head. Alternatively, the beam may be swept by an oscillating acoustic mirror.
- Sequential linear arrays – up to 120 rectangular transducers are used to form an image. Scanning is achieved by switching to different elements in the array and repeating the pulse echo sequences.
- Sequential convex arrays – this is similar to a linear array except that the elements are arranged along a curved surface, giving a wider field view.
- Phased array scanners – the sound beam from an array of transducer elements is steered by introducing electronically controlled small time delays.

Continuous wave ultrasonic Doppler equipment

These are the simplest devices available. The ultrasonic transducer transmits continuously. Returning signals are amplified so that the resultant signal is in the audible frequency range.

Pulsed Doppler

This allows discrimination of Doppler signals from different depths, allowing interrogation of a sample volume anywhere along the axis of the ultrasound beam.

The signal produced by each pulse of a pulsed Doppler instrument is generated from the changes in phase of the echo signal returning from a target, the change varying according to whether the target is receding from or moving towards the transducer.

Duplex ultrasound equipment

Duplex ultrasound instruments are real time B mode scanners with Doppler capabilities. The standard method of combining these two modalities is to use the Doppler equipment to study blood flow in an area localized on the real time image.

Ultrasound transducer properties

An ultrasound transducer provides the communicating link between the imaging equipment and the patient.

Medical ultrasound transducers use piezoelectric ceramic materials to generate and detect sound waves. These materials convert pressure waves into electrical signals and also convert electric signals into mechanical vibrations. As a consequence piezoelectric materials can be used for both the transmission and reception of ultrasonic emissions. Aliasing is the generation of artefactual lower frequency signals which occur when the pulse repetition frequency is less than twice the frequency of the Doppler signal.

COLOUR DUPLEX IMAGING

Colour duplex imaging is done by estimating the mean velocity, relative to the ultrasound beam direction, of scatterers and reflectors in a scanned region. Echo signals from moving reflectors are displayed so that the colour hue and brightness indicates the relative velocity. These data are superimposed on B mode images, and may therefore be displayed in real time. The direction of blood flow, relative to the direction of the beam, is indicated by the display colour, e.g. red towards the transducer and blue away.

Summary

Real time techniques can be used to visualize vessel wall structures. Doppler techniques can be used to determine flow characteristics.

A Doppler instrument can either transmit a continuous or a pulsed wave. The Doppler shift frequency is the difference between the frequency of the transmitted sound and the returning echoes.

Doppler instruments may be directional in terms of determining the direction of blood flow relative to the transducer, or non-directional.

COLOUR DUPLEX SONOGRAPHY

A standard B mode real time ultrasound machine records the time it takes for an echo to return to the transducer and the strength of that echo. Colour duplex instruments provide Doppler information for each echo – the Doppler shift, which is related to the average velocity of blood flow, and the direction of the Doppler shift, which is related to the direction of blood flow relative to the transducer – in addition to the information provided by a standard B mode real time machine.

Advantages of colour duplex imaging

There are several advantages in using colour duplex over standard duplex. Any moving blood will be identified in colour, allowing a larger area to be interrogated more rapidly than with standard duplex. Thus a larger segment of vessel can be assessed.

Limitations of colour duplex imaging

The information provided is based on the average Doppler shift at each point in the vessel, and not the peak Doppler shift which is a more important measurement. Information collected is qualitative and not quantitative, and the shades of colour give only a rough guide to the underlying blood velocity. The contained Doppler information is not corrected for the Doppler angle. The colour ascribed to any vessel is arbitrary and refers to whether flow is toward or away from the transducer.

POWER DOPPLER

This is a recent development in colour flow imaging. In this technique colour is mapped to power rather than the mean frequency. The main advantage of power is that noise is designated a uniform low level and as a result the colour flow is accentuated, with an overall gain of 10–15 dB over conventional imaging. Its chief advantages are that it can detect low volume and low velocity flow, is Doppler angle independent and has good edge detection. The disadvantages are motion artefact and a bias to venous flow. As with standard colour duplex, it gives qualitative and not quantitative information.[26,149,400,422,433,445,446,448]

DUPLEX APPEARANCES OF NORMAL VEINS

The lumen of a normal vein is echo free and the internal surface of the vein wall is smooth. Consequently, a normal wall cannot be identified, and any thickening of the vein wall which makes it detectable implies the presence of underlying pathology. In some instances rouleaux formation of red cells may be seen as mobile echogenic blood. This appearance is readily distinguished from thrombus which is stationary.

Valve cusps, which are more numerous distally, are seen as thin-walled structures that move symmetrically when closing.

Veins are easily compressible. This feature serves to differentiate veins from arteries, which are non-compressible. A vein full of thrombus is not compressible – a very important sign of venous thrombosis. Veins are normally up to twice the size of their accompanying arteries. The diameter of the larger veins increases with deep inspiration or the Valsalva manoeuvre; for example, the diameter of the femoral vein can increase from 50 to 200%. The effect of the Valsalva response diminishes distally if the valves are competent.

Normal venous blood flow has the following characteristics: it is spontaneous, phasic, augmented by distal compression and flows towards the heart.

Spontaneous flow is present in virtually all veins apart from small veins, for example in the calf, where flow is dependent on the calf pump. Here it is necessary to augment the flow physically to demonstrate patency. Absence of spontaneous flow or a response to physical augmentation is a sign of thrombosis.

The velocity of blood flow varies with respiration. When phasic flow caused by respiration is absent and replaced by continuous flow, it is likely that there is thrombus within the vein, either proximal or distal to the point of examination.

Manual compression of a vein distal (upstream) to the site of Doppler examination should increase the flow through the segment under examination. This augmentation also confirms that the segment of vein between the transducer and the point of compression is patent. No augmentation is seen if the segment is totally occluded by thrombus but a normal response can be seen if the thrombus only partly occludes the vein.

Normal venous blood flow is unidirectional, towards the heart. Valves that are incompetent permit retrograde flow. This is best shown ultrasonically during the Valsalva manoeuvre.[107]

Patient examination

Rationale for the full investigation of patients with a suspected diagnosis of deep vein thrombosis

The precise incidence of deep vein thrombosis is not known. In the USA pulmonary emboli contributed to 30 000 deaths in 1982 and was diagnosed 120 000 times in in-patients in 1985.[150] In an autopsy study of 2388 patients who had died while in hospital, pulmonary embolism was found to be the cause of death of 10%. Of the patients with pulmonary emboli, 198 (83%) had deep vein thrombosis at autopsy, but only 45 (19%) had symptoms before death.

Other studies have produced similar results.[254]

A consistent theme reiterated in all studies of the natural history of venous thromboembolism is the high incidence of asymptomatic and undiagnosed cases of deep vein thrombosis and the continuum between deep vein thrombosis and pulmonary embolism.

Clinical assessment of deep vein thrombosis is completely unreliable.[79,260,363] Even in patients suspected of having deep vein thrombosis, the normal phlebogram rates range from 46 to 70%.[79,174]

The consequences of an erroneous diagnosis of deep vein thrombosis are serious. A false-positive diagnosis will result in the patient being given unnecessary, potentially dangerous treatment such as anticoagulants, and a false-negative diagnosis leaves the patient open to the risk of thrombus propagation and pulmonary embolism. The need for a non-invasive, inexpensive test for this diagnosis of deep vein thrombosis has led to the development of duplex ultrasound, and many studies have demonstrated its accuracy and cost effectiveness.[23,105,187,188,363,425,445,449]

The upper limb

The superior vena cava and innominate veins cannot be viewed directly as they are hidden by the bony thorax and lungs, hence information about these veins is obtained by analysing Doppler flow characteristics in the subclavian and axillary veins. When assessing these veins it is important to bear in mind the common normal anatomical variants, the most common deep system variants being duplication of the brachial and subclavian veins.

With the patient lying supine, with the arm by the side, upper limb examination is begun with the subclavian vein. The transducer is placed parallel to the long axis of the vein, which is approached from either a supra- or infra-clavicular direction. The latter approach usually allows more of the vein to be seen. The normal vein is uniform in size and larger than the accompanying artery. All the deep veins of the upper extremity are accompanied by arteries, hence if an artery is not seen near the vein under examination it is likely that it is a superficial vein that is being visualized.

The jugular vein is examined from the mid-neck to its junction with the subclavian vein. It demonstrates considerable variations of flow and diameter with respiration. Next, the cephalic vein is identified at its insertion into the subclavian vein and followed down over the deltoid muscle to the elbow. This is a superficial vein and is easily compressed by the transducer.

The upper end of the axillary vein is detected by placing the transducer high in the axilla. Flow should be spontaneous and phasic. This vessel and the brachial vein below it should have a normal response to the Valsalva manoeuvre. Absence of this response is important evidence of an innominate or superior vena cava obstruction. Care is needed when assessing the brachial vein. It is easily compressed and can be obliterated by excessive pressure. It is often duplicated, so care must be taken to examine both segments for thrombus.

The basilic vein is traced from its junction with the axillary vein in the axilla to the elbow.

The routine described above is usually sufficient for an upper extremity examination, but if clinically indicated the forearm veins can also be examined. This is best done with the arm extended. The duplicated radial and ulnar veins can be detected by using their adjacent arteries as landmarks.

The lower limb (Figures 4.8 and 4.9)

All the deep veins are accompanied by arteries which can be used as landmarks. The superficial veins do not have adjacent arteries.

The common and external iliac veins are often not identified by direct scanning because of overlying gas-filled bowel but indirect evidence of occlusion of these vessels may be obtained from the response to the Valsalva manoeuvre in the ipsilateral femoral vein.

The segment of superficial femoral vein in the adductor canal may be technically difficult to visualize.

As in the upper limb, duplications are often present, notably of the femoral and popliteal veins. What at first looks like popliteal vein duplication is often one of the calf vein trunks with a high termination.

In order to obtain maximum distension, the lower limb is examined in a dependent position, either by elevating the head of the bed or by having the patient seated. Some authors recommend that the calf veins be examined with the patient standing upright to obtain maximum distension.[433]

The examination is commenced at the groin with the identification of the external iliac vein, which is then followed cephalad. A 3 MHz probe often affords more penetration than a 5 MHz probe in

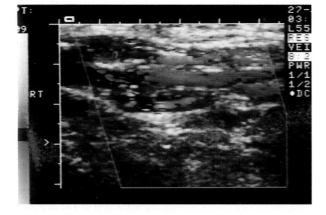

Figure 4.8 The images of the vessels of the upper thigh obtained using colour-coded duplex Doppler ultrasound. Red: superficial and deep femoral veins uniting to form the common femoral vein. Blue: the superficial and deep femoral arteries which originated at a higher level.

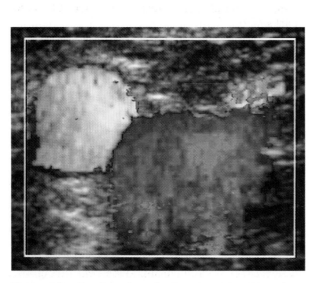 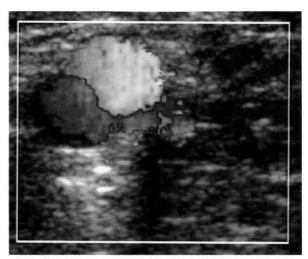

Figure 4.9 Confirmation of vein patency by external compression. Transverse images. Left: at rest; right: external compression. During compression the cross-section of the femoral vein (blue) changes from a circle to a slit.

this region. Whenever possible, images should be obtained of the common iliac vein and lower inferior vena cava , if these segments are not obscured by bowel gas. When the veins cannot be visualized their patency can be deduced from the presence of a normal phasic response during respiration and a normal Valsalva manoeuvre response in the external iliac vein.

Below the groin the leg veins are examined with a 5 MHz probe. The femoral and popliteal veins are examined in both longitudinal and transverse sections. Doppler or colour flow, the phasic response to respiration, the Valsalva manoeuvre response and the response to augmentation by calf compression should all be observed. The profunda femoral vein should also be assessed for patency. Isolated profunda vein thrombosis is a recognized complication of hip surgery.[108,155]

The popliteal vein is first examined at the adductor hiatus with the patient supine, but in the popliteal fossa it is best examined with the patient lying prone or standing. Here the vein lies superficial to the artery. The vein should be traced distally to the origin of the posterior tibial and peroneal trunks.

There are three pairs of crural veins alongside their respective arteries, with frequent horizontal communications between each pair.

The anterior tibial veins pass up the leg between the tibia and fibula on the antero-lateral surface of the interosseous membrane until they reach the level of tibial tuberosity, where they pass over the interosseous membrane into the posterior compartment of the leg to join the tibio-peroneal trunk to form the popliteal vein.

The posterior tibial veins are located distally midway between the medial malleolus and calcaneal tubercle. They are relatively superficial in the calf, but become more lateral and deeper as they approach the tibio-peroneal trunk.

The peroneal veins pass from the inferior tibio-fibula syndesmosis, along the medial crest of the fibula, before passing medially to join the posterior tibial veins.

Identification of each of the pairs of calf veins is best achieved by beginning the scan just below the knee and following the popliteal vein downwards until the termination of each of the three sets of veins is reached. Three different scanning planes are then required for optimal image resolution.

Posterior calf approach

Scanning the proximal calf veins from a posterior approach identifies the confluence of the calf veins and the upper portions of the posterior tibial and peroneal veins. It is not suitable for the anterior tibial veins distal to the confluence as they are anterior to the interosseous membrane.

Postero-medial approach

By placing the transducer on the postero-medial side of the calf it is possible to view the whole length of the posterior tibial and peroneal veins.

Antero-lateral approach

Placing the transducer just lateral to the tibia, diagonally opposite to the postero-medial view, allows examination of the whole length of the anterior tibial veins.

The small anterior tibial veins are rarely involved in isolated thrombosis. When the calf veins are being assessed, colour flow with calf augmentation is a better method for identifying vein patency than compression.[443]

Calf vein thrombosis is often considered to originate in the gastrocnemius and soleal veins and then propagate to the paired calf veins or popliteal vein. The gastrocnemius veins are tributaries of the popliteal vein lying postero-inferior to it. Those in the medial head of the gastrocnemius muscle can usually be easily identified, whereas the smaller veins in the lateral head are not usually seen with ultrasound.

The soleal venous sinuses, embedded in the soleus muscle, cannot usually be seen.

The whole length of the long saphenous vein is not usually examined as part of an examination for deep vein thrombosis. It is best identified at its junction with the femoral vein and then followed down the leg. The presence of two echogenic fascial planes around the vein are helpful landmarks.[41,212,354,443,449]

Ultrasound appearance of a venous thrombus

The appearance of thrombus in a deep vein alters as it develops and then resolves. Recent thrombus is echo poor. After a few days it becomes more echogenic (Figure 4.10a). Colour flow imaging can identify thrombus in a vein which may be otherwise overlooked by using B mode scanning alone (Figure 4.10b). Although thrombus becomes more echogenic with age it is not possible to use this change to deduce its age accurately.

Ultrasonic tissue characterization has been used to distinguish age differences in thrombi in an animal model[354] and has been reported to be able to define acute from chronic deep vein thrombosis in one clinical series, on the basis of higher intercept values in the acute group.[368] These same

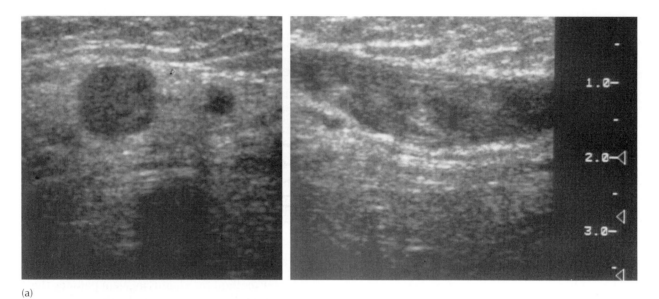

(a)

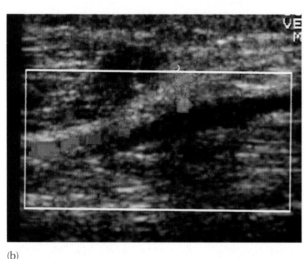

(b)

Figure 4.10   (a) The transverse and longitudinal grey scale ultrasound images of a 7-day-old thrombus in the femoral vein. The thrombus was not compressible and its heterogenous echogenicity almost as great as the surrounding soft tissues. (b) Thrombus in a stem vein of the calf. Blood flow (red) is visible in the veins' accompanying artery but the stem vein, below and parallel to the artery, contains no moving blood and an incompressible material of mixed echogenicity – thrombus.

authors also used ultrasonic tissue characterization to assess thrombus stability.

Recanalization has usually begun in most thrombi within 2–4 weeks. Colour duplex examination may show blood tracking through the thrombus during flow augmentation. Reopened and recanalized veins may be shown to be incompetent.[92] If the deep veins are significantly obstructed, the superficial veins may dilate and treble in diameter as they become collateral routes of venous flow.

The most important features of acute thrombosis are distension of the vein and loss of compressibility. Thrombus does not always adhere to the vessel wall, in which case it can become free floating within the lumen (Figures 4.11–4.13).

Doppler signal changes may be seen proximal or distal to occlusive thrombus. Proximally, flow aug-

mentation is reduced or absent. Distally, phasic flow is lost and becomes continuous.

Late changes

With time thrombus becomes more echogenic and the venous distension diminishes. The thrombus gradually retracts and undergoes lysis, but not all occluded vessels will recanalize.

Complete lysis of thrombus only occurs in 20% of cases.[173] In 80% of cases the residual thrombus becomes converted into fibrous tissue and appears as an echogenic thickening of the vein wall. Permanently occluded veins appear as echogenic strands.

Valve damage is a frequent sequela of venous thrombosis with valve thickening and poor valve

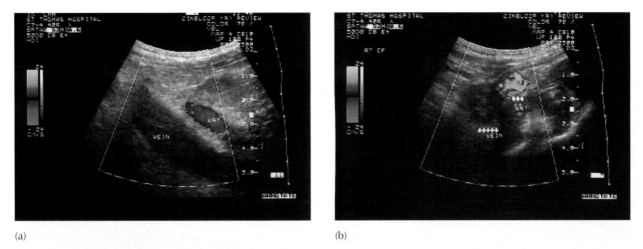

(a)   (b)

Figure 4.11   Longitudinal (a) and transverse (b) images of the iliac veins. There was no blood flow in the vein, it could not be compressed and its contents had a variable echogenicity.

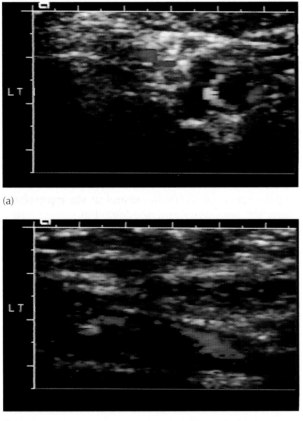

(a)

(b)

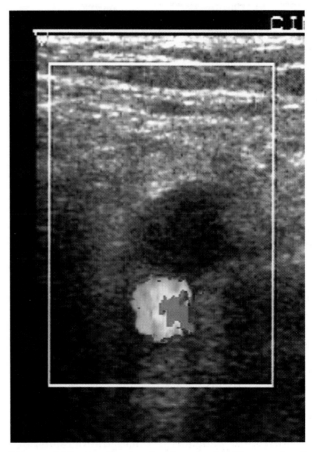

Figure 4.12 A partially occluding thrombus in the femoral vein. The tranverse (a) and longitudinal (b) images show a filling defect in the vein, adherent to one side of the vein, with blood flowing past it (coded red).

Figure 4.13   Popliteal vein thrombosis. The popliteal artery contains fast and slow flowing blood (coded red/yellow/blue). The overlying popliteal vein contains no flowing blood and in spite of external compression remains circular in cross-section. This thrombus is young and relatively echolucent.

motion. These changes may be associated with a reduction of normal phasic respiratory changes, a reduced Valsalva response and a reduced augmentation of flow.[20,105,446,449]

While duplex ultrasound is an accurate method for determining the presence of acute deep vein thrombosis, interpretation of the ultrasonic features of the late changes associated with thrombosis and the post-thrombotic limb can be difficult.[42,106]

In one study, the major errors encountered in the use of ultrasound were in the detection of isolated calf vein thrombosis and inaccurate assessment of the age of the thrombus due to operator inexperience.[446]

One special advantage of an ultrasound examination lies in its ability to reveal alternative diagnoses. Popliteal (Baker's) cysts, haematoma and abscesses can all be identified. This is an advantage over ascending venography in which the study may be normal or only demonstrate extrinsic compression. However, it should be remembered that venous thrombosis may occur in conjunction with any of these conditions if there is venous compression.

Comparison of ultrasound with other imaging techniques

Since its original description there have been numerous studies comparing the accuracy of duplex ultrasound with ascending phlebography. Phlebography has been the gold standard for the diagnosis of deep vein thrombosis for many years.[40,214,249,342] However, it is an invasive procedure, using both ionizing radiation and an intravenous contrast medium. It may also cause patient discomfort and be technically difficult to perform in oedematous limbs of severely ill patients.

The accuracy of both tests depends on the nature of the patient group under evaluation. The distribution of thrombus differs between patients with their first suspected deep vein thrombosis, patients with recurrent thrombosis and asymptomatic patients at high risk for deep vein thrombosis, and the accuracy of each imaging technique similarly varies.

Many patients with a first episode of deep vein thrombosis have thrombus which has extended proximally,[160,192] and many of these patients are at risk of developing pulmonary embolus. In one study of 101 patients, 51% had scintographic evidence of silent pulmonary emboli.[185] Phlebography is better at detecting isolated calf vein thrombus than duplex ultrasonography but both techniques are equally effective at detecting thrombus in the popliteal vein or above, i.e. the 25% of patients with extension into the popliteal vein.[42,184,188]

After their first episode of deep vein thrombosis, 20% of patients will develop recurrent symptoms, but only 30–40% of these will actually have a new recurrent deep vein thrombosis.[183,186] In this group, ascending venography has limitations whether the thrombosis be in the calf or the main axial veins. The diagnosis of a new acute chronic thrombosis in the presence of pre-existing pathological changes in the vessel wall is difficult. Ultrasound has the same difficulty.

Patients who are asymptomatic but have a high risk of deep vein thrombosis often have small and non-occlusive thrombi.[361] Some workers have shown duplex ultrasonography to be useful in this group[112,294,371] but others have not.[92,110,353]

It is still reasonable to regard ascending venography as the gold standard reference method for the assessment of deep vein thrombosis,[40,249,342] when the appearances meet the well defined criteria for the presence of thrombus – notably a persistent intraluminal filling defect that remains constant in at least two projections, or a filling defect in a vein with visible contrast medium both superior and inferior to the defect – but ascending venography has a recognized 20% incidence of inadequate examination and observer disagreement.[183,184,188,189,193,251] Thus, although there have been numerous publications comparing the accuracy of ascending venography with duplex ultrasound,[20,44,45,48,64,72,89,104,122,137,139,155,180,198,216,222,253,259,268,284,294,318,324,340,354,368,385,415,444] it is clear that the accuracy of both techniques depends heavily on the experience of the operator. With high quality apparatus and an experienced operator the sensitivity of both methods is 65–100% and the specificity 72–98%. Using strict objective criteria, the sensitivity and specificity of duplex ultrasound can be raised to 92% and 99%, respectively.[250]

The addition of colour-coded flow, although making the examination technically easier and having the potential advantage of detecting small non-occlusive thrombus, has not been shown to increase the sensitivity above that of Doppler ultrasound alone[75,110,170,253,271,353,354,368,393] in both symptomatic and asymptomatic patients, with the exception of one study which showed an increased sensitivity for the detection of calf vein thrombosis.[354] Early studies suggested that the accuracy of ultrasound was low in detecting calf vein thrombosis – as low as 36% – but more recently other authors have reported a sensitivity of 95% and specificity of 100% for detecting fresh calf vein thrombosis when compared to ascending phlebography.[43,81,94,148,159,201,252,350,353,373,440]

There is currently controversy about the need for bilateral diagnostic imaging in patients with unilateral symptoms. While one study of 206 patients showed no deep vein thrombi in the asymptomatic legs,[155] other studies have shown an incidence of 7–27% in the asymptomatic limb.[40,44,108,368] In view of these latter studies we believe it is prudent clinically and medicolegally to study both lower limbs in patients with unilateral symptoms.

Saphenous vein mapping

The long saphenous vein is often used as a conduit for coronary and lower limb arterial bypass grafting. Duplex ultrasound is a useful tool for assessing whether the vein is suitable, both in terms of its patency, useful length and diameter.

The long saphenous vein should be examined over its whole length and the sites of all communicating veins identified. It is important to identify the site of communicating veins when an in-situ graft is to be performed, as failure to ligate these will result in an arteriovenous fistula.

Whenever the long saphenous vein is being examined, the deep venous system should also be assessed, as removal of the long saphenous vein in the presence of chronic deep vein occlusion is contraindicated if the saphenous vein has become an important collateral conduit for venous return.

PHLEBOGRAPHY

The term phlebography when used alone refers to x-ray contrast phlebography. When it is used to describe other imaging techniques it is conventional to add a prefix, hence for example, isotope phlebography.

Since its description in 1923,[49] phlebography has become one of the most widely used investigations for the investigation of deep vein thrombosis, a position that has only recently been supplanted by the increasing application of duplex ultrasound.

Strontium bromide was initially used as the contrast medium, but was replaced by less toxic compounds, diodone in the 1930s and sodium or meglumine diatrizoate in the 1950s. These agents are hyperosmolar compared to blood. As a consequence, contrast-induced phlebitis, skin necrosis from extravasation of contrast at the injection site and pulmonary oedema due to the hyperosmolar contrast load all became recognized complications.[11,18,19,114,224,227,233,238,246,317]

The introduction of low osmolality contrast virtually eliminated these complications and has made contrast phlebography very safe.

Indications for phlebography

The main indication is for the detection of deep vein thrombosis. Other indications include the assessment of patients with pulmonary emboli in whom there is no demonstrable source for emboli, assessment of the deep veins in patients with post-thrombotic symptoms, and venous trauma.

Contraindications to phlebography

A known history of allergy is considered a contraindication to the use of intravenous contrast. Steroid prophylaxis can be given where phlebography is considered essential, but its use is still controversial in terms of any benefit.[221]

Contrast media are mildly nephrotoxic and patients with renal impairment should be carefully monitored following phlebography. They should be adequately hydrated before the examination and every effort made to reduce the amount of contrast medium used.

Equipment

A standard fluoroscopic screening unit with image intensification is adequate. For lower limb studies a tilting table is helpful. Digital subtraction equipment is helpful for the assessment of venous structures that might be obscured by bone, for example, the thorax and the pelvis. It is also useful as it decreases the patient radiation dose. As with the use of all contrast media, resuscitation facilities must be available at all times.

Technique

Informed patient consent must be obtained. Low osmolar contrast should be used whenever possible.[125,219,278] Warming the contrast medium prior to its use reduces its viscosity and makes its injection easier. Approximately 50 ml of contrast is required to examine a limb.

The upper limb

Most venous abnormalities in the upper limb occur in the axillary, subclavian, innominate veins and the superior vena cava. Indications for demonstrating the veins of the forearm are:

- congenital venous malformations
- assessment of veins for bypass surgery
- renal dialysis fistula formation.

In these cases it is necessary to cannulate a vein in the hand or forearm. Otherwise, cannulation of a vein in the antecubital fossa will suffice. A 20G sheathed cannula is ideal for venepuncture. Preferably the basilic or median cubital vein should be assessed. If the cephalic vein is entered, then the brachial and axillary veins will not be opacified. However, if a tourniquet is placed around the upper forearm, then contrast medium will be directed into the deep veins. If a medial vein is entered then tourniquets are not usually required. Contrast medium is injected by hand. Digital subtraction angiography decreases the contrast load and gives good detail of the intrathoracic veins and should be used wherever possible.

As with ilio-femoral phlebography, venous pressures can be measured by connecting the intravenous cannula to a pressure transducer. In complex cases catheterization of the arm veins may be necessary, for example, when upper limb thrombolysis is undertaken.

Superior venacavography

Assessment of the superior vena cava is required in the evaluation of upper limb thrombosis, suspected obstruction and vascular malformations (see Chapter 25).

With digital subtraction angiography (DSA) often an antecubital fossa injection as part of an upper limb venogram will produce satisfactory images. Bilateral simultaneous arm veins will increase opacification of the superior vena cava, and reduce artefacts due to unopacified blood. As with upper arm phlebography, single or bilateral arm catheterization may be necessary in complex cases. The superior vena cava can be assessed by femoral vein puncture and passage of a catheter through the right atrium. This technique is only usually employed when undertaking metal stent placement for superior vena cava obstruction.

The lower limb

An ankle tourniquet is placed just above the level of the malleoli to distend the superficial veins of the foot. It is useful to palpate an arterial foot pulse before and after tourniquet application as obliteration of the pulse indicates that the tourniquet is too tight. If no suitable vein is visible then immersion of the foot in a bowl of warm water or application of warm packs may produce enough vasodilatation to enable venepuncture.

A 21G needle or sheathed cannula is normally sufficient for peripheral injections. Any vein on the dorsum of the foot is suitable. The medial digital vein of the great toe is often used as it is accessible in the presence of an oedematous foot. In an oedematous foot, finger compression of the oedema will often reveal a vein which can be cannulated. Elevation of an oedematous foot for 24 hours will help to reduce oedema if a vein is not readily accessible.

If there is still no reasonable vein on the foot then any superficial vein in the calf can be used, as long as the tourniquet is applied above the point of injection and a steep foot-down table position is used to encourage the hyperbaric contrast medium to enter the deep veins below the site of puncture.

When percutaneous techniques are impossible a cut down onto the long saphenous vein 2 cm above and anterior to the medial malleolus or an intraosseous injection into the os calcis or the medial malleolus (Figure 4.14) can be used, but the advent of duplex ultrasound has virtually eliminated the need for these invasive measures.

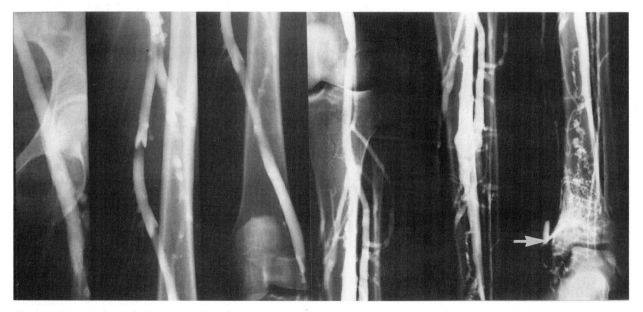

Figure 4.14 A normal phlebograph of the leg obtained by an intraosseous injection. The intraosseous cannula has been introduced into the medial malleolus (arrow).

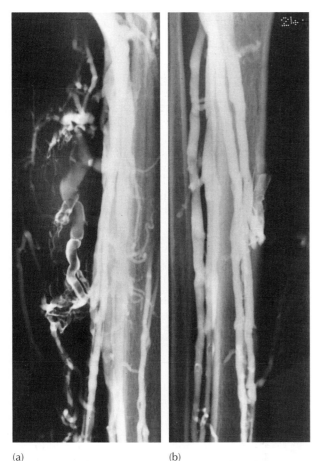

(a)   (b)

Figure 4.15 The importance of taking antero-posterior and lateral views of the calf veins. (a) In the lateral view there is a great deal of thrombus in the stem and muscle veins of the calf. (b) In the postero-anterior view only a little thrombus can be seen because of the overlying bone. This emphasizes the importance of taking a lateral view of the calf in all patients with suspected venous thrombosis.

If the superficial veins are not occluded by the ankle tourniquet, a confusing picture of both superficial and deep systems is produced. The tightness of the ankle tourniquet should therefore be adjusted during screening to prevent filling of the superficial system. If, because of ankle trauma or ulceration, a tourniquet cannot be applied at ankle level, it can be applied higher in the calf and deep venous filling encouraged by a steep foot-down table tilt. A second tourniquet placed above the knee helps to delay calf vein emptying, thus improving their opacification.

With the tourniquets in position, contrast is injected under screening control by hand. Films are taken in the foot-down table position to delay venous return and encourage venous distension.

Films are taken, under flouroscopic control, from the foot to the lower inferior vena cava (Figure 4.14). Postero-anterior, oblique and lateral views of the calf are obtained (Figure 4.15), followed by anterior views of the femoral and iliac veins. Venous distension is assisted if films are taken while the patient is performing the Valsalva manoeuvre (Figure 4.16) which will aid in the assessment of venous valves, which are normally shown as sharply defined bicuspid structures (Figure 4.16c).

During injection of contrast, manual calf compression to produce a sudden increase in axial vein blood flow causes venous distension and increases opacification. This is particularly useful when assessing the iliac veins and gives an adequate demonstration of the iliac veins in 90% of cases, obviating the need for a separate femoral vein puncture.[239] Incompetent communicating veins may also be filled by leg muscle exercise during phlebography.[13,119]

By tilting the table foot down during injection of contrast medium and taking the radiographs while the patient performs a Valsalva manoeuvre, the venous flow is diminished, allowing better visualization of the veins as well as giving an indication of their competence.[121,270]

Exercise phlebography, which involves leg exercise in the tilt down position can be used to assess incompetent perforators.[13,119]

Trauma to the venous system produces less dramatic effects than arterial trauma. Management is usually confined to tying off bleeding veins so emergency phlebography is rarely indicated. However, the adverse late sequelae of tying off major veins, identified by phlebography, has focused attention on immediate and late reconstruction procedures.

In the acute stage, phlebography may be used to assess the site and extent of acutely injured veins. Because of the nature of the patient's injuries, the technique may need to be modified and tourniquets placed at different sites in the limb to direct contrast medium into the deep system.

Varicography (Figure 4.17)

First described in 1929,[282] this technique involves the direct injection of the superficial varicosity. With the patient standing erect, an injection is made into a varicose vein in the group of which the patient complains with a small gauge needle. The patient then lies supine on the fluoroscopic table, and a ruler with radiopaque markers placed behind the leg so that the site of communication of varicose veins with the deep system can be accurately measured. Initially the table is placed foot down during injection of contrast. This allows the hyperbaric

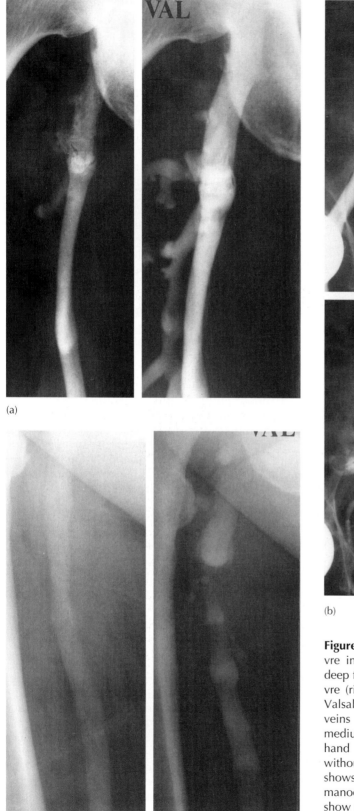

(a)

(c)

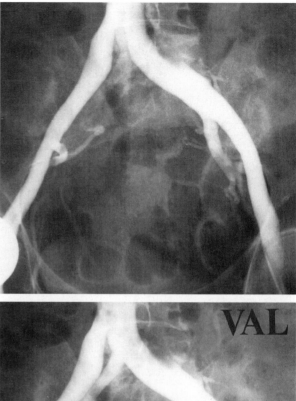

(b)

Figure 4.16   The use and value of the Valsalva manoeuvre in ascending phlebography. (a) Much more of the deep femoral vein is shown during the Valsalva manoeuvre (right-hand panel). (b) The top panel shows how a Valsalva manoeuvre, performed when the common iliac veins are filled with contrast medium, causes contrast medium to reflux into the internal iliac veins. (c) The left-hand panel shows an ascending femoral phlebograph without a Valsalva manoeuvre. The right-hand panel shows competent valves demonstrated by the Valsalva manoeuvre. In this situation a descending phlebograph to show competent valves is not necessary.

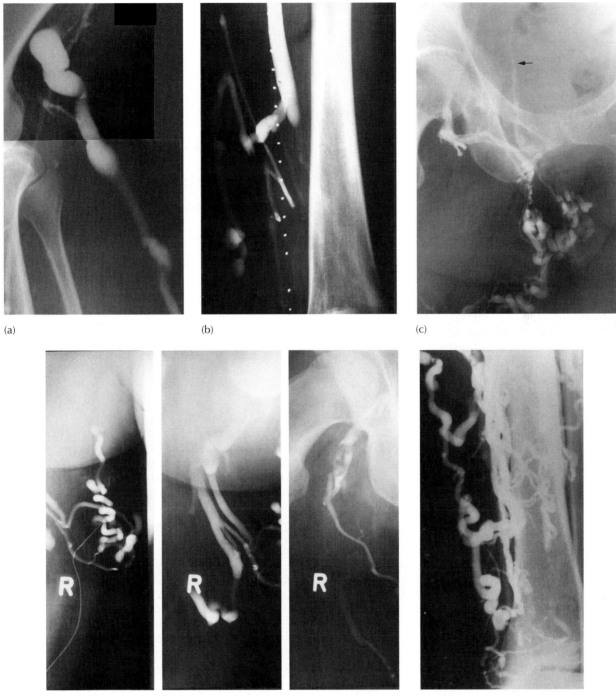

(a) (b) (c)

(d) (e)

Figure 4.17 Varicography. (a) Varicogram showing a varicose short saphenous vein. (b) This varicogram shows a dilated, almost certainly incompetent, communicating vein in the mid-thigh (Hunter's canal). The ruler with metal markers allows the site of the communicating vein to be related to the knee joint. (c) Recurrent varicose veins in region of the vulva. There are connections with the common femoral vein and with the internal pudendal vein (arrow). (d) Recurrent varicose veins in upper thigh and vulva. Varicose veins connect with the obturator vein and then into the internal iliac vein. (e) Medial lower leg (Cockett) communicating veins shown by varicography. Varicography is often a better way of showing the site of the incompetent communicating veins than ascending phlebography. The size and shape of these veins suggests that they are incompetent.

contrast medium to descend the leg and enter incompetent perforators inferiorly, for example in the calf. The table is then placed horizontally to allow contrast to ascend the leg. Radiographs are taken of the superficial veins. Finally, the table is placed head down to enable contrast medium to travel towards the groin, and images taken of the sapheno-femoral junction. If the contrast medium tends to enter the popliteal vein then firm hand pressure behind the knee, while continuing to inject contrast medium, will assist in filling the superficial system. It is important to take early views, as the images can become confusing when many superficial and deep veins are opacified. Frontal exposures with a lateral view of the knee to demonstrate the drainage of the short saphenous vein are the most helpful projections. Oblique projections are confusing and not helpful.

It may be necessary to inject more than one group of varicosities to show all the connections. Tourniquets are not normally applied, as the aim of this technique is to allow the free passage of contrast medium from the superficial to the deep system, although on occasion a tourniquet may be placed above the site of a suspected varicosity, for example in the thigh, to see the incompetent vessel more clearly.

Interpretation of varicograms can be difficult.[99,229,236,245] As mentioned, early images are important before too many vessels are opacified, making identification of the major sites of incompetence problematical.

The normal flow of blood is from the superficial to the deep system. In varicography contrast medium also flows from superficial to deep veins; here the direction of blood flow during varicography is unhelpful as a guide to valvular incompetence. Therefore an assessment is made as to whether a communicating vein is incompetent on its morphological appearances. A dilated (greater then 3 mm) and tortuous communicating vein, which does not taper distally, is likely to be incompetent.[99,229,236,245] While undoubtedly a useful test, an obvious limitation is that the test is wholly dependent on the pathway that the contrast medium follows. Hence it is possible to fail to identify incompetent perforators. This limitation does not apply to duplex ultrasound. Varicography may identify incompetent perforators not seen by ascending venography.[232] Information about the deep system is limited, and ascending venography or colour duplex examination may be necessary to assess deep venous insufficiency.[232] A variation of the technique of varicography is the assessment of congenital venous malformations. The venous malformation is punctured directly. Tourniquet application above the puncture site directs the contrast

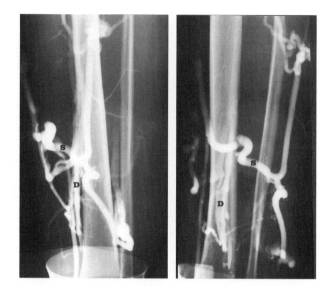

Figure 4.18 Incompetent communicating veins. Sometimes the superficial and deep veins of the calf are difficult to distinguish on a phlebograph. In the left-hand panel the superficial (S) and deep (D) veins are difficult to distinguish because they are superimposed. In the right-hand panel they have been separated by rotating the leg. The deep veins remain close to the bone.

medium into the deep veins and their tributaries. This is then released to identify any further superficial and deep connections more superiorly.

Varicography can be carried out as an operative procedure, with particular reference to short saphenous ligation.[168]

Incompetent communicating veins

Incompetent communicating veins can be assessed by ascending phlebography (Figure 4.18). Tourniquets placed just above the ankle and knee need to be placed tightly enough to prevent superficial vein filling. Incompetent communicators demonstrate retrograde flow from the deep to the superficial system and appear as dilated and valveless veins joining a superficial varicose vein. By placing a ruler with radiopaque markings, the site of any incompetent communicator can be easily referenced to a bony landmark.

Duplex ultrasound is now commonly employed to assess incompetent veins.

Saphenography (Figure 4.19)

The purpose of this investigation is to demonstrate the long saphenous vein and rarely the short saphenous vein for arterial bypass surgery. As in conventional ascending venography, a foot vein or,

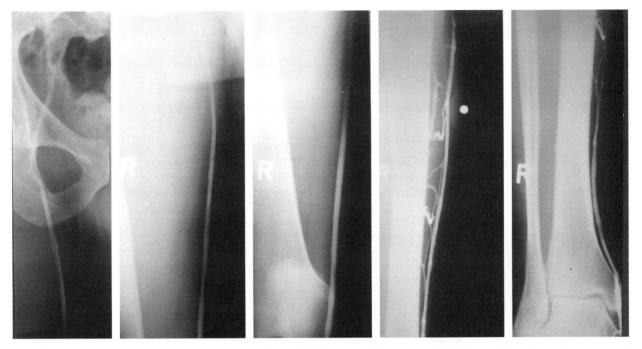

Figure 4.19 Saphenography. Saphenogram performed before arterial bypass surgery. The vein has been demonstrated from the ankle to the groin and has a suitable diameter for bypass surgery. The ball-bearing (fourth panel) enables correction to be made for magnification.

alternatively, the long saphenous vein is cannulated following ankle tourniquet application. The tourniquet is then released and contrast medium injected. By altering the tilt of the table and manual compression of the popliteal vein if necessary, the whole of the long saphenous vein is demonstrated. A ruler with radiopaque marking and a 1 cm ball-bearing placed on at least one projection are useful for calculating the site of communicating veins and the calibre of the vein likely to be used for bypass.[244] A similar technique can be used to demonstrate the cephalic and basilic veins in the upper limb. As with varicography, duplex ultrasound is replacing contrast saphenography in many centres.

Femoral and inferior vena cavography

Direct puncture of the femoral vein is indicated when this segment has not been satisfactorily demonstrated by other means, usually during ascending venography or duplex ultrasound, in the assessment of deep vein thrombosis. Other indications are assessment of femoral vein pressure, for example, in the assessment of patients in whom a Palma reconstruction is contemplated and as part of an inferior vena cavagram.[303]

The femoral vein is punctured by palpating the femoral artery and inserting a needle just medial to this. The vein may be distended by asking the patient to perform the Valsalva manoeuvre. A 19 gauge needle is sufficient and continuous suction applied when inserting the needle to obtain venous blood. Traditionally, contrast medium was then injected into the vein through the needle. However, vein walls are fragile and the walls are easily dissected. For this reason it is often easier to insert a small J guide wire followed by a 5F end hole dilator and perform injections through this. For inferior cavography formal catheterization with a 4 or 5 French pigtail catheter is necessary to delineate the cava from the union of the iliac veins to the right atrium.

While a standard fluoroscopic unit will produce adequate pictures, digital subtraction angiography is preferred as this gives better delineation of the vessels with a reduction in both patient radiation dose and volume of contrast media used.

Anterior and lateral projections are taken. The site of the renal veins is usually demonstrated by a flow void artefact in the vena cava produced by the mixture of unopacified blood from the renal veins with the contrast medium in the vena cava. If the exposures are made during the Valsalva manoeuvre, reflux of contrast medium may occur into the renal veins. This may also demonstrate retrograde flow into the internal iliac veins.

An alternative method to demonstrate the inferior vena cava is by catheterization of an arm vein, and passing the catheter through the right atrium into the inferior vena cava. This technique is particularly useful when the femoral veins are thrombosed.

Indications for inferior vena cavography include assessment of possible obstruction and collateral pathways, presence of thrombus and caval assessment prior to caval filter insertion.

Intraosseous injections (Figure 4.20)

This technique is indicated when conventional techniques are not possible due to venous thrombosis or inaccessible veins, for example in a grossly

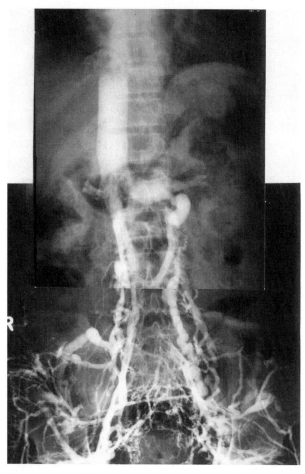

Figure 4.20 Bilateral pertrochanteric intraosseous phlebography to show the iliac veins and inferior vena cava. The iliac veins are grossly narrowed by post-thrombotic changes. The inferior vena cava is totally occluded to just below the left renal vein. The collateral pathways are the ascending lumbar and azygos veins and the left gonadal vein. The advantage of intraosseous phlebography in this situation is that it often displays the vena cava above the obstruction so that separate retrograde cavography is not required.

oedematous leg. The advent of duplex ultrasound has virtually eliminated the demand for this technique. As intraosseous injection is painful, a general anaesthetic is required. The principle of the test is the injection of contrast medium directly into the bone marrow. This subsequently drains to the local venous drainage. If available, digital subtraction angiography should be used to improve image clarity.

Contraindications to the test are the presence of local infection at the injection site, because of the risk of osteomyelitis. Other contraindications include concurrent anticoagulation or a known bleeding disorder, young patients in whom the epiphyses have not formed due to the risk of growth impairment, and a known history of contrast media allergy.

A number of complications are specific to intraosseous phlebography. These include inadvertent puncture of vital structures, for example the aorta or spinal cord. Fat embolism has been reported.[246]

Because contrast medium is hyperbaric, it fills the dependent veins preferentially. Hence when the iliac veins are being studied, injection of contrast while the patient is supine will opacify the internal iliac veins and injection with the patient prone will opacify the external iliac veins.

For bone puncture a cannula with a drill tip is required to penetrate the cortex.[226] Bilateral injections will maximize venous opacification in the pelvis. The usual puncture site to demonstrate the pelvic veins is a pertrochanteric injection. The medial malleolus is used to demonstrate the lower limb. Other access points for intraosseous injection include the pubic rami, the femoral condyles, the tibial tuberosity, the lateral malleolus and the calcaneum. The vertebral plexuses and azygos system can be shown by a vertebral spinous process injection, or into the posterior end of a rib. Injection into the lower radius, olecranon process, or acromion will demonstrate the veins of the arm.[229]

Indirect phlebography

In cerebral angiography the venous phase demonstrates the intracranial vessels extremely well. In peripheral veins, however, the contrast density produced following an arterial injection is usually too poor to be of diagnostic value. An exception to this is where there is an arteriovenous malformation or fistula, with rapid passage of contrast medium from the arterial to venous system.

Descending phlebography (Figure 4.21)

In this technique the femoral vein is punctured and contrast medium injected to assess retrograde

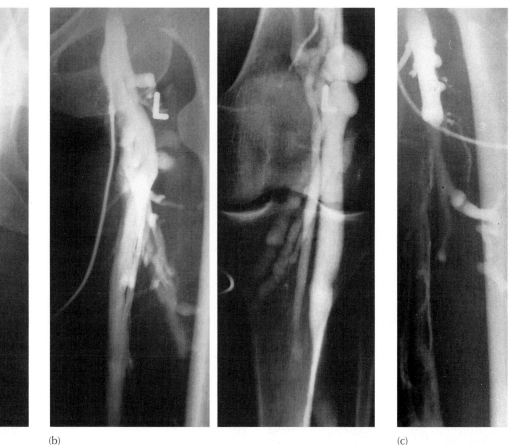

(a)   (b)   (c)

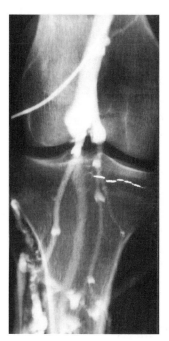

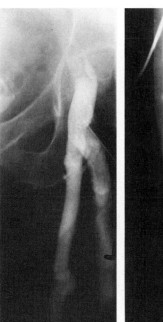

(d)   (e)

Figure 4.21 (a) A normal descending phlebograph. There is grade 1 deep vein reflux with a sharp cut-off at normal valves. (b) This descending phlebograph shows grade 3 deep vein reflux; the contrast medium passes into the calf. The deep veins show post-thrombotic changes. (c) This descending phlebograph shows a competent valve in the common femoral vein, but post-thrombotic changes in the superficial femoral vein below it. There are competent valves in the deep femoral vein. (d) A percutaneous popliteal vein descending phlebograph. The valves in the popliteal vein and the upper calf tributaries are normal. This technique can be used if only the popliteal vein needs to be examined. (e) This descending phlebograph revealed gross long saphenous vein reflux. This is probably the most reliable radiographic way of confirming long saphenous vein incompetence.

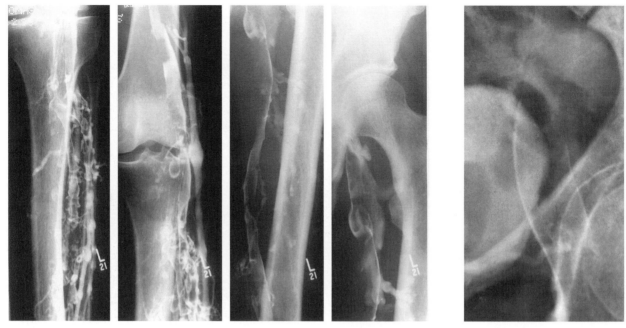

(a)

(b)

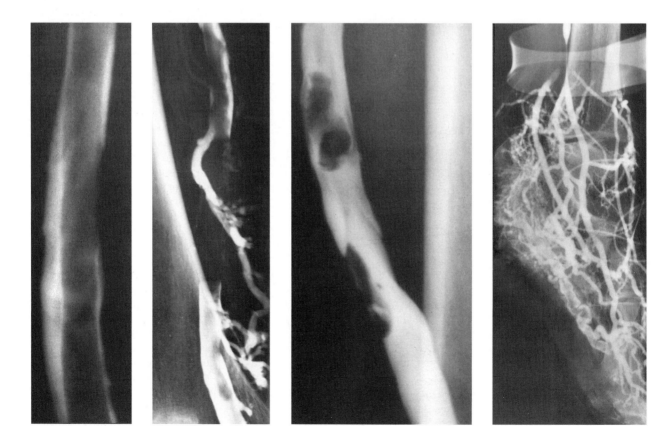

(c)

(d)

(e)

(f)

venous flow. The level of reflux is graded from 0 to 4 (see Chapter 12). While injection can be performed through the needle puncture at the groin, placement of a short 5F dilator by the Seldinger technique eliminates the risk of contrast extravasation during injection. The table is left in the supine position and images taken during an injection with the patient performing a Valsalva manoeuvre. The lower limit of contrast medium reflux is observed fluoroscopically and images taken of this.

Descending phlebography can also assess saphenofemoral incompetence. Any reflux into this vessel is abnormal. Rarely the puncture site may be above a valve in the common femoral vein, thus preventing reflux into an incompetent long saphenous vein. This valve, however, can be readily identified on the images taken. This technique has largely been replaced by duplex ultrasound.

Radiological assessment of deep vein thrombus (Figures 4.22 and 4.23)

When phlebography is undertaken to confirm the presence of deep vein thrombosis, special emphasis should be given to the following points:

- If a lower limb is found to contain thrombus the other limb should be examined as there is an incidence of up to 50% of thrombus in the asymptomatic limb.

Figure 4.22 The phlebographic appearances of deep vein thrombus. (a) This ascending phlebograph shows the calf, popliteal and femoral veins full of fresh non-adherent thrombus. The thrombus has a 'ground glass' appearance and is surrounded by a thin white line of contrast medium. This thrombus is loose and could become an embolus. (b) A loose fresh thrombus in the common femoral and external iliac veins. (c) The thrombus in this femoral vein shows evidence of retraction and adherence. The contrast medium forms a thicker layer on the left-hand side of the vein and the surrounding layer of contrast medium is absent on the right side of the vein. This thrombus is about 10 days old and is becoming adherent to the vein wall. (d) The thrombus in this example is occluding a long segment of the femoral vein in the adductor canal. The thrombus has been demonstrated above and below the occlusion, and the collaterals bridging the obstruction are filled with contrast medium. The thrombus above and below the occlusion shows evidence of some retraction. (e) The thrombi in this phlebograph are adherent, retracted and at least 10 days old. They are beginning to organize and are most unlikely to break free and become emboli. (f) Thrombus in the lateral plantar vein.

- Both the lower and upper limit of any thrombus must be documented. If necessary, additional procedures may be required to demonstrate the upper end of any thrombus.
- More than one image of any thrombus must be taken to confirm that the filling defects produced by any thrombi in the contrast medium column are constant and not artefactual.
- As much of the deep system should be filled as possible, including any collateral channels that may have developed to bypass occluded veins. In suspected superficial vein thrombosis the superficial system can be obtained by loosening the tourniquets and repeating the injection.

Venous thrombosis shows as a constant filling defect in an opacified vein. It should have the same size and shape in at least two images. It is important for accurate diagnosis to try to outline the thrombus itself and not rely on the non-opacification of veins to establish the diagnosis. Artefacts caused by poor mixing of the contrast medium, external venous compression and poor technique are common (Figure 4.23). If the criteria listed above are observed misdiagnoses should not be made.

Fresh thrombus will not be adherent to the vessel wall and will appear as a translucent ground glass defect separated from the wall by a thin white line of contrast medium. The thrombus usually originates from a valve cusp. Obliteration of the thin line indicates adherence of the thrombus to the vessel wall.

In the acute stage of an extensive deep vein thrombosis the pressure in the vascular compartments of the leg may rise to such an extent that opacification of the deep system is prevented and only superficial vein filling seen.[53]

An important feature to identify is a free floating tail of thrombus at the proximal end of a thrombosis, which may pose a particular risk of embolization.

Collateral veins enlarge almost immediately following a thrombosis and their presence gives only a rough indication of the duration of the thrombus. These collaterals may take the form of enlarged venae commitantes, which appear as small veins following the same line as veins they replace. In other instances muscular or superficial veins may form a collateral pathway. Over the next 10–14 days the thrombus retracts and its outline is more clearly defined.

Finally, following the process of organization and retraction of the thrombus, recanalization commences. While this process restores the lumen of the vein, it is often left irregular, with its valves damaged and destroyed. On occasion the veins may return to a normal appearance on phlebography

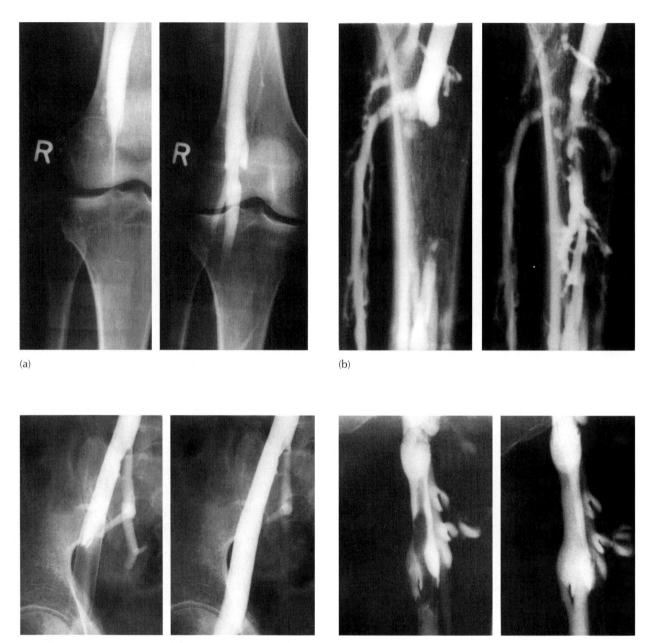

(a) (b)

(c) (d)

Figure 4.23 Phlebographic artefacts that can be misinterpreted as thrombus or pathological stenosis. (a) The popliteal vein can be occluded by hyperextension of the knee (left-hand panel). With the knee slightly flexed the popliteal vein fills (right-hand panel). It is important that this appearance is not attributed to an organic obstruction. (b) There is an unfilled segment of the peroneal vein (left-hand panel) which fills completely when more contrast medium is injected (right-hand panel). Underfilling should not be confused with occlusion by thrombosis. Often a little thrombus can be seen at either end of an unfilled segment if it is occluded by thrombus. (c) Streaming contrast medium along the vein wall can closely mimic a recent thrombus (left-hand panel). The appearance is inconstant (right-hand panel). (d) Streaming of non-opacified blood into a vein filled with contrast medium can closely resemble a thrombus (left-hand panel). It is inconstant in shape and position and disappears with better filling (right-hand panel). (e) Incomplete mixing of hyperbaric contrast medium and blood produces mixing defects which may be confused with post-thrombotic changes. In these examples the defects are present in the superficial femoral vein, the long saphenous vein and the vena cava. These changes are inconstant and, provided more than one film is taken of each segment of the venous system, should not cause confusion.

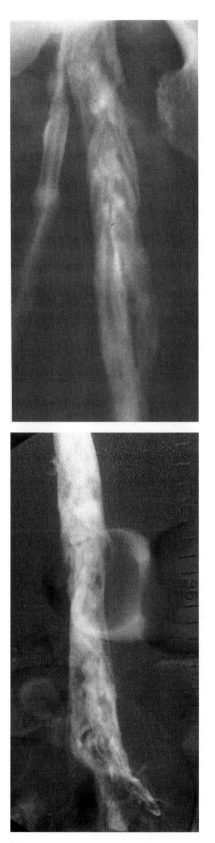

(e)

following previous thrombosis. Digital subtraction is a valuable adjunct for the enhancement of phlebographic images (Figure 4.24).

Complications of phlebography

Contrast media related

Systemic and idiosyncratic reactions

The risk of adverse reaction occurring is reduced by using non-ionic low osmolar contrast media and these agents are recommended for phlebography. Steroid prophylaxis can be given but its effectiveness is controversial.[17,114,221] Minor reactions such as nausea, vomiting and heartburn were seen in up to 5% of patients receiving hyperosmolar agents, but have now virtually disappeared with low osmolar agents. They pass off quickly and require no treatment. Severe reactions, such a bronchospasm, glottic oedema, cardiac arrhythmias and hypotension require intensive resuscitation.

The mortality rate from hyperosmolar contrast media has been calculated at 1 in 40 000 injections.[18,91,233] It is likely that the mortality rate is reduced with non-ionic low osmolar contrast media although no substantiated difference in fatality rates has been demonstrated.[18,374] Overall adverse effects are six times more likely with hyperosmolar agents.[6]

Local complications

Hyperosmolar contrast media can cause local pain on injection, due to the hyperosmolality of the contrast media. These agents may also produce a thrombophlebitis. Low osmolality contrast agents are virtually painless or are virtually non-thrombogenic, reinforcing their use for phlebography.[6,233,238,418] Following the contrast medium injection, saline should be injected to flush the contrast from the veins.

Extravasation of contrast into the skin and soft tissues causes a chemical cellulitis which may progress to ulceration and even gangrene (Figure 4.25).[227,376] This is induced primarily by the hyperosmolality of the contrast agent and in this respect it is reasonable to expect non-ionic low osmolar agents to be less toxic to skin and subcutaneous tissue. Reports of extravasation of non-ionic low osmolar agents have supported this.[56,57,144,260,269,285] If extravasation occurs then application of a cold compress and aspiration of as much of the contrast as possible is advised. Injection of hyaluronidase around the site may be beneficial.[53]

Rarely, with extravasation of large amounts of contrast surgical intervention is required. This should be performed within 6 hours to prevent permanent sequelae.[260,285,374]

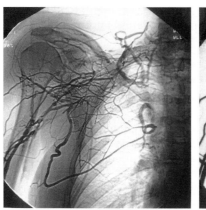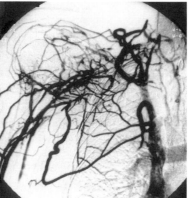

(a)

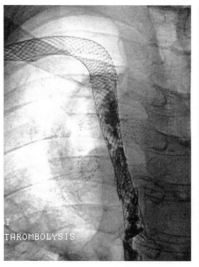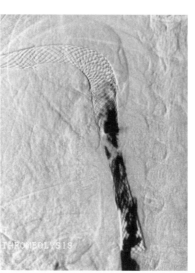

(b)

Figure 4.24 Illustrations of the value of digital subtraction. (a) The left-hand phlebograph shows a subclavian vein thrombosis but many of the vessels are obscured by the images of the bone. The right-hand digitally subtracted image reveals the fine details of the occlusion and collateral vessels. (b) The left-hand phlebograph taken during a course of thrombolysis shows residual thrombus in the stent. The digitally subtracted film (right-hand) shows far more clearly its extent and nature. (c) A normal and subtracted inferior vena cavagraph showing thrombus protruding from the right renal vein. The difference in the definition of the thrombus in the subtracted vein is obvious.

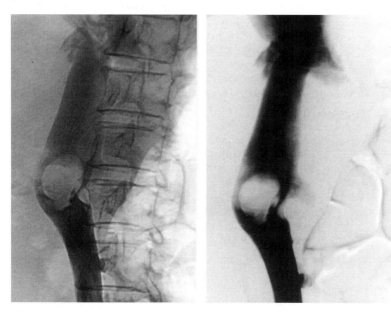

(c)

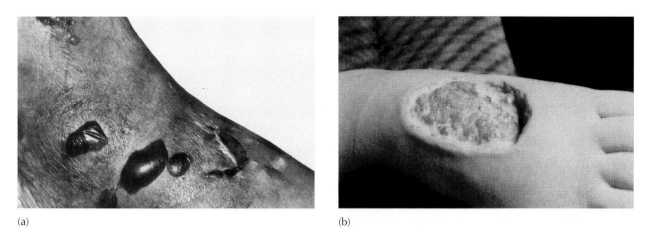

(a) (b)

Figure 4.25 (a) Superficial skin necrosis and blistering following extravasation of conventional hyperosmolar contrast medium into the tissues. Although extravasation should be prevented, its seems likely that serious consequences such as this will not occur with low osmolality media because their osmolality approximates to that of tissue fluid. (b) Full thickness skin loss following the extravasation of an ionic contast medium during phlebography. (We are indebted to Dr L Berlin and the *American Journal of Roentgenology* for permission to publish this illustration.[52])

The issue of obtaining informed consent for the use of contrast media remains controversial.[30,219] However, it seems prudent for the radiologist to obtain informed consent when contrast medium is used in various phlebographic techniques.

Non-contrast media related

Air embolism
Inadvertent injection of air can lead to a fatal air embolism. Meticulous attention to detail should prevent this. In the event of it occurring the patient should be turned onto his/her left side and the table placed 20° head down, so that air will float away from the pulmonary outflow tract.

Pulmonary embolism
There have been very few reports of embolism during phlebography.[423] The possibility of small subclinical embolism occurring during phlebography, either by calf compression or catheter manipulation, exists but it is not possible to assess this risk accurately.

Arteriovenous fistula
This can occur when an artery adjacent to a vein is punctured as well as the vein. The risk of this is increased if large bore catheters are used, or if the patient develops a large haematoma, preventing effective compression after the procedure. It is more commonly seen as a complication of arterial studies.[6]

ISOTOPE PHLEBOGRAPHY

In this technique, technetium-99m (Tc-99m; ^{99m}Tc) labelled radiopharmaceuticals are injected into a peripheral vein and images taken of the limb with a gamma camera (Figure 4.26). Historically, ^{99m}Tc-labelled human albumin microspheres were injected into both feet following application of tourniquets above the ankles and knees. Adherent thrombus results in areas of low radioactivity. The tourniquets were then released and the patient asked to exercise the legs. Further images were then taken. By this time the isotope had become trapped in the thrombus and appeared as an area of 'increased' radioactivity while the isotope passed through the patent veins.[117,228]

Current techniques depend on radiolabelling of erythrocytes with Tc-99m. This is then injected into a peripheral vein, normally an arm vein, and dynamic and static images obtained of the lower limbs. Normally, anterior projections from the level of the inferior vena cava to the knees are taken with posterior, right and left lateral images of the popliteal and calf veins. Using this technique, deep vein thrombosis is diagnosed using the following criteria:

- Abnormal persistence of venous activity on the dynamic phase of the scan.
- Defects or asymmetry in the deep veins.
- Abnormal collateral veins.

Isotope-labelled techniques have been described in clinical use for approximately 20 years. Blood pool

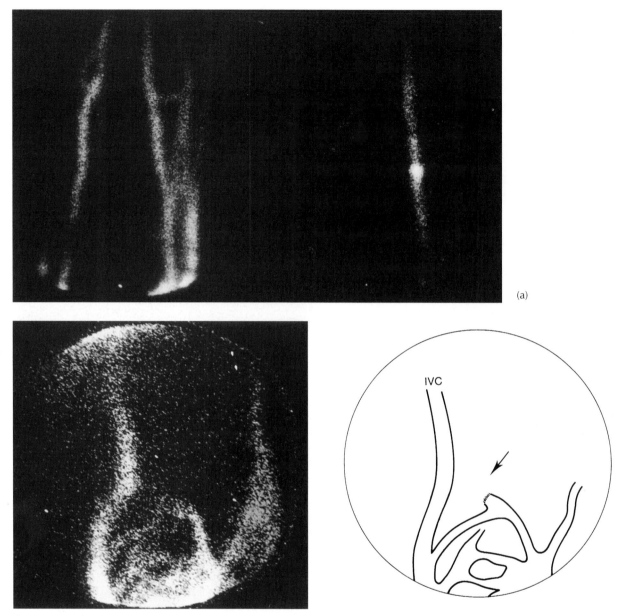

(a)

(b)

Figure 4.26 (a) An isotope phlebograph. The left-hand panel shows the static phase and the right-hand panel shows the appearances after exercise. The accumulation of radioactivity in the calf in the right-hand panel remaining after exercise indicates that this is likely to represent a thrombus rather than stasis below an obstruction. (b) An isotope phlebograph of the pelvis and abdomen. The injection was made into the left foot only. There is an obstruction at the junction of the left common iliac vein with the inferior vena cava (arrowed). There are extensive pelvic collaterals filling the right iliac veins and inferior vena cava. This was an example of left common iliac vein obstruction caused by compression by the overlying artery (see Chapter 13).

scintigraphy has been reported to have a combined sensitivity and specificity of 91% and 88% compared with ascending venography.[54,207,247,255,256] The radiation dose is small (less than 4 mGy total body absorbed dose for a 70 kg person) and the study only requires access to an arm vein rather than to the lower limb. Alternative isotopes used include ^{99m}Tc-labelled synthetic peptides with gamma emitting particles. In one study the sensitivity and specificity for deep vein thrombosis was over 90%.[296]. However, duplex ultrasound has been shown to be more sensitive than blood pool scintigraphy in the diagnosis of acute deep vein thrombosis in the femoropopliteal segment.[349] The need for specialist equipment and the radiation penalty incurred in the performance of isotope phlebography has meant that this test has not been widely adopted into clinical practice.

COMPUTED TOMOGRAPHY VENOGRAPHY

There are preliminary reports on the use of computed tomography (CT) for the detection of deep vein thrombosis, with good results shown in the diagnosis of deep vein thrombosis in the abdomen and pelvis and in recurrent deep vein thrombosis (Figure 4.27).[28,258,381,402,442] In many instances the finding of venous thrombosis is incidental to the main indication for the scan being performed. For example, superior vena cava obstruction may be demonstrated in patients with thoracic malignancies and spiral CT has been used to assess the collateral vessels that develop in superior vena cava obstruction.[39]

Similarly, inferior vena cava thrombosis may be accurately assessed during abdominal CT examinations. In vascular malformations, enhanced CT will

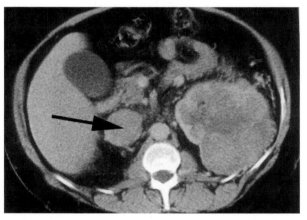

(a)

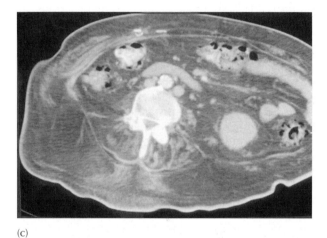

(c)

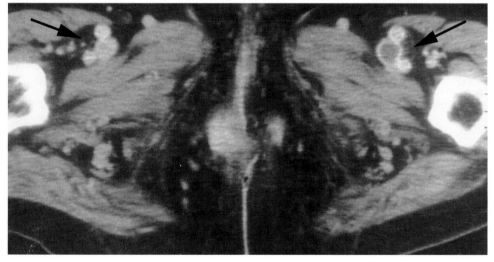

(b)

Figure 4.27 The diagnosis of deep vein thrombosis by computerized tomography. (a) Thrombosis, expansion and infiltration of the vena cava by a large left renal cell carcinoma. (b) The pelvic CT scan of a patient who had had multiple pulmonary emboli showing thrombus filling both femoral veins (arrowed). (c) This CT scan revealed that the patient had a double vena cava. Neither was thrombosed. This abnormality may be missed by conventional phlebography.

show the extent of the lesion and its involvement of adjacent structures, but this has now been largely replaced by magnetic resonance imaging. With spiral CT the veins are optimally enhanced with contrast medium, allowing more accurate assessment than was possible with conventional CT.

Spiral CT scanners employ slip ring technology to acquire data continuously as the patient moves through the gantry. The path of the x-ray beam describes a spinal or helix with its focus passing along the rotational isocentre.

In comparison with conventional incremental CT with multiple breath holds, spiral CT has a number of advantages. The rapidity of the examination means the abdomen can be covered in a single breath-hold, with the abolition of respiratory motion artefacts. High quality reconstructions in any plane can be undertaken from the CT data.

In the technique of spiral CT phlebography, a foot vein is cannulated and tourniquets placed around both ankles as in conventional ascending venography. Diluted contrast is injected and a spiral acquisition obtained. Criteria for the diagnosis of deep vein thrombosis are a filling defect in an opacified vein or a segment of non-opacified vein. Additional findings which support the diagnosis are perivenous fat infiltration due to oedema and the presence of collateral veins. In one study of 103 limbs, correlation between spiral CT phlebography and conventional ascending phlebography was excellent and the sensitivity of CT phlebography was 100% with a specificity of 92%.[29] Compared with ascending phlebography, CT phlebography requires only about 20% as much contrast medium. However, the technique depends on the availability of this type of equipment and, like conventional phlebography, incurs a radiation penalty to the patient. While it appears that spiral CT phlebography is feasible, it is unlikely to become widely used in the assessment of deep vein thrombosis and will probably remain a technique to be used in patients in whom both duplex ultrasound and conventional phlebography have been technically unsatisfactory.

MAGNETIC RESONANCE IMAGING (MRI)

Magnetic resonance phlebography

Magnetic resonance (MR) has been relatively little used in the imaging of veins but this new modality has much to offer. Magnetic resonance phlebography encompasses several different techniques which produce different sorts of images.

Magnetic resonance is the phenomenon by which certain atomic nuclei, notably hydrogen, can absorb electromagnetic radiation at a particular frequency and then re-emit it when placed in a strong magnetic field.

The emitted radiation contains information about the immediate physical environment of the nuclei and can also be spatially encoded. This encoding is achieved by setting up magnetic gradients across the volume to be imaged. This enables cross-sectional images to be reconstructed and these can be obtained in any anatomical plane. More complex reconstructions to give three-dimensional images can also be made.

The strong magnetic field is usually produced by a superconducting magnet. The patient lies within the cylindrical bore of a large coil which is cooled by liquid helium. The radio frequency pulses are received by coils which are in effect radio aerials. These come in many shapes and sizes. In imaging the veins of the legs or abdomen, a body coil is used which is a cylinder built into the bore of the scanner. Surface coils, which are applied to a limb, may also be used. Scanning is a noisy process because of the rapid gradient switching required.

Specific contraindications to MR scanning are patients who have cardiac pacemakers, ferromagnetic cerebral aneurysm clips, prosthetic cardiac valves containing ferromagnetic materials, and patients with a history of metal fragments in the eye, for example, sheet metal workers.

A small number of patients experience claustrophobia as they lie within the coil and will not be able to tolerate the procedure. Mild sedation may alleviate these symptoms. There are no known adverse effects of MR, apart from the specific contraindications already mentioned. Intravenous contrast, in the form of gadolinium compounds can be used in certain instances. Allergic reactions to this are recognized but are much less common than with x-ray contrast media.

The great advantage of MR is the high level of tissue contrast within the images produced. This differs from all x-ray based examinations including CT, where contrast depends only on the tissue attenuation coefficient. MR contrast depends on multiple factors. Essentially the type of contrast within an image is controlled by the pattern of radio frequencies used to excite the hydrogen nuclei in the volume imaged. These are called pulse sequences. The two most commonly used types of contrast are called T1- and T2-weighted. T1 radio frequency decay is due to 'spin-lattice' interactions. Such images have good anatomical detail. Recent haemorrhage or blood clot appears bright on such images. T2 decay is due to 'spin–spin interactions'. Such images are very sensitive to the fluid content of tissues and in particular oedema, which appears bright. Fibrosis and haemorrhage may also be bright.

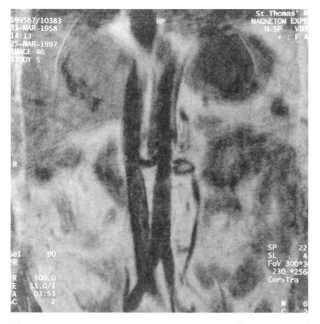

Figure 4.28 A magnetic resonance coronal T1 image of a normal vena cava and aorta.

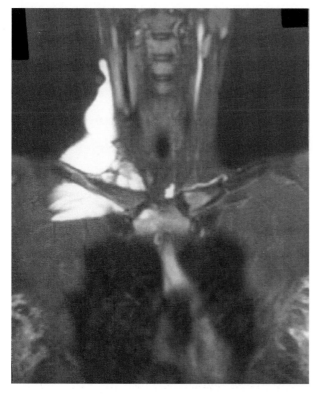

Figure 4.29 A magnetic resonance coronal STIR image of a large venous angioma in the neck and upper chest wall.

The visualization of flowing blood on conventional T1- and T2-weighted images is not straightforward (Figure 4.28). Blood most often appears dark as a flow void within the image but in certain circumstances, such as slow flow or flow in the orientation of the imaging plane, it can also appear bright. Pulse sequences can be designed which are sensitive to flowing blood, where stationary tissues appear dark. These fall into two categories:

1. *Time of flight (TOF) sequences.* Stationary tissues are saturated by repeated radio frequency pulses so that blood flowing into the imaging slice or volume appears bright. The scan can be viewed as sequential multiple slices or the slices or thin volumes can be post-processed, in effect stacked up, using a maximum intensity projection (MIP) algorithm to produce images that resemble those of a contrast phlebogram. Unlike a phlebogram, the vessels are visualized because of blood flow and not injected contrast. Also, unlike contrast phlebograms where a separate exposure has to be made for each projection angle, MIP images in any plane can be reconstructed from a single scan (Figure 4.29). Slowly flowing or static blood will not be visualized and flow which is in the imaging plane, rather than perpendicular to it, can also become saturated and therefore appear dark.

2. *Phase contrast sequences.* The excited nuclei have a frequency and therefore a phase. Flow causes a change in the phase of moving nuclei relative to stationary nuclei and these phase changes can be translated to brightness on images. However, the likely range of velocities within an imaging volume has to be estimated before the scan and the technique are applied for vessels with higher velocities such as the inferior cava.

Use of cross-sectional slices allows visualization of the vessel wall and of surrounding tissues. Perivenous, muscular and subcutaneous oedema can all be demonstrated as can compressive mass lesions such as haematomata or lymphadenopathy. Thrombus retraction, vessel wall thickening, collateral channels and absence of perivenous oedema distinguish chronic from acute venous thrombosis. However, imaging times of 40–50 minutes are required to obtain images from the origin of the popliteal veins to the origin of the IVC. Cross-sectional images are more difficult to assess, and MIP images are usually produced for interpretation (Figure 4.30).

Projectional images using TOF techniques take a long time to acquire since they are built up from a stack of thin slices. They can potentially show vein proximal to a blockage better than a contrast phlebogram since visualization of the vessel depends on blood flow and not on adequate opacification by contrast upstream of a blockage. Interpretation is

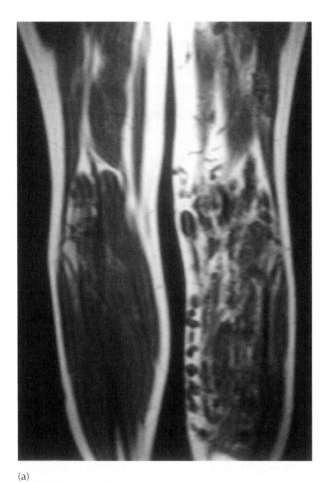

(a)

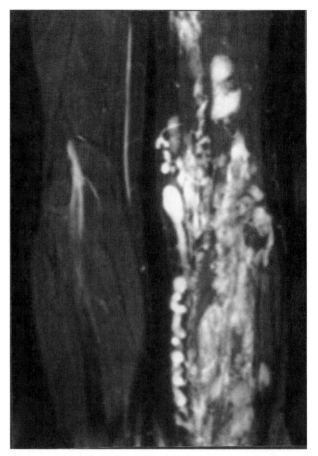

(b)

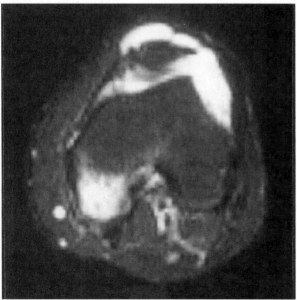

(c)

Figure 4.30   Magnetic resonance phlebography. (a) A coronal T1 MR image of a venous angioma of the lower limb. (b) A coronal STIR MR image of the same angioma. (c) An axial STIR MR image of the same angioma showing extension of the angioma into the knee joint.

based on the same principles as contrast phlebography – notably demonstration of filling defects in veins. The lower limb is well suited to TOF since flow is largely unidirectional (cephalad). The popliteal, superficial and deep femoral, saphenous and iliac veins and IVC are reliably demonstrated. Calf veins are not reliably seen unless some sort of flow augmentation is attempted.

Projectional images of calf veins using fluid-sensitive sequences can be obtained relatively quickly and correlate well with contrast varicography but are not useful for acute deep vein thrombosis, as the presence of oedema, which appears as a bright signal, may obscure underlying vessels.

At present MR phlebography is in its infancy. It is safe, does not involve ionizing radiation as does phlebography and is not operator dependent like duplex ultrasound. Its role will undoubtedly increase in the future.

As it has highly sensitive densitometry characteristics, it will probably prove valuable in discriminating venous abnormalities from those in surrounding tissues. It may also enable measurement of venous blood flow, even in very small veins.

Preliminary experience with MR has been encouraging. Several publications have assessed the efficacy of MR in deep vein thrombosis against duplex ultrasound,[217,343,377] contrast phlebography,[128,142,161,379,380,408] or both[76,77,79,378] using a variety of MR techniques. These studies have shown that in many cases MR can be as effective as or, on occasion, superior to these other imaging modalities.

MR imaging has also been used for saphenous vein mapping prior to bypass surgery.[78] Abdominal

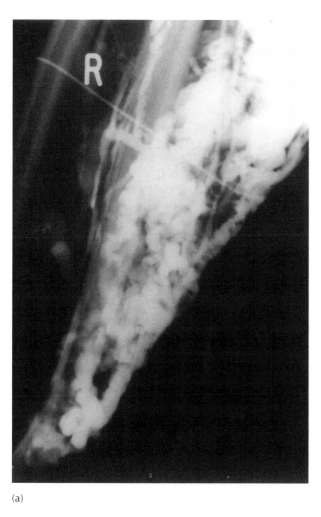

(a)

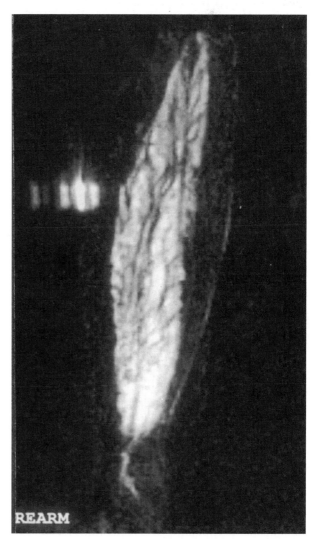

(b)

Figure 4.31 A comparison of the images of a venous angioma provided by (a) peripheral phlebography, (b) a coronal STIR MR scan.

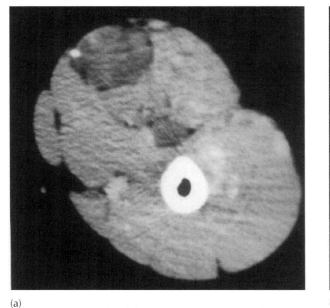

(a)

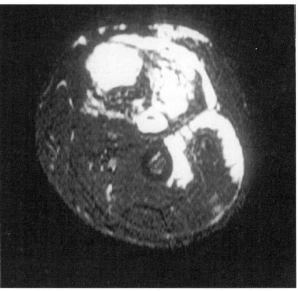

(b)

Figure 4.32 A comparison between the (a) CT and (b) MR images of a venous angioma in the right thigh. The extent of the lesion is better displayed by the MR scan.

vein imaging, including vena cava, renal and portal veins is also possible.[133,403]

A particular use of MR is in the assessment of vascular malformations. Historically, angiography, venography and CT have provided the most specific information. MR, however, depicts the anatomical relationships between vascular malformations and adjacent organs, nerves, tendons and muscles, thereby providing significant help in the assessment of these lesions (Figures 4.31, 4.32).[130,293,359]

Investigations that provide images of thrombus in the lungs

LUNG SCINTIGRAPHY

This is currently the most widely used examination for suspected pulmonary embolism (PE).

The investigation is carried out in two parts. A ventilation (V) scan is normally performed first. The most commonly used agent is xenon-133. Using a gamma camera, the isotope is inhaled and an initial posterior view first breath-hold image is obtained, followed by posterior equilibrium (wash-in) images. Washout images, consisting of posterior and right and left posterior oblique views, then follow. More recently, radiolabelled aerosols have been introduced as alternative agents.

The perfusion (Q) scan is performed with ^{99m}Tc-labelled macroggregates, injected into an antecubital vein over 5–10 respiratory cycles. Anterior, posterior, anterior and posterior oblique and lateral images are obtained.

A gamma camera with a wide field of view mounted with a parallel hole, low energy all purpose collimator is used to acquire the data. Technically satisfactory V–Q scans should be obtained in over 95% of cases.[332]

The V and Q images are reviewed together with a current chest radiograph (Figure 4.33). Images of ventilation are considered normal if the lungs exhibit uniform radioisotope distribution and if all the lung zones are cleared of radioisotope on the washout images. Zones showing delayed washout indicate areas of obstructive pulmonary disease.

Perfusion scans are evaluated for photon-deficient areas or defects. When a perfusion defect is present, comparison is made to the ventilation study. Normal ventilation in a non-perfused area is termed a V–Q mismatch. Abnormal ventilation in the non-perfused areas is termed a V–Q match.

The V–Q scan is most useful if it is clearly normal or demonstrates a pattern suggestive of a high probability of PE. Intermediate or low probability scans in patients for whom there is a strong clinical suspicion of PE does not exclude PE. These patients will require further investigations, such as

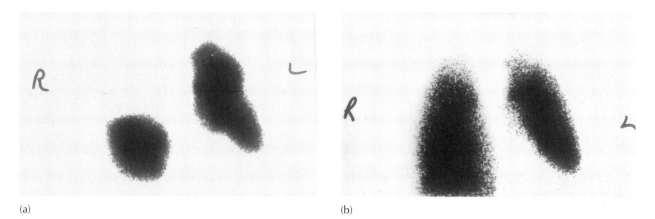

(a)   (b)

Figure 4.33 The ventilation–perfusion scan of a patient with multiple pulmonary emboli. (a) The anterior view of the perfusion scan shows a large defect in the right lung and a small peripheral defect in the left lung. (b) The anterior view of the ventilation scan is normal.

pulmonary angiography or spiral CT, to establish a diagnosis of PE.[151]

A high probability V–Q scan usually indicates the presence of clinically significant PE. A normal or near normal scan in the settling of low clinical suspicion makes diagnosis of PE very unlikely.

An intermediate (indeterminate or low probability) scan with a high clinical suspicion of PE is not helpful in establishing or excluding the diagnosis of PE. Unfortunately, in clinical practice a large number of patients fall into this latter category. In a major study[332] on the usefulness of the V–Q scan, 933 patients were randomly selected out of 1493 patients undergoing lung scintigraphy; 755 underwent pulmonary angiography. Almost all the patients with PE had abnormal scans of high, intermediate or low probability, but so did most of those without PE, giving a sensitivity of 98% and a specificity of 10%. Only 13% (116/775) of patients with PE had a high probability V–Q scan.

A normal, near normal or low probability scan in the setting of low clinical suspicion made the diagnosis of PE very unlikely.

An intermediate/indeterminate or low probability scan with a high clinical suspicion of PE was unhelpful in establishing the diagnosis of PE. More than 60% of the patients in this study were in these categories, indicating further investigations are required in a large proportion of patients undergoing lung scintigraphy to establish or exclude the diagnosis of PE.

It has been suggested that by identifying the location of perfusion defects on the V–Q scan pulmonary angiography could be more directed,[8,407] but this has not been confirmed by others[65] with only 30/185 (16%) of perfusion defects in 68 patients associated with PE at concurrent angiography. In

this study 43 PE identified at angiography were not associated with significant perfusion defects.

Despite its traditional role in the diagnosis of PE, lung scintigraphy does have serious limitations. Spiral CT has been shown to be as sensitive as lung scintigraphy for central PE,[80,124] but not for smaller subsegmental emboli.[124] With the continued improvement of spiral CT techniques this is likely to play a large role in the diagnosis of PE in the future.

PULMONARY ANGIOGRAPHY

Pulmonary angiography is regarded as the definitive study for the detection of pulmonary embolism (PE). Despite multiple publications that include pulmonary angiography in their diagnostic algorithms for the diagnosis of PE, it remains remarkably underused. In one study, 434/600 (72%) patients had an indeterminate/intermediate lung scintigram, yet only 50 (12%) underwent pulmonary angiography.[375] Other studies have shown similar usage of pulmonary angiography with unresolved suspicion for PE after lung scintigraphy.[110,171] This is because of its perceived risk and cost. It is usually reserved for patients in whom more information is needed or other tests have failed to give an adequate diagnosis. The indications for pulmonary angiography have been defined as:

- To assess patients with a high clinical suspicion of PE in whom non-invasive studies have not been diagnostic.
- To establish the diagnosis beyond any doubt in young patients facing long-term anticoagulation.[419]

- To assess patients with an unknown cause of pulmonary hypertension.
- To confirm the presence of PE in patients undergoing aggressive therapy, for example thrombolysis or embolectomy.
- To confirm the presence of PE in patients with a contraindication to anticoagulation.[254]

A clean, preferably sterile room should be set aside for angiographic procedures. Intensification should be available with television monitoring. A rapid serial film changer is required if conventional film is used. Patient positioning is simplified if a C arm unit is used. The introduction of digital subtraction angiography (DSA), which permits computer subtraction of bone and soft tissue while enhancing the opacified artery, offers a reduction in both radiation exposure and the volume of contrast medium needed.

Full resuscitation equipment should be available at all times. Fully informed consent should be obtained from the patient before the procedure. Electrocardiographic and blood pressure monitoring is essential during the procedure.

The femoral vein is the usual point of access. If the use of this vein is precluded by the presence of femoral, iliac or inferior vena caval thrombus, then an arm vein is used. A percutaneous Seldinger technique is used to insert a preshaped pigtail 7F or 8F catheter. The catheter is then passed through the right atrium and ventricle under fluoroscopic control. The catheter tip should be placed midway between the pulmonary artery bifurcation and the pulmonary valve. Pressure recordings can then be taken. Contrast medium is injected via an injector pump and antero-posterior views of both lungs obtained. The catheter can then be advanced into either the left or right pulmonary artery. Selective injections can be made and radiographs taken in anterior, oblique or lateral projections. At the end of the procedure a guide wire should be reinserted to straighten the pigtail catheter to prevent the catheter catching on the chordae tendinae during its removal.

In a normal pulmonary angiogram the arteries follow the distribution of the corresponding bronchi (Figure 4.34). The arteries are smooth and taper as they approach the periphery of the lung fields. A definitive diagnosis of PE can be made if there are persistent intraluminal filling defects in the artery outlined by contrast media. Contrast 'cut-off' is suggestive of pulmonary embolism, but occlusion of small peripheral branches is seen in other pulmonary diseases. Secondary features which are suggestive but not diagnostic of PE include non-filling of the arteries, vascular pruning, vessel tortuosity, decreased vascularity and delayed segmental venous return. In these circumstances comparison with the appearances on other imaging modalities such as chest CT or isotope imaging may be necessary to reach a correct diagnosis.

With good technique the risks of pulmonary angiography are low, with a reported mortality rate of 0.1–0.5% and a morbidity of 2–5%.[182,325,382] Patients at higher risk include those with core pulmonale and pulmonary hypertension. The risk of

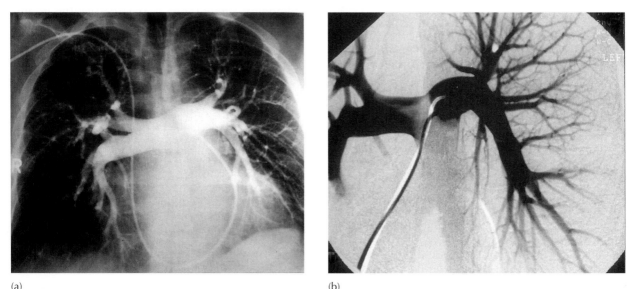

(a) (b)

Figure 4.34 Two normal pulmonary angiographs (a) following injection into the pulmonary trunk, (b) following injection into the left pulmonary artery. The latter technique provides a better image of the small peripheral vessels.

inducing sustained cardiac arrhythmias and cardiac perforations has been reduced with the development of preshaped softer catheters.[382,404,419] The rate of non-diagnostic studies has been reported to be 1–3%.[32]

Non-ionic contrast media have been shown to be safer than ionic contrast media.[182] They have fewer adverse effects than ionic contrast media and are well tolerated by the patient. Pulmonary angiography has a false-negative rate of under 1%.[316,382] The poorer resolution of older digital subtraction units meant that the spatial resolution was inferior to conventional cut film, but newer equipment with higher resolution gives comparable visualization of pulmonary artery branches.[413] The advantages of radiation and contrast media dose reduction with a shorter procedure time makes digital subtraction angiography the technique of choice for pulmonary angiography.

COMPUTED TOMOGRAPHY OF THE PULMONARY ARTERIES

Computed tomography (CT) has emerged as a potentially important diagnostic technique in pulmonary thromboembolic disease. It can provide direct evidence of the obstructing embolus, the associated vascular tree and the pleuroparenchymal space. The observation of pulmonary embolism with incremental CT has been seen as an incidental finding in patients undergoing examination for other cardiopulmonary conditions.

The advent of helical slip-ring CT and electron beam CT have improved the visualization of the pulmonary arteries by reducing scan times and single breath-hold acquisition. In helial CT the lung is scanned following a peripheral injection of a non-ionic contrast medium. A typical protocol would be 5 mm contiguous sections with a 5 mm/s table feed, with reconstruction of overlapped images at 3 mm intervals.

Whereas spiral CT uses the basic gantry design of a conventional CT scanner, in electron beam (ultrafast) CT, an electron gun replaces the x-ray tube. Focused electrons are swept across stationery tungsten rings within the gantry. Opposite the tungsten rings two parallel detector rays operate simultaneously, producing two separate images from a single electron beam sweep.[204]

In acute PE, contrast-enhanced CT has been proven to show thrombi within the central pulmonary vessels and in second to fourth order branches (Figure 4.35). On CT scans the lung parenchyma distal to the emboli may be oligaemic. False-negative and false-positive diagnoses may result from insufficient vascular enhancement of pulmonary arteries, confusing hilar lymph nodes with thrombosed arteries, or involvement of vessels behind the fourth order branches.

In patients with chronic thromboembolic disease, pulmonary arterial thrombus fails to lyse completely, resulting in thrombus organization and varying degrees of vascular occlusion. CT can accurately detect central thrombi as filling defects within the pulmonary vessels. Vascular occlusion of

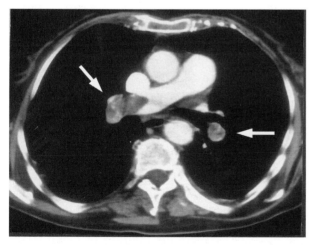

(a)

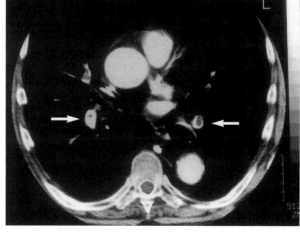

(b)

Figure 4.35   (a) A conventional CT scan showing a large embolus in the right pulmonary artery trunk and another embolus in a branch of the left pulmonary artery (arrowed). (b) Contrast-enhanced spiral CT scan showing emboli in both descending pulmonary arteries (arrowed).

small arteries supplying secondary pulmonary lobules produces an heterogeneous attenuation of the lung paraenchyma called mosaic oligaemia. This must be differentiated from other causes of lung oligaemia such as emphysema and bronchiolitis obliterans.

Pulmonary infarction following pulmonary embolism is uncommon in an otherwise healthy lung, occurring in patients with an impaired bronchial circulation or pulmonary venous hypertension. On CT, pulmonary infarcts appear as pleurally based opacities with an apex directed towards the hilum. This appearance may be mimicked by pneumonia and neoplasm, making the diagnosis of pulmonary infarct on the basis of a pleural mass unreliable. Pleural effusions can be seen in both pulmonary embolism and infarction. They are readily seen with CT but again their detection is non-specific. Cavitation of an infarct usually implies secondary infection of the necrotic lung or septic emboli and can be readily appreciated with CT.

There have been several studies comparing spiral CT with pulmonary angiography and isotope scintigraphy in the detection of PE.[344,345]

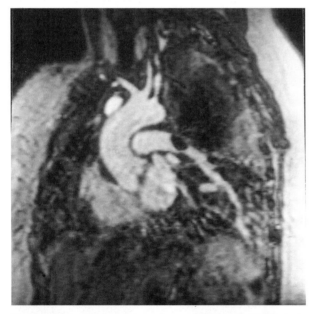

Figure 4.36 A dynamic enhanced MR (3D FISP) study showing a filling defect in the left pulmonary artery. The left subclavian artery is also occluded. There is a large aspergilloma in the left lung. The defect in the pulmonary artery is caused by invasion of the artery by granulation tissue. Pulmonary emboli may be demonstrated equally well and MR may supersede CT scanning for the diagnosis of pulmonary embolism.

MAGNETIC RESONANCE PULMONARY ANGIOGRAPHY (Figure 4.36)

Magnetic resonance (MR) of the pulmonary tree has been facilitated by the development of electrocardiograph-triggering, surface coils and pulse sequences with short echo times.

Initial experience with MR using spin-echo, gradient echo, 2D and 3D time of flight imaging[145,146,265,338,429] showed sixth and seventh order pulmonary arterial branches.[145,146] During the examination patients held their breath for 10–15 seconds during which time up to 10 sections of data were acquired.

In one study of 20 patients suspected of having PE, 14 patients also underwent pulmonary angiography.[158] Pulmonary embolism was detected correctly with both techniques in six patients. There were three false-positive results using MR, giving an overall sensitivity of 100% and a specificity of 62%. In the study overall, however, only 11 patients out of 20 (55%) were deemed to have good quality images; the remainder were considered of marginal quality but interpretable. A further study of 34 patients gave a sensitivity and specificity of MR imaging for diagnosing pulmonary embolism of 90% and 77%, respectively.[129]

Potential sources of error with MR include areas of atelectasis that may be misinterpreted as pulmonary embolism.

Image quality is hampered by patient movement and lack of spatial resolution. However, improved imaging techniques are likely in the near future, with the development of new techniques to differentiate between blood flow and thrombus[165] and the use of contrast media.[261] At present MR is not used in routine clinical practice for the detection of pulmonary embolism, but this position is likely to change in the future.[129]

Investigations of venous function

FOOT VEIN PRESSURE MEASUREMENTS

When the patient stands upright the calf pump plays an important role in assisting the return of blood to the heart by accelerating the flow of blood to the heart from the veins. The effect of calf pump action is to empty and reduce the pressure in the superficial veins. The absence of venous hypotension during exercise damages the microcirculation of the skin and may lead to skin necrosis (ulceration) (see

Chapters 15 and 18). The measurement of the effect of calf muscle exercise on superficial vein pressure is an important test of calf pump function and an indication of the severity of the physiological abnormality.[335] Four of the techniques described in this chapter, photoplethysmography, air plethysmography, strain-gauge plethysmography and foot volumetry, assess the same aspect of calf pump function by measuring the volume of blood in the superficial veins but none correlates perfectly with foot vein pressure which is generally accepted as the gold standard assessment for calf pump function.

A number of studies have shown that the superficial veins constitute a single superficial compartment so that pressure measured in one vein is representative of the pressure throughout the compartment.[22,60,178,263]

Method

A suitable (large and straight) vein on the dorsum of the foot is cannulated. Many modern workers use a 21 gauge butterfly needle. We prefer to use a large cannula to ensure a faster frequency response and avoid the damage that the tip of a needle sometimes causes to the inside of the vein during exercise. The needle is always inserted with the patient lying down because a proportion of patients faint if it is done while they are standing. The needle is connected to a strain gauge which is sensitive enough to detect changes of 2–5 mmHg without excessive amplification and which gives a rapid response (95% +) to changes of at least 10 MHz.

The centre of the transducer is fixed level with the tip of the catheter with the connecting tube as short as is practical to allow exercise.

The system should be checked to ensure that there are no air bubbles. The transducer is connected to a pen recorder and patency and pressure transmission are checked by asking the patient to perform a Valsalva manoeuvre and by putting rapid, brief, high pressure flushes into the system.

The Valsalva manoeuvre should cause a steady rise in foot vein pressure; the flush should produce a vertical rise and fall of pressure. If the rise and, more importantly, the fall are not instantaneous and vertical, the system is either damped by bubbles in the system, or the catheter or vein is too narrow, or the catheter is occluded by the vein wall. Repeated flushes are essential throughout the study to check the patency of the system.

Clotting may be prevented by adding a slow constant infusion of heparinized saline to the system.

The patient exercises by raising both heels off the ground every second in time to a metronome, for 10–20 seconds or until the pressure becomes stable. The patient should hold onto a support throughout

the study so that he/she can fully relax between periods of exercise. An alternative exercise is knee bending but this dorsiflexes the ankle whereas heel raising plantar flexes the ankle and is less likely to disturb or occlude the cannula.

If other tests of calf pump function are being performed, one form of exercise should be used which is suitable for all tests.

The test should be repeated with superficial vein occluding cuffs at different levels on the leg. The resting pressure (the hydrostatic pressure) depends upon the height of the patient, provided there is no cardiac failure, constrictive pericarditis, ascites, abdominal masses, or any other abnormality that will impede venous return.

The fall in pressure during exercise, which is highly reproducible, indicates the efficiency of calf pump function (Figures 4.37 and 4.38). The rise of pressure after exercise which is produced by the arterial inflow and venous reflux can be expressed as the time taken to refill completely, the time taken for 90% refilling, the time for 50% refilling or the maximum rate of refilling.

Provided a laboratory keeps to a standard exercise and standard method of measuring refilling, the way in which the results are expressed is not particularly important. We find that the T½ is the easiest to measure and, as it includes the period of maximum refilling, it is probably the best simple measure of reflux. The maximum refilling rate is frequently difficult to measure as refilling is often not linear.

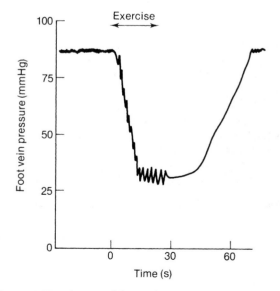

Figure 4.37 A normal foot vein pressure trace. Exercise causes a fall in pressure of 60–80% which takes 25–30 seconds to return to normal.

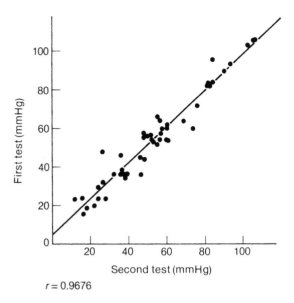

$r = 0.9676$

Figure 4.38 A comparison between repeated tests of the fall in foot vein pressure in 48 limbs.

Application

Foot vein pressures are used to assess calf pump function and detect abnormalities such as chronic deep vein incompetence or obstruction and superficial vein incompetence.[334,408] The use of superficial vein occluding tourniquets can clearly demonstrate the contribution of superficial reflux to pump insufficiency, and the site of incompetent deep-to-superficial vein connections can be detected by moving the tourniquet up and down the leg in the same way as in the simple clinical tourniquet test, provided the deficiencies of tourniquets are remembered.[281,307,387]

Deep vein obstruction is difficult to measure, except when it is so gross that the foot vein pressure rises during exercise.[420]

Foot vein pressure measurements have not been used for detecting deep vein thrombosis, though they would detect a major outflow obstruction, but they have been used to follow changes of calf pump efficiency in the years following thrombosis or operation.[72]

Accuracy

It is assumed that the essential function of the calf pump is to lower foot vein pressure during exercise on the basis of finding a close correlation between symptoms and signs and the inability to reduce pressure (see Figure 15.12, page 459). Pressure has therefore been accepted as the gold standard of calf pump function assessment and other methods have

been compared with it. Provided the technique of measurement is meticulous, the tracing should represent the intravenous pressures without any inaccuracies. The meaning of the changes depends upon our understanding of calf pump physiology. The fact that the surgical correction of pump abnormalities changes the pressure profile in the expected direction suggests that our hypotheses of the causes of pressure profile abnormalities are probably correct. The improvement of the pressure profile is, however, always less than expected which means that either our operations do not fully correct the abnormality or that the abnormalities corrected are not the only cause of the pump inefficiency and the abnormal pressure. Many more studies testing the significance of the abnormal features of foot vein pressure profiles need to be performed.

FEMORAL VEIN PRESSURE MEASUREMENTS

If there is a gross obstruction to the venous outflow from the leg, the venous pressure will rise during muscle exercise.[303] This abnormality can sometimes be observed in the foot vein pressure profile. Lesser degrees of obstruction only limit the reduction of the foot vein pressure during exercise, a change which is not diagnostic as it can also be caused by axial and communicating vein incompetence.

Consequently, lesser degrees of iliac vein obstruction can only be detected by measuring the pressure during exercise in the femoral vein immediately upstream to the obstruction. This is an essential test before considering any type of iliac vein bypass operation (see Chapter 13).[274]

Method

The patient lies supine on a couch, and a fine cannula is inserted into the femoral vein under local anaesthesia. It is helpful to check the position and patency of the femoral vein, before cannulation, with duplex ultrasound. The opposite femoral vein is also cannulated. The precautions required to ensure accurate pressure recordings described in the previous section on foot vein pressure measurement must be observed.

The patient is asked to plantar flex both feet vigorously. Although it is possible to fix the cannulae in place so that the patient can exercise on a bicycle ergometer, this degree of exercise is seldom necessary to reveal a significant obstruction.

If the limbs are normal, the femoral vein pressures will be equal and rise by 2–4 mmHg during calf muscle exercise. If the pressure rises by 5 mmHg or more, and/or if the pressure difference between the abnormal and the normal limb during exercise is greater than 5 mmHg, there is a significant obstruction to outflow.[5,303,304] The rate at which the pressure returns to normal will be delayed in the presence of an iliac vein obstruction.

Application and accuracy

This technique is the only satisfactory method of diagnosing iliac vein obstruction. Phlebography may arouse suspicions but pressure measurements provide physiological proof of obstruction. We combine pressure measurement with bilateral percutaneous common femoral/iliac vein phlebography as a routine part of the phlebography.

In our opinion no iliac vein bypass procedure should be performed without physiological preoperative confirmation of an abnormal femoral vein pressure rise during exercise. It would be a step forward if surgeons were to confirm the adequacy of their bypass operations by showing that the bypass had abolished the pressure rise of exercise by repeating this investigation 3 months and 12 months after the operation, as well as showing that it was patent.

PHOTOPLETHYSMOGRAPHY (PPG)

Photoplethysmography is also known as light reflection rheography.

The density of the skin and its ability to reflect light partly depends upon the volume of blood in the capillaries within the skin.[172,292]

The photoplethysmograph (PPG) contains an infra-red light source (805 nm) and a photoelectric cell which measures the reflectivity of the skin.[82] Many workers have shown that there is sufficient correlation between this indirect method of assessing skin blood volume during exercise and measurements of superficial venous pressure during exercise to justify the use of PPG as an initial quick way of assessing calf pump function,[33,298] but it should always be remembered that the only reliable measurement that can be obtained with this technique is the refilling time after exercise – a measure of the degree of reflux.[33,298]

PPG cannot be used for measuring blood flow. Rapid changes in skin blood volume can be detected if the photoelectric cell is recorded in the a.c. mode because the upslope of each pulse is related to blood flow, but it is extremely difficult to calibrate this in absolute terms. The d.c. mode gives a dampened mean measure of skin reflectivity over a longer course of time and so indicates overall changes of skin blood volume, 70% of which is within the venules and veins, but even this mea-surement will be affected by an unstable vasoactive microcirculation.

Method[288,289]

The probe must be placed parallel to and in complete contact with the skin surface so that it can only receive reflected light from the skin (Figure 4.39). The probe is designed so that its outer part masks the sensor from any back-scattered outside direct light. The probe is fixed to the skin with transparent double-sided adhesive tape.

Although the venous volume changes in any area of skin will reflect changes in the whole leg they will also be affected by local abnormalities such as a nearby incompetent communicating vein or large

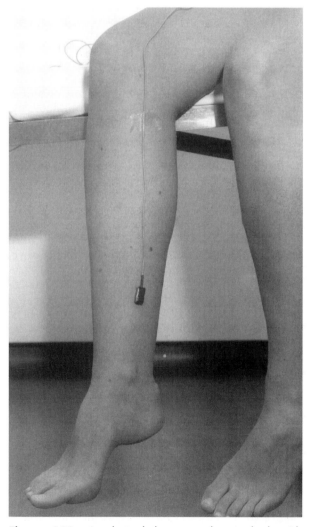

Figure 4.39 A photoplethysmograph attached with double-sided adhesive tape to the skin of the medial side of the leg, 5 in (125 cm) above the medial malleolus.

subcutaneous varix. Refilling times have been shown to vary by as much as 20% in different parts of the leg[357] and will also be affected by the arterial inflow.[329]

Nevertheless, for routine testing the probe is usually fixed on the medial side of the leg, 4–5 inches (10–12.5 cm) above the medial malleolus.

The normal test procedure is to ask the patient to sit with the feet resting on the floor and then to perform regular heel raises, without weight bearing, in time to a metronome. The sitting position prevents the reduction of calf blood volume produced by the calf muscle contractions which are unavoidable when standing.

Alternatively, the patient is asked to stand with all his/her weight on one leg whilst performing the heel raising with the non-weight-bearing leg. The greater hydrostatic pressure when standing gives the maximum initial venous filling and it has been claimed that the correlation between PPG and refilling time is significantly better when measured in the standing position.[310]

Most laboratories use PPG solely for measuring refilling time after exercise because it is not possible to calibrate the PPG tracing in terms of blood volume. A crude calibration can be obtained by adjusting the gain so that the output is zero when the patient is supine and maximal (100%) when standing. The 100% can be equated to the calculated hydrostatic pressure at the site of the probe. The change in reflectivity during exercise can then be expressed as a percentage of the maximum calf volume or as an absolute pressure. Some workers[134,135,206,315] have shown both these methods of calibration to correlate moderately well with simultaneous measurements of foot vein pressure but others[281,412] have described poor correlations. The general view is that PPG should only be used to measure refilling time.

The shape of the PPG tracing (Figure 4.40) is similar to that of the foot vein pressure trace on exercise.[324] It is therefore possible to measure the percentage emptying (provided some attempt has been made at calibration), the refilling time (in seconds) or the 50% refilling time (T½).

Refilling is non-linear, and sophisticated analyses of the refilling curve are not justified.

Application

Venous refilling after exercise normally comes from the arterial circulation. If the superficial or deep veins are incompetent, blood will reflux down the limb and venous refilling will be accelerated. The PPG can therefore be used to assess the degree of venous reflux. Reflux through superficial veins can be prevented with a superficial vein occluding tourniquet. If the application of such a tourniquet restores an abnormally short refilling time to normal, the abnormality must be pure superficial vein incompetence.

If the tourniquet is positioned at various levels on the leg, the site of any superficial-to-deep incompetent connections can be determined in a way similar to the clinical tourniquet test.

These tests depend upon the efficiency of the tourniquets in preventing reflux and modern methods of assessing reflux have shown that tourniquets can be unreliable.[281]

Accuracy

The PPG recovery time correlates well with the foot vein pressure recovery time.[310,324] When a single superficial vein occluding cuff restores an abnormal trace to normal, there is little doubt that the superficial veins are incompetent but when there is only a partial improvement the significance is far less clear. Attempts to define normal ranges of refilling and relate them to disease groups have not been very helpful because of the inherent inaccuracies of PPG and the more fundamental problem – our lack of gold standards for comparison.

PPG is therefore most useful as a test for excluding venous disease. It can identify pure long and/or short saphenous vein incompetence if tourniquets are applied with care and, if possible, this effect checked with a hand-held Doppler flow detector, but gives little information about communicating or deep vein disease apart from indicating its presence. The most sensible way to use this apparatus is to establish your own definition of normal refilling and, when a patient's test is in the abnormal range, measure the effect of superficial vein occluding tourniquets above and then below the knee. This will provide an immediate assessment of the contribution of long and short saphenous vein reflux to the rate of refilling and indicate the possi-

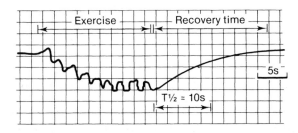

Figure 4.40 A tracing of a normal photoplethysmograph showing a rapid emptying of venous blood from the calf during exercise (Ex) and a half refilling time (T½) of 10 seconds.

bility of deep vein disease. Any attempt to make the PPG tracing provide a more specific and accurate analysis is not worthwhile.

In spite of the relative unreliability of the measurements of venous function obtained with PPG, changes in venous outflow have been used to detect the presence of deep vein thrombosis.[24] Prolongation of emptying has been shown to correlate with the presence of phlebographically proven deep vein thrombosis but, as with other plethysmographic techniques, thrombus which is not causing an obstruction to venous outflow will not be detected.

STRAIN-GAUGE PLETHYSMOGRAPHY (SGP)

If a cross-section of the calf is assumed to be circular, it is possible to calculate its area from a measurement of its circumference and hence calculate its volume.[391] The development of electronics in the 1940s led to the invention of the mercury-in-rubber strain gauge, the resistance of which is directly proportional to its length. When placed around the calf, any change in the length of the gauge caused by a change in calf volume alters its resistance. If the length–resistance relationship has been determined by precalibration, the volume change of a 1 cm slice of calf can be calculated. Strain gauges have now been refined and have become more reliable; silastic is better than rubber, and indium–gallium alloy is better than mercury. Calibration can be carried out electrically, a 1% change in resistance being equivalent to a 1% change in volume.

A strain gauge can only measure the volume change in the plane of the gauge but many studies have shown a close correlation between the volume changes measured with a strain gauge and direct volume measurements obtained with a water-filled plethysmograph. Provided the tube of tissue being studied is horizontal and almost cylindrical, problems caused by uneven filling and irregularities of shape are therefore insignificant. Strain gauges require a temperature compensation circuit and must fit the limb properly. The ideal gauge length should be 90% of the limb circumference, and the gauge should be stretched by 10% when it is applied so that it completely encircles the limb.

Method[73,109,308]

The patient lies supine with the limb elevated above heart level, preferably to 20–30°. This ensures that the veins are as empty as possible before venous congestion is applied.

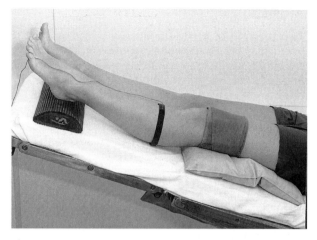

Figure 4.41 A photograph showing a strain gauge around the calf. The limb is elevated to 20°.

A gauge, 90% of the circumference to be studied, is stretched around the limb. It should lie comfortably without compressing the skin or any underlying veins (Figure 4.41).

The leg under examination should be relaxed and not hyperextended as muscle tension and hyperextension of the knee joint have been shown to affect the results.[358]

A large pneumatic tourniquet, at least 20 cm wide, is placed around the thigh. Narrow cuffs and cuffs with bladders that do not encircle the limb will not occlude all the veins in the tissues beneath them. Theoretically, the width of the cuff should be one or two times the diameter of the limb.

The cuff is inflated to 50 mmHg. After 2 minutes, when the volume curve is almost stable, the cuff is released. (The volume will not become absolutely constant as the venous congestion slowly reduces the venous tone and causes tissue oedema.) This procedure provides a measurement of the total calf volume and the venous outflow.

A second narrow cuff in then placed at the top of the thigh and inflated to 300 mmHg. The large thigh cuff is then rapidly inflated to 50 mmHg. This test can be repeated with a superficial vein occluding tourniquet below the knee. These manoeuvres test deep venous reflux.

The cuffs are removed and the patient then stands and performs a series of heel raises in time to a metronome so that the volume changes during and after exercise can be recorded. This test may be repeated with superficial vein occluding tourniquets.

The test may also be performed while the patient walks on a treadmill[132,179] and similar results can be obtained when a strain gauge is placed around the foot.[367]

Application

This method of plethysmography is not as easy to perform as air or impedance plethysmography; it is therefore rarely used in the acute clinical situation presented by venous thrombosis. It is a vascular laboratory investigation most often used to elicit the state of the venous outflow tract and venous reflux.

Calf volume expansion

After 2 minutes of congestion at 50 mmHg, calf volume expansion is usually 2–3%.[36,162] The presence of acute venous thrombosis reduces this to 1–2% because the veins are already full of thrombus and the inflamed vein walls are less distendable. This test is rarely used for the diagnosis of venous thrombosis.

Some patients with chronic venous insufficiency also have a decreased calf volume expansion but measurement of this volume is of no special clinical value.

Maximum venous outflow

The rate at which blood flows out of the calf following venous congestion depends upon the outflow resistance and the pressure gradient, which in turn depends upon the venous tone and the venous distension.[34,200] Some authors have used the maximum rate of outflow, derived from the rate of outflow in the first few seconds after congestion, as a measure of obstructive axial vein damage (Figure 4.42).[37] An outflow less than 20 ml/100 ml/min probably signifies a significant outflow obstruction. Formulae have been devised which incorporate corrections for the degree of venous filling, the volume of the veins under the cuff and the rate of cuff deflation, with the hope that these formulae will make this measurement more discriminatory.[73,200] They have, however, failed. This test only reveals the type of gross

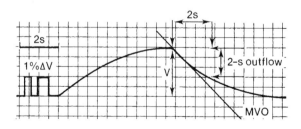

Figure 4.42 The calculations that can be derived from a strain-gauge measurement of calf volume. Calf volume expansion (V), maximum venous outflow (MVO), and 2-second outflow. In this patient, V = 2.5 ml/100 ml, the 2-second outflow = 48 ml/100ml/min and the MVO = 56 ml/100ml/min.

obstruction, acute thrombotic or chronic, that is usually obvious on clinical examination.[163] Moderate and mild obstruction are not detected because the stimulus to outflow – a pressure gradient of 50 mmHg – is too low. This test has a specificity and sensitivity of 84% and 79%, respectively, for femoral and iliac vein occlusion[5] but its specificity for obstruction caused by calf vein thrombosis is only 60%.[37] If the test could be performed with a constant and greater pressure gradient that was reproducible, it might detect lesser degrees of obstruction.

Venous reflux

The inflation of a wide cuff below an arterial occluding cuff will push blood down the leg into the calf if the deep vein valves are incompetent. In a normal limb, thigh cuff inflation expands the calf by 3% whereas in a grossly incompetent venous system the expansion may exceed 10%.[35] Superficial vein incompetence can be distinguished from deep vein incompetence by the addition of a superficial vein occluding tourniquet just above or below the knee. This is an uncomfortable test for the patient, and the scatter of results is so wide that it only detects those patients who have gross abnormalities. It is simpler to measure refilling after erect exercise.[38,179]

The same test can be performed with and without a superficial vein occluding tourniquet to assess superficial vein reflux.

Venous refilling after erect exercise

This measurement is identical in concept to the refilling time measured with PPG, foot volumetry or foot vein pressure. In all these tests it is more informative to look at the recording and see the effect of tourniquets rather than to calculate precise refilling times.

Precise calculations may be misleading if corrections are not made for changes in arterial inflow, especially with tests that involve muscle exercise.[329,330]

We find it difficult to measure venous refilling after erect exercise because of the artefacts caused by movement during exercise. One way of avoiding these artefacts is to squeeze the blood out of the calf manually and then record and measure the rate of reflux, provided you can apply a calf compression of reproducible pressure and rate and release it instantaneously.

AIR PLETHYSMOGRAPHY (APG)

Air-filled plethysmographs, like water-filled plethysmographs, have been used for many

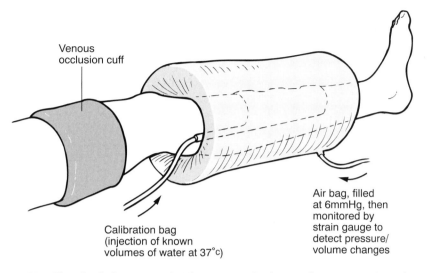

Figure 4.43 The air plethysmograph. The pressure in the air sleeve is monitored continuously after inflating it to a pressure of 6 mmHg. The flat 1-litre bag between the leg and the air sleeve is used to calibrate the changes in pressure in the air sleeve in terms of volume change.

years[67,138,266] but the early devices were difficult to use because of the inflexibility of the available materials and the difficulties of ensuring a good cuff-to-skin seal. Modern materials, and sensitive strain gauges have overcome these problems and air plethysmography has been revived and become a useful method for investigating the function of the veins of the lower limb.

Method (Figure 4.43)

The lower leg is inserted into an inelastic plastic sleeve which is inflated to a pressure of 6–8 mmHg. This pressure is sufficient to keep the inner lining of the sleeve firmly against the skin of the leg without significantly interfering with the volume or tone of the veins beneath it. Changes in the volume of the enclosed calf are then detected by measuring changes in the pressure in the sleeve. To convert these pressure changes to volumes, the system is calibrated by placing a small flat 1 litre capacity PVC bag between the tubular air sleeve and the leg and injecting into it known volumes of water, usually 50 ml at 37°C.[86]

The plethysmograph is applied and calibrated with the patient supine and the leg elevated to 45° to ensure that the venous system is empty.

The patient is then asked to stand up without bearing any weight on the leg being studied, to avoid artefacts caused by calf muscle contractions. This is achieved by asking the patient to hold onto the sides of a walking frame and bear all the weight on the opposite leg.

As the leg fills with blood it swells and the pressure in the air sleeve increases. When the pressure reaches a plateau (the total venous volume, TVV) the patient is asked to make a single tiptoe movement. The reduction in volume observed is the ejection volume (EV) of one calf contraction. After the pressure has returned to the TVV pressure, the patient is asked to make 10 tiptoe movements, one per second. The volume at the end of this exercise, less the original supine baseline volume, is the residual volume (RV). The residual volume and the ejection volume can then be expressed as a percentage of the total venous volume and called the residual volume fraction (RVF) and the ejection fraction (EF), respectively (Figure 4.44).

The rate of refilling on moving from the supine to the erect position and after exercise can also be measured, with and without superficial vein occluding tourniquets at different levels, to obtain an assessment of the degree, site (superficial or deep) and level of any venous reflux.

Because it is sometimes difficult to decide precisely when the total venous volume is reached, the venous filling time (VFT) and venous filling index (VFI) are commonly based on the time taken to reach 90% of the total venous volume.

Application

It has been claimed that air plethysmography can be used to assess most aspects of calf pump function – the ejection volume of a single calf contraction, the ejection volume of sustained activity and the degree

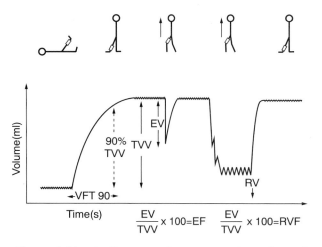

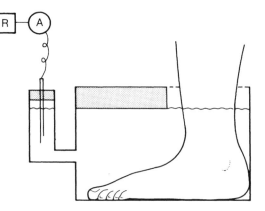

Figure 4.44 A diagrammatic representation of an air plethysmograph trace showing the various divisions of the calf venous volume that can be measured. TVV, total venous volume; EV, expelled volume after one tiptoe; RV, residual volume after 10 tiptoes; VFT 90, time to fill in 90% of TVV; EF, ejection fraction (as a % of TVV); RVF, residual volume fraction (as a % of TVV).

Figure 4.45 The foot volumeter. In this illustration the water level is sensed by the change in resistance between two electrodes in the side arm. A, amplifier; R, recorder.

of superficial and deep reflux.[86,87] Some recent comparisons of air plethysmography with venous pressure measurements have failed to support these claims.[302,323] Some of the published differences may have been caused by errors of methodology. Nevertheless, Payne found the correlation coefficient between residual volume fraction and ambulatory venous pressure to be only 0.04 and the correlation coefficient between refilling times measured by these two methods only 0.58 and although Neglen,[302] when comparing APG against clinical staging found a reasonably good correlation for the filling indices, the correlation with the residual volume fraction was poor. Neglen[302] and Van Bremmelen[411] stress the fact that the APG, like all other forms of plethysmograph, fails to separate clinical groups, because the test results, when subdivided according to the patients' class in the North American Vascular Societies clinical classification, overlap so much. Air plethysmography cannot, therefore, be recommended as being any more reliable a method of assessing venous function than any other form of plethysmography.

FOOT VOLUMETRY

This method is foot plethysmography using an open water-filled plethysmograph.[405] The patient stands in a temperature-controlled water bath, the water reaching up to the narrow part of the ankle, and exercises by performing knee bends in time to a metronome. As the blood is pumped out of the foot so the water level falls. This can be measured precisely with a pressure manometer or an electrical sensor. The method gives an overall indication of calf pump function.

Method[314]

The foot is placed in the plethysmograph. Water at 32°C is added to a marked level on the tank; this volume subtracted from the known volume of the tank gives the volume of the foot (Figure 4.45). The plethysmograph is calibrated by withdrawing 10 ml aliquots of water. The patient holds onto a rail and performs 20 knee bends at intervals of 1 second. The test is then repeated with superficial vein occluding tourniquets. The tracing should show a reduction of volume during exercise followed by refilling. The measurements made from the trace are as follows (Figure 4.46):

- Absolute expelled volume (EV), ml
- Expelled volume relative to resting foot volume (EVr), ml/100 ml
- Refilling or half refilling time (t or tv½)
- Maximum rate of refilling (Q), ml/l00 ml/min
- Ratio of maximum rate of refilling to relative expelled volume (Q/EVr).

Application

The advantage of this technique is its simplicity. The water bath and baffles can be homemade of perspex; it is therefore very cheap, and water put into such a tank at 32°C remains at this temperature ±2°C for 30 minutes so that a heater and thermostat

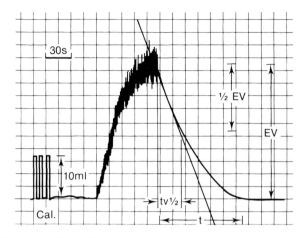

Figure 4.46 A foot volumetry trace showing the calculation of the expelled volume (EV), the half volume refilling time (tv½), and the refilling time (t).

are not necessary. The measurements indicate overall calf pump function (expelled volume – absolute and relative) and the degree of venous reflux, superficial reflux being separated from deep reflux by the use of tourniquets.

Foot volume changes correlate closely with venous pressure changes,[223,321] both of which have been assessed against other forms of diagnosis such as clinical examination and phlebography, though neither are gold standards of peripheral venous physiology.[126] It is easier to use the technique in a qualitative manner by taking note of the shape of the tracing and the effect of the tourniquets rather than the mathematical calculations of expelled volume and refilling time.

ULTRASOUND FLOW DETECTION WITH THE HAND HELD CONTINUOUS WAVE PROBE

The application of ultrasound techniques to the investigation of peripheral vascular disease has produced a significant improvement in our understanding of peripheral vascular physiology. The arteries have yielded some of their secrets more readily than the veins. This is because arterial blood flow is regular and phasic and more susceptible to mathematical analysis than venous blood flow which is irregular and, though ultimately controlled by the heart, is profoundly affected by many other factors (e.g. respiration, abdominal pressure and skeletal muscle contraction).

Doppler flow detection depends upon the principle that the frequency of a sound wave reflected from a moving object is changed in proportion to the speed of movement of the reflecting object.[384]

An object moving away from the source of a sound reflects the sound at a lower frequency; an object moving towards the source of a sound increases the frequency of the sound. The frequency change can be used to detect movement and to measure the velocity of the movement.

The simplest ultrasound probe consists of two piezoelectric crystals; one crystal is excited to transmit ultrasound, the other crystal becomes excited on receipt of the reflected ultrasound. The ultrasound is directed towards a blood vessel by coupling the probe to the tissues with a coupling jelly to stop all the sound being reflected at the air–skin interface. Although other tissue interfaces of different density will reflect some of the sound waves, the majority are reflected from the red cells because they have a much higher density than their surrounding plasma. Any change in reflected frequency indicates movement of the red cells.

Vein patency

Most authorities use a simple hand-held 5 MHz pencil probe with stethoscope ear-pieces without a chart recorder for day-to-day use in the ward or office.[32,390] Better tissue penetration is obtained with 5 MHz than with the 8 MHz, commonly used for arterial studies; 5 MHz is the best frequency to use when examining the deep veins. Superficial veins can be studied using an 8 MHz probe, which gives better spatial discrimination but the 5 MHz probe is the most practical frequency, applicable to all veins in the limbs and to the iliac veins in the lower abdomen.

Position

The patient must lie supine with the head and shoulders above the level of the legs to ensure that the veins are full. The leg should be slightly abducted and externally rotated with the hip and knee slightly flexed. The popliteal vein can usually be examined with the leg in this position but if the signal is poor, the patient must be turned to a prone position.

When the arm is examined, it should be placed at the patient's side, below the level of the right atrium.

The probe

The probe should be placed on the skin within a pool of coupling jelly. When superficial veins are examined the probe should not be pressed hard against the skin, otherwise the veins will be compressed. The probe should be held at 45° to the long axis of the veins. This is usually 45° to the skin surface, except when studying the upper part of the popliteal vein which runs obliquely into the depths of the leg towards the adductor canal. When insonating the upper popliteal vein the probe may have to be held at 90° to the skin.

Finding the vein

The deep veins all run alongside arteries; the simplest way to find a vein is therefore to insonate the artery's pulsatile flow, after feeling the pulse with the fingers, and then move or just angle the probe to that side of the artery where the vein should be found. The sound produced by venous flow has a lower pitch than that of the arterial flow generated by the gentle fluctuations of blood flow caused by respiration. Quick confirmation that the sound is coming from the vein can be obtained by asking the patient to stop breathing. The sounds of venous blood flow should stop immediately and should resume with a rush when breathing recommences. This technique is applicable to the common femoral, superficial femoral, popliteal and posterior tibial veins.

The flow signal

The sound heard through the stethoscope is the amplified combination of the transmitted and reflected ultrasound, the beat frequency. Although ultrasound is inaudible, the beat frequency is audible. You are not actually hearing the blood flow but a noise whose amplitude is proportional to it. It is therefore acceptable to display the sound from a simple pencil probe graphically and call it blood flow, provided the graph is not calibrated.

The effect of respiration

Femoral vein blood flow at rest varies with respiration (Figure 4.47). As the patient inspires, the flow falls; this is caused by the contraction of the diaphragm and the increased abdominal pressure. A few patients breathe without increasing abdominal pressure during inspiration. In these patients the venous flow may increase during inspiration because of the sucking effect of the negative intrathoracic pressure. A deep breath or a Valsalva manoeuvre (a deep breath followed by a forced expiration against a closed glottis to raise both intrathoracic and intra-abdominal pressure) stops the blood flow in the femoral vein (Figure 4.47). When the Valsalva manoeuvre is released, there is a sudden increase in blood flow.

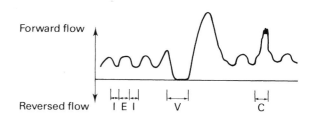

Figure 4.47 The effect of respiration, a Valsalva manoeuvre and upstream compression on femoral vein blood flow detected by ultrasound. Blood flow slows with inspiration (I) and increases during expiration (E). A Valsalva manoeuvre (V) stops femoral vein blood flow. Compression of the vein upstream to the flow detector augments flow (C).

If the blood flow stops in response to a deep breath or a Valsalva manoeuvre, the veins between the heart and the point of examination are patent. The respiratory responses should always be present in the femoral and popliteal veins and can be heard in the posterior tibial veins at the ankle in 80% of patients. The absence of these responses indicates an obstruction between the probe and the chest. The signal just above an obstruction may also have a reduced respiratory fluctuation because the blood flow is reduced by the obstruction.

The effect of venous compression

The blood flow through a vein can be increased by squeezing the vein or the tissues containing the blood that drains into the vein. If manual compression of the calf augments the flow signal in the common femoral vein, it is reasonable to assume that the veins between the compressing hand and the probe are patent;[131,372,386,392] this is not, however, always true (Figure 4.48). Large collateral vessels may conduct sufficient blood around an occluded main vein to augment the flow signal above the block, but the augmentation will be dampened, and the audible signal is often recognizably different from the rapid normal response. Before accepting that there is no augmentation in response to compression, it is important to check the position of the probe and make sure that the upstream veins are full of blood before they are squeezed.

It has been suggested that squeezing a calf containing non-adherent thrombus might cause a pulmonary embolus[68,143] but the experience of many thousands of clinicians world wide who have used this test on countless occasions does not support this view. Squeezing or plantar flexing the foot is an acceptable alternative.[61]

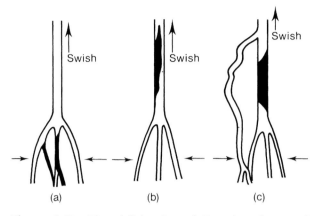

Figure 4.48 The deficiencies of Doppler ultrasound detection of deep vein thrombosis. This figure shows the three situations in which calf compression will augment femoral vein blood flow in the presence of a deep vein thrombosis, thus producing a false-negative test result. (a) A small amount of calf thrombus will not prevent the augmentation of flow produced by squeezing the calf. (b) A non-occluding femoral vein thrombus will not prevent the augmentation of flow produced by squeezing the calf. (c) A large collateral may carry the extra blood flow caused by squeezing the calf into the femoral vein and so mask the presence of a superficial femoral vein occlusion.

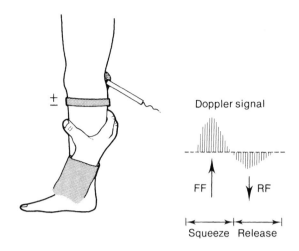

Figure 4.49 The technique for testing for popliteal vein reflux. The vein is insonated with the probe at an angle of 45° to the skin in a pool of coupling jelly. Forward flow (FF) is augmented by squeezing the calf. When the compression is released, flow will stop or, if the popliteal vein is incompetent, flow will occur in the opposite direction (RF). To confirm that the retrograde flow is not in the short saphenous vein, the test is repeated with the short saphenous vein occluded with an assistant's finger or a narrow tourniquet.

Valvular incompetence

When the clinician tests for valvular incompetence (see Figures 4.51–4.54), the patient should be standing upright. If it can be shown that blood can flow downwards (retrogradely) in a vein, its valves cannot be functioning.[279,439]

The two forces commonly used to produce retrograde blood flow are a raised intra-abdominal/intrathoracic pressure (the Valsalva manoeuvre) and venous compression downstream to the probe.

The position of the probe

This test can be applied to superficial veins as well as to deep veins. The long saphenous vein at the groin is detected by finding the common femoral vein and then edging the probe downwards and medially to a point where the vein is visible, or palpable, or where the respiratory fluctuations diminish. Unless the long saphenous vein can be seen or felt, it is difficult to be sure that the probe is insonating the saphenous vein and not a deep vein. This problem can be overcome by using an imaging probe. The source of the signal can then be accurately identified. Unfortunately, such equipment cannot be carried in the pocket for immediate use at the bedside or in the office. The short saphenous vein is easier to find, as it is in the midline below the centre of the popliteal fossa but it is not always possible to be certain whether the superficial vein or the popliteal vein is being insonated (Figure 4.49).

Other superficial veins can only be studied if they are clearly visible or palpable.

The Valsalva manoeuvre

The production of a positive pressure in the chest or abdomen will stop venous blood flow in normal veins but will cause retrograde flow if the valves are incompetent, followed by a sharp increase in flow as the Valsalva manoeuvre is released. The simple Doppler flow detector does not indicate the direction of blood flow but the examiner hears a continuous flow sound during the Valsalva manoeuvre in contrast to the silence (no flow) of a normal limb. A directional flow recording will show that the flow is retrograde (Figure 4.49).

This method may be used over the femoral and the popliteal vein. It is less reliable on the posterior tibial vein at the ankle.

Downstream (cephalad) compression

A similar effect to that caused by the Valsalva manoeuvre can be obtained by compressing the vein downstream (cephalad) to the probe. If the valves are incompetent, there will be retrograde flow; if the valves are competent, the flow will stop – the examiner therefore hears either a louder flow sound during compression or silence, respectively. A directional flow recording will show the retrograde nature of the flow. The advantage of this method over the Valsalva technique is that much shorter segments of vein in many parts of the leg can be tested and in both the superficial and the deep systems. It is, however, essential to know which vein is being insonated and that it is directly continuous with the veins being compressed downstream.

Upstream (caudad) compression

When the patient is standing up it is possible to detect retrograde blood flow by compressing the tissues upstream (caudad) to the probe. For example, if the probe is over the popliteal vein and the calf is squeezed, blood will flow forwards during the compression but run backwards when the compression is released. This is the simplest way to detect popliteal vein reflux when the patient is standing.

This test can be confused by the blood running into the top half of a competent popliteal vein and then down and out through an incompetent short saphenous vein. This cause of false-positive results can be abolished by performing the test with the short saphenous vein occluded by manual compression. We have found this test difficult to perform and unreliable. Popliteal and short saphenous vein incompetence is best assessed with a Duplex imaging system.

Communicating vein incompetence

If flow can be detected in a communicating vein or its immediate tributaries during compression of the deep veins, it is probably incompetent. To detect retrograde flow the examiner must squeeze the leg on one side of a tourniquet which occludes the superficial veins and listen for a flow signal with a Doppler probe over the site of a communicating vein on the other side of the tourniquet (Figure 4.50).[141,290] The tourniquet stops the pressure of the calf squeeze, causing blood flow in the superficial veins so any blood flow in the communicating veins must have come via the deep veins and out through an incompetent communicator. The method has two problems – the identification of the site of the

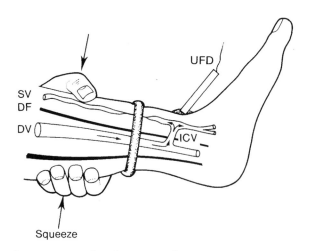

Figure 4.50 The detection of incompetent communicating veins with the ultrasound flow detector. The calf is squeezed on one side of a superficial vein occluding tourniquet and the sites of the communicating veins are insonated with an ultrasound flow detector (UFD) on the other. If blood flow is detected in response to the squeeze, the communicating vein must be incompetent. This test will only work well when performed in this way if the deep vein valves are also incompetent. The effect of the squeeze can be augmented by placing another tourniquet above the knee. If the position of the probe and squeezing hand are reversed, the test will work even when the deep axial veins are competent but the tissues just above the ankle are difficult to squeeze effectively. SV, superficial vein; DV, deep vein; ICV, incompetent communicating vein; DF, deep fascia.

communicating vein for the insonation and the uncertainty that the tourniquet has stopped all blood flow in the superficial compartment. In our hands this technique has not proved to be accurate.

Accuracy

The accuracy of techniques which use a simple Doppler flow detector for detecting venous occlusion depends upon the anatomical complexity of the vein under study. The iliac, femoral and popliteal veins are major axial veins with few collaterals. Occlusion of these vessels by thrombus can be detected with an overall accuracy of 90%, a positive test accuracy of 85% and a negative test accuracy of 95%. Sensitivity (overall ability to detect obstruction) is 95%. Specificity (overall ability to detect normality) is 90%.[390]

The test is less reliable when an occluded vein is part of a plexus of vessels (e.g. in the calf). For detecting deep vein occlusions below the knee the

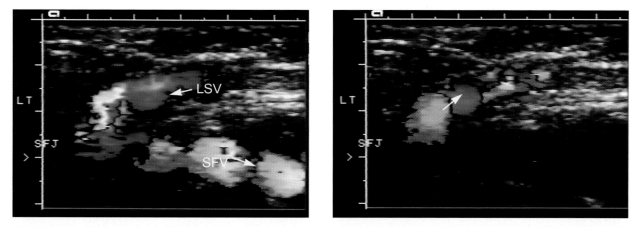

Figure 4.51 Sapheno-femoral vein junction incompetence. At rest (left), there is flow in the normal direction in the long saphenous vein. During a Valsalva manoeuvre (right), flow reverses in the saphenous vein – confirming sapheno-femoral junction incompetence – but stops in the superficial femoral vein (no colour) – confirming superficial femoral vein competence. LSV, long saphenous vein; SFV, superficial femoral vein; → direction of blood flow.

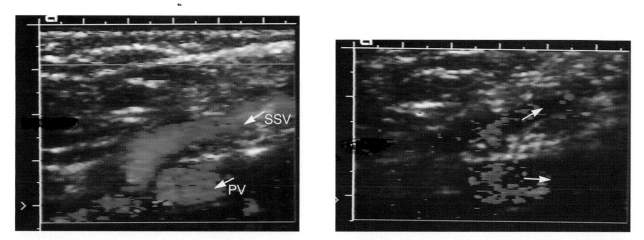

Figure 4.52 Short saphenous popliteal vein junction incompetence. During calf compression (left), colour-coded duplex Doppler ultrasound shows normal forward flow. When the compression is released (right), retrograde flow (coded red) occurs in the popliteal vein, through the sapheno-popliteal junction and down the short saphenous vein. PV, popliteal vein; SSV, short saphenous vein; → direction of blood flow.

overall accuracy in expert hands is claimed to be 80%, the positive test accuracy is 65%, the negative test accuracy is 95%, the sensitivity is 95% and the specificity is 85%,[390] but the published results are very variable, ranging from those quoted above to false-positive rates of 20–50%.[291,372] We find that Doppler techniques are unreliable for the detection of venous thrombosis below the level of the knee joint. Accuracy can be improved by combining Doppler ultrasound with other techniques such as pulse volumetry.[181]

The accuracy of the Doppler flow detector technique for detecting deep vein reflux has not been studied extensively because many investigators are not prepared to perform descending phlebograms on these patients. Studies using foot vein pressure measurements as the gold standard suggest that this technique has a high accuracy[309] but we do not believe that the ability to reduce foot vein pressure during exercise with and without a superficial vein occluding tourniquet is an acceptable gold standard for measuring deep or superficial vein reflux.

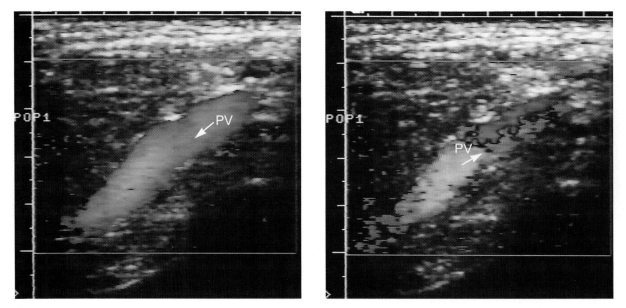

Figure 4.53 Demonstration of popliteal vein reflux with colour-coded Doppler duplex ultrasound. During calf compression (left), blood flows towards the heart (blue). When the compression is released (right) retrograde flow occurs (red) because the popliteal vein is incompetent. PV, popliteal vein; → direction of blood flow.

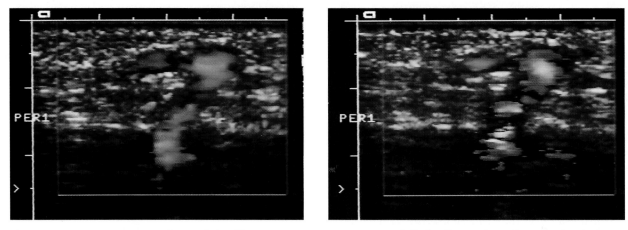

Figure 4.54 Incompetence of a medial calf communicating vein. At rest (left) the flow is from the superficial vein to the deep vein (coded blue). Compression of the upper part of the calf (right) reversed the direction of flow (coded red), confirming that the vein was incompetent.

Our unpublished experience comparing descending venography with Doppler flow detection has revealed a low accuracy rate. The inaccuracies of these techniques stem from our inability to define the precise site of insonation. This problem has been solved by the combination of B mode imaging and directional flow detection.

DUPLEX ULTRASOUND FLOW DETECTION

Duplex ultrasound (see also pages 78–87) provides an extremely accurate and sophisticated method for the assessment of deep vein valvular competence and the detection of incompetent communicating veins.[21,27,28,63,118,164,328,346,364,394,411] (see also Chapter 12).

Deep vein reflux is best assessed by using the colour coded technique to observe the direction of blood flow whilst the patient performs a Valsalva manoeuvre. Normally there is abrupt cessation of flow. Grade I reflux is defined as retrograde flow for 2 seconds, grade 2 for 2–3 seconds, grade 3 for 4–6 seconds and grade 4 is sustained for as long as the Valsalva manoeuvre is maintained. Reflux should be assessed in the femoral vein, both at the groin and in the mid-thigh, in the popliteal vein and in the long and short saphenous veins. The most common finding in patients with chronic venous insufficiency is reflux in both the superficial and the deep systems together with the changes of previous deep vein thrombosis.

Isolated deep reflux is uncommon.[297]

Duplex ultrasound had a predictive value to diagnose severe reflux of 77% compared to 35–44% for descending venography.[301] Another study using duplex ultrasound and ascending venography to assess valvular incompetence, found the accuracy of duplex ultrasound compared with venography to be 70–90% for the femoral, popliteal, and long and short saphenous veins, but only 55–66% for the calf veins.

Duplex ultrasound has been shown to be 80–95% accurate in the assessment of incompetent saphenofemoral and sapheno-popliteal communications, but only 40–63% accurate in assessing communicating vein incompetence.[328]

Duplex ultrasound has been shown to be more accurate in the overall assessment of deep and superficial vein insufficiency than photoplethysmography.[22,281]

PHLEBORHEOGRAPHY (PRG)

Phleborheography is a sophisticated form of whole leg plethysmography using multiple air-filled cuffs to detect the volume changes.[102,103]

Changes in limb blood volume may be caused by respiration and external compression. The fluctuations of volume with respiration, coincident with the flow variations detectable with the Doppler flow meter (see page 123) indicate patent veins. The orthograde transmission of a pulse of blood flow following a foot or calf squeeze also depends upon venous patency. Retrograde flow is prevented by competent valves. The changes of limb volume in response to these stimuli can provide much information about the state of the deep veins.

Method[103]

The patient lies supine on a couch with the legs below the level of the heart (approximately 10°).

This ensures that the limb veins are full of blood.

Pneumatic cuffs are placed around the chest and the lower third of the thigh. Three cuffs are then placed side by side around the upper half of the lower leg and another is placed around the foot – a total of six cuffs.

The cuffs are then inflated to 10 mmHg to ensure that they fit snugly in and around the contours of the limb.

The cuffs are calibrated by the removal of 0.2 ml air from each cuff, the amplification being adjusted so that this change causes a 2 cm deflection of the pen recorder. This is done to ensure that all six cuffs have the same sensitivity, and to allow comparisons between the traces of one patient obtained at different times and between different patients.

After the waveforms from all the cuffs have been recorded, the foot cuff is rapidly inflated three times to 50 mmHg to compress the foot and squeeze blood up the leg.

A similar compression stimulus is then applied to the lower of the calf cuffs or the thigh cuff. A similar technique may be used on the arm.[389]

Application

PRG detects occlusion of the major axial deep veins. It is therefore valuable for the diagnosis of major deep vein thrombosis. An occluded femoral vein will prevent the respiratory waves reaching the calf and will cause the calf volume to rise when the foot is squeezed.

By inflating the thigh cuff to 80 mmHg, the limb can be filled with blood and the time and rate of venous emptying and the maximum venous outflow can be calculated. This can indicate the degree of both acute and chronic venous occlusion, though a chronic occlusion only causes a positive test result when it is causing severe outflow obstruction.

PRG is not suitable for the assessment of superficial venous incompetence but can show retrograde flow in the deep veins if the lower calf expands in response to calf or thigh compression.

Accuracy

There have been many assessments of PRG as a diagnostic tool for deep vein thrombosis. When there is occlusive thrombus in a main axial vein the positive test accuracy is 95% and the negative test accuracy is 90%. A mathematical compilation of eight large studies by Cranley gave an overall accuracy of 92%, a sensitivity of 91% and a specificity of 93%.[93,102] In making this last analysis, however, Cranley, the originator of the method, excluded some of the data of one paper[74] because 56% of the patients studied had thrombus in small veins below

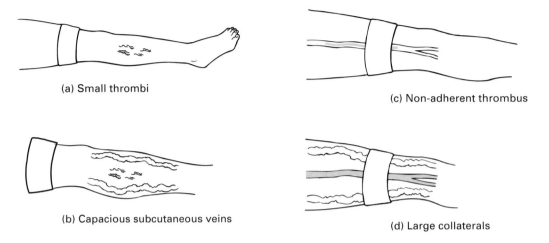

(a) Small thrombi

(c) Non-adherent thrombus

(b) Capacious subcutaneous veins

(d) Large collaterals

Figure 4.55 The reasons why all forms of plethysmography are unable to detect minor calf vein thrombosis. (a) Small thrombi affect neither capacitance nor outflow. (b) Large subcutaneous veins may mask a reduction of venous capacitance. (c) Non-adherent thrombus may not affect the rate of outflow. (d) Large subcutaneous collateral veins may compensate for a deep vein obstruction.

the knee, justifying this with the statement 'PRG cannot detect thrombus not in the mainstream, i.e. veins in the soleus muscle, the deep femoral, internal iliac and saphenous veins'. Many workers consider that this inability to detect thrombosis in small peripheral veins is a serious disadvantage of all forms of plethysmography, not just of PRG and Doppler flow detection (Figure 4.55).

The accuracy of all these methods in detecting thrombus in the calf is 50% or less. Non-occlusive non-obstructing thrombus in major veins may also be missed. The claims for a 90% accuracy must therefore be considered in the context of these exclusions. As a means of diagnosing all forms of venous thrombosis (90% of which is confined to the small calf veins) PRG is only approximately 60% accurate and it has a negative test accuracy of 60–70%.

False-positive readings are usually caused by muscle tension compressing veins in nervous patients – sedation or a change in posture usually corrects this abnormality.[100] Pregnancy also causes false-positive recordings.[306]

IMPEDANCE PLETHYSMOGRAPHY (IPG)

Impedance plethysmography can measure a change in the volume of blood within a limb from the associated change in tissue electrical resistance (impedance).[105,290] A current of low strength (1 mA) and high frequency (22 kHz) is passed through the limb between two circumferential electrodes. This current cannot be felt by the patient and is too high

to stimulate the nerves or muscles. Changes in voltage are recorded from two other electrodes (approximately 10 cm apart) placed inside the first two electrodes. The four electrodes are contained within two Velcro-covered bands. The tissue resistance is principally related to the volume of blood within it so that changes of venous filling and venous emptying can be easily assessed. Other factors which affect tissue impedance are relatively unimportant, and many studies using water, air and strain-gauge plethysmography (SGP) have confirmed the close relationship between tissue impedance and blood volume.

Method[426–428]

The patient lies supine with the hip and knee slightly flexed and the whole limb raised above heart level by elevating the foot of the bed or couch until it is tilted by 20°.

A wide (8 inch, 20 cm) pneumatic tourniquet is placed around the thigh, taking care not to compress the veins and cause distal venous distension. The electrodes are placed around the calf over a conductive jelly, the inner electrodes being approximately 10 cm apart. The chart recorder is adjusted so that an electrically induced 2% change in impedance produces a 5 mm deflection of the recorder.

The cuff is then inflated to 50 mmHg for 2 or 3 minutes, until the venous volume becomes constant. The cuff is then rapidly deflated.

This procedure is repeated four or five times because the ratio between filling and emptying may change as venous congestion alters the venous tone and as the patient relaxes. Ten per cent of normal tests become abnormal and 20% of abnormal tests become normal between the first and fifth inflations.[193,365,399]

False-positive readings are often caused by leg contractions. These subside with repeated testing. It has been suggested that muscle tone should be monitored with an electromyograph during testing.[59] The maximum venous capacitance and the maximum venous outflow in 3 seconds are then measured directly from the tracing in millimetres.

The results can be plotted on a prepared nomogram which indicates whether the ratio of venous volume to the rate of emptying is normal or abnormal.[428] An alternative nomogram gives the ratios for normal legs and legs with venous thrombosis, including the 95% confidence limits.[193]

Venous obstruction slows the rate of emptying disproportionately to the venous filling. Wheeler has also related the venous outflow measurements to the actual diameter of the proximal veins measured with ultrasound.[15,426] This has enabled him to indicate the percentage change in vein diameter that must have caused the observed increase of venous outflow obstruction. These studies suggest that an abnormal test indicates a lumen reduction greater than 50%.

Application and accuracy

Impedance plethysmography was widely used for diagnosing main axial vein thrombosis[16,98,197] but has now been replaced by duplex ultrasonography. Like all forms of plethysmography, it cannot detect thrombus in the calf muscle veins, deep femoral or internal iliac veins and will also miss non-obstructing non-adherent thrombi in large axial veins. IPG can claim the same degree of accuracy as phleborheography for major vein occlusion but is not as good at detecting calf vein thrombosis, though it becomes more accurate if repeated daily.[184] For proximal major vein thrombi the sensitivity and specificity are 95% and 90%, respectively, but for calf vein thrombi the figures are 40% and 85%, respectively.

IPG has not found a place in the investigation of chronic venous insufficiency.[248]

ISOTOPE PLETHYSMOGRAPHY

Isotope plethysmography is a technique which we developed principally for research, which measures the volume of blood within the calf by counting the radioactivity of the calf after labelling the red blood cells with technetium.[430,431]

If stannous pyrophosphate is injected into the bloodstream, it will adhere to the red cells and absorb any radioactive technetium that is subsequently injected. The label remains fixed to the red cells for 2 hours but does not damage them. Calf radioactivity then directly reflects the calf blood volume.

The advantage of this method is that calf blood volume can be measured during calf muscle exercise or passive compression, while the patient is standing, without causing the type of artefacts seen with photoplethysmography and strain-gauge plethysmography.

Method

Stannous pyrophosphate, 3 ml, is injected intravenously followed, 20 minutes later, by 15 mCi (55.5 × 10⁷ Bq) technetium-99m (pertechnate). The patient then stands on an exercise platform and a scintillation counter is loosely fixed to the back of the calf. Exercise is performed by depressing a foot pedal to raise a known weight to a fixed height at a specified rate; thus the work of the exercise is controlled and reproducible. The calf can also be squeezed passively by placing a large pneumatic tourniquet around the whole calf and inflating it to 90 mmHg. Superficial vein occluding tourniquets can be used to eliminate superficial reflux.

Application

This technique can measure the calf blood volume, the percentage expelled volume with exercise and passive compression, the rate of emptying during exercise and passive compression, and the rate of refilling following exercise or passive compression. All these measurements can be made with and without superficial vein occlusion and all can be expressed as a percentage of the total calf volume. These are measurements of calf pump efficiency, outflow obstruction and deep and superficial reflux, respectively. The method therefore measures more aspects of calf pump function than any other technique.

Isotope plethysmography has been tested against clinical assessment, phlebography and foot volumetry. There is general agreement between these tests when the diagnosis is simple but less correlation when there is a combination of abnormalities.

THE FLUORESCEIN TEST

The use of fluorescein to reveal the presence and site of incompetent communicating veins was described by us in 1970.[85] When fluorescein is injected into a foot vein below a tourniquet at the ankle tight enough to occlude the superficial veins, it ascends into the calf through the deep veins and then into the superficial veins if the communicating veins are incompetent. The point where it appears beneath the skin can be seen as a yellow fluorescent area if the leg is illuminated in a darkened room with ultraviolet light. When compared against phlebography, however, this method has a positive test accuracy of only 47%[313] and is no better than many other simpler and less invasive tests; it has never been adopted as a routine investigation.

Commentary

The precise value of the tests described in this chapter are discussed in later chapters when distinct conditions are being described. In the following paragraphs we have drawn together our views of the value of these tests in the clinical context of venous thrombosis and chronic venous insufficiency.

CLINICAL APPLICATION OF THE TESTS FOR DEEP VEIN THROMBOSIS

The clinician needs answers to the following questions.

1. Does the patient have a venous thrombosis?
2. Where is the thrombus?
3. How big is it?
4. Is it fresh or old (i.e. is it likely to fragment or is it stable)?
5. Is it adherent to the vein wall or firmly fixed? (i.e. is it able to float away if it fragments?)

The majority of the tests described in this chapter answer the first and second questions, in part, but do not answer the other three.

Does the patient have a venous thrombosis?

Physical signs are notoriously unreliable – the absence of signs is more unreliable than the presence of positive signs. The clinician cannot, however, afford to ignore anything that suggests the possibility of a thrombus, and therefore, even though it is known that 50% of patients with a tender calf do not have a thrombosis, they must be investigated further.

The simple bedside technique of ultrasound flow detection has serious limitations. Although good at detecting occlusive thrombi in major veins, it can miss non-occlusive thrombi in large veins and often miss small calf vein thrombi. Whilst it is worthwhile detecting adherent thrombi in large veins that may cause serious debilitating late post-thrombotic sequelae, it is more important to detect the non-adherent thrombi which are potentially lethal emboli, and the small calf vein thrombi which can cause serious calf pump damage.

This technique is therefore a useful screening test if the clinician is aware of its deficiencies and repeats the test daily so that any missed calf vein thrombus that extends into the popliteal vein is detected.

In view of these inadequacies most clinicians prefer to use one of the two methods that display the whole of the venous system of the lower limb – duplex ultrasonography or phlebology.

Where is the thrombus?

A test which does not provide an image cannot define the precise limits of a thrombus.

Most of the non-invasive methods can distinguish between popliteal vein and ilio-femoral vein occlusion but none reveals the exact anatomical position of the thrombus, or the presence of thrombus in other parallel veins.

Ultrasound or phlebographic imaging must be used if you wish to know the exact site of the thrombus.

What is the nature of the thrombus?

Phlebography and ultrasound imaging will give some answers to this question.

It is our considered view that the only method currently available in all hospitals that gives the maximum information about deep vein thrombosis is phlebography but as the number of clinicians and technicians skilled in the use of Duplex ultrasound grows, this method is rapidly becoming the investigation of choice.

If a patient has symptoms suggestive of pulmonary embolism, we believe that a full examination of the peripheral veins with ultrasound or phlebography is essential. No other investigations give the information about the site and nature of a thrombus necessary to determine the appropriate treatment. Recurrent pulmonary embolism may be fatal. It must be treated urgently on the basis of the best information available.

CLINICAL APPLICATION OF THE TESTS OF CHRONIC VENOUS INSUFFICIENCY

The clinician needs the answers to the following questions about a patient's chronic venous insufficiency, a condition which he is usually able to suspect following clinical examination.

1. Is there chronic venous insufficiency?
2. Are the superficial veins incompetent?
3. Where are the incompetent superficial-to-deep vein connections?
4. Are the deep veins incompetent?
5. Are the deep veins occluded and obstructing blood flow?

Is there chronic venous insufficiency?

Any of the tests of overall calf pump function will give a crude answer to this question – photoplethysmography, strain-gauge and air plethysmography, foot volumetry and foot vein pressures. In all patients with chronic venous insufficiency the fall of calf or foot vein volume or pressure that should accompany exercise is reduced.

Although direct pressure measurement is the gold standard, photoplethysmography is the simplest qualitative method and foot and air volumetry the simplest quantitative methods.

Superficial veins

All the tests of leg vein blood volume or pressure can be used to test superficial vein valve incompetence by performing the test with and without superficial vein occluding tourniquets, provided the tourniquets are properly applied and their effect checked with a hand held Doppler flow detector.

The precise site of an incompetent superficial-to-deep communicating vein must be deduced by combining the information given by the non-invasive tests about the level of the abnormality and a knowledge of the known anatomical sites of communication.

Doppler flow detection is the quickest and simplest way of demonstrating incompetence in individual superficial veins.

The confirmation of superficial vein incompetence by seeing retrograde blood flow during phlebography is very accurate but no better than Doppler flow detection, but the visualization of retrograde blood flow in incompetent communicating veins by phlebography or duplex ultrasound is a more accurate method of detection than the non-invasive techniques.

Deep vein incompetence

All types of plethysmography can be used to detect deep vein incompetence from measurements of refilling times, with and without superficial vein occlusion. Doppler ultrasound examination of the femoral and popliteal veins is extremely accurate and has replaced descending phlebography.

Deep vein obstruction

This can only be shown by a physiological test. The presence of occluded veins on an ultrasonogram or phlebograph does not mean that the venous outflow from the leg is obstructed, the collateral vessels may be more than adequate.

The physiological tests which reveal obstruction are the maximum venous outflow test (carried out by strain-gauge or air plethysmography), measurement of femoral vein pressures during exercise and foot volumetry during exercise. Femoral vein pressure studies give the best indication of iliac vein obstruction. Unfortunately, none of the other tests is able to detect mild or moderate degrees of obstruction below the groin.

In most patients the function of the calf veins can be assessed with one simple non-invasive test of calf pump function such as photoplethysmography, backed up by careful clinical examination and, careful duplex ultrasonography.

FINAL COMMENT

Chronic venous insufficiency is usually caused by a combination of valvular incompetence and organic or functional obstruction within the complex arrangement of superficial and deep veins of the lower limb.

The comparison of the calf pump with the heart, described in Chapter 3, may help our thinking and understanding but the latter will never be complete until we devise tests which unravel and measure each aspect of calf pump function.

All the function tests described in this chapter are affected simultaneously by more than one aspect of the peripheral circulation. For example, venous refilling is affected by valvular incompetence, passive vein resistance, active venous tone (itself affected by neurogenic and humoral influence), muscle tone, tissue tension and elasticity and arterial inflow. It is not surprising, therefore, that the results of our current testing often fail to distinguish between those with mild, moderate or severe disease[196,301] which they should if the severity of symptoms are a true indication of the severity of the underlying abnormality and if the abnormal function that our tests attempt to detect is the main abnormality.

The symptoms and signs of chronic venous insufficiency are seen in the skin and subcutaneous tissues as well as in the veins themselves. If the abnormality that leads to ulceration lies as much within the microcirculation, as a primary problem not secondary to an abnormality of calf pump function, then our present tests will only reveal part of the problem and never be able to indicate clearly which is the prime abnormality that needs correction.

So it is necessary always to be suspicious of the results of venous function tests. They should be used as aids to understanding and clinical decision but never relied on exclusively or against clinical judgement.

References

1. Abramowitz HB, Queral LA, Flinn WR, *et al.* The use of photoplethysmography in the assessment of venous insufficiency: a comparison to venous measurements. *Surgery* 1979; **86:** 434.
2. Abrams HL. The vertebral and azygos veins. In: Abrams HL, ed. *Abrams' Angiography*, 3rd edition. Boston, MA: Little Brown, 1983.
3. Ackroyd JS, Lea Thomas M, Browse NL. Deep vein reflux: an assessment by descending phlebography. *Br J Surg* 1986; **73:** 31.
4. Adolfsson L, Nordenfelt I, Olsson H, Torstensson I. Diagnosis of deep vein thrombosis with ^{99m}Tc plasmin. *Acta Med Scand* 1982; **211:** 365.
5. Akesson H, Brudin L, Jensen R, *et al.* Physiologic evaluation of venous obstruction in the post-thrombotic leg. *Phlebology* 1989; **4:** 3–14.
6. Albrechtsson U, Olsson CG. Thrombosis after phlebography: a comparison of two contrast media. *Cardiovasc Radiol* 1979; **2:** 9.
7. Albrechtsson U, Olsson CG. Thrombotic side effects of lower limb phlebography. *Lancet* 1976; **1:** 723.
8. Alderson PO, Martin EC. Pulmonary embolism: diagnosis with multiple imaging modalities. *Radiology* 1987; **64:** 297–312.
9. Alderson PO, Ruganavech N, Secker-Walker RH, McKnight RC. The role of ^{133}Xe ventilation studies in the scintigraphic detection of pulmonary embolism. *Radiology* 1976; **120:** 633.
10. Almen T. Contrast agent designs: some aspects of the synthesis of water soluble contrast agents of low osmolality. *J Theor Biol* 1969; **24:** 216.
11. Almen T, Aspelin P, Levin B. Effect of non-ionic contrast media on aortic and pulmonary arterial pressure. *Invest Radiol* 1975; **10:** 519.
12. Almen T, Nylander L. False signs of thrombosis in lower leg phlebography. *Acta Radiol* 1964; **2:** 345.
13. Almen T, Nylander L. Serial phlebography of the normal lower limb during muscular contraction and relaxation. *Acta Radiol* 1962; **57:** 264.
14. Alxesson H, Brudin L, Jensen R, *et al.* Physiologic evaluation of venous obstruction in the post thrombotic leg. *Phlebology* 1989; **4:** 3–14.
15. Anderson FA. Non-invasive quantification of the degree of venous outflow obstruction in the extremities by means of venous occlusion plethysmography.

In: Batel DL, ed. *Advances in Bioengineering*. New York: American Society of Mechanical Engineers, 1983.
16. Anderson FA Jr, Li JM, Wheeler HB. Application of impedance plethysmography to the detection of venous insufficiency. *Bruit* 1983; **7:** 41.
17. Andrews JC, Williams DM, Cho KJ. Digital subtraction venography of the upper extremity. *Clin Radiol* 1987; **38:** 423–4.
18. Ansell G. A national survey of radiological complications: interim report. *Clin Radiol* 1968; **19:** 175–91.
19. Ansell G. Fatal overdose of contrast medium in infants. *Br J Radiol* 1979; **43:** 395–6.
20. Appelman PT, De Long TE, Lampmann LE. Deep venous thrombosis of the leg: US findings. *Radiology* 1987; **163:** 743–6.
21. Araki CT, Back TL Jr, Padberg RVT, Thompson PN, Duran WN, II, Hobson RW. Refinements in the ultrasonic detection of popliteal vein reflux. *J Vasc Surg* 1993; **18:** 742–8.
22. Arnoldi CC. Venous pressure in patients with valvular incompetence of the veins of the lower limb. *Acta Chir Scand* 1966; **132:** 628.
23. Aronen MJ, Suedstrom E, Yrjani J, Bondestam S. Compression sonography in the diagnosis of deep venous thrombosis of the leg. *Ann Med* 1994; **26 (5):** 377–80.
24. Arora S, Lam DJK, Kennedy C, *et al.* Light reflection rheography. A simple non-invasive screening test for deep vein thrombosis. *J Vasc Surg* 1993; **18:** 767–72.
25. Atkins P, Hawkins LA. Detection of venous thrombosis in the legs. *Lancet* 1965; **2:** 1217.
26. Baker D. Application of pulsed Doppler techniques. *Radiol Clin North Am* 1980; **18:** 79–103.
27. Baker SR, Burnand KG, Sommerville KM, Lea Thomas M, Wilson NM, Browse NL. Comparison of venous reflux assessed by duplex scanning and descending phlebography in chronic venous disease. *Lancet* 1993; **341:** 400–3.
28. Baldt MM, Bohler K, Zontsich T, *et al.* Preoperative imaging of lower extremity varicose veins: color coded duplex sonography or venography. *J Ultrasound Med* 1996; **15(2):** 143–54.
29. Baldt MM, Zontsich T, Stumpflen A, *et al.* Deep venous thrombosis of the lower extremity: efficacy of spiral CT venography compared with conventional venography in diagnosis. *Radiology* 1996; **200:** 423–8.
30. Barloon TJ, Shunway JM, Warnock NG. An approach to radiologic quality assurance: analysis of medicolegal claims involving radiologic contrast-media-induced injury. *Acad Radiol* 1995; **2:** 1002–4.
31. Barner HB, DeWeese JA. An evaluation of the sphygmomanometer cuff pain test in venous thrombosis. *Surgery* 1960; **48:** 915.
32. Barnes RW. Doppler ultrasonic diagnosis of venous disease. In: Bernstein EF, ed. *Noninvasive Diagnostic Techniques in Vascular Disease*. St Louis, MO: CV Mosby, 1985.
33. Barnes RW, Collicot RE, Hummell BA, Slaymaker EE, Maixner W, Reinertson JE. Photoplethysmographic assessment of altered cutaneous circulation

in the post-phlebitic syndrome. *Proc Assoc Adv Med Instrum* 1978; **13**: 25.

34. Barnes RW, Collicott PE, Mozersky DJ, Sumner DS, Strandness DE Jr. Noninvasive quantitation of maximum venous outflow in acute thrombophlebitis. *Surgery* 1972; **72**: 971.

35. Barnes RW, Collicott PE, Mozersky DJ, Sumner DS, Strandness DE Jr. Noninvasive quantitation of venous reflux in the postphlebitic syndrome. *Surg Gynecol Obstet* 1913; **136**: 769.

36. Barnes RW, Collicott PE, Sumner DS, Strandness DE Jr. Noninvasive quantitation of venous hemodynamics in the postphlebitic syndrome. *Arch Surg* 1973; **107**: 807.

37. Barnes RW, Hokanson DE, Wu KK, Hoak JC. Detection of deep vein thrombosis with an automatic electrically calibrated strain gauge plethysmograph. *Surgery* 1977; **82**: 219.

38. Barnes RW, Ross EA, Strandness DE Jr. Differentiation of primary from secondary varicose veins by Doppler ultrasound and strain gauge plethysmography. *Surg Gynecol Obstet* 1975; **141**: 207.

39. Bashist B, Parisi A, Frager DH, Suster B. Abdominal CT findings when the superior vena cava, brachiocephalic vein, or subclavian vein is obstructed. *Am J Roentgenol* 1996; **167**: 1457.

40. Bauer G. A venographic study of thromboembolic problems. *Acta Chir Scand Suppl* 1940; **61**: 1–75.

41. Baxter GM, Duffy P. Calf vein anatomy and flow: implications for colour Doppler imaging. *Clin Radiol* 1992; **46**: 84–7.

42. Baxter GM, Duffy P, Mackechnie S. Colour Doppler ultrasound of the post phlebitic limb: sounding a note of caution. *Clin Radiol* 1991; **43**: 301–4.

43. Baxter GM, Duffy P, Partridge E. Colour flow imaging of calf vein thrombosis. *Clin Radiol* 1992; **46**: 198–201.

44. Baxter GM, McKenchnie S, Duffy P. Colour Doppler ultrasound in deep venous thrombosis: a comparison with venography. *Clin Radiol* 1990; **42**: 32–6.

45. Becker D, Gunter E, Cidlinsky K, *et al.* Diagnosis of phlebothrombosis using color-coded duplex sonography. A prospective comparison with phlebography. *Dtsch Med Wochenschr* 1994; **119(14)**: 495–500.

46. Becker J. The diagnosis of venous thrombosis in the legs using I-labelled fibrinogen: an experimental and clinical study. *Acta Chir Scand* 1972; **138**: 667.

47. Beesley WH, Fegan WG. An investigation into the localization of incompetent perforating veins. *Br J Surg* 1970; **57**: 30.

48. Bendick PJ. Pitfalls of the Doppler examination for venous thrombosis. *Am Surg* 1983; **49**: 320–3.

49. Berberich J, Hirsch S. Die rontgenographische darstellung der Arterien und Venen ani lebeneden Menschen. *Klin Wochenschr* 1923; **2**: 2226.

50. Berge T, Berquist D, Efsing HO, Hallbodk T. Local complications of ascending phlebography. *Clin Radiol* 1978; **29**: 691.

51. Bergin CJ, Rios G, King MA, *et al.* Accuracy of high resolution CT in identifying chronic pulmonary thromboembolic disease. *Am J Roentgenol* 1996; **166**: 1371–7.

52. Berlin L. Ionic versus nonionic contrast media. *Am J Roentgenol* 1996; **167**: 1095–7.

53. Bertelli G, Dini D, Forno GB, *et al.* Hyaluronidase as an antidote to extravasation of vinca alkaloids: clinical results. *J Cancer Res Clin Oncol* 1994; **120**: 505–6.

54. Beswick W, Chmiel R, Booth R, *et al.* Detection of deep venous thrombosis by scanning of 99m technetium-labelled red-cell venous pool. *Br Med J* 1979; **1**: 82–4.

55. Bettmann MA. Radiographic contrast agents – a perspective. *N Engl J Med* 1987; **317**: 891–2.

56. Bettmann MA, Robbins A, Braun SD, Wetzner S, Dunnick NR, Finkelstein J. Contrast venography of the leg: diagnostic efficacy, tolerance and complication rates with ionic and nonionic contrast media. *Radiology* 1987; **165**: 113–16.

57. Bettmann MA, Salzman EW, Rosenthal D, *et al.* Reduction of venous thrombosis complicating phlebography. *Am J Roentgenol* 1980; **134**: 1169.

58. Biello DR, Mattar AG, McKnight RC, Siegel BA. Ventilation perfusion studies in suspected pulmonary embolism. *Am J Roentgenol* 1979; **133**: 1033.

59. Biland L, Hull R, Hirsh J, Milner M. The use of electromyography to detect muscle contraction responsible for falsely positive impedance plethysmographic results. *Thromb Res* 1979; **14**: 811.

60. Bjordal RI. Pressure patterns in the saphenous system in patients with venous leg ulcers. *Acta Chir Scand* 1971; **137**: 495.

61. Bracey DW. Hazard of ultrasonic detection of deep vein thrombosis. *Br Med J* 1973; **1**: 420.

62. Bracey DW. Simple device for location of perforating veins. *Br Med J* 1958; **2**: 101.

63. Bradbury AW, Stonebridge PA, Callam MJ, *et al.* Recurrent varicose veins: assessment of the saphenofemoral junction. *Br J Surg* 1994; **81(3)**: 373–5.

64. Bradley DL, James EM, Welch TJ, Joyce JW, Hallett JW, Weaver AL. Diagnosis of acute deep venous thrombosis of the lower extremities: prospective evaluation of color Doppler flow imaging versus venography. *Radiology* 1994; **192**: 651–5.

65. Breslaw BH, Dorfman GS, Noto RB, *et al.* Ventilation/perfusion scanning for prediction of the location of pulmonary emboli: correlation with pulmonary angiographic findings. *Radiology* 1992; **185(P)**: 180.

66. Brodie BC. *Lectures Illustrative of Various Subjects in Pathology and Surgery.* London: Longman, 1846.

67. Brodie TG, Russell AK. On the deterimination of the rate of blood flow through an organ. *J Physiol (Lond)* 1905; **32**: 47.

68. Brown JN, Polak A. Hazard of ultrasonic detection of deep vein thrombosis. *Br Med J* 1973; **1**: 108.

69. Browse NL. The ^{125}I-fibrinogen uptake test. *Arch Surg* 1972; **104**: 160.

70. Browse NL. Venous pressure measurements. In: Bernstein EF, ed. *Non-invasive Diagnostic Techniques in Vascular Disease*. St Louis, MO: CV Mosby, 1985.

71. Browse NL, Clapham WF, Croft DN, Jones DJ, Lea Thomas M, Williams OJ. Diagnosis of established deep vein thrombosis with the ^{125}I fibrinogen uptake test. *Br Med J* 1971; **4**: 325.

72. Burnand KG, O'Donnell TF, Lea Thomas M, Browse NL. The relative importance of incompetent communicating veins in the production of varicose veins and venous ulcers. *Surgery* 1977; **82**: 9.

73. Bygdeman S, Aschberg S, Hindmarsh T. Venous plethysmography in the diagnosis of chronic venous insufficiency. *Acta Chir Scand* 1971; **137**: 423.

74. Bynum LJ, Wilson JE, Crotty CM, Curry TS, Smitson HL. Non-invasive diagnosis of deep venous thrombosis by phleborheography. *Ann Intern Med* 1978; **89**: 162.

75. Cameron JD. Pulmonary edema following drip-infusion urography. Case report. *Radiology* 1974; **111**: 89–90.

76. Carpenter JP, Holland GA, Bauma RA. Magnetic resonance venography for the detection of deep venous thrombosis: comparison with contrast venography and duplex Doppler ultrasonography. *JVIR* 1994; **5**: 535.

77. Carpenter JP, Holland GA, Baum RA. Magnetic resonance venography for the detection of deep venous thrombosis: comparison with contrast venography and duplex Doppler ultrasonography. *Radiology* 1994; **191**: 880.

78. Carpenter JP, Holland GA, Baum RA, Riley CA. Prelminary experience with magnetic resonance venography: comparison with findings at surgical exploration. *J Surg Res* 1994; **57**: 373–9.

79. Carpenter JP, Holland GA, Baum RA, Owen RS, Carpenter JT, Cope C. Magnetic resonance venography for the detection of deep venous thrombosis: comparison with contrast venography and duplex Doppler ultrasonography. *J Vasc Surg* 1993; **18**: 734–41.

80. Cauvain O, Remy-Jardin M, Remy J, *et al.* Spiral CT angiography in the diagnosis of central pulmonary embolism: comparison with pulmonary angiography and scintigraphy. *Rev Mal Respir* 1996; **13(2)**: 141–53.

81. Cavaye D, Kelly AT, Appleberg M, Briggs GM. Duplex ultrasound of lower limb deep venous thrombosis. *Aust N Z J Surg* 1990; **60**: 283–8.

82. Challoner AVJ. Photoelectric plethysmography for estimating cutaneous blood flow. In: Rolfe P, ed. *Non-invasive Physiological Measurements*. Vol. I. New York: Academic Press, 1979.

83. Charnsangavej C, Carrasco CH, Wallace S, *et al.* Stenosis of the vena cava: preliminary assessment of treatment with expandable metallic stents. *Radiology* 1986; **161**: 295–8.

84. Chevrier L. De l'examin aux reflux veineux dans les varices superficielles. *Arch Gen Chir* 1908; **2**: 44.

85. Chilvers AS, Thomas MH. Method for the localization of incompetent ankle perforating veins. *Br Med J* 1970; **2**: 577.

86. Christopolous D, Nicolaides AN. Air plethymosgraphy in the assessment of the calf muscle pump. *J Physiol* 1986; **374**: 11P.

87. Christopoulos D, Nicolaides AN, Szendro G. Venous reflux: quantification and correlation with the clinical severity of chronic venous disease. *Br J Surg* 1988; **75**: 352–6.

88. Coelho JC, Sigel B, Ryva JC, Machi J, Rerigers SA. B Mode sonography of blood clots. *JCU* 1982; **10**: 323.

89. Cogo A, Lensing AWA, Prandoni P, *et al.* Comparison of real-time B-mode ultrasonography and Doppler ultrasound with contrast venography in the diagnosis of venous thrombosis in symptomatic outpatients. *Thromb Haemost* 1993; **70**: 404–7.

90. Cohan RH, Dunnick NR, Leder RA, Baker ME. Extravasation of nonionic radiologic contrast media: efficacy of conservative treatment. *Radiology* 1990; **176**: 65–7.

91. Cohan RH, Ellis JH, Garner WL. Extravasation of radiographic contrast material: recognition, prevention, and treatment 1. *Radiology* 1996; **200**: 593–604.

92. Coleridge Smith JH, Scurr JH. Duplex scanning for venous disease. *Curr Pract Surg* 1995; **7**: 182–8.

93. Comerota AJ, Cranley JJ, Cook SE, Sipple P. Phleborheography: results of a ten-year experience. *Surgery* 1982; **91**: 573.

94. Connerta AJ, Katz ML, Hashemi HA. Venous duplex imaging for the diagnosis of acute venous thrombosis. *Haemostasis* 1993; **23(1)**: 61–71.

95. Cooke ED. Thermography. In: Nicolaides AN, Yao JST, eds. *Investigation of Vascular Disorders*. New York: Churchill Livingstone, 1981; 416.

96. Cooke ED, Bowcock SA. Investigation of chronic venous insufficiency by thermography. *Vasc Diagn Ther* 1982; **3**: 25.

97. Cooke ED, Pilcher MF. Deep vein thrombosis. Preclinical diagnosis by thermography. *Br J Surg* 1974; **61**: 971.

98. Cooperman M, Martin EW Jr, Satiani B, Clark M, Evans WE. Detection of deep venous thrombosis by impedance plethysmography. *Am J Surg* 1979; **137**: 252.

99. Corbett CR, McIrvine AJ, Aston NO, Jamieson CW, Lea Thomas M. The use of varicography to identify the sources of incompetence in recurrent varicose veins. *Ann R Coll Surg Engl* 1984; **66**: 412.

100. Cranley JJ. Air plethysmography in venous disease, the phleborheograph. In: Bernstein EF, ed. *Non-invasive Diagnostic Techniques in Vascular Disease*. St Louis, MO: CV Mosby, 1985.

101. Cranley JJ. Phleborheography in the diagnosis of deep venous thrombosis. In: Hershey FB, Barnes RW, Sumner DS, eds. *Non-invasive Diagnosis of Vascular Disease*. Pasadena: Appleton Davies, 1984.

102. Cranley JJ, Flanagan LD, Sullivan ED. Diagnosis of deep vein thrombosis by phleborheography. In: Bernstein EF, ed. *Non-invasive Diagnostic Techniques in Vascular Disease*. St Louis, MO: CV Mosby, 1985.

103. Cranley JJ, Gay AY, Grass AM, Simeone FA. A plethysmographic technique for the diagnosis of deep venous thrombosis of the lower extremities. *Surg Gynecol Obstet* 1973; **136:** 385.

104. Cranley JJ, Higgins RF, Berry RE, Ford CR, Comerota AJ, Griffen LH. Near parity in the final diagnosis of deep venous thrombosis by duplex scan and plebography. *Phlebology* 1989; **4:** 71–4.

105. Cremer H. Über die registrierung mechnischer voranje auf electrischen veg. speziell mit hilfa des salt engalvonometers und saitendektromelers. *MMW* 1907; **54:** 1629.

106. Cronan J, Gentone E, Hall R. Recurrent deep venous thrombosis. Limitations of ultrasound. *Radiology* 1989; **177:** 739–42.

107. Cronan JJ. Venous thromboembolic disease: the role of US. *Radiology* 1993; **186:** 619–30.

108. Cronan JJ, Froelich JA, Dorfman GS. Image directed Doppler ultrasound: a screening technique for patients at high risk to develop deep vein thrombosis. *JCU* 1991; **19:** 133–8.

109. Dahn I, Eiriksson E. Plethysmographic diagnosis of deep venous thrombosis of the leg. *Acta Chir Scand Suppl* 1968; **398:** 33.

110. Davidson BL, Elliott CG, Lensing AW. Low accuracy of color Doppler ultrasound in the detection of proximal leg vein thrombosis in asymptomatic high risk patients. *Ann Intern Med* 1992; **117:** 735–8.

111. Davidson BL, Elliott CG, Lensing AWA. Low accuracy of color Doppler ultrasound in the detection of proximal leg vein thrombosis in asymptomatic high risk patients. *Ann Intern Med* 1992; **117:** 735–8.

112. Davidson HC, Mazzu D, Gage BF, Jeffrey RB. Screening for deep venous thrombosis in asymptomatic postoperative orthopedic patients using color Doppler sonography: analysis of prevalence and risk factors. *Am J Roentgenol* 1996; **166:** 659–62.

113. Davies P, Roberts MB, Roylance J. Acute reactions to urographic contrast media. *Br Med J* 1975; **2:** 434–7.

114. Dawson P, Sidhu P. Is there a role for corticosteroid prophylaxis in patients at increased risk of adverse reactions to intravascular contrast agents? *Clin Radiol* 1993; **48:** 225–6.

115. Day TK, Fish PJ, Kakkar VV. Detection of deep vein thrombosis by Doppler angiography. *Br Med J* 1976; **1:** 618.

116. Deacon JM, Ell PJ, Anderson P, Khan O. Technetium 99m plasmin: a new test for the detection of deep vein thrombosis. *Br J Radiol* 1980; **53:** 673.

117. Dean RH. Radionuclide venography and simultaneous lung scanning: evaluation of clinical application. In: Bernstein EF, ed. *Non-invasive Diagnostic Techniques in Vascular Disease.* St Louis, MO: CV Mosby, 1978.

118. De Maeseneer MG, De Hert SG, Van Schil PE, Vanmaele RG, Eyskens EJ. Preoperative colour-coded duplex examination of the saphenopopliteal junction in recurrent varicosis of the short saphenous vein. *Cardiovasc Surg* 1993; **1(6):** 686–9.

119. De Weese JA, Rogoff SM. Functional ascending phlebography of the lower extremity by serial long film technique. *Am J Roentgenol* 1959; **81:** 841.

120. Dodd H, Cockett FB. *The Pathology and Surgery of the Veins of the Lower Limb.* Edinburgh: Livingstone, 1965.

121. Dohn K. Tilt phlebography; retrograde Phlebography by ascending injection. *Acta Radiol* 1958; **50:** 293.

122. Dosick SM, Blakemore WS. The role of Doppler ultrasound in acute deep vein thrombosis. *Am J Surg* 1978; **136:** 256–68.

123. Dow JD. Retrograde phlebography in major pulmonary embolism. *Lancet* 1973; **2:** 407.

124. Dresel S, Stabler A, Schiedler J, Holzknecht N, Tatsch K, Hahn K. Diagnostic approach in acute pulmonary embolism: perfusion scintigraphy versus spiral computed tomography. *Nucl Med Commun* 1995; **16(12):** 1009–15.

125. Dunnick NR. Patient outcome from ionic versus nonionic contrast agents (answer to question). *Am J Roentgenol* 1995; **164:** 1547.

126. Eiriksson E. Plethysmographic studies of venous diseases of the legs. *Acta Chir Scand* 1986; **Suppl 398**.

127. Elem B, Shorey BA, Lloyd Williams K. Comparison between thermography and fluorescein test in the detection of incompetent perforating veins. *Br Med J* 1971; **4:** 651.

128. Erdman WA, Jayson HT, Redman HC, Miller GL, Parkey RW, Peshock RW. Deep venous thrombosis of extremities: role of MR imaging in the diagnosis. *Radiology* 1990; **174:** 425–31.

129. Erdman WA, Peschock RM, Redman HC, *et al.* Pulmonary embolism: comparison of MR images with radionuclide and angiographic studies. *Radiology* 1994; **190(2):** 499–508.

130. Evans AJ, Sostman HD, Witty LA, *et al.* Detection of deep venous thrombosis: prospective comparison of MR imaging and sonography. *JMRI* 1996; **1:** 44–51.

131. Evans DS. The early diagnosis of thromboembolism by ultrasound. *Ann R Coll Surg Engl* 1971; **49:** 225.

132. Fernandes FJ, Homer J, Needham T, Nicolaides A. Ambulatory calf volume plethysmography in the assessment of venous insufficiency. *Br J Surg* 1979; **66:** 327.

133. Finn JP, Longmaid HE. Abdominal magnetic resonance venography. *Cardiovasc Intervent Radiol* 1992; **15:** 51–9.

134. Fischer M, Wupperman T. A new method of non-invasive estimation of ambulatory venous pressure. *Surgery* 1985; **97:** 247.

135. Fischer M, Wupperman T. Vergleich der Wertigkeit der Phlebodynamometrie mittels unblutiger Infrarot-Photoplethysmographie und blutiger Druckmessung. *Phlebol Proktol* 1982; **11:** 259.

136. Fischgold H, Adam H, Ecoiffier J, Plquet J. Opacification of spinal plexuses and azygos veins by osseus route. *J Radiol Electrol Med Nucl* 1952; **33:** 37.

137. Flanagan LD, Sullivan ED, Cranley JJ. Venous imaging of the extremities using real-time B mode ultrasound. In: Bergan JJ, Yao JST, eds. *Surgery of the Veins*. Orlando, FL: Grune & Stratton, 1985.

138. Flanc C, Kakkar VV, Clark MB. The detection of venous thrombosis of the legs using ^{125}I-labelled fibrinogen. *Br J Surg* 1968; **55:** 742.

139. Flanigan DP, Goodreau JJ, Burnham SJ, *et al.* Vascular laboratory diagnosis of clinically suspected acute deep vein thrombosis. *Lancet* 1978; **2:** 331–4.

140. Flemmer L, Chan JSL. A pediatric protocol for management of extravasation injuries. *Pediatr Nurs* 1993; **19:** 355–8.

141. Folse R, Alexander RH. Directional flow detection for localizing venous valvular incompetency. *Surgery* 1970; **67:** 114.

142. Francis CW, Foster TH, Totterman S, Brenner B, Marder VJ, Bryant RG. Monitoring of therapy for deep vein thrombosis using magnetic resonance imaging. *Acta Radiol* 1989; **30:** 445.

143. Froggatt DL, Tibbutt DA. Hazard of ultrasonic detection of deep vein thrombosis. *Br Med J* 1973; **1:** 614.

144. Gault DT, Extravasation injuries. *Br J Plast Surg* 1993; **46:** 91–6.

145. Gefter WB, Gupta KB, Holland GA. MR, CT enhance diagnosis of pulmonary emboli. *Diagn Imaging* 1993; **15:** 80–5.

146. Gefter WB, Hatabu H. Evaluation of pulmonary vascular anatomy and blood flow by magnetic resonance. *J Thorac Imaging* 1993; **8:** 122–36.

147. Geraghty JJ, Stanford W, Landas SK, Galvin JR. Ultrafast computed tomography in experimental pulmonary embolism. *Invest Radiol* 1992; **27:** 60–3.

148. Gibson RN. Lower limb deep venous thrombosis: a critical view of ultrasound. *Australas Radiol* 1995; **39:** 168–70.

149. Gill RW. Pulsed Doppler with B mode imaging for quantitative blood flow measurement. *Ultrasound Med Biol* 1979; **5:** 223–35.

150. Gillum RF. Pulmonary embolism and thrombophlebitis in the United States 1970-1985. *Am Heart J* 1987; **114:** 1262–4.

151. Goldhaber SZ. Recognition and management of pulmonary embolism. *Heart Dis Stroke* 1993; **2:**142–6.

152. Goodman LR, Curtin JJ, Mewissen MW, *et al.* Detection of pulmonary embolism in patients with unresolved clinical and scintigraphic diagnosis: helical CT versus angiography. *Am J Roentgenol* 1995; **164:** 1369–74.

153. Goodman LR, Lipchik RJ. Diagnosis of acute pulmonary embolism: time for a new approach. *Radiology* 1996; **199:** 25–7.

154. Gorney RL, Wheeler B, Belko JS, Warren R. Observations on the uptake of radioactive fibrinolytic enzyme by intravascular clots. *Ann Surg* 1963; **158:** 905.

155. Grady-Benson JC, Oishi CS, Hanson PB, Colwell CW, Otis SM, Walker RH. Routine postoperative duplex ultrasonography screening and monitoring for the detection of deep vein thrombosis. A survey of 110 total hip arthroplasties clinical orthopaedics and related research. *Clin Orthop* 1994; **307:** 130–41.

156. Grant EG. Sonography for deep vein thrombosis. *Am J Roentgenol* 1995; **164:** 257.

157. Greaves SM, Hart EM, Brown K, Young DA, Batra P, Aberle DR. Pulmonary thromboembolism: spectrum of findings on CT. *Am J Roentgenol* 1995; **165:** 1359–63.

158. Grist TM, Sostman HD, MacFall JR *et al.* Pulmonary angiography with MR imaging; preliminary clinical experience. *Radiology* 1993; **189:** 523–30.

159. Habscheid W, Hohmann M, Wilhelm T, Epping J. Real-time ultrasound in the diagnosis of acute deep venous thrombosis of the lower extremity. *Angiology* 1990; **41:** 599–608.

160. Haeger K. Problems of acute deep venous thrombosis. The interpretation of signs and symptoms. *Angiology* 1969; **20:** 219.

161. Haire WD, Lynch TG, Lund GB, Lieberman RP, Edney JA. Limitations of magnetic resonance imaging and ultrasound-directed (duplex) scanning in the diagnosis of subclavian vein thrombosis. *J Vasc Surg* 1991; **13:** 391–7.

162. Hallbook T, Gothlin J. Strain gauge plethysmography and phlebography in the diagnosis of deep venous thrombosis. *Acta Chir Scand* 1971; **137:** 37.

163. Hallbook T, Ling L. Pitfalls in plethysmographic diagnosis of deep venous thrombosis. *J Cardiovasc Surg* 1973; **14:** 427.

164. Hanrahan LM, Araki CT, Fisher JB, *et al.* Evaluations of the perforating veins of the lower extremity using high resolution duplex imaging. *J Cardiovasc Surg* 1991; **32:** 89–97.

165. Hatabu H, Gefter WB, Axel L, *et al.* MR imaging with spatial modulation of magnetization in the evaluation of chronic central pulmonary thromboemboli. *Radiology* 1994; **190:** 791–6.

166. Heckler FR. Current thoughts on extravasation injuries. *Clin Plast Surg* 1989; **16:** 557–63.

167. Heijboer H, Cogo A, Büller HR, Prandoni P, ten Cate JW. Detection of deep vein thrombosis with impedance plethysmography and real-time compression ultrasonography in hospitalized patients. *Arch Intern Med* 1992; **152(9):** 1901–3.

168. Hemingway AF. Venography. In: Grainger RG, Allison DJ, eds. *Diagnostic Radiology*. Edinburgh: Churchill Livingstone, 1986.

169. Henderson HP, Cooke ED, Bowcock SA, Hackett ME. After-exercise thermography for predicting postoperative deep vein thrombosis. *Br Med J* 1978; **1:** 1020.

170. Hennequin LM, Fade O, Fays JG, *et al.* Superior vena cava stent placement: results with wallstent endoprosthesis. *Radiology* 1995; **196:** 353–61.

171. Henschke CI, Mateescu I, Yankelvitz DF. Changing practice patterns in the workup of pulmonary embolism. *Chest* 1995; **107:** 940–5.

172. Hertzmann AB. The blood supply of various skin areas as estimated by the photo-electric plethysmograph. *Am J Physiol* 1938; **124:** 328.

173. Hirsh J, Genton E, Hall R. *Venous Thrombo-embolism*. New York: Grune & Stratton, 1981; 1–4.

174. Hirsh J, Hull RD. Thromboembolism: natural history, diagnosis and management. In: *Diagnosis of Venous Thrombosis*. Boca Raton, FL: CRC Press, 1987; 23–8.

175. Hirshfield JW. Low-osmolality contrast agents: who needs them? *N Engl J Med* 1992; **326:** 482–4.

176. Hobbs JT. Per-operative venography to ensure accurate sapheno-popliteal vein ligation. *Br Med J* 1980; **2:** 1578.

177. Hobbs JT, Davies JWL. Detection of venous thrombosis with ^{131}I-labelled fibrinogen in the rabbit. *Lancet* 1960; **2:** 134.

178. Hojensgard JC, Sturup H. Static and dynamic pressures in superficial and deep veins of the lower extremity in man. *Acta Physiol Scand* 1953; **27:** 49.

179. Holm JSE. A simple plethysmographic method for differentiating primary from secondary varicose veins. *Surg Gynecol Obstet* 1976; **143:** 609.

180. Holmes MCG. Deep venous thrombosis of the lower limbs diagnosed by ultrasound. *Med J Aust* 1973; **4:** 210–11.

181. Howe HR, Hansen KJ, Plonk GW. Expanded criteria for the diagnosis of deep vein thrombosis. Use of the pulse volume recorder and Doppler ultrasonography. *Arch Surg* 1984; **119:** 1167.

182. Hudson ER, Smith TP, McDermott VG, *et al.* Pulmonary angiography performed with iopamidol: complications in 1,434 patients. *Radiology* 1996; **198(1):** 61–5.

183. Huisman MV, Büller HR, ten Cate JW, *et al.* Management of clinically suspected acute venous thrombosis in outpatients with serial impedance plethysmograpy in a community hospital setting. *Arch Intern Med* 1989; **149:** 511–13.

184. Huisman MV, Buller HR, Cate JW, Vrecken J. Serial impedance plethysmography for suspected deep venous thrombosis in out patients. *N Engl J Med* 1986; **314:** 823–9.

185. Huisman MU, Buller HR, Ten Cate JW, *et al.* Unexpected high prevalence of silent pulmonary embolism in patients with deep vein thrombosis. *Chest* 1989; **95:** 498–502.

186. Hull RD, Carter CJ, Jay RM. The diagnosis of acute recurrent deep-vein thrombosis: a diagnostic challenge. *Circulation* 1983; **67:** 901–6.

187. Hull RD, Feldstein W, Pineo GF, Raskob GE. Cost effectiveness of diagnosis of deep vein thrombosis in symptomatic patients. *Thromb Haemost* 1995; **74(1):** 189–96.

188. Hull RD, Hirsh J, Carter CJ, *et al.* Diagnostic efficacy of impedance plethysmography for clinically suspected deep vein thrombosis: a randomised trial. *Ann Intern Med* 1985; **102:** 21–6.

189. Hull RD, Hirsh J, Sackett DL, *et al.* Clinical validity of a negative venogram in patients with clinically suspected venous thrombosis. *Circulation* 1981; **64:** 622–5.

190. Hull R, Hirsh J, Sackett DL, Powers P, Turpie AG, Walker I. Combined use of leg scanning and impedance plethysmography in suspected venous thrombosis. An alternative to venography. *N Engl J Med* 1977; **296:** 1497.

191. Hull R, Hirsh J, Sackett DL, *et al.* Replacement of venography in suspected venous thrombosis by impedance plethysmography and ^{125}I-fibrinogen leg scanning: a less invasive approach. *Ann Intern Med* 1981; **94:** 12.

192. Hull RD, Secker-Walker RH, Hirsh J. Diagnosis of deep vein thrombosis. In: *Hemostasis and Thrombosis*. Philadelphia, PA: Lippincott, 1987; 1220–39.

193. Hull R, Taylor DW, Hirsh J, *et al.* Impedance plethysmography: the relationship between venous filling and sensitivity and specificity for proximal vein thrombosis. *Circulation* 1978; **58:** 898.

194. Hull R, van Aken WG, Hirsh J, *et al.* Impedance plethysmography using the occlusive cuff technique in the diagnosis of venous thrombosis. *Circulation* 1976; **53:** 696.

195. Hyman C, Winsor T. History of plethysmography. *J Cardiovasc Surg* 1961; **2:** 506.

196. Iafrati MD, Welch H, O'Donnell F, Belkin M, Vumphrey S, McLaughlin R. Correlation of venous non-invasive tests with the Society of Vascular Surgery / International Society for Cardiovascular Surgery) clinical classification of chronic venous insufficiency. *J Vasc Surg* 1994; **19:** 1001–7.

197. Irvine AT, Burnand KG, Lea Thomas M. Arteriography. *Curr Pract Surg* 1996; **8:** 72–83.

198. Irvine AT, Thomas ML. Colour-coded duplex sonography in the diagnosis of deep vein thrombosis: a comparison with phlebography. *Phlebology* 1991; **6:** 103–9.

199. Jacobson PD, Rosenquist CJ. The diffusion of low osmolality contrast agents: technological change and defensive medicine. Rand Corporation Report, Washington, DC: Office of Technology Assessment, 1994, DRU 826-OTA.

200. Johnston KW, Kakkar VV. Plethysmographic diagnosis of deep vein thrombosis. *Surg Gynecol Obstet* 1974; **138:** 41.

201. Jongbloets LM, Lensing AW, Koopman MM, Büller HR, ten Cate JW. Limitations of compression ultrasound for the detection of symptomless postoperative deep vein thrombosis. *Lancet* 1994; **343:** 1142–4.

202. Kakkar VV. The diagnosis of deep vein thrombosis using the ^{125}I-fibrinogen test. *Arch Surg* 1972; **104:** 152.

203. Kakkar VV, Nicolaides AN, Renney JT, Friend JR, Clarke MB. ^{125}I-labelled fibrinogen test adapted for routine screening for deep-vein thrombosis. *Lancet* 1970; **1:** 540.

204. Kalbhen CL, Pierce KL. Fast CT scanning: applications of helical and electron beam CT. *Appl Radiol* 1993; **22:** 47–51.

205. Kanterman RY, Witt PD, Hsieh PS, Picus D. Klippel–Trenaunay syndrome: imaging findings and percutaneous intervention. *Am J Roentgenol* 1996; **167:** 989–95.

206. Kempczinski RF, Berlatzky Y, Pearce WH. Semiquantitative photoplethysmography in the

diagnosis of lower extremity venous insufficiency. *J Cardiovasc Surg* 1986; **27:** 17.

207. Kempi V, van der Linden W. Diagnosis of deep vein thrombosis with in vivo 99mTc labelled red blood cells. *Eur J Nucl Med* 1981; **6:** 5–9.

208. Keogan MT, Paulson EK, Paine SS, Hertzberg BS, Carroll BA. Bilateral lower extremity evaluation of deep venous thrombosis with color flow and compression sonography. *J Ultrasound Med* 1994; **13:** 115–18.

209. Kistner RL. Surgical repair of the incompetent femoral vein valve. *Arch Surg* 1975; **110:** 1336.

210. Kistner RL. Transvenous repair of the incompetent femoral vein valve. In: Bergan JJ, Yao JST, eds. *Venous Problems.* Chicago, IL: Year Book Medical Publishers Inc., 1978.

211. Kistner RL, Kamida CB. 1994 update on phlebography and varicography. *Dermatol Surg* 1995; **21(1):** 71–6.

212. Kliewer MA, Sandridge BK, Hertzberg BS, Bowie JD. Deep vein thrombosis: value of self augmentation US evaluation. *Radiology* 1994; **190:** 576–9.

213. Kolecki RV, Sigel B, Justin J, *et al.* Determining the acuteness and stability of deep venous thrombosis by ultrasonic tissue characterization. *J Vasc Surg* 1995; **21:** 976–84.

214. Koopman MMW, Van Beek EJR, Ten Cate JW. Diagnosis of deep vein thrombosis. *Prog Cardiovasc Dis* 1994; **37:** 1–12.

215. Kriessmann A. Ambulatory venous pressure measurements. In: Nicolaides AN, Yao JST, eds. *Investigation of Vascular Disorders.* New York: Churchill Livingstone, 1981.

216. Kristo DA, Perry ME, Kollef MH. Comparison of venography, duplex imaging, and bilateral impedance plethysmography for diagnosis of lower extremity deep vein thrombosis. *South Med J* 1994; **87(1):** 55–60.

217. Laissy JP, Cinqualbre A, Loshkajian A, *et al.* Assessment of deep venous thrombosis in the lower limbs and pelvis: MR venography vs duplex Doppler sonography. *Am J Roentgenol* 1996; **167:** 971–5.

218. Lalli AF. Urography, shock reaction and repeated urography. *Am J Roentgenol* 1975; **125:** 264–8.

219. Lambe HA, Hopper KD, Matthews MA. Use of informed consent for ionic and nonionic contrast media. *Radiology* 1992; **184:** 145–8.

220. Lambie JM, Mahaffy RG, Barber DC, Karmody AM, Scott MM, Matheson NA. Diagnostic accuracy in venous thrombosis. *Br Med J* 1970; **2:** 142.

221. Lasser E, Berry C, Talner L, *et al.* Pre-treatment with corticosteroids to alleviate reactions to intravenous contrast material. *N Engl J Med* 1987; **317:** 845–9.

222. Lausen I, Jensen R, Wille-Jorgensen P, *et al.* Colour Doppler flow imaging ultrasonography versus venography as screening method for asymptomatic postoperative deep venous thrombosis. *Eur J Radiol* 1995; **20(3):** 200–4.

223. Lawrence D, Kakkar VV. Venous pressure measurement and foot volumetry in venous disease. In:

Verstraete M. *Techniques in Angiology.* The Hague: Martinus Nijhoff, 1979.

224. Lea Thomas M. *Phlebography of the Lower Limb.* Edinburgh: Churchill Livingstone, 1982.

225. Lea Thomas M. Pelvic phlebography. In: McLaren JW, ed. *Modern Trends in Diagnostic Radiology.* London: Butterworths, 1970; 201–9.

226. Lea Thomas M. An improved intraosseous phlebography cannula. *Br J Radiol* 1969; **42:** 395.

227. Lea Thomas M. Gangrene following peripheral phlebography of the legs. *Br J Radiol* 1970; **43:** 528.

228. Lea Thomas M. Phlebography of the limb veins. In: Partridge JB, ed. *A Textbook of Radiological Diagnosis.* Vol. 2, 5th edition. London: HK Lewis, 1985.

229. Lea Thomas M. *Phlebography of the Lower Limb.* Edinburgh: Churchill Livingstone, 1982.

230. Lea Thomas M. Pulmonary angiography. In: Dodd H, Cockett FB, eds. *The Pathology and Surgery of the Veins of the Lower Limbs.* Edinburgh: Churchill Livingstone, 1976.

231. Lea Thomas M, Bowles J N. Descending phlebography in the assessment of long saphenous vein incompetence. *Am J Roentgenol* 1985; **145:** 1255.

232. Lea Thomas M, Bowles JN. Incompetent perforating veins. Comparison of varicography and ascending phlebography. *Radiology* 1985; **154:** 619.

233. Lea Thomas M, Briggs GM. Low osmolality contrast media for phlebography. *Int Angiol* 1984; **3:** 73.

234. Lea Thomas M, Browse NL. Internal iliac vein thrombosis. *Acta Radiol* 1972; **12:** 660.

235. Lea Thomas M, Carty H. The appearances of artefacts on lower limb phlebograms. *Clin Radiol* 1975; **26:** 527.

236. Lea Thomas M, Keeling FP. Varicography in the management of recurrent varicose veins. *Angiology* 1986; **37:** 570.

237. Lea Thomas M, Keeling FP, Ackroyd JS. Descending phlebography: a comparison of three methods and an assessment of the normal range of deep vein reflux. *J Cardiovasc Surg* 1986; **22:** 27.

238. Lea Thomas M, MacDonald LM. Complications of ascending phlebography of the leg. *Br Med J* 1978; **2:** 317.

239. Lea Thomas M, MacDonald L. The accuracy of bolus ascending phlebography in demonstrating the ilio-femoral segment. *Clin Radiol* 1977; **28:** 165.

240. Lea Thomas M, Macfie GB. Phlebography in the Klippel–Trenaunay syndrome. *Ann Surg* 1974; **162:** 303.

241. Lea Thomas M, McAllister V. The radiological progression of deep vein thrombosis. *Radiology* 1971; **99:** 37.

242. Lea Thomas M, McAllister V, Rose DH, Tonge K. A simplified technique for phlebography for the localization of incomplete perforating veins of the legs. *Clin Radiol* 1972; **23:** 486.

243. Lea Thomas M, O'Dwyer JA. A phlebographic study of the incidence and significance of venous thrombosis. *Am J Roentgenol* 1978; **130:** 751.

244. Lea Thomas M, Posniak HV. Saphenography. *Am J Roentgenol* 1983; **141:** 812.

245. Lea Thomas M, Posniak HV. Varicography. *Int Angiol* 1985; **4:** 475.

246. Lea Thomas M, Tighe JR. Death from fat embolism, a complication of intraosseous phlebography. *Lancet* 1973; **2:** 1415.

247. Leclerc JR, Wolfson T, Rush C, *et al.* The role of Tc-99m red blood cell (RBC) venography in patients with clinically suspected deep vein thrombosis. *J Nucl Med* 1987; **28:** 649 (Abstr).

248. Lee BY, Kavner D, Thoden WR, Trainor FS, Lewis JM, Madden JL. Technique of venous impedance plethysmography for quantitation of venous reflux. *Surg Gynecol Obstet* 1982; **154:** 49.

249. Lensing AWA, Buller HR, Prandoni P. Contrast venograpy, the gold standard for the diagnosis for deep vein thrombosis: improvement in observer agreement. *Thromb Haemost* 1992; **67:** 8–12.

250. Lensing AWA, Levi MM, Büller HR, *et al.* An objective Doppler method for the diagnosis of deep vein thrombosis. *Ann Intern Med* 1990; **113:** 9–14.

251. Lensing AWA, Prandoni P. Distribution of venous thrombi in symptomatic patients. *Thromb Haemost* 1991; **65:** 1176(abstr).

252. Lensing AWA, Prandoni P, Brandjes D, *et al.* Detection of deep vein thrombosis by real-time B-mode ultrasonography. *N Engl J Med* 1989; **320:** 342–5.

253. Lewis BD, James EM, Welch TJ, Joyce JW, Hallett JW, Weave AL. Diagnosis of acute deep venous thrombosis of the lower extremities: prospective evaluation of color Doppler flow imaging versus venography. *Radiology* 1994; **192:** 651–5.

254. Lindblad B, Sternby NH, Bergquist D. Incidence of venous thromboembolism. Verified by necropsy over 30 years. *Br Med J* 1991; **302:** 709–12.

255. Lisbona R, Stern J, Derbekyan V. 99mTc red blood cell venography in deep vein thrombosis of the leg: a correlation with contrast venography. *Radiology* 1982; **143:** 771–3.

256. Littlejohn GO, Brand CA, Ada A, *et al.* Popliteal cysts and deep venous thrombosis. Tc99m red blood cell venography. *Radiology* 1985; **155:** 237–40.

257. Lohr JM, Hasselfeld KA, Byrne MP, Deshmuki RM, Cranley JJ. Does the asymptomatic limb harbor deep venous thrombosis? *Am J Surg* 1994; **168:** 184–7.

258. Lomas DJ, Britton PD. CT demonstration of acute and chronic iliofemoral thrombosis. *J Comput Assist Tomogr* 1991; **15:** 861–2.

259. Losch W, Beyer-Enke S, Rompel O, Schlick J, Zeitler E. Color-coded duplex sonography (angiodynography) in comparison with phlebography. *Bildgebung* 1993; **60(4):** 297–300.

260. Loth TS, Jones DEC. Extravasations of radiographic contrast material in the upper extremity. *J Hand Surg (Am)* 1988; **13:** 395–8.

261. Loubeyre P, Revel D, Douek P, *et al.* Dynamic contrast-enhanced MR angiography of pulmonary embolism; comparison with pulmonary angiography. *Am J Roentgenol* 1994; **162:** 1035–9.

262. Lowenberg RI. The sphygmomanometer cuff pain test. *Community Med* 1958; **22:** 287.

263. Ludbrook J. *Aspects of Venous Function in the Lower Limbs.* Springfield, IL: Charles C Thomas, 1966.

264. Lynn TN, Blakenship JB, Bottomley R. Semiquantified constriction of the leg; a test for deep venous thrombosis. *Geriatrics* 1963; **18:** 713.

265. MacFall JR, Sostman HD, Wu JJ, *et al.* MR imaging of pulmonary embolism in a dog model with 3D white blood fast gradient-echo sequences. *Radiology* 1992; **185(P):** 217.

266. MacKay IFS, McCathy G. Measurement of valvular competence in the legs. *J Appl Physiol* 1957; **12:** 329–33.

267. Malins AF. Pulmonary oedema after radiological investigation of peripheral occlusive vascular disease. Adverse reaction to contrast media. *Lancet* 1978; **1:** 413–15.

268. Markel A, Weich Y, Gaitini D. Doppler ultrasound in the diagnosis of venous thrombosis. *J Vasc Dis* 1995; **6(1):** 65.

269. Martin PH, Carver N, Petros AJ. Use of liposuction and saline washout for the treatment of extensive subcutaneous extravasation of corrosive drugs. *Br J Anaesth* 1994; **72:** 702–4.

270. Mathieson FR. Tilt phlebography of normal legs. *Acta Radiol* 1958; **50:** 493.

271. Mattos MA, Londrey GL, Leutz DW, *et al.* Color-flow duplex scanning for the surveillance and diagnosis of acute deep venous thrombosis. *J Vasc Surg* 1992; **15:** 366–76.

272. Mavor G, Galloway JMD. The ilio-femoral segment as a source of pulmonary emboli. *Lancet* 1967; **1:** 871.

273. May R. Thrombophlebitis nach Phlebographic. *Vasa* 1977; **6:** 169.

274. May R, DeWeese JA. Surgery of the pelvic veins. In: May R, ed. *Surgery of the Veins of the Legs and Pelvis.* Stuttgart: Georg Thieme, 1974.

275. McAllister WH, Palmer K. The histological effects of four commonly used contrast media for excretory urography and an attempt to modify the response. *Radiology* 1971; **99:** 511.

276. McAllister WH, Siegel MJ, Shackeford GD. Pulmonary edema following intravenous urography in a neonate. *Br J Radiol* 1979; **52:** 410.

277. McBride KD, Gaines PA, Beard JD. Pneumatic phlebography: a possible new technique for the assessment of recurrent varicose veins. *Eur J Radiol* 1993; **17(2):** 101–5.

278. McClennan BL, Stolberg HO. Intravascular contrast media: ionic versus nonionic – current status. *Radiol Clin North Am* 1991; **29:** 437–54.

279. McIrvine AJ, Corbett CCR, Aston NO, Sherriff EA, Wiseman PA, Jamieson CW. The demonstration of saphenofemoral incompetence. Doppler ultrasound compared with standard clinical tests. *Br J Surg* 1984; **71:** 509.

280. McLachlin J, Richards T, Paterson JC. An evaluation of clinical signs in the diagnosis of venous thrombosis. *Arch Surg* 1962; **85:** 738.

281. McMullin GM, Scott HJ, Coleridge Smith PD, Scurr JH. A comparison of photoplethysmography,

Doppler ultrasound and duplex scanning in the assessment of venous insufficiency. *Phlebology* 1989; **4**: 75–82.

282. McPheeters HO, Rice CO. Varicose veins – the circulation and direction of the venous flow. *Surg Gynecol Obstet* 1929; **49**: 29.

283. Meaney TF, Weinstein MA. Digital subtraction angiography. In: Grainger RG, Allison DJ, eds. *Diagnostic Radiology*. Edinburgh: Churchill Livingstone, 1986.

284. Medway J, Nicholaides AN, Walker CJ, *et al.* Value of Doppler ultrasound in diagnosis of clinically suspected deep vein thrombosis. *Br Med J* 1975; **4**: 552–4.

285. Memolo M, Dyer R, Zagoria RJ. Extravasation injury with nonionic contrast material. *Am J Roentgenol* 1993; **160**: 203.

286. Mesereau WA, Robertson HR. Observations on venous endothelial injury following the injection of venous radiographic contrast media in the rat. *J Neurosurg* 1961; **18**: 289.

287. Meyers S, Neiman HL, Mintzer RA. Pulmonary angiography. In: Neiman HL, Yao JST, eds. *Angiography of Vascular Disease*. New York: Churchill Livingstone, 1985.

288. Miles C, Nicolaides AN. Photophlethysmography: principles and development. In: Nicolaides AN, Yao JST, eds. *Investigation of Vascular Disorders*. New York: Churchill Livingstone, 1981; 501.

289. Miles C, Nicolaides AN. Photoplethysmography: principles and development. In: Nicolaides AN, Yao JST, eds. *Investigation of Vascular Disorders*. New York: Churchill Livingstone, 1981; 516.

290. Miller SS, Foote AV. The ultrasonic detection of incompetent perforating veins. *Br J Surg* 1974; **61**: 653.

291. Milne RM, Gunn A, Griffiths JMT, Ruckley CV. Postoperative deep vein thrombosis, a comparison of diagnostic techniques. *Lancet* 1971; **2**: 445.

292. Molitor H, Kniajuk M. A new bloodless method for continuous recording of peripheral circulatory changes. *J Pharmacol Exp Ther* 1936; **57**: 6.

293. Morrison J, Rubin DA, Tomaino MM. Venous aneurysm of the distal forearm. MR imaging findings. *Am J Roentgenol* 1996; **167**: 1552–4.

294. Mostafa A, Herba MJ, Reinhold C, *et al.* Accuracy of sonography in the evaluation of calf deep vein thrombosis in both postoperative surveillance and symptomatic patients. *Am J Roentgenol* 1996; 166: 1361–7.

295. Mullick S, Wheeler H, Songster G. Diagnosis of deep venous thrombosis by measurement of electrical impedance. *Am J Surg* 1970; **119**: 417.

296. Muto P, Lastoria S, Varella P, *et al.* Detecting deep venous thrombosis with technetium-99m-labeled synthetic peptide P280. *J Nucl Med* 1995; **36(8)**: 1384–91.

297. Myers KA, Ziegenbein RW, Zeng GH, Matthews PG. Duplex ultrasonograpy scanning for chronic venous disease: patterns of venous reflux. *J Vasc Surg* 1995; **21(4)**: 605–12.

298. Nachbur B. Die periphere Venendruckmessung: eine Methode zur Bestimmung der vendsen Leistungsreserve der unteren Extremitaten. *Zentralbl Phlebol* 1971; **10**: 224.

299. Naidich JB, Torre JR, Pellerito JS, Smalberg IS, Kase DJ, Crystal KS. Suspected deep venous thrombosis: is US of both legs necessary? *Radiology* 1996; **200**: 429–31.

300. Nanson EM, Palko PD, Dick AA, Fedoruk SO. Early detection of deep venous thrombosis of the legs using human fibrinogen. A clinical study. *Ann Surg* 1965; **162**: 438.

301. Neglen P, Raju S. A comparison between descending phlebography and duplex Doppler investigation in the evaluation of reflux in chronic venous insufficiency: a challenge to phlebography as the 'gold standard'. *J Vasc Surg* 1992; **16(5)**: 687–93.

302. Neglen P, Raju S. A rational approach to detection of significant reflux with duplex Doppler scanning and air plethysmography. *J Vasc Surg* 1993; **17**: 590–5.

303. Negus D, Cockett FB. Femoral vein pressures in post-phlebitic vein obstruction. *Br J Surg* 1967; **54**: 522.

304. Negus D, Edwards JM, Kinmonth JB. The iliac veins in relation to lymphoedema. *Br J Surg* 1969; **56**: 481.

305. Negus D, Pinto DJ, Le Quesne LP, Brown N, Chapman H. ^{125}I-labelled fibrinogen in the diagnosis of deep vein thrombosis and its correlation with phlebography. *Br J Surg* 1968; **55**: 835.

306. Nicholas GG, Loreny RP, Botti JJ, Chez RA. The frequent occurrences of false positive results in phleboreography during pregnancy. *Surg Gynecol Obstet* 1985; **161**: 133.

307. Nicolaides A, Hoare M, Miles C. The value of ambulatory venous pressure in the assessment of venous insufficiency. *Vasc Diagn Ther* 1982; **3**: 41.

308. Nicolaides AN, Fernandes JF, Schull K, Miles C. Calf volume plethysmography. In: Nicolaides AN, Yao JST, eds. *Investigation of Vascular Disorders*. New York: Churchill Livingstone, 1981.

309. Nicolaides AN, Fernandes JF, Zimmerman H. Doppler ultrasound in the investigation of venous insufficiency. In: Nicolaides AN, Yao JST, eds. *Investigation of Vascular Disorders*. New York: Churchill Livingstone, 1981.

310. Nicolaides AN, Miles C. Photoplethysmography in the assessment of venous insufficiency. *J Vasc Surg* 1987; **5(3)**: 405–12.

311. Nicolaides AN, Olsson CG. The 99mTc plasmin test. In: Bernstein EF, ed. *Non-invasive Diagnostic Techniques in Vascular Disease*. St Louis, MO: CV Mosby, 1985.

312. Nielson PE, Kirchner PT, Gerber GH. Oblique views in lung perfusion scanning; Clinical utility and limitations. *J Nucl Med* 1977; **18**: 967.

313. Noble J, Gunn AA. Varicose veins. Comparative study of methods for detecting incompetent perforators. *Lancet* 1972; **1**: 1253.

314. Norgren L. Functional evaluation of chronic venous insufficiency by foot volumetry. *Acta Chir Scand* 1973; **Suppl 444**.

315. Norris CS, Beyrau A, Barnes RW. Quantitative photoplethysmography in chronic venous insuffi-

ciency: a new method of noninvasive estimation of ambulatory venous pressure. *Surgery* 1983; **94**: 758.

316. Novelline RA, Baltarowich OH, Athanasoulis CA, *et al*. The clinical course of patients with suspected pulmonary embolism and a negative pulmonary arteriogram. *Radiology* 1978; **126**: 561–7.

317. Nylander G. Phlebographic diagnosis of acute deep leg thrombosis. *Acta Chir Scand* 1968; **397 (suppl)**: 30.

318. O'Leary DH, Kane RA, Chase BM. A prospective study of the efficacy of B-scan sonography in the detection of deep venous thrombosis in the lower extremities. *JCU* 1988; **16**: 1–8.

319. Palko PD, Nauson EM, Fedornk SO. The early detection of deep venous thrombosis using ^{131}I tagged human fibrinogen. *Can J Surg* 1964; **7**: 215.

320. Parsons RE, Sigel B, Feleppa EJ, *et al*. Age determination of experimental venous thrombi by ultrasonic tissue characterization. *J Vasc Surg* 1993; **17**: 470–8.

321. Partsch H. Simultane venendruckmessung und plethysmographie am Fuss. In: May R, Kriessmann A, eds. *Periphere Venendruckmessung*. Stuttgart: Georg Thieme, 1978.

322. Patil KD, Williams JR, Lloyd Williams K. Thermographic localization of incompetent perforating veins in the leg. *Br Med J* 1970; **1**: 195.

323. Payne SPK, Thrush AJ, London NJM, Bell PRF, Barrie WW. Venous assessment using air plethysmography, a comparison with clinical examination, ambulatory venous pressure and duplex scanning. *Br J Surg* 1993; **80**: 967–70.

324. Pearce WH, Ricco J-B, Queral LA, Flinn WR, Yao JST. Haemodynamic assessment of venous problems. *Surgery* 1983; **93**: 715.

325. Perimutt LM, Braun SD, Newman GE, *et al*. Pulmonary arteriography in the high-risk patient. *Radiology* 1987; **162**: 187–9.

326. Perrin M, Bolot JE, Genevois A, Hiltbrand G. Dynamic popliteal phlebography. *Phlebography* 1988; **3**: 227–35.

327. Perthes G. Uber die Operation der Unterschenkelvaricen nach Trendelenburg. *Dtsch Med Wochenschr* 1895; **21**: 253–7.

328. Phillips GW, Paige J, Molan MP. A comparison of colour duplex ultrasound with venography and varicography in the assessment of varicose veins. *Clin Radiol* 1995; **50(1)**: 20–5.

329. Pierce EC, Chiang K, Schanzer H. Volume tests for chronic venous insufficiency. An appraisal. *Surgery* 1991; **109**: 567–74.

330. Pierce EC, Premus G, Martinelli G, Schanzer H. Foot flood flow measurements improve venous plethysmographic studies. *Surgery* 1987; **101**: 422–9.

331. Pilcher R. Postoperative thrombosis and embolism. *Lancet* 1939; **2**: 629.

332. Pioped investigators. Value of the ventilation/perfusion scan in acute pulmonary embolism. *JAMA* 1990; **263(20)**: 2753.

333. Pochaczevsky R, Pillari G, Feldman F. Liquid crystal contact thermography of deep venous thrombosis. *Am J Roentgenol* 1982; **138**: 717.

334. Pollack AA, Taylor BE, Myers TT, Wood EH. The effect of exercise and body position on the venous pressure at the ankle in patients having venous valvular defects. *J Clin Invest* 1949; **28**: 559.

335. Pollack AA, Wood EH. Venous pressure in the saphenous vein at the ankle in man during exercise and changes in posture. *J Appl Physiol* 1949; **1**: 649.

336. Polak JF. Venous thrombosis. In: *Peripheral Vascular Sonography*. Baltimore, MD: Williams & Wilkins, 1992; 155–214.

337. Porter JM, Rutherford RB, Claggett GP. *et al*. Reporting standards in venous disease. *J Vasc Surg* 1988; **8**: 172–81.

338. Posteraro RH, Sostman HD, Spritzer CE, *et al*. Cine gradient-refocused imaging of central pulmonary emboli. *Am J Roentgenol* 1989; **152**: 465–68.

339. Putnam JS, Uchida BT, Antonovic R, Rösch J. Superior vena cava syndrome associated with massive thrombosis: treatment with expandable wire stents. *Radiology* 1988; **167**: 727–8.

340. Quintavalla R, Larini P, Miselli A, *et al*. Duplex ultrasound diagnosis of symptomatic proximal deep vein thrombosis of lower limbs. *Eur J Radiol* 1992; **15(1)**: 32–6.

341. Rabinov K, Paulin S. Venography of the lower extremities. In: Abrams HL, ed. *Abrams' Angiography*, 3rd edition. Boston, MA: Little Brown, 1983.

342. Rabinov K, Paulin S. Roentgen diagnosis of venous thrombosis in the leg. *Arch Surg* 1972; **104**: 134–44.

343. Rak KM, Yakes WF, Ray RL, *et al*. MR imaging of symptomatic peripheral vascular malformations. *Am J Roentgenol* 1992; **159**: 107–112.

344. Remy-Jardin M, Remy J, Deschildre F, *et al*. Diagnosis of pulmonary embolism with spiral CT: comparison with pulmonary angiography and scintigraphy. *Radiology* 1996; **200(3)**: 699–706.

345. Remy-Jardin M, Remy J, Wattinne L, Giraud F. Central pulmonary thromboembolism diagnosis with spiral volumetric CT with the single-breath-hold technique – comparison with pulmonary angiography. *Radiology* 1992; **185**: 381–7.

346. Richardson GD, Beckwith T. Duplex scanning of recurrent varicose veins. *Phlebology* 1990; **5**: 281–4.

347. Ritchie W, Lapayowker MS, Soulen RL. Thermographic diagnosis of deep venous thrombosis. Anatomically based diagnostic criteria. *Radiology* 1979; **132**: 321.

348. Ritchie WGM, Lynch RR, Stewart GJ. The effect of contrast media on normal and inflamed canine veins. *Invest Radiol* 1974; **9**: 444.

349. Robertson PL, Berlangieri SU, Goergen SK, *et al*. Comparison of ultrasound and blood pool scintigraphy in the diagnosis of lower limb deep venous thrombosis. *Clin Radiol* 1994; **49**: 382–90.

350. Robertson PL, Georgen SK, Waugh JR, Fabiny RP. Colour-assisted compression ultrasound in the diagnosis of calf deep venous thrombosis. *Med J Aust* 1995; **163(10)**: 515–18.

351. Rooke TW, Nicolaides AN, Clement DL. Laboratory assessment of circulation in limbs. In: Clement DL, Shepherd JT, eds. *Vascular Diseases*

in the Limbs. Chicago, IL: Mosby-Yearbook Inc., 1993; 118.

352. Rösch J, Putnam JS, Uchida BT. Modified Gianturco expandable wire stents in experimental and clinical use. *Ann Radiol* 1988; 31: 100–3.

353. Rose SC, Zwiebel WJ, Murdock LE, *et al.* Insensitivity of color Doppler flow imaging for detection of acute calf deep venous thrombosis in asymptomatic postoperative patients. *J Vasc Intervent Radiol* 1993; **4:** 111–17.

354. Rose SC, Zwiebel WJ, Nelson BD. Symptomatic lower extremity deep venous thrombosis: accuracy, limitations, and role of color-duplex flow imaging in diagnosis. *Radiology* 1990; 175: 639–44.

355. Rosenberg ER, Trought WS, Kirks DR, Sumner TE, Grossman H. Ultrasonic diagnosis of renal vein thrombosis in neonates. *Am J Roentgenol* 1980; **134:** 35.

356. Rosenberg N, Marchese FP. Perforator vein localization by heat emission detection. *Surgery* 1963; **53:** 575.

357. Rosfors S. Venous photoplethysmography. Relationship between transducer position and regional distribution of venous insufficiency. *J Vasc Surg* 1990; **11:** 436–40.

358. Rouweler BJF, Bakkee AJM, Kuijper JP. Plethysmographic measurement of venous flow resistance and venous capacity in the human leg. *Phlebography* 1989; **4:** 241–50.

359. Saks AM, Paterson FC, Irvine AI, Ayers BA, Burnand KG. Improved MR venography. Use of fast short inversion time inversion-recover technique in evaluation of venous angiomas. *Radiology* 1995; **194(3):** 908–11.

360. Salzman EW. Venous thrombosis made easy. *N Engl J Med* 1986; **314:** 847–8.

361. Salzman EW, Hirsh J. Prevention of venous thromboembolism. In: *Hemostasis and Thrombosis*. Philadelphia, PA: Lippincott, 1987; 1252–65.

362. Sandler DA, Martin JF. Liquid crystal thermography as a screening test for deep vein thrombosis. *Lancet* 1985; **2:** 665.

363. Sandler A, Mitchell JRA. How do we know who has had deep vein thrombosis? *Postgrad Med J* 1989; **65:** 16–19.

364. Sarin S, Sommerville K, Farrah J, Scurr JH, Coleridge Smith PD. Duplex ultrasonography for assessment of venous valvular function of the lower limb. *Br J Surg* 1994; **81:** 1591–5.

365. Satiani B, Paoletti D, Henry M, Burns R, Smith D. A critical appraisal of impedance plethysmography in the diagnosis of acute deep venous thrombosis. *Surg Gynecol Obstet* 1985; **161:** 25.

366. Sawadas S, Fujiwara Y, Koyama T, *et al.* Application of expandable metallic stents in the venous system. *Acta Radiol* 1992; **33:** 156–9.

367. Schanzer H, Lande L, Premus G, Pierce EC III. Non-invasive evaluation of chronic venous insufficiency. Use of foot mercury straingauge plethysmography. *Arch Surg* 1984; **119:** 1013.

368. Schindler JM, Kaiser M, Gerber A, *et al.* Colour coded duplex sonography in suspected deep vein thrombosis of the leg. *Br Med J* 1991; **301:** 1369–70.

369. Schobinger RA. *Intraosseous Phlebography*. New York: Grune & Stratton, 1960.

370. Shehadi WH. Contrast media adverse reactions: occurrence, recurrence, and distribution patterns. *Radiology* 1982; **143:** 11–17.

371. Sheiman RG, McArdle CR. Bilateral lower extremity US in the patient with unilateral symptoms of deep venous thrombosis: assessment of need. *Radiology* 1995; **194:** 171–3.

372. Sigel B, Felix WR, Popky GL, Ipsen J. Diagnosis of lower limb venous thrombosis by Doppler ultrasound technique. *Arch Surg* 1972; **104:** 174.

373. Simons GR, Skibo LK, Polak JF, Greager MA, *et al.* Utility of leg ultrasonography in suspected symptomatic isolated deep calf vein thrombosis. *Am J Med* 1995; **99:** 43–7.

374. Sistrom CL, Gay SB, Peffley L. Extravasation of iopamidol and iohexol during contrast-enhanced CT: report of 28 cases. *Radiology* 1991; **180:** 707–10.

375. Sostman HD, Ravin CE, Sullivan DC, Mills SR, Glickman MG, Dorfman GS. Use of pulmonary angiography for suspected pulmonary embolism: influence of scintigraphic diagnosis. *Am J Roentgenol* 1982; **139:** 673–7.

376. Spigos DG, Thane TT, Capek V. Skin necrosis following extravasation during peripheral phlebography. *Radiology* 1977; **123:** 605.

377. Spritzer CE, Craig Evans A, Kay HH. Magnetic resonance imaging of deep venous thrombosis in pregnant women with lower extremity edema. *Obstet Gynecol* 1995; **85(4):** 603–7.

378. Spritzer CE, Norconk JJ, Sostman HD, Coleman RE. Detection of deep venous thrombosis by magnetic resonance imaging. *Chest* 1993; **104:** 54–60.

379. Spritzer CE, Sostman HD, Wilkes DC, Coleman RE. Deep venous thrombosis: experience with gradient-echo MR imaging in 66 patients. *Radiology* 1990; **177:** 235–41.

380. Spritzer CE, Sussman SK, Blinder RA, Saeed M, Herfkens RJ. Deep venous thrombosis evaluation with limited-flip-angle, gradient-refocused MR imaging: Preliminary experience. *Radiology* 1988; **166:** 371–5.

381. Stehling MK, Rosen MP, Weintraub J, Kim D, Raptopoulos V. Spiral CT venography of the lower extremity. *Am J Roentgenol* 1994; **163:** 451–453.

382. Stein PD, Athanasoulis C, Alavi A, *et al.* Complications and validity of pulmonary angiography in acute pulmonary embolism. *Circulation* 1992; **85:** 462–8.

383. Stonebridge PA, Chalmers N, Beggs I, Bradbury AW, Ruckley CV. Recurrent varicose veins: a varicographic analysis leading to a new practical classification. *Br J Surg* 1995; **82(1):** 60–2.

384. Strandness DE. Doppler ultrasonic techniques in vascular disease. In: Bernstein EF, ed. *Non-invasive Diagnostic Techniques in Vascular Disease*. St Louis, MO: CV Mosby, 1985.

385. Strandness DE Jr, Diagnostic approaches for detecting deep vein thrombosis. *Am J Cardiac Imaging* 1994; **8(1):** 13–17.

386. Strandness DE, Sumner DS. Ultrasonic velocity detector in the diagnosis of thrombophlebitis. *Arch Surg* 1972; **104:** 180.

387. Sturup H, Hojensgard IC. Venous pressure in varicose veins in patients with incompetent communicating veins. *Acta Chir Scand* 1950; **99:** 518.

388. Sullivan ED, Peter DJ, Cranley JJ. Real-time B-mode venous ultrasound. *J Vasc Surg* 1984; **1:** 465.

389. Sullivan ED, Reece C, Cranley JJ. Phleborheography of the upper extremity. *Arch Surg* 1983; **118:** 1134.

390. Sumner DS. Diagnosis of deep venous thrombosis by Doppler ultrasound. In: Nicolaides AN, Yao JST, eds. *Investigation of Vascular Disorders*. New York: Churchill Livingstone, 1981.

391. Sumner DS. Strain gauge plethysmography. In: Bernstein EF, ed. *Non-Invasive Diagnostic Techniques in Vascular Disease*. St Louis, MO: CV Mosby, 1985.

392. Sumner DS, Baker DW, Strandness DF. The ultrasonic velocity detector in a clinic study of venous disease. *Arch Surg* 1968; **97:** 75.

393. Sumner DS, Londrey GL, Spadone DP, *et al.* Study of deep venous thrombosis in high-risk patients using color flow Doppler. In: Bergan JJ, Yao JST, eds. *Venous Disorders*. Philadelphia, PA: WB Saunders, 1991; 63–76.

394. Szendro G, Nicholaides AN, Zukowski AJ, *et al.* Duplex scanning in the assessment of deep venous incompetence. *J Vasc Surg* 1986; **4:** 237–42.

395. Taheri SA, Lazar L, Elias S, Marchand P, Heffner R. Surgical treatment of postphlebitic syndrome with vein valve transplant. *Am J Surg* 1982; **144:** 221.

396. Talbot SR. Use of real-time imaging in identifying deep venous obstruction: a preliminary report. *Bruit* 1982; **6:** 41.

397. Taplin GV, Johnson DE, Dore EK. Suspensions of radioalbumin aggregates for photoscanning of the liver, spleen, lung and other organs. *J Nucl Med* 1964; **5:** 259.

398. Tardivon AA, Musset D, Maitre S, *et al.* Role of CT in chronic pulmonary embolism. Comparison with pulmonary angiography. *J Comput Assist Tomogr* 1993; **17:** 345–51.

399. Taylor DW, Hull R, Sackett DL, Hirsch J. Simplification of the sequential impedance plethysmograph technique without loss of accuracy. *Thromb Res* 1980; **17:** 561.

400. Taylor KJW, Holland S. Doppler US: Part 1. Basic principles, instrumentation and pitfalls. *Radiology* 1990; **174:** 297–307.

401. Teigen CL, Maus TP, Sheedy PF, *et al.* Pulmonary embolism: diagnosis with electron-beam CT. *Radiology* 1993; **188:** 839–45.

402. Tello R, Scholz E, Finn JP, Costello P. Subclavian vein thrombosis detected with spiral CT and three-dimensional reconstruction. *Am J Roentgenol* 1993; **160:** 33–4.

403. Tempany CMC, Morton RA, Marshall FF. MRI of the renal veins: assessment of nonneoplastic venous thrombosis. *J Comput Assist Tomogr* 1992; **16(6):** 929–34.

404. Tempkin DL, Ladika JE. New catheter design and placement technique for pulmonary arteriography. *Radiology* 1987; **163:** 275–6.

405. Thulesius O, Norgren L, Gjores JE. Foot volumetry, a new method for objective assessment of oedema and venous function. *Vasa* 1973; **2:** 325.

406. Trendelenburg F. Uber die Unterbindung der Vena saphena magna bei Unterschenkelvaricen. *Beitr Z Klin Chir* 1891; **7:** 195.

407. Tulchinsky M, Eggli DF, Kotlyarov EV, *et al.* V/Q lung scanning in pulmonary embolism. *Appl Radiol* 1992; **21:** 60–70.

408. Tyson MD, Goodlett WC. Venous pressures in disorders of the venous system of the lower extremities. *Surgery* 1945; **18:** 669.

409. Urigo F, Pischedda A, Pinna L, Rovasio SS, Maiore M, Canalis GC. Role of phlebography in the study of recurrent leg varices. *Radiol Med* 1993; **85(6):** 764–72.

410. Utility of leg ultrasonography in suspected symptomatic isolated calf deep venous thrombosis. *Am J Med* 1995; **99(1):** 43–7.

411. Van Bemmelen PS, Bedford G, Beach K, Strandness DE. Quantitative segmental evaluation of venous valvular reflux with duplex ultrasound scanning. *J Vasc Surg* 1989; **10:** 425–31.

412. Van de Broek TAA, Rauwerda JA, Kuijper CF, *et al.* Comparison of strain gauge and photo-cell venous function testing with invasive pressure measurements. *Phlebography* 1989; **4:** 223–30.

413. Van Rooij WJ, den Heeten GJ. Intra-arterial digital subtraction angiography of the pulmonary arteries using a flow-directed balloon catheter in the diagnosis of pulmonary embolism. *Rofo Fortschr Geb Rontgenstr Neuen Bildgeb Verfahr* 1992; **156:** 333–7.

414. Van Sonnenberg E, Neff CC, Pfister RC. Life-threatening hypotensive reactions to contrast media administration: comparison of pharmacologic and fluid therapy. *Radiology* 1987; **162:** 15–19.

415. Vogel P, Laing FC, Jeffrey RB Jr, Wing VW. Deep venous thrombosis of the lower limb: US evaluation. *Radiology* 1987; **163:** 747–51.

416. Vukov LF, Berquist TH, King BF. Magnetic resonance imaging for calf deep venous thrombophlebitis. *Ann Emerg Med* 1991; **20:** 497–9.

417. Wagner HN, Sabiston DC, McAfee JG. Diagnosis of massive pulmonary embolism in man by radioisotope scanning. *N Engl J Med* 1964; **271:** 377.

418. Walters HL, Clemenson J, Browse NL, Lea Thomas M. [125]I fibrinogen uptake following phlebography of the leg. *Radiology* 1980; **135:** 619.

419. Waltman AC, Geller SC. Pulmonary arteriography: questions you are afraid to ask. A diagnostic categorical course in interventional radiology. *RSNA Syllabus* 1991; 179–184.

420. Warren R, White EA, Beicher CD. Venous pressures in the saphenous system in normal, varicose and post phlebitic extremities. Alterations following femoral vein ligation. *Surgery* 1949; **26:** 435.

421. Webb IJ, Berger LA, Sherlock S. Greyscale ultrasonography of portal vein. *Lancet* 1977; **2:** 675.

422. Wells, PNT. Doppler equipment. In: Fullerton G, Zagzebski J, eds. *Medical Physics of CT and Ultrasound.* New York: American Institute of Physics, 1980; 343–66.

423. Werner H, Otto K. Hazards and complications in roentgenological venous diagnosis. *Fortschr Roentgenstr* 1962; **96:** 655.

424. Wester JP, Holtkamp M, Linnebank ER, *et al.* Non-invasive detection of deep venous thrombosis: ultrasonography versus duplex scanning. *Eur J Vasc Surg* 1994; **8(3):** 357–61.

425. Wheeler BH, Hirsh J, Wells P, Anderson F. Diagnostic tests for deep vein thrombosis. *Arch Intern Med* 1994; **154:** 1921–8.

426. Wheeler HB, Anderson FA. The diagnosis of venous thrombosis by impedance plethysmography. In: Bernstein EF, ed. *Non-invasive Diagnostic Techniques in Vascular Disease.* St Louis, MO: CV Mosby, 1985.

427. Wheeler HB, Mullick SC, Anderson JN, Pearson D. Diagnosis of occult deep vein thrombosis by a non-invasive bedside technique. *Surgery* 1971; **70:** 20.

428. Wheeler HB, O'Donnell JA, Anderson FA, Penney BC, Penra RA, Benedict CJP. Bedside screening for venous thrombosis using occlusive impedance phlebography. *Angiology* 1975; **26:** 199.

429. White RD, Winkler ML, Higgins CB. MR imaging of pulmonary arterial hypertension and pulmonary emboli. *Am J Roentgenol* 1987; **149:** 15–21.

430. Whitehead SM. Quantitative assessment of calf pump function using ^{99m}technetium labelled red blood cells. *Br J Surg* 1981; **68:** 366.

431. Whitehead S, Clemenson G, Browse NL. The assessment of calf pump function by isotope plethysmography. *Br J Surg* 1983; **70:** 675.

432. Widmer LK. *Peripheral Venous Disorders. Basle Study 111.* Berne: Hans Huber, 1978.

433. Winsberg F. Real time scanners. *Med Ultrasound* 1979; **3:** 99.

434. Witten DM, Hirsch FD, Harman GW. Acute reactions to urographic contrast medium. *Am J Roentgenol* 1973; **119:** 823.

435. Witten DM, Hirsch FD, Harman GW. Acute reactions to urographic contrast medium. *Am J Roentgenol* 1973; **119:** 823.

436. Wojciechowski J, Holm J, Zachrisson BT. Thermography and phlebography in the detection of incompetent perforating veins. *Acta Radiol (Diag) (Stockh)* 1982; **23:** 199.

437. Wolfe GI, Mishkin M, Roux S, *et al.* Comparison of the roles of adverse drug reaction – ionic agents, ionic agents combined with steroids and non-ionic agents. *Invest Radiol* 1991; **36:** 404–10.

438. Wright DJ, Shepard AD, McPharlin M, Ernst CB. Pitfalls in lower extremity venous duplex scanning. *J Vasc Surg* 1990; **11:** 675–9.

439. Wupperman T, Exler U, Mellman J, Kestila M. Noninvasive quantitative measurement of regurgitation in insufficiency of the greater saphenous vein by Doppler ultrasound. A comparison with clinical examination and phlebography. *Vasa* 1981: **10:** 24–7.

440. Yucel EK, Fisher JS, Egglin TK, Geller SC, Waltman AC. Isolated calf venous thrombosis: diagnosis with compression US. *Radiology* 1991; **179:** 443–6.

441. Zenk KE, Dungy CI, Greene GR. Nafcillin extravasation injury: use of hyaluronidase as an antidote. *Am J Dis Child* 1981; **135:** 1113–14.

442. Zerhouni EA, Barth KH, Siegelman SS. Demonstration of venous thrombosis by computed tomography. *Am J Roentgenol* 1980; **134:** 753–8.

443. Ziegenbein RW, Myers KA, Matthews PG, Zeng GH. Duplex ultrasound scanning for chronic venous disease: 1. Techniques for examination of the crural veins. *Phlebology* 1994; **9:** 108–13.

444. Zielinsky A, Hull R, Carter C, *et al.* Doppler ultrasonograpy in patients with clinically suspected deep vein thrombosis: improved sensitivity by inclusion of posterior tibial vein examination site. *Thromb Haemost* 1983; **50:** 153 (abstr).

445. Zwiebel WJ. Colour duplex imaging and Doppler spectrum analysis: principles, capabilities and limitations. *Semin Ultrasound CT MR* 1990; **11(2):** 84–96.

446. Zwiebel WJ. Color-encoded blood flow imaging. *Semin Ultrasound CT MR* 1988; **9:** 320–5.

447. Zwiebel WJ. *Introduction to Vascular Ultrasonography.* Philadelphia, PA: WB Saunders, 1983.

448. Zwiebel WJ. Sources of error in duplex venography and an algorithmic approach to the diagnosis of deep venous thrombosis. *Semin Ultrasound CT MR* 1988; **9:** 286–94.

449. Zwiebel WJ, Priest DL. Color-duplex sonography of extremity veins. *Semin Ultrasound CT MR* 1990; **11:** 136–67.

CHAPTER 5

Varicose veins: pathology

Epidemiology	145	Pathology	156
Aetiology	147	References	158

Definitions

The World Health Organization (WHO)[112] defines varicose veins as:

'Saccular dilatation of the veins which are often tortuous.'

This definition specifically excludes:

- Dilatation of small intradermal subcutaneous veins called 'venectasis'
- Any tortuous dilated veins that are secondary to previous thrombophlebitis or an arteriovenous fistula.

The Basle study[40,46,148] separated varicose veins into:

1. Dilated saphenous veins (trunk veins)
2. Dilated superficial tributaries (reticular veins)
3. Dilated venules (hyphenwebs).

Groups 1 and 2 of the Basle definition are definitely varicose veins, but the WHO definition would exclude group 3, as it is difficult to define when a small vessel is a venule rather than a vein.

It has been suggested[64] that a varicose vein is defined as a subcutaneous vein in which the valves have become incompetent. While this definition may be etymologically satisfactory, valvular incompetence of a superficial vein is difficult to detect on clinical examination, and in this book the descriptive definition of varicose veins will be used (i.e. veins which have become excessively tortuous and dilated) because, though this definition is imprecise and open to considerable observer variation,[146] it has the major advantage of simplicity (Figure 5.1a and b).

The advent of duplex scanning has allowed easy assessment of superficial vein reflux, making it possible to include valvular incompetence within the definition of a varicose vein (see Chapter 4) but a standard stimulus to reflux and the duration of retrograde flow to that stimulus still needs to be defined and accepted for superficial as well as deep veins [75,144] (see Chapters 4 and 12).

Epidemiology

The *incidence* of a condition is the estimated number of patients in whom the condition has developed in a specified time period.

The *prevalence* of a condition is the estimated number of patients in whom the condition exists at a specified time or within a specified interval of time.

The prevalence of varicose veins (the incidence in the whole population) has been studied in a number of national surveys and by three local population surveys.[19]

The USA National Surveys of 1935–36 and 1959–61[143]

The first survey was part of the United States of America National Health Survey of 1935–36. It was based on a house-to-house questionnaire conducted by lay interviewers on 2.8 million people. One and three-quarter million people stated that they had varicose veins, making this the seventh commonest condition. A subsequent survey between 1959 and 1961, of severe chronic disabling conditions, produced an estimated rate (prevalence) of 2.25 patients with varicose veins per 100

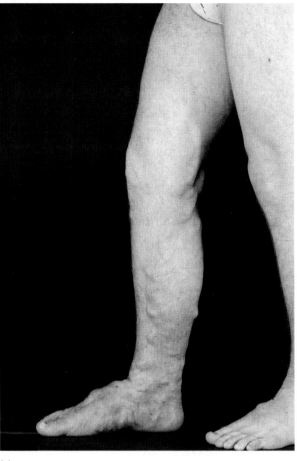

(a)

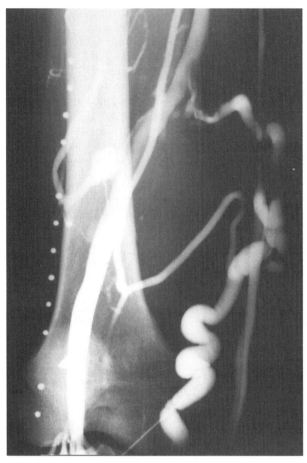

(b)

Figure 5.1 (a) A number of tortuous dilated 'varicose' veins, all tributaries of the long saphenous vein. (b) A varicogram showing tortuous dilated tributary veins draining into a long saphenous vein of normal size.

of the population per year, comprised of 0.8% in men and 3.5% in women.

The UK Survey of Sickness (England and Wales 1950)[83]

This was also based on interviews conducted by non-medical personnel, and showed that 1.41% of men and 3.74% of women had varicose veins. It was estimated that 2.25% of the population had varicose veins.

The Sickness Survey of Denmark 1952–53[130]

This survey of patients attending hospital with varicose veins found an incidence of 1.7% of males and 2.0% females attending in 1 year.

The Canadian Sickness Survey 1950–51[66]

This survey showed a lower incidence of varicose veins than the others (0.53% overall), but was poorly organized and is of doubtful value.

Summary

All these surveys were conducted by questionnaire, administered by untrained non-medical personnel, and therefore probably underestimate the prevalence of varicose veins.[19]

Regional surveys

There have now been at least 20 regional surveys[26] on the prevalence of varicose veins within defined populations. Most suffer methodological defects and problems with definition so the picture is confused.

Three of the best studies are still those of Bobek *et al.*[18], Widmer[148] and Baglehole *et al.*,[15] though the recent Bochumer studies of Shultz-Ehrenburg are also very instructive.[124-126] Bobek *et al.*[18] surveyed a defined population over the age of 15 years in Czechoslovakia using a questionnaire and a medical examination. He found an incidence of varicose veins of 14% in women and 6.6% in men.

Widmer *et al.*,[148] in a survey carried out in 1974 in Basle, Switzerland, showed that 4.2% of 4376 chemical workers had evidence of severe varicose veins. They found that 5.2% of the men and 3.2% of the women were affected. Widmer's team took photographs of all the subjects in the survey which was carried out entirely by medical personnel. The Basle study showed that 10% of the population between the ages of 25 and 34 years had varicose veins, while 50% of those between the ages of 64 and 75 years were affected.

Beaglehole *et al.*[15] looked at the prevalence of varicose veins in New Zealand in 1976. They showed that 36.3% of Maori men and 47.4% of Maori women had varicose veins. After standardizing the prevalence for the different age distribution within the two races, in the white population the incidence was 21.5% in men and 40.4% in women.

Schultz-Ehrenburg[124] found evidence of venous reflux was already present in a cohort of 10- and 12-year-old school children but there was no evidence of visible veins at this stage. He found an increased incidence of venous reflux in 16-year-olds, some of whom had developed varicose veins. By the age of 20, 20% had developed saphenous reflux and 8% had varicose veins. He felt that these studies showed that saphenous reflux predated the development of varicose veins. A number of other studies have suggested that the incidence of varicose veins increases to about 50% or more in the over-50s. Many of these are very mild, however, and patients do not feel that they require treatment.[1,33,52]

Comment

The national surveys in both Europe and North America have shown a remarkably consistent prevalence of varicose veins of approximately 2%. Local surveys have shown a greater prevalence with levels varying between 4 and 15%. The problem with all these surveys is the varying diagnostic criteria and knowledge of the observers. The Basle study is the only survey in which the prevalence of severe varicose veins was found to be higher in males than in females.

If it is accepted that 2% of the population has varicose veins and that a proportion of these subjects will develop problems that need treatment, the

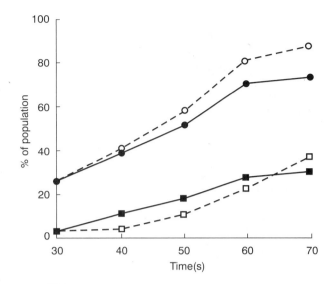

Figure 5.2   The prevalence of varicose veins according to age. ● Men (all veins); ○ women (all veins); ■ men (trunk veins); □ women (trunk veins). (Based on data from Widmer.[148])

size of the problem on an international or even a national basis is enormous.

It is also important to recognize that the incidence of varicose veins increases with age (see Figure 5.2) and as the average age of the population increases so will the incidence of venous problems.

Aetiology

Valvular deficiency

The concept that varicose veins are caused by descending valvular incompetence has been accepted ever since Trendelenburg introduced the high saphenous ligation for long saphenous vein incompetence. He suggested that the venous valves normally protect the wall of the vein below each valve from the pressure in the vein above it. He believed that varicose veins began when the highest valve in the long saphenous vein gave way and that if the vein was ligated and divided, preventing retrograde flow of blood downwards, the saphenous vein would regain its former dimensions and the varicosities in the tributaries would regress.

Anatomical studies[13,48,109] on the distribution of venous valves in cadavers have shown that between 20 and 40% of apparently 'normal' individuals have an absent valve in and above the common femoral vein on one or both sides (Figure 5.3).

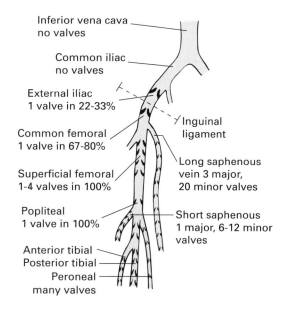

Inferior vena cava
no valves

Common iliac
no valves

External iliac
1 valve in 22-33%

Common femoral
1 valve in 67-80%

Superficial femoral
1-4 valves in 100%

Popliteal
1 valve in 100%

Anterior tibial
Posterior tibial
Peroneal
many valves

Inguinal
ligament

Long saphenous
vein 3 major,
20 minor valves

Short saphenous
1 major, 6-12 minor
valves

Figure 5.3 Diagram of the distribution of the valves in the veins of the lower limb and pelvis collated from the cadaver dissection studies of Eger and Casper,[48] Powell and Lynn,[109] and Basmajian.[13]

These studies suggested that an absence of ilio-femoral valves exposes the highest valve in the long saphenous vein to thoraco-abdominal pressures and that on standing upright the hydrostatic pressure produced by the vertical column of venous blood between the groin and the heart would be resisted only by a single important saphenous valve. Basmajian,[13] however, failed to show a convincing association between the absence of ilio-femoral valves and the presence of long saphenous incompetence.

The greater incidence of left-sided varicose veins that has been reported by some[91] may be related to left common iliac vein compression because the venous return from the leg is always partially impeded where the right common iliac artery compresses the left common iliac vein in front of the sacral promontary.[31,91]

One study in the 1950s suggested that almost half the patients with varicose veins had defective valves in the deep veins.[96] The technique by which the absence of the deep venous valves was judged was, however, disputed,[99] and our own studies of descending phlebography and duplex scanning in patients with varicose veins contradict these earlier findings.

In 1963, Ludbrook[86] re-examined the theory of descending incompetence. He set out to discover if valvular incompetence in the long saphenous vein

preceded the development of its varicose tributaries. He found that the reduction of venous pressure on exercise was equally poor in patients with both severe and mild varicose veins, and consequently thought that incompetence of the long saphenous valve preceded the development of severe distal varicosities. But the pressure falls found in the patients with long saphenous incompetence were in fact significantly worse than those found in the patients with mild disease, in whom no attempt was made to exclude the presence of long saphenous incompetence. Incompetence of the long saphenous valve could just as well be the result as the cause of venous dilation. The recent studies of Schultz-Ehrenburg do, however, lend this theory some support (see page 147).

In order to prove that the descending valvular incompetence theory is correct, an attempt must be made to show that ligating the long saphenous vein reverses the changes in existing varicose veins or prevents the development of new varicose veins. Our clinical experience indicates that neither of these events occurs. Varicograms, descending phlebography and duplex ultrasound examinations show that tributary veins may become varicose and incompetent before there is any evidence of long saphenous incompetence (Figures 5.1 and 5.4), whilst others may become incompetent after long saphenous reflux has been abolished by sapheno-femoral junction ligation.

A recent paper[2] showed that 63 of 190 limbs with duplex ultrasound confirmation of reflux in the saphenous veins in the thigh or calf had no reflux through the sapheno-femoral junction.

There are a few patients who have a congenital absence of all venous valves (congenital valve aplasia)[80,82] who often do develop severe secondary varicose veins. These patients may also have an absence of valves in their arm veins and in other veins, such as the foot (see Chapter 24, Figure 24.7).

The function of venous valves is thought to protect the capillaries and venules from sudden excessive rises in pressure during muscular exercise. Foote[53] was unable to find evidence of the existence of varicose veins in any members of the animal kingdom other than man, except for one poor donkey. It appears that varicose veins are a human condition unrelated directly to the presence or absence of venous valves.

Defective structure of the vein wall

It is difficult to know who first suggested that a defect in the tissues of the wall of the vein was responsible for the development of varicosity. In an influential article written in 1950, King[71] made the following points.

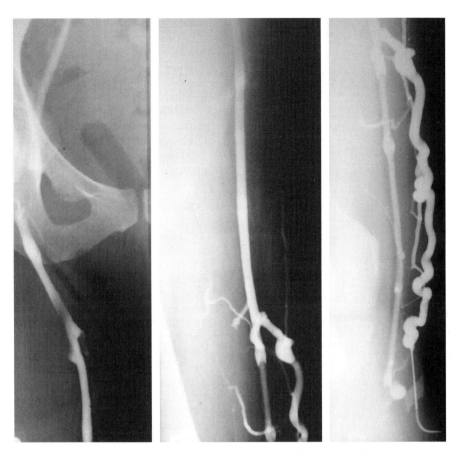

Figure 5.4   A varicogram showing a long saphenous vein of normal calibre containing normal valves, with an obviously varicose tributary that is tortuous and dilated.

- Varicose veins usually make their first appearance as a sharply circumscribed group of veins which communicate with other veins of normal calibre. These varices often communicate with a saphenous vein of normal calibre in which there is no evidence of valvular incompetence (Figure 5.4).
- The early 'swelling' of the vein is distal not proximal to the valve, making the position of the dilation difficult to explain by the theory of 'back-pressure'.
- The extent of the varicosities may vary from time to time without any obvious mechanical alteration. The veins may be larger on some occasions and smaller on others.
- Histological examination of the vein wall in the early stages of varicosis shows it to be thickened with hypertrophy of the muscle coat and increased vascularity of the adventitia.

Having made these observations, King did not suggest a local abnormality of the vein wall but instead proposed that the venous dilatation was caused by a haemodynamic alteration in blood flow brought about by a chemical stimulus.

The position of the dilatation in relation to the valve is of critical importance in refuting the theory of descending valvular incompetence. The site of the venous dilatation has been addressed by several investigators (Table 5.1).

Table 5.1   Site of dilatation in varicose veins[37]

Dilatation proximal to the valve
    Callender 1862[27]
    Rindfleisch 1867[116]
    Bennett 1890[16]
Proximal and distal to the valve
    Löwenstein 1908[84]
No relation to the valve
    Schwartz 1934[127]
Below the valve
    Trendelenburg 1891[141]
    Slawinski 1899[132]
    Ledderhose 1906[79]
    Hasebroek 1916a, b[59,60]

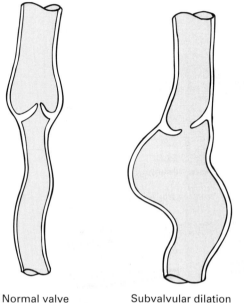

Normal valve   Subvalvular dilation
causing incompetence

Figure 5.5 Diagram of the eccentric dilatation causing valvular incompetence found by Cotton[37] beneath the valve in casts taken of varicose veins. A normal valve is shown for comparison.

In 1961, Cotton[37] published a detailed study of the relationship between the venous dilation and the valves. He examined saphenous veins which had been removed by stripping at operation, veins removed from cadavers and the whole venous system in amputated limbs. The veins were either opened to inspect the valve distribution or resin casts were made of the whole system.

Inspection of the veins was carried out at operation and venograms were also obtained. From these studies Cotton drew the following conclusions.

1. The number of valves in varicose long saphenous veins was significantly less than the number found in normal long saphenous veins.
2. There was no evidence of primary valvular disease to be found on naked eye inspection.
3. The number of valves did not diminish with age.
4. Prominent dilations occurred below the cornua of the valve cusps (Figure 5.5).

5. The long saphenous vein showed little evidence of lengthening while the varicose tributaries were greatly elongated and tortuous.
6. The varicose tributaries showed sacculations projecting from alternate sides of the vein (Figure 5.6).
7. Tributaries joining communicating veins were also very tortuous (Figure 5.7).
8. There were no varicosities in the deep veins of the leg.

Points 1 and 2 of Cotton's conclusions appear to be contradictory, though the number and function of the valves may be independent features. He did, however, definitely show that the site of dilatation was below rather than above the valves, though this had previously been disputed by others (see Table 5.1), but he also pointed out that this cannot be taken as unequivocal evidence of a wall abnormality as opposed to a valvular defect, because valvular incompetence might allow regurgitant blood to impinge on the wall of the vein below the valve and so weaken it and cause it to dilate. This would be akin to the post-stenotic dilation seen beyond a narrowed artery. Arguing against this hypothesis, Cotton pointed out that the dilatation of varicose veins is always eccentric (see Figures 5.5 and 5.6) whereas the cusps are always concentric, making the possibility of dilatation caused by the valvular reflux less likely.

Rokitansky[117] suggested that venous valves 'increase to a certain degree with dilatation of the vein but, after a time, cease to increase and are no longer capable of closing the enlarged vessel'. Edwards and Edwards[47] described separation and shortening of the valves cusps as a result of venous dilatation. Cotton postulated that the venous dilatation so increased the tension in the valves that it led to sclerosis and contraction of the valve cusps with the eventual disappearance of the whole valve.

Detailed histological and electron-microscopic examination of the venous valves of varicose veins has demonstrated depression of the commissures and expansion of the space between the valves. The valve cusps are reversed and tortuous. Intimal thickening of the vein wall is present in almost all cases.[104]

Thus there are a number of studies which support the hypothesis that the valvular incompetence follows rather than precedes a change in the vein wall.

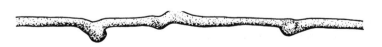

Figure 5.6 Diagram of the spiral arrangement of the dilatations found along the course of a varicose long saphenous vein. (After Cotton.[37])

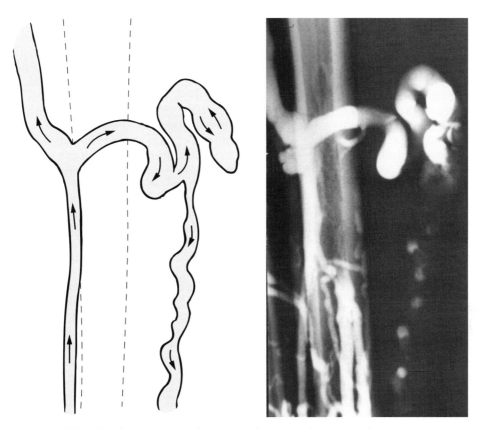

Figure 5.7 A dilated surface varicosity lying directly over and connected to an incompetent communicating vein. The diagram shows the direction of blood flow.

Collagen, elastin and hexosamine content of varicose veins

In 1963, Svejcar *et al.*[134,135] analysed the content of collagen, elastin, muscle and hexosamine in the vein wall because their perceived association between varicose veins, flat feet, hernias and haemorrhoids made them postulate that there was a common tissue abnormality. They took veins from normal subjects and compared them with varicose veins and 'normal' veins from a group of patients with varicose veins at other sites. This last group they called 'potential varicose veins'. They found the following.

- The collagen content was significantly lower in the varicose veins and the potential varicose veins' than in normal veins.
- Varicose veins contained relatively more muscle than normal veins.
- The hexosamine content was significantly higher in actual and potential varicose veins than in normal veins.
- There was a much greater variation of water and hexosamine content in different segments of varicose veins when compared with different segments of normal veins which showed relatively little variation.

From these results Svejcar *et al.* proposed that the similarity between varicose veins and potential varicose veins might be the result of an inherited abnormality of collagen metabolism.

This is a very important study but is heavily dependent upon the methods used to assess the constituents of the vein wall. Barbaro *et al.*[11] repeated this work and reported completely different results, but Andreotti *et al.*[8] in a later study confirmed a significantly lower content of collagen and elastin in varicose veins compared with controls.

A recent study from Nottingham also failed to show any difference in the collagen and elastin content of varicose veins but did find an increase in the muscle density with a corresponding decrease in the collagen and elastin density. This suggested that an increase in the smooth muscle rather than a decrease in the collagen is responsible for the development of varicosity.[28,140] Others[34] have, however, confirmed an increase in collagen types I and III and a reduction in elastin in varicose vein biopsies. This is only seen in those parts of the vein that are 'varicose', where it is also associated with smooth muscle atrophy and collagen infiltration. This results in an increase in the collagen/elastin ratio. There was an increase in collagen even in 'normal' areas of the varicose veins.

The presence of a localized dilatation in one area of the vein wall suggests that a local fault must be present because back pressure would be likely to produce uniform dilatation.

Recently, a number of studies have suggested that oxygen free radicals,[49] infiltration by mast cells,[151] a reduction in antiperoxidant activity,[41] antikinase activity[55] and increased levels of circulating noradrenaline[38] may all have a role in the development of varicose veins. Further studies are necessary to confirm these individual reports.

Rose has made a number of clinical observations which support the concept of a defect in the vein wall.[118]

- Sixty per cent of varicose veins occur below a competent saphenous valve (not all investigators would agree with this observation).
- A normal saphenous vein inserted as an arterial substitute has no difficulty in withstanding arterial pressure without becoming varicose.
- When varicose veins are used as a conduit or patch in the arterial system they invariably dilate or develop localized aneurysms.
- *In situ* saphenous vein bypass grafts in which all the valves have been deliberately destroyed before they are attached to the arterial system do not show any increased evidence of aneurysmal dilatation.

All these clinical 'experiments' make the theory of descending valvular incompetence as a cause of varicose veins untenable.

A primary valvular defect cannot explain why there are normal segments in continuity with 'varicose' segments, when the whole vein wall is subjected to the same pressure changes, or that the inevitable rise in superficial venous pressure that occurs after a deep vein thrombosis is not always associated with the development of superficial varicosities.

Valve cusps have been shown to have twice the tensile strength of the vein wall,[4] again indicating that the venous valve is less likely to give way under pressure than the venous wall.

Two studies published in 1989 suggested that change in venous elasticity, perhaps as a result of changes in the collagen/elastin ratio within the vein wall, might be the final pathway in the development of varicose veins.[29,113]

Haemodynamic effects

Varicose veins certainly develop upstream of an arteriovenous fistula.[65] This response was always seen after an arteriovenous fistula was formed in the hind-limb of a dog to produce venous hypertension.[24]

In 1916 Hasebroek[59,60] developed a vein model made from a thin-walled latex tube containing three single flap non-return valves. This model was attached to a pulsatile fluid pump at pressures which were comparable to those within the venous system. 'Blow-outs' occurred in the side of the latex tubing at certain critical frequencies of pulsation.

Cotton[37] attempted to repeat these experiments but could not obtain the blow-outs unless the tubing was deliberately narrowed at the 'valve sites'. He concluded that reflection of the pulse waves at the sites of valvular narrowing might be responsible for the development of dilatation. Nylander[103] has shown that varicosities assume the shape of a sine wave which is the wave form that results from an increase in blood flow.

Pigeaux[107] was the first person to observe that blood in varicose veins may be as red as that found in arteries, and he noted that an arterial pulsation could occasionally be felt over the veins. Pratt[110] also suggested that some primary varicose veins could be felt to pulsate, and he called these 'arterial varices'; it is possible, however, that Pratt was looking at limbs with the Parkes–Weber syndrome.

Raised oxygen tensions have been found in blood taken from varicose veins as compared with blood taken from normal veins;[20,114] this suggested that arteriovenous shunts might be responsible for the development of varicose veins.

Schalin, and others, have consistently championed the role of arteriovenous fistulae in the development of varicose veins and has produced a series of publications [12,61,115,121–123] which support his hypothesis. The methodology of many of these reports can be challenged, and there is little evidence for the existence of functioning pathological arteriovenous shunts in every patient with varicose veins. A lower oxygen content of blood samples taken from saphenous varicosities has been found when compared with popliteal vein blood from the same level.[115] It is conceivable that the arteriovenous shunts which are normally present in the skin to allow temperature regulation open intermittently in response to changes in temperature or venous pressure.[74,119]

Fegan suggested that retrograde flow occurring through incompetent valves in the ankle communicating veins causes turbulent flow in the superficial system.[50,51] An asymmetrical fine jet of high velocity retrograde flow might affect the overlying vein wall. There is, however, no experimental or clinical evidence to support this hypothesis.[63] Although the concept of an increased blood flow giving rise to turbulence which in turn causes venodilatation is an attractive hypothesis, more studies are required to prove this association.

Table 5.2 Predisposing factors

Age	Side (left or right)
Sex	Bowel habit
Race	Occupation
Weight	Heredity
Height	Alcohol
Pregnancy	Clothes
Diet	Erect stance

Table 5.3 Effect of gender on prevalence of varicose veins in five Western countries

Survey	Reference	M:F ratio
Switzerland	Widmer[148]	1:1.0
	Bobek[18]	1:2.1
UK	Survey of Sickness[83]	1:2.5
Denmark	Sickness Survey[130]	1:2.9
USA	National Health Survey[143]	1:4.0

Secondary aetiological factors (predisposing factors) (Table 5.2)

Age

The surveys which have been described earlier in this chapter have all shown that the prevalence of varicose veins increases with age. There appears to be a peak frequency between 50 and 60 years of age[40] with a declining frequency in old age. This latter observation may, however, be incorrect because elderly patients with varicose veins are rarely referred for surgery. Varicose veins are unusual in subjects less than 20 years of age and are most common in people between 45 and 65 years of age.

The Basle study of Widmer showed a steady increase in prevalence with age for all types of varicosity.[148] This has been confirmed by a number of other reports.[1,33,62,87] The recent continuing epidemiological studies by Schultz-Ehrenburg and his colleagues[124–126] have shown that a cohort of school children did not develop varicose veins until they entered their teenage years. The follow-up of these children will provide important information on the influence of age in the development of varicose veins.

Gender

The Basle survey[148] is the only study that shows a male-to-female preponderance for the prevalence of varicose veins. Studies on patients presenting to doctors for treatment are biased because women are more likely to complain of 'unsightly veins' (especially in those parts of the world where they expose their legs by wearing short dresses) than men.[53] All the other large surveys show a female-to-male excess of between 2:1 and 4:1 (Table 5.3).[26]

Pregnancy

This factor is obviously closely associated with the difference in sex incidence of varicose veins. Lake *et al.*[76] examined the prevalence of varicose veins in a group of 536 employees, all over 40 years of age,

in a New York department store. They found an increased incidence in women who had been pregnant compared to the nulliparous group (Table 5.4) (79.5% vs 66.9%).

When they compared the male and female employees, they found a greater prevalence of varicose veins in the women but even when a correction was made for gender, the effect of pregnancy persisted. This suggests that pregnancy and gender influence the development of varicose vein independently.

The incidence of varicose veins developing during pregnancy varies between 8 and 20%.[44,70,101] In a group of 405 women with varicose veins, Mullane[97] found that 13% were primiparous, 30% were secundiparous, 57% were multiparous; Donato and Nejamkin[45] found similar rates, and Berge and Feldthusen[17], who reviewed 908 pregnancies, found that the risk of developing varicose veins after two or more pregnancies was significantly greater than the risk after the first pregnancy.

It is possible that the development of varicose veins during pregnancy is related to the changing hormone levels, particularly oestrogens, which encourage venous distension by causing smooth muscle relaxation.[92] Compression of the iliac veins by the enlarging uterus may also contribute to their development.

The results of the Basle survey[148] which failed to confirm any relationship between childbirth and the prevalence of varicose veins again contradicts most of the other studies.

Table 5.4 Prevalence of varicose veins related to parity

	Total examined	No. with varicose veins	%
Nulliparous	133	89	66.9
Multiparous	98	78	79.5

Adapted from Lake *et al.*, 1942.[76]

Race, diet and bowel habit

It is easier to consider these factors together. The figure for the overall prevalence of varicose veins of 2% is based on the European and American surveys. A comparison between German and Japanese soldiers, however, showed a sixfold increase in varicose veins in the Germans.[95] It was suggested that this difference in prevalence was caused by a difference in height.

Both Pirner[108] and Foote[53] stated that varicose veins are uncommon in Africans, and Dodd[43] found only three cases of varicose veins in 11 000 in-patient admissions in a tribal reserve in Zululand. Dodd also reported that black people living in eastern Africa in Western conditions developed varicosities as often as their white counterparts.

These racial differences in prevalence are supported by two studies reported in 1986 where different rates were found between the white and native populations of Brazil[87] and the Siberian and Mongolian populations of Siberia.[81]

Cleave[30] suggested that a lack of fibre in the Western diet prolongs faecal transit time, which results in compression of the iliac veins by the distended sigmoid colon and caecum, whereas Burkitt[21] claimed that the lack of fibre combined with straining at defaecation on Western style lavatory seats raises the venous pressure. He suggested that the squatting position and the relative ease of defaecation achieved by Africans on a high fibre diet protected them from the ill effects of a raised abdominal venous pressure. As it now seems likely that descending valvular incompetence is not the cause of varicosities, these hypotheses are probably incorrect.

Two investigators actually measured venous pressures in the sitting and squatting position during straining[90] and showed that the squatting position was no more effective than the sitting position in preventing the transmission of intra-abdominal pressure to the veins of the lower leg.

Alexander[5] has re-examined the published work concerning the influence of race on varicose veins. He felt that there was good evidence that the prevalence is greater in Western than in Eastern communities, and is very low in both Africa and India.

The influence of race is probably multifactorial and cannot easily be separated from genetic factors, dietary factors, body build and other extraneous factors such as clothing and occupation.

Height and weight

Both excessive height and increased weight have been thought to be associated with a greater risk of developing varicose veins. In 1913 Miyauchi[95] originally suggested that the high prevalence of varicose veins in German soldiers compared with their Japanese counterparts was a result of their greater height. Dodd, however, noted a very low incidence in the Zulus who are a very tall race.[43] There is a significant correlation between the height of the individual and the resting venous pressure in the lower limb[23] (Figure 5.8) but it is doubtful if this correlation is of any clinical importance. Widmer[148] found that 4.5% of the very tall people in his survey developed varicose veins compared with 5% of the very short people, indicating little effect of height.

Both Myers[100] and Ludbrook[85] found that patients with varicose veins were heavier than age- and sex-matched controls without varicose veins, but the Basle study[148] again failed to reveal any significant differences in prevalence between fat and thin subjects. Widmer did find evidence of an increased prevalence of dilated intradermal venules in obese women but no association with trunk vein varicosities. There appears to be an inverse relationship between the waist/hips and waist/thigh fat ratios and the incidence of varicose veins, suggesting that fat storage in the hips and thighs might increase the risk of varicose veins.[128]

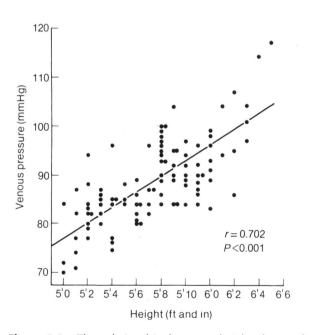

Figure 5.8 The relationship between height (feet and inches) and the resting venous pressure measured in the foot (mmHg) of 100 subjects. There is a highly significant correlation between height and foot vein pressure.[23]

Table 5.5 Incidence of a positive family history in patients with varicose veins

1921	Magnus[88]	50–75%
1927	Nicholson[102]	55%
1930	de Takats and Quint[42]	65%
1932	Jensen[68]	50%
1936	Payne[106]	50%
1943	Larsen and Smith[77]	43%
1946	McPhetters and Anderson[93]	6–10%
1950	Pratt[111]	80%
1978	Widmer[148]	63–67%
1994	Cornu-Thenard[35]	25–62%

Occupation, posture and clothing

In the same way that the height of the patient was thought to influence the development of varicose veins, so occupations which involve prolonged periods of standing have also been thought to increase the risk of varicose veins. Policemen and shop assistants, in addition to surgeons, were regarded as high risk occupations. Santler *et al.*[120] reviewed 2854 patients with varicose disease and found 6.3% were required to walk in their occupation, 29.2% spent their time sitting, and 64.5% stood still at work. Lake *et al.*,[76] in their New York department store survey, found that 74% of the employees who stood had varicose veins compared with 57% who sat. In one of the analyses of the Basle study[148] a weak correlation was found between the type of occupation, standing or sitting, and the risk of varicose veins.

Mekky *et al.*[94] reported a different incidence of varicose veins in two matched populations of cotton workers in Egypt and England. The prevalence of the condition was much higher in the English workers than in the Egyptians, and this was significantly related to age, parity, body weight, type of corsetry, and occupation (namely standing at work).

Taken together, these studies suggest that occupations which involve prolonged standing may carry an increased risk of varicose veins. The case against tight corsetry requires further support! This has not been forthcoming to our knowledge since the first edition of this book.

Heredity

Foote[53] reported that the majority of patients who sought medical attention for their varicose veins proffer information that 'one or other of their parents was a sufferer'. Virchow[145] recognized the influence of heredity in the development of varicose veins, and Gay[56] reported two affected families in some detail. Ottley[105] examined 50 families with varicose veins and claimed that inheritance was of a simple dominant type. The prevalence of relatives affected in eight studies up to 1950 is given in Table 5.5.

A review by Gundersen and Hauge in 1963[58] found that 43% of the relatives of women and 19% of the relatives of men had varicose veins. Although this prevalence is higher than that expected in the general population, it is far less than that expected from a true dominant inheritance. These authors conclude that the inheritance of varicose veins is polygeneric. Munn *et al.*[98] have reported a family history of varicose veins in almost 80% of their patients admitted for surgery for long saphenous vein incompetence. Surprisingly, we have been unable to find any evidence in the medical literature of the incidence of varicose veins in twins, where detailed studies might help to elucidate the mechanism of inheritance.

Cornu-Thenard and his co-workers[35,36] found similar hereditary tendencies in 134 familes and have also reported that there was a higher incidence of blood group A in patients with varicose veins, and this appeared to be an independent variable.

Side

Although the left common iliac vein passes behind the right common iliac artery in the pelvis and there is a higher incidence of ilio-femoral thrombosis in the left leg, there is no evidence that the incidence of varicose veins is higher in the left leg.

Summary of factors responsible for primary varicose veins

Inherited structural weakness with a possible but a still as yet unidentified haemodynamic factor appears to be the main cause of primary varicose veins. Age, female gender, parity, race and occupation may all contribute to the development of varicose veins. A much weaker case exists for other factors.

Secondary varicose veins are caused by post-thrombotic damage, pelvic tumours, especially pregnancy, congenital abnormalities (Klippel–Trenaunay syndrome, and congenital valvular agenesis) (see Chapter 24) and acquired or congenital arteriovenous fistulae (Figure 5.9).

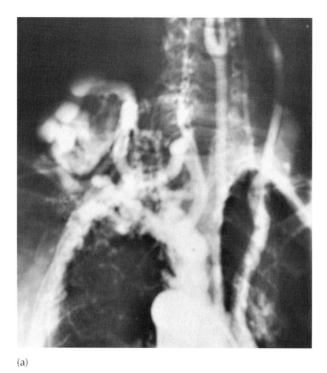

(a)

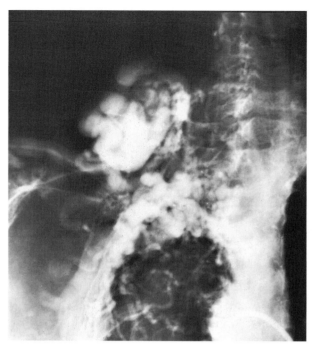

(b)

Figure 5.9   An arch aortogram (a) of a massive acquired arteriovenous fistula in the root of the neck. The venous phase (b) shows a large mass of secondary varicose veins.

Pathology

Histological studies on varicose veins[118,152] have shown that the most striking change is an increase in fibrous tissue which invades the media, breaking up the smooth muscle layers into a number of separate bundles. Collagen and fibrous tissue also accumulate in the subintima, and the elastic fibres tend to be spread throughout the layers of the vein wall instead of being restricted to the internal and external elastic laminae (Figure 5.10). All these changes have a patchy distribution.

On electron microscopy the smooth muscle cells are seen to contain excessive numbers of granules but the significance of these granules is not known. It has been suggested[118] that the granules contain collagenase and elastase which when secreted by the smooth muscle cells, may cause weakening of the wall which in turn leads to dilatation. Other enzymes and free radicals may also be released. The loss of muscle cells and their replacement by connective tissue appears to be the main pathological process associated with varicosity. The loss of elastin fibres may also be important.[28]

Smooth muscle hypertrophy has also been found in the wall of varicose veins.[139,140] Histochemical studies performed on varicose veins with smooth muscle hypertrophy suggest that the hypertrophic muscle depends on anaerobic glycolysis for its metabolic requirements.[147] When, however, the reaction of venous smooth muscle to distension was studied in the walls of normal and varicose veins, no significant differences could be found.[137] This appears to exclude a primary abnormality of the smooth muscle as a cause of varicosity.

Valves

The valves of varicose veins become stretched and, in the later stages of vein distension, atrophic.[37,104] In grossly dilated varices there is often evidence of thrombosis on the valve cusps which together with the walls of the veins may become calcified (Figure 5.11).

The anatomical distribution of the varices

Although the long saphenous system of veins is most frequently affected, the main trunk (stem) vein only rarely becomes varicose, and it is the tributaries of the long saphenous vein that usually dilate (Figure 5.12). The long saphenous vein itself

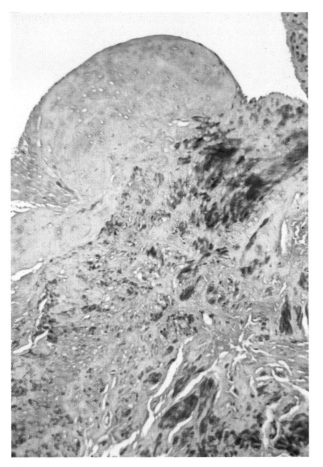

Figure 5.10 A photomicrograph of the wall of a varicose vein showing collagen fibres extending throughout all layers of the wall breaking up the muscle of the media. (We are indebted to Mr S Rose for this illustration.)

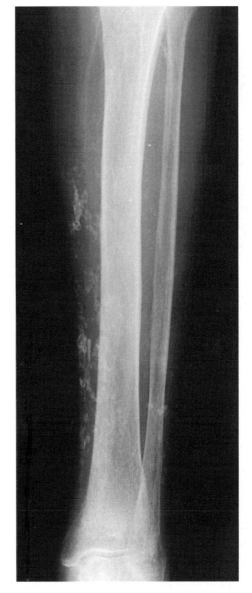

Figure 5.11 A plain x-ray showing calcification in the walls of long-standing varicose veins.

is probably protected by its well-developed muscular media and a layer of fibrous tissue which binds it to the deep fascia.[137]

The tributaries of the long saphenous vein contain relatively less muscle in their walls and lie unsupported in the subcutaneous fat close to the skin. This combination of a lack of support with relative weakness of the muscle wall probably explains the frequency with which the tributaries dilate.

Enzymatic changes in the wall

Collagenase, elastase, maleate dehydrogenase, non-specific esterases, adenosine triphosphate and 5-nucleotidases[134,135] are all said to be reduced in varicose veins when compared with normal veins, while acid phosphatase and lactic dehydrogenase

have been found to be elevated.[142] The level of tissue plasminogen activator is reduced in varicose veins compared with normal controls[78,150] and recently it has been shown that monoclonal and polyclonal plasminogen activator antibodies localize to the smooth muscle of vein wall in addition to the endothelial cells.[78] It is unlikely that low levels of plasminogen activator are the cause of varicosities, and a recent paper[129] has shown that urokinase levels are increased within the walls of varicose veins. Free radicals[49] and mast cells[151] may also be increased.

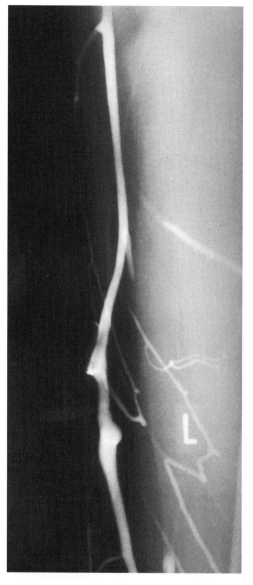

Figure 5.12 A varicogram showing saccular dilatations of the long saphenous vein itself, a relatively unusual finding.

Lysozymes

It has been suggested that an increase in lysosomal enzymes[73] may dissolve ground substance and so cause varicosity. Blood levels of proteoglycans have been found to be raised in the serum of patients with varicose veins compared with the levels in normal controls.

Changes in the calf muscle

Makitie[89] has found changes in the striated muscle of the calf pump in patients with varicose veins. He

has not shown whether these changes are primary or secondary to the varicose veins.

THE COMPLICATIONS OF VARICOSE VEINS

The pathology of the complications such as superficial thrombophlebitis, eczema, pigmentation, lipodermatosclerosis, haemorrhage, ulceration and an increased risk of deep vein thrombosis are discussed in detail in Chapters 8, 15 and 23.

References

1. Abramson JH, Hopp C, Epstein LM. The epidemiology of varicose veins. A survey in Western Jerusalem. *J Epidemiol Community Health* 1981; **35:** 213–17.
2. Abu-own A, Scurr JH, Coleridge-Smith PD. Saphenous vein reflux without incompetence at the sapheno-femoral junction. *Br J Surg* 1994; **81:** 1452–4.
3. Ackroyd JS, Lea Thomas M, Browse NL. Deep vein reflux: an assessment by descending phlebography. *Br J Surg* 1986; **73:** 31–3.
4. Ackroyd JS, Pattison M, Browse NL. A study of the mechanical properties of fresh and preserved human femoral vein wall and valve cusps. *Br J Surg* 1985; **72:** 117–19.
5. Alexander CJ. The epidemiology of varicose veins. *Med J Aust* 1972; **1:** 215–18.
6. Alexander CJ. Chair sitting and varicose veins. *Lancet* 1972; **2:** 822–3.
7. Andreotti L, Cammelli D. Connective tissue in varicose veins. *Angiology* 1979; **30:** 798–805.
8. Andreotti L, Cammelli D, Banchi G, Guarnieri M, Serantoni C. Collagen, elastin and sugar content in primary varicose veins. *Ric Clin Lab* 1978; **8:** 273–85.
9. Arnoldi CC. The heredity of venous insufficiency. *Dan Med Bull* 1958; **5:** 169–75.
10. Arnoldi CC. The aetiology of primary varicose veins. *Dan Med Bull* 1957; **4:** 102–7.
11. Barbaro G, Guerrina G, Traverso G, Vota L. Determinazione quantitativa del collagene e delle frazioni del connettivo nella varice idiopatica. *Pathologica* 1967; **59:** 87–90.
12. Baron HC, Cassaro S. Role of a-v shunts in the pathogenesis of varicose veins. *J Vasc Surg* 1986; **4:** 124–8.
13. Basmajian JV. The distribution of valves in the femoral, external iliac and common iliac veins and their relationship to varicose veins. *Surg Gynecol Obstet* 1952; **95:** 537–42.
14. Beaglehole R. Epidemiology of varicose veins. *World J Surg* 1986; **10:** 898–902.
15. Beaglehole R, Salmond CE, Prior IAM. Varicose veins in New Zealand. Prevalence and severity. *N Z Med J* 1976; **84:** 396–9.

16. Bennett WH. Congenital sacculations and cystic dilations of veins. *Lancet* 1890; **1:** 788.

17. Berge TH, Feldthusen U. Varicer hos kvinnor. Faktorer av betydelse for deras uppkomst. *Nord Med* 1963; **69:** 744–9.

18. Bobek K, Cajzl L, Cepelak V, Slaisova V, Opatzny K, Barcal R. Etude de la fréquence des maladies phlébologiques et de l'influence de quelques facteurs étiologiques. *Phlébologie* 1966; **19:** 217–30.

19. Borschberg E. *The Prevalence of Varicose Veins of the Lower Extremity*. Basle: S Karger, 1967.

20. Brewer AC. Arteriovenous shunts. *Br Med J* 1950; **2:** 270.

21. Burkitt DP. Varicose veins, deep vein thrombosis, and haemorrhoids: epidemiology and suggested aetiology. *Br Med J* 1972; **2:** 556–61.

22. Burkitt DP, Townsend AJ, Patel K, Skacig K. Varicose veins in developing countries. *Lancet* 1976; **2:** 202–3.

23. Burnand KG. *Studies on the Cause of Venous Ulceration*. London University, MS Thesis, 1981.

24. Burnand KG, Clemenson G, Whimpster I, Gaunt J, Browse NL. The effect of sustained venous hypertension on the skin capillaries of the canine hind limb. *Br J Surg* 1982; **69:** 41–4.

25. Butterworth DM, Rose SS, Clark P, Rowland P, Knight S, Baboubi NY. Light microscopy, immunohistochemistry and electronmicroscopy of the valves of the lower limb veins and jugular veins. *Phlebology* 1992; **7:** 27–30.

26. Callam MJ. Epidemiology of varicose veins. *Br J Surg* 1994; **81:** 167–73.

27. Callender GW. Diseases of the veins, In: Holmes T, ed. *System of Surgery*. London: Parker and Bourn, 1862.

28. Chello M, Mastroroberto P, Romano R, Crillo F, Cusano T, Marchese AR. Alteration in collagen and elastin content in varicose veins. *J Vasc Surg* 1994; **28:** 23–7.

29. Clarke H, Smith SRG, Vasdekris SN, Hobbs JT, Nicolaides AN. Role of venous elasticity in the development of varicose veins. *Br J Surg* 1989; **76:** 577–80.

30. Cleave TL. *On the Causation of Varicose Veins and their Prevention and Arrest by Natural Means*. Bristol: Wright, 1960.

31. Cockett FB, Lea Thomas M, Negus D. Iliac vein compression: its relation to ilio-femoral thrombosis and the post thrombotic syndrome. *Br Med J* 1967; **2:** 14–19.

32. Coles RW. Varicose veins in Tropical Africa. *Lancet* 1974; **2:** 474–5.

33. Coon WW, Willis PW, Keller JB. Venous thromboembolism and other venous disease in the Tecumseh Community Health Study. *Circulation* 1973; **48:** 839–46.

34. Corcos L, Peruzzi G, Romeo V, Procacci T, Dini S. Peripheral venous biopsy: significance, limitations, indications and clinical applications. *Phlebology* 1989; **4:** 271–4.

35. Cornu-Thenard A, Bolvin P, Baud JM, Vincenzi I, Carpentier PH. Importance of the familial factor in varicose disease. Clinical study of 134 families. *J Dermatol Surg* 1994; **20:** 318–26.

36. Cornu-Thenard A, Dab W, de Vinconzi I, Valty J. Relationship between blood groups (ABO) and varicose veins. A case control study. *Phlebology* 1989; **4:** 37–40.

37. Cotton L. Varicose veins: gross anatomy and development. *Br J Surg* 1961; **48:** 589–98.

38. Crotty TP. Is circulating noradrenaline the cause of varicose veins? *Med Hypotheses* 1991; **34:** 243–51.

39. Dalrymple J, Crofts T. Varicose veins in developing countries. *Lancet* 1975; **1:** 808–9.

40. DaSilva A, Widmer LK, Martin H, Mall TH, Glaus L, Schneider M. Varicose veins and chronic venous insufficiency. *Vasa* 1974; **3:** 118–25.

41. Deby C, Hariton C, Pincemail J, Coget J. Decreased tocopherol concentration of varicose veins is associated with a decrease in antilipoperoxidant activity without similar changes in plasma. *Phlebology* 1989; **4:** 113–21.

42. de Takats G, Quint H. The injection treatment of varicose veins. *Surg Gynecol Obstet* 1930; **50:** 545.

43. Dodd HJ. The cause, prevention and arrest of varicose veins. *Lancet* 1964; **2:** 809–11.

44. Dodd H, Wright HP. Vulval varicosities in pregnancy. *Br Med J* 1959; **1:** 831–2.

45. Donato VM, Nejamkim J. Varices y embarazo. Su tratamiento. *Prensa Med Argent* 1952; **43:** 551.

46. Duchosal F, Allemann H, Widmer LK, Breil H, Leu HJ. Varikosis – Alter - Körpergewicht. *Z Kreislaufforsch* 1968; **57:** 380.

47. Edwards JE, Edwards EA. The saphenous valves in varicose veins. *Am Heart J* 1940; **19:** 338–51.

48. Eger SA, Casper SL. Etiology of varicose veins from an anatomic aspect based on dissections of 38 adult cadavers. *JAMA* 1943; **123:** 148–9.

49. Farbiszewski R, Glowinski J, Makarewicz-Plonska M, Chwiecko M, Ostapowicz R, Glowinski S. Oxygen-derived free radicals as mediators of varicose vein wall damage. *Vasc Surg* 1996; **30:** 47–52.

50. Fegan WG. Anatomy and pathophysiology of varicose veins. In: *Venous Diseases Medical and Surgical Management*. Montreux: Foundation International Corporation, Medical Sciences, 1974.

51. Fegan WG, Kline AL. The cause of varicosity in superficial veins of the lower limb. *Br J Surg* 1972; **59:** 798–801.

52. Fischer H. *Venenleiden – Eine representative Undersuchung in der Bundesrepublik Deutschland*. Munich: Urban & Schwarzenberg, 1981.

53. Foote RR. *Varicose Veins*. London: Butterworths, 1954.

54. Franks PJ, Wright DDI, McCollum CN. Epidemiology of venous disease. A review. *Phlebology* 1989; **4:** 143–51.

55. Garcia-Rospide V, Penafiel-Marfil R, Moreno-Padilla F, Gonzalez-Rios J, Ramos Bruno JJ, Ros Die E. Enzymatic and isoenzymatic study of varicose veins. *Phlebology* 1991; **6:** 187–98.

56. Gay J. *On Varicose Diseases of the Lower Extremities. The Lettsomian Lectures of 1867*. London: Churchill, 1868.

57. Gjores JE. The incidence of venous thrombosis and its sequelae in certain districts of Sweden. *Acta Chir Scand* 1956; **Suppl 206**.

58. Gundersen J, Hauge M. Hereditary factors in venous insufficiency. *Angiology* 1969; **20**: 346–55.

59. Hasebroek K. Uber die Bedeutung der Arterienpulsationen für die Stromung in den Venen und die Pathogenese der Varicen. *Pflugers Arch ges Physiol* 1916; **163**: 191–238.

60. Hasebroek K. Eine physikalisch-experimentell begründete neue Auffassung der Pathogenese der Varicen. *Dtsch Z Chir* 1916; **136**: 381.

61. Hehne HJ, Locher J Th, Waibel PP, Fridrich R. Zur Bedeutung arteriovenoser Anastomosen bei der primaren Varicosis und der chronisch-venosen Insuffizienz. *Vasa* 1974; **4**: 396–8.

62. Hirai M. Prevalence and risk factors of varicose veins in Japanese women. *Angiology* 1990; **3**: 228–2.

63. Hobbs J. Surgery and sclerotherapy in the treatment of varicose veins. A random trial. *Arch Surg* 1974; **109**: 793–6.

64. Hobsley M. *Pathways in Surgical Management*, 2nd edition. London: Edward Arnold, 1986; 196.

65. Holman EF. Development of arterial aneurysms. *Surg Gynecol Obstet* 1955; **100**: 599.

66. *Illness and Health Care in Canada. Canadian Sickness Survey 1950–1951*. Ottawa: The Department of National Health and Welfare and the Dominion Bureau of Statistics, 1960.

67. Jager A. Venenklappen und muskelkontraktion. *Pflugers Arch ges Physiol* 1936; **238**: 508.

68. Jensen DR. Varicose veins and their treatment. *Ann Surg* 1932; **95**: 738.

69. Jurukova Z, Milenkov C. Ultrastructural evidence for collagen degradation in the walls of varicose veins. *Exp Mol Pathol* 1982; **37**: 37–47.

70. Kilbourne NJ. Varicose veins in pregnancy. *Am J Obstet Gynecol* 1933; **25**: 104–6.

71. King ESJ. The genesis of varicose veins. *Aust N Z J Surg* 1950; **20**: 126–33.

72. Klotz K. Untersuchungern. Über die Saphena Magna beim Menschen besonders zücksichtlich ihrer Klappenverhaltnisse. *Arch Anat Physiol (Lpz)* 1887; **3**: 159.

73. Kreysel HW, Nissen HP, Enghofer E. A possible role of lysosomal enzymes in the pathogenesis of varicosis and the reduction in their serum activity by Venostasin. *Vasa* 1983; **12**: 377–82.

74. Kulka JP. In: Hill AGA, ed. *Modern Trends in Rheumatology*. Vol. 1. London: Butterworths, 1966.

75. Lagatolla NRF, Donald A, Lockhart S, Burnand KG. Retrograde flow in the deep veins of subjects with normal venous function. *Br J Surg* 1997; **84**: 36–9.

76. Lake M, Pratt GH, Wright IS. Arteriosclerosis and varicose veins: occupational activities and other factors. *JAMA* 1942; **119**: 696–701.

77. Larsen RA, Smith FL. Varicose veins: evaluation of observations in 491 cases. *Proc Mayo Clin* 1943; **18**: 400–6.

78. Layer GT, Pattison M, Evans B, Davies DR, Burnand KG. Tissue fibrinolytic activity is reduced in varicose veins. In: Negus D, Jantet G, eds. *Phlebology '85*. London: John Libbey, 1986.

79. Ledderhose G. Studien über den Blutlauf in der Hautvenen unter physiologischen und Pathologischen Bedingungen. *Mitt Grenzgeb Med Chir* 1906; **15**: 355.

80. Lindvall N, Lodin A. Congenital absence of venous valves. *Acta Chir Scand* 1962; **124**: 310–19.

81. Listitsyn KM. Epidemiology of disease of the veins of the lower extremities in various climato geographic conditions. *Vestn Khir* 1986; **137**: 71–2.

82. Lodin A, Lindvall N, Gentele H. Congenital absence of venous valves as a cause of leg ulcers. *Acta Chir Scand* 1959; **116**: 256–71.

83. Logan WPD, Brooke EM, eds. *Studies on Medical and Population Subjects. Number 12. The Survey of Sickness 1943–52*. London: General Register Office, 1957.

84. Löwenstein A. Über die Venenklappen und Varicenbildung. *Mitt Grenzgeb Med Chir* 1907; **18**: 161.

85. Ludbrook J. Obesity and varicose veins. *Surg Gynecol Obstet* 1964; **118**: 843.

86. Ludbrook J. Valvular defect in primary varicose veins. Cause or effect? *Lancet* 1963; **2**: 1289–92.

87. Maffei FHA, Magaldi C, Pinho SZ, *et al*. Varicose veins and chronic venous insufficiency in Brazil. Prevalence among 1755 inhabitants of a country town. *Int J Epidemiol* 1986; **15**: 210–17.

88. Magnus G. Zirkulationsverhaltnisse in varicen. *Dtsch Z Chir* 1921; **162**: 71.

89. Makitie J. Muscle changes in patients with varicose veins. *Acta Pathol Microbiol Scand (A)* 1977; **85**: 864–8.

90. Martin A, Odling-Smee W. Pressure changes in varicose veins. *Lancet* 1976; **1**: 768–70.

91. May R, Thurner J. The cause of the predominately sinistral occurrence of thrombosis of the pelvic veins. *Angiology* 1957; **8**: 419.

92. McCausland AM. Influence of hormones upon varicose veins. *West J Surg* 1943; **51**: 199.

93. McPhetters HO, Anderson JK. *Injection Treatment of Varicose Veins and Haemorrhoids*. Philadelphia, PA: Davis, 1946.

94. Mekky S, Schilling RSF, Walford J. Varicose veins in women cotton workers. An epidemiological study in England and Egypt. *Br Med J* 1969; **2**: 591–5.

95. Miyauchi K. Die Haufigkeit der varizen am unterschenkel bei Japanem und der Erfolg einiger operativ beihandelter Falle. *Arch Klin Chir* 1913; **100**: 1079–85.

96. Moore HD. Deep venous valves in the aetiology of varicose veins. *Lancet* 1951; **2**: 7–10.

97. Mullane DJ. Varicose veins of pregnancy. *Am J Obstet Gynecol* 1952; **63**: 620–3.

98. Munn SR, Morton JB, Macbeth WAAG, McLeish AR. To strip or not strip the long saphenous vein? A varicose vein trial. *Br J Surg* 1981; **68**: 426–8.

99. Murley RS. Deep venous valves in the aetiology of varicose veins. *Lancet* 1951; **1**: 176.

100. Myers TT. Varicose veins. In: Barker, Hines, eds. *Barker and Hines's Peripheral Vascular Diseases*, 3rd edition. Philadelphia, PA: Saunders, 1962.
101. Nabatoff RA. Varicose veins of pregnancy. *JAMA* 1960; **174:** 1712.
102. Nicholson BB. Varicose veins etiology and treatment. *Arch Surg* 1927; **15:** 351.
103. Nylander G. Meanders of the great saphenous vein. *Angiology* 1969; **20:** 587–91.
104. Obitsu Y, Ishimaru S, Furukawa K, Yoshihama I. Histopathological studies of the valves of varicose veins. *Phlebology* 1990; **5:** 245–54.
105. Ottley C. Heredity and varicose veins. *Br Med J* 1934; **1:** 528.
106. Payne RT. The treatment of varicose diseases of the lower limb. *Br Med J* 1936; **1:** 877–8.
107. Pigeaux ALJ. *Traite Practique des Maladies des Vaisseaux Contenant des Recherches Historiques Speciales.* Paris: Labe et Rouvier, 1843.
108. Pirner F. *Der varikose Symptomen-komplex.* Stuttgart: F Enke, 1957.
109. Powell T, Lynn RB. The valves of the external iliac, femoral and upper third of the popliteal veins. *Surg Gynecol Obstet* 1951; **92:** 453–5.
110. Pratt GH. Arterial varices: a syndrome. *Am J Surg* 1949; **77:** 456.
111. Pratt GH. Differential diagnosis and treatment of pathologically enlarged veins. *Med Clin North Am* 1950; **34:** 897–905.
112. Prerovsky I. *Diseases of the Veins.* World Health Organization, internal communication. MHO-PA 10964.
113. Psaila JV, Melhuish J. Viscoelastin properties and collagen content of the long saphenous vein in normal and varicose veins. *Br J Surg* 1989; **76:** 37–40.
114. Puilacks P, Vidal Barraquer F. Pathogenic study of varicose veins. *Angiology* 1953; **4:** 59–100.
115. Reikeras O, Sorlie D. The significance of arteriovenous shunting for the development of varicose veins. *Acta Chir Scand* 1983; **149:** 479–81.
116. Rindfleisch E. *Lehrbuch der Pathologischen Gewebelehre*, 6th edition. Leipzig: Engelmann, 1867.
117. Rokitansky C. *A Manual of Pathological Anatomy.* Vol. 4. London: Sydenham Society, 1852.
118. Rose SS, Ahmed A. Some thoughts on the aetiology of varicose veins. *J Cardiovasc Surg* 1986; **27:** 534–43.
119. Ryan TJ, Copeman PWM. Microvascular pattern and blood stasis in skin disease. *Br J Dermatol* 1969; **81:** 563–73.
120. Santler R, Ernst G, Weiel B. Statistisches über der varikosen Symptomenkomplex. *Hautarzt* 1956; **10:** 460.
121. Schalin L. AV communications in varicose veins localised by thermography and identified by operative microscopy. *Acta Chir Scand* 1981; **147:** 409–20.
122. Schalin L. Arteriovenous communication to varicose veins in the lower extremity studied by dynamic angiography. *Acta Chir Scand* 1980; **146:** 397–406.
123. Schalin L. Role of arteriovenous shunting in the development of varicose veins. In: Eklof B, Gjores JE, Thulesius O, Bergqvist D, eds. *Controversies in the Management of Venous Disorders.* London: Butterworth, 1989; 182–92.
124. Schultz-Ehrenburg U, Weindorf N, VonUslar D, Hiche H. Prospective epidemiologiche Studie uber die Entstehungsweise der Kramptadern bei Kindern und Jugendlichen (Bochumer Studie I und II). *Phlebol Proktol* 1989; **18:** 3–11.
125. Schultz-Ehrenburg U, Weindorf N, VonUslar D, Hiche H. Prospective epidemiological investigations in early and preclinical stages of varicosis. In: Davy A, Stemmer R, eds. *Phlebology 89.* Paris: John Libbey, Eurotext, 1989; 163–5.
126. Schultz-Ehrenburg U, Weindorf N, Mattes U, Hirche H. New epidemiological findings with regard to initial stages of varicose veins. Bochum study I to III. *Phlebologie* 1992; 234–6.
127. Schwarz E. Die Krampfadern der unteren Extre mitat mit besonderer Berücksichtigung ihrer Entstehung und Behandlung. *Ergebn Chir Orthop* 1934; **27:** 256.
128. Seidell JC, Oosterlee A, Deurenberg P, Hautvast JGAJ. What causes varicose veins? *Lancet* 1986; **1:** 321.
129. Shireman PK, McCarthy WJ, Pearce WH, *et al.* Plasminogen activator levels are influenced by location and varicosity in greater saphenous vein. *J Vasc Surg* 1996; **24:** 719–24.
130. *The Sickness Survey of Denmark.* The committee on the Danish national morbidity survey. Copenhagen, 1960.
131. Sinzinger H, Fitscha P. Prostacyclin (PGI^2) contracts normal and varicose human saphenous veins. *Vasa* 1984; **13:** 228–30.
132. Slawinski Z. Przyczynek do anatomii zylakow konczyny dolnej; o umiejscowieniu rozszerzen woreczkowatych zyly podskornej uda wielkiej. *Gaz Lek Warsz* 1899; **19:** 1355.
133. Somerville J, Byrne P, King D. Turbulence in the causation of varicose veins. *Br J Surg* 1973; **60:** 311–12.
134. Svejcar J, Prerovsky I, Linhart J, Kruml J. Content of collagen, elastin, and water in walls of the internal saphenous vein in man. *Circ Res* 1962; **11:** 296.
135. Svejcar J, Prerovsky I, Linhart J, Kruml J. Content of collagen, elastin and hexosamine in primary varicose veins. *Clin Sci* 1963; **24:** 325–30.
136. Tannyol A, Menduke H. Alcohol as a possible etiological agent in varicose veins. *Angiology* 1961; **12:** 382.
137. Thompson H. The surgical anatomy of the superficial and perforating veins of the lower limb. *Ann R Coll Surg Engl* 1979; **61:** 198.
138. Thulesius O, Gjores JE. Reactions of venous smooth muscle in normal men and patients with varicose veins. *Angiology* 1974; **25:** 145–54.
139. Thulesius O, Ugaily-Thulusius L, Gjores JE, Neglen P. The varicose saphenous vein, functional and ultrastructural studies, with special reference to smooth muscle. *Phlebology* 1988; **3:** 89–95.
140. Travers JP, Dalton CM, Baker DM, Makin GS. Biochemical and histological analysis of collagen

and elastin content and smooth muscle density in normal and varicose veins. *Phlebology* 1992; **7:** 92–100.

141. Trendelenburg F. Ueber die unterbindung der vena saphena magna bie unterschenkel varicen. *Beitr Klin Chir* 1890–1; **7:** 195–210.

142. Urbanova D, Prerovsky I. Enzymes in the wall of normal and varicose veins. Histochemical study. *Angiologia* 1972; **9:** 53–61.

143. US Department of Health, Education and Welfare. *National Health Survey 1935–1936.* Washington, DC: 1938.

144. Van Bemmelen PS, Bedford G, Beach KW, Strandness DE. Quantitative segmental evaluation of venous valvular reflux with ultrasonic duplex scanning. *J Vasc Surg* 1989; **10:** 425–31.

145. Virchow R. *Cellular Pathology.* London: Churchill, 1860.

146. Wedell JM. Varicose veins pilot study. *Br J Surg* 1969; **23:** 179–86.

147. Wegmann R, El Samannoudy FA, Olivier C, Rettori R. Histochemical studies on the wall of human varicose veins: the saphenous varicose vein. *Ann Histochim* 1974; **19:** 285–92.

148. Widmer LK. *Peripheral Venous Disorders. Prevalence and Socio-medical Importance. Observations in 4529 apparently Healthy Persons. Basle 111 Study.* Bern: Hans Huber, 1978.

149. Williams AF. A comparative study of venous valves in the limbs. *Surg Gynecol Obstet* 1954; **99:** 676.

150. Wolfe JHN, Morland M, Browse NL. The fibrinolytic activity of varicose veins. *Br J Surg* 1979; **66:** 185–7.

151. Yamada T, Tomita S, Mori M, Sasatomi E, Suenaga E, Itoh T. Increased mast cell infiltration in varicose veins of the lower limbs: a possible role in the development of varices. *Surgery* 1996; **119:** 494–7.

152. Zancani A. Über die Varicen der unteren Extremitaten; experimentelle und klinische Untersuchungen. *Arch Klin Chir* 1911; **96:** 91.

153. Zwillenberg LO, Laszt L, Zwillenberg H. Die Fienstruktur der Venenwand bei Varikose. [Possible influence of smooth muscle on collagen.] *Angiologica* 1971; **8:** 318–46.

CHAPTER 6

Varicose veins: diagnosis

The symptoms caused by varicose veins	163	Definition of the extent and connections of		
History	169	varicosities		182
Physical signs of varicose veins	169	Special investigations of the deep veins		183
Summary	177	Suggested diagnostic pathways		185
Special investigations of the superficial veins	178	References		187

The symptoms caused by varicose veins

The major symptoms caused by varicose veins are summarized in Table 6.1; other conditions which may give similar appearances are listed in Table 6.2.

UNSIGHTLINESS

Many patients with varicose veins complain of the unsightliness produced by tortuous dilated veins in their lower limbs. O'Leary *et al.* in 1996 found 33% of women made this complaint compared with 8% of men.[52] Women are more aware of varicose veins

than men, because even today, with the exception of a few countries, men tend to cover their legs with long trousers while women expose their legs by wearing skirts. The desire to have legs without blemish, whether for personal 'body image' or sexual motives, is the main cause of the increasing demand for the treatment of varicose veins.

Patients concerned with the unsightly appearance of their varicose veins often complain of discomfort but the severity of this discomfort is difficult to assess and does not seem to be related to the size of the varices.[8] Massive varicosities in men often cause few symptoms while minor varicosities in women may be the source of intractable

Table 6.1 Symptoms caused by varicose veins

Unsightliness
Aches and pains
'Cramps'
Mild ankle oedema
'Itching'
Superficial thrombophlebitis
Haemorrhage
Eczema
Pigmentation
Lipodermatosclerosis
Ulceration

Table 6.2 Differential diagnosis of varicose veins

Visible non-varicose veins
Post-thrombotic collateral veins
Klippel–Trenaunay syndrome
Parkes–Weber syndrome
Arteriovenous fistula or fistulae (congenital or acquired)
Avalvular disease of the deep veins (congenital absence)
Dilated cutaneous venules
Pelvic tumours causing venous obstruction
Venous angiomata
Herniation of the anterior tibial muscle through the fascia
Dilated veins of pregnancy

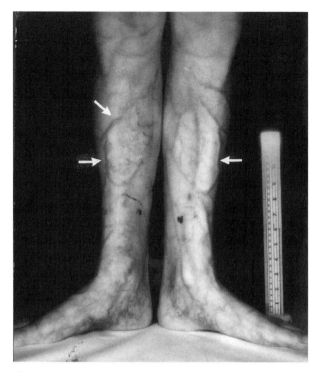

Table 6.3 Some of the causes of discomfort in the leg which must be differentiated from varicose vein pain

Osteoarthritis of the hip
Osteoarthritis of the knee
Sciatica and spinal claudication
Sarcomata of soft tissue or bone
Osteomyelitis
Osteoid osteoma
Tears of the menisci of the knee joint
Achilles tendonitis
Torn Achilles tendon
Rheumatoid arthritis
Intermittent claudication (arterial)
Venous claudication
Cramp
Myalgia
Peripheral neuropathy
Meralgia paraesthetica
Neuromas
Lymphoedema

Figure 6.1 An infra-red photograph which shows many visible but straight subcutaneous veins. One vein on the front of the left shin is dilated but straight (arrowed) whereas another on the right shin (arrowed) is tortuous but not dilated. Varicose veins are both tortuous and dilated.

pain. Perhaps patients wishing treatment for cosmetic reasons assuage their conscience by convincing themselves that they are suffering pain, or perhaps pain is unrelated to the size of the varicosities.

Some patients without any obvious tortuosity or elevation of their subcutaneous veins ask for treatment, and it is sometimes difficult to decide when a 'visible vein' becomes a 'varicose vein' (Figure 6.1). These patients often state, on the day when they attend the clinic, that the veins have 'gone down' and do not represent their true appearance. In women the size of the varices may alter with the menstrual cycle and varices may also increase in size in very warm weather. It is best to ask such patients to return for review in 3–6 months' time when the veins may have become more obvious. This is especially true in winter as a return visit in the summer may show a completely different picture.

The other group of patients who complain of severe disfigurement are those with dilated intra-dermal venules ('spider veins', 'venous stars', 'sunburst veins', or 'cutaneous arborizing telangiectases') (Figure 6.2). These are not true varicose veins. They are frequently associated with varicose veins but are a separate, distinct, independent entity. They often develop during pregnancy or at the menopause, which suggests that they may be caused by a change in hormone levels. They are far more common in women and may extend to cover the whole leg, turning the skin a deep blue–purple colour. Their exact cause remains obscure.

ACHES AND PAINS

This is the most common symptom to accompany the complaint of unsightliness (39% in O'Leary's series).[52] Many patients will admit, on close questioning, that their pain is minor and infrequent and that the real reason for consultation is because they dislike the appearance of their legs.

Many patients do, however, experience considerable discomfort which is sometimes localized to the main varices, but is often a diffuse dull ache felt throughout the leg which gets worse as the day passes and is exacerbated by prolonged standing. Worsening of the pain before a period is characteristic and pain is sometimes accompanied by a severe 'itch' over the veins. Pain that is present at rest or in bed is unlikely to be caused by varicose veins, and another source must be sought. The typical description of 'venous' pain is an 'ache' or 'discomfort'. The presence of a sharp or acute pain should suggest an alternative diagnosis.

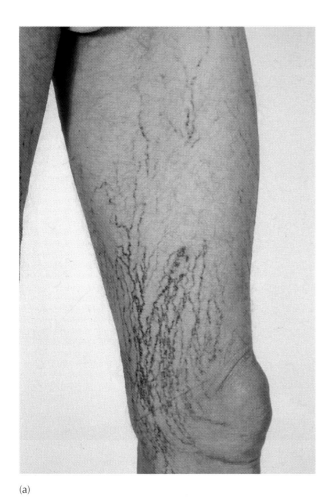

(a)

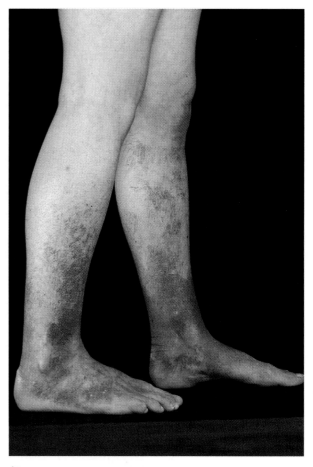

(b)

Figure 6.2 (a) Cutaneous telangiectases in the skin of the thigh. These dilated skin venules are more common in women than in men and may develop during pregnancy. They have been called 'spider veins', 'venous stars' and 'sunburst veins' and a number of other descriptive terms including 'birch-twigs' . This is a severe example. (b) Cutaneous arborizing telangiectasis. These intradermal veins are gradual spreading over the whole of both lower legs turning them blue/purple in colour. This patient had no large visible varicose veins.

Relief of the discomfort by wearing an elastic stocking provides good circumstantial evidence that the pain is of venous origin. We sometimes use this as a diagnostic test when uncertain if varicose veins are the cause of leg pain. Elevation of the legs, bed rest and walking all relieve venous pain, while standing still for prolonged periods invariably makes it worse.

A history of a bursting pain during exercise (venous claudication) may indicate venous outflow obstruction but is a rare symptom in patients with uncomplicated varicose veins.

Night cramps are a common complaint and appear to be particularly frequent in patients with varicose veins, especially after a long day of standing without exercise.

Table 6.3 lists the other causes of leg pain that may be incorrectly ascribed to varicose veins. A careful history of the nature of the leg pain, followed by a meticulous clinical examination, will often help to indicate its cause. It is especially important to examine the hips, knees and back, which are the main causes of leg pain in the middle aged or elderly. The peripheral pulses should also be carefully palpated. Some leg pains, however, defy all attempts at diagnosis in spite of phlebography, venous duplex, calf pump measurements, exercise Doppler ultrasound, arteriography, radiculography, electromyography, computerized tomography and magnetic resonance of the spine and limbs. Compartment pressure measurements are the unhelpful refuge of the diagnostically destitute!

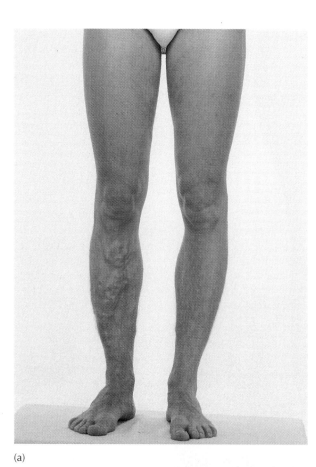

(a)

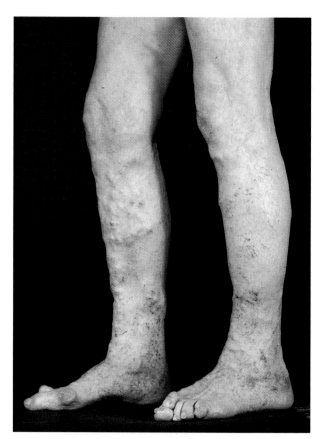

(b)

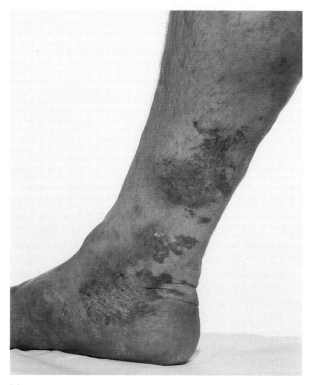

(c)

Figure 6.3 These photographs show the minor swelling of the calf and ankle that is often caused by varicose veins. Severe swelling is not a common symptom of uncomplicated varicose veins. (a) The varicose veins of the right leg are clearly causing mild swelling of the calf, ankle and forefoot. (b) Swelling of the left ankle caused by extensive varicose veins. (c) Swelling around the ankle associated with pigmentation and mild chronic lipodermatosclerosis. In each of these examples the oedema does little more than fill in the hollows of the ankle and mildly distort the normal contours of the lower leg.

ANKLE OEDEMA

Oedema is not a common or prominent feature of varicose veins. It is usually mild and only becomes noticeable at the end of the day. Other causes of oedema, such as deep vein obstruction or lymphatic obstruction, must be excluded if there is marked oedema and the patient complains of swelling of the lower leg as well as the ankle. Incompetence of the lower leg communicating veins in isolation or in association with post-thrombotic damage of the deep veins can cause moderate oedema of the ankle and lower leg (Figure 6.3), especially in elderly obese patients who take little exercise.

Table 6.4 lists the causes of ankle swelling. Lymphoedema is the condition most commonly misdiagnosed as venous oedema (Figure 6.4) and isotope or radiographic contrast lymphangiography is often

Table 6.4 Causes of ankle oedema

Local	General
Acute deep vein thrombosis	Cardiac failure
Post-thrombotic deep vein damage	Nephrotic syndrome
Venous obstruction	Hypoalbuminaemia
Venous valvular agenesis	Fluid overload
Lymphoedema	Fluid retention syndromes
Lipodystrophy	
Hemihypertrophy	

needed to confirm the diagnosis. The general causes of oedema must not be forgotten. Fat does not pit with digital pressure (Figure 6.5). Hemihypertrophy, which may be suspected when the limb and foot are

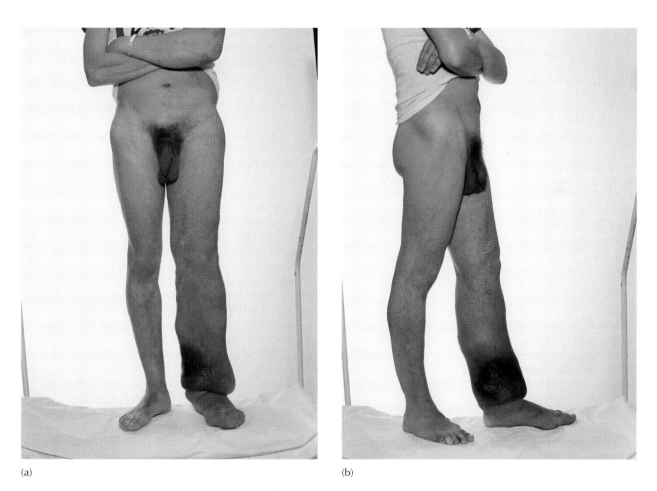

(a) (b)

Figure 6.4 (a, b) This swollen limb shows evidence of lipodermatosclerosis (pigmentation, induration and inflammation). A few varicose veins are visible, but phlebography was essentially normal. Radiographic lymphography showed peripheral lymphatic obliteration. All the visible changes were caused by the lymphoedema.

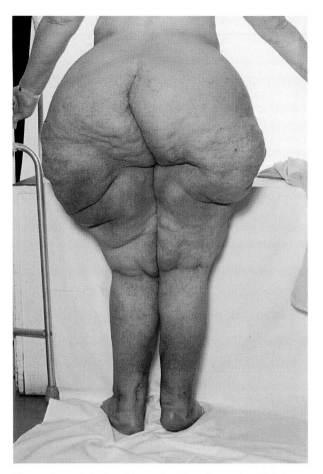

Figure 6.5 A lady with marked lipodystrophy. This is an abnormal and excessive deposition of fat in the lower half of the body causing apparent swelling, in this patient mainly of the thighs and buttocks. There is mild secondary lymphoedema and lipodermatosclerosis. Fat does not pit on pressure.

enlarged, can be confirmed by computerized tomography. Any capillary naevus or limb lengthening should suggest the diagnosis of Klippel–Trenaunay syndrome (see Chapter 24).

SUPERFICIAL THROMBOPHLEBITIS

This is a common complication of varicose veins but must be differentiated from superficial thrombophlebitis caused by other conditions (see Chapter 23). Thrombophlebitis usually presents as a tender, hot, red thickening on the course of a varicose vein. Patients usually know that they have varicose veins, and they may have had previous episodes of thrombophlebitis. The attack may be initiated by an episode of minor trauma or period of bed rest, but in many instances no predisposing cause is found, other than the presence of a varicose vein. The inflamed vein is usually extremely painful and tender, and the patient may be pyrexial and feel unwell.

HAEMORRHAGE

A varicose vein may bleed after injury and can occasionally bleed spontaneously. Large veins are easily knocked or cut and, if this occurs, they can bleed profusely for a short time. Despite their apparent vulnerability, it is surprising how well the overlying skin protects most varicose veins from injury.

'Spontaneous' rupture of a varix may cause bleeding from the skin surface or into the subcutaneous tissues. Elderly patients with thin-walled veins are particularly at risk. The bleeding usually comes from one of the small intradermal veins near the ankle and may be profuse and even life threatening. The high venous pressure at the ankle during standing is presumably responsible for a 'true' spontaneous rupture of a surface varix, but minor trauma is invariably involved. Patients may be unaware of the rupture until they feel a sensation of 'wetness' as blood runs down the leg or they begin to feel faint.

Subcutaneous bleeding in elderly people with weak veins, causing bruises and petechiae, is common but rarely of clinical importance, though it may frighten and distress the patient.

Ulcers overlying subcutaneous varicosities near the ankle can bleed in a similar manner to the spontaneous variceal rupture already described,[30] and it has been suggested that local steroidal medications applied to an ulcer may increase the risk of bleeding.[3] It is important to ensure that another cause in the leg is not responsible for the bleeding and to exclude any haematological abnormality which could be responsible for a bleeding tendency. These patients are usually old and, if they are unfortunate enough to faint in a sitting position, the bleeding continues, whereas if they fall to the ground, so lowering the venous pressure in the ruptured varix, the bleeding usually stops spontaneously. The mistaken application of a tourniquet to the leg which is not tight enough to occlude the arteries but which is sufficient to cause venous congestion may enhance rather than reduce the rate of bleeding.

In a survey published in 1974,[30] 23 deaths were reported as the result of haemorrhage from varicose veins.

ECZEMA, PIGMENTATION, LIPODERMATOSCLEROSIS AND ULCERATION

These complications of varicose veins are discussed in detail in Chapters 15, 16 and 19, which describe the post-thrombotic syndrome and venous ulceration.

It is important to ask patients if they have ever had a deep vein thrombosis or leg ulcer and also to question them about the duration of skin discoloration or induration around the ankle. Many patients who complain of varicose veins fail to notice minor skin changes in the lower leg because they develop so slowly.

Fear of deterioration

O'Leary *et al.* found that this was an important reason for referral (14%).[52]

History

FAMILY HISTORY

The age of onset of the varicosities should be recorded and any family history of varicose veins noted. Varicose veins occurring in patients under 20 years of age suggest the possibility of a congenital abnormality such as the Klippel–Trenaunay syndrome, valvular agenesis, or a congenital arteriovenous fistula (see Chapter 24). More than a third of patients presenting with varicose veins have relatives who are also affected (see Chapter 5).

PAST HISTORY

All patients presenting with varicose veins must be closely questioned about the possibility of a previous deep vein thrombosis. It is often necessary to ask additional direct questions about leg swelling after childbirth, previous operations, injuries (including fractures), or prolonged periods of bed rest. A history of chest pain, haemoptysis, or anticoagulant therapy provides good circumstantial evidence of a previous thrombosis but confirmation by duplex study, phlebogram or lung scan obtained at the time of the event is even better proof.

Previous episodes of haemorrhage, superficial thrombophlebitis, acute lipodermatosclerosis, skin irritation and ulceration must also be recorded.

All past treatments for varicose veins and their complications must be documented with the dates and places where the treatment was given.

All past operations, serious injuries and illnesses must be noted together with a history of previous medication and known allergies.

GENERAL HEALTH

It is essential to enquire about the patient's general health and fitness as this will be important if surgical treatment of the varicose veins is contemplated, and it may also influence the method of treatment that is selected.

COMMENT

The history is of critical importance both in detecting conditions masquerading as varicose veins and in drawing attention to other systems that deserve examination. The overall picture of the patient's present and past health may have considerable bearing on the method of treatment that is selected. If the history suggests previous thromboembolism, particular care must be taken to record this in a prominent place so that the need for anti-thrombosis prophylaxis will not be forgotten if the patient is admitted to hospital.

Physical signs of varicose veins

A general examination of the patient, paying special attention to any system which the history indicates might be abnormal, is followed by a detailed examination of the lower limbs. This examination is best described in the traditional manner of 'inspection', 'palpation', 'percussion' and 'auscultation', but most clinicians quickly develop their own technique for examining varicose veins which does not necessarily follow this rigid pattern. The examination should take place in a warm and well lit room which should preserve the privacy and respect the modesty of the patient.

A vaginal or rectal examination should always be performed, especially if there is ankle oedema or any suspicion of a pelvic tumour.

INSPECTION

The legs should be examined with the patient standing on a low stool or platform, suitably undressed to expose the whole of both lower limbs from the groins to the toes. Shoes, socks, stockings, trousers, dresses, skirts, shirts or blouses must be removed to ensure adequate exposure of the lower limbs, and

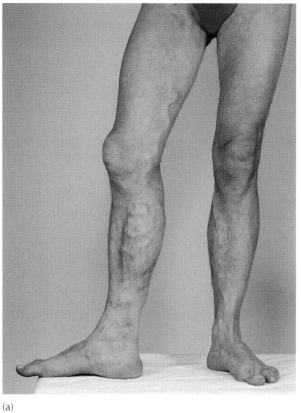

(a)

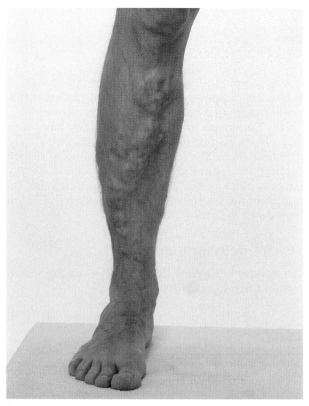

(b)

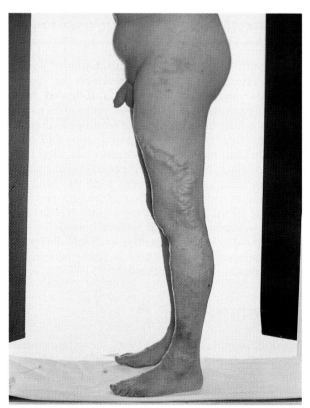

(c)

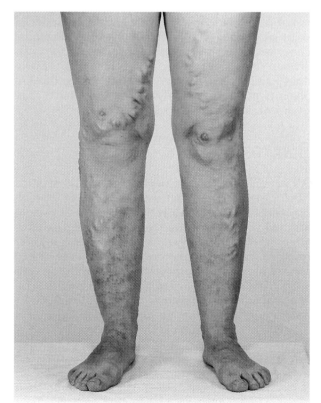

(d)

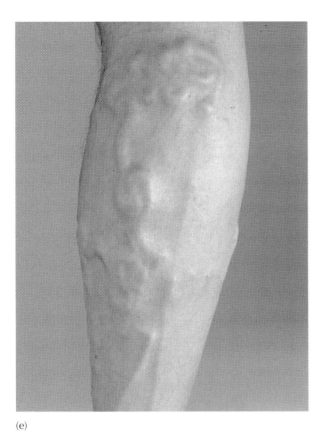

(e)

Figure 6.6 The common distribution of varicose veins. (a) A varicose tributary lying over the course of the long saphenous vein on the medial side of the thigh and calf. Varicosities in this position suggest long saphenous incompetence. (b) Large varicose veins mainly below the knee, on the medial and antero-medial aspect of the lower leg, all draining into an incompetent long saphenous vein. (c) A varicose antero-lateral thigh vein. This is one of the two major tributaries of the long saphenous vein that join it near its termination. It may become varicose without any evidence of long saphenous incompetence. It usually runs across the upper thigh and then down the outer aspect of the thigh or, as in (d) crosses the thigh lower down just above the patella and then runs down the outer aspect of the lower leg. (e) Varicosities on the back of the lower leg in a limb with incompetence of the short saphenous vein.

enable the examiner to at least look at and palpate the lower abdomen.

The presence or absence of the following abnormalities should be recorded.

1. The distribution of all major subcutaneous varicosities (Figure 6.6a–d). Both limbs must be inspected from all aspects (front, back and side) to ensure varicosities in the short saphenous territory or abnormal axial veins are not missed. The distribution of the varicosities should be recorded on stamps or outline drawings of the leg, showing both the anterior and the posterior surfaces (Figure 6.7). Particular note should be made of varicose veins in unusual positions (e.g. a large vein on the lateral side of the limb is often present in the Klippel–Trenaunay syndrome (Chapter 24, Figure 24.12).

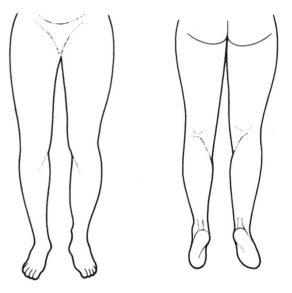

Figure 6.7 Outline 'stamps' of the legs used in our clinic to record the distribution of the varicosities.

2. The presence of a saphena varix (Figure 6.8).
3. The presence of a capillary naevus (Chapter 24, Figure 24.11).
4. The presence of dilated intradermal venules ('spider veins', or 'venous stars') (Figure 6.2).
5. The presence of any angiomatous malformations (Chapter 27, Figure 27.2).
6. The presence of ankle oedema or limb swelling (Figures 6.3 and 6.4).
7. The presence of an 'ankle flare' (corona phlebectatica) (Figure 6.9)
8. The presence of large varicosities, 'blow-outs', over known sites of communicating veins (Figure 6.10).

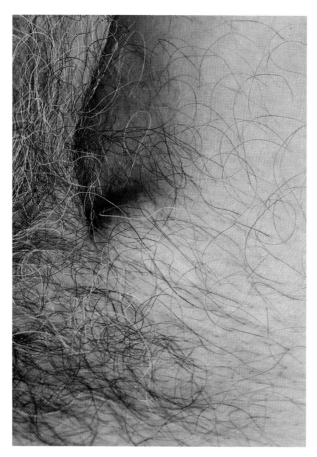

Figure 6.8 A swelling over the termination of the long saphenous vein. The swelling disappeared on lying down and had a marked 'cough impulse'. A saphena varix.

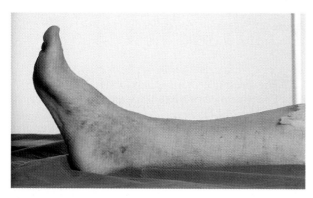

Figure 6.9 The 'ankle flare' of dilated small venules in the skin beneath the malleolus. It is also called the corona phlebectatica. It is usually most noticeable on the medial side of the ankle, below the medial malleolus. In this example there is some early pigmentation and a small healed ulcer at its apex.

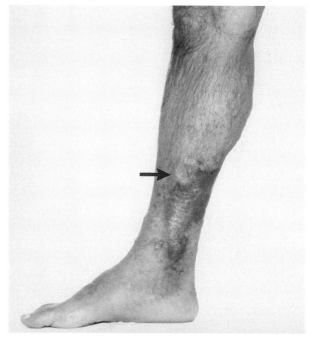

(a)

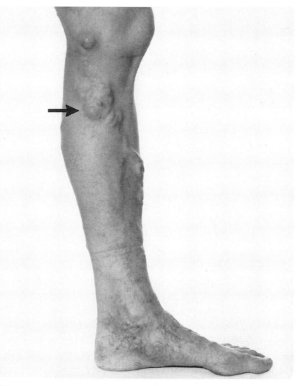

(b)

Figure 6.10 (a) A limb with lipodermatosclerosis; a large 'blow-out' is situated just above the abnormal skin. This is over Cockett's 'middle calf' communicating vein. (b) A limb with dilated varicosities overlying Boyd's communicating vein.

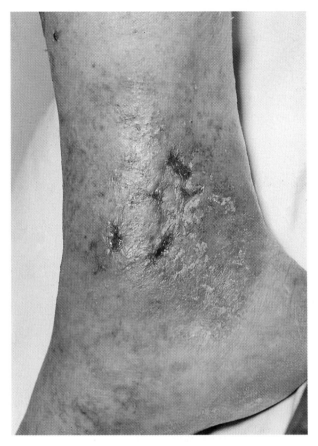

Figure 6.11 Venous eczema over the gaiter region with small areas of superficial ulceration.

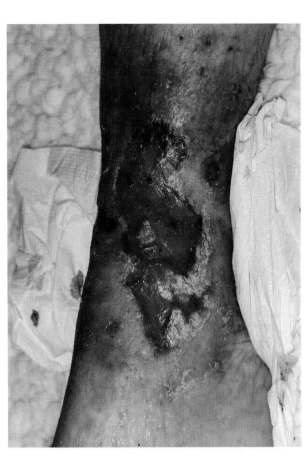

Figure 6.12 A large irregularly shaped venous ulcer situated over the gaiter region of the leg. There is severe chronic and acute lipodermatosclerosis in the skin around the ulcer; causing constriction of gaiter region – a champagne-bottle leg.

9. The presence of acute and chronic lipodermatosclerosis (see Figure 6.10).
10. The presence of eczema (Figure 6.11).
11. The presence of ulceration (Figure 6.12).
12. The presence of atrophie blanche or livedo reticularis (Figure 6.13).
13. An increase in the length or circumference of the limb (Chapter 24, Figures 24.13, 24.16 and 24.17).
14. Shortening of the limb or muscle wasting (Chapter 24, Figure 24.25).
15. Evidence of swollen or deformed knee or hip joints (Chapter 24, Figure 24.13).
16. Evidence of distended veins in the groin, pubic region or abdominal wall (Figure 6.14).

It is helpful to have either a specially designed record card with a printed outline of the front and back of a pair of lower limbs, or re-usable ink stamps, of the same design, that can be stamped on the records and on which the distribution of the abnormalities found by inspection can be noted

(Figure 6.7). Individual varicosities and their connections (see Figure 6.6a–d) should be accurately recorded on these charts.

PALPATION AND PERCUSSION

Some varicose veins are more easily felt than seen. For example, the upper end of a dilated long saphenous vein can often be felt along its course in the thigh between the groin and a lower dilated visible varicose tributary, even when it cannot be seen. A dilated short saphenous vein is invariably easier to feel than to see because it lies beneath the layer of fascia covering the popliteal fossa. The short saphenous vein is easier to palpate if the knee is slightly flexed to relax the deep fascia.

After palpating the terminal segments of the long and short saphenous veins, the hand should be gently passed over the inner side of the thigh and

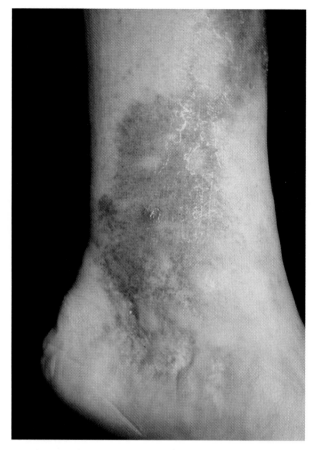

Figure 6.13 This patient has a number of patches of 'atrophie blanche', as white scars, in a larger area of chronic dermatitis, lipodermatosclerosis, and pigmentation.

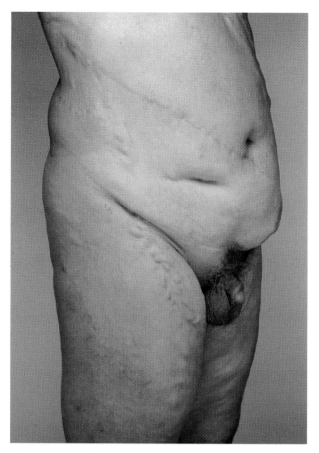

Figure 6.14 The importance of performing a full clinical examination. This patient presented with an area of lipodermatosclerosis in the right calf but examination of the abdomen revealed dilated superficial inferior epigastric veins suggesting diagnosis of ilio-caval obstruction, which was confirmed on phlebography.

Table 6.5 Compilation of 11 studies on locating incompetent calf communicating veins

Method	Number of studies	Number of studies with false-positive results	% of false-positive results* (range)	Number of studies with false-negative results	% of false-negative results† (range)
Clinical	8	5	16–95%	3	46–70%
Doppler	3	3	12–50%	1	52%
Fluorescein	3	2	8–92%	1	53%
Thermography	3	2	15–150%	1	36%
Phlebography	5	3	13–97%	2	27–30%

* $\dfrac{\text{(Number of positive tests – Number of true positives)}}{\text{(Number of true positives)}} \times 100.$

† $\dfrac{\text{(Number of true positives – Number of test positives)}}{\text{(Number of true positives)}} \times 100.$

leg and up the posterior surface of the calf to detect other sites of venous dilatation that might not have been detected by inspection.

Any difference in the temperature of the two limbs should also be recorded, and any firm subcutaneous cords, which are usually felt if there have been past episodes of superficial thrombophlebitis, should be noted.

Palpation of the 'gaiter' region may confirm the edge of a plaque of indurated subcutaneous fat in an area of lipodermatosclerosis. This is not always obvious on inspection and may only be found by careful palpation. The degree of tenderness should also be recorded.

The cough impulse test[21]

A visible or palpable venous expansion that occurs on coughing indicates the absence of competent valves between the right atrium and the vein under examination. When this sign is detected in the groin over a large saphena varix (Figure 6.8), it indicates long saphenous incompetence and may be accompanied by a palpable 'thrill', indicating turbulent retrograde flow. The presence of a 'thrill' is clear evidence of reflux, but patients who jerk or cough overvigorously can make the detection of an expansile venous cough impulse extremely difficult. A cough impulse is very difficult to detect in the very obese.

The percussion test (Schwartz test)[13,21,27]

This consists of 'tapping' a varix with the fingertip of one hand while the other hand palpates the termination of the long or short saphenous veins. The vein must be distended with blood for the impulse (or shock wave) to travel up the vein. The test should then be repeated in the opposite direction with the tap applied to the main vein and the examining hand placed over the varices. The valves must be incompetent for the impulse to be conducted down through them. This downward impulse is, however, often difficult to elicit except in the most severe cases.

Palpation of fascial defects

Cockett[15] originally suggested that large 'blow-out' veins in the calf indicated underlying incompetent communicating veins. The site at which a dilated communicating vein pierces the deep fascia can sometimes be felt as a 'gap' or 'defect' in the deep fascia.[39] This is an inaccurate method of locating incompetent communicating veins (see Tables 6.5–6.8). Many of the palpable 'defects' are simply

Table 6.6 Accuracy of tests in predicting the presence or absence of incompetent communicating veins in 39 limbs[47]

	Present	Absent	False-positive	False-negative
Operation	31	8	0	0
Clinical examination	31	0	8	0
Phlebography	25	7	1	6
Ultrasound	31	2	6	0

Table 6.7 Accuracy of tests in predicting the site of incompetent calf communicating veins in 39 limbs[47]

Test	Total number predicted	Number correctly predicted	False-negatives	False-positives
Operation	55	55 (100%)	0	0
Clinical examination	64	33 (60%)	22 (40%)	31
Phlebography	40	33 (60%)	22 (40%)	7*
Ultrasound	83	34 (62%)	21 (38%)	49*

*The difference between these two figures is significant ($\chi^2 = 18.8$, $P = 0.000\ 25$).

Table 6.8 Accuracy of a combination of tests in predicting the site of incompetent communicating veins in 39 limbs[47]

Test	Total number predicted	Number correctly predicted	False-negatives	False-positives
Operation	55	55 (100%)	0	0
Clinical examination and phlebography	83	48 (58%)	7 (8%)	35
Clinical examination and ultrasound	108	48 (45%)	6 (6%)	59
Ultrasound and phlebography	98	48 (49%)	7 (9%)	50
All three tests combined	115	53 (22%)	2 (2%)	62

depressions or spaces in thickened subcutaneous fat occupied by a varix. For this reason many other techniques, including Doppler ultrasound, thermography, phlebography and now duplex scanning, have been used in an attempt to improve accurate localization (see below).

Sliding finger control

Both Hobbs and Fegan[5,24,33] have suggested that incompetent communicating veins should be suspected if the veins, which have been emptied by leg elevation, can be prevented from refilling by one or more fingers placed over the suspected sites of communicating vein incompetence. The suspected sites of incompetence are confirmed if rapid venous refilling occurs when the fingers are slid away from the 'points of control'; control should be regained when the fingers are slid back to their original positions.

This test is difficult to perform and interpret, and it only achieves acceptable accuracy when complete control is achieved by pressure at one site, indicating a single incompetent communicating vein.

AUSCULTATION

A bruit coming from a superficial vein usually indicates the presence of an arteriovenous fistula in the limb. When either a single fistula or multiple fistulae are present, the veins can often be seen to pulsate if they are carefully watched for 10–15 seconds.

THE TOURNIQUET TEST (THE BRODIE–TRENDELENBURG TEST)[6,65]

This simple bedside test (see Chapter 4, page 71) was designed to assess the direction of blood flow and the source of refilling of the superficial veins. Its accuracy depends upon the skill of the investigator who performs the test, and the results improve with experience.

The patient must be laid flat on the couch or bed and the limb elevated to at least 45° to empty all the subcutaneous veins. This may be helped by stroking the limb with the hand from the foot upwards along the course of the major veins. When the veins have been emptied, a narrow rubber tourniquet is applied around the thigh as close to the groin as possible.

We use a simple piece of 1 cm diameter red rubber tubing or a short length of rubber bandage and a strong pair of artery forceps or fingers to hold it in place (Figure 6.15). It must be applied tightly to prevent all superficial vein reflux. Sapheno-femoral incompetence is indicated if the varices below the tourniquet remain collapsed for between 15 and 30

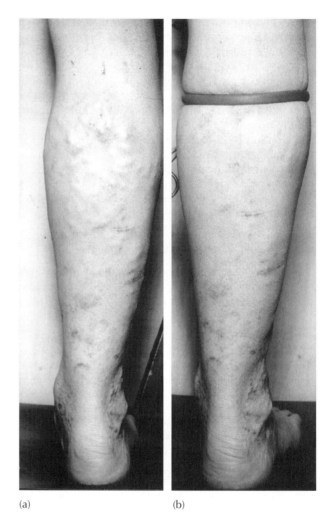

(a)   (b)

Figure 6.15 The tourniquet test. Large calf varicosities (a), which were not controlled by a thigh tourniquet, are controlled by a below knee tourniquet (b).

seconds after the patient stands up, and rapidly refill when the tourniquet is removed (Figure 6.16). The test should be repeated if the results are equivocal.

Errors also result from inadequate venous emptying, releasing the tourniquet too soon, and failure to appreciate that natural venous refilling always occurs; natural venous refilling is more obvious after periods of exercise or in hot weather. If the tourniquet is applied too tightly, it can cause pain, but if it is not applied tightly enough, saphenous reflux will not be controlled and the test will give incorrect results. Venous reflux may be particularly difficult to control in fat limbs.

When sapheno-femoral incompetence is associated with other sites of deep-to-superficial incompetence, the varices quickly refill on standing but the venous distension may still increase when the

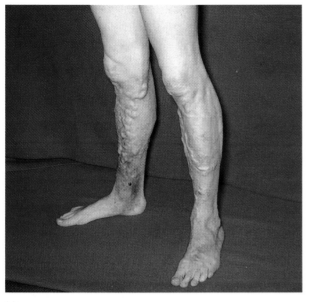
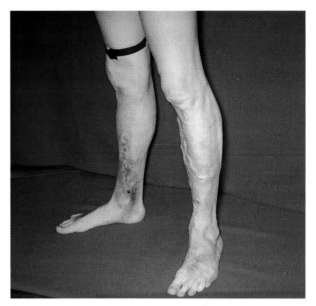

(a)   (b)

Figure 6.16   The tourniquet test. Large varicosities in the lower leg (a) which have been controlled by a thigh tourniquet (b).

tourniquet is released. This additional refilling can best be detected by palpating the increased tension in the varices on release of the tourniquet.

If the high thigh tourniquet fails to control venous refilling, the tourniquet should be placed just above the patella, to exclude an incompetent mid-thigh communicating vein (a rare occurrence in isolation), and then below the knee to detect sapheno-popliteal incompetence. Incompetence of individual lower leg communicating veins may be detected by applying the tourniquet around the lower leg, but the lower the level, the fewer the varices that are controlled and the more difficult it is to interpret the results. The presence of incompetent communicating veins in the lower leg should be suspected if a below-knee tourniquet fails to control the varices. Tourniquet testing is a poor way of discovering the precise sites at which incompetent lower leg communicating veins pierce the deep fascia.[41]

Ochsner and Mahorner[50] advocated a triple tourniquet test, with tourniquets placed around the upper thigh, the lower thigh and below the knee. This test sometimes helps to distinguish between sapheno-femoral and sapheno-popliteal incompetence when both are present, but usually gives no more information than repeated single tourniquet tests at different levels.

Foote described a modification (a double tourniquet test) in which the tourniquets are placed above and below a collection of prominent varices while

they are full of blood.[27] Emptying of the varicosities when the leg is elevated implies that there is a superficial to deep communication between the two tourniquets. If the leg is lowered and the veins between the tourniquets refill, this communicating vein must be incompetent. This test is often difficult to interpret and is rarely used because there are now more accurate methods of identifying the site of incompetent communicating veins.

Perthes suggested that, if a tourniquet was placed below the knee and the patient either walked or heel-raised on the spot, the veins would collapse if the communicating veins and the deep veins were competent and unobstructed.[54] Failure of the superficial veins to empty may be caused by incompetence of valves in the communicating or deep veins or by deep venous obstruction. This test is an inaccurate but simple way of detecting a deep vein abnormality, and it may be used as a screening test to reveal a severe deep venous abnormality.

Summary

After taking the history and completing the physical examination (including the tourniquet tests) the clinician should know the answers to the following questions, and this will dictate the patients' further management.

Are the varicose veins the cause of the patient's symptoms?

If the history or the physical signs fail to convince the examiner that the varicose veins are the cause of the patient's symptoms, additional examination and tests of the spine, abdomen, hip and knee joints, peripheral arteries and nervous system may be indicated.

If the varicose veins are the cause of the symptoms, are they primary varicose veins or secondary to another condition?

The history and examination may reveal the possibility of a post-thrombotic syndrome, a congenital venous abnormality or a pelvic tumour, that requires investigation.

If the patient has primary varicose veins which are responsible for the symptoms, which veins are dilated and incompetent?

The possibilities are:

- sapheno-femoral incompetence
- sapheno-popliteal incompetence
- incompetence of lower leg communicating veins
- mid-thigh communicating vein incompetence
- gastrocnemius communicating vein incompetence
- tributary varicosity without major superficial vein incompetence.

An attempt should be made to categorize the cause of the varicose veins under one or more of these headings. Sapheno-femoral incompetence is by far the most common abnormality. Sapheno-popliteal incompetence is said to be responsible for only 6–14% of all varicosities,[31,41] but it has been suggested that these figures are underestimations.[19,32,59] Additional tests are required, if categorization is difficult or impossible on the basis of clinical evaluation.

Has the patient any associated diseases that will prejudice or influence treatment?

The patient's general health may preclude active treatment. Unsightly varicose veins in a 90-year-old with heart failure, are best left untreated! Varicose veins in a leg which is ischaemic should not be treated, and the long saphenous vein should not be stripped out of a lymphoedematous limb (see Chapter 7).

Has the patient developed any complications as a result of the varicose veins that make treatment imperative?

Lipodermatosclerosis, incipient or past ulceration, eczema, haemorrhage or recurrent attacks of superficial thrombophlebitis are all indications for active treatment.

Does the patient need any treatment at all?

Intradermal spider veins or very small visible veins in women are often best treated by reassurance. Symptomless veins for which an unwilling patient has been encouraged to seek treatment by relatives or the family practitioner also should be left alone.

Is the available information sufficient to plan treatment?

If not, further investigations are necessary.

Special investigations of the superficial veins

The techniques that are available for investigating varicose veins have been described in Chapter 4. The indications and accuracy of the special investigations which are of value in the further management of varicose veins are discussed below and listed in Table 6.9.

Note: *The majority of patients with straightforward varicose veins require nothing more than a full history and the careful examination described above.*

DIRECTIONAL DOPPLER ULTRASOUND

Confirmation of sapheno-femoral or sapheno-popliteal reflux using a simple hand-held 8 mHz directional Doppler ultrasound probe in the clinic is a valuable adjunct to clinical examination[11,23,26,28,32,36,42–45,56,69] (see Chapter 4, page 67).

Table 6.9   Methods used for investigating varicose veins

Ultrasound
  Direction of flow
    Superficial vein reflux*
    Communicating vein reflux
    Deep vein reflux*
  Duplex imaging – the direction of flow in the deep, superficial and communicating veins*
Contrast phlebography
  Varicography – site, extent and connections of varices*
  Ascending phlebography – state of deep veins and detection of incompetent communicating veins*
  Descending phlebography – function of deep vein valves and long saphenous incompetence
  Dynamic cine phlebography – direction of blood flow during exercise
  Percutaneous femoral phlebography – anatomy of iliac veins and vena cava
  Retrograde caval phlebography – anatomy of the inferior vena cava above an iliac or caval occlusion and the
    function of femoral vein valves
  Intra-operative venography – sites of superficial to deep communication
Foot volumetry – calf pump function*
Foot vein pressure measurements – calf pump function
Strain gauge, impedance, isotope or photoplethysmography – calf pump function
Thermography – sites of incompetent communicating veins
Fluorescein angiography – site of incompetent communicating veins

---

*Tests commonly used to assess varicose veins by the authors.

Comparisons have been made between the clinical tests of reflux during a Valsalva manoeuvre and after tourniquet release and the same tests with the Doppler flow detector. The results have been compared with reflux provoked by positive pressure ventilation before and after operative division of the long saphenous vein.[11,32,42] These studies have shown a better correlation between operatively confirmed or absent valvular incompetence and the Doppler tests of reflux than any of the clinical tests. Reflux at open operation is, however, a poor reference investigation for assessing sapheno-femoral incompetence, and in a study in which the Doppler test was compared with clinical examination, descending phlebography, varicography, and intraoperative testing, we found the Doppler ultrasound test gave a number of false-positive and false-negative results.[9]

The Doppler ultrasound test of long saphenous incompetence is, however, quick and easy to perform and helpful when clinical tests are equivocal. If this test is to be considered a valuable guide to management, it must be shown to help avoid operations that would have been performed had it not been used, and to detect valvular incompetence that would have been missed by simple clinical examination. Finally, the 'expected' improvement in patient management should result in a lower rate of recurrent varicose veins after treatment. A massive prospective study would be needed to assess this improvement because the end point is so diffuse. Most clinicians believe that Doppler testing of superficial vein reflux is of considerable value, particularly in fat legs.

The directional Doppler ultrasound flow detector may also be used to detect sapheno-popliteal reflux down the short saphenous vein,[32,56,59] and it has been used to determine the exact site of the sapheno-popliteal junction[56] which may vary considerably in position (see Chapter 2). Short saphenous incompetence is confirmed if retrograde flow after calf squeezing is abolished by digital or tourniquet compression which occludes the upper end of the short saphenous vein.

ADDITIONAL TESTS OF SAPHENOUS REFLUX

Duplex scanning is now accepted as the best method of investigating doubtful cases of saphenous reflux and for that matter perforating vein incompetence.[16] The same workers have even suggested that all patients with varicose veins require a duplex examination. The value of duplex in assessing recurrent veins,[20,55,57] short saphenous incompetence[55,66] and perhaps incompetent communicating veins[29] is becoming established but its role in assessing *all* patients with varicose veins is debatable. It is unlikely to be cost effective.[34,46]

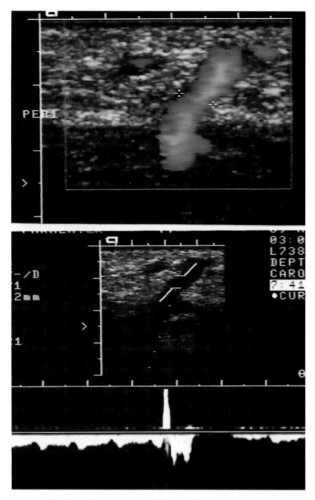

Figure 6.17 The duplex ultrasound image of an incompetent communicating vein showing flow (blue) between the superficial and deep systems. The lower panel shows reversal of flow through the communicating vein when the upper calf was squeezed.

DUPLEX ULTRASOUND

Although some investigators have claimed an 80% accuracy[26,44] for simple directional Doppler detection of incompetent communicating veins, others have not been able to achieve this high level of accuracy[35,51] (Tables 6.5–6.8), probably because blood refluxing through an incompetent communicating vein then passes some distance along an incompetent superficial tributary, so making it difficult to define the exact site at which the actual incompetent communication pierces the deep fascia (see Chapter 4).

None of the other techniques which include thermography,[49,53,67] fluorescein dye injection[10,14,40,49] and

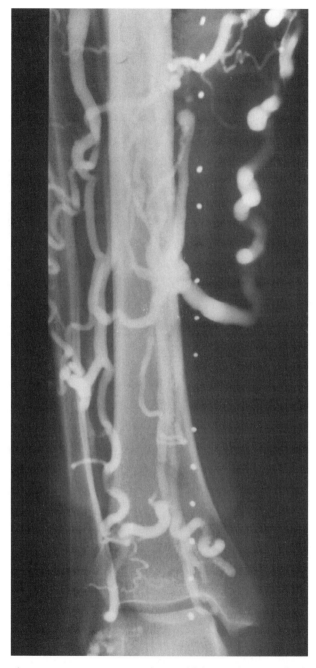

Figure 6.18 An ascending phlebograph in which incompetent calf communicating veins are seen filling with contrast, which has passed from the deep veins to the surface varicosities.

isotope plethysmography[68] (see Chapter 4) is any better at determining the exact sites of incompetent calf communicating veins; calf pump function tests simply indicate their likely presence (see Tables 6.5–6.9).[2]

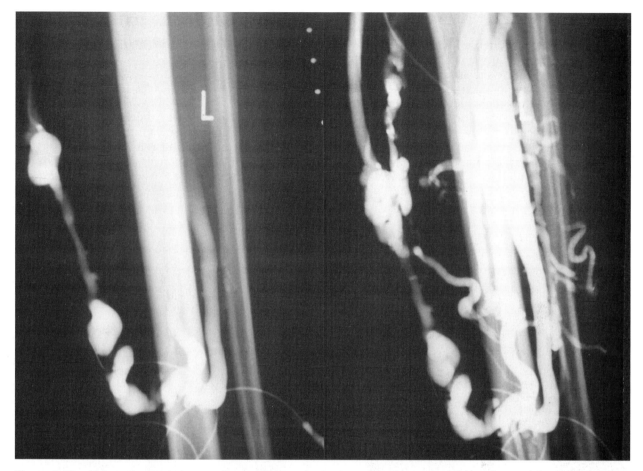

Figure 6.19 This varicogram shows a large calf communicating vein. It is not possible to know if this vein is incompetent as the contrast medium in a varicogram passes from the superficial to the deep veins.

By contrast, duplex ultrasound scanners are capable of imaging the superficial and deep veins of the leg and the communications between these two systems and is now accepted as the best method of investigating doubtful cases of saphenous reflux and communicating vein incompetence.[16] Many have suggested that, before deciding upon treatment, all patients with varicose veins should have a full Duplex examination.[16,18,55,58,62,63] Directional Doppler signals can then be obtained from specific anatomical locations during Valsalva manoeuvres and calf squeezing, and the presence of venous reflux in different veins can be determined (see Chapter 4). This represents a considerable advance over the simple hand-held Doppler flow detector because it is often very difficult to know exactly from which vessel the reflected ultrasound is coming. This is not only very valuable in the groin and popliteal fossa, where the deep and superficial systems meet, but especially helpful in

the calf where duplex ultrasound can be used to assess incompetence of the communicating veins and localize their position (Figure 6.17; see also Figure 4.12).

Duplex ultrasound scanning has a good specificity but needs further assessment against a reliable 'gold standard'.[29,45,46,70] Ascending phlebography is now no longer used to assess the size and incompetence of calf communicating veins because, although its specificity is good, its sensitivity is poor. It is unusual for phlebography to fail to detect any incompetent communicating veins when more than one is present (Figure 6.18) but duplex ultrasound has now largely replaced it because it is easier to obtain.

Communicating veins are sometimes revealed by varicography (Figure 6.19), but varicography cannot demonstrate reflux.

The detection of one incompetent communicating vein in a patient with lipodermatosclerosis or ulceration is an indication to explore all the known sites of incompetent calf communicating veins endoscopically or through a long incision, providing the deep veins are normal. The alternative is to use the duplex ultrasound scan to determine the site and competence of each of the calf communicating veins so that incompetent communicating veins can be selectively explored and ligated. If this selective approach is followed, it must be recognized that in more than one-third of the limbs managed in this way, incompetent communicating veins will pass undetected and will therefore be untreated.

Definition of the extent and connections of varicosities

VARICOGRAPHY

Varicography is the direct injection of radiopaque contrast medium into surface varicosities followed by screening and radiographs to determine their connections (see Chapter 4). This investigation is particularly useful in assessing recurrent varicose veins (Figure 6.20).[4,7,12,17,22,38,60,61] We have also found

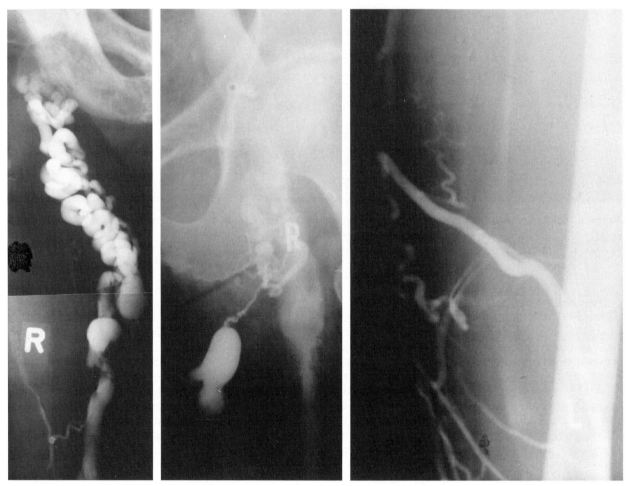

(a)　　　　　　　　　(b)　　　　　　　　　(c)

Figure 6.20 Varicography. (a) A varicogram showing a large mass of veins reconnecting a previously divided long saphenous vein to the femoral vein. (b) A varicogram showing a minute vein reconnecting a previously divided long saphenous vein to the femoral vein. (c) A varicogram showing a large recurrent varicose vein crossing the thigh and draining into a long saphenous vein, which had been ligated in the groin and then into the superficial femoral vein through a Hunterian communicating vein which duplex ultrasound showed was incompetent.

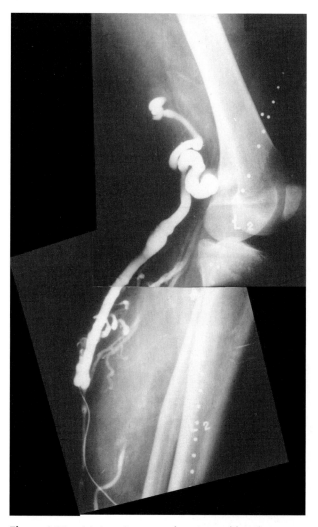

Figure 6.21 (a) A varicogram showing a dilated tortuous termination of the short saphenous vein. (b) A varicogram showing dilated varicosities connected to the short saphenous vein near its termination, which is situated high in the popliteal fossa.

it to be of value in examining veins that cannot be classified by clinical examination and the tourniquet tests.[7] It can also be used to determine the exact position of the termination of the short saphenous vein (Figure 6.21). There is no published direct comparison between varicography and duplex ultrasound scanning but Ruckley believes that varicography is superior to duplex in assessing possible groin varices.[61]

The information obtained from a varicogram depends upon the site chosen for the injection. One injection will not reveal all the sites of the superficial-to-deep venous connections, and sometimes three or four injections must be made for one study.

Varicograms show the superficial connections, the communicating veins,[33] the tortuosity, the dilatation and the extent of the varicose veins (Figure 6.22) but they do not give any information about valve function or venous reflux which must be assessed separately by duplex scanning or descending phlebography.

Special investigations of the deep veins

DIRECTIONAL DOPPLER ULTRASOUND

Some investigators have found that the test of deep vein reflux using this technique is accurate[22,42] but we have found that it does not correlate well with reflux demonstrated by descending venography.[1]

DUPLEX ULTRASOUND SCANNING

This technique allows the operator to identify the source of the flow signal. Individual valves may be visualized and the direction of venous flow observed; it has greatly improved the detection and measurement of deep venous reflux (see Chapter 4).[54,58,59]

DESCENDING PHLEBOGRAPHY

Descending phlebography has now been replaced by duplex ultrasound because the latter gives the same information without any need for groin venepunctures and contrast injection (see Chapters 4 and 12).[1]

PHYSIOLOGICAL TESTS OF VENOUS OBSTRUCTION

Venous obstruction can only be demonstrated by a test of venous function. The presence of a venous occlusion on a phlebogram should not be equated with functional obstruction. Obstruction must be confirmed by detecting an increase in distal venous pressure or venous volume during exercise or reactive hyperaemia, by measuring the venous pressure directly or with some form of plethysmography.

TESTS WHICH DETECT POST-THROMBOTIC DEEP VEIN DAMAGE

We still routinely obtain ascending phlebograms if we suspect that a patient's varicose veins are secondary

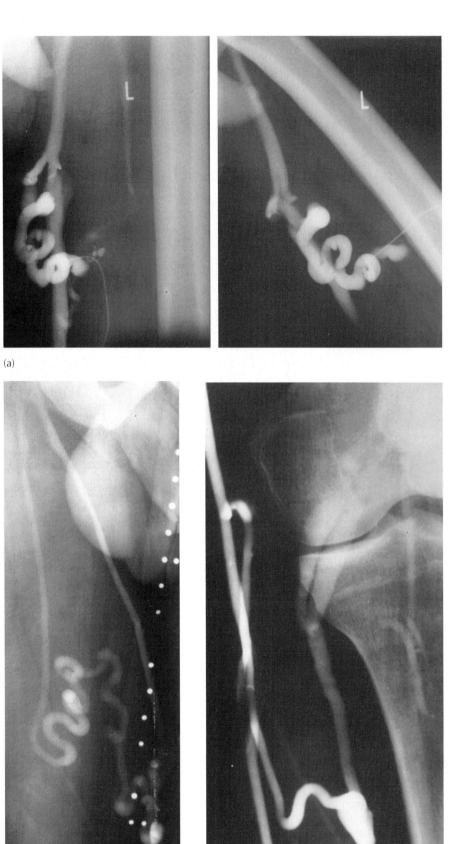

(a)

(b)

(c)

Figure 6.22 A selection of varicograms showing different connections. (a) Varicosities connecting with a 'normal' long saphenous vein in the thigh which contains valves of normal appearance. (b) Varicosities draining into an 'undilated' long saphenous vein via an antero-lateral thigh vein, which is dilated. (c) Varicosities connecting the long saphenous vein to a paired gastrocnemius communicating vein. An undilated short saphenous vein can be seen passing up behind the tibia. (d) A varicose vein passing up on the lateral side of the calf and thigh which is connected by a series of paired communicating veins to the peroneal veins. (e) A large, and probably incompetent, communicating vein on the medial side of the calf connecting subcutaneous varicosities to the posterior tibial veins.

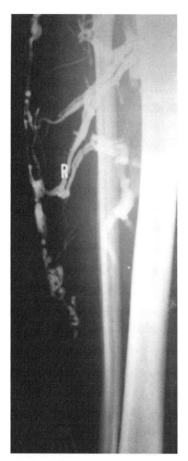

Figure 6.22 (d)

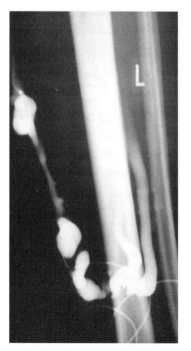

Figure 6.22 (e)

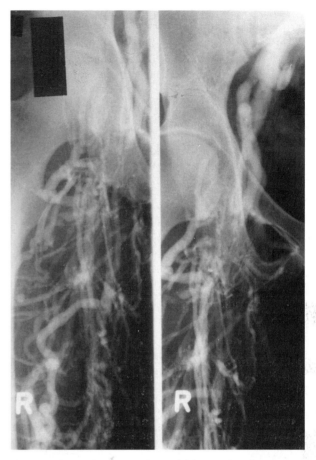

Figure 6.23 The ascending phlebograph of a young male who was stabbed in the groin and sustained a total femoral vein occlusion during the surgery which was required to stop the haemorrhage.

to deep vein damage (Figure 6.23). We perform foot volumetry to establish the anatomy and functional severity of the damage. Foot vein pressure measurements and the other forms of plethysmography are alternative and equally efficacious tests. We find foot volumetry the most simple and reliable quantitative method; photoplethysmography is just as simple but is only qualitative. Duplex scanning may suggest deep vein obstruction but is not always accurate, especially if the iliac veins are occluded.

Suggested diagnostic pathways

After a thorough clinical examination, including the tourniquet tests, it is usually possible to place the patient into one of several categories. The diagnostic pathway is then complete and treatment can be planned. The following section summarizes our use of the special investigations in patients who have been placed in one of these clinical categories, when the information available from clinical examination is not sufficient to proceed with treatment.[3]

Sapheno-femoral incompetence with long saphenous vein tributary dilatation

- No lipodermatosclerosis, ulceration, or ankle flare.
- All the veins controlled by a high thigh tourniquet.
- Perthes' test shows superficial veins empty with exercise.

Action

1. Confirmation of sapheno-femoral reflux with hand-held or duplex ultrasound is optional.
2. No further tests are required – proceed to treat.

Note: This is the most common situation seen in a varicose vein clinic.

Sapheno-popliteal incompetence with short saphenous vein tributary dilatation

- No clinical evidence of sapheno-femoral incompetence.
- No lipodermatosclerosis, ulceration or ankle flare.
- All varicosities controlled by a below-knee tourniquet.
- Perthes' test shows superficial veins of calf empty with exercise.

Action

1. Confirm sapheno-femoral competence with an ultrasound test.
2. Confirm sapheno-popliteal incompetence with ultrasound test.
3. Varicogram to define the anatomy of sapheno-popliteal junction (optional but valuable if the termination of the short saphenous cannot be easily felt).
4. Duplex ultrasound imaging is now the method of choice as it detects the site of the sapheno-popliteal junction.
5. Proceed to treat.

Sapheno-femoral and sapheno-popliteal incompetence with tributary dilatation of both saphenous veins

- No lipodermatosclerosis, ulceration or ankle flare.
- All varicosities controlled by a below-knee tourniquet.

- Perthes' test shows superficial veins empty with exercise.

Action

1. Confirm sapheno-femoral and sapheno-popliteal incompetence with ultrasound.
2. Varicogram to confirm that varices connect to both saphenous systems and to define the anatomy of the sapheno-popliteal junction (optional).
3. Proceed to treat.

Sapheno-femoral or sapheno-popliteal incompetence or both but varices below the knee not controlled by a below-knee tourniquet

- No lipodermatosclerosis or ulceration.
- An ankle flare may be present.
- No past history of deep vein thrombosis.
- Perthes' test shows the veins remain distended during exercise.

Action

1. Clinical examination of the sites of possible incompetent communicating veins in the lower leg (probably not of much value).
2. Confirm presence of sapheno-femoral and sapheno-popliteal incompetence with ultrasound.
3. Test for sapheno-femoral and sapheno-popliteal reflux with ultrasound.
4. Varicography of superficial veins to examine the communications of the superficial veins (optional). Look for medial calf communicating vein incompetence with ultrasound.
5. Assess function of deep veins and define site of incompetent communicating veins with foot volumetry (or photophlethysmography), ascending phlebography, and/or duplex ultrasound.
6. Proceed to treat.

Both duplex scanning and ascending venography are helpful in this type of patient.

Sapheno-femoral or sapheno-popliteal incompetence or both, but varices below the knee not controlled by a below-knee tourniquet with skin changes, ankle flare, lipodermatosclerosis, past or present ulceration

- History of deep vein thrombosis unreliable.
- Perthes' test shows superficial veins remain distended during exercise.

Action

1. As above.

Skin changes and calf varices with no clinical evidence of long or short saphenous incompetence

- No history of deep vein thrombosis.

Action

1. Test the competence of the sapheno-popliteal and sapheno-femoral junctions with duplex ultrasound.
2. Varicography of the superficial veins (optional).
3. Duplex ultrasound study of the deep veins (ascending phlebography helpful but optional).
4. Foot volumetry.

Varicosities of tributary veins but no evidence of sapheno-femoral or sapheno-popliteal incompetence

- No lipodermatosclerosis, ankle flare or ulceration.

Action

1. Confirm competence of sapheno-femoral and sapheno-popliteal junction with ultrasound.
2. Varicograms if mid-thigh communicating vein or gastrocnemius communicating vein is suspected (optional).
3. Proceed to treat.

Recurrent varicose veins after previous surgery

If clinical examination does not clearly indicate the cause of the recurrence (e.g. the site of the superficial to deep vein incompetence), varicography, ultrasound and ascending phlebography are very helpful investigations, followed by calf pump function studies (foot volumetry) if the ascending phlebogram shows any deep vein damage. Varicography is probably the most useful test.

References

1. Ackroyd JS, Lea Thomas M, Browse NL. Deep vein reflux: an assessment by descending phlebography. *Br J Surg* 1986; **73:** 31–3.
2. Anon. The hidden perforating veins. *Br Med J* 1970; **1:** 186–7.
3. Baker SR, Burnand KG, Sommerville KM, Lea Thomas M, Wilson NM, Browse NL. Comparison of venous reflux assessed by duplex scanning and descending phlebography in chronic venous disease. *Lancet* 1993; **341:** 400–3.
4. Barabas AP, MacFarlane R. The use of varicography to identify the sources of incompetence in recurrent varicose veins. *Ann R Coll Surg Engl* 1985; **67:** 208.
5. Beesley WH, Fegan WG. An investigation into the localization of incompetent perforating veins. *Br J Surg* 1970; **157:** 30–2.
6. Brodie B. *Lectures Illustrative of Various Subjects in Pathology and Surgery*. London: Longmans, 1846.
7. Burnand KG. Intéret de la varicographie dans l'appréciation des varices essentielles des membres inférieurs. In: *Phlebologie '83*. Brussels: Medical Media International, 1984; 269–70.
8. Burnand KG. Management of varicose veins of the legs. *Nurs Mirror* 1977; **144(11):** 45.
9. Burnand KG, Pattison M, Powell S, Lea Thomas M, Browse NL. Can we diagnose long saphenous incompetence correctly? In: Negus D, Jantet G, eds. *Phlebology '85*. London: John Libbey, 1985; 101–5.
10. Callum KG, Gray LJ, Lea Thomas M. An evaluation of the flourescein test and phlebography in the detection of incompetent perforating veins. *Br J Surg* 1973; **60:** 699–702.
11. Chan A, Chisholm I, Royle JP. The use of directional Doppler ultrasound in the assessment of sapheno femoral incompetence. *Aust N Z J Surg* 1983; **53:** 399–402.
12. Chant ADB, Jones HO, Townsend JCF, Williams JE. Radiological demonstration of the relationship between calf varices and sapheno-femoral incompetence. *Clin Radiol* 1972; **23:** 519–23.
13. Chevrier L. De l'examin aux reflux veinaux dans les varices superficielles. *Arch Gen Chir* 1908; **2:** 44.
14. Chilvers AS, Thomas MH. Methods for the localization of incompetent ankle perforating veins. *Br Med J* 1970; **2:** 577–9.
15. Cockett FB. Diagnosis and surgery of high pressure venous leaks in the leg. A new overall concept in the surgery of varicose veins and venous ulcer. *Br Med J* 1953; **2:** 1399–403.
16. Coleridge-Smith PD, Scurr JH. Duplex scanning for venous disease. *Curr Pract Surg* 1995; **7:** 182–8.
17. Corbett CR, McIrvine AJ, Aston NO, Jamieson CW, Lea Thomas M. The use of varicography to identify the sources of incompetence in recurrent varicose veins. *Ann R Coll Surg Engl* 1984; **66:** 412–15.
18. Corcos L, Peruzzi GP, Romeo V, Fiori C. Considerations of the anatomical variations in the venous system of the lower limbs in varicose disease. *Phlebology* 1989; **4:** 259–70.
19. Corcos L, Peruzzi GP, Romeo V, Fiori C. Intraoperative phlebology of the short saphenous vein. *Phlebology* 1987; **2:** 241–8.
20. De Maeseneer MG, De Hert SG, Van Schil PE, Vanmaele RG, Eyskens EJ. Preoperative colour-coded duplex examination of the saphenopopliteal

junction in recurrent varicosis of the short saphenous vein. *Cardiovasc Surg* 1993; **1(6):** 686–9.

21. Dodd H, Cockett FB. *The Pathology and Surgery of the Veins of the Lower Limb.* London: Churchill Livingstone, 1976.

22. Doran FS, Barkat S. The management of recurrent varicose veins. *Ann R Coll Surg Engl* 1981; **63:** 432–6.

23. Evans GA, Evans DMD, Seal RME, Craven JL. Haemorrhage from varicose veins. *Lancet* 1973; **2:** 1359–61.

24. Fegan WG. *Varicose Veins: Compression Sclerotherapy.* London: Heinemann, 1967.

25. Folse R, Alexander RH. Directional flow detection for localizing venous valvular incompetency. *Surgery* 1970; **67:** 114–21.

26. Foote AV, Miller SS, Grossman JA. The ultrasonic detection of incompetent perforating veins. *Br J Surg* 1971; **58:** 872.

27. Foote RR. *Varicose Veins.* London: Butterworths, 1954.

28. Goren G, Yellin AE. Primary varicose veins: topographic and hemodynamic correlations. *J Cardiovasc Surg* 1990; **31:** 672–7.

29. Hanrahan LM, Araki CT, Fisher JB, *et al.* Evaluation of the perforating veins of the lower extremity using high resolution duplex imaging. *J Cardiovasc Surg* 1991; **32:** 87–97.

30. Harman RR. Haemorrhage from varicose veins. *Lancet* 1974; **1:** 363.

31. Helmig L, Stelzer G. Haufigkeit der operativen Behandlung der insuffizienten Vena saphena parve. *Vasa* 1983; **12:** 159–65.

32. Hoare MC, Royle JP. Doppler ultrasound detection of saphenofemoral and saphenopopliteal incompetence and operative venography to ensure precise saphenopopliteal ligation. *Aust N Z J Surg* 1984; **54:** 49.

33. Hobbs J. Surgery and sclerotherapy in the treatment of varicose veins. A random trial. *Arch Surg* 1974; **109:** 793–6.

34. Labropoulos N, Leon M, Nicolaides AN, Giannoukas AD, Volteas N, Chan P. Superficial venous insuffficiency: correlation of anatomic extent of reflux with clinical symptoms and signs. *J Vasc Surg* 1994; **20(6):** 953–8.

35. Lamont P, Bavin D, Woodyer A, *et al.* Accuracy of clinical versus Doppler examination for detecting incompetent perforating veins. *Br J Surg* 1986; **73:** 493.

36. Large J. Doppler testing as an important conservation measure in the treatment of varicose veins. *Aust N Z J Surg* 1984; **54:** 357–9.

37. Lea Thomas M, Bowles JN. Incompetent perforating veins: comparison of varicography and ascending phlebography. *Radiology* 1985; **154:** 619–23.

38. Lea Thomas M, Keeling FP. Varicography in the management of recurrent varicose veins. *Angiology* 1986; **37:** 570–5.

39. Lofgren KA. Management of varicose veins: Mayo Clinic experience. In: Bergan JJ, Yao JST, eds. *Venous Problems.* Chicago, IL: Year Book Medical Publishers, 1971.

40. Lofqvist J, Jansson I, Thomsen M, Elfstrom J. Evaluation of the fluorescein test in the diagnosis of incompetent perforating veins. *Vasa* 1983; **12:** 46–50.

41. Massell TB, Ettinger J. Phlebography in the localization of incompetent communicating veins in patients with varicose veins. *Ann Surg* 1948; **127:** 1217–25.

42. Mclrvine AJ, Corbett CRR, Aston NO, Sherriff EA, Wiseman PA, Jamieson CW. The demonstration of saphenofemoral incompetence; Doppler ultrasound compared with standard clinical tests. *Br J Surg* 1984; **71:** 509–10.

43. Miller SS. Investigation and management of varicose veins. *Ann R Coll Surg Engl* 1974; **55:** 245–52.

44. Miller SS, Foote AV. The ultrasonic detection of incompetent perforating veins. *Br J Surg* 1974; **61:** 653–6.

45. Myers KA. Special investigations prior to surgery for varicose veins. *Aust N Z J Surg* 1983; **53:** 394–6.

46. Myers KA, Ziegenbein RW, Zeng GH, Matthews PG. Duplex ultrasonography scanning for chronic venous disease: patterns of venous reflux. *J Vasc Surg* 1995; **21(4):** 605–12.

47. Nabatoff RA. 3000 stripping operations for varicose veins on a semi-ambulatory basis. *Surg Gynecol Obstet* 1970; **130:** 497–500.

48. Nicolaides AN, Fernandes JF, Zimmerman H. Doppler ultrasound in the investigation of venous insufficiency. In: Nicolaides AN, Yao JST, eds. *Investigations of Vascular Disorders.* Edinburgh: Churchill Livingstone, 1981.

49. Noble J, Gunn AA. Varicose veins: comparative study of methods for detecting incompetent perforators. *Lancet* 1972; **1:** 1253–5.

50. Ochsner A, Mahorner HR. The modern treatment of varicose veins. *Surgery* 1937; **2:** 889–902.

51. O'Donnell TF, Burnand KG, Clemenson G, Lea Thomas M, Browse NL. Doppler examination vs clinical and phlebographic detection of the location of incompetent perforating veins: a prospective study. *Arch Surg* 1977; **112:** 31–5.

52. O'Leary DP, Chester JF, Jones SM. Management of varicose veins according to reason for presentation. *Ann R Coll Surg Engl* 1996; **78:** 214–16.

53. Patil KD, Williams JR, Lloyd-Williams K. Thermographic localization of incompetent perforating veins in the leg. *Br Med J* 1970; **1:** 195–7.

54. Perthes G. Uber die Operation der Unterschenkel varicen nach Trendelenburg. *Dtsch Med Wochenschr* 1895; **21:** 253–7.

55. Quigley FG, Raptis S, Cashman M. Duplex ultrasonography of recurrent varicose veins. *Cardiovasc Surg* 1994; **2(6):** 775–7.

56. Roberts AK, Hoare MC, Royle JP. The detection of sapheno-popliteal incompetence using Doppler ultrasound and operative venography. *J Cardiovasc Surg* 1985; **26:** 400–1.

57. Scott HJ, Coleridge Smith PD, McMullin GM, Scurr JH. Venous disease: investigation and treatment, fact or fiction? *Ann R Coll Surg Engl* 1990; **72:** 188–92.

58. Semrow C, Ryan TJ, Buchbinder D, Rollins DL. Assessment of valve function using real-time B-mode ultrasound. In: Negus D, Jantet G, eds. *Phlebology '85*. London: John Libbey, 1986.

59. Sheppard M. Sapheno-popliteal incompetence. *Phlebology* 1986; **1:** 23–32.

60. Starnes HF, Vallance R, Hamilton DNH. Recurrent varicose veins: a radiological approach to investigation. *Clin Radiol* 1984; **35:** 95–9.

61. Stonebridge PA, Chalmers N, Begg I, Bradbury AW, Rudkley CV. Recurrent varicose veins: a varicographic analysis leading to a new practical classification. *Br J Surg* 1995; **82:** 60–2.

62. Sullivan ED, David JP, Cranley JJ. Real-time B-mode venous ultrasound. *J Vasc Surg* 1984; **1:** 465–71.

63. Szendro G, Nicolaides AN, Zukowski AJ, *et al.* Duplex scanning in the assessment of deep venous incompetence. *J Vasc Surg* 1986; **4:** 237–42.

64. Townsend J, Jones H, Williams JE. Detection of incompetent perforating veins by venography at operation. *Br Med J* 1967; **3:** 583–5.

65. Trendelenburg F. Uber die Unterbildung der Vena saphena magna bei unterschenkel Varicen. *Beitr Klin Chir* 1891; **7:** 195–210.

66. Vasdekis SN, Clarke GH, Hobbs JT, Nicolaides AN. Evaluation of non-invasive and invasive methods in the assessment of short saphenous vein termination. *Br J Surg* 1989; **76:** 929–32.

67. Vuori J, Inberg MV, Koskinen R, Rasanen O, Vanttinen E. Pre-operative localization of incompetent perforating veins. *Ann Chir Gynaecol* 1972; **61:** 20–2.

68. Whitehead SM, Clemenson G, Browse NL. The assessment of calf pump function by isotope plethysmography. *Br J Surg* 1983; **70:** 675–9.

69. Zelikovski A, Zamir B, Hadar H, Urea I. Saphenofemoral valve insufficiency in varicose veins of the lower limb. *Angiology* 1981; **32:** 807–11.

70. Zukowski AJ, Nicolaides AN, Szendro G, *et al.* Haemodynamic significance of incompetent calf perforating veins. *Br J Surg* 1991; **78:** 625–9.

CHAPTER 7

Varicose veins: natural history and treatment

The natural history of untreated and uncomplicated varicose veins	191	Results of treatment	237
Treatment: general	193	Varicose veins of pregnancy and vulval varicosities	239
Surgical treatment of varicose veins	195	Treatment of dilated intradermal venules	241
Injection sclerotherapy	231	Treatment of the complications of varicose veins	241
Alternative treatments of varicose veins	237	References	241

The natural history of untreated and uncomplicated varicose veins

It is commonly assumed that if varicose veins are left untreated they will continue to enlarge and the 'varicose process' will spread to involve other previously 'normal' veins. This is supported by the natural history study of Schultz-Ehrenburg in school children which showed this process to be progressive.[226–228]

There is anecdotal evidence that long saphenous vein incompetence can regress. This certainly seems to occur after pregnancy,[86,132,213] and regression of thigh vein varices may follow the injection of incompetent lower leg communicating veins,[81] though this latter claim has been disputed.[117,118] Other investigators have observed that simple ligation and division of the sapheno-femoral junction causes regression of distal varices.[154]

The influence of prolonged external elastic compression on the natural history of varicosities has still not, to our knowledge, been specifically examined, but it is interesting to note that many patients with primary varicose veins who have been given elastic stockings to wear while they await operation, subsequently decline hospital admission for surgery on the grounds that they are so much better that they no longer require treatment.[39] Little is known, therefore, about the rate of progression of varicose veins or about the factors that modify this, although the German natural history study may be valuable in providing this type of information. Watts[265] stated that the propensity to develop varicose veins is a progressive incurable disease that can be satisfactorily palliated, *but not cured*, by a number of different techniques.

THE SKIN COMPLICATIONS OF PRIMARY VARICOSE VEINS

It is frequently argued that varicose veins must be treated to prevent the development of skin changes but little is known about the magnitude of the risk that patients with uncomplicated varicose veins have of developing the skin changes that lead to ulceration.

Some authors[82,105,181,182] have suggested that all patients with skin changes or venous ulceration in the 'gaiter' area of the leg have incompetent lower leg communicating veins, and Haegar[105] has stated that 'no venous ulcer can exist without perforator incompetence'; this is unlikely to be true. Hoare only detected evidence of incompetent communicating veins with Doppler ultrasound in a small proportion of a large series of patients with venous ulceration,[112] and Bjordal [22–26] has shown that incompetence of the calf communicating veins has less of an effect on calf pump function than incompetence of the saphenous vein; we have confirmed his findings.[34] Cockett found no evidence of incompetent calf communicating veins at operation in 18 out of 54 limbs with skin changes and long saphenous incompetence,[71] and we too have explored legs looking for incompetent communicating veins in patients with grossly abnormal venous pressures and healed venous ulcers and on some occasions found no large communicating veins crossing the deep fascia.

The problem with all these studies and observations is the definition of communicating vein incompetence. The accepted proof of communicating vein incompetence remains the presence of significant back bleeding on transection of the communicating vein during forcible foot dorsiflexion at the time of operative exploration. This is the Turner Warwick bleed-back test.[44,150,259] This test does not take account of the diameter of the communicating vein. A large vein of 4–5 mm diameter, which bleeds profusely when divided, is obviously incompetent and important, whereas a small vein which only just bleeds on forcible dorsiflexion is of doubtful significance. Nevertheless, retrograde flow through a small vessel is considered to be significant, even though the vein is so small that the quantity of blood that is capable of passing through it is of no haemodynamic significance (though of course it may be hydrostatically important). The method of division of the vessel and forcible dorsiflexion of the foot varies from surgeon to surgeon, and reflux may be abolished if there is traumatic venospasm caused by clumsy dissection and rough division of the vein. The very act of opening the deep fascia and dissecting the vein away from the surrounding tissues that may normally hold it open, may render an incompetent vein competent or vice versa. Finally, a surgeon who has made an extensive incision in the leg has a bias in favour of finding incompetent communicating veins, as have junior surgeons instructed by their consultants to 'ligate this patient's incompetent communicating veins'.

A satisfactory method for diagnosing incompetent communicating veins and measuring their effect on calf pump haemodynamics is still needed urgently. Until we can do this satisfactorily, we cannot investigate the precise role of superficial and communicating vein incompetence in the genesis of skin changes and venous ulceration. We have to rely on our clinical experience, which suggests that only a small number of patients with simple long saphenous incompetence will develop skin changes and ulceration; most patients with skin complications have incompetent calf communicating veins or post-thrombotic damage (see Chapter 15).

Therefore all patients with varicose veins must either be advised to have treatment in the hope of avoiding ulceration or they must be watched carefully and treated if skin changes appear. Large prospective studies on the natural history of varicose veins, documented with anatomical and physiological, as well as clinical, measures are required so that the true relationship between the presence of varicose veins, their progression and the development of skin changes can be defined.

Fletcher and Tibbs,[252] using dynamic phlebography, have been able to distinguish between two groups of incompetent communicating veins. One group allows re-entry into the deep system of blood refluxing down the saphenous vein; in the other group the direction of blood flow is chiefly outward. The first group of veins does not appear to be related to skin changes; the second group of veins does seem to be related to skin changes.

This has been confirmed by J Large[138] who found that some calf communicating veins which show evidence of retrograde flow preoperatively have this abolished by saphenous vein surgery.

Another study[272] has suggested that patients with communicating vein incompetence can be divided into three groups: one in which they have no haemodynamic significance; and two in which they have either moderate or major significance. The last group are indistinguishable from limbs with deep venous disease.

Not every incompetent communicating vein is associated with proof of post-thrombotic damage in the deep veins,[33] and we find it difficult to accept that a localized thrombosis can occur on so many occasions solely within a communicating vein, to account for all the patients whose communicating veins have become incompetent in the presence of normal deep veins. It is more likely that communicating vein incompetence is part of the involvement of these veins in the generalized inherited varicose process.[71,124,252] Confirmation of this hypothesis awaits the development of better tests for assessing incompetence of the calf communicating veins. The magnitude of the risk of developing skin changes and ulceration from primary varicose veins can only be assessed by well organized prospective long-term studies, which still have not been organized since the first edition of this book.

Should varicose veins be treated?

- Yes – if the patient wishes to be treated for symptomatic or cosmetic reasons.

- No – if the patient does not wish to be treated and has perfectly normal skin.
- Yes – when recognizable changes appear in the skin of the lower leg, however minor.
- No – if the object of treatment is solely to stop progression of varicosis and to avoid treatment later.
- Yes – if there are problems with haemorrhage or recurrent superficial thrombosis.

Can we cure varicose veins?

- No. Every patient should be told that all treatment is palliative, not curative.[93,127]

Treatment: general

CLINICAL OBJECTIVES OF TREATMENT

The treatment of varicose veins has five main objectives:

1. Satisfactory cosmesis
2. Relief of symptoms
3. Treatment of complications
4. Prevention of complications
5. Prevention of recurrence.

Satisfactory cosmesis

A perfect cosmetic result is achieved if all varices are removed without leaving visible evidence of their removal and at the same time future recurrences are prevented. Neither of these aims has ever been realized though some remarkably low 5-year and 10-year recurrence rates have been claimed for surgical treatment.[139,209] Reviews by Gillies and Ruckley[92] and Juhan *et al.*[127] reveal that reported recurrence rates vary from 7% to 70%, the variation depending upon the form of treatment and the lack of an agreed definition of recurrence. The median recurrence rate at 5 years of the 30 publications in the aforementioned reviews is approximately 25%, rising to at least 50% by 10 years.

Relief of symptoms

All forms of treatment that successfully eradicate or compress varicose veins have been claimed to relieve pain and discomfort,[39,71,81,202] but it has been pointed out, in a report of a comparative trial of sclerotherapy and surgical treatment,[38] that the level of agreement on the severity of symptoms within a group of observers varied between 50 and 70%. This lack of correlation has been confirmed by other investigators.[202] A score based on the number of symptoms and signs may give no indication of the severity of the discomfort or disability experienced by the patient. Symptom relief is almost impossible to quantify; requests for additional treatment may be a better indication of a patient's dissatisfaction. The results of clinical trials based on symptomatology must be viewed with considerable scepticism.

Relief and prevention of complications

The major complications of varicose veins are skin changes, ulceration, haemorrhage and superficial thrombophlebitis. When there is definite evidence of communicating vein incompetence, treatment should relieve symptoms and reverse some of the skin changes (see Chapter 15). We do not know whether the treatment of saphenous vein incompetence prevents the development of skin changes, though eradication of surface varices does prevent haemorrhage and superficial thrombophlebitis (see below).

Prevention of complications

Skin changes and ulceration

The role of varicose vein surgery in preventing and alleviating skin changes and ulceration is discussed in detail in Chapter 15.

Superficial thrombophlebitis

This is common in patients with varicose veins (see Chapter 22), and removal of varicose subcutaneous veins prevents its development. Once thrombophlebitis has occurred, it can usually be treated conservatively by support and analgesia, followed later, if the veins remain visible, by elective surgery to prevent further attacks. Surgical ligation of the long saphenous vein or short saphenous vein is indicated to prevent the development of deep vein thrombosis if the superficial thrombophlebitis is extending upwards towards the femoral or popliteal veins. If an acute attack of superficial thrombophlebitis fails to resolve, symptomatic relief may be provided by expelling the intravascular thrombus through a small incision or needle puncture into the vein.

Prevention of recurrence

This is the second main aim of treatment. Reports of success following sclerotherapy vary from approximately 80% at 2–3 years[39,74] to 50% at 3 years[176] and to as little as 8% at 5 years.[93,118,127] Eighty-five per cent success at 10 years and 93% success at 6–10 years postoperatively have been claimed by Larsson[139] and Rivlin,[209] respectively. In these studies the assessment was through the subjective and unacceptable method of 'surgeons' appraisal', which was not submitted to any form of external audit.

METHODS OF RELIEVING SYMPTOMS FROM VARICOSE VEINS

1. Eradication of all visible varices by excision or obliteration.
2. Disconnection of the connections between the superficial veins and the deep veins.
3. Reduction of transmural pressure by external elastic compression.
4. Combinations of all three techniques.

Eradication of all visible varices by excision or obliteration

The superficial venous system of the lower limb is extensive and cannot be completely obliterated even by extensive surgery or repeated sclerotherapy, though Lofgren's[90] postoperative pictures show that this can almost be achieved at the cost of multiple extensive incisions (Figure 7.1).

Stripping, direct excision, avulsion, sclerotherapy, diathermy coagulation and infra-red coagulation are methods which have been used to eradicate or obliterate surface varices. These techniques will be discussed in detail in the subsequent sections.

Eradication of the connections between the superficial and deep veins

This forms the basis of surgical treatment and sclerotherapy, both of which are designed to occlude

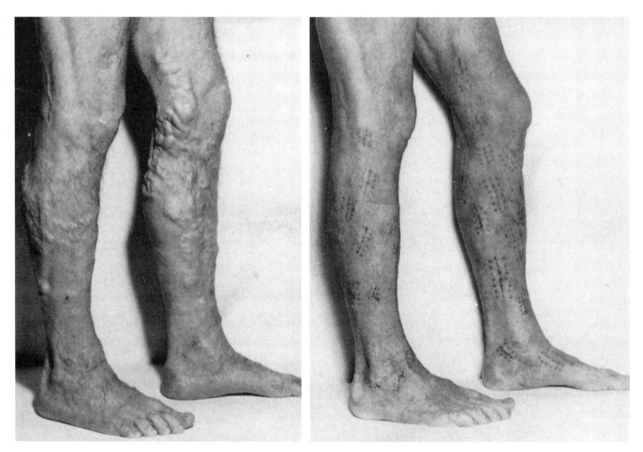

Figure 7.1 Lofgren's method[153] of radical excision of superficial varicosities. It can be seen that this method, though very effective at eradicating the varicose veins, leaves many large scars, some of which are unsightly. We therefore prefer to remove surface varicosities through multiple minute stab incisions. (Reproduced from Lofgren[153] with kind permission.)

the connections between the superficial and deep veins. Some believe that this eradication prevents descending valvular incompetence,[154] while others think that it prevents high pressure in the deep veins being transmitted to the superficial veins.[48,81,150] Although primary valvular incompetence may only rarely be the cause of varicose veins (see Chapter 5), once it has developed it must be stopped to prevent recurrence of varicose veins.

Reduction of the transmural pressure with external elastic compression

The role of elastic compression is discussed in detail in Chapters 17 and 20. Support stockings have been recognized for many years as an alternative method of relieving symptoms in patients with varicose veins;[71,86] it has also been suggested that elastic support may produce a prolonged reduction in ambulatory venous pressure.[240] We were unable to confirm this, however, in a similar study which used foot volumetry rather than venous pressure to measure calf pump function.[242] Nevertheless, elastic stockings can be so effective that some patients will voluntarily withdraw themselves from a surgical waiting list for varicose vein surgery, preferring to continue with external support.[39]

No treatment

One-third of all patients attending a varicose vein clinic are said to require no treatment,[165] and certainly there is a group of patients who have visible veins, spider veins or varicose veins of such small proportions that active treatment is inappropriate. Some patients may be considered too old or unfit to be treated by any method other than elastic support and in other patients the symptoms may be the result of another abnormality. Failure to obtain relief of discomfort by wearing support hose indicates that the pain is unlikely to be of venous aetiology. Lightweight tights provided relief of symptoms in 74% of a group of 461 women employed in occupations where they stood for long periods.[65] Unfortunately this study had no control group so an important placebo effect may have been missed.

Surgical treatment of varicose veins

Most varicose vein operations are performed under general anaesthesia. There are, however, a number of surgeons who practise all their vein surgery under local or regional anaesthesia[99,179,203] and financial

Table 7.1   Contraindications to varicose vein surgery

General ill-health affecting fitness for anaesthesia
Arterial ischaemia of the lower limb
Pregnancy
Contraceptive pill ingestion
Severe coexistent skin infection
Lymphoedema
Bleeding diatheses

pressures have made this and day case surgery much more attractive.[17,43,75,204,216,246] Patients seem well satisfied with these options[246] but major saphenous stripping can only be comfortably performed using a spinal block.[8] These operations have a low mortality and morbidity, but do have some contraindications, which are listed in Table 7.1. The different types of operation are listed below and are then discussed in detail.

1. Flush ligation of the sapheno-femoral junction, also called high saphenous ligation
2. Stripping of the long saphenous vein
3. Sapheno-popliteal junction ligation, also called short saphenous ligation
4. Stripping of the short saphenous vein
5. Ligation of the medial lower leg communicating veins
6. Ligation of other communicating veins (i.e. gastrocnemius, lateral calf, Hunterian and miscellaneous veins)
7. Avulsion of varicosities, ligation of tributaries and local excision of tributaries
8. Operations on recurrent varicose veins.

LIGATION AND DIVISION OF THE LONG SAPHENOUS VEIN AND ITS TRIBUTARIES AT THE SAPHENO-FEMORAL JUNCTION

Although a number of surgeons suggested ligation of the long saphenous vein near its termination, it was Homans,[123] not Trendelenburg,[258] who first suggested that this vein and its tributaries should be ligated *flush* with the femoral vein in the groin. This prevents the reflux of blood into the origin of the long saphenous vein and any of the four or five tributaries that join it near its termination. Recurrent varicose veins are common if the saphenous vein is ligated below these tributaries or if they are left untied. The additional procedure of stripping the long saphenous vein was introduced by Mayo[172] and refined by Babcock[7] and Myers,[177] with the introduction of better intraluminal and flexible strippers.

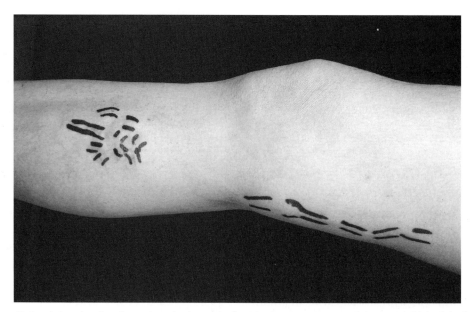

Figure 7.2   A leg that has been 'marked out' before varicose vein surgery. An indelible, black felt-tip pen is used to mark the course of the subcutaneous varicose veins on the overlying skin. Separate marks (crosses inside circles) maybe used to indicate specific sites for exploration for incompetent communicating veins.

Preoperative preparation

If the operation is being performed under general anaesthesia, the patient's general fitness must be confirmed by a full history and clinical examination. The skin of the groin and leg must be shaved before the operation, and the sites of all the prominent varicosities must be carefully marked on the skin with an indelible pen (Figure 7.2). There is a theoretical advantage in marking each vein with two parallel lines on either side of it, as stab wounds through the indelible marker have been reported to result in tattooing.

The sites of incompetent superficial-to-deep connections are also carefully located and marked. Care must be taken to ensure that these marks are not removed or obliterated before the patient reaches the operating theatre. Some surgeons seal the marks with a plastic wound dressing to prevent their removal, but this is not necessary if a pen with waterproof ink is used.

Anaesthesia

General anaesthesia is preferred if sapheno-femoral ligation is to be combined with long saphenous vein stripping, and multiple avulsions. Local anaesthesia[178] and regional anaesthesia,[8,21] usually a spinal anaesthetic with bupivacaine (Marcain) through a fine bore needle, are preferred by others.

Local anaesthesia is more than adequate, if the sapheno-femoral ligation is the sole procedure.

Position

The patient lies supine with each leg abducted by 20–30°, and with the heels supported on a padded vein board (Figure 7.3). The leg veins are emptied by applying a 15–30° of head-down foot-up tilt, which reduces intraoperative haemorrhage. Dale[60] recommends additional elevation of the legs on a slotted rack attached to the end of the operating table, but we have not used this technique. A diathermy electrode is placed under the patient's buttocks.

Skin preparation and drapes

All surfaces of the limb from the heel to the groin, including the anterior surface of the abdomen and pubis to the level of the umbilicus, are prepared with chlorhexidene in water to which edicol dye can be added. Two per cent iodine or Betadine may be used as an alternative but this occasionally produces skin reactions and the colour tends to obscure the preoperative markings. When the limb has been fully painted, with the exception of the foot which is being held by an unsterile assistant, large sterile towels are placed beneath one or both legs on the surface of the operating table (Figure 7.4). The surgeon or the assistant then holds each limb in turn, supporting it with a sterile swab or towel

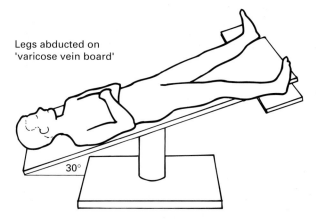

Legs abducted on 'varicose vein board'

30°

Figure 7.3 Diagram to show the position of the patient on the operating table for long saphenous vein surgery. Note the 'foot-up' tilt of the operating table and the use of a padded board to allow abduction of both lower limbs. The 'foot-up' tilt reduces venous engorgement and therefore haemorrhage. The abduction of both limbs allows easier access to the medial side of the leg for long saphenous vein stripping, multiple avulsions and exposure of the medial calf communicating veins.

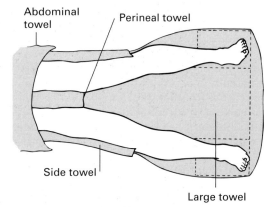

Abdominal towel

Perineal towel

Side towel

Large towel

Figure 7.4 The positions of the sterile towels used to cover all the non-sterile skin and still provide a sufficiently wide sterile field for access to the whole limb.

placed beneath the prepared skin of the calf. The skin of the foot and heel is then prepared, taking care to 'paint up' all parts of the foot and toes and especially the interdigital spaces. Alternatively, the foot can be wrapped in a towel or covered with a sterile surgical glove, taking care not to contaminate the outer surfaces of the glove when it is applied. It is important to remove the glove after the operation, as the wrist ring can cause ischaemia of the toes if it is accidentally left around the foot. Sterile towels are then laid over the abdomen and chest and on either side of the patient to screen off

the abdomen and buttocks (Figure 7.4). A narrow towel is placed between the legs to cover the unsterile skin of the genitalia and perineum (Figure 7.4).

Incision

An oblique incision is made just below the crease of the groin, centred over the sapheno-femoral junction which is 2.5 cm lateral to and below the pubic tubercle. The incision should be straight or curved slightly downwards at its medial end to improve the exposure of the upper end of the long saphenous vein and reach the upper end of the postero-medial thigh vein. We have not found vertical incisions, or the long 'hockey stick' incision suggested by Dodd[69] helpful (Figure 7.5). These incisions do not follow Langer's or Kraissl's lines (see Figure 7.38, page 223) and do not give as good a scar as an incision

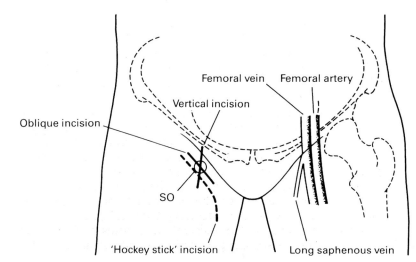

Femoral vein   Femoral artery

Vertical incision

Oblique incision

SO

'Hockey stick' incision   Long saphenous vein

Figure 7.5 The incisions that can be used to approach the sapheno-femoral junction which lies approximately 2 cm below and lateral to the pubic tubercle. The relationship of the sapheno-femoral junction to the other anatomical structures is also shown. We favour the oblique incision placed in or just below the groin crease centred over the sapheno-femoral junction. FA, femoral artery; FV, femoral vein; LSV, long saphenous vein; SO, saphenous opening.

which is placed in or just below the groin crease. The edges of an incision placed exactly in the groin crease tend to 'invert' easily and are more susceptible to superficial infection.

The length of this incision has been the subject of much debate.[60,71,157,170,178] Although it is desirable for cosmetic reasons that the length of the incision should be kept to a minimum, adequate exposure is essential and must not be compromised. It is important to be able to see the anatomy of the subcutaneous veins so that a satisfactory operation can be performed. The size of the leg and the thickness of the subcutaneous fat are factors that must be considered when deciding on the length of the incision. We usually make a 4–6 cm incision but make a shorter incision in a thin, young subject, or increase it to as much as 10 cm in a very obese patient. Incisions are rarely placed too high, and the majority of errors occur when the incision is placed too low or is made too short.

Procedure

The subcutaneous tissues are divided with a scalpel through both the fatty and fibrous layers until the first large vein is seen; this is often the long saphenous vein itself. The skin and subcutaneous tissues are then swept upwards and downwards with a swab to improve the exposure (Figure 7.6a). This dissection is extended by inserting a self-retaining retractor (Cockett's, Traver's, or West's retractors are ideal) into the subcutaneous fat and opening its blades as far as the skin will allow. It is then left in place, retracting the edges of the wound.

Any remaining subcutaneous tissue covering the veins is then divided until the trunk of the long saphenous vein is found running in a vertical direction towards the sapheno-femoral junction. The trunk of the vein is traced upwards using both sharp and blunt dissection until its junction with the femoral vein is displayed (Figure 7.6b). This dissection is simple and bloodless if the correct plane of cleavage is found between the subcutaneous fat and the adventitia of the vein. The plane is easy to recognize because until it is opened the veins are held down flat and compressed by the subcutaneous tissue. Once the fascia has been divided, the veins bulge and are easy to dissect. If the incision is placed too low, or if the patient is very fat, the upper edge of the incision may need to be retracted by an assistant using an additional right-angle retractor as the vein is traced upwards. The right angle retractor can be held by a holder which can be attached to the operating table if an assistant is not available.

The main trunk of the vein should never be divided until the sapheno-femoral junction has been clearly seen (Figure 7.6b). It is possible to mistake

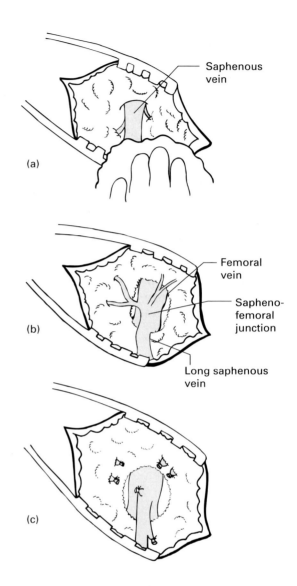

Figure 7.6 (a) After the skin and subcutaneous tissues have been incised the subcutaneous fat is separated by blunt dissection or is pushed gently apart by two gauze swabs to reveal the long saphenous vein passing up towards the sapheno-femoral junction. Tributaries can be seen entering the vein from either side. A self-retaining retractor is inserted into the wound and is opened widely to provide a better view of the vein. (b) The long saphenous vein is traced upwards until the sapheno-femoral junction is clearly identified. Neither the main trunk of the vein nor any of its major tributaries should be divided until this junction has been clearly identified. Small tributaries can be ligated and divided if they interfere with the dissection. (c) Once the sapheno-femoral junction has been identified, all the tributaries of the long saphenous vein are ligated and divided. Small veins joining the femoral vein near the sapheno-femoral junction are also ligated and divided.

the femoral vein r artery for the long saphenous vein,[76,156,192] with astrous consequences if either of these vessels is divided. The only foolproof method of avoiding such a complication is to display the whole anatomy of the long saphenous vein, its tributaries and its junction with the femoral vein, before any large vessels are divided or ligated.

The surgical anatomy of the sapheno-femoral junction

A variable number of tributaries join the long saphenous vein as it approaches the femoral vein. The normal anatomy, the anomalies, and their approximate incidences are shown in Figures 7.7–7.11. These diagrams are derived from two studies of the normal anatomy found in a series of cadaver dissections and a comparable number of operations.[62,111] It can be seen that the 'normal' anatomy described in a 'student textbook' is found in less than one-third of the dissections. Few sapheno-femoral junctions are similar, and this makes knowledge of the possible variations very important before undertaking operations in this area. Tortuosity and saccular dilatation of the termination of the tributaries sometimes makes them appear more prominent than the long saphenous vein itself, for which they may be mistaken, thus making the dissection even more difficult.

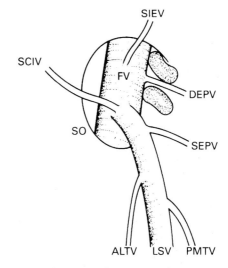

Figure 7.7   The 'normal' anatomical arrangement of tributaries that are found near the sapheno-femoral junction. All these vessels must be defined, ligated and divided at the time of a saphenous vein ligation. ALTV, antero-lateral thigh vein (lateral accessory saphenous vein); DEPV, deep external pudendal vein; FV, femoral vein; LSV, long saphenous vein; PMTV, postero-medial thigh vein (medial accessory saphenous vein); SEPV, superficial external pudendal vein; SCIV, superficial circumflex iliac vein; SIEV, superficial inferior epigastric vein; SO, saphenous opening.

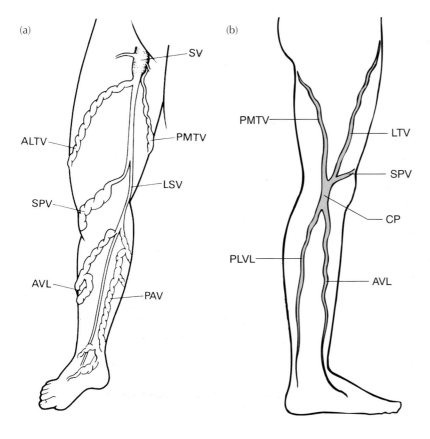

Figure 7.8   (a) The major superficial tributaries of the long saphenous vein which become varicose. Note that the long saphenous vein itself rarely becomes varicose. (b) The superficial veins of the lateral aspect of the leg. These usually drain into the long saphenous system and are a common site for postoperative recurrences. ALTV, antero-lateral thigh vein; AVL, anterior vein of leg (accessory saphenous vein); CP, crossing point; LSV, long saphenous vein; PAV, posterior arch vein; PLVL, postero-lateral vein of the leg; PMTV, postero-medial thigh vein; SPV, suprapatellar vein; SV, saphena varix.

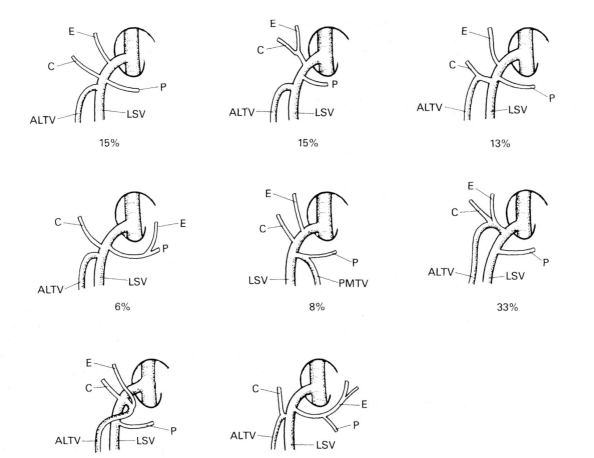

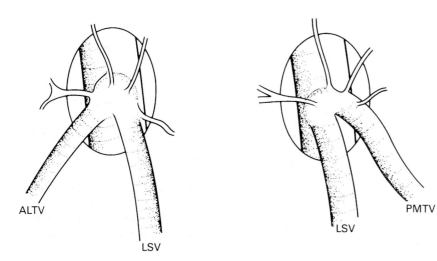

Figure 7.9 The different appearances and terminations (and their incidences) of the long saphenous vein and its main tributaries that were found by Daseler *et al.*[62] and Hilty[111] at operation and at autopsy dissections. (Modified from Foote.[86]) ALTV, antero-lateral thigh vein; C, circumflex iliac; E, epigastric; LSV, long saphenous vein; P, pudendal; PMTV, postero-medial thigh vein.

Figure 7.10 Dilatation and a high termination of either of the two main thigh tributaries, the antero-lateral (ALTV) or the postero-medial (PMTV) thigh veins, may be mistaken for the long saphenous vein, or raise the suspicion that there is a bifid or double long saphenous vein (LSV).

There are six named veins that join the long saphenous vein at or near its termination (Figure 7.7), but they are variable in both number and position. The postero-medial and antero-lateral veins of the thigh enter the long saphenous vein on its medial and lateral side, respectively, at various points between 0 and 20 cm below its termination (Figures 7.7 and 7.8). The superficial inferior epigastric, the superficial circumflex iliac and the superficial external pudendal veins usually join the long saphenous vein just before its termination, but all the variations shown in Figure 7.9 are frequently encountered. The deep external pudendal vein usually joins the medial side of the femoral vein near the sapheno-femoral junction, but this vein quite often joins the saphenous vein at its termination.

Independent terminations of the antero-lateral and postero-medial thigh veins into the femoral vein may give the appearance of a double saphenous vein (Figure 7.10), or the long saphenous vein may be truly double with one channel joining the femoral vein lower down the leg, below the level of the real saphenous opening (Figure 7.11). This is the variation that even an experienced surgeon is likely to miss. It is an important cause of excessive bleeding during vein stripping and may be responsible for the early recurrence of varicose veins.

The other structure that is encountered during the dissection of the sapheno-femoral junction is the external pudenal artery, which may pass either in front or behind the saphenous vein (Figure 7.12). Care should be taken to avoid damaging this vessel, as the resulting haemorrhage can be annoying. If this vessel is inadvertently injured, it can be ligated and divided with impunity.

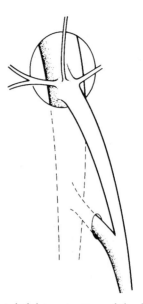

Figure 7.11 A bifid termination of the long saphenous vein. One division joins the femoral vein in the normal position, the other division joins the femoral vein lower down the thigh. If this anomaly is not detected, considerable haemorrhage may follow stripping, or, if only the upper vein is ligated, varicosities may rapidly recur because of the missed lower branch.

Once all the tributaries of the saphenous vein have been clearly displayed they can be doubly ligated in continuity with fine chromic catgut (or polyglycolic acid absorbable sutures) and divided. Division of each tributary between artery forceps is an alternative method but is more likely to cause damage and lead to haemorrhage. It is important to re-emphasize that *no major tributaries should be*

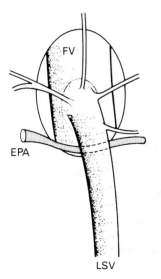

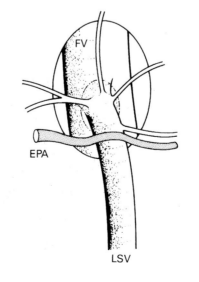

Figure 7.12 The relation of the external pudendal artery (EPA) to the sapheno-femoral junction. This vessel normally passes between the termination of the long saphenous vein (LSV) and the femoral vein (FV), but it sometimes passes in front of the long saphenous vein, making it more susceptible to damage during the dissection.

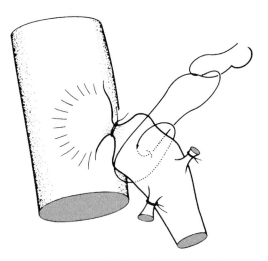

Figure 7.13 Ligation of the sapheno-femoral junction. After all the branches of the long saphenous vein have been ligated and divided, the long saphenous vein is itself ligated in continuity, and is divided. Two ligatures are usually placed on the proximal end as a precautionary measure. A transfixion suture may be used for the second ligature if the vein is exceptionally large. It is important to place these ligatures between the junction and all the major tributaries of the saphenous vein. The stumps of the tributaries then prevent the ligature from 'rolling off'.

divided before the site of the sapheno-femoral junction has been clearly identified.

Both sides of the femoral vein should then be dissected free for 1–2 cm above and below the sapheno-femoral junction. The deep external pudendal vein and any other tributaries joining the femoral vein must be ligated and divided. The long saphenous vein itself can then be ligated, in continuity, with absorbable ligatures, and divided. Non-absorbable sutures carry the risk of stitch sinuses but are used by some.

If the vein is particularly large, the proximal stump is ligated and a transfixion stitch can be used for the second ligature (Figure 7.13). If these ligatures are placed between the sapheno-femoral junction and some of the divided tributaries, there is less chance of them slipping off (Figure 7.13). Care should be taken to ensure that all the tributaries are ligated and divided between the long saphenous stump and its ligature, as any tributaries that are left intact may be responsible for recurrence (Figure 7.14).

The distal segment of the long saphenous vein is dissected downwards for 5–10 cm. A right-angled retractor is inserted under the lower skin flap to expose the saphenous vein more clearly. If the antero-lateral and postero-medial thigh veins can

easily be seen, they should be freed, doubly ligated and divided, even if the saphenous vein is not going to be stripped out. At least 5–10 cm of the long saphenous vein should be resected if a sapheno-femoral ligation is the only operation to be performed.

Care must be taken to:

1. avoid damaging the femoral vein or tearing off small tributaries that enter this vein;
2. ligate all small tributaries entering the femoral vein directly (particularly the deep external pudendal vein);
3. make sure that all sutures are properly tied and do not come undone or slip off the long saphenous vein or its tributaries;
4. ensure that when the long saphenous vein is tied flush with the femoral vein it does not narrow the femoral vein;
5. avoid dividing any vein assumed to be the long saphenous vein until its junction with a normal femoral vein has been confirmed.

Closure

The incision should be closed using catgut, polyglycolic and or polydioxone sulphate (PDS) sutures to approximate the fatty layers and fine nylon or an intradermal absorbable 4/0 PDS suture to close the skin. The latter sutures may be used in conjunction with adhesive tapes.

Alternatives

A number of surgeons have now attempted to restore competence to the highest long saphenous valve by plicating it or wrapping it in a synthetic cuff[12,13,57,137]. These operations are experimental and at present have only been tried by individual surgeons. A multicentre trial with external audit might help to determine their value. The present studies[12,13,57,137] unfortunately do not have a control limb, were not randomized and have had no external audit or assessment. There is currently a study taking place in North America which compares ligation and banding, but the series is small and the follow-up short.[224]

Technical problems

Bleeding

Sudden massive bleeding from a slipped ligature or direct damage to a major vein should be controlled by applying direct pressure to the bleeding point with a finger or swab. A junior surgeon should obtain help from an experienced senior colleague (preferably one who has had vascular training).

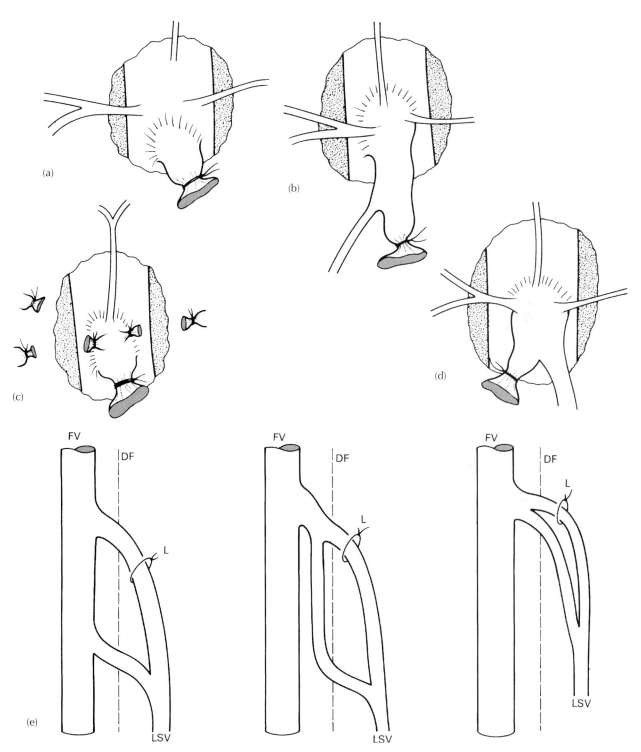

Figure 7.14 Reasons for the development of recurrent connections between the deep and superficial veins at the saphenous opening. (a) Failure to ligate 'normal' tributaries of the long saphenous vein which join the common femoral vein directly. (b) A low ligation of the long saphenous vein, which produces the same circumstances as (a). (c) Failure to ligate all the tributaries. Usually, either the superficial inferior epigastric or the superficial external pudendal veins are not ligated. (d) Ligation of the antero-lateral or postero-medial thigh vein in the mistaken belief that it is the long saphenous vein, thus leaving the long saphenous vein intact. (e) Three variations of a double termination of the long saphenous vein which may result in the placement of the ligature around only one limb of the termination. DF, deep fascia; FV, femoral vein; L, site of ligature; LSV, long saphenous vein.

After applying pressure for several minutes (a minimum of 2 minutes) the swabs or finger may be gently removed. The bleeding is usually much reduced, and using suction to remove any blood and provide a clear view of the bleeding point, the damaged vein can be closed with a direct vascular suture (5/0 polypropylene).

Pressure should be reapplied if the bleeding cannot be controlled in this way, and the wound should be enlarged to allow the femoral vein to be exposed some distance above and below the saphenous opening. Direct digital compression of the femoral vein above and below the saphenous junction will always control the bleeding, allowing further dissection of the damaged vein and the placement of sutures to close the defect. It is only necessary to apply clamps to the femoral vein when it has been severely damaged and requires some form of reconstruction. In these circumstances 5000 units of heparin should be given to the patient before the vein is clamped. A vein patch may be used to repair the femoral vein if necessary (see Chapter 26).

Artery forceps must never be applied to a bleeding point without a good view of the damaged vessel and should never be applied to a side hole in a large vein – such unthinking precipitous action will often make the venous injury worse.

Damage to the femoral artery

The femoral artery should not be injured during straightforward varicose vein surgery; if, however, it is damaged, and the damage is recognized, it should be repaired by direct suture, a vein patch or a vein graft. The three common ways of injuring the femoral artery are: tearing off a small side branch, inadvertent ligation and inadvertent stripping.

In a review of arterial complications associated with varicose vein surgery Cockett[46] has pointed out that the majority are caused by inexperienced surgeons (GPs or trainees) who fail to recognize the problem at the time of injury. The inexperience of the operating surgeon was confirmed by Redmond *et al.*[205] who reported a similar experience in Ireland.

Damage to the femoral vein

Damage to the femoral vein which causes bleeding is discussed above. The femoral vein may also be inadvertantly ligated, and if this is recognized, the ligature should be carefully removed and the vein wall be inspected (see Figure 26.5, page 716). If there is a circumferential disruption of the intima, the vein may have to be resected and repaired with an end-to-end anastomosis or an interposition vein graft (see Chapter 26). This accident is responsible for 11% of cases coming to legal action.[248]

STRIPPING THE LONG SAPHENOUS VEIN

We routinely strip the long saphenous vein to a point just below the knee to prevent recurrence developing through the Hunterian communicating veins[53] and to remove a vein in the thigh which is difficult to treat later by sclerotherapy. Vascular and cardiac surgeons have complained that unnecessary stripping of the long saphenous vein removes a potential vascular conduit,[47,121] but other surgeons have pointed out that a grossly distended incompetent long saphenous is probably of little use in bypass surgery. Both arguments are probably valid but most authorities agree that a combination of a high saphenous ligation with long saphenous stripping reduces the incidence of upper thigh recurrences.[60,71,139,153,177,178,209] We only strip the long saphenous vein to just below the knee to avoid damaging the saphenous nerve whose branches lie close to the vein in the lower leg.[58,67] This also has the potential advantage that it leaves a reasonable length of vein below the knee for use by the cardiac surgeons at a later date.[10] The sapheno-femoral junction can be ligated under local anaesthesia as a day case but stripping under local anaesthesia is not acceptable.[220]

Technique

After ligating and dividing the long saphenous vein (as described above), a long silk ligature is passed around the lower part of the vein and a transverse venotomy is made in the vein above the ligature (Figure 7.15). The ligature is 'held up' to occlude the vein and prevent haemorrhage from the venotomy, but it is not tied down until the stripper has been inserted.

Sarin[218,219] has reviewed all the comparison trials of sapheno-femoral ligation versus stripping that have been performed and conducted a further study which suggests that stripping of the long saphenous vein reduces recurrences.

A flexible intraluminal stripper is selected and attached to an 'olive' of appropriate size. We prefer a flexible wire stripper (Figure 7.16) because we find that it is easier to direct through the kinks and lateral sacculations of a varicose vein; other surgeons, however, prefer the modern stiff plastic disposable strippers with reversible heads (Figure 7.17).

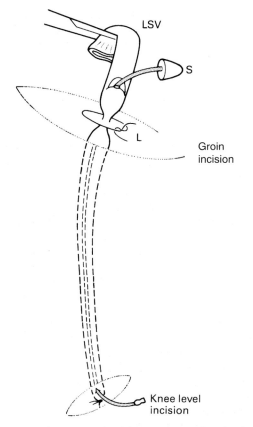

Figure 7.15 The insertion of the stripper. After the long saphenous vein (LSV) has been ligated and divided, the distal end of the vein is freed from the surrounding sub-cutaneous tissues for several centimetres and the termination of both the antero-lateral and postero-medial thigh veins are ligated and divided. An artery forceps is placed on the end of the vein for counter-traction, and a ligature (L) is passed around the vein and pulled taut to prevent bleeding when the venotomy is made. The stripper (S) is then inserted and manipulated down to the knee. The stripper is retrieved from the vein at the knee level, through a small incision, to allow the vein to be avulsed from above downwards.

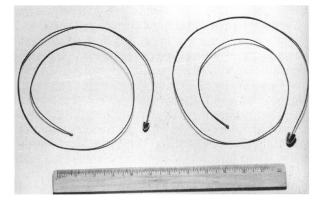

Figure 7.16 Two flexible Myers' wire strippers with olives of different sizes. The tips also come in different shapes and sizes. These strippers must be carefully handled and stored to avoid kinking the wire.

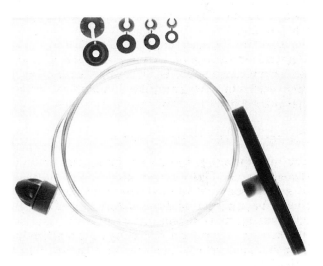

Figure 7.17 A disposable, flexible, intraluminal, plastic stripper with removable heads of different sizes (shown above) and handle.

In a recent study, Corbett[51] showed no real difference in the passage of either type of stripper although the passage of the plastic stripper was quicker. We are more persuaded by the economic argument that favours the reusable (metal) stripper. A metal stripper costs £100–150 and lasts a lifetime; each disposable plastic stripper costs £8.00. It is important to use a handle on the stripper to avoid kinking of the wire and to reserve a set of wire strippers for each individual surgeon.

The blunt pointed tip of the stripper (Figure 7.16) is inserted into the venotomy and pushed downwards.

The ligature is then tied down to prevent bleeding from around the stripper, and an artery forceps is placed on the proximal end of the divided vein to allow counter-traction to be exerted on the vein as the stripper is advanced down the limb. On many occasions the stripper will pass without difficulty to below the knee, but if resistance is met during insertion, the stripper should be withdrawn a few centimetres and then reinserted while a rotatory movement is applied to the free portion which is still protruding outside the vein. The passage of the stripper may be made easier if an assistant takes over the counter-traction on the divided vein, to allow the surgeon to use his free hand to feel and direct the stripper head down the main vein and, by applying gentle external pressure over its tip, prevent it passing into varicose tributaries. The passage of the stripper may be facilitated at knee level by flexing and extending the knee joint with external pressure applied over the tip of the stripper, accompanied by further rotation of the stripper wire and intermittent insertion and withdrawal. As the surgeon's experience in the use of the stripper increases, more successful passages of the stripper to the knee will be achieved.[51]

When the stripper has been successfully passed beyond the level of the knee joint, a short oblique incision is made in the direction of Kraissl's (Langer's) lines (see Figure 7.38) over the palpable tip. The vein containing the stripper (it may be the long saphenous, the anterior leg vein, or the posterior arch vein) is isolated by blunt dissection, and the distal end of the vein ligated with a catgut or polyglycolic acid suture. A venotomy is then made and the stripper extracted from the lumen of the vessel. A further ligature is passed around the proximal part of the vein containing the stripper wire and the vein is divided.

A handle is attached to the stripper and the vein is removed by steady firm traction applied in the long axis of the vein. The vein and its tributaries are avulsed as it concertinas up against the undersurface of the mushroom-shaped olive on the end of the stripper (Figure 7.18). The incision at the knee must be long enough to allow the mass of vein on the stripper and the stripper head to pass through it, but if a small incision is required at knee level, the stripper head can be pulled back up its track by attaching a silk or nylon ligature to it [130,212] so that it can be removed, with the vein, through the groin incision. The plastic disposable strippers have removable heads, which can be attached at either end, thus the direction of stripping is optional.

A flexible metal stripper has now been produced with a threaded hole in the top of the head to which a second wire can be attached, allowing the stripper to be easily pulled back up the stripper track.

If the stripper will not pass down the vein, an incision must be made just below the medial condyle of the tibia to expose the long saphenous vein, which is always quite deep at this point, lying on the deep fascia. A segment of vein is dissected out, ligated distally and the stripper is passed up to the groin (Figure 7.19a). Upward passage of the stripper is unavoidable in some operations. We prefer to strip the vein downwards, not simply because it allows a smaller incision below the knee, but also because greater lengths of tributary veins are usually avulsed when the stripper is pulled downwards rather than upwards, and there is a lower incidence

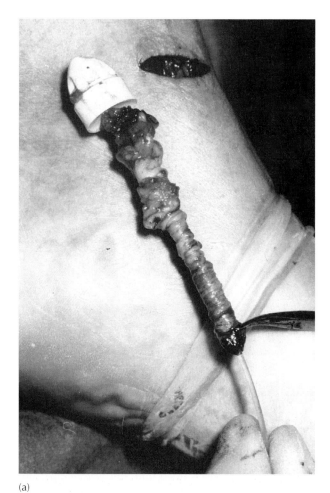

(a)

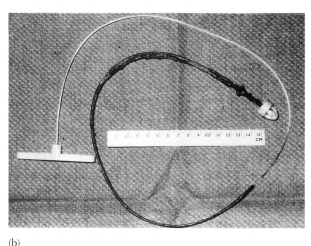

(b)

Figure 7.18 Stripping the long saphenous vein. (a) As the stripper head is pulled through the leg, the vein 'concertinas up' on the wire below the olive so that when the stripper is removed from the lower incision, the concertina'd vein appears to be quite short. (b) The vein should be pulled out, to check that the full length of the long saphenous vein and short lengths of its tributaries have been removed.

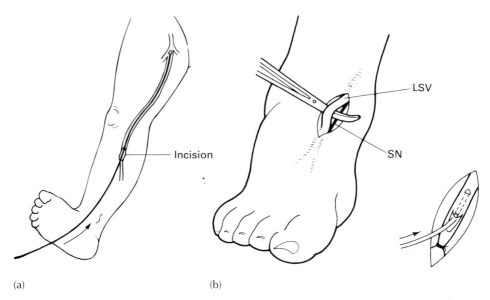

Figure 7.19 (a) Passage of the stripper through the long saphenous vein from the knee upwards. The long saphenous vein is isolated near the knee and, after it has been ligated distally, the stripper is inserted and passed up to the groin. (b) Passage of the stripper from the ankle. The vein is isolated where it crosses the anterior aspect of the medial malleolus, taking care to separate it from the saphenous nerve. The stripper is inserted into the vein and then passed up to the groin (insert). LSV, long saphenous vein; SN, saphenous nerve.

of saphenous nerve damage when the stripper is pulled downwards.[50,58,67]

May[170] has emphasized the dangers of passing a stripper from the ankle to the groin to help to locate the sapheno-femoral junction; he pointed out that the stripper may enter the deep veins through a communicating vein in the thigh or an accessory low sapheno-femoral junction (Figure 7.11), thus making inadvertent ligation or stripping of the femoral vein more likely. He has also suggested that thrombus can form on a stripper which is left in place for a long time during the groin dissection. Small pulmonary emboli may then occur, if the long saphenous vein is not ligated early in the dissection. The only advantage of passing a stripper from the ankle is the ease with which the vein can be found as it crosses the subcutaneous surface of the medial malleolus and the fact that it will pass up to the groin unimpeded in most cases (Figure 7.19b). The disadvantages, which have already been mentioned, are the loss of a potentially useful normal vein below the knee which might be used as an arterial graft at a later date[47,121] and an increased risk of skin anaesthesia secondary to saphenous nerve damage.[58,67]

Stripping the long saphenous vein below the knee does *not* correct any lower leg communicating vein incompetence as most of these veins do not drain directly into the long saphenous vein (see Chapter 2), whereas the Hunter Canal thigh communicating vein does drain directly into the saphenous vein.

Furthermore, the long saphenous vein below the knee is quite often normal in size with competent valves, even when the upper thigh segment is dilated and incompetent. For these reasons (lack of abnormality and no worthwhile physiological effect), we do not strip the long saphenous vein below the knee. We have not found problems with retrograde passage of the stripper to the knee, because if the operation is being done for the correct indications there should be few, if any, competent valves to obstruct its passage. Nevertheless, we do not persist for a prolonged time with our attempts at retrograde passage; if any difficulty is experienced, a cut-down is made behind the knee, the vein is found and the stripper is passed upwards.

Alternative methods of stripping

Baccalini[8] has developed an external stripper which is pushed over a stiff wire which is passed down the long saphenous vein to just below the knee. The external stripper cuts off the tributaries as it is manoeuvred to the knee and a rotation of its handle divides the long saphenous vein beyond the wire, allowing it to be pulled out of the groin incision, thus avoiding the need for a second long incision at the knee to retrieve the stripper sleeve. PIN stripping is a newer technique developed by Oesch[184] in which the long saphenous vein is deliberately invaginated after passage of a pin stripper up the

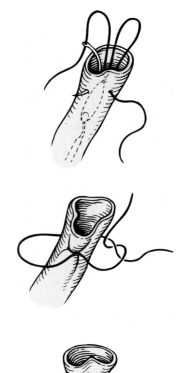

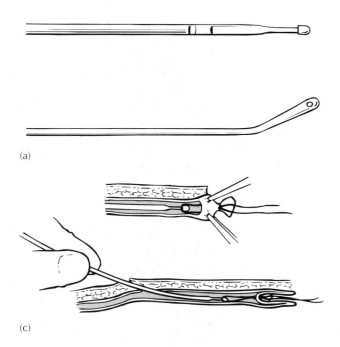

Figure 7.20 The pin stripper for invagination stripping. (a) The small stripper head for insertion through a small incision with 'eye' for the attachment of the invaginating suture. (b) Technique for attaching vein to stripper head which will ensure that the vein invaginates when the stripper is pulled. (c) Invagination and stripping.

lumen of the long saphenous vein (see Figure 7.20). This is a modification of other techniques of inverted stripping.[243,262] It is claimed that this technique reduces haematoma formation and postoperative pain but two recent controlled trials have failed to demonstrate any clear-cut benefits. There is a greater incidence of the vein breaking during inversion, resulting in the loss of what can amount to a considerable segment.

Another technique of multiple cut-downs on the long saphenous vein with complete excision is reported to reduce the incidence of bruising.[85] The vein may also be selectively stripped as far as the reflux has been measured.[136] Cryostripping is yet another method of removing the long saphenous vein but it may cause skin and nerve damage.[41,89]

Technical problems

Failure to pass the stripper

Occasionally, varicosities of the long saphenous vein itself (Figure 7.21) prevent the passage of a stripper in both directions. If this happens, two strippers are passed, one from above, the other from below, to the point of obstruction (Figure 7.22). An incision is made at this point and the tips of both strippers are extracted. Both segments of the vein are then avulsed. Alternatively, the heads of the strippers can be tied together so that either one can be used to guide the other stripper through the opposite segment of vein. Occasionally, all these manoeuvres fail and the vein has to be stripped 'piecemeal' through a number of separate incisions. These incisions should be as small as possible, and they should be placed in the direction of Langer's/Krassl's lines (Figure 7.38).[88,98,184,262]

Haemorrhage from the track

Stripping of the vein is best left to the end of the operation. The limb may then be bandaged as the stripper is removed to minimize haematoma formation in the track. This means a reversal of the olives and the vein being stripped upwards. Alternatively, stripping can be performed at an early stage so that any collections of blood can be expelled by gentle compression produced by rolling

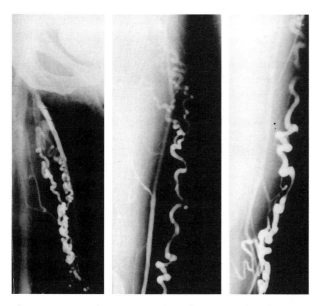

Figure 7.21 This varicogram shows a double long saphenous vein. One vein is straight and the stripper would pass along it easily (this is the normal finding). The other vein is so tortuous that the stripper would not pass through it.

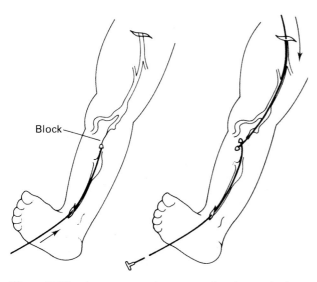

Figure 7.22 A narrow portion or a varicosity on the long saphenous vein may prevent the passage of the stripper. In these circumstances it may be helpful to pass the stripper from each direction to the level of the block. The second stripper may occasionally pass through the block and down the full length of the vein but if this does not happen, a cut-down should be made over the obstruction to allow the strippers to be tied together and pulled through the full length of the vein or the vein should be stripped out in two halves.

a gauze swab, made into a ball, up and down the leg along the course of the vein. The haemorrhage soon stops, if the leg is elevated, providing the uppermost major branches (the antero-lateral and postero-medial thigh veins) have been ligated before the vein is stripped. Severe bleeding can invariably be controlled by external pressure and increased elevation of the leg. It is almost never necessary to explore the track of a stripped vein to arrest bleeding. An arterial injury or a coincidental bleeding diathesis must be suspected if bleeding persists.

Inversion of the vein

If the olive of the stripper that is selected is too small, it may pass into the lumen of the vein which is then invaginated as the vein is stripped (Figure 7.23). This technique is preferred by some[88,98,184,262] to reduce the trauma. The vein can usually be delivered satisfactorily from below by gentle traction, but if this fails, the silk ligature or wire threaded through the olive may be used to pull the stripper back so that a stripper with a larger olive may be substituted.

Perforation of the vein

If the stripper cannot be passed (despite the techniques described above) and excessive force is used during its insertion, the tip may pierce the vein wall before passing down the leg in a false passage alongside rather than inside the vein. This is often recognized when the cut-down over the tip finds the stripper lying outside the lumen of the vein. The whole of the vein may be satisfactorily avulsed if an attempt is made to strip the vein, but often only part of the vein is stripped out. It is wiser to pass a second stripper from below, by the method described above, and to strip the vein upwards or use the lower stripper to guide the upper stripper down the correct path (Figure 7.22).

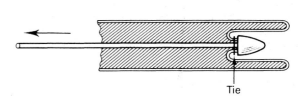

Figure 7.23 Inversion of the vein by the stripper. This happens when the olive that has been selected is too small for the diameter of the vein being stripped. The vein often slips off the stripper or breaks when this happens.

Damage to the saphenous nerve

This is a well recognized complication when the long saphenous vein is stripped from the ankle,[58,67,122,140] but it seldom occurs if the vein is only stripped to just below the knee. Stripping below the knee serves little purpose and should be avoided.

Arterial injury

Although this has already been discussed in the section on high saphenous ligation (page 204), there are also reports that the major arterial supply of the lower limb can be avulsed.[77,192] Such an injury is difficult to comprehend and is indefensible.

Contraindications to stripping

Patients with recognized *bleeding disorders* are best treated by high saphenous ligation without stripping the long saphenous vein, unless the defect can be corrected before operation.

In patients with *lymphoedema*, ankle swelling can be exacerbated by stripping, perhaps as a result of damage to the lymphatics which surround the vein.[260] A high saphenous ligation and avulsion of the tributaries is the treatment of choice.

In patients with evidence of *arterial insufficiency*, varicose vein surgery is almost always contraindicated and light support stockings should be used as an alternative. The surgeon should especially avoid making incisions in the lower leg which may not heal satisfactorily and stripping a vein which, even if dilated, may act as a useful bypass.

Postoperative management

Patients should be encouraged to get up and walk as soon as possible (i.e. the same evening or the following morning). They can be discharged from hospital the same or the following day, depending upon the extent of the surgery providing there are no social contraindications to discharge and no complications. Mild oral analgesic drugs are provided for the first few days. Sutures are removed 5–7 days after the operation, but firm compression bandages should be worn at all times during the first week, and for the next 3 weeks they should only be removed at night. Compression bandages reduce postoperative bruising and oedema, and may also reduce the risk of deep vein thrombosis.[146,147] We use a combination of Elastocrepe (Smith & Nephew), Setopress (Seton) or Tensopress bandages (Smith & Nephew) covered with Tubigrip stockinette because the heavier Blue or Red Line[10] bandages tends to slip down after a few hours of activity. Alternatively, patients can be provided with elastic stockings[48] but these are expensive and patients find them painful to pull on and off when they have tender incisions on the legs. Antiembolism stockings (TED, Kendall) are used by a number of surgeons but these do not apply sufficient compression to reduce haematoma formation and cannot be recommended, even though one study[235] has shown no difference between high and low compression stockings after vein surgery. Patients should be told to discard their bandages when they feel comfortable and there is no ankle swelling.

LIGATION AND DIVISION OF THE SAPHENO-POPLITEAL JUNCTION AND STRIPPING OF THE SHORT SAPHENOUS VEIN

The position of the sapheno-popliteal junction is extremely variable (see Chapter 2); a summary of the anatomical variations is shown in Figure 7.24. Haeger[106] and Kosinski[134] have shown that the short saphenous vein only joins the popliteal vein a few centimetres above the level of the knee joint in 57% of all limbs. In approximately one-third (33%) of limbs, the short saphenous vein has a high termination, joining either the long saphenous vein or connecting with one of the intermuscular communicating veins to empty into the deep femoral vein.[173] In 10% of limbs the short saphenous vein has a low termination, joining either the long saphenous vein in the calf or one of the deep veins in the centre of the calf.[171,174] Some surgeons advocate routine stripping of the short saphenous vein; others think the short saphenous vein should be disconnected and never stripped. The short saphenous vein operation should be carried out first, if a long saphenous vein operation is to be performed under the same anaesthetic.

Preoperative preparation

Particular care must be taken to identify the termination of the short saphenous vein.[31] Clinical examination is notoriously inaccurate; better information can be provided by the Doppler flow detector,[113] duplex scanning,[208] preoperative varicography,[32,141] or intraoperative phlebography.[55,114,169,233] Just over one-half of short saphenous veins join the popliteal vein in the popliteal fossa at the level of the knee joint. Very few – approximately 10% – join at a lower level, but a significant 30% join at the top of, or above, the popliteal fossa (Table 7.2). The termination of the vein must be carefully marked preoperatively if duplex scanning is used to locate it.

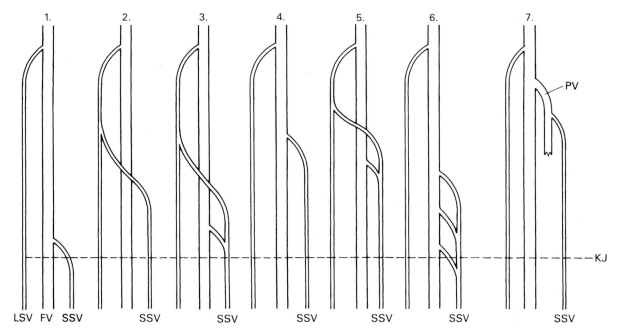

Figure 7.24 Some of the variations that are found at the termination of the short saphenous vein. 1. The 'normal' (only found in 60% of all short saphenous terminations) terminations. 2. The short saphenous vein drains into the long saphenous vein rather than into the popliteal vein. 3. A connection between the short saphenous vein and long saphenous vein. 4. A high termination. 5. A high termination and a connection with the long saphenous vein. 6. Multiple terminations and connections, at different levels, with the femoro-popliteal vein. 7. The short saphenous vein may be connected to a tributary of the deep femoral vein or may terminate in the deep femoral vein.[173] FV, femoral vein; KJ, level of knee joint; LSV, long saphenous vein; PV, deep femoral vein; SSV, short saphenous vein.

Table 7.2 The level of the sapheno-popliteal vein junction

Study	Method	Level of termination (% incidence)		
		Mid-popliteal fossa	High	Low
Kosinski 1926[134]	Dissection	57%	33%	10%
Haeger 1962[106]	Surgery	60%	32%	8%
May 1978[171]	Phlebography	85%	14%	1%
Hobbs 1980[114]	Phlebography	60%	30%	10%
Sheppard 1986[233]	Phlebography	60%	30%	10%
Corcos 1987[55]	Phlebography	44%	33%	23%

Based upon Corcos *et al.*[56]

Position

If the operation is to be performed under a general anaesthetic, the patient must be intubated, before being placed in a prone position on the operating table. Two pillows are placed under the patient's hips and chest to prevent abdominal compression and to allow free movement of the diaphragm. Abduction of the limbs is not essential but is often quite helpful.

Skin preparation and towelling

When the patient has been placed in a prone position on the operating table an assistant grasps the foot and bends the knee to 90°, to allow the lower part of the leg (with the exception of the foot) to be painted with Hibitane in water (1 in 10 000) or iodine. The assistant then lifts the whole leg off the table so that the knee and lower part of the anterior surface of the thigh can be painted. A large towel is slipped beneath the knee to cover the upper surface of the operating table. The surgeon grasps the painted area of the calf in a swab before painting the foot with antiseptic or enclosing it in a towel or glove. The upper part of the limb is covered by another large sterile towel. The operating table is placed with a 15-30° head-down tilt to reduce venous congestion and lessen bleeding.

Short saphenous vein stripping

We routinely strip the short saphenous vein because there are communicating veins which drain directly into it, and the presence of the stripper within the vein helps us to identify the vein in the popliteal fossa. We begin by making a short vertical or transverse incision midway between the Achilles tendon and the lower part of the fibula over the lower end of the short saphenous vein (Figure 7.25). It is important to make the incision high enough as two tributaries commonly join to form the short saphenous and neither is usually large enough to allow the stripper to pass. The main vein is found in the subcutaneous tissue deep to this incision. Care must be taken to define the sural nerve which is occasionally mistaken for the vein and is always closely applied to its surface. Careful inspection will reveal that the nerve is composed of a number of nerve bundles without branches, whereas the vein is usually formed from one or two tributaries just below this level.

When the vein has been separated from the nerve, a non-absorbable ligature is tied around the distal end of the vein. Another ligature is passed around the vein, proximally, but is not tied. A transverse venotomy is then made in the vein between the two ligatures; the upper ligature is held taut to prevent back-bleeding, and a flexible wire stripper is inserted into the vein, as for long saphenous vein stripping. After the stripper has been passed a short distance, the upper ligature is tied to prevent back-bleeding. The stripper is then gently passed up the vein from below in a manner similar to that already described in long saphenous vein stripping (see page 204).

The popliteal incision can be made directly over the sapheno-popliteal junction if the sapheno-popliteal junction has been defined by one of the methods already described and if the stripper passes easily up to the expected level. Careful palpation of the stripper tip as it enters the popliteal fossa may help to define the level of the junction, if preoperative localization of the junction has not been attempted. The short saphenous vein can pass beneath the deep fascia at any point as it ascends the leg (Figure 7.26)[174] but it bends sharply inwards before it joins the popliteal vein. The stripper tip can often be felt to disappear at this point and it may give a little kick or jump as it enters the popliteal vein. This is a useful indication (but no more than an indication) of the site of the termination of the short saphenous vein, which can be used if other methods of sapheno-popliteal localization are not available.

As short saphenous incompetence is relatively rare[178] (see Chapter 6), we still prefer to perform preoperative ultrasound scans varicograms on all

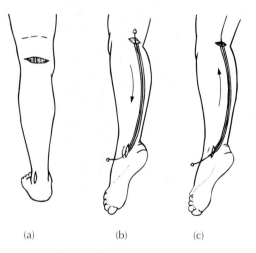

(a)   (b)   (c)

Figure 7.25   Short saphenous vein stripping. (a) The incisions used for stripping the short saphenous vein. A second incision, higher in the popliteal fossa, may be required if there is a high termination of the vein. (b, c) The vein may be stripped upwards or downwards. (Modified from May.[170])

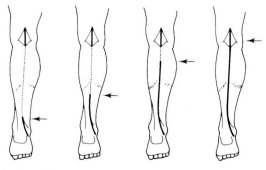

Distal third   Middle third   Proximal third   Popliteal fossa
7%   51.5%   32.5%   9%

Figure 7.26   The positions where the short saphenous vein may pierce the deep fascia as it ascends the leg. The relative incidences are based on Moosman *et al.*[174] (Modified from May.[170])

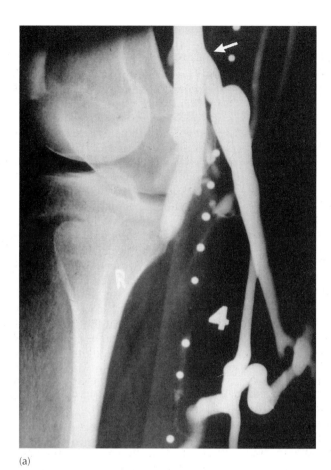

(a)

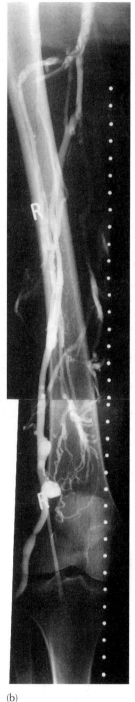

(b)

Figure 7.27 (a) A varicogram showing a dilated short saphenous vein with a termination (arrowed) 4 cm above the knee joint. The metal ball-bearings (1 cm apart) are incorporated in a plastic ruler which is placed on the surface of the leg There are varicose veins connecting the long and short saphenous veins. The calibre of the long saphenous vein is normal. (b) A high termination of the short saphenous vein. The short saphenous vein is normal size and competent at the level of the knee. It is joined by an incompetent varicose tributary 5 cm above the knee joint and above this is itself incompetent. It ultimately joins a tributary of the deep femoral vein in the middle of the thigh.

patients with short saphenous incompetence to confirm the diagnosis and ascertain the exact anatomy (Figure 7.27 and Table 7.2). Many surgeons now use the Doppler ultrasound scanner in preference to varicography to determine the exact location of the sapheno-popliteal junction. This may be more cost-effective but requires a skilled duplex operator.[78] Intraoperative venography, as suggested by Hobbs,[114] provides a satisfactory alternative but does add time to the operation. The vein is stripped after the sapheno-popliteal junction has been dissected and divided.

Exploration of the popliteal fossa

A transverse incision is made over the termination of the short saphenous vein. The length of the incision depends upon the size of the patient and the amount of subcutaneous fat surrounding the limb, but it should always err on the generous side and should be at least 5–8 cm long.

The subcutaneous fat is split beneath the line of the incision down to the deep fascia, which is also opened in a similar direction although there are those who feel a vertical incision through the deep fascia is preferable to allow better access and avoid damaging the sural nerve.[36]. Care must be taken because the vein and the sural nerve may occasionally lie within the layers of fascia rather than deep to it. A self-retaining retractor is inserted to open the skin, fat and the deep fascia (Figure 7.28). The short saphenous vein should be found passing vertically upwards. It can easily be felt if it contains the stripper, but *great care must be taken to ensure that the stripper is not in the popliteal vein having entered it through a connecting vein in the lower calf.*

The stripper is withdrawn to allow dissection of the sapheno-popliteal junction. The short saphenous vein should never be ligated until the surgeon has clearly demonstrated its junction with the popliteal vein (Figure 7.28). Sometimes this dissection is difficult, especially when the short saphenous vein dips down into a deep and fatty popliteal fossa. Visibility can sometimes be improved by inserting two Langenbeck retractors to pull the fat and the heads of the gastrocnemius muscle apart.

A large tributary, the vein of Giacomini,[91] commonly joins the short saphenous vein from above,

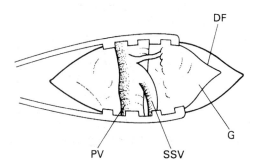

Figure 7.28   The dissection of the termination of the short saphenous vein in the popliteal fossa. The short saphenous vein is usually found lying beneath the deep fascia (see Figure 7.26) and can be traced to its termination in the popliteal vein. All the tributaries joining the short saphenous vein should be ligated and divided once the site of the sapheno-popliteal junction has been confirmed. The vein may then be stripped out, if stripping is indicated. DF, deep fascia; G, gastrocnemius muscle; PV, popliteal vein; SSV, short saphenous vein.

before it turns deeply to join the popliteal vein or one of the paired venae comitantes that pass up on either side of the popliteal artery. This tributary must be carefully divided between ligatures before the short saphenous vein is ligated flush with the popliteal vein. Occasionally the vein of Giacomini acts as an extension of the short saphenous vein and passes up to join the posterior branch of the long saphenous vein or even the profunda femoris vein. Dodd and Cockett[71] recommend flexion of the knee during dissection of the popliteal fossa to relax the popliteal fascia, but we have not found this to be of any particular benefit. The popliteal dissection is, however, difficult, and it is essential that the popliteal vein is not damaged because this can have disasterous consequences.

Large veins from the gastrocnemius muscle and other large tributaries may also join the undersurface of the short saphenous vein near its termination, making the anatomy difficult to define.[36,232,233] All the tributaries of the short saphenous vein must be carefully ligated. A young surgeon in training should look at an anatomical dissection of the popliteal fossa before undertaking this operation, as this provides a salutary reminder of the important structures within the popliteal fossa that can be damaged by inexpert dissection (Figure 7.29). It is better to leave a stump of short saphenous vein, rather than damage the popliteal vein in an attempt to perform a perfect flush ligation, but if a small stump of vein is left, it must not be left with any patent tributaries, otherwise it may allow recurrent incompetent veins to develop which can be extremely difficult to manage.

If the popliteal incision is placed too low, a second incision may be required at a higher level, which may be gauged by pulling down on the vein and seeing where this produces a dimple in the skin. After ligating and dividing the short saphenous vein in the popliteal fossa, it is also divided at the ankle and stripped out.

The fascia of the popliteal fossa is closed with 2/0 chromic catgut and the skin is closed with interrupted 4/0 nylon stitches or a subcuticular suture with adhesive skin tapes.

If no other procedure is to be performed, the foot and lower leg are firmly bandaged. Alternatively, after the short saphenous incisions have been covered by sterile gauze and the leg has been wrapped in a sterile towel to prevent contamination, the patient can be turned onto his/her back for long saphenous vein ligation and stripping.

Postoperative care

This is identical to that following the long saphenous operation.

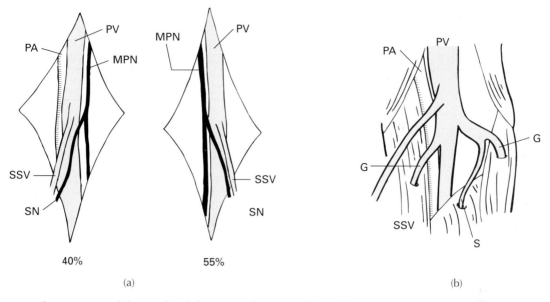

Figure 7.29   The anatomy of the popliteal fossa. (a) There is a close relationship between the short saphenous vein and the medial popliteal nerve in the popliteal fossa. The vein can lie either medial or lateral to the nerve. LPN, lateral popliteal nerve; MPN, medial popliteal nerve; PA, popliteal artery; PV, popliteal vein; SN, sural nerve; SSV, short saphenous vein. (b) The 'normal' venous anatomy. The gastrocnemius veins may join the short saphenous vein before it joins the popliteal vein.[170] G, medial and lateral tributaries from gastrocnemius muscle; PA, popliteal artery; PV, popliteal vein; S, tributaries from the soleus muscle; SSV, short saphenous vein.

Technical problems

The problems associated with this operation are similar to those already described for the long saphenous vein operation, except that the popliteal artery, vein and nerve are all at risk during the popliteal fossa dissection. The sural nerve is easily damaged if it is not dissected free from the vein at the ankle and if it is not found and preserved in the popliteal fossa. For this reason a considerable number of surgeons[36,232,233] feel that the short saphenous vein should never be stripped. There is no controlled trial to settle this controversy and the subject remains a matter of opinion.

LIGATION OF THE MEDIAL LOWER LEG COMMUNICATING VEINS

Surgery for these veins is usually required in patients with lipodermatosclerosis or ulceration, but as Tibbs and Fletcher have shown[252] (see Chapter 6) some 're-entry' communicating veins may exist with superficial venous incompetence. Large [138] also reports that incompetent 're-entry' calf communicating veins may become competent after the saphenous incompetence has been corrected. Failure to ligate these veins may, however, account for recurrence despite satisfactory saphenous surgery, and Sherman,[234] Massel,[168] and May[170] have all emphasized the value of accurate 'perforator' ligation in preventing recurrent varicosities. In order to prevent the unsightly scar of a full ankle communicating operation (see below), 'on-table'[168,170] or preoperative varicography[32,142] may allow local ligations to be carried out.

Duplex scanning[249] is another method for communicating vein identification but we are only aware of one study which shows the sensitivity and specificity of this technique.[108] A full exploration should be carried out in patients with incompetent communicating veins and venous skin complications; this is described below. The newer endoscopic technique for ligation of the calf communicating veins is still being evaluated and is described later.

Subfascial ligation of the medial communicating veins (Linton's operation)[150]

The patient is prepared and positioned as if for long saphenous vein surgery. The suspected sites of 'communicating vein incompetence' are carefully marked on the skin with an indelible pen in a manner which distinguishes them from the other

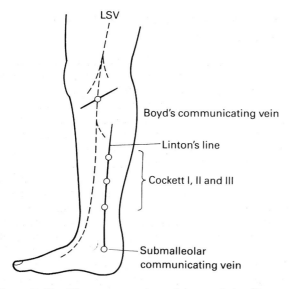

Figure 7.30 The common sites of the medial calf communicating veins and the incision used to explore them (Lipton's line). LSV, long saphenous vein.

marks placed over the superficial varices that are to be avulsed.

A vertical incision is made 2 cm (1 inch) behind the posterior border of the subcutaneous surface of the tibia from the tip of medial malleolus to a point at least three hand's breadths above the malleolus which is usually just above the midpoint of the leg (Figure 7.30).

Some surgeons perform this operation in a bloodless field (having expelled the blood with an Esmarch bandage or Rhys Davis exsanguinator and inflated an arterial occlusion tourniquet above the knee),[214,215] but we have not found it necessary to adopt this technique.

The incision should pass straight down through the subcutaneous tissues to the deep fascia which is vertically incised in line with the skin incision. The subcutaneous fat is often sclerotic and contains many large veins, which may bleed copiously when they are divided; this bleeding can be controlled by digital pressure on either side of the incision or by applying an artery forceps to the deep fascia and everting it over the edge of the wound. Small curved artery forceps can then be directly applied to the cut ends of the divided subcutaneous veins which are then carefully ligated with 2/0 or 3/0 chromic catgut.

Alternatively, the veins in the subcutaneous fat can be dissected and clamped before they are divided. This is possible if the fat is relatively soft and pliable but can be very difficult if it is fibrotic. The veins can be under-run with fine catgut sutures

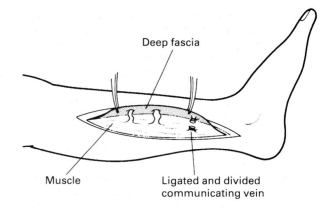

Figure 7.31 Subfascial ligation of incompetent medial calf communicating veins.[34] A long vertical incision is made through the skin and subcutaneous fat down to the deep fascia, approximately 1 cm behind the subcutaneous posterior border of the tibia. Any subcutaneous veins that are divided are ligated. The deep fascia is incised in the same line as the skin incision and is held open gently with a self-retaining retractor. As the subfascial space is opened, leashes of communicating vessels (usually two veins and one artery) can be seen passing from the posterior tibial vessels between the muscles to the undersurface of the deep fascia. These vessels are isolated, divided and ligated. If necessary, their incompetence can be tested by a Turner Warwick test.[259] When all the communicating veins have been ligated, the deep fascia and skin are carefully approximated.

if the surrounding tissues are too firm to allow the veins to be picked up with artery forceps. It is important not to undercut or dissect beneath the skin but to make a vertical incision down to the deep fascia to avoid damaging the blood supply of the skin.

After the deep fascia has been incised and the bleeding has been controlled, artery forceps are placed on the cut edges of the fascia to help elevate it from the underlying muscles which are gently dissected free with a gauze swab or by a gentle sweep of an index finger. As the muscles are separated from the deep surface of the fascia, the communicating veins will be seen crossing the subfascial plane, between the flexor digitorum longus and the free border of the soleus muscle, to enter the undersurface of the deep fascia (Figure 7.31). These veins should be isolated, doubly ligated and divided. If the Turner Warwick test[259] is to be performed, the superficial end of the vein should be clamped and tied before the vein is divided at a point that leaves a good stump protruding from the muscle. The stump will bleed if the communicating vein valve is incompetent. This is made more obvious if the ankle is forcibly dorsiflexed to encourage flow up the deep veins and produce a jet of blood out of the incompetent vein. The distance of the communicating vein above the tip of medial malleolus and the presence or absence of venous reflux should be recorded.

The subfascial dissection should continue until the whole of the subfascial space has been explored and all the vessels which cross it, between the subcutaneous border of the tibia and the midline posteriorly, have been ligated and divided. The communicating veins most likely to be missed are those which come out in front of flexor digitorum longus, close to the posterior border of the tibia and any vein which comes out below the level of the medial malleolus.

When the dissection is complete, a finger must be pushed up beneath the deep fascia under the upper end of the incision to explore the subfascial space to the level of the medial condyle of the tibia. Sometimes other large communicating veins may be found in this area and these must be ligated and divided. The positions of the main calf communicating veins are shown in Figure 2.31 (page 43). Further small communicating vessels may be found in other positions[201,263] but these are almost all indirect communicating veins which are of doubtful clinical significance.

When the whole of the subfascial space on the medial side of the leg has been separated from the muscles and cleared of communicating veins, haemostasis is achieved and the deep fascia may be closed with an interrupted or continuous 2/0 chromic catgut suture. Alternatively, the deep fascia may be left open. The skin is closed with a minimum of carefully placed nylon mattress stitches or simple sutures, between adhesive skin tapes or with adhesive tape alone. Although closure with a subcuticular suture may produce a more satisfactory result cosmetically; it should be resisted because it increases the chances of skin necrosis.

Postoperative care

After subfascial communicating vein ligation, the patient should be kept in bed with the leg bandaged and elevated to 30° for 24 hours. Mobilization must be gradual as the leg is painful and skin is slow to heal. Patients may be discharged after 4 or 5 days if the wound is healing well but the sutures are left in place for 10 days. The patient should be kept in hospital if the wound becomes infected or the skin edges look unhealthy until the infection is under control and the incision is showing signs of healing. The scar of the incision will eventually become almost invisible (Figure 7.32).

Subfascial endoscopic ligation of the perforating veins

This is the Linton operation performed through an endoscope to avoid the long, unattractive and often poorly healing wound (Figure 7.33). The operation can be performed under general or spinal anaesthesia. The exploration of the subfascial space through a small incision in the upper part of the medical aspect of the lower leg was first described in 1972,[14] using a Magill laryngoscope, malleable probes with lights and long-handled silver clip applicators. The method was not developed until the advent of laparoscopic surgery and its attendant instrumentation. The first modern paper on the endoscopic subfascial dissection of the communicating veins was published in 1985.[109] Hauer used a rigid bronchoscope or short oesophagoscope with a cold light source for illuminating its apex, but there is now a host of specially designed instruments that are commercially available.

After the leg has been exsanguinated, a small transverse incision is made in the upper fleshy part of the calf two centimetres or so behind the posterior border of the tibia. The incision is deepened through the fascia and the index finger inserted to develop the subfascial space. The endoscope is then inserted and pushed down towards the ankle. By angulating the tip of the endoscope away from the muscle, the space is opened and perforating vessels can be seen crossing the space. These are defined by blunt dissection and occluded by Ligaclips. They may then be divided between the clips although not all surgeons divide the veins. The whole of the subfascial space of the medial compartment is opened up by frequent passage of the instrument. All of the communicating vessels, both arteries and veins, are divided. The instrument is withdrawn, the wound is sutured and the leg bandaged before the tourniquet is released.

A large series has been reported from Rotterdam using this technique.[198] It was reported to speed ulcer healing and prevent recurrences. However, there was no control group. The technique is already being modified by using two trochars and opening the space, and inflating a balloon and insufflating the subfascial space with gas.[191,221] Diathermy coagulation may be used as an alternative to liga-clipping. Time may be saved if the site of the incompetent communicating veins is carefully located with duplex ultrasound before the endoscope is inserted. We await the long-term results of the American registry and the United Kingdom trial for a clearer idea of whether this technique is durable and effective. [84,109,110,197,221]

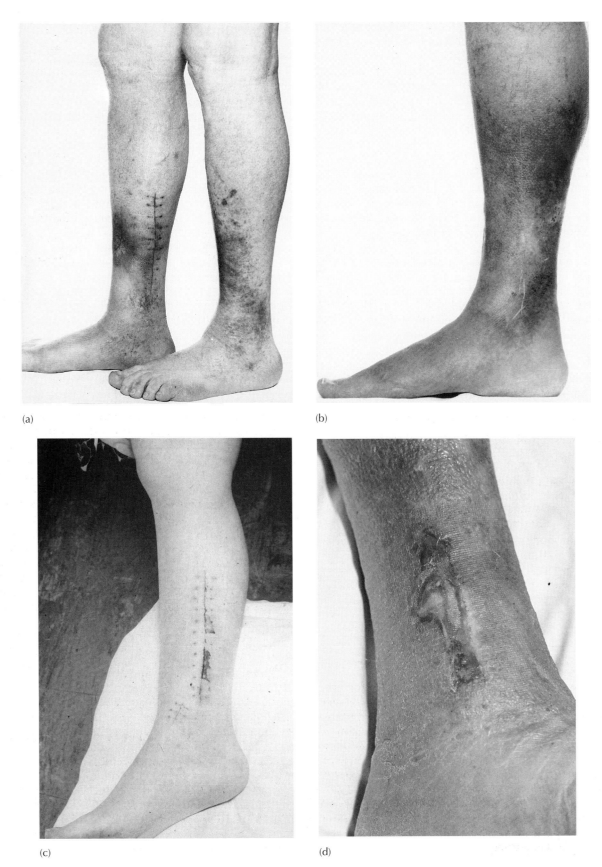

(a)

(b)

(c)

(d)

Figure 7.32

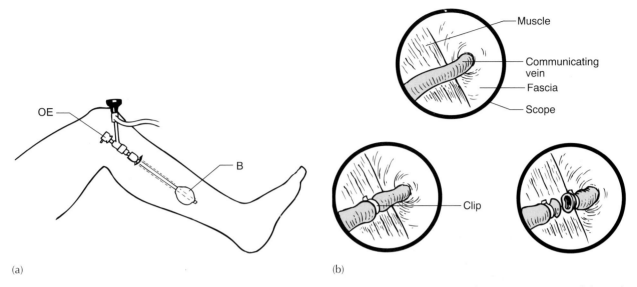

Figure 7.33 Subfascial endoscopic ligation of communicating veins. (a) The operating endoscope (OE) inserted through a small incision, tissue dissection by balloon (B) dilation. (b) The view through the endoscope.

Extrafascial ligation of the medial communicating veins (Cockett's operation)[71]

In patients who have had venous ulceration or in those who have severe lipodermatosclerosis, this operation is more difficult to perform than the subfascial operation because the sclerosis of the subcutaneous fat makes dissection of the subcutaneous layer extremely difficult.

Figure 7.32 (facing page)   The scars of communicating vein exploration. (a) A young (1 month) wound that is healing well. (b) An old (5 years) wound that is just visible as a thin white line in the pigmentation. (c) A recent (3 weeks) wound. At its posterior edge the superficial layers have become necrotic. The necrosis is usually the result of undercutting the skin edges or pulling the skin sutures too tight. Sometimes the skin is so unhealthy that any wound made within it will heal badly. (d) A recent (3 weeks) wound showing full-thickness necrosis of the anterior and posterior flaps. This had to be treated by excision and split skin grafting.

The initial preparation and incision are the same as for the subfascial procedure, but when the deep fascia is reached the skin and subcutaneous tissues are stripped from it by blunt dissection. The communicating veins are found as they appear through defects in the fascia and can be tested for incompetence by the bleed-back test (see above). Care must be taken to prevent the deep end of the vein retracting beneath the fascia when it is tested for incompetence. An area of deep fascia should be exposed which is of similar size to that undermined in the subfascial procedure. The skin closure and postoperative care are identical to that for the subfascial ligation operation.

As this operation is more difficult to carry out than the subfascial procedure and is, in our experience, associated with a higher incidence of skin necrosis, we never use it.

Alternative methods of ablating the medial lower leg communicating veins

The stocking-seam incision

Dodd[68–70] recommended that a vertical incision be made down the back of the calf – the 'stocking-seam' incision. Subfascial flaps are then elevated on both sides of the calf to expose the medial and lateral communicating veins.

This incision has two possible advantages. Both sides of the lower leg can be explored through a single incision and, because the tissues on the back of the leg are often healthier, there may be a lower incidence of wound edge necrosis.[71,181,182] The scar of the procedure is often more obvious and unsightly than a medial incision. As the operation has to be carried out with the patient in the prone position, it is less convenient to combine with surgery on the long saphenous vein. Incompetence of the lateral communicating veins is uncommon and seldom of clinical importance, making this approach unnecessary.

Multiple transverse incisions

De Palma[63] recommended an extrafascial exploration through three or four oblique incisions placed in the direction of Langer's lines (Figure 7.34) to reduce the incidence of wound edge necrosis. We have not found that the appearance of the resulting scars is markedly superior to the vertical incision, and access to the communicating veins can be difficult. The advent of duplex ultrasound localization of incompetent communicating veins may make this approach more attractive and an alternative to the endoscopic procedure, especially in patients without skin changes or ulceration. It is not known how many incompetent communicating veins this selective approach misses.

Subfascial shearing

Albanese,[1,2] Edwards,[76] and Petrov and Pennin[194] all invented blunt instruments to cut through or 'shear off' the communicating veins. Albanese[1,2] produced a series of chisels, Petrov and Pennin[194] a 'communicatome' and Edwards[76] a 'phlebotome' (Figure 7.35). These techniques are the forerunner to the endoscopic approach (see above). Their advantage is that the skin can be incised some distance from the area of lipodermatosclerosis or previous ulceration, which reduces the chance of poor healing.

A transverse or oblique incision is made on the medial side of the upper calf, below the knee, often at the site of the lower incision used for stripping the long saphenous vein. The deep fascia is incised and the subfascial space is opened by gentle finger dissection. The 'chisel' or 'shearer' can then be inserted and pushed down beneath the deep fascia to the level of the malleolus to separate the fascia from the muscle; this should open up the same area of subfascial space as that explored in the Linton operation. The shearer must be thrust down through the subfascial space to ensure that all the communicating veins are divided. Considerable bleeding usually appears from the track of the

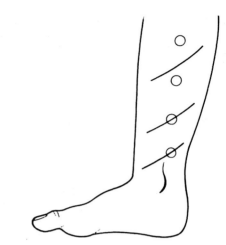

Figure 7.34 An alternative approach to the medial calf communicating veins. De Palma[63] suggested using multiple oblique incisions as an alternative to the long vertical incision. If ulcers are present, skin grafts can be applied to them simultaneously.

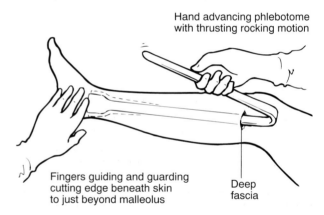

Figure 7.35 Technique for shearing calf communicating veins. The Edwards' phlebotome (this is similar to the phlebotome of Petrov and Pennin.[194]) The instrument is inserted beneath the deep fascia[76] and is then pushed down to the ankle in the subfascial space to divide any veins that are crossing this space. The blade must be held up against the deep fascia to avoid damaging the muscles and the posterior tibial vessels. (Modified from Edwards.[76])

shearer when large incompetent perforating veins have been divided. Care must be taken to keep the instrument close against the deep fascia to avoid damaging the posterial tibial vessels which lie near to the surface at the ankle.

There is no objective evidence that these methods do divide all the communicating veins, but one study has reported good long-term results after shearing.[238] Shearing may cause extensive bruising of the lower leg and more precise techniques are now used (see below).

Complications of communicating vein ligation

Necrosis of the wound edges

This is the most common and troublesome complication of both the subfascial and extrafascial operations. It appears to occur more frequently after the extrafascial operation. The incidence of this complication is reduced if the skin edges are not undercut or forcibly retracted. Careful skin closure is essential. More than 50% of the wounds following the Linton operation heal within 14 days of surgery, but some wounds take more than 6 weeks to heal.[83] Prolonged healing usually occurs where there has been ulceration and extensive fibrosis. Haeger[105] quotes a wound infection and skin necrosis rate of 15%; this should be less than 5% if great care is taken when handling the tissues.

Haemorrhage

This may occur if the posterior tibial vessels are damaged and the foot may become ischaemic if the posterior tibial artery is inadvertently ligated. Unless there is pre-existing arterial insufficiency, this is extremely rare. A large subfascial haematoma may cause considerable pain and can make walking difficult. If the haematoma is not evacuated, the skin becomes stretched, oedematous and more ischaemic. The risk that the wound will break down is increased if the tension is not relieved.

OPERATIONS TO LIGATE OTHER COMMUNICATING VEINS

Raivio[201] and Van Limborgh[263] have shown that more than 150 veins cross the deep fascia in every lower limb. Most of these veins are, however, considered unimportant. Some authors make a distinction between direct and indirect communicating veins.[45,144] Direct communicating veins pass directly from the superficial veins to the main trunks. Indirect communicating veins pass from a superficial vein to a vein within a muscle before draining to a deep vein.

The sites of the direct communicating veins on the medial side of the leg are shown in Figure 2.31

(page 43). The communicating veins discussed below are of clinical significance and must be ligated if they become incompetent.

Boyd's vein

The vein known as Boyd's communicating vein[28] joins the termination of the posterior arch vein or the long saphenous vein just below the knee (see Figure 6.11b, page 173). It is relatively constant and connects the superficial veins with the posterior tibial vein.

Lateral communicating vein

There is a single constant large lateral[45] communicating vein which joins the short saphenous vein to the peroneal vein. Occasionally, there is a second smaller communicating vein which joins the same veins a little lower down the calf.

Mid-calf communicating vein

This is an inconstant vein which joins the tributaries of the short saphenous vein to the soleal muscle sinusoids.

Gastrocnemius communicating veins

Varicosities close to the popliteal fossa may drain into the veins in the bellies of the gastrocnemius muscle and then into the popliteal vein, often via the termination of the short saphenous vein (Figure 7.36). These veins have been underestimated and are an important cause of recurrent varicosities.[119,250,261] They are, strictly speaking, indirect communicating veins but their course and length within the muscle is so straight and short that they are, in effect, direct communications.

Hunterian communicating veins (Dodd's communicating veins)[68,69]

These veins connect the long saphenous vein with the femoral vein as it lies in the lower part of Hunter's subsartorial canal. They are often multiple[190] (Figure 7.37), but occasionally a single vein or a pair of vessels is found on varicography (see Figure 2.30c, page 42).

Operations

Each of the veins described above can be ligated and divided through an incision placed directly over the point where the vein traverses the deep fascia. The vein should subsequently be traced to its deep connection and ligated.

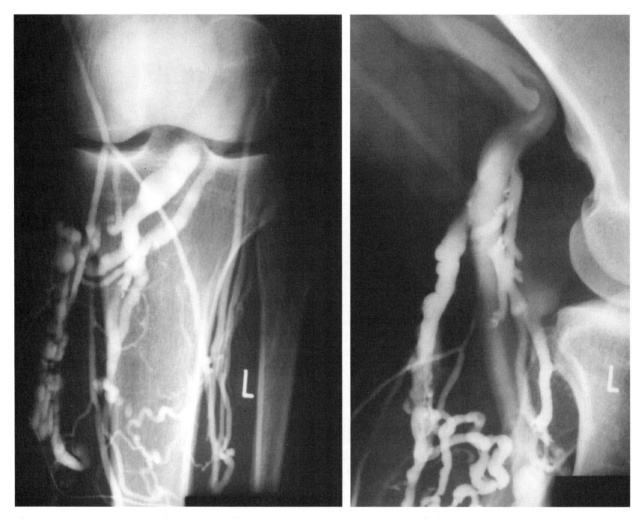

Figure 7.36 A varicogram showing superficial varicosities connecting to a medial gastrocnemius communicating vein.

The Boyd and the Hunterian communicating veins are usually avulsed during long saphenous vein stripping. The lateral communicating vein is avulsed when the short saphenous vein is stripped, and the mid-calf communicating vein is rarely important.

The gastrocnemius communicating veins should be ligated on the superficial surface of the gastrocnemius and again where they appear from the deep surface of the gastrocnemius muscle to join the short saphenous vein, before it enters the popliteal vein. A full popliteal exploration for recurrent varices caused by an incompetent gastrocnemius communicating vein may require a vertical incision in the popliteal fossa to allow the anatomy to be properly displayed. The site of these unusual communicating veins must be precisely defined by phlebography, varicography or duplex ultrasound scanning before an operation is undertaken.

AVULSION, LIGATION OR EXCISION OF VARICOSE VEINS

Lofgren[153] made a vast number of large incisions to excise superficial varicosities (see Figure 7.1). This is a very effective method of extirpating all the varicose veins and preventing recurrence but it invariably leaves unsightly scars. Many surgeons have independently developed a technique whereby the tributaries are exposed and then avulsed or ligated through multiple minute (2–3 mm long) incisions. With meticulous marking, careful planning and great perseverance, it is possible to remove virtually all the subcutaneous varicosities of a leg through tiny incisions. The incisions should be made carefully in the direction of Langer's lines to ensure good healing (Figure 7.38). The incisions are made with a narrow scalpel, the vein is then gently freed by lifting it through the wound with a hook

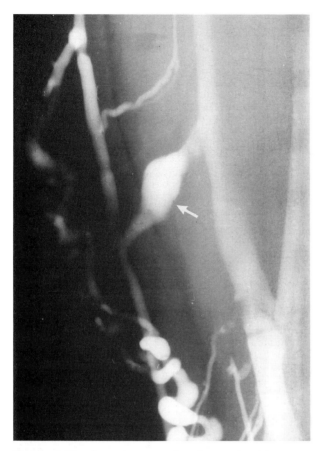

Figure 7.37 A varicogram showing varicosities connecting to a normal size long saphenous vein which is connected to the femoral vein by three Hunterian communicating veins. One of these (arrowed) is large and obviously abnormal.

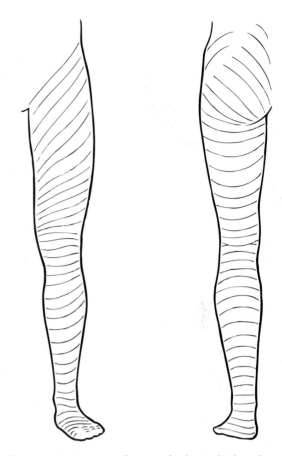

Figure 7.38 Langer's lines in the lower limb. Whenever possible, skin excisions should be placed parallel to these lines to achieve the best cosmetic result. This is particularly important when multiple incisions are being made for local avulsions.

(Figure 7.39a) or very fine pointed mosquito artery forceps (Figure 7.39b). The loop of vein which is pulled through the wound is then doubly clamped and divided (Figure 7.39b). Each end of the vein is gently teased out through the incision as the areolar tissue on its surface is dissected off using another pair of fine mosquito forceps (Figure 7.39b). As the vein is delivered, new forceps are placed upon it, near the wound, to prevent it breaking (Figure 7.39b). A gentle circular motion on the forceps sometimes helps to free the vein from the tethering areolar tissue and delivers a longer length of vein.

When the veins are thick-walled and appear 'white' they avulse well, but if they are thin-walled and 'blue' they often tear easily and the operation is frustrating and often quite bloody. When the vein is strong it can be rolled around the jaws of the forceps by twisting the handles. The forceps are then pulled down onto the wound and a longer length of vein is obtained without stretching the incision.

A number of devices have now been produced for hooking up the tributaries from beneath the skin rather than using the fine mosquitos to tease them out (Figure 7.39a). They may allow shorter skin incisions to be made and have as a consequence been taken up with enthusiasm by many surgeons.[42,166]

When a suitable length of vein has been freed, another incision may be placed 5–10 cm further along its course through which the intervening length of vein may be successfully teased out. The distance between incisions should be reduced if the veins are thin-walled and tear easily. This technique can be used to remove a long unsightly vein through three or four small incisions; this gives satisfaction to the surgeon and provides a very acceptable cosmetic result for the patient.

The varicosities avulsed by this technique are usually major tributaries of one of the saphenous veins, which will require stripping at the same

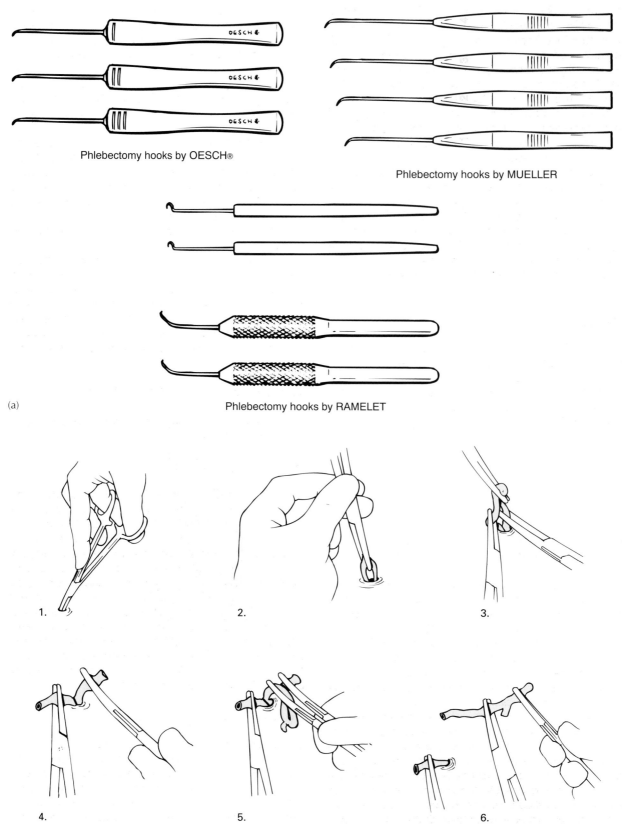

Phlebectomy hooks by OESCH®

Phlebectomy hooks by MUELLER

Phlebectomy hooks by RAMELET

(a)

1.

2.

3.

4.

5.

6.

(b)

operation. The lower end of the vein can be ligated with a fine absorbable material to prevent excessive bleeding. Some surgeons prefer to ligate each segment of vein, while other surgeons reduce bleeding by performing the avulsions after the limb has been exsanguinated by using a tourniquet.[214,215] There is some evidence that this reduces blood loss and it is definitely more aesthetically pleasing.[52,251] In most patients the bleeding that occurs after avulsion can be controlled by firm external pressure applied by an assistant.

The tiny stab incisions can be left unsutured or may be closed with a subcuticular stitch, adhesive skin strips, or a single 4/0 nylon suture.

The cosmetic results of this method of removing varices are very good, providing it is accompanied by appropriate surgery to the saphenous veins if these are incompetent. It can be used as an alternative to injections for the varices of a single tributary.

Comment

Many limbs in which there are varicose veins have a combination of long saphenous, short saphenous and calf communicating vein incompetence with multiple varicosities all over the leg. Often both lower limbs are affected. Careful preoperative evaluation followed by careful marking of the major

Figure 7.39 (facing page) (a) Four of the many forms of hooks that have been invented for avulsing varicose veins. (b) The technique of vein avulsion using fine artery forceps. 1. A small incision (2–3 mm) is placed in Langer's lines over a varicosity and is gently enlarged by inserting fine artery forceps and opening the blades to expose the varix lying in the subcutaneous fat. Careful preoperative marking is important if the vein is to be easily found. 2. A loop of the vein is pulled out of the wound. 3. Once a sufficient length of vein has been delivered, the vein is divided between forceps. 4. Both ends of the divided vein are gradually pulled out of the wound by gentle traction and rotation of the forceps. 5. As the vein appears, the forceps are reapplied close to the wound to allow traction to be applied on the stronger piece of vein close to the incision. 6. The vein eventually tears off. The spasm caused by stretching and tearing of the vein reduces the haemorrhage. Alternatively, the vein can be ligated with a very fine absorbable material before it tears. The other end of the vein is then avulsed towards the next cut-down incision.

sites of incompetence and of all surface varicosities is essential. Varicosities cannot be seen when the patient is anaesthetized and the leg veins are collapsed. We still try to treat all the veins in both limbs at one operation, though this is sometimes extremely time consuming and precludes day case surgery. Occasionally, it is advisable to treat legs with large numbers of varicose veins at separate operations.

It is easiest to start with the patient in the prone position and to treat short saphenous incompetence or varicosities on the posterior surface of the limb first. When the surgery on these veins has been completed, the patient is turned over so that the long saphenous vein, the calf communicating veins and the varicosities in the anterior aspect of the leg can be excised.

Very occasionally, it is necessary to replace the blood loss from bilateral, multiple, combined operations. A blood sample should be taken preoperatively for blood grouping and the serum should be saved for cross-matching. During the last 30 years we have only had to give blood transfusions to two patients both of whom were anaemic before surgery.

RECURRENT VARICOSE VEINS

It is important to distinguish between residual veins and recurrent veins.

Residual veins

These are veins that were not treated at the original operation, because they were not detected preoperatively, not found during the operation or were deliberately left untreated. Residual veins can be treated by further surgery or sclerotherapy. Surgery is relatively straightforward because it is unhampered by the scar tissue that complicates the surgery of recurrent veins. A failure to remove the full length of a tortuous tributary is the most common cause of residual varicosities, but short saphenous vein incompetence may only become obvious when long saphenous vein incompetence has been treated, especially if it has not been carefully excluded before the first operation.

Recurrent varicose veins

Recurrent varicose veins are veins which have become varicose after the original treatment, having been 'normal' at the time of that treatment. This occurs when all the visible varicosities were treated but the underlying abnormality was not corrected; the remaining 'normal' veins therefore continue to be subjected to abnormal pressures and subsequently dilate. Failure to correct the underlying abnormality is caused by:

- an inadequate or incorrect original operation;
- failure to occlude an 'incompetent' superficial-to-deep communication;
- the development of new sites of superficial-to-deep incompetence, often as a result of a deep vein abnormality.

It is easy to treat an incompetent superficial-to-deep communication once the site of the communication has been diagnosed. Similarly, new sites of superficial-to-deep incompetence can be easily corrected if the new abnormality is in a site previously untouched by surgery. Surgical problems arise from the first category, and sometimes from the third category, when the recurrence is at the site of a previous operation.

Sapheno-femoral recurrence

Incompetent communications between the femoral vein and the superficial veins in the upper thigh may cause recurrent varicose veins under the following conditions.

- The original long saphenous ligation was not made 'flush' with the femoral vein.
- Terminal tributaries of the saphenous vein were left intact (Figure 7.11).
- There were two terminations of the long saphenous and only one was ligated (Figure 7.14).
- There were two separate long saphenous veins and only one was ligated.
- The long saphenous vein was ligated but not stripped so that recurrence develops from dilatation of the Hunterian communicating veins (Figure 7.37).
- After simple ligation of the long saphenous vein, collaterals may develop to reconnect the common femoral vein with the long saphenous veins (Figure 6.20, page 182).

Ruckley and his colleagues[244] have recently analysed their 'groin' recurrences on the basis of varicography and the surgical findings. They produced a simplified classification of the six headings listed above. They have added in neovascularization and also put in a separate heading for cross-groin collaterals (see Figure 7.40b). They have not found a problem with a double long saphenous although anatomical variables are well recognized.[57]

They found that unsatisfactory primary surgery on the sapheno-femoral junction was the most important factor (66%) and failure to remove the long saphenous vein in the thigh was responsible for 60% of the recurrences.[244]

Lofgren and Lofgren,[152] however, on the basis of their clinical experience, also believe that the main cause of recurrence in the groin is improperly performed initial surgery.

Sheppard[232] also reported that 90% of 204 legs that developed recurrent varicose veins had recurrent sapheno-femoral incompetence as a result of new collateral veins. He suggested that 'neovascularization' of granulation tissue around the sapheno-femoral junction leads to the formation of new channels between the saphenous stump on the femoral vein and the residual saphenous vein or its tributaries, even when the original surgery has been correctly performed. Sheppard thought that a flap of pectineus fascia should be sutured over the stump of the long saphenous vein to separate the femoral vein from the superficial veins after saphenofemoral ligation to prevent this happening (Figure 7.40a). Unfortunately, there is no prospective data to show whether this modification is worthwhile, but there is some support for Sheppard's theory in a number of reports by Glass[93,94] who found that recurrent varicose veins that developed after a sapheno-femoral ligation connected with the femoral vein through vessels with a 'primitive' structure. Similar primitive vessels were found bridging sections of locally excised saphenous vein at the knee level. Glass concluded that recurrences would be less frequent if the ligated sapheno-femoral junction was covered by fascia or a synthetic mesh. He subsequently described an individual unaudited series claiming lower recurrence rates because the cribiform fascia was closed with sutures or a mesh.[94]

There are now a number of trials comparing the incidence of recurrent varicosities in patients who have been randomly treated either by sapheno-femoral ligation alone or by ligation combined with long saphenous vein stripping.[53,176,180,218,271] They have all shown that recurrences were reduced by the addition of the vein stripping. This suggests that the development of incompetence in the Hunterian communicating vein may be an important cause of recurrent varicosities after sapheno-femoral ligation without stripping.

Diagnosis

An old scar, some distance from the groin crease, should make you suspect that a proper flush ligation of the long saphenous vein was probably not performed at the first operation and that a groin recurrence is therefore a strong possibility.

The likelihood of sapheno-popliteal incompetence must also be considered in any patient with new varices developing over the medial side of the leg after a sapheno-femoral ligation.

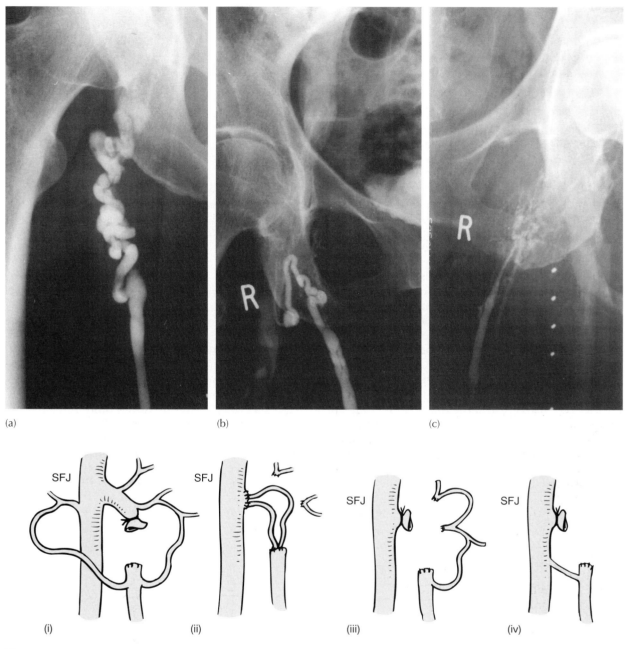

(a)   (b)   (c)

(i)   (ii)   (iii)   (iv)

(d)

Figure 7.40 Recurrent incompetence at the sapheno-femoral junction may be caused by single large vessels (a and b) or a mass of fine vessels in the scar tissue (c). (d) Four of the common patterns of sapheno-femoral recurrence: (i) interconnecting tributaries; (ii) neovascularization; (iii) connections across the groin to the iliac vein or contralateral femoral vein; (iv) mid-thigh connections. SFJ, sapheno-femoral junction.

A cough impulse or thrill can rarely be felt in the groin when it is scarred but the varicosities are often seen extending up towards the groin. Clinical suspicions are confirmed if a high thigh tourniquet controls all the varicosities in the limb.

We always attempt to confirm the diagnosis by obtaining varicograms (see Figure 6.20, page 182); these demonstrate single or multiple connections between a residual segment of long saphenous vein or one of its major tributaries and the femoral vein, and thus help to clarify the abnormal anatomy before the subsequent dissection. Ruckley also feels that varicography rather than duplex ultrasound is the investigation of choice.[30]

Re-exploration of the groin

We favour the direct approach in which the old scar is excised and usually extended both medially and laterally. The femoral vein can then be approached from either the medial[146] or the lateral side (Figure 7.41).[107] It is better to approach the junction from the lateral side through relatively normal tissues. The femoral artery is found first and the scar tissue can be dissected from its anterior surface before the femoral vein is displayed lying on the medial side of artery. The dissection can then continue over the front of the vein to expose the sapheno-femoral junction. The stump of the long saphenous vein is usually found entering the anterior surface of the femoral vein. This stump is freed on all surfaces until a Lahey forceps can be passed around it, followed by a strong ligature (Figure 7.42). Once the sapheno-femoral junction has been ligated, the main tributary veins are dissected and individually ligated and divided. If the incision is deepened medially down to the fascia covering the pectineus muscle, the medial aspect of the femoral vein can be identified just before its anterior aspect is cleaned to expose the sapheno-femoral junction.

An alternative approach (Figure 7.41) is to make an incision above the previous groin incision down to the lower edge of the external oblique aponeurosis before dissecting downwards to find the ante-

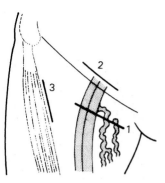

Figure 7.41 The three approaches that can be used to explore recurrent sapheno-femoral varicosities: 1, the approach of Li;[146] 2, the approach of Luke;[155] 3, the lateral approach, now rarely used. (Modified from May.[170])

rior surface of the femoral vein immediately below the inguinal ligament.[71,155] This approach may be awkward if the original scar is high, but it does allow the femoral vein and artery to be found and protected before the difficult dissection of the small recurrent branches attached to the sapheno-femoral junction is undertaken and it avoids dividing any lymphatics.

Second operations are always more difficult, and if the anatomy is not displayed first, it is easy to damage the major vessels. Care must be taken not to damage the femoral nerve during the lateral approach.

Two particular problems may follow a second extensive dissection. A lymphocele or lymph fistula

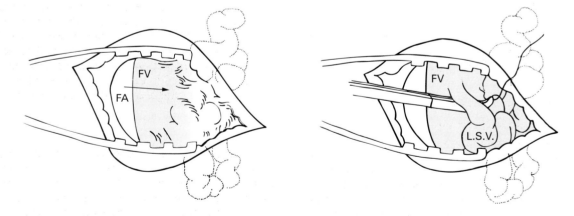

Figure 7.42 The ligation of groin recurrences using the approach of Li.[146] (a) The lateral end of the incision is deepened to find the femoral artery (FA). The dissection then continues in the direction of the arrow over the front of the femoral vein. (b) When the stump of the long saphenous vein is found on the front of the femoral vein, a ligature is passed around the stump and tied. This can be carried out using an aneurysm needle or by passing a Lahey forceps behind the stump as shown. When the upper ligature has been tied the mass of small varices draining into the stump can be ligated. (Modified from Li.[146]) FV, femoral vein; LSV, long saphenous vein.

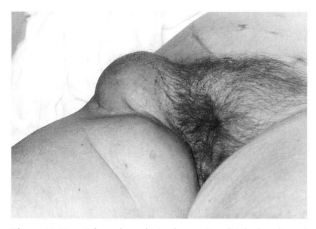

Figure 7.43 A lymphocele in the groin which developed after the re-exploration of the groin for a recurrent hernia.

may appear in the early postoperative period and lymphoedema of the leg may, very occasionally, appear months later.

It is important not to disturb the lymphatic channels during the dissection. May[170] has recommended that patent blue–violet dye should be injected subcutaneously in the thigh to reveal the lymphatics before beginning the dissection. The lateral approach is more likely to damage lymphatics than the medial approach.

Lymphocele (Figure 7.43) and lymph fistulae usually resolve spontaneously but occasionally they have to be aspirated or excised. Lymphoedema probably only occurs if there is a pre-existing congenital or acquired lymphatic deficiency. Acquired lymphatic deficiency is common in geographical areas where the people do not wear shoes and get repeated subclinical episodes of cellulitis and lymphadenitis. There is a higher incidence of leg swelling after varicose vein surgery in these areas. The swelling sometimes has to be treated with lymphatic bypass operations.[126,133]

Sapheno-popliteal recurrence

Although recurrent short saphenous vein incompetence in the popliteal fossa is less common than groin recurrence (because of the lower frequency of primary sapheno-popliteal incompetence), when it does occur it is as difficult, if not more difficult, to correct than sapheno-femoral recurrence. The same factors that cause recurrences in the groin cause recurrences in the popliteal fossa, but because of the variable entry of the short saphenous termination, technical errors are much more common. Recurrences develop from collaterals in the scar tissue, trans-gastrocnemius communicating veins which were not ligated at the initial operation, and

muscle communications that connect short saphenous tributaries with an incompetent long saphenous vein system.

The diagnosis is usually suspected on clinical grounds, confirmed by tourniquet testing and defined by varicography.

Re-exploration of the popliteal fossa is best carried out through a vertical or S-shaped incision. The popliteal vein and artery are found well above the previous scarring and are traced down until the stump of the short saphenous vein and any other vessels connecting to the superficial veins are found and ligated. All the tributaries of the short saphenous vein in the popliteal fossa are then dissected, ligated and divided.

Communicating vein recurrence

This is discussed in detail in Chapter 15. Some patients definitely develop recurrent varicose veins from incompetent communicating veins that were missed at the initial operation. Also, some previously competent communicating veins may later become incompetent. The clinical diagnosis should always be confirmed by varicography and ascending phlebography. A second subfascial exploration with ligation of the incompetent vein or veins is then performed through the original incision.

Isolated recurrent superficial varicosities

Most recurrent varicosities are the result of missed or new superficial-to-deep communicating vein incompetence, but they can also develop as a result of localized venous dilatation in a previously normal subcutaneous vein. If there is no evidence of new superficial-to-deep incompetent connections, recurrent varicosities can either be avulsed through multiple small incisions under local or general anaesthesia or be treated by injection sclerotherapy. Recurrences in the lower part of the leg are best treated by injection compression; recurrences within the thigh are best avulsed.[86,170,178]

Comment

Not all recurrences are caused by inadequate operations. Perhaps one in every two recurrences is the result of poor technique (the surgeon sometimes fails to ligate the saphenous vein itself) but in nearly half the cases the second exploration of the groin or popliteal fossa reveals abnormal veins that have clearly developed since the first operation. An accurate knowledge of the anatomical variations that can exist, combined with a careful exploration of the common sites of superficial-to-deep connections, will undoubtedly reduce the incidence of recurrent varicosities. The role of the separation of the deep veins from the subcutaneous tissues with a layer of fascia or prosthetic material, which is aimed at reducing the incidence of recurrence, has yet to be established.

Short saphenous vein incompetence is often overshadowed by a more obvious long saphenous vein incompetence and will only be found if the surgeon searches diligently for it; the same is true for communicating vein incompetence.

All the possible sites of superficial-to-deep communication must be carefully re-examined in patients with recurrent varicosities. Phlebography and varicography are extremely helpful investigations for the assessment of these patients.

A deep vein abnormality must be considered a possibility in all patients who have recurrent varicose veins after apparently satisfactory primary surgery. Clinical suspicion may be confirmed by physiological tests of calf pump function, and by duplex ultrasound studies or bipedal ascending phlebography (see Chapter 4).

Recurrent varicose veins in the presence of a deep vein abnormality are best treated by elastic compression. Further surgery may be beneficial but should not be expected to be curative and must always be followed by life-long elastic compression.

GENERAL COMPLICATIONS OF VARICOSE VEIN SURGERY

The complications which are specific to each operation have been discussed under the headings of individual operations. They include: recurrence; haemorrhage; damage to the deep veins – femoral, popliteal, crural; damage to the arteries – femoral, popliteal and posterior tibial; damage to the superficial nerves – saphenous or sural; wound necrosis, haematoma formation; lymphoedema and lymphocele; unsightly or keloid scars and recurrent ulceration (Chapter 20).

As operations on varicose veins are common, rare complications do occur with some frequency. In the UK an average of 34 patients bring a legal action after vein surgery each year. Femoral artery damage and major vein injuries account for 2% and 7%, respectively, of these claims.[248]

Chest infection

Chest infection rarely occurs after varicose vein surgery, even though some operations are lengthy, because most patients are fit, many are young, the level of anaesthesia is light and there are no wounds which restrict chest movement.

Wound infection

Infection of the groin wound is uncommon. Some obese patients have intertrigo, and in these patients it is worthwhile treating the skin preoperatively to reduce the risk of sepsis. Lower leg wounds may become infected if they are in the vicinity of an open ulcer. In general, infection is more often a sequel of haematoma formation than an event in its own right.

Deep vein thrombosis and pulmonary embolism

Deep vein thrombosis seldom occurs after varicose vein surgery. Cockett and Dodd[71] observed one case of pulmonary embolism in 204 varicose vein operations at St Thomas's Hospital performed between 1949 and 1954, and Keith[129] reported that three deep vein thromboses occurred in 544 operations, an incidence of 0.6%. Lofgren *et al.*[151] reported 16 patients out of 4000 who were suspected, on clinical grounds, to have had a pulmonary embolism (PE), a risk of 0.39%. More recently, studies by Bounameaux and Huber[27] have suggested that pulmonary emboli occurred in 0.56% after varicose vein surgery. This incidence of PE is high and fits poorly with the absence of thrombosis found by duplex ultrasound scanning. Some deep vein thromboses undoubtedly pass undetected but the incidence of pulmonary embolism does appear to be very low. The bandages that are used to reduce haematoma and swelling and the early mobilization of patients that is encouraged after operation may be important prophylactic factors.

Our own practice includes many patients who have varicose veins which complicate the post-thrombotic syndrome. We give these patients 5000 units of heparin subcutaneously, twice daily, starting on the day of their admission. Before beginning this routine, we saw a number of these patients develop deep vein thrombosis, not only postoperatively but even during the preoperative period.

Campbell[37] has recently surveyed a large number of vascular surgeons to discover what form of prophylaxis they use during varicose vein surgery. Only 12% use subcutaneous heparin routinely; 71% use it selectively in high risk cases.

GENERAL POSTOPERATIVE CARE

The special aspects of aftercare have been discussed with the individual operations. The general aspects of postoperative care are summarized here.

Compression bandages

The legs are elevated to 20 or 30° and compression is maintained by elasticated bandages. This reduces the incidence of haematoma formation[257] and may reduce the incidence of deep vein thrombosis.

Analgesia

Opiates may be needed during the first 24 hours after surgery but milder oral analgesics (e.g. soluble aspirin, Panadol, DF 118, co-proxamol or codeine) will usually suffice thereafter.

Mobilization

Patients should be encouraged to get up and walk[179] as soon as they are wide awake, which is usually within 4–6 hours of surgery unless they have had a full exploration of the medial leg communicating veins, when they should rest in bed for at least 24 hours. When the patient gets up, an additional supporting bandage (Blue Line, Bisgaard, Elastocrepe, Tensopress or Thusane) must be worn over the bandages which were put on in the operating theatre. The patient must either walk or sit with the legs elevated when not in bed. Standing still or sitting with dependent legs is discouraged. Thromboembolism prevention stockings do not apply adequate compression to prevent bruising.

Duration of admission

Most patients can be discharged the day after the operation, though if surgery is performed under local anaesthesia, they may go home on the day of the operation. There is evidence that the in-patient stay after vein surgery has dropped dramatically in the last 15 years.[210]

Patients who have had an open exploration of the medial calf communicating veins must stay in hospital longer. They can usually be discharged after 5–7 days but if the skin is red and tender or if the wound shows any signs of slow healing (e.g. a serous discharge), they should be treated as if they had a venous ulcer and should be confined to bed until the wound is dry and the inflammatory response has subsided. Strong supporting bandages should be applied, sometimes Calaband or Viscopaste, and the patient should be told to rest as much as possible and only increase daily exercise when the leg feels comfortable. This is a major advantage of endoscopic surgery when the patient can usually be discharged after a couple of days.

After discharge from hospital

The sutures should be removed from the multiple tiny avulsion incisions, and from the groin and popliteal incisions 5–7 days after the operation, unless absorbable subcutaneous sutures or adhesive skin tapes have been used. At least 10 days should elapse from the time of operation before the sutures are removed from the vertical incisions used to ligate the medial leg communicating veins. These wounds may be treated by compression bandaging if their healing is slow.

Elastic bandages or stockings should be worn for at least 1 month after surgery to reduce haematoma formation and prevent ankle oedema.

Review

Patients should be seen 1 month after the operation to review the state of the wounds, to look for oedema and to record the presence of any residual varices. A second review at 6 months allows a more complete examination when the wounds have fully healed and the bruising has disappeared; residual varices are easily detected at this review. This is the council of perfection. Many purchasing health authorities in the UK and HMGs in the United States will no longer pay for follow-up visits.

Small recurrent or residual varicosities may be obliterated by injection sclerotherapy or by local excisions at the second follow-up. If the results satisfy both the surgeon and the patient, the patient is discharged back to the family doctor with the advice that he/she should return if new varicosities develop. Patients are not encouraged to return with minor varicosities, and we do not recommend long-term elastic compression stockings for patients with normal skin, as the purpose of the surgery is to eradicate the veins and to obviate the necessity for wearing stockings permanently.

However, there is now some evidence that compression stockings do reduce the incidence of recurrent varicose veins – so perhaps patients should be given the choice.[256]

Injection sclerotherapy

The invention of the hypodermic syringe[125] in the 1840s allowed Chassaignac[40] in 1855 to try to obliterate varicose veins by injecting a solution of ferric chloride. Foote[86] lists a series of clinicians who attempted to sclerose veins with ferric chloride, iodotannin, phenol, mercury bichloride, alcohol and Lugol's iodine.

Surgical ligation was, at one stage, combined with a distal injection of sclerosant to obliterate varices,[225,247] and in 1916 Linser[147–149] described the use of compression bandages after the injection of hypertonic saline; this probably makes Linser the father of modern compression sclerotherapy. Unfortunately, his choice of sclerosant did not prove ideal, as it caused considerable pain and, if injected outside the vein, gave rise to a severe inflammatory reaction which often resulted in skin necrosis.

A number of safer sclerosants were developed after the First World War. A mixture of quinine and urothane was introduced by Génévrier,[90] sodium salicylate was first used by Sicard,[236] and Maingot[164] injected both these substances using a twin injection technique. Sodium morrhuate[211] and monoethanolamime oleate[18] were introduced in the 1930s, and at the same time, Tournay[253,254] in Paris used a number of different solutions including sodium tetradecyl sulphate (STD), which was reintroduced in 1946 and is still the most popular sclerosant in use. It is essentially a detergent which produces a local chemical phlebitis with minimal systemic complications.[207] All sclerosants are toxic if given in large quantities, causing haemolysis and renal damage; all cause catastrophic thrombosis if they are injected by mistake into an artery,[46] and all cause local skin necrosis if a sufficiently large quantity is injected between a vein and the overlying skin.

Other sclerosant solutions have been introduced, for example, oxypolyethoxydodeconate (Aethoxysclerol) 1%, a mixture of iodine and benzyl alcohol (Variglobin) 0.5% and Chromeglycerne (Sclérémo) 1–2% (Table 7.3). The exact concentration at which each sclerosant is used varies between 0.5% and 5% depending upon the size and type of vein that is being sclerosed.

Aim of treatment

The aim of compression sclerotherapy is to produce a sterile inflammation on the inner surface of the vein wall. Clinicians who believe that compression is an essential part of the treatment[80,81,116,117,188,212] think that it occludes the lumen by making opposing surfaces stick together without any intervening thrombus. The vein is theoretically converted into a thin fibrosed cord (the sclerosis), not a vein full of red thrombus which can recanalize. The evidence that this always occurs is poor and usually minor or extensive thrombus results. Many veins do recanalize after sclerotherapy, and some clinicians consider that prolonged compression is unnecessary and have abandoned it altogether. The effectiveness of sclerotherapy depends upon the intensity of the inflammatory response. A severe response causes venospasm and vein wall swelling; both these effects reduce the size of the lumen, thus decreasing the quantity of intraluminal thrombus. We have considerable doubts that external compression always reduces the amount of thrombosis, though we recognize that a superficial vein which becomes full of red thrombus will almost certainly recanalize.

Some radiographic investigations[29] have suggested that sclerosants which are injected into the superficial veins quickly disperse into the deep veins; this casts doubt on the effectiveness of sclerotherapy and implies that injections increase the risk of deep vein thrombosis. Other studies[128] have shown that sclerosants can remain in the superficial veins for a considerable time. These variations make the results of injection sclerotherapy less reliable than the results of surgery.

Indications

Many advocates of injection sclerotherapy use it to treat all types of varicose veins. The French school[61,188,264] even inject sclerosant directly into the uppermost portion of the long saphenous vein to obliterate its termination. The British school[38,81,116,117] concentrate on the distal veins of the limb and treat sapheno-femoral and saphenopopliteal incompetence by surgical ligation. We support the latter approach, as we are very concerned that deep vein thrombosis may be initiated if sclerosant is injected into the upper part of the long saphenous vein.

Table 7.3 Some of the chemicals that have been used for venous sclerotherapy

Physical property	Chemical composition	Trade name
Hypertonic	Sodium chloride, glucose	Varicophtin, Variko, Calorose
Anionic	Fatty acids	Varicoid
Detergent	Sodium tetradecyl sulphate	Thrombovar
Non-ionic	Oxypolyethoxydodecane	Aethoxysklerol, Sotravaric
Corrosive	Iodine with benzyl alcohol	Variglobin
	Glycerin with chrome alum	Sclérémo

Studies in the UK have shown that only 60% of long saphenous veins are obliterated by two injections into the upper end of the long saphenous vein. Bishop[20] found that the sapheno-femoral junction remained patent on duplex ultrasound scanning even after successful placement of sclerosant.

Compression sclerotherapy is ideal for solitary varicose tributaries in the absence of main saphenous vein incompetence. It is also ideal for obliterating small varicose veins that were not avulsed at the time of saphenous surgery. We do not consider compression sclerotherapy to be suitable or effective for the treatment of incompetent lower leg communicating veins, although others[117] are in favour. It is the treatment of choice for patients who are very old or unfit, or for those who refuse operation. Intradermal spider veins can also be treated by injection sclerotherapy.[167]

Contraindications to sclerotherapy

Sclerotherapy is contraindicated under the following circumstances:

- Women on the contraceptive pill
- Pregnancy
- Patients with a strong history of allergy, especially if this has been to previous sclerosant injection
- Foot veins should not be injected because of the risk of intra-arterial injections
- Patients with very fat legs, because compression is very difficult.

Technique

We use a modification of the technique described by Hobbs,[117] rather than that of Fegan.[80,81] After a decision has been taken to treat the varicose veins by compression sclerotherapy, the patient is re-examined standing on a stool in a good light. The surface varices are carefully marked with an indelible pen. The patient then lies down horizontally on a couch. A sufficient number of 2 ml syringes fitted with 25 gauge (16 mm) needles are filled with 0.5 ml of STD to cater for the number of injections that are planned (Figure 7.44). The maximum volume of STD that can be given during one treatment is 20 ml but many clinicians would regard this as excessive and would prefer to give less than 10 ml of sclerosant.[160] The skin is cleaned with chlorhexidene and venepunctures are made at approximately 5 cm intervals along the course of each vein, beginning at either end. A total of 10–15 injections can be given into one, or both limbs, at one time. If many more injections are required, it is best to treat one leg at a time.

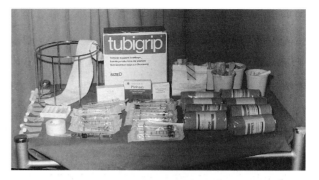

Figure 7.44   The trolley we use for sclerotherapy. The syringes, needles, dental rolls, and sclerosant (STD) are shown. Hydrocortisone, adrenaline and Piriton are kept on the trolley to treat anaphylactic shock.

When the patient is lying on the couch, the veins are partially collapsed but are not completely empty. This allows the doctor to confirm the position of the needle by withdrawing blood into the syringe. The simplest technique is to transfix the vein with the needle and then gradually pull it back through the vein whilst simultaneously withdrawing the plunger of the syringe (Figure 7.45a, b). When the tip of the needle is located in the lumen of the vein, blood will appear in the barrel of the syringe. At this moment the fingers of the injector's free hand empty the vein by gentle simultaneous movement, on either side of the needle away from its point, combined with downward pressure so that the sclerosant is injected into an 'empty' vein. When the injection has been completed, an assistant should press the compression dressing on to the injection site as the needle is withdrawn. We use cotton wool balls, which are recommended by Hobbs,[117] held in place by micropore tape. We do not use the foam rubber pads advocated by Fegan, except occasionally over the course of the long saphenous vein if the injections are put close to, or into this vein at knee level or in the lower thigh.

When all the injections have been completed, the leg is bandaged with Setopress and covered with Tubigrip. Many other bandaging methods and elastic stockings are equally effective.[230] The patient is encouraged to walk immediately afterwards to clear any sclerosant from the deep veins and thus reduce the risk of thrombosis.

Fegan originally recommended[80,81] that the bandages should be worn for 6 weeks but more recent studies[11,87] have suggested that shorter periods of compression give identical results. Hobbs has argued that the compression time should vary with the size of the legs and veins injected (e.g. longer

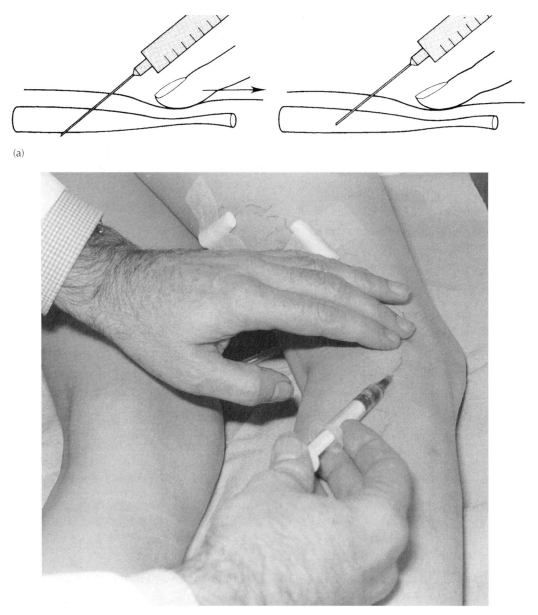

(a)

(b)

Figure 7.45 (a, b) The technique of injecting a varicose vein. The varicosity is transfixed. The needle is then slowly withdrawn while exerting suction through the needle by pulling on the plunger of the syringe. When blood appears in the syringe, the sclerosant is injected. The vein is kept as empty as possible by the fingers of the free hand, which also stretches the vein to prevent it from kinking. The vein is compressed as the needle is withdrawn. Cotton wool balls are used to keep the vein compressed beneath the bandage.

periods of compression for large varices in fat legs than for those in thin legs).[115]

In the absence of any firm evidence to guide us, we compromise by asking our patients to wear their bandages for 3 weeks. Patients are instructed not to remove or loosen the bandages and to keep their legs dry when bathing by putting them on the rim of the bath or covering them with a plastic bag. On the weekend before they return to the clinic they are asked to remove the bandages and cotton wool balls and have a full normal bath; this allows the legs to be examined without bandage marks or compression dents. The legs are carefully inspected and palpated and untreated varices or failed injection sites are re-injected.

Extravascular haematoma and veins full of red thrombus are evacuated by making a puncture into the vein with a large needle and expelling the thrombus by gentle finger pressure.[117,237] It is important to do this to avoid the risks of skin discoloration and to prevent the thrombus persisting as a tender palpable or sometimes visible thickened cord. The veins of the opposite leg may be injected at this time, if this was the original intention. Throughout the whole period of treatment the patient is encouraged to work and walk normally.

Alternative techniques of injection sclerotherapy

Sigg[237] recommended inserting a number of needles into the veins selected for injection with the patient standing. The positions of the needles are confirmed by allowing blood to flow into a kidney dish. The patient then lies down and the leg is elevated before syringes are attached to the needles and the injections are made. Sigg used up to 15 injections of 0.5 ml of Variglobin (4%) in one session.

Fegan[80,81] punctured the vein with needles which were already attached to syringes while the patient sat on a couch with the legs dependent. When blood was successfully sucked back into the syringe, it was taped to the leg. The leg was then elevated and the vein was occluded above and below the site of injection by the ring and index fingers, before the sclerosant was injected. The syringe was then withdrawn but the fingers kept in place to hold the sclerosant in the isolated segment of vein. The free hand was used to apply a bandage over a sorbo-rubber pad which was placed over the course of the injected vein; further turns of the bandage are applied over the pad and along the leg until the next site of injection is reached. Fegan recommended that injections should be started distally to avoid the development of venous congestion as a result of the bandaging. Each injection site was bandaged in an identical manner until all the veins which had been injected had been compressed. Fegan inspected the leg after 3 weeks, and gave further injections if required. He used multiple injections and gave up to 1 ml of sodium tetradecyl sulphate in each injection.

Davy and Ouvry[61,188] give only one or two injections at each session and spend many weeks treating a single limb. They inject the long saphenous vein right up to its termination, and have not reported many problems (e.g. venous thrombosis) from their high thigh vein injection technique.

Comment

Sigg's technique is time consuming and upsetting to the patient, and carries a high risk of vasovagal attacks. Fegan's technique is more difficult to use than Hobbs' method, because the needles often slip out of the vein as the patient changes position. Although Fegan's method keeps the veins empty at the time of injection, the number of injections is limited by the instant application of the bandage. We have not yet been bold enough to try injecting the upper end of the long saphenous vein.

We would support the opinion of Goren that sclerotherapy has little or no part in treating truncal varicosity unless the patient refuses surgery or accepts a high risk of recurrence.[99]

ECHO-SCLEROTHERAPY (DUPLEX ULTRASOUND-GUIDED SCLEROTHERAPY)

Duplex ultrasound has been used in conjunction with sclerotherapy to provide more accurate placement of the needle in deeper veins and to confirm that sclerosis has occurred. Early reports of the technique[222] have been followed by claims for improved success.[102,205,223]

The improved results of this technique await external audit by others and future clinical trials.

COMPLICATIONS OF SCLEROTHERAPY[161]

Vasovagal attacks

Fainting during the venepuncture is reported to occur once in every 100 patients.[270] It is much more frequent when using the technique of Fegan or Sigg[80,81,237] in which the needles are inserted while the patient is sitting or standing.

Allergic or anaphylactic reactions

These reactions are reported to occur in 2 of every 1000 patients treated[270] but only one fatality has been recorded in a series of over one million patients injected with sodium tetradecyl sulphate.[161] MacGowan attributes allergic reactions to overdosage (more than 5 ml per sitting) but also recommends care in patients with a long history of allergy.[161] Piriton (chlorpheniramine maleate), adrenaline, hydrocortisone and salbutamol should be kept on the injection trolley to treat these reactions instantly if they occur.

Toxic reactions

These reactions consist of shivering, loin pain and haematuria; they are usually caused by the haemolysis of red cells. Such reactions rarely occur if less than 5 ml of sclerosant is used[160] but they are occasionally seen with smaller doses.

Skin necrosis and ulceration

There are no published statistics that indicate how often this complication occurs. Skin necrosis and ulceration should be suspected when the patient complains of severe pain after a course of injections. When the bandages are removed there is usually an inflammatory reaction and signs of skin necrosis. Large ulcers may follow a misplaced injection and are difficult to treat and slow to heal; they are the main source of the medico-legal problems associated with injection sclerotherapy.[161]

Venous thrombosis

Although Winstone[270] claimed that the incidence of this complication is low (1 in 1000 treatments), other investigators[268] found evidence of thrombosis in 9 out of 67 extremities treated by sclerotherapy. The former estimate, based on clinical evidence, is definitely too low, the latter estimate, based on impedence plethysmography, which is not a very sensitive method of detecting calf vein thrombosis, may be more accurate. A definitive study is still required to ascertain the true incidence of thrombosis after sclerotherapy.

Pulmonary embolism

This complication is reported to occur in 8 out of every 10 000 patients (0.1%);[104] this is a lower incidence than that reported after operations on varicose veins.

Intra-arterial injection

Five examples of this complication had been reported to the Medical Defence Union in Great Britain by 1985.[160] Cockett[46] discovered 18 such accidents by 1986. All had occurred from attempting to inject a vein on the medial side of the ankle. MacGowan also reported that injections around the medial malleolus at the ankle were particularly dangerous, with the posterior tibial artery being especially at risk.[160] The anterior tibial artery may be inadvertently punctured when injections are made on the front of the lower leg and ankle. The femoral

artery may be at risk if the upper end of the long saphenous is injected.

An accidental intra-arterial injection causes severe burning pain, often with tingling sensations in the foot.[46,160] Patients should always be asked if the injection is causing pain as it is being given. The injection should be stopped immediately any pain is experienced, *but the needle should not be withdrawn*. Blood should be drawn back into the syringe to empty the needle (and vessel) of sclerosant, and the syringe should then be replaced with a syringe containing 10 000 units of heparin, which is injected slowly into the artery. The needle should then be removed and the leg watched carefully for 2 or 3 hours, monitoring the distal vessel at regular intervals with a Doppler ultrasound probe. If the pulses remain palpable and the skin of the leg remains warm, the patient can be allowed to go home, but if there is any suggestion of arterial thrombosis or distal ischaemia, the patient must be admitted to hospital for full anticoagulation and observation. Delay will result in inevitable tissue ischaemia and amputation (14 of 18 of Cockett's cases and two of five of MacGowan's). Both these authors caution against injecting veins around the ankle or the foot.

Injection of a nerve

The saphenous and sural nerves may be injected with sclerosant. This is very painful, and if continued may cause anaesthesia and sometimes a permanent interruption of nerve function.

Skin discoloration

This is a common side-effect of injection sclerotherapy. All patients should be warned that they may develop some brown pigmentation over a thrombosed vein. The pigment is haemosiderin and is caused by the perivenous inflammatory response. Hobbs[117] considers that discoloration is caused by the injection of too much sclerosant at a single site but it can occur after a perfect injection of a small amount of sclerosant. It usually fades after 1–2 years.

Telangiectatic matting

These are the fine red 'spider vessels' that occasionally develop profusely after sclerotherapy. They may be the result of inflammation produced by the sclerosant or some angiogenic factor produced by mast cells. There is no guaranteed method of avoiding this complication. Small amounts of low concentration sclerosant may reduce its incidence.[96]

Alternative treatments of varicose veins

Out-patient percutaneous ligation[229,269]

This is an alternative to sclerotherapy or excision of local varices under local anaesthesia. There is no evidence to suggest that it is any better than other established techniques.

Diathermy sclerosis[185,186]

This is another way of producing a vigorous thrombophlebitis. A fine electrode is threaded down the vein to allow endovenous percutaneous diathermy destruction of the intima. It can be used as an alternative to sclerotherapy. O'Reilly has reported diathermy skin burns after this form of treatment, and it has not been widely adopted.

Light coagulation[187]

The equipment for light coagulation is expensive, and the technique has only been used in a few patients.

Elastic stockings

Graduated compression stockings are effective in relieving symptoms in many patients. They have been shown to improve venous function[239] and improve the elasticity of developing veins.[145] Stockings also appear to reduce the incidence of recurrent veins.[256] They are therefore an effective symptomatic treatment in the old or infirm or in those who do wish for surgery.

Pharmacological palliation

A number of studies have investigated the benefit of rutosides on the symptoms of varicose veins. These drugs do not reduce the size of the varicosities but, by altering capillary permeability, they are said to relieve the aching, swelling and nocturnal cramps that are commonly experienced by patients with varicose veins. The evidence supporting these claims is slender, principally because symptoms such as aching are impossible to measure accurately. Some controlled trials have shown a significant improvement in symptoms in patients taking the active drug compared with patients taking a placebo,[117] but this form of treatment can only be regarded as palliation because there is no effect on the veins themselves. There is good evidence that these drugs do reduce oedema and improve tissue oxygenation.[35,183] For this reason rutosides may be of value in patients who decline other methods of treatment or who continue to complain of symptoms after other treatments have eradicated the veins. A controlled crossover trial which compared elastic compression with the effect of rutosides on symptom relief found that both treatments produced modest improvement in symptoms and a combination of the two produced the best results.[3]

Other drugs that have been used to alleviate symptoms in patients with varicose veins include dihydroergotamine flavonoids, calcium dobesilate, homoeopathic medicines and horse chestnut extract.[79] There is some anecdotal evidence that all do some good.

Results of treatment

Measurement of recurrence

The measurement and classification of recurrence after variocse vein treatment is extremely difficult because there is always a considerable difference of opinion between observers on what constitutes a recurrence.[38,202] Very few patients, if any, have a totally perfect, 'normal' leg 1 year after treatment, let alone after 20 years. Some new varicose veins invariably develop but these may not require further treatment. Probably the best way of determining the success of treatment is to count the number of patients who have further treatment,[61] but it is difficult to follow patients for 10 or 20 years, because many move house and have second and third courses of treatment elsewhere. Almost every published long-term study lacks credibility because of the large proportion of patients who cannot be followed up and the absence of a clearly defined anatomical or physiological assessment by an independent observer.

The first aim of treatment must be the eradication of the veins that exist when the patient presents. The second aim is to prevent recurrence. Proof that the first aim has been achieved needs careful extensive documentation of the site and size of the original varices – this is rarely done. Proof that the second objective has been achieved needs a 100% independent follow-up and even then the incidence depends upon the length of the follow-up. It might be better to express recurrence as a yearly rate rather than as an absolute number.[61,179]

Surgery

Lofgren's 10-year review[153] of radical surgical obliteration of the veins (the ligation of sites of superficial-to-deep incompetence and the removal of sub-cutaneous varicosities) showed that 44% had excellent results, 41% had good results and 15% had a fair result. No patients reported poor results. These results were obviously open to considerable observer bias, as 15% had definite recurrences requiring further treatment which most clinicians would classify as poor results.

Rivlin[209] claimed that only 7% of patients developed residual or recurrent varicosities between 6 years and 10 years after operation, but these results have not been confirmed by any form of external audit, and they may also be affected by observer bias. There are now, however, a number of studies which show that recurrences are quite frequent.

Sclerotherapy

Fegan[80,81] claimed that 82% of his patients were satisfied with the result of sclerotherapy. Similar results have been published by Stother *et al.*[245] in a study of 348 legs. Stother claimed 89% success between 1 year and 4 years and 68% success at 3–4 years.

Reid and Rothnie[206] treated 1080 legs with primary varicose veins and claimed that 90% had good results at 1 year.

Dejode[64] treated 146 patients and followed them for between 1 and 5 years. The results were very good in 83% but in 3% the veins were not improved.

Raj and Makin[202] found that 80% of patients had good results at 6 weeks, as assessed by the surgeon, but there was only a 40% agreement between the surgeon and the patient as to what constituted a good result!

Sigg,[237] Davy,[61] Ouvry,[188] Nabatoff[179] and Dale[60] all recognized that a significant number of recurrences occur after sclerotherapy and they recommend regular follow-up examinations with further courses of injections whenever these are indicated.

Comparisons between sclerotherapy and surgery

In 1968, Hobbs[116] reported the 2-year results of a controlled trial comparing compression sclerotherapy with surgery. This showed that all the veins in the legs could be treated by injection sclerotherapy but Hobbs felt that patients with sapheno-femoral incompetence were best treated by surgery because the recurrence rate after sclerotherapy was greater. Injections below the knee cured 60% and improved 40% of patients and were more effective than

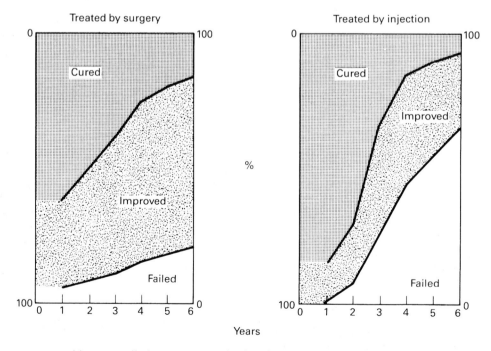

Figure 7.46   Hobbs' controlled comparison of sclerotherapy with surgery. It can be seen that many more patients were improved or cured 5 years after the initial treatment in the surgical group than in the injection group, but at 2–3 years the results of the two forms of treatment were comparable. (Modified from Hobbs.[118])

surgery. However, the 5-year results[118] showed that the sclerotherapy 1-year 'cure' rate of 82% had fallen to only 7% and only 30% were still improved (Figure 7.46). By contrast, 20% of the surgical group remained 'cured' and 80% were still improved at 5 years.

In a randomized study of 155 patients treated by injection compression sclerotherapy compared with 100 patients treated surgically (Figure 7.47), Chant *et al.* found that 14% of the surgical group and 22% of the injection group required further treatment by 3 years.[38] This difference was not found to be statistically different, and patients were said to express a preference for injection compression therapy. Analysis of the same patients after 5 years showed that the patients treated by sclerotherapy had fared less well.[15]

In 1973, Seddon[231] also showed no statistically significant differences between the results of surgery and sclerotherapy, 12–18 months after treatment.

In 1975, Doran and White[74] concluded that the long-term results of Fegan's method were uncertain but suggested that the cost saving was so great that it should always be used as a first procedure. Piachaud and Weddell[196] had already commented on the savings accruing to the economy if a policy of injection compression was followed by all, but their estimate was based on

the 3-year results of Chant's study[38] not on the 5-year results of Hobbs' study.[118]

Comment

Two editorials in the *British Medical Journal*[4,5] and one in the *Lancet*[6] presented a rational case for combining surgery and injections in the treatment of varicose veins, surgery being reserved for major long and short saphenous vein incompetence, and sclerotherapy being the treatment of choice for veins of the lower leg and isolated varicosities. The place of surgery versus sclerotherapy in the treatment of incompetent lower leg communicating veins is still debatable. In our opinion, the combined approach is sensible and logical. We continue to find that most of our patients require surgery because they present with advanced disease involving long or short saphenous vein incompetence, and we consider that the only effective treatment for incompetent communicating veins is surgical ligation, especially if there are already signs of skin abnormality. If our patients presented earlier, many of them would be treated initially by injection sclerotherapy before their saphenous system became incompetent. If surgery is to be undertaken, it is obviously reasonable to avulse as many of the varicosities as possible at the same time. Injections are helpful to obliterate residual varices after surgery.

One study of simple high saphenous ligation showed that this failed to abolish reflux in the long saphenous vein of many patients and persistent reflux was associated with poor calf pump function.[163] More studies like this on differing forms of treatment are required to determine the best forms of treatment.

Patient satisfaction

A number of studies have now been published which try to assess outcome by health assessment questionnaires.[9] These not surprisingly show that vein surgery improves the quality of life. Despite this, the costs of treatment are increasing and even day case varicose vein surgery may prove too expensive for a state to provide. It is not known if this will increase the risks of venous ulceration in those who cannot pay for their treatment.

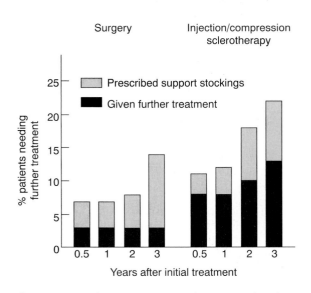

Figure 7.47 Chant's comparison between sclerotherapy and surgery. There was no statistical difference in the number of requests for further treatment in either group at 3 years, though in the sclerotherapy group the percentage of patients needing further treatment was greater throughout the trial. (Modified from Chant *et al.*[38])

Varicose veins of pregnancy and vulval varicosities

These are two subgroups of varicose veins that deserve special mention.

Pregnancy

The aetiology of these veins has already been discussed (see Chapter 5, page 153). During pregnancy new varicose veins may appear or existing varicose veins may enlarge. Twenty per cent of mothers develop varicose veins in pregnancy.[66] The treatment is always expectant and should await the completion of the pregnancy. Support stockings may help both symptomatically and prophylactically. Surgery should not be carried out until after breast-feeding has been completed, and even sclerotherapy should be delayed for several months to ensure maximum regression of the veins after parturition. It is better, if possible, to delay definitive treatment until no further pregnancies are envisaged. Compression sclerotherapy may provide a useful interim measure. A recent communication by De Cossart showed that veins increased in diameter during pregnancy but this was not associated with long saphenous vein reflux.

Vulval varicosities

Dixon and Mitchell[66] found that 33% of women who developed varicose veins in pregnancy had vulval varicosities but Dodd and Payling-Wright[72] found that the incidence was only 2%. Both these studies suggested that vulval varicosities regressed after parturition, but Craig and Hobbs[59] have reported a group of 12 women in whom the veins persisted after childbirth. Contrast radiology of these veins[59,69] has shown that many of them are connected to tributaries of the internal iliac vein (Figure 7.48). Craig and Hobbs[59] associate the continued presence of vulval varicosities with 'the pelvic congestion syndrome' (dyspareunia, dysmenorrhoea and menorrhagia) but the exact aetiology of this syndrome remains obscure. Hobbs reported that 4% of a series of nearly 5000 women seen in a varicose vein clinic presented with vulval varicosities.[120] Dixon and Mitchell[66] advocated that the following measures could be taken to eradicate vulval varicosities:

- Ligation of the internal pudendal vein
- Ligation of the obturator vein
- Ligation of the veins of the round ligament
- Ligation of the upper tributaries of the long saphenous vein.

Fifty cases treated by resection of the gonadal veins, ligation of the uterine veins with excision of the vulval and leg varicosities reported excellent results.[143] This represents a very radical solution and simpler procedures may be more appropriate.

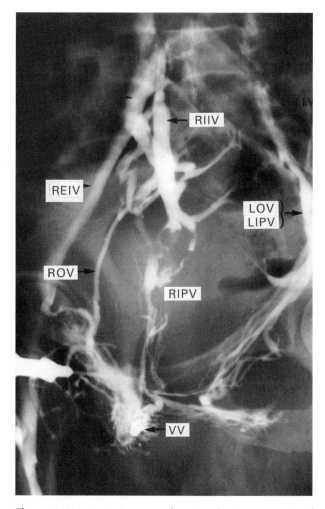

Figure 7.48   A varicogram showing the connections of vulval varicosities. Vulval varicosities drain to the pudendal veins, the vaginal veins and the internal iliac veins. LIPV, left internal iliac vein; LOV, left ovarian vein; REIV, right external iliac vein; RIIV, right internal iliac vein; RIPV, right internal pudendal vein; ROV, right ovarian vein; VV, vulval varices.

Detailed varicography is essential before determining what approach will be used.

Craig and Hobbs have also suggested that hysterectomy may be helpful.[59]

Comment

Treatment of vulval varicosities should be aimed at ligating the sites of superficial-to-deep communication that are shown on contrast radiology.[59] Hysterectomy is a draconian option for most women with this condition.

Treatment of dilated intradermal venules

The physical findings of dilated intradermal venules have already been described in Chapter 6. A number of descriptive terms have been given to these veins, including: spider veins, tache bleu, brush veins, blue shoots, birch sprig, spider webs, spider bursts, sunburst veins, angetids, thread veins and hair veins.[86,103]

Dilated intradermal venules may be associated with varicose veins or they may occur independently.[86,103] They are symptomless but patients complain of their unsightliness. They were thought to be more common after pregnancy[50] but this has not been confirmed.[103] They are more common in women and increase with age,[103] and they may be related to occupation and diet.

Treatments for dilated intradermal venules include:

- reassurance
- camouflage creams
- injection of sclerosant through a microneedle[54]
- electrocautery
- surgical intracuticular or subcuticular lancing
- laser photocoagulation.[195]

Many of these treatments carry a considerable risk of scarring, especially laser and microsclerotherapy.

Treatment of the complications of varicose veins

These are thrombophlebitis (see Chapter 23), haemorrhage and skin changes. Haemorrhage can usually be stopped by lying the patient flat and elevating the leg. Death occasionally results from remaining vertical after a faint. Many bleeds occur at the site of a small ulcer, but occasionally a thin-walled ankle varicosity simply bursts. The site of bleeding can be treated by local excision and ligation with removal of any associated major venous incompetence. Occasionally local sclerotherapy may be very effective.[158]

References

1. Albanese AR. New instruments of varicose vein surgery. *J Cardiovasc Surg* 1965; **6:** 65–9.
2. Albanese AR, Albanese AM. Radical and esthetic surgery for varicose veins of the legs. *Vasc Surg* 1969; **3:** 194–9.
3. Anderson JH, Geraghty JG, Wilson YT, Murray GD, McArdle CS, Anderson JR. Paroven and graduated compression hosiery for superficial venous insufficiency. *Phlebology* 1990, **5:** 271–6.
4. Anon. Economics of varicose veins. *Br Med J* 1973; **2:** 626–7.
5. Anon. Tailored treatment for varicose veins. *Br Med J* 1975; **1:** 593–4.
6. Anon. The treatment of varicose veins. *Lancet* 1975; **2:** 311–12.
7. Babcock WW. A new operation for the extirpation of varicose veins of the leg. *N Y Med J* 1907; **86:** 153–6.
8. Baccaglini U, Spreatico G, Sorrentino P, *et al.* Outpatient surgery of varices of the lower limbs: experience of 2568 cases at 4 universities. *Int Angiol* 1995; **14:** 397–9.
9. Baker DM, Turnbull NB, Pearson JCG, Makin GS. How successful is varicose vein surgery? A patient outcome study following varicose vein surgery using the SF-36 Health Assessment Questionnaire. *Eur J Endovasc Surg* 1995; **9:** 299–304.
10. Barabas AP. The long saphenous in primary varicose veins. *Br J Surg* 1986; **73:** 320.
11. Batch AJG, Wickremesinghe SS, Gannon ME, Dormandy JA. Randomized trial of bandaging after sclerotherapy for varicose veins. *Br Med J* 1980; **2:** 423.
12. Belcaro GV. Plication of the sapheno-femoral junction: effects on incompetence after two years. *Phlebology* 1991; **6:** 159–65.
13. Belcaro G, Errichi BM. Selective saphenous vein repair: a 5 year follow-up study. *Phlebology* 1992; **7:** 121–4.
14. Bentley RJ. The obliteration of perforating veins of the leg. *Br J Surg* 1972; **59:** 199.
15. Beresford SAA, Chant ADB, Jones HO, Poachaud D, Widdell JM. Varicose veins: a comparison of surgery and injection compression sclerotherapy – 5 year follow up. *Lancet* 1978; **1:** 921–4.
16. Bergan JJ. New developments in the surgical treatment of venous disease. *Cardiovasc Surg* 1993; **6:** 624–31.
17. Berridge DC, Makin GS. Day case surgery: a viable alternative to surgical treatment of varicose veins. *Phlebology* 1987; **2:** 103–8.
18. Biegeleisen HI. La cronicidad de las venas varicosas. Un estudio estadistico de cirugia vs escleroterapia. *Medicina (Mexico)* 1953; **33:** 193–8.
19. Bisgaard H. *Ulcers and Eczema of the Leg. Sequels of Phlebitis: Studies on Stasis Diseases of the Lower Limbs and their Treatment.* Copenhagen: Munksgaard, 1948.
20. Bishop CC, Fronek HS, Fronek A, Dilley RB, Bernstein EF. Real time colour duplex scanning after sclerotherapy of the greater saphenous vein. *J Vasc Surg* 1991; **14:** 505–8.
21. Bishop CCR, Jarrett PEM. Outpatient varicose vein surgery under local anaesthesia. *Br J Surg* 1986; **73:** 821–2.
22. Bjordal RI. Blood circulation in varicose veins of the lower extremities. *Angiology* 1972; **23:** 163–73.

23. Bjordal RI. Circulation patterns in incompetent perforating veins in the calf and in the saphenous system in primary varicose veins. *Acta Chir Scand* 1972; **138:** 251–61.

24. Bjordal RI. Circulation patterns in the saphenous system and the perforating veins of the calf in patients with previous deep venous thrombosis. *Vasa Suppl* 1974; **3:** 1–41.

25. Bjordal RI. Pressure patterns in the saphenous system in patients with venous leg ulcers. *Acta Chir Scand* 1971; **137:** 495–501.

26. Bjordal RI. Simultaneous pressure and flow recordings in varicose veins of the lower extremity. *Acta Chir Scand* 1970; **136:** 309–17.

27. Bounameaux H, Huber O. Postoperative deep vein thrombosis and surgery for varicose veins (letter). *Br Med J* 1996; **312:** 1158.

28. Boyd AM. Discussion on primary treatment of varicose veins. *Proc R Soc Med* 1948; **41:** 633–9.

29. Boyd AM, Robertson DJ. Treatment of varicose veins. Possible dangers of injection of sclerosing fluids. *Br Med J* 1947; **2:** 452–4.

30. Bradbury AW, Stonebridge PA, Callam MJ, *et al.* Recurrent varicose veins: assessment of the saphenofemoral junction. *Br J Surg* 1994; **81:** 373–5.

31. Bradbury AW, Stonebridge PA, Ruckley CV, Beggs I. Recurrent varicose veins. Correlation between preoperative clinical and hand held Doppler ultrasonographic examination and findings at Surgery. *Br J Surg* 1993; **80:** 849–51.

32. Burnand KG. Intéret de la varicographie dans l'appréciation des varices essentielles des membres inférieurs. *Phlebologie* 1984; **1:** 269–70.

33. Burnand KG, O'Donnell TF, Lea Thomas M, Browse NL. Relation between post phlebitic changes in the deep veins and results of surgical treatment of venous ulcers. *Lancet* 1976; **1:** 936–8.

34. Burnand KG, O'Donnell TF, Lea Thomas M, Browse NL. The relative importance of incompetent communicating veins in the production of varicose veins and venous ulcers. *Surgery* 1977; **82:** 9–14.

35. Burnand KG, Powell S, Bishop C, Stacey M, Pulvertaft T. Effect of Paroven on skin oxygenation in patients with varicose veins. *Phlebology* 1989; **4:** 15–22.

36. Campbell WB. Short saphenous varicose veins. *Curr Pract Surg* 1995; **7:** 195–9.

37. Campbell WB, Ridler BMF. Varicose vein surgery and deep vein thrombosis. *Br J Surg* 1995; **82:** 1494–7.

38. Chant ADB, Jones HO, Weddell JM. Varicose veins: a comparison of surgery and injection/compression sclerotherapy. *Lancet* 1972; **2:** 1188–91.

39. Chant ADB, Magnussen P, Kershaw C. Support hose and varicose veins. *Br Med J* 1985; **290:** 204.

40. Chassaignac E. *Nouvelle Méthode pour la Traitement des Tumours Haemorhoidales.* Paris: Baillière, 1885.

41. Cheatle TR, Kayombo B, Perrin M. Cryostripping the long and short saphenous veins. *Br J Surg* 1993; **80:** 1283.

42. Chester JF, Taylor RS. Hookers and French strippers: a technique for varicose vein surgery. *Br J Surg* 1990; **77:** 560–1.

43. Clinton O, Negus D. Suitability for day-case varicose vein surgery. *Phlebology* 1990; **5:** 277–9.

44. Cockett FB. Diagnosis and surgery of high pressure venous leaks in the leg: a new overall concept of the surgery of varicose veins. *Br Med J* 1956; **2:** 399.

45. Cockett FB. The pathology and treatment of venous ulcers of the leg. *Br J Surg* 1955; **43:** 260–78.

46. Cockett FB. Arterial complications during surgery and sclerotherapy of varicose veins. *Phlebology* 1986; **1:** 3–6.

47. Cole DS. 'Save our saphenous veins'. *Medical Tribune International Edition* Scandinavia 1973; **5:** 3.

48. Coleridge-Smith PD, Scurr JH, Robinson KP. Optimum methods of limb compression following varicose vein surgery. *Phlebology* 1987; **2:** 165–72.

49. Conrad P. Endoscopic exploration of the subfascial space of the lower leg with perforator vein interruption using laparoscopic equipment: a preliminary report. *Phlebology* 1994; **9:** 154–7.

50. Conrad P. Groin to knee downward stripping of the long saphenous vein. *Phlebology* 1992; **7:** 20–2.

51. Corbett CRR, Harries WJ. Which vein stripper, metal or plastic disposable? *Phlebology* 1991; **6:** 149–51.

52. Corbett R, Jayakumar KN. Clean up varicose vein surgery – use a tourniquet. *Ann R Coll Surg Engl* 1989; **71:** 57–8.

53. Corbett CR, McIrvine AJ, Aston NO, Jamieson CW, Lea Thomas M. The use of varicography to identify the sources of incompetence in recurrent varicose veins. *Ann R Coll Surg Engl* 1984; **66:** 412–15.

54. Corcos L, Longo L. Combined laser and sclerotherapy for telangiectasis of the lower limbs. *Phlebology* 1989; **4:** 51–3.

55. Corcos L, Peruzzi GP, Romeo V, Fiori C. Intraoperative phlebography of the short saphenous vein. *Phlebology* 1987; **2:** 241–8.

56. Corcos L, Peruzzi GP, Romeo V, Fiori C. Considerations of the anatomical variations in the venous system of the lower limbs in varicose disease. *Phlebology* 1989; **4:** 259–70.

57. Corcos L, Peruzzi GP, Romeo V, Procacci T. Preliminary results of external valvuloplasty in saphenofemoral junction insufficiency. *Phlebology* 1989; **4:** 197–202.

58. Cox SJ, Wellwood JM, Martin A. Saphenous nerve injury caused by stripping of the long saphenous vein. *Br Med J* 1974; **1:** 415–17.

59. Craig O, Hobbs JT. Vulval phlebography in the pelvic congestion syndrome. *Clin Radiol* 1975; **26:** 517–25.

60. Dale WA. Ligation, stripping, and excision of varicose veins. *Surgery* 1970; **67:** 389–93.

61. Davy A, Ouvry P. Possible explanation for recurrence of varicose veins. *Phlebology* 1986; **1:** 15.

62. Daseler EH, Anson BJ, Reimann AF, Beaton LE. Saphenous venous tributaries and related structures in relation to technique of high ligation, based

chiefly upon study of 550 anatomical dissections. *Surg Gynecol Obstet* 1946; **82:** 53–63.

63. De Palma RG. Surgical therapy for venous stasis. *Surgery* 1974; **76:** 910–17.

64. Dejode LR. Injection compression treatment of varicose veins. A follow up study. *Br J Surg* 1970; **57:** 285–6.

65. Dinn E, Henry M. Value of lightweight elastic tights in standing occupations. *Phlebology* 1989; **4:** 45–9.

66. Dixon JA, Mitchell WA. Phlebographic and surgical observations in vulval varicose veins. *Surg Gynecol Obstet* 1970; **130:** 458–64.

67. Docherty JG, Morrice JJ, Bell G. Saphenous neuritis following varicose vein surgery. *Br J Surg* 1994; **81:** 698.

68. Dodd H. The diagnosis and ligation of incompetent perforating veins. *Ann R Coll Surg Engl* 1964; **34:** 186–96.

69. Dodd H. Varicose veins. *Br J Hosp Med* 1968; 1101–2.

70. Dodd H, Calo AR, Mistry M, Rushford A. Ligation of the ankle communicating veins for the treatment of the venous ulcer syndrome of the leg. *Lancet* 1957; **2:** 1249–52.

71. Dodd H, Cockett FB. *The Pathology and Surgery of the Veins of the Lower Limb.* London: Churchill Livingstone, 1956.

72. Dodd H, Payling-Wright H. Vulval varicose veins in pregnancy. *Br Med J* 1959; **1:** 831–2.

73. Donini I, Corcos L, De Anna D, Gasbarro V, Pozza E, Zamboni P. Preliminary results of external sapheno-femoral valvuloplasty: a trial by the Italian Society of Phlebolymphology. *Phlebology* 1991; **6:** 167–79.

74. Doran FSA, White M. A clinical trial designed to discover if the primary treatment of varicose veins should be by Fegan's method or by an operation. *Br J Surg* 1975; **62:** 72–6.

75. Doran FS, White M, Drury M. The scope and safety of short stay surgery in the treatment of groin hernia and varicose veins. *Br J Surg* 1972; **59:** 333–9.

76. Edwards JM. Shearing operation for incompetent perforating veins. *Br J Surg* 1976; **63:** 885–6.

77. Eger M, Golcman L, Torok G, Hirsch M. Inadvertent arterial stripping in the lower limb: problems of management. *Surgery* 1973; **73:** 23–7.

78. Engel AF, Davies G, Keenan JN. Preoperative localisation of the sapheno-popliteal function with Duplex scanning. *Eur J Vasc Surg* 1991; **5:** 507–9.

79. Ernst E, Saradeth T, Resch KL. Complementary treatment of varicose veins – a randomized, placebo-controlled, double-blind trial. *Phlebology* 1990; **5:** 157–63.

80. Fegan WG. Continuous compression technique for injecting varicose veins. *Lancet* 1963; **2:** 109–12.

81. Fegan WG. Injection with compression as a treatment for varicose veins. *Proc R Soc Med* 1965; **58:** 874–6.

82. Field ES, Kakkar VV, Stephenson G, Nicolaides AN. The value of cinephlebography in detecting incompetent venous valves in the postphlebitic state. *Br J Surg* 1972; **59:** 304.

83. Field P, Van Boxel P. The role of the Linton flap procedure in the management of stasis, dermatitis and ulceration of the lower limb. *Surgery* 1971; **70:** 920–6.

84. Fischer RH. Diagnosis and treatment of incompetent Cockett's perforator veins by endoscopy: present status. In: Martinbeau P, Prescott R, Zummo M, eds. *Phlebologie 92* Paris: J Libbey, Eurotext 92.

85. Fliegelstone LJ, Salaman RA, Oshodi TO. Flush saphenofemoral ligation and multiple stab phlebectomy preserve a useful greater saphenous vein four years after surgery. *J Vasc Surg* 1995; **22:** 588–92.

86. Foote RR. *Varicose Veins.* London: Butterworths, 1954.

87. Fraser IA, Perry EP, Hatton M, Watkin DFL. Prolonged bandaging is not required following sclerotherapy of varicose veins. *Br J Surg* 1985; **72:** 488–90.

88. Fullerton GM, Calvert MH. Intraluminal long saphenous vein stripping: a technique minimizing perivenous tissue trauma. *Br J Surg* 1987; **74:** 255.

89. Garde C. Cryosurgery of varicose veins. *J Dermatol Surg Oncol* 1994; **20:** 56–8.

90. Génévrier M. Du traitement des varices par les injections coagulantes concentrées de sels de quinine. *Soc Med Mil Franc* 1921; **15:** 169.

91. Giacomini C. *Giron Accad Med Torino* 1893; 14.

92. Gillies TE, Ruckley CV. Surgery for recurrent varicose veins. *Curr Pract Surg* 1996; **8:** 22–7.

93. Glass GM. Regrowth of veins in recurrence of varicose veins after surgical treatment. *Br J Surg* 1984; **71:** 991.

94. Glass GM. Prevention of recurrent saphenofemoral incompetence after surgery for varicose veins. *Br J Surg* 1989; **76:** 1210.

95. Gloviczki P, Cambria RA, Rhee RY, Canton LG, McKusick MA. Surgical technique and preliminary results of endoscopic subfascial division of perforating veins. *J Vasc Surg* 1996; **23(3):** 517–23.

96. Goldman MP, Sadick NS, Weiss RA. Cutaneous necrosis, telangiectatic matting, and hyperpigmentation following sclerotherapy. *Dermatol Surg* 1995; **21:** 19–29.

97. Goren G. Injection sclerotherapy for varicose veins: history and effectiveness. *Phlebology* 1991; **6:** 7–11.

98. Goren G. Invaginated pin-stripping (letter). *Phlebology* 1994; **9:** 173–4.

99. Goren G, Yellin AL. Ambulatory stab avulsion phlebectomy for truncal varicose veins. *Am J Surg* 1991; **162:** 166–74.

100. Goren G, Yellin AE. Invaginated axial stripping and stab avulsion (hook) phlebectomy: a definitive out patient procedure for primary varicose veins. *Ann Surg* 1994; **2:** 27–35.

101. Goren G, Yellin AE. Invaginated axial saphenectomy by a semirigid stripper: perforate-invaginate stripping. *J Vasc Surg* 1994; **20:** 970–7.

102. Goudin L, Soriano J. Echosclerotherapy. A Canadian study. In: Martinbeau R, Prescott R, Zummo M, eds. *Phlebologie 92.* Paris: J Libbey, Eurotext 92.

103. Gubéran E, Widmer LK, Rougement A, Glaus L. Epidemiology of spider webs. *Vasa* 1974; **4**: 391–5.

104. Hadfield GJ. In: *The Treatment of Varicose Veins by Injection and Compression*. Proceedings of the Stoke Mandeville Symposium. Hereford: Pharmaceutical Research STD Ltd, 1971; 52.

105. Haeger K. Indications for surgery in ankle perforator insufficiency. *Zentralbl Phlebol* 1969; **8**: 158–63.

106. Haeger K. The surgical anatomy of the saphenofemoral and sapheno-popliteal junctions. *J Cardiovasc Surg* 1962; **6**: 420–7.

107. Haliday P. Repeat high ligation. *Aust N Z J Surg* 1970; **39**: 354–6.

108. Hanrahan LM, Araki CT, Fisher JB, *et al.* Evaluation of the perforating veins of the lower extremity using high resolution duplex imaging. *J Cardiovasc Surg* 1991; **32**: 87–97.

109. Hauer G. Die endoscopische Sub fascica diszision der Perforensvenen – vorlaufige Mitteilung. *Vasa* 1985; **14**: 59–61.

110. Hauer G, Borkun J, Willer I, Diller S. Endoscopic subfascial ligation of perforating veins. *Surg Endosc* 1988; **2**: 5–12.

111. Hilty H. *Die makroskopiche Gefässvaribilität im Mandungsgebiet der Vena saphena magna des Menschen*. Basel: Schwabe, 1955.

112. Hoare MC, Nicolaides AN, Miles CR, *et al.* The role of primary varicose veins in venous ulceration. *Surgery* 1983; **82**: 450–3.

113. Hoare MG, Royle JP. Doppler ultrasound detection of saphenofemoral and saphenopopliteal incompetence and operative venography to ensure precise saphenopopliteal ligation. *Aust N Z J Surg* 1984; **54**: 49–52.

114. Hobbs JT. Peroperative venography to ensure accurate sapheno-popliteal ligation. *Br Med J* 1980; **2**: 1578–9.

115. Hobbs JT. In: Negus D, Jantet G, eds. *Phlebology '85*. London: J Libbey, 1986; 143.

116. Hobbs JT. Treatment of varicose veins. A random trial of injection compression therapy versus surgery. *Br J Surg* 1968; **55**: 777–80.

117. Hobbs J. Compression sclerotherapy of varicose veins. In: Bergan JJ, Yao JST, eds. *Venous Problems*. Chicago, IL: Year Book Medical Publishers, 1976.

118. Hobbs J. Surgery and sclerotherapy in the treatment of varicose veins. A random trial. *Arch Surg* 1974; **109**: 793–6.

119. Hobbs J. The enigma of the gastrocnemius vein. *Phlebology* 1988; **3**: 19–30.

120. Hobbs JT. The pelvic congestion syndrome. *Br J Hosp Med* 1990; **43**: 200–6.

121. Holm J, Nilsson NJ, Schersten T, Sivertsson R. Elective surgery for varicose veins; a simple method for evaluation of the patients. *J Cardiovasc Surg* 1974; **15**: 565–71.

122. Holme JB, Skajaa K, Holme K. Incidence of lesions of the saphenous nerve after partial or complete stripping of the long sapehenous vein. *Acta Chir Scand* 1990; **156**: 145–8.

123. Homans J. Operative treatment of varicose veins and ulcers. *Surg Gynecol Obstet* 1916; **22**: 143–58.

124. Homans J. The etiology and treatment of varicose ulcers of the leg. *Surg Gynecol Obstet* 1917; **24**: 300–11.

125. Howard Jones N. Critical study of origins and early development of hyperdermic medication. *J Hist Med Allied Sci* 1947; **2**: 201–49.

126. Hurst PA, Kinmonth JB, Rutt DL. A gut and mesentery pedicle for bridging lymphatic obstruction. *J Cardiovasc Surg* 1978; **19**: 589–96.

127. Juhan C, Haupert S, Miltgen G, Barthelemy P, Eklof B. Recurrent varicose veins. *Phlebology* 1990; **5**: 201–11.

128. Kakkar VV, Howe CT, Flank C. Compression sclerotherapy for varicose veins: a phlebographic study. *Br J Surg* 1969; **56**: 620.

129. Keith LM, Smead WL. Saphenous vein stripping and its complications. *Surg Clin North Am* 1983; **63**: 1303–12.

130. Kent SJS. Personal communication, 1985.

131. Kilbourne NJ. Varicose veins in pregnancy. *Am J Obstet Gynecol* 1933; **25**: 104–7.

132. King ESJ. The genesis of varicose veins. *Aust N Z J Surg* 1950; **20**: 126–33.

133. Kinmonth JB, Hurst PA, Edwards JM, Rutt DL. Relief of lymph obstruction by use of a bridge of mesentery and ileum. *Br J Surg* 1978; **65**: 829–53.

134. Kosinski C. The anatomy of the veins of the lower limb. *J Anat (Lond)* 1926; **60**: 131.

135. Kosinski C. Obstructions in the superficial venous system of the lower extremity. *J Anat* 1926; **60**: 131–42.

136. Koyano K, Sakaguchi S. Selective stripping operation based on Doppler ultrasonic findings for primary varicose veins of the lower extremities. *Surgery* 1988; **6**: 615–19.

137. Lane RJ, McMahon C, Cuzilla M. The treatment of varicose veins using the venous valve cuff. *Phlebology* 1994; **9**: 136–45.

138. Large J. Surgical treatment of saphenous varices, with prevention of the main great saphenous trunk. *J Vasc Surg* 1985; **2**: 886–91.

139. Larsson RH, Lofgren E, Myers TT, Lofgren KA. Long term results after vein surgery: study of 1000 cases after 10 years. *Mayo Clin Proc* 1974; **49**: 114–117.

140. Laurikka V, Sisto T, Tarkka M, Auvinen O. Long term saphenous nerve lesions after varicose vein stripping operation. *Surg Res Commun* 1992; **12**: 343–5.

141. Lea Thomas M, Bowles JN. Incompetent perforating veins: comparison of varicography and ascending phlebography. *Radiology* 1985; **154**: 619–23.

142. Lea Thomas M, Fletcher EWL, Andreas MR, Cockett FB. The venous connections of vulval varices. *Clin Radiol* 1967; **18**: 313–17.

143. Lechter A, Alvarez A, Lopez G. Pelvic varices and gonadal veins. *Phlebology* 1987; **2**: 181–8.

144. Ledentu A. *Recherches anatomiques a considerations physiologiques sur la circulacion veineuse du pied et de la jambe*. Thesis, Paris, 1867.

145. Leon M, Volteas N, Labropoulos N, *et al.* The effect of elastic stockings on the elasticity of varicose veins. *Int Angiol* 1993; **12(2)**: 173–7.

146. Li AKC. A technique for re-exploration of the saphenofemoral junction for recurrent varicose veins. *Br J Surg* 1975; **62:** 745–6.

147. Linser P. Die Behandlung der Krampfadern mit intravarikosen Kochsalzinjektionen. *Dermatol Wochenschr* 1925; **81:** 1345–51.

148. Linser P. Die Behandlung der Varizen mit Künstlicher Thrombosierung. *Dermatol Z* 1925; **45;** 22.

149. Linser P. Über die konservative Behandlung der Varicen. *Med Klin* 1916; **12:** 847.

150. Linton RR. The communicating veins of the lower leg and the operative technique for their ligation. *Ann Surg* 1938; **107:** 582–93.

151. Lofgren EP, Coates HLC, O'Brien PC. Clinically suspect pulmonary embolism after vein stripping. *Mayo Clin Proc* 1976; **51:** 77–80.

152. Lofgren EP, Lofgren KA. Recurrence of varicose veins after the stripping operation. *Arch Surg* 1971; **102:** 111–14.

153. Lofgren KA. Management of varicose veins: Mayo Clinic experience. In: Bergan JJ, Yao JST, eds. *Venous Problems*. Chicago, IL: Year Book Medical Publishers, 1978.

154. Ludbrook J. Valvular defect in primary varicose veins. Cause or effect? *Lancet* 1963; **2:** 1289–92.

155. Luke JC. The management of recurrent varicose veins. *Surgery* 1954; **35:** 40–4.

156. Luke JC, Miller GG. Disasters following operation of ligation and retrograde injection of varicose veins. *Ann Surg* 1948; **127:** 426–31.

157. Lumley JSP. Surgical treatment of varicose veins. *Br J Hosp Med* 1977; **17(5):** 508–17.

158. McCarthy WJ, Dann C, Pearce WH, Yao JST. Management of sudden profuse bleeding from varicose veins. *Surgery* 1993; **113(2):** 178–83.

159. McFarland RJ, Scott HJ, Kay DN, Scott RAP. High injection sclerotherapy for varicose veins in the presence of femoro-saphenous reflux. *Phlebology* 1988; **3:** 49–54.

160. MacGowan WAL. Sclerotherapy: prevention of accidents. A review. *J R Soc Med* 1985; **78:** 136–7.

161. MacGowan WAL, Holland PDJ, Browne HI, Byrnes D. The local effects of intra-arterial injections of sodium tetradecyl sulphate (S.T.D.) 3%. An experimental study. *Br J Surg* 1972; **59:** 101–4.

162. McIrvine A, Corbett R, Aston NO, Sherriff EA, Wiseman PA, Jamieson CW. The demonstration of saphenofemoral incompetence: Doppler ultrasound compared with standard clinical tests. *Br J Surg* 1984; **71:** 509–10.

163. McMullin GM, Coleridge Smith PD, Scurr JH. Objective assessment of high ligation without stripping the long saphenous vein. *Br J Surg* 1991; **78:** 1139–42.

164. Maingot R, Carlton CH. Injection treatment of varicose veins; estimate of its place in practice. *Lancet* 1928; **1:** 806–7.

165. Marston A. Treatment of varicose veins. *Lancet* 1975; **2:** 453.

166. Martin AG, Wainwright AM, Lear PA. Crochet hooks in varicose vein surgery. *Ann R Coll Surg Engl* 1995; **7:** 460–1.

167. Martinet JD. *Traitment des Maladies Veineuses de Membres Inférieurs*. Paris: Doin, 1965.

168. Massel TB. Problem of adequate therapy for varicose veins: new procedure. *West J Surg* 1950; **58:** 112–15.

169. May R. *La Chirurgia delle Vene degli Arti Inferiori e del Bacino*. Padova: Eds Piccin, 1978.

170. May R. Varicose veins. In: May R, ed. *Surgery of the Veins of the Leg and Pelvis*. Stuttgart: Georg Thieme, 1979.

171. May R, Nissl R. Phlebographic Studien zur Anatomie der Beinvenen. *Fortschr Roentgenstr* 1966; **104:** 171.

172. Mayo CH. Treatment of varicose veins. *Surg Gynecol Obstet* 1906; **2:** 385–8.

173. Mercier R, Fouques PH, Portal N, Vanneuville G. Anatomie chirurgicale de la veine saphene externe. *J Chir* 1967; **93:** 59–70.

174. Moosman A, Hartwell W. The surgical significance of the subfascial course of the lesser saphenous vein. *Surg Gynecol Obstet* 1964; **118:** 761–6.

175. Mosquera DA, Manns RA, Duffield RGM. Phlebography in the management of recurrent varicose veins. *Phlebology* 1995; **10:** 19–22.

176. Munn SR, Morton JB, Macbeth WAG, McLeish AR. To strip or not to strip the long saphenous vein? A varicose veins trial. *Br J Surg* 1981; **68:** 426–8.

177. Myers TT, Cooley JC. Varicose vein surgery in the management of the post-phlebitic limb. *Surg Gynecol Obstet* 1954; **99:** 733–44.

178. Nabatoff RA. Surgical technique for stripping the long saphenous vein. *Surg Gynecol Obstet* 1977; **145:** 81–7.

179. Nabatoff RA. Three thousand stripping operations for varicose veins on a semi-ambulatory basis. *Surg Gynecol Obstet* 1970; **130:** 497–500.

180. Neglen P. Treatment of varicosities of saphenous origin. Comparison of ligation sclerotherapy and selected stripping. In: Bergan JT, Goldman MP, eds. *Varicose Veins and Telangiectasias: Diagnosis and Management*. St Louis, MO: Quality Medical, 1993.

181. Negus D. Prevention and treatment of venous ulceration. *Ann R Coll Surg Engl* 1985; **67:** 144–8.

182. Negus D, Friedgood A. The effective management of venous ulceration. *Br J Surg* 1983; **70:** 623–7.

183. Nocker W, Diebschlag W, Lehmacher W. Three month, randomised, double-blind, dose response study with O-(beta-hydroxyethyl)-rutosides drinking solution. *Vasa* 1989; **18(3):** 235–8.

184. Oesch A. Pin stripping a novel method of a traumatic stripping. *Phlebology* 1993; **8:** 171–3.

185. O'Reilly K. A technique of diathermy sclerosis of varicose veins. *Aust N Z J Surg* 1981; **51:** 379–82.

186. O'Reilly K. Endovenous diathermy sclerosis of varicose veins. *Aust N Z J Surg* 1977; **47:** 393–5.

187. Otsu A, Mori N. Therapy of varicose veins. The lower limb spy light calculator. *Angiology* 1971; **22:** 107–13.

188. Ouvry PA, Davy A. Traitement sclérosant de la saphène externe variqueuse. In: Negus D, Jantet G, eds. *Phlebology '85*. London: J Libbey, 1986; 115.

189. Owen ERTC, Pflug JJ. Endoscopic ligation of perforator leg veins (letter). *Lancet* 1991; **338:** 248.

190. Papadakis K, Christodoulou C, Christopoulos D, *et al.* Number and anatomical distribution of incompetent thigh perforating veins. *Br J Surg* 1989; **76:** 581–4.

191. Paraskeva PA, Cheshire N, Stansby G, Darzi AW. Endoscopic subfascial division of incompetent perforating calf veins. *Br J Surg* 1996; **83:** 1105–6.

192. Pegoraro M, Baracco C, Ferrero E, Palladino F. Successful vascular reconstruction after inadvertant femoral artery 'stripping'. *J Cardiovasc Surg* 1987; **28:** 440–4.

193. Peruzzi G, Corcos L, Romeo V. Structure and use of the external phlebo-extractor. *Phlebology* 1989; **4:** 275–8.

194. Petrov ML, Pennin BA. Khirurgicheskoe Lechenie pri posttromboflebiticheskom sindrome. *Vestn Khir* 1976; **116:** 48–50.

195. Pfeifer JR, Hawtof GD. Injection sclerotherapy and CO_2 laser sclerotherapy in the ablation of cutaneous spider veins of the lower extremity. *Phlebology* 1989; **4:** 231–40.

196. Piachaud D, Weddell JM. The cost of treating varicose veins. *Lancet* 1972; **2:** 1191–2.

197. Perhoniemi V, Salo JA, Haapianien R, Salo H. Strain gauge plethysmography in the assessment of venous reflux after subfascial closure of perforating veins: a prospective study of twenty patients. *J Vasc Surg* 1990; **12:** 34–7.

198. Pierik EGJM, Wittens CHA, Van Urk H. Subfascial endoscopic ligation in the treatment of incompetent perforating veins. *Eur J Vasc Surg* 1995; **9:** 38–41.

199. Price C. The anatomy of the saphenous nerve in the lower leg with particular reference to its relationship to the long saphenous vein. *J Cardiovasc Surg* 1990; **31:** 294–7.

200. Pulvertaft TB. General practice treatment of symptoms of venous insufficiency with oxerutins. *Vasa* 1983; **12:** 373–6.

201. Raivio E. Untersuchungen über die Venen der unteren extremitaten mit besonderer berucksichtigung der gegenseit igen verbindungen zwischen den oberflachigen und tiefen Venen. *Ann Med Exp Finn* 1948; **26:** 1–127.

202. Raj TB, Makin GS. A random controlled trial of two forms of compression bandaging in outpatient sclerotherapy of varicose veins. *J Surg Res* 1981; **31:** 440–5.

203. Ramelet AA. La phlebectomie amblatoire selon Muller: technique, avantages, desavantages. *J Mal Vasc* 1991; **16:** 119–22.

204. Ramesh S, Umeh N, Galland RB. Day case varicose vein operations: patient suitability and satisfaction. *Phlebology* 1995; **10:** 103–5.

205. Redmond HP, Broe PJ, Bouchier-Hayes DJ. Vascular complications of varicose vein surgery in Ireland. *Phlebology* 1988; **3:** 251–3.

206. Reid RG, Rothnie NG. Treatment of varicose veins by compression sclerotherapy. *Br J Surg* 1968; **55:** 889–95.

207. Reiner L. Activity of anionic surface active compounds in producing vascular obliteration. *Proc Soc Exp Biol Med* 1946; **62:** 49–54.

208. Richardson, Beclewith, Royle JP. Duplex scanning of recurrent varicose veins. *Phlebology* 1990; **5:** 281–4.

209. Rivlin S. The surgical cure of primary varicose veins. *Br J Surg* 1975; **62:** 913–17.

210. Robbins MA, Frankel SJ, Nanchahal K, Coast J, Williams MH. *Health Care Needs Assessment Booklet.* London: HMSO, 1995.

211. Rogers L, Winchester AH. Intravenous sclerosing solutions. *Br Med J* 1930; **2:** 120–1.

212. Rose SS. Personal communication, 1985.

213. Rose SS, Ahmed A. Some thoughts on the aetiology of varicose veins. *J Cardiovasc Surg* 1986; **27:** 534–43.

214. Royle JP. Operative treatment of varicose veins. *Hosp Update* 1984; 941–9.

215. Royle JP. Operative treatment of varicose veins. In: Greenhalgh RM, ed. *Vascular Surgical Techniques.* London: Butterworths, 1984.

216. Ruckley CV, Cuthbertson C, Fenwick N, Prescott RJ, Garraway WM. Day care after operations for hernia or varicose veins: a controlled trial. *Br J Surg* 1978; **65:** 456–9.

217. Saradeth T, Resch KL, Ernst E. Placebo treatment for varicosity: don't eat it, rub it! *Phlebology* 1994; **9:** 63–6.

218. Sarin S, Scurr JH, Coleridge-Smith P. Assessment of stripping the long saphenous vein in the treatment of primary varicose veins. *Br J Surg* 1992; **79:** 889–93.

219. Sarin S, Scurr JH, Coleridge-Smith P. Stripping the long saphenous vein in the treatment of primary varicose veins. *Br J Surg* 1994; **81:** 1455–8.

220. Sarin S, Shields DA, Abu-Owen A, Scurr JH, Coleridge-Smith PD. Is the normal limb normal in unilateral varicose veins. *Phlebology* 1988; **3:** 261–4.

221. Sattler G, Mossler K, Hagedorn M. Paratibial endoscopic perforator interruption. In: *Advances in Medical and Surgical Treatment of Venous Disorders.* 6th American Congress of the North American Society for Phlebology, 1993; Abst.

222. Schadeck M. Doppler and echotomography in sclerosis of the saphenous veins. *Phlebology* 1987; **2:** 221–40.

223. Schadeck M. Echoslcerose de la grand vein saphene. *Phlebologie* 1993; **4:** 665–7.

224. Schanzer H, Skladany M. Varicose vein surgery with preservation of the saphenous vein: a comparison between high ligation-avulsion versus saphenofemoral banding valvuloplasty-avulsion. *J Vasc Surg* 1994; **20:** 684–7.

225. Schiassi B. La Cure des varices par l'injection d'une solution d'iode. *Semin Méd Paris* 1908; **28:** 601.

226. Schultz-Ehrenberg U, Weindorf N, Mattes H, Hirche C. New epidemiological findings with regard to initial stages of varicose veins. Bochum Study I to III. *Phlebology* 1992; 234–6.

227. Schultz-Ehrenberg U, Weindorf N, VonUslar D, Hirche H. Prospective epidemiological investigations

in early and preclinical stages of varicosis. In: Davy A, Stemmer R, eds. *Phlebology 1989*. Paris: John Libbey, Eurotext 1989; 163–5.

228. Schultz-Ehrenberg U, Weindorf N, VonUslar D, Hirche H. Prospective epidemiologiche Studie uber die Entstehungsweise der Kramptadern bei Kindern und Jugendlichen (Bochumer Studie I and II). *Phlebol Proktol* 1989; **18:** 3–11.

229. Scott A, Dormandy J. Outpatients ligation of varicose veins. *Proc R Soc Med* 1976; **69:** 22–3.

230. Scurr JH, Coleridge-Smith P, Cutting P. Varicose veins: optimum compression following sclerotherapy. *Ann R Coll Surg Engl* 1985; **67:** 109–11.

231. Seddon J. The management of varicose veins. *Br J Surg* 1973; **60:** 345–7.

232. Sheppard M. A procedure for the prevention of recurrent saphenofemoral incompetence. *Aust N Z J Surg* 1978; **48:** 322–6.

233. Sheppard M. The incidence, diagnosis and management of sapheno-popliteal incompetence. *Phlebology* 1986; **1:** 23–32.

234. Sherman RS. Varicose veins: further findings based on anatomic and surgical dissections. *Ann Surg* 1949; **130:** 218–32.

235. Shouler PJ, Runchman PC. Varicose veins: optimum compression after surgery and sclerotherapy. *Ann R Coll Surg Engl* 1989; **71:** 401–4.

236. Sicard JA, Gaugier L. *Le Traitement des Varices par les Injections Locales Sclérosantes*. Paris: Masson, 1927.

237. Sigg K. Treatment of varicosities and accompanying complications (ambulatory treatment of phlebitis with compression bandage). *Angiology* 1952; **3:** 355–79.

238. Simpson CJ, Smellie GD. The phlebotome in the management of incompetent perforating veins and venous ulceration. *J Cardiovasc Surg* 1987; **28:** 279–80.

239. Sjoberg T, Einarsson E, Norgren L. Functional evaluation of four different compression stockings in venous insufficiency. *Phlebology* 1987; **2:** 53–8.

240. Somerville JF, Brow GO, Byrne PJ, Quill RD, Fegan WG. The effect of elastic stockings on superficial venous pressures in patients with venous insufficiency. *Br J Surg* 1974; **61:** 979–81.

241. Speakman MJ, Collins J. Are swelling and aching of the legs reduced by operating on varicose veins? *Br Med J* 1986; **293:** 105–6.

242. Stacey MC, Burnand KG, Layer GT, Pattisson M. Calf pump function in patients with healed venous ulcers is not improved by surgery to the communicating veins or elastic stockings. *Br J Surg* 1988; **75:** 436–9.

243. Staelens I, Van der Stricht J. Complication rate of long stripping of the greater saphenous vein. *Phlebology* 1992; **7:** 67–70.

244. Stonebridge PA, Chalmers N, Beggs I, Bradbury AW, Ruckley CV. Recurrent varicose veins: a varicographic analysis leading to a new practical classification. *Br J Surg* 1995; **82:** 60–2.

245. Stother IG, Bryson A, Alexander S. Treatment of varicose veins by compression sclerotherapy. *Br J Surg* 1974; **61:** 387–90.

246. Sugrue M, Mehigan D, Hederman WP. Acceptability and safety of out-patient saphenofemoral ligation under local anaesthesia. A report of 100 consecutive cases. *Phlebology* 1988; **3:** 261–4.

247. Tavel E. Die Behandlung der varicen durch die künstliche Thrombose. *Dtsch Z Chir* 1912; **116:** 735.

248. Tennant WG, Ruckley CV. Medicolegal action following treatment for varicose veins. *Br J Surg* 1996; **83:** 291–2.

249. Thibault PK, Lewis WK. Recurrent varicose veins: evaluation using Duplex 'imaging'. *J Dermatol Surg Oncol* 1992; **18:** 618–24.

250. Thiery L. La vena fossa poplitea. *Phlebologie* 1983; **2:** 649–51.

251. Thompson JF, Royle GT, Farrands PA, Najmaldin A, Clifford PC, Webster JHH. Varicose vein surgery using a pneumatic tourniquet: reduced blood loss and improved cosmesis. *Ann R Coll Surg Engl* 1990; **72:** 119–22.

252. Tibbs DJ, Fletcher EWL. Direction of flow in superficial veins as a guide to venous disorders of the lower limbs. *Surgery* 1983; **93:** 758–67.

253. Tournay R. Indications et résultats de la méthode sclérosante dans le traitement des varices. *Bull Méd Paris* 1931; **45:** 73–7.

254. Tournay R. Traitement des varices: chirurgie ou injections sclérosantes. *Bull Soc Méd Pract Lille* 1937.

255. Tournay R. How should resistant varicose veins be sclerosed? *Phlebology* 1990; **5:** 151–5.

256. Travers JB, Machin GS. Reduction of varicose vein recurrence by the use of post operative compression stockings. *Phlebology* 1994; **9:** 204–7.

257. Travers JP, Rhodes JE, Hardy JG, Makin GS. Postoperative limb compression in reduction of haemorrhage after varicose vein surgery. *Ann R Coll Surg Engl* 1993; **75:** 119–22.

258. Trendelenburg F. Uber die Unterbildung der Vena saphena magna bei unterschenkel Varicen. *Beitr Klin Chir* 1891; **7:** 195–210.

259. Turner Warwick W. *The Rational Treatment of Varicose Veins and Varicocele (with notes on the obliterative method of treatment of other conditions)*. London: Faber & Faber, 1931.

260. Van Bellen B, Gross WS, Verta Jr MJ, Yao JST, Bergan JJ. Lymphatic disruption in varicose vein surgery. *Surgery* 1977; **82(2):** 257–9.

261. Vandendriessche M. Association between gastrocnemial vein insufficiency and varicose veins. *Phlebology* 1989; **4:** 171–84.

262. Van Der Strict J. Saphenectomie par invagination sur fil. *Presse Med* 1963; **71:** 1081–2.

263. Van Limborgh J. L'anatomie du système veineux de l'extrémité inférieux en relation avec la pathologie variqueuse. *Folia Angiol* 1961; **8:** 3.

264. Wallois P. The condition necessary to achieve an effective sclerosant therapy. *Phlebologie* 1982; **35:** 337–98.

265. Watts GT. The treatment of varicose veins. *Lancet* 1973; **1:** 435.

266. Wilkins RW, Mixter G, Stanton JR, Litter J. Elastic stockings in the prevention of pulmonary embolism: preliminary report. *N Engl J Med* 1952; **246:** 360–4.

267. Wilkins RW, Stanton JR. Elastic stockings in the prevention of pulmonary embolism; progress report. *N Engl J Med* 1953; **248:** 1087–90.
268. Williams RA, Wilson SE. Sclerosant treatment of varicose veins in deep vein thrombosis. *Arch Surg* 1984; **119:** 1283–5.
269. Wilson MG. Method of treatment for varicose veins. *Lancet* 1953; **1:** 1273–5.

270. Winstone N. In: *The Treatment of Varicose Veins by Injection and Compression.* Proceedings of the Stoke Mandeville Symposium. Hereford: Pharmaceutical Research STD Ltd, 1971; 41.
271. Woodyer AB, Dormandy JA. Is it necessary to strip the long saphenous vein? *Phlebology* 1986; **1:** 221–4.
272. Zukowski Z, Nicolaides AN, Szendro G, *et al.* Haemodynamic significance of incompetent perforating veins. *Br J Surg* 1991; **78:** 625–9.

CHAPTER 8

Deep vein thrombosis: pathology

Prevalence and incidence of deep vein thrombosis 249
Aetiology of deep vein thrombosis 254

Temporal changes in a deep vein thrombosis 273
References 276

Definition

A thrombus is a semi-solid mass formed from the components of flowing blood, within the heart or blood vessels. A clot is blood which has coagulated *in vitro* (i.e. in a test tube). A deep vein thrombosis is a thrombus which has formed in the veins beneath the deep fascia of the leg. Thrombus within the pelvic or abdominal veins that carry blood from the legs is also commonly classified as 'deep vein thrombosis' and some would include thrombus in the communicating veins of the lower limb within the definition (Figure 8.1).

Prevalence and incidence of deep vein thrombosis

The true prevalence of deep vein thrombosis in the population is unknown as many cases without symptoms pass undetected (see also Chapter 11).[465]

Clinical evidence

The computerization of hospital deaths and discharges has allowed the prevalence of individual conditions to be obtained from national databases. These suggest a prevalence of deep vein thrombosis of 79 per 100 000 of the population.[151]

A number of the early studies on the incidence of deep vein thrombosis in the population relied on a diagnosis based upon a clinical history and examination.[93,154,337] and many were based on patients presenting to doctors with leg symptoms or attending hospital for other disorders. It soon became apparent from these studies that there was a poor relationship between clinical symptoms and signs and objective tests[138,150,195,314,327,399,465] and they are now therefore not considered to be valid; nevertheless, two community-based population studies have found similar results, namely that 2.5–5% of the population had had a 'clinical' venous thrombosis.

Phlebographic evidence

In 1976, Nylander and Olivecrona[333] performed phlebograms on all patients presenting to the only hospital in Malmö with any symptoms in the legs which were suggestive of deep vein thrombosis. Evidence of thrombosis was present in 231 of these phlebographs. The population served by this hospital was 263 000 and therefore the incidence of deep vein thrombosis presenting to their hospital was of 0.9/1000/year (0.09%). Because the indications for phlebography were clinical signs, this study suffered from the same defects as the other clinical studies mentioned above, but it did give an indication of the incidence of 'clinical' deep vein thrombosis in the 'normal' population.

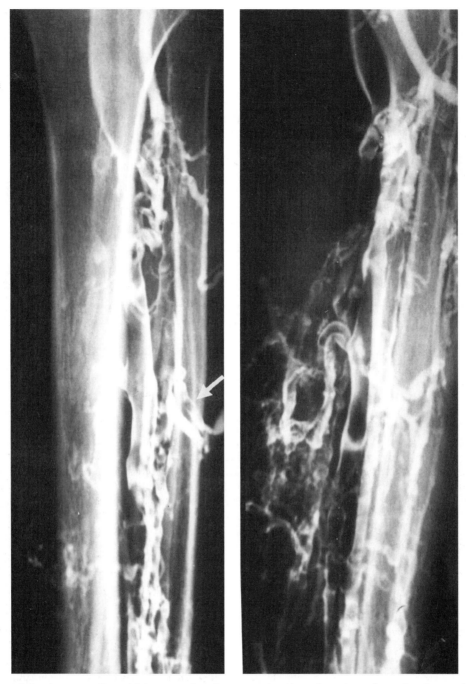

Figure 8.1 An ascending phlebogram showing extensive thrombus throughout the deep veins of the calf. Thrombus is seen in the tibial and peroneal veins, and on the lateral projection there is extensive thrombus within the soleal sinusoids. The arrow points to a small thrombus within a calf communicating vein which is seen as a small circular filling defect.

Extrapolating from all the postoperative surveys that have been made,[43,89] it is reasonable to assume that at least twice as many patients are having silent thromboses and that the true incidence of deep vein thrombosis is nearer 0.27%. This figure takes no account of all the patients who are admitted to hospital with a serious illness or for an operation, one-third of whom will develop a thrombosis, if prophylactic measures are not taken.

In 1977, Nylander and his colleagues[334] found that 24% of the phlebographs which showed evidence of recent or old thrombosis came from patients who had had an operation and 8% came from patients who had had a major injury. These percentages agree surprisingly well with the survey by Gjöres[154] of patients with 'clinical' thrombosis. Surgery and trauma have therefore been shown to be responsible for approximately one-third of all deep vein thromboses in Scandinavia over the last 30 years.

The prevalence of thrombosis in the general population is dependent upon the number of patients having operations and sustaining major injuries. Approximately a third of these patients used to develop a deep vein thrombosis but this proportion is now much less since the advent of effective prophylaxis. It is hoped that improvements in prophylaxis (see Chapter 11) will continue to drive this figure down.

Death certificate and hospital discharge surveys

Hume *et al.*[208] used centralized records to obtain an estimate from the number of death certificates in 1967 in England and Wales where pulmonary embolism was given as the cause of death. They found that 21 000 deaths in England and Wales were estimated to be the result of pulmonary embolism, giving an incidence of 40/100 000 deaths per annum. The majority of these death certificates relied on a clinical diagnosis and the association with other fatal disease could not be determined. Many other deaths where pulmonary embolism may have contributed to death must have been missed by this survey. Others have looked at the final discharge from hospital and and have deduced prevalence rates of approximately 50 per 100 000 for pulmonary embolism and 80 per 100 000 for deep vein thrombosis.[152,259]

Recent population surveys

There have been three recent studies which have reported on the incidence of venous thromboembolism within defined local populations. The first was based on an urban population of 380 000 in Worcester, USA. International Classification of Disease codes were used retrospectively to obtain hospital discharges where a diagnosis of deep vein thrombosis was made. Individual records were then obtained and reviewed. Postal codes were used to exclude patients from outside the community but patients from within the community who went outside for treatment were not included. The major value of this survey was that more than 80% of the coded patients had had objective tests to confirm the diagnosis. The incidence of venous thrombosis was found to be a little lower than in the previous clinical studies – 56/100 000 (vs 80/100 000) and the incidence of pulmonary embolism was half – 23/100 000 (of 50/100 000). This study confirmed that age, recent surgery, malignancy, obesity, heart failure, pulmonary disease and injury were all in-patient risk factors.[12]

A similar prospective study was reported from Malmö, Sweden, in 1992.[328] The study population was 281 000, and 1009 patients in whom the diagnosis of deep vein thrombosis was suspected were referred for phlebography. The diagnosis was confirmed in 366 patients. This gives an incidence of 1.6/1000 inhabitants per year or 160 per 100 000. Pulmonary embolism was suspected in 5% of the patients but confirmed by lung scanning in only 2%. Age, injury and known or subsequent malignancy were all recognized risk factors.

The third study was the Olmstead County Study which was part of the Rochester epidemiology project being run by the Mayo clinic.[403] Initial results from 1966 to 1970 demonstrated that the annual incidence of thrombembolism was approximately 120 cases per 100 000 of the population.

Pooling all these studies suggests that the incidence of deep vein thrombosis is between 50 and 150 cases per 100 000 of the population per year.[81]

Autopsy evidence

Autopsy only provides the incidence of deep vein thrombosis in patients who have died as a result of pulmonary embolism or other causes. Autopsy does not determine the prevalence of thrombosis in those patients with the same diseases who have not died. In 1961, Sevitt and Gallagher[399] reported that 60% of all patients who had died after injuries or burns had thrombosis in their deep veins at autopsy. Pulmonary embolism was found in 20% of these examinations and in 16% the emboli were considered to be large enough to have caused death.

Morrell and Dunhill[304] found an incidence of pulmonary embolism at autopsy of 63% in surgical patients and 45% in medical patients. Havig[182] found a similar incidence (55%) of macroscopic pulmonary embolism in a randomly selected group of autopsies, and evidence of microscopic emboli was found in another 14% of autopsies; the overall incidence was therefore 69%. Pulmonary embolism was thought to be the cause of death in 33% of patients and to be a major factor in 19%. These figures must be accepted with caution because it is extremely difficult for a pathologist to estimate the pathophysiological significance of an autopsy finding. In Havig's study, two-thirds of the deep vein thrombi were within the ilio-femoral segment, and only one-third were confined to the calf or foot. Embolism appeared to be the immediate cause of death in seven of the 31 patients who died postoperatively.

The incidence of fatal pulmonary embolism after surgery, based on a few large series of patients who had autopsies because they died after a surgical operation,[23,217,241,378] has been found to lie between 0.4% and 1.6%.

Two studies in 1981 suggested that the incidence of pulmonary embolism was beginning to decline.[115,375] It is not clear whether this decline was the result of effective prophylactic regimens which have been used with increasing vigour over the past 20 years or the result of a real change in the natural history of the disease.

All the autopsy studies show that pulmonary embolism complicates at least one in every 30 cases of deep vein thrombosis (see Chapter 22).

In 1991, Lindblad, Sternby and Bergqvist[260] reported a longitudinal analysis of the incidence of venous thromboembolism in all the necropsies done in one hospital in 1957, 1964, 1975 and 1987. The incidence of thromboembolism was remarkably stable at between 31 and 35% of all autopsies apart from that associated with orthopaedic surgery which fell from 60.7% in 1975 to 32.2% in 1987. They concluded that the incidence of fatal embolism had not changed, but also noted that beneficial effects from the use of prophylaxis may have been masked by a doubling of the population aged over 65 years. Another paper published in 1994[377] on a continuous series of over 4000 post mortems between 1979 and 1989 had an incidence of thromboembolism of 23.7%. The fatal embolism rate was judged to be 14.6%.

DEEP VEIN THROMBOSIS AND SURGERY

Incidence of postoperative deep vein thrombosis

Our knowledge of the incidence of postoperative deep vein thrombosis is much better than our knowledge of the incidence of deep vein thrombosis in the general population who may be forming and lysing small thrombi all the time. The incidence of postoperative thrombosis varies with the method used for its detection (see Chapter 4).

The radioactive fibrinogen uptake test was extensively employed as a screening test but has now been abandoned. Bipedal ascending phlebography remains the gold standard for diagnosis, especially after orthopaedic surgery. The fibrinogen uptake test,[77,228] plethysmography,[99,473] Doppler ultrasound[384] and thermography[383] are all unreliable methods for detecting small established thrombi in the calf muscles and vena comes and even phlebography relies on interpretation.

The ideal method for assessing the incidence of postoperative thrombosis is preoperative and postoperative phlebography but only a few such studies, involving small numbers of patients, have been carried out.[44] Several studies have used postoperative phlebography alone,[43] and in many past studies phlebography was employed to confirm the accuracy of a positive fibrinogen uptake test.[43,231]

Unfortunately, the clinical significance of very small calf thrombi is not known,[52,120] though there is a correlation between the risk of pulmonary embolism and a positive fibrinogen uptake test.[67,373,378,461] It is possible that improvements in the quality of duplex scans may make it feasible to use this technique to determine the incidence of small postoperative thrombi below the knee but it is not sufficiently accurate at present.

Incidence of preoperative deep vein thrombosis

The majority of thrombi develop in the deep veins of the calf in the first 5 days after an operation but some thrombi start even before the operation. Four studies have used phlebography to screen patients awaiting an operation. Thrombi were found in five of 60 patients awaiting prostatectomy,[37] in three of 40 patients awaiting hip replacement,[44] in 10 out of 50 patients awaiting operations on the gastrointestinal tract[184] and in seven of 47 patients awaiting operation on hip fractures.[420] Thus between 5 and 20% of patients begin their operation with a thrombus already present in their calf veins.

Deep vein thrombosis after general surgery

Bergqvist[43] has summarized the published data and has computed an average incidence of thrombosis of 29% from 28 studies on 1081 general surgical patients in whom the fibrinogen uptake test was used for screening. This figure of 29% for general surgical patients not given any form of prophylaxis has been confirmed by others.[36,89] Malignant disease increases the risk of developing a postoperative thrombosis[45] but the effect of splenectomy, which was thought to be associated with a higher incidence of thrombosis, remains unproven.[73,107] Recently, there has been interest in discovering whether laparoscopic cholecystectomy has a higher or lower incidence of deep vein thrombosis than open cholecystectomy. One report from Australia has suggested that there is a very high incidence (55%), perhaps as a result of the pneumoperitoneum reducing venous return.[345] This figure seems excessive and does not agree with our experience, or that of others.

Deep vein thrombosis after urological surgery

There is a significantly greater incidence of thrombosis after open prostatectomy (38%) than after general surgical operations,[43,90] but a much lower incidence (11%) after transurethral resection of the prostate.[70,185,287,314,318] The administration of epsilon-aminocaproic acid, an antifibrinolytic agent which used to be given commonly after prostatectomy to reduce bleeding, does not appear to increase the risk of deep vein thrombosis or pulmonary embolism.[453] Very few patients now have an open prostatectomy and therefore the incidence of thrombosis after urological surgery has fallen. The incidence after renal transplantation is, however, as high as 8%.[8]

Deep vein thrombosis after gynaecological surgery

The incidence of thrombosis after gynaecological surgery varies between 29%[30] and 14%.[460] Thrombosis appears to be less common after gynaecological operations than after general surgical operations (19%),[43] even after making an allowance for the younger age of many of the gynaecological patients. Malignancy increases the risk of thrombosis. This was confirmed when thrombosis was found in 35% of a group of patients who had a hysterectomy for carcinoma, compared with 12% when the hysterectomy was performed for benign disease.[460]

Deep vein thrombosis after vascular surgery

In a group of patients who had phlebograms after femoro-popliteal bypass surgery, 43% had evidence of a deep vein thrombosis;[172] other investigators have found a lower incidence of approximately 8%.[214,309]

The incidence of thrombosis, estimated by the fibrinogen uptake test, following aorto-iliac surgery has varied between 21% and 32%.[15,39,178] When Doppler flow detection was combined with the fibrinogen uptake test, the incidence was 13%.[361] This figure is closer to the 4% incidence reported by Satiani *et al.*,[387] who used a combination of the fibrinogen uptake test with impedance plethysmography, and reported that the fibrinogen uptake test gave many false-positive results. A study comparing low molecular weight and standard heparin in prophylaxis after vascular surgery found a 7.5% incidence of deep vein thrombosis despite heparin treatment.[133] Another study on the incidence of thrombosis after abdominal aortic aneurysm surgery found an 18% incidence when phlebography was carried out 5 days after operation.[341] No prophylaxis was administered in this study.

Operations on varicose veins are reported to carry a low incidence of deep vein thrombosis[116,285] but objective studies have not been performed, perhaps because of the fear of inducing venous thrombosis in a recently traumatized venous system. This lack of knowledge has recently been highlighted by Campbell.[75] The incidence after compression sclerotherapy is also reputed to be low.[194]

Deep vein thrombosis after fractures and orthopaedic surgery

Most of the studies that have tried to determine the incidence of thrombosis after orthopaedic surgery used phlebography rather than the fibrinogen uptake test because leg wounds made the fibrinogen uptake tests inaccurate. It has been recognized that patients with fractures of the lower limb have an increased risk of thrombosis. Bauer in 1944[33] showed a relationship between the site of thrombosis and the site of the fracture and Sevitt and Gallagher[398] showed that 29 (83%) of 35 patients on whom an autopsy was performed after a fractured hip had evidence of deep vein thrombosis (Figure 8.2).

A recent study suggested that the incidence was 40% after femoral shaft fractures, 43% after tibial plateau fractures and 22% after tibial shaft fractures.[1] With the advent of total hip replacement and the vast increase in hip surgery, it has been recognized that planned orthopaedic surgery also carries a high risk of thrombosis (see Chapter 11). It has been suggested that the increased incidence of femoral vein thrombosis on the side of a hip replacement operation is caused by local trauma to the femoral vein when the hip is dislocated during the operation.[322,415] The incidence of thrombosis beginning in the calf is, however, similar in both legs and Bergqvist's compilation,[43] based on nine studies of the risk of venous thrombosis after hip fracture, showed that though 40% of the thrombi occurred on the side of the fractured limb, 23% developed in the opposite limb. A recent study in which aspirin and warfarin (relatively ineffective agents) were used for thrombosis prophylaxis, has again shown that the incidence of deep vein thrombosis is between 47 and 50% after cemented and uncemented hip replacement, respectively.[253]

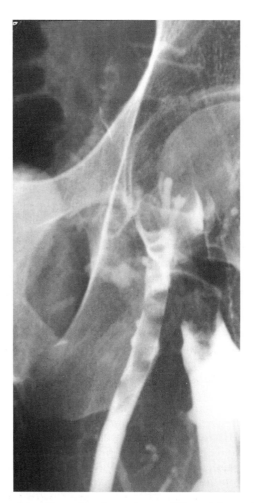

Figure 8.2 Thrombus is seen as a filling defect within the common femoral and long saphenous vein in relation to a fracture of the neck of the femur (not visible on this film). The thrombus was localized to the area of the injury, the calf and popliteal veins did not contain any filling defects.

Deep vein thrombosis after neurosurgery

The incidence of thrombosis after neurosurgical operations is said to be approximately 30%.[43] This is a high figure, others have suggested that the incidence may be lower (20%).[419,445]

Deep vein thrombosis during pregnancy

Venous thrombosis remains the most common cause of maternal death.[444] The overall risk of thromboembolism in pregnancy is six times greater than in the non-pregnant state. Factors increasing this risk are obstruction of venous return by the enlarging uterus and prothrombotic haemostatic changes. The incidence of thromboembolism is higher in those who have had a previous thrombosis.[25] Women at highest risk are those with an inherited or acquired thrombophilia such as activated protein C resistance, antithrombin III, protein C and S deficiency and anti-phospholipid syndrome. The incidence may, however, be as low as 1 in 1000 or less.[368]

Major injury

A prospective study on 716 patients admitted to a regional trauma unit and who had routine phlebography without prophylaxis showed that 58% developed deep vein thrombosis. Of these patients, 50% had suffered major injuries of the chest and abdomen; 53.8% had major head injuries alone. The incidence of thrombosis in those with spinal injuries was 62% and in those with major orthopaedic injuries 69%.[156] Others have found a lower incidence after spinal cord injury of 5–10%,[240,248] and this may be reduced still further by adequate prophylaxis.[365]

Amputees

One study, using duplex scanning, has shown that the incidence of postoperative deep vein thrombosis in amputees is 12.5%.[486]

Burns

The incidence of deep vein thrombosis in patients with burns has been estimated to be between 0.6 and 5%, which suggests that routine prophylaxis is unnecessary.[376]

Medical patients

There is quite a high incidence of thrombosis in certain groups of medical patients in hospital. High-risk conditions include stroke, heart failure and myocardial infarction. Incidences vary between 20 and 80%!

Aetiology of deep vein thrombosis

The preceding section on the incidence of thrombosis shows the important influence of surgery, trauma and intercurrent illness on the development of thrombosis. These factors, together with a number of other factors which will be discussed at the end of this section, are contributory to thrombus development rather than truly causative.

The mechanisms that cause blood to coagulate *in vivo* have been widely investigated in the last decade. The mechanism responsible for thrombosis in arteries appears to be different from that responsible for thrombosis in veins, and there may even be differences in the composition of thrombi in various parts of the vascular system.[349] Thrombus in arteries with little or no blood flow consists of a fibrin mesh and red cells, whereas the thrombus in a free-flowing system consists of a laminate of platelets and fibrin (the white head) with fibrin and red cells in its propagating tail.

Wiseman described pulmonary embolism in 1676[480] and Hunter[213] described 'phlebo-thrombosis' in his 'Treatise on the blood, inflammation and gun-shot wounds', but it was Rudolph Virchow[454] who recognized the association between the two conditions and went on to propose his famous 'triad' of causes for thrombosis:

1. Changes in the lining of the vessel wall (wall damage)
2. Changes in the flow of blood (stasis or low flow)
3. Changes in the constituents of the blood (hypercoagulability).

Much time and energy has been expended to try to discover which of these mechanisms, alone or in combination, is the most important in the generation of a thrombus.

It was known as early as 1922 that the blood fibrinogen increased in response to trauma[141] but it was not until the discovery of the coagulation cascade[49,273] that the modern era of thrombosis research began. Early experimental work showed that platelets accumulated on the walls of damaged vessels,[50,467] particularly during periods of low blood flow.[88]

Von Recklinghausen[458] suggested that the deposition of thrombus was related to eddy currents, a fact that was confirmed when deposits of platelets were found at sites of turbulent flow in arteriovenous shunts.[372] In 1929, Evans[131] associated the postoperative increase in circulating platelets with an increased risk of thrombosis.

In 1922, Aschoff[19] described the pathological changes that occurred in a developing thrombus and suggested that this process could only exist if there was an associated slowing of blood flow. He chose to ignore a considerable number of earlier studies[34,155,189,261,394] which showed that blood trapped in a vessel between two ligatures did not clot immediately but remained fluid for several hours.

In 1934, Homans[199] recognized the high incidence of thrombosis in the deep veins of the lower limb and suggested that stasis was an important factor in these veins. He produced a thrombosis by injecting a mixture of saline and 'muscle juice' into a segment of a dog's femoral vein that had been occluded by ligatures, but observed that thrombus did not form if a collateral vein draining the occluded segment was left untied.

In 1942, Wright[484] reported that the number of circulating platelets and their adhesiveness increased in the postoperative period, and several other workers described postoperative increases in blood coagulability that were associated with a clinical deep vein thrombosis.[112,297,338,400,401,464]

In 1950, Ochsner, DeBakey and Decamp,[337] in their large survey of venous thrombosis, suggested that shortened prothrombin times and raised antithrombin levels found in some of their patients might lead to thrombosis when combined with 'circulatory stasis'.

In 1956, Wright *et al.*,[483] using a radioisotope clearance technique, showed that the velocity of venous flow was reduced in limbs that were horizontal at rest, and increased with elevation or movement. This provided a rationale for the practice of early ambulation after operation[53,76,257,350] and the wearing of elastic stockings.[475,476] Both these practices have been reported to reduce the incidence of thrombosis.

At the end of the 1950s two important autopsy studies on the location of thrombi in the deep veins of the lower limb were carried out.[150,399] These investigations demonstrated that the majority of thrombi developed in the venous sinusoids of the soleus muscle.

By the end of the 1950s most investigators believed that stasis was the major factor responsible for the development of venous thrombosis, but, apart from some simple studies on coagulation factors, the relationship between coagulation and thrombosis remained largely unexplored. The role of vein wall damage was largely discredited by the failure to find any endothelial abnormalities beneath the origins of thrombi, even though the limitations of the histological techniques available at the time were clearly recognized.[289,343,382]

ENDOTHELIAL CELL INJURY

It is readily accepted that ulceration or rupture of an atheromatous plaque in an artery leads to exposure of the blood to collagen and macrophages laden with tissue factor. This stimulates platelet and fibrin deposition.[20,142,306–308,349] There is little evidence, however, that endothelial damage and subendothelial collagen exposure occur in veins, leading to thrombosis.[210,346,454] Many of the attempts to discover venous endothelial changes beneath thrombus, have, in the past used standard transmission microscopy. This technique is now accepted to be severely limited.[289,343,382]

The high incidence of thrombosis found in the veins of the lower limbs of patients who have sustained tibial fractures[193,335] supports the hypothesis that endothelial injury can cause deep vein thrombosis. The distortion of the femoral vein that occurs during total hip replacement is also associated with a high incidence of femoral vein thrombosis close to the site of injury.[415]

Many of the experimental systems for producing deep vein thrombosis in animals have relied on causing severe endothelial damage, often by introducing noxious materials into the vein.[212,300] Some systems produce a red propagating thrombus;[108,173] other systems induce a platelet thrombus[18,41,204,205,490] and their relevance to human deep vein thrombosis is therefore questionable. Ligation of the femoral vein of rabbits rarely induces thrombosis, unless it is combined with local or distant trauma, the incidence of thrombosis being proportional to the extent of the trauma.[56] The animal models of Day *et al.*[108] and Hamer and Malone[173] appear to relate more closely to clinical deep vein thrombosis, and may be more suitable for detailed studies of the role of endothelial changes in thrombogenesis.

We have recently developed a number of animal models in which thrombosis occurs without venous injury and these may enable us to discover the initial stages of thrombus development. A human thrombus model has also been developed that produces standard thrombosis in flowing blood.[353]

In a series of studies using scanning electron microscopy, Stewart *et al.* re-examined the role of the endothelium in thrombosis.[421,422] Stasis was produced in the jugular and femoral veins of the dog by gentle finger occlusion of the vein[424] and in some experiments coincidental trauma was applied to another distant part of the animal.[426] It was found that neither distant trauma nor stasis alone were capable of producing consistent changes in the endothelium but a combination of the two factors caused large numbers of white blood cells to adhere to the endothelial surface of the occluded vein.[424] These white cells migrated through the intercellular junctions to accumulate between the endothelium and basement membrane. This migration was followed by patchy endothelial desquamation, exposing large areas of subendothelial collagen.

White cell migration in response to acute inflammation has been recognized for many years,[77,88,139,482] but it had never before been ascribed a role in the production of venous thrombosis. The endothelial cells appeared to be intact on scanning electron microscopy suggesting that the damage was produced by the white cells, rather than the endothelial cell injury or activation (see below) resulting in white cell invasion.

Stewart *et al.*[423] also studied the consequences of white cell invasion at 6 and 24 hours, and at 3, 7, 15 and 28 days after the initial insult. At 6 hours white cell invasion was still apparent and amorphous material had accumulated on the areas of vein wall denuded of epithelium. One vein was said to contain a 'typical' venous thrombus consisting of red cells enmeshed with fibrin. By 24 hours the subendothelial white cells were no longer visible but the endothelium was extensively damaged with amorphous material scattered over its surface. After 28 days the appearances were returning to normal but the amorphous material and giant cells could still be seen.

Stewart[421] has emphasized the importance of 'early' examination of experimentally thrombosed veins, as many of the minor changes which she observed could easily have been missed because they disappeared within 24 hours. These changes were only clearly seen with scanning electron microscopy and would not have been detected by standard histological preparations. The endothelial damage is patchily distributed, and leucocytes have a short life span and rapidly disappear.[82]

The jugular vein that had not been occluded showed a few adherent white cells without evidence of migration or endothelial shedding. This indicated that extensive distant tissue damage was capable of producing only minor local vessel wall changes if stasis was absent. Stewart suggested[421] that the leucotactic stimulus might be a component of the complement system activated by the release of antigen–antibody complexes[61] or endotoxins,[148,204,422] though any factor capable of increasing endothelial permeability might be responsible. She felt that the stasis effect was not the result of ischaemic damage,[421] but that stasis increased the leucotactic gradient, thus enhancing white cell migration. Stasis may also alter the activity of coagulation and adhesion factors and, if these factors accumulate on the vessel wall as a result of the injury, stasis may promote thrombosis.

Collagen is one of the best known stimuli of platelet activation and adhesion.[20,59,60,142,201,202,204,206,369,370,411,412,491] The small gaps in the endothelium described by Stewart *et al.*,[424] which may also be caused by the venous distension, may be sufficient to initiate thrombosis.

Anoxia is also known to produce endothelial activation and/or injury.[220] It has been suggested that a hypoxia may be produced within the valve cusps which may lead to endothelial malfunction or shedding.[174]

Regardless of whether thrombosis is the result of venous distension, mild anoxia or leucocyte

Table 8.1 Agents which are noxious to endothelium

Anoxia
Distension
Antibodies against endothelium
Sensitized lymphocytes
Circulating immune complexes
Complement and leucocytes
Oxygen free radicals
Platelet aggregations
Serotonin (5-hydroxytryptamine)
Adenosine diphosphate
Histamine
Prostaglandins
Increased wall shear
Thrombin

migration, it may develop without overt macroscopic or histological signs of endothelial damage (Table 8.1).

Stewart has provided further support for her theory by showing that white cells are capable of binding fibrin and producing a red 'fibrin' venous type of thrombus rather than the platelet (arterial) thrombus that usually occurs on exposed collagen.

Doubt has been cast on Stewart's theory by Thomas *et al.*,[437] who re-examined the effect of a severe local venous crushing injury on the development of thrombosis in the jugular veins of rabbits. They found that though platelets rapidly adhered to the damaged surface, there was no fibrin formation at the injured site and the subsequent addition of stasis failed to generate stasis thrombi. They therefore failed to confirm Stewart's findings and concluded that even severe vessel wall injury was a poor stimulus to fibrin formation at the site of injury.

We have not found any evidence of white cell adherence in those of our human or animal models of thrombosis where the wall is not damaged by finger compression. There is also no evidence that local blood levels of soluble adhesion molecules are raised during early thrombosis, although expression of soluble vascular cell adhesion molecule-1 (VCAM-1) is increased in patients who present with a deep vein thrombosis.[354]

Comment

Stewart's experiments have given considerable support to the concept of endothelial injury but there remain misgivings about the role of this mechanism in the genesis of human deep vein thrombosis, and a more subtle change of endothelial cell function remains a credible alternative. Improved

methods of producing experimental thrombi may help to define the role of endothelial injury.[229]

ENDOTHELIAL CELL ACTIVATION

The endothelium is far from the inert lining to blood vessels that it was once considered to be, but is instead a highly specialized, metabolically active organ. Resting endothelial cells form a monolayer maintaining a barrier between blood constituents and the extravascular space, but they also exert homeostatic effects (see Table 8.2).

The quiescent endothelium maintains the status quo, but under the stimulation of certain cytokines such as interleukin-1 (IL-1) and tumour necrosis factor (TNF) it undergoes a series of metabolic changes and participates in the inflammatory process. This process, known as endothelial cell activation, may have an important pathophysiological role in the development of atherosclerosis, the systemic inflammatory response, the vasculitidies, transplant rejection and diabetes, but its role in the development of deep vein thrombosis has been poorly studied. The work of Stewart (see above) suggests that it may be a factor in the development of deep vein thrombosis.

The term endothelial cell activation was proposed in the late 1960s by Willms-Kretshmer[477] to describe the vascular response in hapten-specific delayed hypersensitivity and contact dermatitis. In delayed hypersensitivity reactions it was observed that venules became leaky and their endothelial cell linings became plump, protruding into the lumen. These endothelial cells also displayed increased quantities of endoplasmic reticulum. Willms-Kretshmer referred to these endothelial cells as being 'activated', implying that there was a functional consequence of the altered morphology. This theory that the endothelium had a dynamic function was ignored in the 1970s because the endothelium was considered to be inert and passive. There was, however, a growing realization that when endothelial cells were exposed, *in vitro*, to cytokines that mediate the inflammatory

Table 8.2 Functions of the vascular endothelium

Maintenance of selective permeability
Integration and transduction of blood-borne signals
Regulation of inflammatory and immune reactions
Regulation of vascular tone
Maintenance of thromboresistance
Modulation of leucocyte interactions with tissues
Regulation of vascular growth

response, they developed new surface molecules and biological functions. To emphasize that this process did not represent a severe injury with consequent dysfunction, Pober reintroduced the term endothelial cell activation with the following definition: 'a quantitative change in the level of expression of certain gene products (i.e. proteins) that, in turn, endow endothelial cells with new capacities that allow endothelial cells to perform new functions'.[347]

Agents that are capable of inducing endothelial cell activation include the cytokines interleukin-1 and tumour necrosis factor, bacterial endotoxin/lipopolysaccharide, complement, viral infections and immune complexes. Knowledge concerning endothelial cell activation is largely based on in-vitro stimulation of these cells by interleukin-1, tumour necrosis factor or lipopolysaccharide. Pober and Cotran[348] have distinguished two types of endothelial cell response; the first, 'endothelial cell stimulation', does not require protein synthesis or gene upregulation (e.g. the release of von Willebrand factor) and the second, 'endothelial cell activation', which does. Thus endothelial cell activation requires a period of time for the stimulating agent to cause its effect. For instance, expression of tissue factor by endothelial cells in culture occurs after 4–6 hours, whereas in endothelial cell stimulation the response occurs within seconds.[26]

Endothelial cell stimulation causes retraction of endothelial cells from one another, exposing the underlying subendothelium. This is accompanied by translocation of P-selectin, release of von Willebrand factor and secretion of platelet activating factor.[26] Endothelial cell activation *in vitro* causes progressive transcription of many genes including leucocyte adhesion molecules (E-selectin, ICAM-1, and VCAM-1), cytokines (IL-1, IL-6, IL-8) and monocyte chemoattractant protein, and tissue factor which is the main initiator of coagulation. Thrombomodulin and other important molecules are lost from the surface of endothelial cells.[27]

The changes in endothelial cell activation

There are five main changes associated with endothelial cell activation: loss of vascular integrity; expression of leucocyte adhesion molecules; secretion of cytokines; prothrombotic changes and upregulation of human leucocyte antigen molecules.

Loss of vascular integrity

After endothelial cells are stimulated by agents such as thrombin or histamine, they retract from one another, leaving gaps that allow cells and proteins to pass from the intravascular space into the underlying tissue space.[26]

Expression of leucocyte adhesion molecules

Leucocyte–endothelial interactions involve four sequential steps of tethering, triggering, strong adhesion and migration.[4,78]

Tethering of circulating leucocytes to the endothelium results in their rolling along the vessel wall. Tethering is mediated by the selectins. E-selectin is synthesized and expressed by endothelial cells when activated by cytokines.[4,78] P-selectin is expressed by activated endothelium and by platelets. It is present on the inner surface of intracellular storage bodies, known as Weibel–Palade bodies, in the cytoplasm of endothelial cells and by the alpha granules of the platelets[4,78] These bodies also store von Willebrand factor. On stimulation of endothelial cells the Weibel–Palade bodies fuse with the endothelial cell surface membrane, discharging their contents and exposing P-selectin.[4,78] Surface expression of P-selectin is rapid and transient, peaking at 10 minutes and returning to normal by 20–30 minutes.[4,78] L-selectin is constitutively expressed on most leucocytes.[4,78] Each selectin recognizes specific carbohydrate motifs on either endothelial cells or leucocytes. The endothelial cell selectins extend beyond the surrounding glycocalyx, so allowing capture of circulating leucocytes that express the appropriate receptor.

This loose association of leucocyte and endothelium allows exposure to triggering factors which activate leucocyte integrins. Activation of leucocytes triggers an increase in avidity caused by a conformational change in the integrin heterodimer. Once activated, the leucocyte integrins bind to counter receptors on the endothelium – endothelial cell adhesion molecules, which are members of the immunoglobulin gene superfamily. The β2 integrins bind to intercellular adhesion molecules 1 and 2 (ICAM-1) and ICAM-2. ICAM-2 is constitutively expressed on the endothelium, but ICAM-1 is increased by endothelial cell activation and inflammation. The β1 integrin mediates binding of lymphocytes and monocytes to vascular cell adhesion molecule 1 (VCAM-1), which is induced by proinflammatory cytokines. Important triggering factors are IL-8, produced by the endothelium itself or underlying inflammatory cells; platelet activating factor, a phospholipid that is rapidly produced by endothelium in response to thrombin, histamine or leukotrienes; monocyte inhibiting protein-1β bound to endothelial proteoglycans; bacterial wall components; and complement activation products. Leucocytes migrate into the tissues following strong adhesion to the endothelium. Many of the cytokines that trigger strong adhesion are also chemotactic. Interleukin-8 induces adhesion and chemotaxis of neutrophils and monocyte inhibiting protein-1β induces adhesion and migration of T lymphocytes.

Diseases characterized by acute inflammation and neutrophil infiltration show increased expression of E- and P-selectin, whereas in chronic lymphocytic inflammation there is increased VCAM-1 expression. Different combinations of cytokines alter the type of inflammatory response that develops. There are also differences in the ability to express these molecules between the endothelium of large vessels and that of the microvasculature.

Cytokine production

Cytokines are important mediators of inflammation. They promote immunity and host defence in infectious disease, and also augment the response to non-infectious inflammatory states contributing to tissue injury. The endothelium is an important source as well as a target of these molecules. Endothelial cells synthesize large amounts of IL-6 that affects the proliferation of T and B lymphocytes and regulates production of acute phase proteins in the liver. Stimulation of the endothelium with lipopolysaccharides, tumour necrosis factor and IL-1 induces interleukin production by endothelial cells, which amplifies the inflammatory response.[266] The endothelium also releases chemoattractants such as IL-8 and monocyte chemoattractant protein 1.[280]

Prothrombotic changes

The antithrombotic activity of the resting endothelium can be separated into antiplatelet, anticoagulant and fibrinolytic actions. The prothrombotic activity of the endothelium is caused by a loss of antithrombotic activity and the expression of prothrombotic molecules.

Antiplatelet/vasodilator effects

Endothelial cells prevent thrombosis by synthesizing and releasing prostacyclin, nitric oxide, and also ecto-adenosine diphosphatase, all of which reduce platelet activity.[27,105,276,281]

Prostacyclin

Prostacyclin is a potent inhibitor of platelet aggregation and a powerful vasodilator.[302] Prostacyclin is a very unstable prostaglandin with a half-life in serum of approximately 2 minutes. It was first isolated, from arterial walls in 1976 by Moncada and his colleagues.[301] It prevents platelet aggregation by

increasing the intracellular concentration of cyclic adenosine diphosphate,[435] which in turn blocks the synthesis of thromboxane by the platelets. There is a report[252] of a single patient with prostacyclin deficiency who experienced recurrent deep vein thromboses and spontaneous abortions and who later developed ovarian infarction and aortic thrombosis. No prostacyclin activity was detectable in tissue biopsies of this patient's arterial wall, and a sample of the patient's plasma abolished prostacyclin production by a rat aorta. Further studies are required to determine whether prostacyclin plays an important role in the aetiology of venous thrombosis.

Nitric oxide

Nitric oxide is a potent inhibitor of platelet aggregation and works synergistically with prostacyclin.[105] The vascular relaxant and platelet inhibitory action of nitric oxide are produced by stimulation of soluble guanylate cyclase, which raises cyclic guanidine monophosphate levels in smooth muscle and platelets. This contrasts with the actions of prostacyclin, many of which are the result of a rise in cyclic adenosine monophosphate levels. Unlike prostacyclin, nitric oxide also inhibits platelet adhesion to subendothelium.

Nitric oxide synthetase is the enzyme responsible for synthesizing nitric oxide. There are two main classes of this enzyme: one is constitutively expressed by endothelial cells, neuronal cells and several other cell types and is regulated by calcium and calmodulin. Nitric oxide is released from the endothelium under basal conditions, and also released by a number of physiological stimuli such as shear stress. It is also released by the action of circulating hormones, such as noradrenaline, vasopressin, bradykinin and various autacoids such as acetylcholine, histamine and substance P. Shear stress, in particular, appears to be a major stimulus for its release, for nitric oxide activity is highest in large arteries that are subject to greater variation in pulsatile flow and shear stress.

The other class of nitric oxide synthetase is an inducible enzyme which is found in macrophages and neutrophils. It is induced by cytokine exposure and is capable of generating far greater quantities of nitric oxide than the constitutively expressed form. In high concentrations nitric oxide is cytotoxic and plays a key role in eliminating bacteria and other pathogens.

Platelet activation

Platelet activating factor is rapidly produced by many of the agonists that induce prostacyclin synthesis and causes platelet secretion and aggregation.

Activated platelets release adenosine triphosphate and adenosine diphosphate from their dense granules. Adenine nucleotides are relatively stable and are degraded by ectonucleotidases present at the endothelial cell surface. Thus endothelial cells can inhibit platelet aggregation, in part, by an increase in ecto-adenosine diphosphatase activity. Endothelial cells also convert adenosine monophosphate to adenosine which also inhibits platelet aggregation.

Adenosine diphosphatase is the enzyme which converts adenosine diphosphate to adenosine monophosphate and adenosine, both of which inhibit platelet aggregation.[190,191] When endothelial cells are activated *in vitro*, platelet aggregation occurs and there is an associated loss of ecto-adenosine diphosphatase activity, which permits accumulation of adenosine diphosphate, a potent stimulus to platelet thrombosis.

Endothelin

Endothelin is the most potent vasoconstrictor known at present, and is capable of causing contraction of isolated arteries and veins. It is released in response to hypoxia, thrombin, transforming growth factor β and noradrenaline. After binding to specific receptors, endothelin promotes influx of calcium ions and release of calcium from intracellular stores, resulting in phosphorylation of myosin light chains which initiates smooth muscle contraction. It also has mitogenic properties, stimulating DNA synthesis in vascular smooth muscle, and more recently has been shown to stimulate neutrophil adhesion to endothelial cells.

Anticoagulant pathways

Heparin sulphate

The endothelium of the aorta, veins and microcirculation exerts an important anticoagulant effect by expressing glycosaminoglycans.[160,220,321] Approximately 80% of the glycosaminoglycans are in the form of heparan sulphate.[72,244,305] Smaller quantities of hyaluronic acid, chondroitin sulphate and heparin are also present in the vessel wall and are of doubtful significance. Heparan sulphate potentiates antithrombin, which is a major physiological anticoagulant. Antithrombin is an irreversible inhibitor, not only of thrombin as the name suggests, but of the majority of intrinsic coagulation proteases. Heparan sulphate acts by accelerating the inactivation of thrombin by antithrombin, but it also carries a strongly negative surface charge (as does heparin), and this may help to maintain the ability of the endothelium to act as a continuous membrane and to resist thrombus forming on its

surface.[388] There is at present insufficient information to attribute a role to surface glycosaminoglycans in the development of venous thrombosis.

Heparan sulphate proteoglycans are the main proteoglycans found in the endothelium. Cytokines stimulate synthesis of the glycosaminoglycans whilst physical injury, hypoxia and viral infection decrease their synthesis.[216]

During inflammation heparan sulphate is released from the endothelium. Cleavage of the glycosaminoglycan chains by heparanases, produced by many cells including activated platelets, activated endothelial cells and activated T cells is one of the mechanisms for its release. Proteases from activated T cells and neutrophil elastase may also cause its release through proteolysis of the protein core. The binding of antibodies to endothelial cells and the activation of complement also causes rapid release of heparan sulphate.

Apart from its anticoagulant function, heparan sulphate is also important in maintaining vascular integrity and its loss from the endothelial cell surface may result in oedema and the exudation of plasma proteins. There is also some evidence that heparan sulphate can influence cellular immune responses through interactions with antigen presenting cells. Heparan sulphate tethers extracellular superoxide dismutase, an important naturally occurring free radical scavenger, to the vessel wall. The loss of heparan sulphate during endothelial cell activation thus results in the loss of its anticoagulant and anti-free radical actions.

Thrombomodulin

Thrombomodulin is another glycoprotein which is expressed on the endothelial cell surface. This glycoprotein is an important receptor in the protein C anticoagulant system.[130] This system is activated when coagulation is initiated and thrombin is generated. Thrombin bound to thrombomodulin on the surface of endothelial cells activates protein C. Thrombin once bound to thrombomodulin loses its coagulant activity and is no longer able to convert fibrinogen to fibrin, or activate platelets. Activated protein C, together with its cofactor protein S, acts as an anticoagulant by inactivating factors Va and VIIIa, thus limiting further thrombin generation.

Endothelial activation results in the loss of thrombomodulin from the endothelial cell surface. This is the result of thrombomodulin being internalized in the cells and by decreased transcription of mRNA with a subsequent decrease in thrombomodulin synthesis.[303] Thrombomodulin is absent from the human cerebral endothelium and other anticoagulant pathways such as protease nexin II may be important here.

Tissue factor pathway inhibitor

Tissue factor pathway inhibitor is produced by the endothelium and inhibits the first steps of the extrinsic coagulation pathway by inhibiting factor and the tissue factor/VIIa complex.[355] Much of circulating tissue factor pathway inhibitor is bound to lipoprotein, and platelets carry about 10% of the circulating tissue factor pathway inhibitor, which they release upon activation. This inhibitor is also released into the circulation in response to heparin and other glycosaminoglycans, although to a lesser degree.[385] It has been suggested that tissue factor pathway inhibitor is bound to endothelial cell glycosaminoglycans, but this has not been confirmed. The main physiological role of tissue factor pathway inhibitor appears to be in the inhibition of small amounts of tissue factor and it is thus probably essential for maintaining a normal haemostatic balance.

Procoagulant effects: von Willebrand factor

Von Willebrand factor (vWF) is stored in Weibel–Palade bodies of endothelial cells and in alpha granules in platelets. It is also present free in plasma and anchored in the subendothelium.[54,197,221] When platelets are activated, this factor acts as the ligand for platelet adhesion by binding to a specific receptor, glycoprotein Ib. Following endothelial cell stimulation, Weibel–Palade bodies fuse with the endothelial cell membrane, releasing von Willebrand factor.[153] The inner surface of the Weibel–Palade bodies is coated with P-selectin, which is thus expressed on the endothelial cell surface.[288] In the plasma, von Willebrand factor also acts as the carrier for factor VIII; thus, in von Willebrand's disease, levels of factor VIII are reduced. Plasma levels are increased by its release from endothelial cells and platelets at sites of thrombosis, endothelial cell activation and injury. Levels also increase as part of the acute phase response.[73,324] This elevation may be important in the development of postoperative thrombosis but this has not yet been confirmed.

Tissue factor

Tissue factor is an important membrane component that serves as the essential cofactor for coagulation factor VII/VIIa, which subsequently activates factor X and has also been shown to activate factor IX.[315] Tissue factor is strongly expressed in all solid tissues, especially vascular adventitial cells, forming a haemostatic envelope around blood vessels; thus, if a vessel is injured, extra-endothelial tissue factor initiates coagulation.[121] It is not expressed on endothelium, but in-vitro expression can be induced on monocytes and endothelium 2–6 hours after stimulation with IL-1, tumour necrosis factor or lipopolysaccharide, and it may cause activation of coagulation and clot formation.[48]

Stimulation of platelets or endothelium by complement results in deposition of C5–9 and subsequent vesiculation of platelet membranes. These vesicles are endowed with prothrombinase activity. This phenomenon also occurs with endothelial cell activation.

Fibrinolytic system

The fibrinolytic system is responsible for thrombus and clot breakdown and may therefore be important in wound healing. Plasmin is produced from its inactive precursor plasminogen by the action of tissue plasminogen activator which, with its inhibitor, plasminogen activator inhibitor type I, is produced by the endothelium.[127] Tissue plasminogen activator is released in response to a number of different stresses including stasis, adrenaline, desmopressin, and exercise.[22,61,134,327] Stimulation of endothelial cells with cytokines such as tumour necrosis factor or lipopolysaccharides leads to unaltered or decreased secretion of tissue plasminogen activator, but enhanced plasminogen activator inhibitor 1 release.[312] This results in an overall reduction of fibrinolytic activators and reduced fibrinolytic potential.[127,312,390]

Defective production or release of activator from the vein wall has been found to be associated with recurrent deep vein thrombosis,[92,218,226,237,262,417,427,430] but production and release is increased by other types of injury.[485] Reduced levels of vein wall activator are found in patients with severe lipodermatosclerosis or post-thrombotic deep vein damage. It is not clear, however, if this is the cause or the result of the initial thrombotic episode[68,481] (see Chapter 15).

Reduced levels of fibrinolytic activity have been detected in the soleal veins which are often the first veins to develop thrombus,[316] but this finding has not been confirmed.[109,263] The fibrinolytic activity of the vein wall declines with age,[227] as the risk of postoperative deep vein thrombosis increases.

Nilsson *et al.*[326] studied plasminogen activator release in a group of patients with recurrent deep vein thromboses and found reduced levels of activator production in some patients and normal levels of activator release with elevated levels of inhibitor in others. They have suggested that high levels of tissue plasminogen activator inhibitor might be responsible for recurrent thromboses in some patients. Doubt has been cast on the validity of this study because activator and inhibitor levels were measured after the thrombosis had occurred and might be an effect of repeated thromboses rather than the cause.[255]

High levels of plasminogen activator inhibitor 1 have not been clearly shown to relate to an increased risk of venous thrombosis.[352,429] All these observations on the association between alterations in fibrinolysis and venous thrombosis support the hypothesis that endothelial cell activation or injury may therefore be an important cause of venous thrombosis.

The intracellular mechanisms underlying endothelial cell activation

Endothelial cell activation is under the control of gene transcription.[29] After a stimulating agent attaches to its receptor on the endothelial cell surface, the message is transmitted into the cell cytoplasm to a transcription factor nuclear factor κB (NF-κB). Most inducible transcriptional activators are stimulated by a limited number of physiological agents, but NF-κB, however, is activated by a large variety of agents and represents a major threat to the organism. The genes that are upregulated during endothelial cell activation *in vitro* (e.g. tissue factor, plasminogen activator inhibitor, E-selectin) contain binding sites for NF-κB in their promoter area. NF-κB is stored in an inactive form in the cytoplasm, and is activated by the removal of an inhibitory subunit, IκB.[188] In the absence of IκB, exposed sequences on the NF-κB dimer composed of p50 and p65 (RelA) subunits are recognized by a receptor and transported into the nucleus, where binding to DNA regulatory sequences initiates transcription of the genes involved in endothelial cell activation. NF-κB binding sites are found in the regulatory region of all the genes that are induced as part of endothelial cell activation.[91]

Comment

Endothelial cell activation appears to be an effector mechanism in the inflammatory response and is thus an important component of the pathophysiological response to injury. Endothelial cell activation may also play a role in the pathogenesis of venous thrombosis. There is considerable scope, for future research and further evidence must be produced before this mechanism is generally accepted. Alterations in the the antithrombotic effect of the endothelium may initiate or occur during the pathogenesis of deep vein thrombosis.

Table 8.3 Techniques that have been used for measuring venous blood flow

Sodium-24 clearance[482]
[125]I Hippuran clearance[180]
Xenon clearance[43]
Thermodilution[43]
Plethysmographic venous emptying[43]
Serial phlebography[321]
Arterial inflow[70]

STASIS

There are a number of clinical conditions in which obstructed or defective venous drainage is known to be associated with an increased risk of thrombosis, supporting the hypothesis that stasis is a causal agent for thrombosis. These conditions include partial caval obstruction during pregnancy,[236] iliac vein obstruction by a transplanted kidney,[225] the left common iliac vein compression syndrome[87,286] and paralysed calf muscles.[95,149,462]

Any assessment of the role of postoperative venous stasis in the genesis of deep vein thrombosis is affected by the technique used to measure venous blood flow. All the techniques shown in Table 8.3 have been used to measure the velocity of venous return from the lower limbs after surgery. Most of these techniques, however, measure superficial vein blood flow from the skin and subcutaneous tissues which may not be the same as deep vein blood flow. In an attempt to separate blood flow changes in the deep and superficial veins, Nicolaides *et al.*[317,321] combined serial phlebography with isotope clearance studies. They found a rapid rate of flow in the major limb veins and a reduced flow from the soleal sinusoids. This study has, however, been criticized on the grounds that flow measured by the serial phlebography is affected by the density of the contrast medium.[43]

After drawing attention to the development of thrombi in the apices of the valve pockets (Figure 8.3), McLachlin and his colleagues,[293] using cinephlebography, showed that contrast medium remained in the valve sinuses for 30–60 minutes if the calf muscles were not exercised. This finding was confirmed by Cotton and Clark[96] who suggested that eddy currents within the valve pocket might encourage the deposition of platelets and thrombus (Figure 8.4). The presence of vortices within the valve pockets is known to increase the risk of thrombus deposition.[232,409,418] Although McLachlin[293] and Sevitt[396] found that thrombi may develop in any valve sinus of the lower limb, the fibrinogen uptake test has shown that the majority of

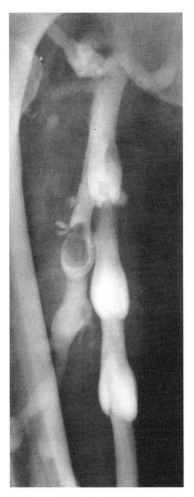

Figure 8.3 A phlebograph showing a thrombus within a valve cusp. The valve sinus was thought, by McLachlin *et al.*[293] to be the site of origin of all deep vein thrombi.

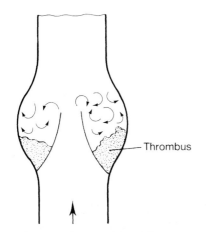

Figure 8.4 A diagram showing blood flow past a venous valve with the arrows showing the 'vorticeal' flow setting up 'eddy currents' which allow platelet and thrombus deposition within the valve cusp.

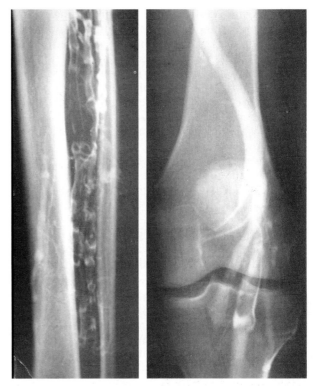

Figure 8.5 Extensive thrombosis in the calf veins extending up to the popliteal vein. There is no thrombus within the femoral vein.

thrombi begin in the calf veins or soleal sinusoids below the knee; this observation has been confirmed by phlebography (Figures 8.1 and 8.5).[71,320]

The calf pump does not function during general anaesthesia with muscle relaxation, calf blood flow, and consequently venous velocity falls. The reduction of calf blood flow may persist for 7 days after an operation,[65,270] and any increase in blood viscosity reduces the flow rate still further.[119,466]

The studies of Wessler,[470,471] and those of Stewart,[421,422] have shown that stasis is not the prime cause of experimental venous thrombosis, but stasis is undoubtedly a strong potentiating factor which, when combined with one of the other two major mechanisms, will cause thrombosis.

ABNORMALITIES OF HAEMOSTASIS

Although intravascular thrombosis does not readily occur in an occluded segment of vein, Wessler[470] showed that thrombosis did accompany stasis if it was preceded by activation of the clotting mechanism; he achieved this experimentally by infusing heterologous serum before producing venous stasis. Thrombus was not produced by either the serum infusion or the stasis alone, but only by their combination and then only if the serum infusion preceded the stasis. The thrombi that formed within the veins in response to these combined stimulae bore a closer resemblance to red propagated thrombus than to the laminated platelet/fibrin thrombus that appears to initiate deep vein thrombosis in man. Fibrin, platelets and leucocytes adhered to the surface of these 'stasis thrombi' if they were left in a free-flowing circulation.[438]

The results of these experiments suggest that hypercoagulability, at either a local or distant site, is an essential factor in the initiation of deep vein thrombosis. Abnormalities of the blood such as polycythaemia rubra vera, leukaemia, multiple myeloma and other macroglobulinaemias, all of which raise blood viscosity, are associated with an increased risk of deep vein thrombosis.

Changes in the coagulation factors and their inhibitors perioperatively

Macfarlane originally observed in 1937 that increased fibrinolytic activity occurs during and shortly after an operation.[272] He observed that blood removed from a patient immediately after a cholecystectomy clotted normally but was 'quite fluid' when inspected the following day.

Haemostatic activation is thought to occur intraoperatively as a result of physiological stress. The type of anaesthetic technique used can indirectly alter the haemostatic balance as levels of von Willebrand factor and factor VIII are increased by plasma levels of arginine vasopressin. The latter can be increased by an anaesthetic agent such as enflurane.[245] The procoagulant activity of monocytes is directly inhibited by anaesthetics.[85]

Postoperatively there is an acute phase response which results in an increase in the concentration of coagulation factors including fibrinogen, prothrombin and factors V, VII and XII.[141] The fibrinogen half-life also decreases, presumably a reflection of the increased turnover of coagulation factors.[106,192] The levels of fibrinopeptide A and thrombin–antithrombin complexes increase, indicating that thrombin activation is taking place. The rise in plasma fibrinogen concentration increases blood viscosity which in turn slows venous blood.[284]

Postoperatively there is a coincidental rise in the platelet count[125,157,487] and a decrease in fibrinolytic potential as part of the acute phase response - 'the postoperative shut down'.[185] The blood levels of any of the haemostatic factors are unable to predict the development of postoperative thrombosis.[432] The preoperative blood level of fibrinopeptide A, which is released in the late stages of the coagulation, also

appears to be unrelated to the development of thrombosis.[440] Levels of factor XII (Hageman factor) have been reported to be reduced postoperatively.[186]

Blood fibrinolytic activity rapidly increases after trauma[13,40,192,336] and then falls over the next 24–48 hours.[279,336,487] The extent of this fall was shown by Browse *et al.*[68] to relate to the presence of malignancy and to the presence, rather than the development, of a thrombosis. Becker[35] and Reilly *et al.*[358] were unable to correlate the preoperative fibrinolytic status of the blood with the risk of postoperative thrombosis but in retrospective and prospective studies other workers have found that patients developing postoperative thrombi have significantly lower levels of blood fibrinolytic activity.[2,140,158,279]

THROMBOPHILIA

During the last 30 years more information about haemostasis and the endothelium has appeared and, though the role of stasis is still widely accepted as a major contributory factor in the development of venous thrombosis, most of the current arguments concern the relative significance of endothelial abnormalities and hypercoagulability of the blood.

Familial clustering of venous thromboembolic events was observed at the start of this century, but it was not until the 1970s when a better understanding of haemostasis allowed the genetic defects associated with familial thrombosis to be unravelled. This led to the definition of a new group of haemostatic disorders collectively categorized as thrombophilia (Table 8.4). Thrombophilia is the

Table 8.4 The known abnormalities associated with thrombophilia

Defect	Approximate incidence (%)
Antithrombin deficiency	0.05
Protein C deficiency	0.2
Protein S deficiency	<0.2
Activated protein C resistance/factor V Leiden	5.0
Hereditary dysfibrinogenaemia	?
Thrombomodulin deficiency	?
Hyperhomocysteinaemia	0.0003
Plasminogen deficiency	?
Factor XII deficiency	?
Elevated factor VIII levels	?
Antiphospholipid syndrome	Variable

term applied when there is an increased tendency to develop thrombosis as the result of a primary disorder of the coagulation system.[362] The predisposing defects do not necessarily cause continuous impairment, but they weaken the ability to cope with prothrombotic stimuli induced by enviromental changes such as surgery. Clinicians usually apply the term thrombophilia to a subset of patients who tend to have thrombosis at an early age of onset, who have frequent recurrences when not treated and often have a strong family history.[436] The thromboses are usually episodic, separated by long, trouble-free periods, suggesting that there is a trigger for each event.

Thrombophilia can either be inherited or acquired. Inherited thrombophilia is a genetically determined tendency to venous thrombosis. Dominant abnormalities or combinations of less severe defects may be clinically apparent from an early age of onset, frequent recurrence and a significant family history. Milder traits may be discovered only by laboratory investigation. During a 3-year period in 1992, 392 adult patients were screened for thrombophilia[296] and a congenital deficiency state was present in nearly a third. With the discovery of activated protein C (APC) resistance, this figure is now likely to be even higher as Dahlbeck[101–103] showed that this was present in 40% of a population with deep vein thromboses. All the genetic influences and their interactions are not yet understood.

Each condition is reviewed below and the conditions causing thrombophilia are summarized in Table 8.4.

Antithrombin deficiency (formally known as antithrombin III deficiency)

In 1965, Egeberg[124] described a Norwegian family that had suffered from recurrent venous thromboses in whom low levels of antithrombin were found. The antithrombin levels in those members of the family (and some of their near relatives) who had had a thrombosis were found to be half the normal value. Antithrombin deficiency appears to be transmitted as an autosomal dominant. Since the original report many other families who have this deficiency have been described[167,168,277,386,456,457] and the abnormality has been estimated to occur in one in every 2000 families.[366,367]

Acquired antithrombin deficiency can develop in patients with the nephrotic syndrome (as the result of loss of the protein in the urine). It can also be caused by increased consumption: in patients with an acute venous thrombosis and in those receiving heparin.[456] It can develop postoperatively[342,416] and in women who are taking the contraceptive pill.[455]

All these conditions are known to predispose to venous thrombosis.

Like other causes of thrombophilia, a second 'insult', such as an operation,[471] in the presence of antithrombin deficiency, increases the risk of thrombosis. It may account for up to 4% of familial thromboses and by the age of 50 years, 85% of those affected have suffered a thrombosis.

Antithrombin deficiency is a heterogenous disorder. There are two types of the disorder: type I antithrombin deficiency in which there is a reduction of both the functional and immunological antithrombin; and type II antithrombin deficiency where there is a functional defect but no immunological defect. From a clinical viewpoint the mutations causing type II deficiency have a lesser risk of thrombosis.[251]

Antithrombin is a single chain glycoprotein (58 kDa) which belongs to the superfamily of serine protease inhibitors (serpins). It is synthesized by the liver and its concentration in the plasma is 2.5 μM. It is a primary inhibitor of thrombin formation and also inhibits most of the other activated serine proteases in the blood such as factor IXa, Xa, XIIa and kallikrein by forming a 1:1 bond with the active site of the protease. Inhibition is relatively slow but can be accelerated at least 1000-fold by heparin and heparin-like substances.[249]

The gene coding for antithrombin III is on chromosome 1 between 1q23 and 1q25. Several sequence variations or polymorphisms have been described within the human gene including a highly polymorphic trinucleotide repeat in intron 4, which is useful for haplotype analysis.[250] A 1993 database of mutations lists 39 distinct mutations and nine whole or partial gene deletions (>30 base pairs).

The presence of antithrombin deficiency appears to constitute a greater risk for thrombosis than congenital deficiencies of either protein C or protein S.[111,136]

Protein C deficiency

Protein C is a vitamin K-dependent plasma glycoprotein which is the inactive precursor of the serine proteinase-activated protein C (APC). Protein C is activated by thrombin and this reaction is accelerated by the binding of thrombin to thrombomodulin, a receptor on endothelial cells. Activated protein C, once formed, inactivates the cofactors factor Va and VIIIa by proteolytic cleavage. To do this efficiently it needs to form a complex with protein S on a suitable membrane surface. Apart from these anticoagulant properties it also has antifibrinolytic and anti-inflammatory effects. Protein C is synthesized in the liver, and its concentration in the plasma is 65 nM, which is reduced during treatment with oral anticoagulants.[129]

Protein C deficiency is a risk in 3–8% of a group of selected patients with recurrent venous thrombosis but it is also present in one in 500 of the normal population where it does not appear to represent a thrombosis risk.[433] It is a heterogenous disorder. Like antithrombin, it has two categories of deficiency: type I is a deficiency of both functional and immunogenic levels and type II is a deficiency of functional but not immunological levels. In 1995, an update of protein C mutations was published reporting 160 different mutations described so far.[359] Members of the family of a symptomatic heterozygote proband who are heterozygous for the mutation in protein C gene have an increased risk of venous thrombotic events compared with normal family members (4% vs 9%).[6]

Protein S deficiency

Protein S is another vitamin K-dependent plasma glycoprotein. It is synthesized in the liver, but also in endothelial cells, megakaryocytes and Leydig cells in the testis. It is a non-enzymatic cofactor of activated protein C, taking part in the inactivation of factors Va and VIIIa. In plasma, protein S circulates both free (40%) and in a 1:1 stoichiometric complex with its carrier protein C4b-binding protein.[103] Only the free form of protein S is active.

Deficiencies of protein S can be either type I (reduced levels of both functional and antigenic protein S or type II (functional abnormalities). The majority of type I deficiencies are the result of a single nucleotide substitution by insertion or deletion. So far 33 mutations have been reported.[250] Four mutations have been reported to give the type III deficiency. It tends to have a less severe outcome than protein C deficiency.

Activated protein C resistance/factor V Leiden

Activated protein C (APC) resistance was a term derived by Dahlback to describe a new thrombophilic defect he found in patients with recurrent venous thrombosis.[102] Protein C is a serine protease with potent anticoagulant properties which is activated by contact with thrombomodulin, a protein on the endothelium. During normal haemostasis, APC limits thrombus formation by protolytic inactivation of factors Va and VIIIa. The anticoagulant response to APC (APC resistance) is decreased in patients with a strong personal or family history of thrombosis.[47] Factor V is synthesized in the liver and megakaryocytes. Once activated, when it is known as FVa, it serves as a non-enzymatic cofactor in prothrombinase

(the combination of factor Xa, phospholipid, calcium), by increasing the catalytic efficiency 2000-fold. Factor Va is inactivated by proteolytic degradation by activated protein C. In activated protein C resistance there is a single point mutation in factor V in nucleotide 1691 involving a glutamine → arginine substitution. This new factor V variant is known as factor V Leiden after the town where the group discovered it.[459] The presence of factor V Leiden appears to confer a considerably increased risk of venous thrombosis.[360,431]

This discovery has far-reaching implications, as the prevalence of factor V Leiden is up to 7% in Caucasian populations, although it has a lower frequency in Japanese and other Eastern ethnic groups.[357] It is almost totally absent in Eskimos and appears to have its origin in the European Caucasian population.[110]

It appears to impart a sevenfold increase in the risk of deep vein thrombosis[243] and this increased to a 100-fold increase in homozygous cases.[101] Inherited resistance to activated protein C increases the risk of thrombosis in oral contraceptive users and also increases the risk of a thrombosis occurring during pregnancy.[187,446]

Other defects

Other defects are rare causes of thrombophilia. They include the following.

Hereditary dysfibrinogenaemia

Depending on the defect in the gene these patients have clinical symptoms which vary from none to bleeding or venous or arterial thrombosis. Only five families from five different countries have been described to have venous thromboses. Thrombosis occurred in the homozygote in only one family.[181]

Thrombomodulin

This is a transmembrane protein synthesized by endothelial cells that acts as a cofactor for the activation of protein C. Deficiencies or defects might therefore be expected to be associated with thrombosis. To date four mutations have been described.[339]

Hyperhomocysteinaemia

This is a disorder of methionine metabolism and two large studies have shown that hyperhomocysteinaemia is a rare but important risk factor for recurrent thrombosis.[11,113,114] It can lead to a two- or threefold increase in the risk of developing deep vein thrombosis, but the mechanism of thrombogenesis is unclear. It may damage endothelium clinically, it may activate factor V, inhibit thrombolysis or increase the activation of platelets. Severe hyperhomocysteinaemia occurs in approximately 1:300 000 of the population and is usually the result of homozygous cystathionine synthetase deficiency. A recently described mutation of methylenetetrafolate reductase may be a significant and frequent cause for mild hyperhomocysteinaemia.[143]

Plasminogen deficiency

This was reported to be associated with thrombophilia but this has not been confirmed in subsequent studies. Type II plasminogen deficiency associated with a point mutation at Ala601 is a common variant in the Japanese population and is not associated with an increased risk of thrombosis.[215] Another Japanese study suggests that dysplasminogenaemia is an important role factor for venous thrombosis.[234]

Heparin cofactor II deficiency

A few families have been reported where this deficiency is associated with a thrombophilic defect.[404]

Factor XII deficiency

Initial reports suggested this was associated with thrombophilia but subsequent reports have not confirmed this.[242]

Factor VIII levels

Elevated factor VIII levels have been identified as a risk factor for thrombosis. The inheritance of this has not been investigated.[243] This study suggested that blood groups other than group O and higher levels of von Willebrand factor in blood are associated with the high levels of factor VIII.

ANTIPHOSPHOLIPID ANTIBODIES

The antiphospholipid or Hughes' syndrome is the association of thromboses, recurrent abortion and thrombocytopenia with antiphospholipid antibodies. It was identified 15 years ago in a subset of patients with systemic lupus erythematosus (SLE) who were noted to have thrombotic events and false-positive serological tests for syphilis.[203] Today it is recognized that the syndrome can occur independently from other autoimmune disease, when it is designated as the primary antiphospholipid syndrome (primary

APS).[238] Secondary antiphospholipid syndrome is the term used when it is associated with other autoimmune disease, usually systemic lupus erythematosus. Antiphospholipid antibodies can be detected by assaying for the lupus anticoagulant and anticardiolipin antibodies.

Patients with antiphospholipid syndrome have many presentations and signs but the underlying pathology is always thrombosis. Histological examination of the thrombus shows it to be organized with platelets and fibrin. There is no evidence of vasculitis, which differentiates it from systemic lupus erythematosus and other autoimmune disorders where inflammatory changes are seen.[258] Thus the management of the disorder is based on antithrombotic, rather than anti-inflammatory, treatment. Unlike the congenital thrombophilias (factor V Leiden mutation, deficiencies of protein C, protein S, and antithrombin), which predispose to venous thrombosis, antiphospholipid syndrome is almost unique in predisposing patients to both venous and arterial thrombosis. Any size of vessel may be affected and no part of the circulation is spared. Clinical presentations do not seem to differ between anticardiolipin antibody and lupus anticoagulant, but, generally speaking, patients having the highest titres of antibody, particularly of the IgG isotype, have been observed to have the severest disease.

The nomenclature surrounding antiphospholipid syndrome has always been confusing. The term lupus anticoagulant is a misnomer which arose because the anticoagulant was first identified in patients with systemic lupus erythematosus. The vast majority of those with lupus anticoagulant do not, in fact, have systemic lupus erythematosus. Furthermore, the antiphospholipid antibodies detected by the assay are anticoagulant *in vitro* but are procoagulant *in vivo* and associated with thrombosis. Moreover, recent research has shown that antiphospholipid antibodies are not actually directed against phospholipid alone. The term Hughes' syndrome has been used, as Dr Graham Hughes' group originally described the condition. Some prefer terms which reflect more accurately the pathogenesis of the syndrome, such as the phospholipid-cofactor syndrome.

It is important to ask any woman with an unusual thrombotic event about her obstetric history. Recurrent fetal loss in patients with the syndrome is thought to be caused by recurrent thrombosis within the placenta, which causes intrauterine growth retardation secondary to placental insufficiency, leading eventually to intrauterine death during the second trimester.[265] Some women have recurrent first trimester miscarriages. A normal obstetric history, however, does not preclude a diagnosis of the disorder because a 'full house' of symptoms is not always present. There are some women who have recurrent pregnancy loss without having systemic thrombosis and vice versa. This may reflect the heterogeneity of antigens against which an individual's antiphospholipid antibodies are directed. Occasionally antiphospholipid develops following viral infections with Epstein–Barr virus, HIV, hepatitis C virus and syphilis.

Laboratory diagnosis

The diagnosis of antiphospholipid syndrome is based on the presence of thrombosis and/or recurrent pregnancy loss and antiphospholipid antibodies detected on at least two occasions. Antiphospholipid antibodies are detected by two laboratory assays: anticardiolipin antibodies and the lupus anticoagulant. It is important to note that an individual patient may have only one of these two types of antibodies and therefore both assays must be performed.[132]

Anticardiolipin antibody

Cardiolipin, an anionic phospholipid (diphosphatidylglycerol), is a membrane constituent found in high concentration on the inner leaflet of the mitochondrial membrane. The anticardiolipin antibody is detected using an ELISA where patient serum is added to microtitre plates coated with cardiolipin.[269]

Lupus anticoagulant

The lupus anticoagulant can produce a prolongation of the activated partial thromboplastin time.[235] Mixing lupus anticoagulant plasma with normal plasma does not correct this prolongation. This is a most important feature of the disorder because it distinguishes the lupus anticoagulant from clotting factor deficiencies, in which the addition of normal plasma corrects the coagulation abnormality. A more specific test is also performed in most laboratories, the commonest in use (in the UK) being the dilute Russell viper venom test.[442] In this assay, the anticoagulant activity of the antibody *in vitro* is accentuated by lowering the phospholipid concentration and inhibited by raising the phospholipid concentration. The latter is achieved by adding a source of phospholipid such as platelet fragments, and this procedure is known as platelet neutralization.

The mechanism by which antiphospholipid antibodies cause thrombosis

Some antibodies have been shown to have inhibitory effects on the protein C and S pathway, which is a physiological anticoagulant pathway.[371] Others have prothrombotic effects on endothelial cell surface proteins such as thrombomodulin, heparan sulphate, tissue factor and the production of prostacyclin;[196] still others enhance platelet activation.[196]

The exact mechanism by which the antibodies cause thrombosis remains unclear despite an enormous amount of research.[371] It was originally thought that the antibodies were solely directed at phospholipid, a ubiquitous constituent of cell membranes. Recent studies showed that a cofactor, β_2-glycoprotein I (β_2-GPI), is required for binding of anticardiolipin antibody. β_2-GPI has also been termed apolipoprotein H, as approximately 40% is bound to lipoproteins, but it bears no structural similarity to other apolipoproteins.[256] Human β_2-GPI is a non-complement member of the complement control protein family, a plasma glycoprotein with a molecular mass of 50 kDa. The amino acid sequence is thought to be arranged as five consensus repeats, or so-called 'sushi domains', the fifth domain containing a phospholipid-binding region.[211] It appears that anticardiolipin antibodies bind to a modified form of β_2-GPI which has been conformationally changed by binding to a microtitre plate, leading to the exposure of a previously hidden epitope. Studies of anticardiolipin antibodies and this cryptic epitope using deletional mutants of β_2-GPI and synthesized peptides have defined it as the fifth domain of β_2-GPI.

The lupus anticoagulant effect is thought to be caused by antibodies that are directed against immobilized or phospholipid-bound prothrombin. These antibodies may be directed against cryptic epitopes which are exposed when prothrombin binds to phospholipid. A small subset of patients have hypoprothrombinaemia, suggesting that their antibodies either have particularly high affinity for prothrombin or recognize circulating prothrombin in addition to bound prothrombin.

This confusing spectrum of antigenic specificities may explain the variation of clinical manifestations of the syndrome, or it may be that these mechanisms are 'red herrings' and that there is an underlying common mechanism in all cases of thrombosis which is yet to be discovered. It is not known what finally precipitates the development of thrombosis. The antibodies are known to persist for many years, and most of the time the patient is symptom free. Some believe in a 'two-hit hypothesis' – that several insults need to occur in a particular sequence in order to result in coagulation.

Clinical manifestations

Skin

Livedo reticularis occurs in 19% of individuals with the disorder.[5] The presence of livedo reticularis in a patient with a previous thrombosis is considered to be almost pathognomonic of the syndrome, so it is essential that the entire skin is examined in a good light. It is usually present on the upper arms and thighs but may be widely distributed.

Thrombocytopenia

This is a common feature of the disorder.[274] Usually patients have mild thrombocytopenia (platelet count $> 100 \times 10^9$/l), and occasionally the count falls further, but rarely below 50×10^9/l. This produces no clinical problems other than bruising but is of concern when the patient is receiving anticoagulant therapy.

Thrombocytopenia probably results from cross-reactivity of some antibodies with epitopes on the platelet membrane.[145] This causes a chronic immune-mediated thrombocytopenia as the result of increased peripheral destruction of platelets.

Clinical presentation

Venous thrombosis commonly occurs as a simple deep vein thrombosis (DVT) of the lower limb, either in conjunction with a predisposing factor such as the oral contraceptive pill[451] or without an apparent trigger.

Changes in the platelets

Platelets do not appear to play such a dominant role in the development of venous thrombosis as they do in arterial thrombosis,[306,308,396,490] Antiplatelet drugs have been shown to reduce the risk of venous thrombosis in the postoperative period[69,207] but the reduction in the incidence is small and requires a massive meta-analysis to confirm any significant effect (see Chapter 11).

After any injury there is an initial fall in the platelet count but this then rises above normal levels.[40,463] This increase in platelets is accompanied by an increase in platelet activity.[128,463,484] Despite these changes, no relationship has been found between the alteration in platelet behaviour and the risk of developing a postoperative thrombosis.[36,313] The platelet specific β-thromboglobulin, which can be measured in blood samples, does not rise significantly with the onset of thrombosis.[408]

Although thrombocytosis is frequently stated to be associated with an increased risk of deep vein thrombosis,[170] the association has not been proven[74] and the role of the platelet in the genesis of deep vein thrombosis remains obscure.

Comment

Interest in the genesis of venous thrombosis is now moving away from the relatively simple concepts of stasis, damage to the vessel wall, and changes in coagulation. More attention is being focused on the balance between activator and inhibitor substances secreted by the vessel wall and circulating levels of procoagulants and anticoagulants. Many of these compounds exist in a delicate balance in which inhibition and activation are evenly matched. Alteration of this balance may encourage thrombosis. The development of methods capable of measuring minute quantities of activators and inhibitors will allow the role of these compounds in the development of thrombosis to be determined. The factors discussed above are the prime elements in the initiation of thrombosis. These effects are potentiated by many well recognized risk factors which are discussed in the next section.

FACTORS THAT INCREASE THE RISK OF DEEP VEIN THROMBOSIS

The factors that increase the risk of deep vein thrombosis are listed in Table 8.5.

Table 8.5 Risk factors for deep vein thrombosis

Age
Sex
Season
Race
Occupation
Type of operation
Type of anaesthetic
Length of operation
Pregnancy and puerperium
General injury
Local injury
Immobilization
Bedrest
Malignancy
Previous venous thrombosis
Varicose veins
Obesity
Cardiac failure
Myocardial infarction
Arterial ischaemia
Contraceptive pill
Intravenous saline (haemodilution)
Haemostatic drugs
Other drugs
Vasculitis (Buerger's disease, Behçet's syndrome)
Congenital venous abnormalities, Klippel–Trenaunay syndrome

Age and gender

Many studies have shown that the risk of deep vein thrombosis increases with age[31,154,337,402] but the majority of large series show that the incidence of deep vein thrombosis is equal in men and women.[179]

The risk of thrombosis occurring in children is very small.[364]

Climate

It is difficult to separate the geographical and climatic factors which may influence deep vein thrombosis from racial factors but some studies suggest that thrombosis is less common in warmer countries[163,254] and during the summer months. Other investigators have suggested that there is a seasonal variation in the incidence of deep vein thrombosis with peaks in the spring and autumn,[7,337] and more pulmonary emboli have been reported during these periods.[135,182] These observations have not, however, been confirmed by studies using more objective forms of diagnosis.[14,58]

Race

There are definite differences in the incidence of deep vein thrombosis between racial groups (e.g. between the Caucasians of the USA and the Japanese,[159] and between the Negroes and Caucasians of South Africa).[224] The reason for these differences is not known; perhaps activated protein C resistance is responsible (see p. 266).

Occupation

Little is known about the influence of occupation on deep vein thrombosis but prolonged episodes of sitting during airplane flights, watching television, or being confined in an air-raid shelter have been reported to predispose to thrombosis.[198,310,319,406] (We have all seen patients who have suffered a pulmonary embolism as they walked away from an aeroplane.)

The association between sitting in cramped conditions and death from pulmonary embolism was first described in civilians sheltering in air-raid shelters during the Second World War.[406] Since the advent of air travel, long haul flights in particular, there have been many reports suggesting that people who travel long distances by air are at higher risk of deep vein thrombosis and pulmonary emboli, even in the absence of a previous history of cardiovascular problems.[126,239,298] This condition has recently been termed the 'economy class syndrome'.[100]

It has been postulated that during air travel deep vein thrombosis may occur as a result of stasis of the lower limbs exacerbated by cramped conditions and dehydration. Relative hypoxia caused by a decrease in blood oxygen tension at the lower cabin pressures used at high altitudes is also thought to contribute to the initiation of venous thrombosis in these travellers.[38,222] Others, however, believe that dehydration and cabin pressures are not predisposing factors.[28]

No prospective investigations of this phenomenon have as yet been reported. Our current understanding is therefore based on data obtained anecdotally,[51] from case reports[100,137,381] and from retrospective studies of patients who were admitted to hospitals diagnosed as having a deep vein thrombosis and who developed symptoms during or after a flight.[126,239] It is therefore not certain whether these patients already had existing symptomless thromboses prior to starting their journeys, or whether the cramped conditions during the flights precipitated the thromboses.

Operations

The type and length of surgical operations affects the incidence of postoperative deep vein thrombosis.[43]

Pregnancy

The high incidence of deep vein thrombosis during pregnancy and the puerperium has been recognized for many years.[17,443,484]

Vein trauma

The role of local vein damage and of distant trauma in deep vein thrombosis has been confirmed by a number of studies which have already been discussed (see page 255).

Prolonged immobility

The adverse effect of prolonged immobility and bedrest has been well documented.[65,76,150]

Malignant disease

In a series of autopsies in which a deep vein thrombosis was found,[414] 10% had a coincidental carcinoma of the pancreas. In 1941, Barker *et al.*[31] also found an increased risk of venous thrombosis in patients with malignant disease. These clinical studies have been confirmed by studies using the fibrinogen uptake test.[230,363]

A large study in 1992[351] found that of 263 patients with a phlebographically proven deep vein thrombosis, 29% had a coincidental cancer at the time of presentation and 7.6% of the cohort with 'idiopathic' DVTs defined at presentation went on to develop cancers, mostly within 1 year.

Previous thrombosis

A history of a previous episode of venous thrombosis and embolism is associated with an increased risk of a further deep vein thrombosis.[230,389] This is particularly apparent if it is combined with another risk factor (e.g. operation or pregnancy).

Varicose veins

The association of varicose veins and deep vein thrombosis is probably the result of superficial thrombophlebitis (a recognized risk in patients with varicose veins) spreading through communicating veins into the deep veins (see Chapter 23). This association is not universally accepted because the published evidence is conflicting.[75]

Obesity

Obesity has been shown to confer an additional risk of thrombosis on patients taking the contraceptive pill,[447] and increases the risk of postoperative deep vein thrombosis.[182,230] In three studies of predictive indices, obesity has consistently appeared as a major indicator increasing the chance of thrombosis.

Medical illness

Ochsner *et al.*[337] reported a high incidence of deep vein thrombosis in medical patients, and Short[402] subsequently drew attention to the increased incidence of deep vein thrombosis in patients with heart failure. Patients suffering from an acute myocardial infarction also have a high incidence of deep vein thrombosis and pulmonary embolism;[176,461] this may explain the reduction in mortality effected by treatment with anticoagulants.[299]

Oral contraceptives

In the 1960s it was recognized that the contraceptive pill increases the risk of thromboembolic disease.[447–449] Large scale prospective epidemiological studies have continued to confirm this association.[294,413,450] Oestrogens are known to increase the permeability of rabbit aortic wall, and this suggests that they may initiate a thrombosis by causing endothelial damage.[9] Low levels of antithrombin have also been found in patients taking oestrogen-based oral contraceptives[379] (see page 265) Oral

contraception users who are carriers of the factor V Leiden mutation or protein S deficiency are at increased risk of thrombosis.[446,452]

Hormone replacement therapy

Three papers published in the *Lancet* in 1996 all showed that there was an increased risk of deep vein thrombosis and pulmonary embolism in women currently taking this therapy.[104,162,223]

Haemodilution

It has been suggested that the administration of intravenous saline may increase the risk of deep vein thrombosis.[183]

Vasculitis

In Buerger's disease (thromboangiitis obliterans) and in Behçet's syndrome there is a vasculitis of unknown aetiology. Both conditions are associated with superficial and deep vein thrombosis, and patients with these conditions who are undergoing surgical operations probably have a higher risk of thrombotic complications. The incidence of deep venous thrombosis in patients with Behçet's syndrome was 76% in one survey.[380] Patients with Behçet's syndrome have an increased incidence of protein S deficiency.

Congenital venous abnormalities

Patients with the Klippel–Trenaunay syndrome (and probably venous angioma) have an increased incidence of spontaneous venous thromboembolism and a higher incidence of postoperative deep vein thrombosis.[32] The same is true of patients with cystic disease of the popliteal vein and thrombosis has also been reported following compression by a femoral exostosis.[237]

Hyperlipidaemia

One report suggests that this is a possible aetiological factor in deep vein thrombosis.[234]

Comment

All the conditions discussed in this section are accepted risk factors for deep vein thrombosis and are not primary causes. They are important because recognition of these factors in the presence of other major risk factors (e.g. surgery) may affect the type of prophylactic measures that are considered. Whenever possible, the summation of risk factors should be avoided. For example, patients should probably stop taking the contraceptive pill before surgery,[16,165] obese patients should try to lose weight before surgery, and a prolonged period of bedrest before an operation should be avoided if possible.

A number of predictive indices of deep vein thrombosis have been developed; these are based on the risk factors and laboratory tests of coagulability and fibrinolytic capacity. The purpose of these indices is to identify patients at increased risk so that they can be given suitable prophylaxis and if possible avoid giving unnecessary prophylaxis to patients who are unlikely to develop a thrombosis.

PREDICTIVE INDICES

Lister in 1862[261] and Ochsner *et al.* in 1951[337] recognized that a number of factors (e.g. age, operations, fractures and cardiac disease) increased the risk of deep vein thrombosis. In the 1960s, Hume[209] attempted to predict thrombosis from a series of coagulation tests but in 1973, Gallus[146] found that the partial thromboplastin time was the only coagulation test of predictive value. Nilsen *et al.*[323] showed that a high plasma fibrinogen and a low antithrombin level were indicative of an increased risk of deep vein thrombosis, and they produced a formula from these tests to aid prediction. Breneman[62,63] devised a predictive assessment from a discriminate analysis of retrospective data.

Clayton *et al.*[86] developed an extremely complicated scoring system from an analysis of the results of a number of tests of coagulation and fibrinolysis which had been carried out on a large cohort of patients undergoing operations. The presence or absence of postoperative thrombosis was diagnosed in these patients by the fibrinogen uptake test. Clayton found that the five variables which had the best predictive value were: the euglobulin clot-lysis time, age, the presence of varicose veins, fibrin-related antigen (fibrin degradation products) and the percentage overweight. This index was then examined prospectively. Nine out of 10 patients who developed a deep vein thrombosis were correctly identified[97] but the index incorrectly identified seven patients to be at 'high' risk who did not subsequently develop a thrombosis. The index was then used to determine prophylaxis;[22] patients who were predicted to develop a thrombosis were given subcutaneous heparin. The incidence of thrombosis in the 'high-risk' group who were treated with 5000 units of heparin twice a day was 3.8%; this was similar to the incidence of 4% which was found in the 'low-risk' group who were not given heparin. This was the first study to test the efficacy of a predictive index in a prospective study. It shows that this approach can be highly effective but it has not been generally adopted because of the time and cost involved in performing the laboratory tests.

Another study, by Lowe *et al.*[268] on 63 patients who had upper gastrointestinal surgery, found that five clinical variables had predictive value whereas the laboratory tests were unhelpful. The useful predictors were age, percentage overweight for age, sex, the presence of varicose veins and cigarette smoking. Lowe *et al.* also tested their index prospectively on 41 patients, and then used it to give selective prophylaxis to a further 40 patients. Deep vein thrombi developed in two of the 24 'high-risk', treated patients (8%) and in two of 16 'low-risk', untreated patients (14%). This study shows that anthropomorphic measurements can be used to predict deep vein thrombosis.

Sue-Ling *et al.*[428] identified seven factors which were then used to construct a predictive index. In descending order of predictive power these factors were: age, the euglobulin clot-lysis time, previous abdominal surgery, varicose veins, antithrombin concentration, cigarette smoking and the platelet count. Preoperatively, the predictive index correctly indentified 91% of patients who developed a deep vein thrombosis and wrongly allocated 19% of patients who did not. A shortened version of this index, based on age and euglobulin lysis time, was 91% sensitive and 63% specific. In a prospective study of 43 patients, this shortened predictive index correctly identified 93% of the patients who developed a thrombosis and wrongly allocated 17% of those who did not.

Comment

It is interesting that each of these studies searching for predictive indices has found different risk factors to be of value. The main object of these studies has been to find a way of abandoning universal deep vein thrombosis prophylaxis and replacing it by selective prophylaxis for those patients who are really at risk.

The concept is financially attractive and has the ability to reduce the incidence of side-effects of treatment. Few surgeons have, however, introduced any of these indices to their clinical practice, and most rely on clinical experience (the clinical factors of the various indices). Another interesting feature of these studies has been the regular appearance of a test of fibrinolysis among the useful tests of predictive value. This suggests that an abnormality of the control of coagulation is of major importance in the aetiology of deep vein thrombosis.

Temporal changes in a deep vein thrombus

The pathological features of a deep vein thrombus have been described in detail by Aschoff, Hadfield and Sevitt (Figure 8.6).[19,169,395]

Aschoff described the initial platelet cluster on the vessel wall as a grey amorphous thickening.[19] The next stage is the development of Aschoff's 'coral reef' or corralline thrombus produced by the deposition of more platelets on the surface of the initial platelet clump, presumably in response to adenosine diphosphate or thromboxane release. The thrombus then grows towards the centre of the vessel lumen; alternate layers of fibrin and red cells are trapped between layers consisting mainly of platelets, giving the laminated appearance known as the 'lines of Zahn' (Figure 8.6).[489] As the thrombus grows out into the bloodstream it is bent in the direction of flow, making the lines of Zahn appear curved or oblique. If this type of thrombus is viewed from its surface, it appears to have a number of ridges which are the platelet layers; the troughs in between correspond to the 'red thrombus' which is made up from fibrin and red cells and is slower to develop and earlier to retract. White cells, primarily polymorphonuclear leucocytes, are also located with the platelets.

As the coralline thrombus extends across the lumen, the flow beyond it becomes turbulent and gradually decreases. Red thrombus, a mixture of fibrin and red cells, then forms on the surface of the coralline thrombus and extends in the direction of flow (Figure 8.6). This 'propagated' thrombus develops when blood flow in the vessel is critically reduced. Propagated thrombus can form in flowing blood but when the vein is completely occluded there is usually rapid extension of this jelly-like red thrombus up to the mouth of the next major tributary. If this tributary becomes occluded, the propagated thrombus continues to extend proximally and may reach several feet in length.

When a vein becomes totally occluded by a thrombus, the thrombus begins to adhere to the endothelium and stimulate an hyperaemic inflammatory response in the vein wall (Figure 8.7). This is the origin of the subsequent processes of organization, invasion with granulation tissue, and replacement of the fibrin by fibrous tissue. If the thrombus remains loose within the lumen, the polymerization and maturation of the fibrin within the thrombus causes it to retract (Figure 8.8). Thrombus retraction and organization eventually leads to some form of recanalization and re-endothelialization.[164,391,434] This process destroys all

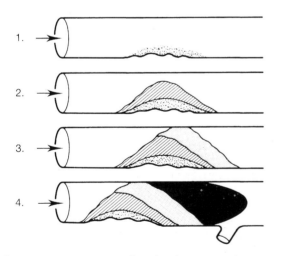

Figure 8.6 Stages in the development of a venous thrombosis. 1. The initial platelet cluster adheres to the vein wall as a grey amorphous thickening. 2. Laminated coralline thrombus develops on the surface of the platelet cluster, with alternate layers of fibrin and red cells trapped between layers of fibrin and platelets (the lines of Zahn).[489] 3. As the thrombus grows across the flowing blood, it bends in the direction of the blood flow, making the lines of Zahn oblique. 4. When the vein is totally occluded, non-adherent, jelly-like, soft, propagated thrombus spreads up the vessel as far as the next major tributary.

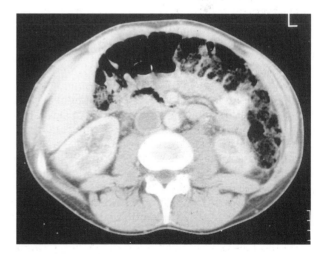

Figure 8.7 An enhanced CT scan showing marked enhancement of the wall of the vena cava around a totally occlusive adherent vena cava thrombosis. This enhancement is caused by the hyperaemic inflammation that occurs in the vein wall in response to thrombus adhesion. This inflammatory process initiates the organization and subsequent dissolution or fibrosis of the thrombus.

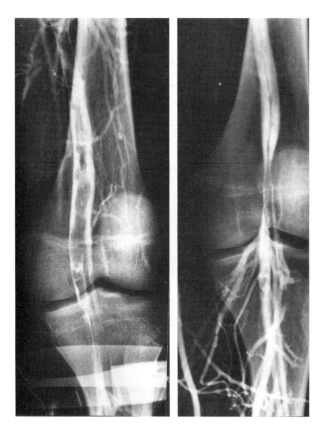

Figure 8.8 Contraction and retraction of a thrombus. The phlebograph on the left shows a large, 7–10-day-old popliteal vein thrombus which is beginning to retract and adhere to the vein wall. The phlebograph on the right was performed on the same limb 1 month later. The thrombus has contracted considerably but remains as a central strand in the centre of the vein lumen.

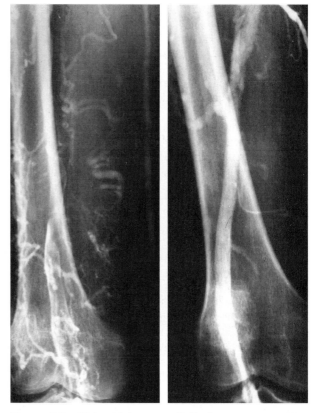

Figure 8.9 This phlebograph (left) shows an extensive superficial femoral vein thrombus. A second phlebograph obtained 6 months later (right) shows good reopening but a totally valveless channel.

the valves in the affected segment of vein[123] (Figure 8.9) and is accompanied by an enlargement of the collateral venous channels. There is a considerable danger of embolization until a non-adherent non-occlusive thrombus begins to contract. Contraction normally occurs 5–10 days after thrombus formation and is caused by the contraction of polymerizing strands of fibrin. If a thrombus has not fragmented by this stage, it usually becomes adherent to one side of the vein, and organization occurs as if the thrombus was fully adherent.

Natural thrombus dissolution has long been thought to be dependent on a fibrinolytic response by the local endothelium. In studies in a rat model of thrombosis that did not involve endothelial damage, developed to test this hypothesis,[329] we have been unable to demonstrate an increase in local plasminogen activator activity in the vessel wall adjacent to the thrombus.[330] Indeed, the

endothelium beneath the forming thrombus almost completely disappeared within 48 hours and this corresponded to a reduction in the concentration of tissue plasminogen activator activity in the vessel wall, which continued for several days.

Nevertheless, plasminogen activity was detected in the isolated thrombus and this activity increased as thrombus organization proceeded. Urokinase was present in significantly greater amounts in the thrombus than was tissue-type plasminogen activator, and the difference increased as lysis progressed.[330] The intensity of staining for tissue plasminogen activator increased as the thrombus became organized and was predominantly located within a developing monocyte infiltrate.[410] In-situ hybridization with a specific tissue plasminogen activator ribo-probe demonstrated increased message within monocyte infiltrate, implying that these cells, which appeared to have been actively recruited, were producing tissue plasminogen activator within the thrombus. The origin of these cells was confirmed by their positive staining with a monocyte/macrophage marker. These cells have not as yet been shown to be responsible for thrombus dissolution, and their source remains unidentified. They may have migrated through the vessel wall, or have been derived directly from the blood. More recently we have shown that injection of a monocyte chemoattractant, monocyte chemotactic protein 1, accelerates the maturation of experimental venous thrombi.[291]

It is known that extracted peripheral blood monocytes have the ability to synthesize tissue plasminogen activator, urokinase and the urokinase receptor, all of which may be influenced by thrombin, cytokines and lipopolysaccharide.[175,177,246,247,271,332] Monocytes also produce inhibitors of fibrinolytic activation in response to the same stimulus and at the same time.[246,247,271,332] Furthermore, these cells have been recently shown to actively degrade fibrin in the absence of plasmin.[405] It is therefore possible that the fibrinolytic/procoagulant balance of these cells may determine the clinical outcome of venous thrombi and reasonable to postulate from these findings that monocytes play an important role in the natural resolution of thrombosis in veins.

There is no value in distinguishing phlebothrombosis from thrombophlebitis[395] because septic thrombophlebitis, although common during the last century,[213] is rarely seen today. Any inflammatory changes that are found in a thrombosed deep vein are almost certainly the result of the thrombosis and not the cause of the thrombosis. A venous thrombus is usually sterile and is only mildly irritant.

Site of origin of deep vein thrombosis

In extensive autopsy studies on the occurrence of deep vein thrombosis, Gibbs[150] drew attention to the large number of thrombi that appear to involve or originate in the calf veins. Sevitt and Gallagher[399] confirmed Gibb's findings but observed that in burnt and injured patients thrombus could also develop in isolation in the iliac, femoral (superficial and deep), and popliteal veins (Figure 8.10). The advent of phlebography and the use of the fibrinogen uptake test has confirmed both these postmortem observations.[71,138,314,320,415] Most deep vein thrombi develop in the calf veins but they can develop at other sites, particularly if there is local tissue damage. The soleal sinusoids and the valves of the calf veins are the common sites of origin of deep vein thrombi. Sevitt has suggested that the eddy currents that occur as blood passes a valve[397] encourage the deposition of thrombus within the valve cusp with the 'formed elements', especially

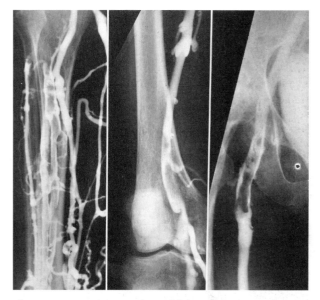

Figure 8.10 An ascending phlebograph showing separate and distinct areas of thrombosis – in the calf, in the popliteal vein and in the femoral vein. There is no connection between the thrombi at these different sites.

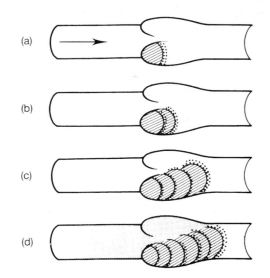

Figure 8.11 This diagram illustrates Sevitt's platelet clumps with fibrin fringes (building blocks). The first diagram shows thrombus being laid down in the valve sinus. The subsequent diagrams show the thrombus extending across the vessel wall to occlude flow and allow propagation of thrombus. (Modified from Sevitt.[395])

the red cells, being sifted out into the valve pocket by the turbulence (see Figure 8.4). Compression by exercising muscles may wash these small deposits away but if thromboxane (which stabilizes the aggregation of any platelet clumps) is released, the nidus for the growth of thrombus will persist. The subsequent chain reaction, with the generation of thrombin and fibrin, produces a growing thrombus.

Sevitt[395] described the platelet clump with its fibrin fringe as the foundation stone and building blocks of the growing thrombus (Figure 8.11). Propagation then depends on the balance between the coagulation and fibrinolytic mechanisms; the coagulation mechanisms favour extension and the fibrinolytic mechanisms favour thrombolysis. Growth is by the deposition of layers of aggregated platelets and fibrin containing red and white cells; this becomes the visible propagating head and tail of the thrombus. The original platelet nidus is usually transformed into a fibrin thrombus containing many red cells and a few platelets. Duplex studies[295] suggest that thrombus can commonly propagate to new venous segments and this adversely affects the ultimate function of the limb.

References

1. Abelseth G, Buckley RE, Pineo GE, Hull R, Rose MS. Incidence of deep-vein thrombosis in patients with fractures of the lower extremity distal to the hip. *J Orthop Trauma* 1996; **10(4):** 230–5.
2. Aberg M, Isacson S, Niisson IM. The fibrinolytic system and postoperative thrombosis following operation of rectal carcinoma. A preliminary report. *Acta Chir Scand* 1974; **140:** 352.
3. Aberg M, Nilsson IM, Hedner U. Antithrombin III after operation. *Lancet* 1973; **2:** 1337.
4. Adams DH, Shaw S. Leucocyte-endothelial interactions and regulation of leucocyte migration. *Lancet* 1994; **343:** 831–6.
5. Alarcon-Segoria D, Deleze M, Oria CV, Sanchez-Guerrero J, Pacheco L, Cabledo J. Antiphospholipid antibodies and the antiphospholipid syndrome in systemic lupus erythemetosis. A prospective analysis of 500 consecutive patients. *Medicine (Baltimore)* 1989; **68:** 353–6.
6. Allaart CF, Poort SR, Rosendaal FR, Reitsma PH, Bertina RM, Briet E. Increased risk of venous thrombosis in carriers of hereditary protein C deficiency defect. *Lancet* 1993; **341:** 134–8.
7. Allen A, Linton R, Donaldson G. Venous thrombosis and pulmonary embolism. *JAMA* 1945; **12X:** 397.
8. Allen RDM, Mitchell CA, Murie JA, Morris PJ. Deep venous thrombosis after renal transplantation. *Surg Gynecol Obstet* 1987; **164:** 137–42.
9. Almen T, Hartel M, Nylander G, Olivecrona H. Effect of estrogen on the vascular endothelium and its possible relation to thrombosis. *Surg Gynecol Obstet* 1975; **140:** 938.
10. Almen T, Nylander G. Serial phlebography of the normal lower leg during muscular contraction and relaxation. *Acta Radiol* 1962; **57:** 264.
11. Amundsen T, Ueland PM, Waage A. Plasma homocysteine levels in patients with deep venous thrombosis. *Arteriosclerosis, Thromb Vasc Biol* 1995; **15(9):** 1321–3.
12. Anderson FA, Wheeler HB, Golberg RJ, *et al.* A population based perspective of the hospital incidence and case-fatality rates of deep vein thrombosis and pulmonary embolism: The Worcester DVT Study. *Arch Intern Med* 1991; **151:** 933–8.
13. Anderson L, Nilsson IM, Olow B. Fibrinolytic activity in man during surgery. *Thromb Diath Haemorrh* 1962; **7:** 391.
14. Andreasen C, Krieger-Lassen H. Fatal pulmonary embolism in a surgical department during a period of 15 years. *Acta Chir Scand Suppl* 1965; **343:** 42.
15. Angelides NS, Nicolaides AN, Fernandes J, Gordon-Smith I, Bowers R, Lewis JD. Deep venous thrombosis in patients having aortoiliac reconstruction. *Br J Surg* 1977; **64:** 517.
16. Anon. Elective surgery and the pill. *Br Med J* 1976; **2:** 546.
17. Anon. Thromboembolism in pregnancy. *Br Med J* 1979; **1:** 1661.
18. Apitz K. Die Bedeutung der Gerinnung und Thrombose für die Blutstillung. *Virchows Arch Pathol Anat* 1942; **308:** 540.
19. Aschoff L. Thrombose und Sandbankbildung. *Beitr Pathol Anat* 1912; **52:** 207.
20. Ashford TP, Freiman DG. The role of the endothelium in the initial phases of thrombosis. *Am J Pathol* 1967; **50:** 257.
21. Astedt B, Pandolfi M. On release and synthesis of fibrinolytic activators in human organ culture. *Eur J Clin Biol Res* 1972; **17:** 261.
22. Astrup T. Tissue activators of plasminogen. *Fed Proc* 1966; **25:** 42.
23. Atik N. Broghamer W. The impact of prophylactic measures in fatal pulmonary embolism. *Arch Surg* 1979; **114:** 366.
24. Awbrey BJ, Hoak JC, Owren WG. Binding of human thrombin to cultured human endothelial cells. *J Biol Chem* 1979; **254:** 4092.
25. Babaracco MA, Vessey M. Recurrence of venous thromboembolism and the use of oral contraceptives. *Br Med J* 1974; **2:** 215–17.
26. Bach FH, Robson SC, Winkler H, *et al.* Barriers to xenotransplantation. *Nat Med* 1995; **1:** 869–73.
27. Bach FH, Robson SC, Ferran C, *et al.* Endothelial cell activation and thromboregulation during xenograft rejection. *Immunol Rev* 1994; **141:** 5–30.
28. Bagshaw M. Jet lag, pulmonary embolism and hypoxia. *Lancet* 1996; **348:** 415.
29. Baldwin AS. The NF-κB and IκB proteins: new discoveries and insights. *Annu Rev Immunol* 1996; **14:** 649–81.
30. Ballard RM, Bradley-Watson PJ, Johnstone FD, *et al.* Low doses of subcutaneous heparin in the prevention of deep vein thrombosis after gynaecological surgery. *J Obstet Gynaecol Br Commonw* 1973; **80:** 469.
31. Barker NU, Nygaard K, Walters W, Priestly JT. A statistical study of postoperative venous thrombosis

and pulmonary embolism. III. Time of occurrence during the postoperative period. *Proc Mayo Clin* 1941; **16:** 17.

32. Baskerville PA, Ackroyd JS, Lea Thomas M, Browse NL. The Klippel–Trenaunay syndrome: clinical, radiological and haemodynamic features and management. *Br J Surg* 1985; **72:** 232.

33. Bauer G. Thrombosis following leg injuries. *Acta Chir Scand* 1944; **90:** 229.

34. Baumgarten P. *Die sogennaute Organization des Thrombus*. Leipzig: O Wigand, 1877.

35. Becker J. Fibrinolytic activity of the blood and its relation to postoperative venous thrombosis of the lower limbs. A clinical study. *Acta Chir Scand* 1972; **138:** 787.

36. Becker J. The relation of platelet adhesiveness to postoperative venous thrombosis in the legs. *Acta Chir Scand* 1972; **138:** 781.

37. Becker J, Borgstrom S, Saltzman CF. Incidence of thrombosis associated with epsilon-aminocaproic acid administration and with combined epsilon-aminocaproic acid and subcutaneous heparin therapy. II A clinical study with the aid of intravenous phlebography. *Acta Chir Scand* 1970; **136:** 167.

38. Beighton PH, Richards PR. Cardiovascular disease in air travellers. *Br Heart J* 1968; **30:** 367–72.

39. Belch JJF, Lowe GDO, Pollock JG, Forbes CD, Prentice CRM. Subcutaneous heparin in the prevention of venous thrombosis after elective aortic bifurcation graft surgery. *Thromb Haemost* 1979; **42:** 303.

40. Bergentz S-E, Nilsson IM. Effect of trauma on coagulation and fibrinolysis in dogs. *Acta Chir Scand* 1961; **122:** 21.

41. Berman HJ, Fulton GP. Platelets in the peripheral circulation. In: Johnson SA, ed. *The Henry Ford Hospital Symposium on Blood Platelets*. Boston: Little Brown, 1961.

42. Berqvist A, Berqvist D, Hedner U. Clinical manifestations of thrombosis during pregnancy. *Lakartidningen* 1982; **79:** 901.

43. Berqvist D. *Postoperative Thromboembolism*. Berlin: Springer, 1983.

44. Berqvist D, Elvelin R, Eriksson U, Hjelmstedt A. Thrombosis following hip arthroplasty; a study using phlebography and the ^{125}I fibrinogen test. *Acta Orthop Scand* 1976; **47:** 549.

45. Berqvist D, Hallbook T. Prophylaxis of postoperative venous thrombosis in a controlled trial comparing dextran 70 and low-dose heparin. A study with the ^{125}I fibrinogen test. *World J Surg* 1980; **4:** 239.

46. Bertina RM, Broekmans AW, Van Der Linden IK, Mertens K. Protein C deficiency in a Dutch family with thrombotic disease. *Thromb Haemost* 1982; **48:** 1.

47. Bertina RM, Koeleman BP, Koster T, *et al*. Mutation in blood coagulation factor V associated with resistance to activated protein C. *Nature* 1994; **369:** 64–7.

48. Bevilacqua MP, Pober JS, Majeau GR, *et al*. Interleukin-1 induces biosynthesis and cell surface expression of procoagulant activity in human vascular endothelial cells. *J Exp Med* 1984; **160:** 618–23.

49. Biggs R. *Human Blood Coagulation, Haemostasis and Thrombosis*. Oxford: Blackwell Scientific Publications, 1972.

50. Bizzozero J. Uber einen neuen formbestandtheil des bluts und dessen rolle bei der Thrombose und der Blutgerinnung. *Virchows Arch Pathol Anat* 1882; **90:** 261.

51. Black J. Deep vein thrombosis and pulmonary embolism. *Lancet* 1993; **342:** 352–3.

52. Blaisdell FW. Low dose heparin prophylaxis of venous thrombosis. *Am Heart J* 1979; **97:** 685.

53. Blodgett JB, Beattie EJ. Early post-operative rising: a statistical study of hospital complications. *Surg Gynecol Obstet* 1946; **82:** 485.

54. Bloom AL, Giddings JC, Wilks CJ. Factor VIII on the vascular intima: possible importance in haemostasis and thrombosis. *Nature* 1973; **241:** 217.

55. Boey LM, Colaco CB, Gharavi AK, Elkon KB, Loizou S, Hughes GRV. Thrombosis in systemic lupus erythematosus: striking association with the presence of circulating 'lupus anti-coagulant'. *Br Med J* 1983; **287:** 1021.

56. Borgström S, Gelin E. The formation of vein thrombin following tissue injury. An experimental study in rabbits. *Acta Chir Scand Suppl* 1959; **247**.

57. Botti RE, Ratnoff OD. The clot promoting effect of long chain saturated fatty acids. *J Clin Invest* 1963; **42:** 1569.

58. Bounameaux H, Hicklin L, Desmarais S. Seasonal variation in deep vein thrombosis. *Br Med J* 1996; **312:** 284.

59. Bounameaux Y. The adherence of blood platelets to subendothelial fibers. *Thromb Diath Haemorrh* 1961; **6:** 504.

60. Bounameaux Y. The coupling of platelets with subendothelial fibers. *C R Soc Biol* 1959; **153:** 865.

61. Boyden S. The chemotactic effect of mixtures of antibody and antigen on polymorphonuclear leucocytes. *J Exp Med* 1962; **115:** 453.

62. Breneman J. A formula for predicting and a device for preventing postoperative thromboembolic disease. *Angiology* 1963; **14:** 437.

63. Breneman J. Postoperative thromboembolic disease. Computer analysis leading to statistical prediction. *JAMA* 1965; **193:** 576.

64. Broekmans AW, Veltkamp JJ, Bertina RM. Congenital protein C deficiency and venous thromboembolism. A study of three Dutch families. *N Engl J Med* 1983; **309:** 340.

65. Browse NL. Effect of bedrest on resting calf blood flow of healthy adult males. *Br Med J* 1962; **1:** 1721.

66. Browse NL. The ^{125}I fibrinogen uptake test. *Arch Surg* 1972; **104:** 160.

67. Browse NL, Clemenson G, Croft D. Fibrinogen detectable thrombosis in the legs and pulmonary embolism. *Br Med J* 1974; **1:** 603.

68. Browse NL, Gray L, Morland M, Jarrett PEM. Blood and vein wall fibrinolytic activity in health and vascular disease. *Br Med J* 1977; **1:** 478.

69. Browse NL, Hall JH. Effect of dipyridamole on the incidence of clinically detectable deep vein thrombosis. *Lancet* 1969; **2:** 718.

70. Browse NL, Jackson BT, Mayo ME, Negus D. The value of mechanical methods of preventing postoperative calf vein thrombosis. *Br J Surg* 1974; **61:** 219.

71. Browse NL, Lea Thomas M. Source of non-lethal pulmonary emboli. *Lancet* 1974; **1:** 258.

72. Buonassisi V. Sulfated mucopolysaccharide synthesis and secretion in endothelial cell cultures. *Exp Cell Res* 1973; **76:** 363.

73. Butler MJ, Britton BJ, Smith M, Hawkey C, Irving MH. Coagulation and fibrinolytic response during operative surgery. *Br J Surg* 1975; **62:** 666.

74. Butler MJ, Mathews F, Irving MH. The incidence of post-operative deep vein thrombosis after splenectomy. *Clin Oncol* 1977; **3:** 51.

75. Campbell B. Thrombosis, phlebitis and varicose veins. *Br Med J* 1996; **312:** 198–9.

76. Canavarro K. Early post-operative ambulation. *Ann Surg* 1946; **124:** 180.

77. Cappell DF. Chapter 3. In: *Muir's Textbook of Pathology*. London: Edward Arnold, 1958.

78. Carlos TM, Harlan JM. Leukocyte-endothelial adhesion molecules. *Blood* 1994; **84:** 2068–101.

79. Carreras LO, Defreyn G, Makin SJ, *et al*. Arterial thrombosis, intrauterine death and 'lupus' anticoagulant: detection of immunoglobulin interfering with prostacylin formation. *Lancet* 1981; **1:** 244.

80. Carreras LO, Vermylen JG. 'Lupus' anticoagulant and thrombosis: possible role of inhibition of prostacyclin formation. *Thromb Haemost* 1982; **48:** 38.

81. Carter CJ, Anderson FA, Wheeler HB. Epidemiology and pathophysiology of venous thromboembolism. In: Hull R, ed. *Venous Thromboembolism*. New York: Futura, 1996; Chapter 1.

82. Cartwright GE, Athens JW, Boggs DR, Wintrobe MM. The kinetics of granulopoiesis in normal man. *Blood* 1965; **24:** 780.

83. Chan V, Chan TK. Antithrombin III in fresh and cultured human endothelial cells: a natural anticoagulant from the vascular endothelium. *Thromb Res* 1979; **15:** 209.

84. Chesterman CN, McGready JR, Doyle DJ, Morgan FJ. Plasma levels of platelet factor 4 measured by radio-immunoassay. *Br J Haematol* 1978; **40:** 489.

85. Chu AJ. Inhibition of the endotoxin-induced monocytic procoagulant activity by n-alcohols and anaesthetics. *Comp Biochem Physiol* 1991; **99c:** 451–6.

86. Clayton JK, Anderson JA, McNichol GP. Preoperative prediction of post-operative deep vein thrombosis. *Br Med J* 1976; **2:** 910.

87. Cockett FB, Lea Thomas M. The iliac compression syndrome. *Br J Surg* 1965; **52:** 816.

88. Cohnheim J. In: McKee AB, ed. *Lectures in General Pathology*. London: New Sydenham Society, 1889.

89. Colditz GA, Tuden RA, Oster G. Rates of venous thrombosis after general surgery: combined results of randomized clinical trials. *Lancet* 1986; **2:** 143.

90. Collins R, Klein L, Skillman J, Salzman E. Thromboembolic problems in urologic surgery. *Urol Clin North Am* 1976; **3:** 393.

91. Collins T, Palmer HJ, Whitley MZ, Neish AS, Williams AJ. A common theme in endothelial activation – insights from the structural analysis of the genes for E-selectin and VCAM-1. *Trends Cardiovasc Med* 1993; **3:** 92–7.

92. Conard J, Veuillet-Duval A, Horellou MH, Samama M. Etude de la coagulation et de la fibrinolyse dans 131 cas de thromboses veineuses récidivants. *Nouv Rev Fr Hematol* 1982; **24:** 205.

93. Coon WW, Willis PW, Keller JB. Venous thromboembolism and other venous disease in the Tecumseh Community Health Study. *Circulation* 1973; **48:** 839–46.

94. Cooper DR, Lewis GP, Lieberman GE, Webb H, Westwick J. Adenosine diphosphate metabolism in vascular tissue, a possible thrombo-regulating mechanism. *Thromb Res* 1979; **14:** 901.

95. Cope C, Reyes T, Skversky N. Phlebographic analysis of the incidence of thrombosis in hemiplegia. *Radiology* 1973; **109:** 581.

96. Cotton LT, Clarke C. Anatomical localization of venous thrombosis. *Ann R Coll Surg Engl* 1965; **36:** 214.

97. Crandon AJ, Peel KR, Anderson JA, Thompson V, McNichol GP. Post-operative deep vein thrombosis: indentifying high risk patients. *Br Med J* 1980; **281:** 343.

98. Crandon AJ, Peel KR, Anderson JA, Thompson V, McNichol GP. Prophylaxis of postoperative deep vein thrombosis: selective use of low-dose heparin in high-risk patients. *Br Med J* 1980; **281:** 345.

99. Cranley JJ, Canos AJ, Sull WJ, Grass AM. Phleborheographic technique for diagnosis of deep vein thrombosis of the lower extremities. *Surg Gynecol Obstet* 1975; **141:** 331.

100. Cruickshank JM, Gorlin BJ, Jennet B. Air travel and thrombotic episodes; the economy class syndrome. *Lancet* 1988; **2:** 497–8.

101. Dahlbach B. New molecular insights into the genetics of thrombophilia. Resistance to activated protein C caused by Arg506 to Gin mutation in factor V as a pathogenic risk factor for venous thrombosis. *Thromb Haemost* 1995; **74(1):** 139–48.

102. Dahlbach B, Carlsson M, Svensson PJ. Familial thrombophilia due to a previously unrecognized mechanism characterized by poor anticoagulant response to activated protein C. *Proc Natl Acad Sci USA* 1993; **90:** 1004–8.

103. Dahlbach B, Stonflo J. High molecular weight complex in human plasma between vitamin-K dependent protein S and complement protein C4b-binding protein. *Proc Natl Acad Sci USA* 1981; **78:** 2515–26.

104. Daly E, Vessey MP, Hawkins MM, Carson JL, Gough R, Marsh S. Risk of venous thromboembolism in users of hormone replacement therapy. *Lancet* 1996; **348:** 977–80.

105. Davies MG, Fulton GJ, Hagen PO. Clinical biology of nitric oxide. *Br J Surg* 1995; **82:** 1598–610.

106. Davies JWL, Liljedahl SO, Reizenstein P. Fibrinogen metabolism following injury and its surgical treatment. *Injury* 1970; **1:** 178.

107. Dawson AA, Bennett B, Jones PF, Munro A. Thrombotic risks of staging laparotomy with splenectomy in Hodgkin's disease. *Br J Surg* 1981; **68:** 842.

108. Day TK, Cowper SV, Kakkar VV, Clarke KGA. Early venous thrombosis: a scanning electron microscopic study. *Thromb Haemost* 1977; **37:** 477.

109. de Cossart L. Plasminogen activator in soleal veins. *Phlebology* 1986; **1:** 119.

110. De Maat MPM, Kluft C, Jespersen J, Gram J. World distribution of factor V Leiden mutation. *Lancet* 1996; **347:** 58.

111. De Stefano V, Finazzi G, Mannucci PM. Inherited thrombophilia, pathogenesis, clinical syndromes, and management. *Blood* 1996; **87:** 3531–44.

112. de Takats G. Heparin tolerance. A test of the clotting mechanism. *Surg Gynecol Obstet* 1943; **77:** 31.

113. den Heijer M, Blom HJ, Gerrits WBJ, *et al.* Is homocysteinaemia a risk factor for recurrent thrombosis. *Lancet* 1995; **345:** 882–5.

114. den Heijer M, Koster T, Blom HJ, *et al.* Hyperhomocysteinemia as a risk factor for deep vein thrombosis. *N Engl J Med* 1996; **334:** 759–62.

115. Dismuke SE. Declining mortality from pulmonary embolism in surgical patients. *Thromb Haemost* 1981; **46:** 17.

116. Dodd H, Cockett F. *The Pathology and Surgery of the Veins of the Lower Limb.* Edinburgh: Churchill Livingstone, 1976.

117. Donati MB, Poggi A, Mussoni L, de Gaetano G, Garattini S. Hemostasis and experimental cancer dissemination. In: Day SB, Myers WPL, Stansly P, Garratini S, Lewis MG, eds. *Cancer Invasion and Metastasis: Biologic Mechanisms and Therapy.* New York: Raven Press, 1977.

118. Doran FSA, Drury M, Sivyer A. A simple way to combat the venous stasis which occurs in the lower limb during surgical operations. *Br J Surg* 1964; **51:** 486.

119. Dormandy J, Edelman J. High blood viscosity: an aetiological factor in venous thrombosis. *Br J Surg* 1973; **60:** 187.

120. Douss TW. The clinical significance of venous thrombosis of the calf. *Br J Surg* 1976; **63:** 377.

121. Drake TA, Morissey JH, Edgington TS. Selective cellular expression of tissue factor in human tissues. Implications for disorders of haemostasis and thrombosis. *Am J Pathol* 1989; **134:** 1087–97.

122. Eberth CJ, Schimmelbusch C. *Die Thrombose nach Versuchen und Leichenbefunden.* Stuttgart: F Enke, 1888.

123. Edwards AK, Edwards JE. The effect of thrombophlebitis on the venous valve. *Surg Gynecol Obstet* 1937; **65:** 310.

124. Egeberg O. Inherited antithrombin deficiency causing thrombophilia. *Thromb Diath Haemorrh* 1965; **13:** 516.

125. Egeberg O. Changes in the coagulation system following major surgical operations. *Acta Med Scand* 1962; **171:** 679.

126. Eklof B, Kistner RL, Masuda EM, *et al.* Venous thromboembolism in association with prolonged air travel. *Dermatol Surg* 1996; **22:** 637–41.

127. Emeis JJ, Kooistra T. IL1 and lipopolysaccharide induce an inhibitor of tissue type plasminogen activator in vivo and in cultured endothelial cells. *J Exp Med* 1986; **163:** 1260–6.

128. Emmons PR, Mitchell JRA. Postoperative changes in platelet-clumping activity. *Lancet* 1965; **1:** 71.

129. Esmon CT. The protein C anticoagulant pathway. *Arterioscler Thromb* 1992; **12:** 135–45.

130. Esmon CT, Owen WG. Identification of an endothelial cell cofactor for the thrombin-catalysed activation of protein C. *Proc Natl Acad Sci USA* 1981; **78:** 2249–54.

131. Evans WH. Discussion on post-operative thrombosis. *Proc R Soc Med* 1929; **22:** 729.

132. Exner T, Tripiett DA, Taberner D, Machin SJ. Guidelines for testing and revised criteria for lupus anticoagulants. SSC Subcommittee for standardization of lupus anticoagulants. *Thromb Haemost* 1989; **65:** 320.

133. Farkas JC, Chapuis C, Combe S, *et al.* A randomised controlled trial of a low-molecular-weight heparin (Enoxaparin) to prevent deep-vein thrombosis in patients undergoing vascular surgery. *Eur J Vasc Surg* 1993; **7(5):** 554–60.

134. Fearnley GR. *Fibrinolysis.* London: Edward Arnold, 1965.

135. Feinleib M. Venous thrombosis in relation to cigarette smoking, physical activity and seasonal factors. *Millbank Med Fund Q* 1972; **50:** 123.

136. Finazzi G, Barbui T. Difference incidence of venous thrombosis in patients with inherited deficiencies of antithrombin III, protein C and protein S. *Thromb Haemost* 1994; **71(1):** 15–18.

137. Finch PJ, Ransford R, Hill-Smith A. Thromboembolism and air travel. *Lancet* 1988; **2:** 1025.

138. Flanc C, Kakkar VV, Clarke MB. The detection of venous thrombosis of the legs using ^{125}I labelled fibrinogen. *Br J Surg* 1968; **55:** 742.

139. Florey HW. *General Pathology.* London: Lloyd Luke, 1962.

140. Flute PT, Kakkar VV, Renney JTG, Nicolaides AN. The blood and venous thromboembolism. In: Kakkar VV, Jonhar AJ, eds. *Thromboembolism.* Edinburgh: Churchill Livingstone, 1972.

141. Foster DP, Whipple CH. Blood fibrin studies. Fibrin influenced by cell injury, inflammation, intoxication, liver injury and the Eck fistula. Notes connecting the origin of fibrin in the body. *Am J Physiol* 1922; **58:** 407.

142. French JE, Macfarlane RG, Sanders AG. The structure of haemostatic plugs and experimental thrombi in small arteries. *Br J Exp Pathol* 1964; **45:** 467.

143. Frosst P, Blom HJ, Milos R, *et al.* A candidate genetic risk factor for vascular disease: a common mutation on methylenetetrafolate. *Nat Genet* 1995; **10:** 111–13.

144. Gaffney PJ, Joe F, Mahmoud M. Giant fibrin fragments derived from cross-linked fibrin: structure and clinical application. *Thromb Res* 1980; **20:** 647.

145. Galli M, Daldossi M, Barbui T. Antiglycoprotein Ib/IX and IIb/IIIa antibodies in patients with

antiphospholipid antibodies. *Thromb Haemost* 1994; **71:** 571–5.

146. Gallus AS, Hirsh J, Gent M. Relevance of preoperative and postoperative blood tests to postoperative leg vein thrombosis. *Lancet* 1973; **2:** 806.

147. Gasic GJ, Boettiger D, Catalfamo JL, Gasic TB, Stewart GJ. Platelet interactions in malignancy and cell transformation: functional and biochemical studies. In: de Gaetano G, Garattini S, eds. *Platelets: a Multidisciplinary Approach.* New York: Raven Press, 1978.

148. Gaynor E. The role of granulocytes in endotoxin induced vascular injury. *Blood* 1973; **41:** 797.

149. Gibbard FB, Gould SR, Marks P. Incidence of deep vein thrombosis and leg oedema in patients with strokes. *J Neurol Neurosurg Psychiatry* 1976; **39:** 1222.

150. Gibbs NM. Venous thrombosis in the lower limbs with particular reference to bedrest. *Br J Surg* 1957; **45:** 209.

151. Gillum RF. Pulmonary embolism and thrombophlebitis in the United States 1970–1985. *Am Heart J* 1990; **120:** 392–5.

152. Gillum RF. Pulmonary embolism and thrombophlebitis in the United States 1970-1985. *Am Heart J* 1987; **114:** 1262–4.

153. Girma J, Meyer D, Verweiij C, Pannekogk H, Sikmc J. Structure–function relationship of human von Willebrand factor. *Blood* 1987; **70:** 605–11.

154. Gjöres J-E. The incidence of venous thrombosis and its sequelae in certain districts of Sweden. *Acta Chir Scand Suppl* 1956; **206:** 1.

155. Glennard F. *Contribution à l'étude des causes de la coagulation spontanée du sang à son issue de l'organisme application à la transfusion.* Paris: Thesis, 1875.

156. Glerts WH, Code KI, Jay RM, Chen E, Szalai JP. A prospective study of venous thromboembolism after major trauma. *N Engl J Med* 1994; **331(24):** 1601–6.

157. Godal HC. Quantitative and qualitative changes in fibrinogen following major surgical operations. *Acta Med Scand* 1962; **171:** 687.

158. Gordon-Smith IC, Hickman JA, LeQuesne LP. Postoperative fibrinolytic activity and deep vein thrombosis. *Br J Surg* 1974; **61:** 213.

159. Gore I, Hirst A, Tanaka K. Myocardial infarction and thromboembolism. A comparative study in Boston and in Kyushu, Japan. *Arch Intern Med* 1964; **113:** 323.

160. Gore I, Larkey BJ. Functional activity of aortic mucopolysaccharides. *J Lab Clin Med* 1960; **56:** 839.

161. Griffin JH, Evatt B, Zimmerman TS, Kleiss AJ, Widemann C. Deficiency of protein C in congenital thrombotic disease. *J Clin Invest* 1981; **68:** 1370.

162. Grodstein F, Stampfer MJ, Goldhaber SZ, Manson JE, Colditz GA, Speizer FE. Prospective study of exogenous hormones and risk of pulmonary embolism in women. *Lancet* 1996; **348:** 983–7.

163. Groote Schuur Hospital Thromboembolus Study Group. Failure of low-dose heparin to prevent significant thromboembolic complications in high-risk surgical patients. Interim report of a prospective trial. *Br Med J* 1979; **1:** 1447.

164. Gryner L. Activity of anchonitic surface compounds in producing vascular obliteration. *Proc Soc Exp Biol Med* 1946; **62:** 49.

165. Guillebaud J. Surgery and the pill. *Br Med J* 1985; **291:** 498.

166. Gunn I. Anti-Xa factor as a predictor of postoperative deep vein thrombosis in general surgery. *Br J Surg* 1979; **66:** 636.

167. Gyde OHB, Littler WA, Stableforth DE. Familial antithrombin III deficiency. *Br Med J* 1978; **1:** 508.

168. Gyde OHB, Middleton MD, Vaughan GR, Fletcher DJ. Antithrombin III deficiency hypertriglyceridaemia and venous thromboses. *Br Med J* 1978; **1:** 621.

169. Hadfield C. Thrombosis. *Ann R Coll Surg Engl* 1950; **6:** 219.

170. Hamberg M, Svensson J, Samuelsson B. Thromboxanes: a new group of biologically active compounds derived from prostaglandin endoperoxides. *Proc Natl Acad Sci USA* 1975; **72:** 2994.

171. Hamblin TJ. Endothelins. *Br Med J* 1990; **301:** 568.

172. Hamer JD. Investigation of oedema of the lower limb following successful femeropopliteal bypass surgery: the role of phlebography in demonstrating venous thrombosis. *Br J Surg* 1972; **59:** 979.

173. Hamer JD, Malone PC. Experimental deep venous thrombogenesis by a non-invasive method. *Ann R Coll Surg Engl* 1984; **66:** 416.

174. Hamer JD, Malone PC, Silver IA. The PO2 in venous valve pockets: its possible bearing on thrombogenesis. *Br J Surg* 1981; **68:** 166–70.

175. Hamilton JA, Hart PH, Leizer T, Vitti GF, Campbell IK. Regulation of plasminogen activator activity on arthritic joints. *J Rheumatol* 1991; **S27:** 106–9.

176. Handley A. Low-dose heparin after myocardial infarction. *Lancet* 1972; **2:** 623.

177. Hart PH, Burgess DR, Vitti GF, Hamilton JA. Interleukin-4 stimulates human monocytes to produce tissue-type plasminogen activator. *Blood* 1989; **74:** 1222–5.

178. Hartsuck J, Greenfield L. Postoperative thromboembolism. A clinical study with ^{125}I fibrinogen and pulmonary scanning. *Arch Surg* 1973; **107:** 733.

179. Harvey-Kemble JV. The incidence of deep vein thrombosis. *Br J Hosp Med* 1971; **6:** 721.

180. Harvey-Kemble JV. The effect of surgical operation on leg venous flow measured with radioactive hippuran. *Postgrad Med J* 1971; **47:** 773.

181. Haveerkate F, Samama M. Familial dysfibrinogenaemia and thrombophilia. Report on a study of the SSC Subcommittee on fibrinogen. *Thromb Haemost* 1995; **73:** 151–61.

182. Havig O. Deep vein thrombosis and pulmonary embolism. An autopsy study with multiple regression analysis of possible risk factors. *Acta Chir Scand Suppl* 1977; **478:** 1–120.

183. Heather B, Jennings S, Greenhalgh R. The saline dilution test – a preoperative predictor of DVT. *Br J Surg* 1980; **67:** 63.

184. Heatley RV, Hughes LE, Morgan A, Okwonga W. Preoperative or postoperative deep-vein thrombosis? *Lancet* 1976; **1:** 437.

185. Hedlund PO. Postoperative venous thrombosis in benign prostatic disease. A study of 316 patients with the ^{125}I fibrinogen uptake test. *Scand J Urol Nephrol* 1975; **(27 suppl):** 1–100.

186. Hedner U, Martinsson G, Bergqvist D. Influence of operative trauma on factor XII and inhibitor of plasminogen activator. *Haemostasis* 1983; **13:** 219.

187. Hellgren M, Svensson PJ, Dahlback B. Resistance to activated protein C as a basis for venous thromboembolism associated with pregnancy and oral contraceptives. *Am J Obstet Gynecol* 1995; **173(1):** 210–13.

188. Henkel T, Machleidt T, Alkalay I, Kronke M, Benneriah Y, Baeuerle PA. Rapid proteolysis of IκBα is necessary for activation of transcription factor NF-κB. *Nature* 1993; **365:** 182.

189. Hewson W. *Experimental Enquiries: I An Enquiry into the Properties of Blood with Some Remarks on its Morbid Appearances and an Appendix relating to the Discovery of the Lymphatic System in Birds, Fish and the Animals called Amphibians.* London: T Cadell, 1771.

190. Heyns AP, Badenhorst CJ, Retief FP. Adenosine diphosphatase activity of normal and atherosclerotic human aorta intima. *Thromb Haemost* 1977; **37:** 429.

191. Heyns AP, Van Den Berg DJ, Potgieler FP, Retief FP. The inhibition of platelet aggregation by an aorta intima extract. *Thromb Diath Haemorrh* 1974; **32:** 417.

192. Hickman JA. A study of the metabolism of fibrinogen after surgical operations. *Clin Sci* 1971; **41:** 141.

193. Hjelmstedt A. *Deep Venous Thrombosis in Tibial Fracture. A Clinical Phlebographic and Physiological Study.* Thesis. Uppsala: Almquist and Wiksell, 1968.

194. Hobbs JT. Compression sclerotherapy of varicose veins. In: Bergan JJ, Yao JST, eds. *Venous Problems.* Chicago, IL: Year Book Medical Publishers, 1978.

195. Hobbs JT, Davis JWL. Detection of venous thrombosis with ^{131}I labelled fibrinogen in the rabbit. *Lancet* 1960; **2:** 134.

196. Hoffman M. From anti α phospholipid syndrome to antibody mediated thrombosis. *Lancet* 1997; **350:** 1491–2.

197. Holmberg L, Mannucci BM, Turesson I, Ruggeri ZM, Nilsson IM. Factor VIII antigen in the vessel wall in von Willebrand's disease and haemophilia A. *Scand J Haematol* 1974; **13:** 33–8.

198. Homans J. Thrombosis of deep leg veins due to prolonged sitting. *N Engl J Med* 1954; **250:** 148.

199. Homans J. Thrombosis of the deep veins of the leg, causing pulmonary embolism. *N Engl J Med* 1934; **211:** 993.

200. Horellou MH, Conard J, Bertina RM, Samama M. Congenital protein C deficiency and thrombotic disease in nine french families. *Br Med J* 1984; **289:** 1285.

201. Hovig T. The effect of calcium and magnesium on rabbit blood platelet aggregation *in vitro. Thromb Diath Haemorrh* 1963; **12:** 179.

202. Hovig T. The ultrastructure of rabbit blood platelet aggregates. *Thromb Diath Haemorrh* 1962; **8:** 455.

203. Hughes GRV. The antiphospholipid syndrome: ten years on. *Lancet* 1993; **342:** 341–4.

204. Hugues J. Accolement des plaquettes aux structures conlonctives perivasculaires. *Thromb Diath Haemorrh* 1962; **8:** 241.

205. Hugues J. Contribution à l'étude des facteurs vasculaires et sanguine dans l'hémostase spontanée. *Arch Int Physiol* 1953; **61:** 565.

206. Hugues J, Lapiere M. Nouvelles researches sur l'accolement des plaquettes aux fibères de collagère. *Thromb Diath Haemorrh* 1964; **11:** 327.

207. Hull R, Hirsh J. Prevention of venous thrombosis and pulmonary embolism with particular reference to the surgical patient. In: Joist JH, Sherman LA, eds. *Venous and Arterial Thrombosis. Pathogenesis, Diagnosis, Prevention and Therapy.* New York: Grune & Stratton, 1979.

208. Hume M. The incidence and importance of thromboembolism. In: Hume M, Sevitt S, Thomas DP, eds. *Venous Thrombosis and Pulmonary Embolism.* Cambridge, MA: Harvard Clinical Press, 1970.

209. Hume M, Chan YK. Examination of the blood in the presence of venous thrombosis. *JAMA* 1967; **200:** 747.

210. Hume M, Sevitt S, Thomas DP. *Venous Thombosis and Pulmonary Embolism.* Cambridge, MA: Harvard University Press, 1970.

211. Hunt JE, Simpson RJ, Krilis SA. Identification of a region of beta-2-glycoprotein I critical for lipidbinding and anti-cardiolipin cofactor activity. *Proc Natl Acad Sci USA* 1993; **90:** 2141.

212. Hunt PS, Reeves TS, Hollings RM. A 'standard' experimental thrombus: observations on its production, pathology, response to heparin and thrombectomy. *Surgery* 1966; **59:** 812.

213. Hunter J. In: Palmer JF, ed. *A Treatise on Blood, Inflammation and Gunshot Wounds.* London: Longman, 1834.

214. Husni EH. The oedema of arterial reconstruction. *Circulation* 1967; **35(Suppl 1):** 169.

215. Ichinose A, Espling ES, Takamatsu J, *et al.* Two types of abnormal plasminogen genes in families with a predisposition for thrombosis. *Proc Natl Acad Sci USA* 1991; **88:** 115–19.

216. Ihrcke NS, Wrenshall LE, Lindman BJ, Platt JL. Role of heparan sulphate in immune system–blood vessel interactions. *Immunol Today* 1996; **14:** 500–5.

217. International Multi-centre Trial. Prevention of fatal post-operative pulmonary embolism by low doses of heparin. *Lancet* 1975; **2:** 45.

218. Isacson S, Nilsson IM. Defective fibrinolysis in blood vein walls in recurrent 'idiopathic' venous thrombosis. *Acta Chir Scand* 1972; **138:** 313.

219. Ishak M, Morley K. Deep venous thrombosis after total hip arthroplasty: a prospective controlled study to determine the prophylactic effect of graded pressure stockings. *Br J Surg* 1981; **68:** 429.

220. Izuka K, Murata K. Inhibitory effects of human aortic and venous acid glycosaminoglycans on thrombus formation. *Atherosclerosis* 1972; **16:** 217.

221. Jaffe EA, Hoyer LW, Nachman RL. Synthesis of antihemophilic factor antigen by cultured human endothelial cells. *J Clin Invest* 1973; **52**: 2757.

222. James PB. Jet 'leg', pulmonary embolism and hypoxia. *Lancet* 1996; **347**: 1697.

223. Jick H, Derby LE, Myers MW, Vasilakis C, Newton KM. Risk of hospital admission for idiopathic venous thromboembolism among users of postmenopausal oestrogens. *Lancet* 1996; **349**: 981–3.

224. Joffe SN. Racial incidence of postoperative deep vein thrombosis in South Africa. *Br J Surg* 1974; **61**: 982.

225. Joffe SN. Deep vein thrombosis after renal transplantation. *Vasc Surg* 1976; **10**: 134.

226. Johansson L, Hedner U, Nilsson IM. A family with thromboembolic disease associated with deficient fibrinolytic activity in vessel wall. *Acta Med Scand* 1978; **203**: 477.

227. Johnson RH, Mansfield A. A new method for the detection of plasminogen activator content of vein walls. *Acta Haematol* 1978; **60**: 243.

228. Kakkar VV. The diagnosis of deep vein thrombosis using fibrinogen test. *Arch Surg* 1972; **104**: 152.

229. Kakkar VV, Day TK. The vessel wall and venous thrombosis. In: Neville Wolfe, ed. *Biology and Pathology of the Vessel Wall*. New York: Praeger, 1983.

230. Kakkar VV, Howe CT, Nicolaides AN, Renney JTG, Clarke MB. Deep vein thrombosis of the leg: Is there a 'high-risk' group? *Am J Surg* 1970; **120**: 527.

231. Kakkar VV, Sasahara AA. Diagnosis of venous thrombosis and pulmonary embolism. In Bloom AL, Thomas DP, eds. *Haemostasis and Thrombosis*. Edinburgh: Churchill Livingstone, 1981.

232. Karino T, Motomiya M. Vortices in the pockets of a venous valve. *Microvasc Res* 1981; **21**: 247.

233. Kawasaki T, Kambayashi J, Sakon M. Hyperlipidaemia: a novel etiologic factor in deep vein thrombosis. *Thromb Res* 1995; **79(2)**: 147–51.

234. Kawasaki T, Kambayashi J, Uemara Y, *et al.* Involvement of dysplasminogenemia in occurrence of deep vein thrombosis. *Int Angiol* 1995; **14(1)**: 65–8.

235. Kelsey PR, Stevenson KJ, Poller L. The diagnosis of lupus anticoagulants by the activated partial thromboplastin time – the central role of phospletidyl senna. *Thromb Haemost* 1984; **52**: 172–5.

236. Kerr MG, Scott DB, Samuel E. Studies of the inferior vena cave in late pregnancy. *Br Med J* 1964; **1**: 532.

237. Khaira HS, Parnell A, Crowson MC. Femoral exostosis presenting with deep vein and arterial thrombosis. *Br J Surg* 1995; **82**: 911.

238. Khamashta MA, Asherson RA. Hughes syndrome: antiphospholipid antibodies move closer to thrombosis in 1994. *Br J Rheumatol* 1995; **34**: 493–7.

239. Khan FS. *The Curse of Icarus: the Health Factor in Air Travel*. London: Routledge, 1990.

240. Kim SW, Charallel JT, Park KW, *et al.* Prevalence of deep venous thrombosis in patients with chronic spinal cord injury. *Arch Phys Med Rehabil* 1994; **75(9)**: 965–8.

241. Klein A, Hughes LE, Campbell H, Williams A, Zlosnick J, Leach KG. Dextran 70 in prophylaxis of thrombo-embolic disease after surgery: a clinically orientated randomized double blind trial. *Br Med J* 1975; **2**: 109.

242. Koster T, Rosendaal FR, Briet E, Vandenbrouke JP. John Hagemann's factor and deep vein thrombosis: Leiden thrombophilia study. *Br J Haematol* 1994; **87**: 422–4.

243. Koster T, Rosendaal FR, de Ronde H, Briet H, Vandenbroucke JP, Bertina RM. Venous thrombosis due to poor anticoagulant response to activated protein C: Leiden thrombophilia study. *Lancet* 1993; **342**: 1503–6.

244. Kraemer PM. Heparin releases heparan sulfate from the cell surface. *Biochem Biophys Res Commun* 1977; **78**: 1334.

245. Kuitnen A, Hynynen M, Salmenpera M, *et al.* Anaesthesia affects plasma concentrations of vasopressin, von Willebrand factor and coagulation factor VIII in cardiac surgical patients. *Br J Anaesth* 1993; **70**: 173–80.

246. Kung SKP, Lau HKF. Modulation of the plasminogen activation system in murine macrophages. *Biochim Biophys Acta* 1993; **1176**: 113–22.

247. Kuraoka S, Campeau JD, Rodgers KE, Nakamura RM, DiZerega G. Effects of IL-1 on postsurgical macrophage secretion of protease and protease inhibitor activities. *J Surg Res* 1992; **52**: 71–8.

248. Lamb GC, Tomski MA, Kaufman J, Maiman DJ. Is chronic spinal cord injury associated with increased risk of venous thromboembolism? *J Am Paraplegia Soc* 1993; **16(3)**: 153–6.

249. Lane DA, Caso R. Antithrombin: structure, genomic organisation, function and inherited deficiency. *Ballière's Clin Haematol* 1989; **2**: 961–98.

250. Lane DA, Mannucci PM, Bauer KA, et al. Inherited thrombophilia: part 1. *Thromb Haemost* 1996: **76**: 651–62.

251. Lane DA, Olds RJ, Bosiclair M, *et al.* Antithrombin III mutation database: first update. *Thromb Haemost* 1993; **70**: 361–9.

252. Lanham JG, Levin M, Brown Z, Gharavi AK, Thomas PA, Hanson GC. Prostacyclin deficiency in a young woman with recurrent thrombosis. *Br Med J* 1986; **292**: 435.

253. Laupacis A, Rorabeck C, Bourne R, *et·al.* The frequency of venous thrombosis in cemented and non-cemented hip arthroplasty. *J Bone Joint Surg Br* 1996; **78(2)**: 210–12.

254. Lawrence JC, Xabregas A, Gray L, Ham JM. Seasonal variation in the incidence of deep vein thrombosis. *Br J Surg* 1977; **64**: 777.

255. Layer G, Burnand KG. Two different mechanisms in patients with venous thrombosis and defective fibrinolysis. *Br Med J* 1985; **291**: 56.

256. Lee NS, Brewer BH, Osborne JC. Beta-2-glycoprotein I: molecular properties of an unusual apolipoprotein, apolipoprotein H. *J Biol Chem* 1983; **258**: 4765.

257. Leithauser OJ. *Early Ambulation and Related Procedures in Surgical Management*. Springfield, IL: Charles C Thomas, 1946.

258. Lie JT. Vasculopathy in the antiphospholipid syndrome: thrombosis or vasculitis, or both? *J Rheumatol* 1989; **48:** 362–7.

259. Lilenfeld DE, Godbold JH, Burke GL, *et al.* Hospitalization and case fatality for pulmonary embolism in the twin cities 1979–1984. *Am Heart J* 1990; **120:** 392–5.

260. Lindblad B, Erickson A, Bergqvist D. Autopsy verified pulmonary embolism in a surgical department: analysis of the period from 1951 to 1988. *Br J Surg* 1991; **78:** 849–52.

261. Lister J. On the coagulation of blood. Croonian Lecture. *Proc R Soc Lond* 1862; **12:** 580.

262. Ljungnér H, Berqvist D, Isacson S. Plasminogen activator activity of superficial veins in acute deep venous thrombosis. *Vasa* 1982; **11:** 174.

263. Ljungnér H, Berqvist D, Isacson S, Nilsson IM. Comparison between the plasminogen activator activity in walls of superficial, muscle and deep veins. *Thromb Res* 1981; **22:** 295.

264. Ljungnér H, Isacson S. The fibrinolytic activity in vein walls in patients undergoing prostatectomy. *Sven Lakaresallsk Forh* 1979; **88:** 23.

265. Lockshin MD, Qammar T, Druziun M, Goesi S. Antibody to cardiolipin, lupus anticoagulant and fetal death. *J Rheumatol* 1987; **14:** 259–62.

266. Loppnow H, Libby P. Proliferating or interleukin-1 activated human vascular smooth muscle cells secrete copious Interleukin 6. *J Clin Invest* 1990; **85:** 731–8.

267. Loskutoff DJ, Edgington T. Synthesis of a fibrinolytic activator and inhibitor by endothelial cells. *Proc Natl Acad Sci USA* 1977; **74:** 3903.

268. Lowe GDO, Osborne DH, McArdle BM, *et al.* Prediction and selective prophylaxis of venous thrombosis in elective gastrointestinal surgery. *Lancet* 1982; **1:** 409.

269. Lozou S, McCrea JD, Rudge AC, Reynolds R, Boyle CC, Harris EN. Measurements of anticardiolipin antibodies by enzyme-linked immunoassay. Standardization and quantitation of results. *Clin Exp Immunol* 1986; **62:** 739.

270. Ludlam CA, Cash JD. β3-Thromboglobulin: a new tool for the diagnosis of hypercoagulability? In: Neri Serner GG, Prentice CRM, eds. *Haemostasis and Thrombosis*. London: Academic Press, 1978; 159.

271. Lundgren CH, Sawa H, Soble BE, Fujii S. Modulation of expression of monocyte/macrophage plasminogen activator activity and its implications for attenuation of vasculopathy. *Circulation* 1994; **90:** 1927–34.

272. Macfarlane RG. Fibrinolysis following operation. *Lancet* 1937; **1:** 10–12.

273. MacFarlane RG. An enzyme cascade in the blood clotting mechanism and its function as a biochemical amplifier. *Nature* 1964; **202:** 498.

274. Machin SJ. Platelets and antiphospholipid antibodies. *Lupus* 1996; **5:** 386–7.

275. Macintyre IMC, Webber RG, Crispin JR, *et al.* Plasma fibrinolysis and postoperative deep vein thrombosis. *Br J Surg* 1976; **63:** 694.

276. Marcus AJ, Safier LB, Hajjar KA, *et al.* Inhibition of platelet function by an aspirin-insensitive endothelial cell membrane adenosine diphosphatase. Thromboregulation by endothelial cells. *J Clin Invest* 1991; **88:** 1690.

277. Mackie M, Bennett B, Ogston D, Douglas AS. Familial thrombosis inherited deficiency of antithrombin III. *Br Med J* 1978; **1:** 136.

278. Malone PC, Morris CJ. Margination and sequestration of platelets and leucocytes on hypoxic endothelium. *J Pathol* 1978; **125:** 119.

279. Mansfield A. Alteration in fibrinolysis associated with surgery and venous thrombosis. *Br J Surg* 1972; **59:** 754.

280. Mantavani A, Dejana E. Cytokines as communication signals between leucocytes and endothelial cells. *Immunol Today* 1989; **10:** 370–5.

281. Marcus AJ. Thrombosis and inflammation as multicellular processes: significance of cell-cell interaction. *Semin Haematol* 1994; **31:** 261–9.

282. Marlar RA, Endres-Brooks J. Recurrent thromboembolic disease due to heterozygous protein C deficiency. *Thromb Haemost* 1983; **50:** 331.

283. Mason R, Sharp D, Chuang H, Mohammed F. The endothelium. Roles in thrombosis and haemostasis. *Arch Pathol Lab Med* 1977; **101:** 61.

284. Matsuda T, Murakami M. Relationship between fibrinogen and blood viscosity. *Thromb Res* 1976; **8 (2 Suppl):** 25–33.

285. May R. *Surgery of Veins of the Leg and Pelvis.* Stuttgart: Thieme, 1979.

286. May R. Thurner J. Ein Gefasssporn in der Vena iliaca com. sin. als wahrscheinliche Ursache der Überwiegend linksseitigen Beckenvenenthrombosen. *Z Kreislaufforsch* 1956; **45:** 912.

287. Mayo ME, Halil T, Browse NL. The incidence of deep vein thrombosis after prostatectomy. *Br J Urol* 1971; **43:** 738.

288. McCarrol D, Levin E, Montgomery R. Endothelial cell synthesis of von Willebrand antigen. *J Clin Invest* 1985; **75:** 1089–95.

289. McGovern VJ. Reactions to injury of vascular endothelium with special reference to the problems of thrombosis. *J Pathol Bacteriol* 1955; **69:** 283.

290. McGrath JM, Stewart GJ. The effects of endotoxin on vascular endothelium. *J Exp Med* 1969; **129:** 833.

291. McGuinness CL, Humphries J, Smith A, Burnand KG. Monocyte chemotactic protein-1 accelerates thrombus resolution. *Surg Res Soc* 1998; in press.

292. McLachlan MSF, Thompson JG, Taylor DW, Kelly M, Sackett DL. Observer variation in the interpretation of lower leg venograms. *Am J Radiol* 1979; **132:** 227.

293. McLachlin AD, McLachlin JA, Jory TA, Rawling EG. Venous stasis in the lower extremities. *Ann Surg* 1960; **152:** 678.

294. McPherson K. Third generation oral contraception and venous thromboembolism. *Br Med J* 1996; **312:** 68–9.

295. Meissner MH, Caps MT, Bergelin RO, Manzo RA, Strandness DE Jr. Propagation, rethrombosis and new thrombus formation after acute deep venous thrombosis. *J Vasc Surg* 1995; **22(5):** 558–67.

296. Melissari E, Monte G, Lindo VS, *et al.* Congenital thrombophilia among patients with venous thromboembolism. *Blood Coagul Fibrinolysis* 1992; **3(6):** 749–58.

297. Meyers L, Poindexter CH. A study of the prothrombin time in normal subjects and in patients with arteriosclerosis. *Am Heart J* 1946; **31:** 27.

298. Milne R. Venous thromboembolism and travel: is there an association? *J R Coll Phys (Lond)* 1992; **26:** 47–9.

299. Mitchell JRA. Can we really prevent postoperative pulmonary emboli? *Br Med J* 1979; **1:** 1523.

300. Mitchell JRA. Experimental thrombosis. In: Chalmers DG, Gresham GA, eds. *Biological Aspects of Occlusive Vascular Disease.* London: Cambridge University Press, 1964.

301. Moncada S, Gryglewski R, Bunting S, Vane JR. An enzyme isolated from arteries transforms prostaglandin endoperoxides to an unstable substance that inhibits platelet aggregation. *Nature* 1976; **263:** 663.

302. Moncada S, Vane JR. Unstable metabolites of arachidonic acid and their role in haemostasis and thrombosis. *Br Med Bull* 1978; **34:** 129.

303. Moore KL, Esmon CT, Esmon CL. Tumour necrosis factor leads to the internalization and degradation of thrombomodulin from the surface of bovine endothelial cells in culture. *Blood* 1989; **73:** 159–65.

304. Morrell MT, Dunhill MS. The post mortem incidence of pulmonary embolism in a hospital population. *Br J Surg* 1968; **55:** 347.

305. Murata K, Nakazawa K, Hamai A. Distribution of acidic glycosaminoglycans in the intima, media and adventitia of bovine aorta and their anticoagulant properties. *Atherosclerosis* 1975; **21:** 93.

306. Mustard JF. Function of blood platelets and their role in thrombosis. *Trans Am Clin Climatol Assoc* 1976; **87:** 104.

307. Mustard JF, Hegardt B, Rowsell HC, MacMillan RL. Effect of adenosine nucleotides on platelet aggregation and clotting time. *J Lab Clin Med* 1964; **64:** 548.

308. Mustard JF, Murphy EA, Rowsell HC, Downie HG. Factors influencing thrombus formation in vivo. *Am J Med* 1962; **33:** 621.

309. Myhre HO, Storen EJ, Ongre A. The incidence of deep venous thrombosis in patients with leg oedema after arterial reconstruction. *Scand J Thorac Cardiovasc Surg* 1974; **8:** 73.

310. Naide M. Spontaneous venous thrombosis in the legs of tall men. *JAMA* 1952; **148:** 1202.

311. Nakazawa K, Murata K. Acidic glycosaminoglycans in three layers of human aorta: their different constitution and anticoagulant function. *Paroi Arterielle* 1975; **2:** 203–11.

312. Nawroth PP, Stern DM. Modulation of endothelial cell haemostatic properties by tumour necrosis factor. *J Exp Med* 1986; **163:** 740–5.

313. Negus D, Pinto DJ, Brown N. Platelet adhesiveness in postoperative deep vein thrombosis. *Lancet* 1969; **1:** 220.

314. Negus D, Pinto DH, LeQuesne LP, Brown N, Chapman M. [125]I labelled fibrinogen in the diagnosis of deep vein thrombosis and its correlation with phlebography. *Br J Surg* 1968; **55:** 835.

315. Nemerson Y. Tissue factor and haemostasis. *Blood* 1988; **71:** 1–8.

316. Nicolaides AN, Clark CT, Thomas RD, Lewis JD. Soleal veins and local fibrinolytic activity. *Br J Surg* 1972; **59:** 914.

317. Nicolaides AN, Fernandez JF, Pollack AV. Intermittent sequential compression of the legs in prevention of venous stasis and postoperative DVT. *Surgery* 1980; **87:** 69.

318. Nicolaides AN, Field ES, Kakkar VV, Yates-Bell AJ, Taylor S, Clarke MB. Prostatectomy and deep-vein thrombosis. *Br J Surg* 1972; **59:** 487.

319. Nicolaides AN, Irving D. Clinical factors and the risk of deep venous thrombosis. In: Nicolaides AN, ed. *Thromboembolism, Aetiology, Advances in Prevention and Management.* Lancaster: MTP, 1975.

320. Nicolaides AN, Kakkar VV, Field ES, Fish P. Soleal veins, stasis and prevention of deep vein thrombosis. In: Kakkar VV, Jouhar AJ, eds. *Thromboembolism.* Edinburgh: Churchill Livingstone, 1972.

321. Nicolaides AN, Kakkar VV, Field ES, Renney JTG. The origin of deep vein thrombosis: a venographic study. *Br J Radiol* 1971; **44:** 653.

322. Nillius AS, Nylander G. Deep vein thrombosis after total hip replacement: a clinical and phlebographic study. *Br J Surg* 1979; **66:** 324.

323. Nilsen D, Jeremic M, Weisert O. An attempt at predicting postoperative deep vein thrombosis by preoperative coagulation studies in patients undergoing total hip replacement. *Thromb Haemost* 1980; **43:** 194.

324. Nilsson IM. Biochemical and clinical aspects of factor VIII. In: Saldeen T, ed. *The Microembolism Syndrome.* Stockholm: Almqvist & Wiksell, 1979.

325. Nilsson IM, Krook H, Sternby N-H, Soderberg E, Soderstrom N. Severe thrombotic disease in a young man with bone marrow skeletal changes and with a high content of an inhibitor in the fibrinolytic system. *Acta Med Scand* 1961; **169:** 323.

326. Nilsson IM, Ljungner H, Tengborn L. Two different mechanisms in patients with venous thrombosis and defective fibrinolysis: low concentration of plasminogen activator or increased concentration of plasminogen activator inhibitor. *Br Med J* 1985; **290:** 1453.

327. Nilsson IM, Pandolfi M. Fibrinolytic response of the vascular wall. *Thromb Diath Haemorrh (Suppl)* 1970; **40:** 231.

328. Nordstrom M, Lindblad B, Bergquist D, Kjellstrom T. A prospective study of the incidence of deep vein thrombosis within a defined urban population. *J Int Med* 1992; **232:** 155–60.

329. Northeast ADR, Creighton LJ, Gaffney PJ, Burnand KG. Vein wall fibrinolysis: the response to thrombosis. *Ann NY Acad Sci* 1992; **667:** 127–40.

330. Northeast ADR, Soo KS, Bobrow LG, Gafney PJ, Burnand KG. The tissue plasminogen activator and urokinase response in vivo during natural resolution of venous thrombosis. *J Vasc Surg* 1995; **22:** 573–9.

331. Nossel HL. Radioimmunoassay of fibrinopeptides in relation to intravascular coagulation and thrombosis. *N Engl J Med* 1976; **295:** 428.

332. Nykjaer A, Peterson CM, Christensen EI, Davidsen O, Gliemann J. Urokinase receptors in human monocytes. *Biochim Biophys Acta* 1990; **1052:** 399–407.

333. Nylander G, Olivecrona H. The phlebographic pattern of acute leg thrombosis within a defined urban population. *Acta Chir Scand* 1976; **142:** 505.

334. Nylander G, Olivecrona H, Hedner U. Earlier and concurrent morbidity of patients with acute lower leg thrombosis. *Acta Chir Scand* 1977; **143:** 425.

335. Nylander G, Semb H. Veins of the lower part of the leg after tibial fractures. *Surg Gynecol Obstet* 1972; **134:** 974.

336. O'Brien TE, Woodford M, Irving MH. The effect of intermittent compression of the calf on the fibrinolytic responses in the blood during a surgical operation. *Surg Gynecol Obstet* 1979; **149:** 380.

337. Ochsner A, DeBakey ME, DeCamp PT. Venous thrombosis. Analysis of 580 cases. *Surgery* 1951; **29:** 24.

338. Ogura JH, Fetter NR, Blankenhorn MA, Glueck HI. Changes in blood coagulation following coronary thrombosis measured by the heparin retarded clotting test (Waugh and Ruddick test). *J Clin Invest* 1946; **25:** 586.

339. Ohlin A-K, Marlar RA. Mutations in the thrombomodulin gene associated with thromboembolic disease. *Thromb Haemost* 1995; **73:** 1096.

340. Olds RJ, Lane DA, Chowdhury V, *et al.* (ATT) trinucleotide repeats in the antithrombin gene and their use in determining the origin of repeated mutations. *Hum Mut* 1994; **4:** 31–41.

341. Olin JW, Graor RA, O'Hara P, Young JR. The incidence of deep venous thrombosis in patients undergoing abdominal aortic aneurysm resection. *J Vasc Surg* 1993; **18(6):** 1037–41.

342. Olsson P. Variations in antithrombin activity in plasma after major surgery. *Acta Chir Scand* 1963; **126:** 24.

343. O'Neill JF. The effects on venous endothelium of alterations in blood flow through the vessels in vein walls, and the possible relation to thrombosis. *Ann Surg* 1947; **126:** 270.

344. Pabinger-Fasching I, Bertina RM, Lechner K, Niessner H, Korininger CH. Protein C deficiency in two Austrian families. *Thromb Haemost* 1983; **50:** 180.

345. Patel MI, Hardman DT, Nicholls D, Fisher CM, Appleberg M. The incidence of deep venous thrombosis after laparoscopic cholecystectomy. *Med J Aust* 1996; **164(11):** 652–4.

346. Paterson JC. The pathology of venous thrombi. In: Sherry S, Brinkhous KM, Genton E, Stengle JM, eds. *Thrombosis.* Washington, DC: National Academy of Sciences USA, 1969.

347. Pober JS. Cytokine-mediated activation of vascular endothelium. *Am J Pathol* 1988; **133:** 426–33.

348. Pober JS, Cotran RS. The role of endothelial cells in inflammation. *Transplantation* 1991; **50:** 536–44.

349. Poole JCF, French JE. Thrombosis. *J Atheroscler Res* 1961; **1:** 251.

350. Powers JH. Post-operative thromboembolism: some remarks on the influence of early ambulation. *Am J Med* 1947; **3:** 224.

351. Prandoni I, Lensing AWA, Buller HR, *et al.* Deep vein thrombosis and the incidence of subsequent symptomatic cancer. *N Engl J Med* 1992; **327:** 1128–33.

352. Prisco D, Chiarantini E, Boddi M, Rostagno C, Colella A, Gensini GF. Predictive value for thrombotic disease of plasminogen activator inhibitor-1 plasma levels. *Int J Clin Lab Res* 1993; **23(2):** 78–82.

353. Quarmby JW, Smith A, Collins M, Eastham D, Burnand KG. A human model of venous thrombosis. *Phlebology Society of America 16th Annual Congress*, New York: 1996.

354. Quarmby JW, Smith A, Humphries J, Burnand KG, Collins M, McGuinness CL. Increased expression of soluble VCAM-1 in venous thrombosis. *SVS & ISCVS Joint Annual Meeting*, Boston, MA: 1997.

355. Rapaport SI. The extrinsic pathway inhibitor: a regulator of tissue factor-dependent blood coagulation. *Thromb Haemost* 1991; **66:** 6–15.

356. Ratnoff OD, Busse RJ, Sheon RP. The demise of John Hageman. *N Engl J Med* 1968; **279:** 760.

357. Rees DC, Cox M, Clegg JB. World distribution of factor V Leiden. *Lancet* 1995; **346:** 330–6.

358. Reilly DT, Burden AC, Fossard DP. Fibrinolysis and the prediction of postoperative deep vein thrombosis. *Br J Surg* 1980; **67:** 66.

359. Reitsma PH, Poort SR, Bernardi F, *et al.* Protein C deficiency: a database of mutations. 1995 update. *Thromb Haemost* 1995; **73:** 876–89.

360. Ridker PM, Hennekens CH, Lindpaintner K, Stampfner MJ, Eisenberg PR, Miletich JP. Mutation in the gene coding for coagulation factor V and the risk of myocardial infarction, stroke and venous thrombosis in apparently healthy men. *N Engl J Med* 1995; **332(14):** 912–17.

361. Riley KN, McCabe CJ, Abbott WM, *et al.* Deep venous thrombophlebitis following aortoiliac reconstructive surgery. *Arch Surg* 1982; **17:** 1210.

362. Roberts J, ed. *The Haemostasis and Thrombosis Task Force of the Investigation and Management of Thrombophilia in Standard Haematology Practice.* Oxford: Blackwell Scientific Press, 1991; 112–27.

363. Roberts VC, Cotton LT. Prevention of postoperative deep vein thrombosis in patients with malignant disease. *Br Med J* 1974; **1:** 358.

364. Rohrer MJ, Cutler BS, MacDougall E, Herrmann JB, Anderson FA Jr, Wheeler HB. A prospective study of the incidence of deep venous thrombosis in hospitalized children. *J Vasc Surg* 1996; **24(1):** 46–9.

365. Rokito SE, Schwartz MC, Neuwirth MG. Deep vein thrombosis after major reconstructive spinal surgery. *Spine* 1996; **21(7):** 853–8.

366. Rosenberg RD. Actions and interactions of antithrombin and heparin. *N Engl J Med* 1975; **292:** 146.

367. Rosenberg RD. Heparin, antithrombin and abnormal clotting. *Annu Rev Med* 1978; **29:** 367.

368. Rosenfeld JC, Estrada FP, Orr RM. Management of deep venous thrombosis in the pregnant female. *J Cardiovasc Surg* 1990; **31:** 678–82.

369. Roskam J. Role of platelets in the formation of a hemostatic plug. In: Johnson SA, ed. *The Henry Ford Hospital Symposium on Blood Platelets.* Boston, MA: Little Brown, 1961.

370. Roskam J, Hughes J, Bounameaux Y, Salmon J. The part played by platelets in the formation of an efficient hemostatic plug. *Thromb Diath Haemorrh* 1959; **3:** 510.

371. Roubey RAS. Autoantibodies to phospholipid-binding plasma proteins: a new view of lupus anticoagulants and other 'antiphospholipid' autoantibodies. *Blood* 1994; **84:** 2854–67.

372. Rowntree LG, Shionya T. Studies on experimental extracorporeal thrombosis. I – A method for direct observation of extracorporeal thrombosis formation. *J Exp Med* 1927; **45:** 7.

373. Ruckley CV. ¹²⁵I fibrinogen test in the diagnosis of deep vein thrombosis. *Br Med J* 1975; **2:** 498.

374. Ruckley CV. A multi-unit controlled trial of heparin and dextran in the prevention of venous thromboembolic disease. In: Kakkar VV, Thomas DP, eds. *Heparin, Chemistry and Clinical Usage.* London: Academic Press, 1976.

375. Ruckley CV. Pulmonary embolism; trends in Edinburgh surgical units over twenty years. *Thromb Haemost* 1981; **46:** 18.

376. Rue LW 3d, Cioffi WG Jr, Rush R, McManus WF, Pruitt BA Jr. Thromboembolic complications in thermally injured patients. *World J Surg* 1992; **16(6):** 1151–4.

377. Saeger W, Genzkow M. Venous thromboses and pulmonary embolisms in post-mortem series: probable causes by correlations of clinical data and basic diseases. *Pathol Res Pract* 1994; **190(4):** 394–9.

378. Sagar S, Massey J, Sanderson JM. Low dose heparin prophylaxis against fatal pulmonary embolism. *Br Med J* 1975; **4:** 257.

379. Sagar S, Stamatakis JD, Thomas DP, Kakkar VV. Oral contraceptives antithrombin 111 activity and post-operative deep vein thrombosis. *Lancet* 1976; **1:** 509.

380. Sagdic K, Ozer ZG, Saba D, Ture M, Cengiz M. Venous lesions in Behcet's disease. *Eur J Vasc Endovasc Surg* 1996; **11(4):** 437–40.

381. Sahiar F, Mohler SR. Economy class syndrome. *Aviat Space Environ Med* 1994; **65:** 957–60.

382. Samuels PB, Webster DR. The role of venous endothelium in the inception of thrombosis. *Ann Surg* 1952; **136:** 422.

383. Sandler DA, Martin JF. Liquid crystal thermography as a screening test for deep-vein thrombosis. *Lancet* 1985; **1:** 665.

384. Sandler D, Martin JF, Duncan JS, *et al.* Diagnosis of deep-vein thrombosis: comparison of clinical evaluation, ultrasound, plethysmography and venoscan with X-ray venogram. *Lancet* 1984; **2:** 716.

385. Sandset PM, Abildgaard U, Larsen ML. Heparin induces release of extrinsic pathway inhibitor (EPI). *Br J Haematol* 1988; **72:** 391–6.

386. Sas G, Blasko G, Bankegyi D, Jako J, Palos A. Abnormal antithrombin III (antithrombin III 'Budapest') as a cause of a familial thrombophilia. *Thomb Diath Haemorrh* 1974; **32:** 105.

387. Satiani B, Kuhns M, Evans WE. Deep venous thrombosis following operations upon the abdominal aorta. *Surg Gynecol Obstet* 1980; **151:** 241.

388. Sawyer PN, Srinivasan S. The role of surface phenomena in intravascular thrombosis. *Bibl Anat* 1973; **12:** 106.

389. Schaub N, Duckert F, Fridrich R, Gruber UF. Haufigkeit postoperative tiefer Venenthrombosen bei Patienten der allgemeinen Chirurgie und Urologie. *Langenbecks Arch Chir* 1975; **340:** 23.

390. Schleef RR, Bevilacqua MP, Sawdey M, *et al.* Cytokine activation of vascular endothelium: effects on tissue type plasminogen activator and type one plasminogen activator inhibitor. *J Biol Chem* 1988; **263:** 5797–803.

391. Scott GBD. Venous intimal thickenings and thrombosis. *J Pathol Bacteriol* 1956; **72:** 543.

392. Seeger WH, Marciniak E. Inhibition of autoprothrombin C activity with plasma. *Nature* 1962; **193:** 1188.

393. Seigel DG. Pregnancy, the puerperium and the steroid contraceptive. In: Foster D, ed. *The Epidemiology of Venous Thrombosis. Milbank Mem Fund Q* 1972; **50(Suppl 2):** 15–23.

394. Senftleben W. Uber den verschluss der blutgefasse nach unterbindung. *Arch Pathol Anat Physiol* 1879; **77:** 421.

395. Sevitt S. Pathology and pathogenesis of deep vein thrombi. In: Bergan JJ, Yao JST, eds. *Venous Problems.* Chicago, IL: Year Book Medical Publishers, 1978.

396. Sevitt S. The structure and growth of valve pocket thrombi in femoral veins. *J Clin Pathol* 1974; **27:** 517.

397. Sevitt S. Venous thrombosis and pulmonary embolism. Their prevention by oral anticoagulants. *Am J Med* 1962; **33:** 703.

398. Sevitt S, Gallagher NG. Prevention of venous thrombosis and pulmonary embolism in injured patients. *Lancet* 1959; **2:** 981.

399. Sevitt S, Gallagher NG. Venous thrombosis and pulmonary embolism. A clinico-pathological study in injured and burned patients. *Br J Surg* 1961; **48:** 475.

400. Shapiro S. Hyperprothrombinemia, a premonitory sign of thromboembolization (description of a method). *Exp Med Surg* 1944; **2:** 103.

401. Shapiro S, Sherwin B, Gordimer H. Postoperative thrombo-embolization. *Ann Surg* 1942; **116:** 175.

402. Short DS. A survey of pulmonary embolism in a general hospital. *Br Med J* 1952; **1:** 790.

403. Silverstein MD, Mohr DN, Heit JA, Petterson T, O'Fallon WM. Incidence of deep vein thrombosis and pulmonary embolism. A population based study. *Soc Gen Int Med* 1993; 6 (Abstract).

404. Simioni P, Lazarro AR, Corer E, Salmiistraro G, Girolami A. constitutional heparin cofactor II deficiency and thrombosis. *Blood Coagul Fibrinolysis* 1990; **1:** 351–6.

405. Simon DI, Ezratty AM, Francis SA, Rennke H, Lascalzo J. Fibrinogen is internalized and degraded by activated human monocytoid cells via Mac-1 (CD11b/CD18): a non-plasmin fibrinolytic pathway. *Blood* 1993; **82:** 2414–22.

406. Simpson K. Shelter deaths from pulmonary embolism. *Lancet* 1940; **2:** 744.

407. Sinclair J, Forbes CD, Prentice CRM, Scott R. The incidence of deep vein thrombosis in prostatectomised patients following the administration of the fibrinolytic inhibitor, aminocaproic acid (EACA). *Urol Res* 1976; **4:** 129.

408. Smith RC, Duncancson J, Ruckley CV, *et al.* β-Thromboglobulin and deep vein thrombosis. *Thromb Haemost* 1978; **39:** 338.

409. Smith R, Thick E, Coalston J, Stein P. Thrombus production by turbulence. *J Appl Physiol* 1972; **32:** 261.

410. Soo KS, Northeast ADR, Happerfield LC, Burnand KG, Bobrow LG. Tissue plasminogen activator production by monocytes in venous thrombolysis. *J Pathol* 1998; **178:** 190–4.

411. Spaet TH, Erichson RB. The vascular wall in the pathogenesis of thrombosis. *Thromb Diath Haemorrh (Suppl)* 1966; **21:** 67.

412. Spaet TH, Ts'Ao CH. Vascular endothelium and thrombogenesis. In: Sherry S, Brinkhous KM, Genton E, Stengle JM, eds. *Thrombosis.* Washington, DC: National Academy of Sciences USA, 1969.

413. Spitzer WO, Lewis MA, Heinemann LAJ, Thorogood M, MacRae KD. Third generation oral contraceptives and risk of venous thromboembolic disorders: and international case-control study. *Br Med J* 1996; **312:** 83–8.

414. Sproul EE. Carcinoma and venous thrombosis: the frequency of association of carcinoma in the body or tail of the pancreas with multiple venous thrombosis. *Am J Cancer* 1938; **34:** 566.

415. Stamatakis JD, Kakkar VV, Sagar S, Lawrence D, Nairn D, Bentley PG. Femoral vein thrombosis and total hip replacement. *Br Med J* 1977; **2:** 223.

416. Stathatkis N, Papayannis AG, Gardikas CD. Postoperative antithrombin III concentration. *Lancet* 1973; **1:** 430.

417. Stead NW, Bauer KA, Kinney TR, *et al.* Venous thrombosis in a family with defective release of vascular plasminogen activator and elevated plasma factor VIII, von Willebrand's factor. *Am J Med* 1983; **74:** 33.

418. Stein P, Sabbah H. Measured turbulence and its effect on thrombus formation. *Circ Res* 1974; **35:** 608.

419. Stephens PH, Healy MT, Smith M, Jewkes DA. Prophylaxis against thromboembolism in neurosurgical patients: a survey of current practice in the United Kingdom. *Br J Neurosurg* 1995; **9(2):** 159–63.

420. Stevens J, Fardin R, Freeark R. Lower extremity thrombophlebitis in patients with femoral neck fractures. A venographic investigation and a review of the early and late significance of the findings. *J Trauma* 1968; **8:** 527.

421. Stewart GJ. The role of the vessel wall in deep venous thrombosis. In: Nicolaides AN, ed. *Thromboembolism. Aetiology, Advances in Prevention and Management.* Lancaster: MTP, 1975.

422. Stewart GJ, Anderson MJ. An ultrastructural study of endotoxin induced changes in mesenteric arteries. *Br J Exp Pathol* 1971; **52:** 75.

423. Stewart GJ, Ritchie WGM, Lynch PR. A scanning and transmission electron microscopic study of canine jugular veins. Scanning electron microscopy (Part III). In: *Proceedings of the Workshop on Scanning Electron Microcopy in Pathology.* Chicago, IL: II T Research Institute, 1973.

424. Stewart GJ, Ritchie WGM, Lynch PR. Venous endothelial damage produced by massive sticking and emigration of leukocytes. *Am J Pathol* 1974; **74:** 507.

425. Stewart GJ, Stern HS, Lynch PR, Malmud LS, Schaub RG. Response of the canine jugular veins and carotid arteries to hysterectomy: increased permeability and leukocyte adhesions and invasion. *Thromb Res* 1980; **20:** 473.

426. Stewart GJ, Stern HR, Schaub RG. Endothelial alterations, deposition of blood elements and increased accumulation of ^{131}I-albumin in canine jugular veins following abdominal surgery. *Thromb Res* 1978; **12:** 555.

427. Stormorken H, Lund M, Holmsen I. Vessel wall activator (tPA) as evaluated by poststasis euglobulin lysis time (PELT) in recurrent deep vein thrombosis. In: Jespersen J, Kluft C, Korsgaard O, eds. *Clinical Aspects of Fibrinolysis and Thrombolysis.* Esbjerg: South Jutland University Press, 1983.

428. Sue-Ling HM, Johnston D, McMahon MJ, Phillips PR, Davis JA. Pre-operative identification of patients at high risk of deep venous thrombosis after elective major abdominal surgery. *Lancet* 1986; **1:** 1173.

429. Sue-Ling HM, Johnston D, Verheijen JH, Kluft C, Philips PR, Davies JA. Indicators of depressed fibrinolytic activity in preoperative prediction of deep venous thrombosis. *Br J Surg* 1987; **74:** 275–8.

430. Sundqvist S-B, Hedner U, Kullenberg HKE, Bergentz S-E. Deep venous thrombosis of the arm: a study of coagulation and fibrinolysis. *Br Med J* 1981; **283:** 265.

431. Svensson PJ, Dahlbach B. Resistance to activated protein C as a basis for venous thrombosis. *N Engl J Med* 1994; **330(8):** 517–22.

432. Taberner DA, Poller L, Burslem RW. Antiplasmin concentration after surgery: failure of alpha2-antiplasmin to rise in patients with venous thrombosis. *Br Med J* 1979; **1:** 1122.

433. Tait RC, Walker ID, Reitsma PH, *et al.* Prevalence of protein C deficiency in the healthy population. *Thromb Haemost* 1995; **73(1):** 87–93.

434. Tanaka K, Hirst AK, Smith LL. Rate of endothelialization in venous thrombi: an experimental study. *Arch Surg* 1982; **117:** 1045.

435. Tateson JE, Moncada S, Vane JR. Effect of prostacyclin (PGX) on cyclic AMP concentration in human platelets. *Prostaglandins* 1977; **13:** 389.

436. The British Society of Haematology 1988. *Thrombophilia: Diagnosis and Management.* International Symposium, 19 February, 1988. London: Royal Society of Medicine.
437. Thomas DP, Merton RE, Wood RD, Hockley DJ. The relationship between vessel wall injury and venous thrombosis: an experimental study. *Br J Haematol* 1985; **59:** 449.
438. Thomas DP, Wessler S. Stasis thrombi induced by bacterial endotoxin. *Circ Res* 1964; **14:** 486.
439. Todd AS. The histological localization of fibrinolysis activator. *J Pathol Bacteriol* 1959; **78:** 281.
440. Törngren S, Norén I, Savidge G. The effect of low-dose heparin on fibrinopeptide A, platelets, fibrinogen degradation products and other haemostatic parameters measured in connection with intestinal surgery. *Thromb Res* 1979; **14:** 871.
441. Tran TH, Marbet GA, Duckert F. Association of hereditary heparin co-factor 2 deficiency with thrombosis. *Lancet* 1985; **2:** 413.
442. Triplett DA. Coagulation assays for the lupus anticoagulant: review and critique of current methodology. *Stroke* 1992; **23:** 11.
443. Trousseau A. *Phlegmatia alba dolens. In Clinique médicale de l'Hotel-Dieu de Paris*, 2nd edition. Vol. 3. Paris: Baillière, 1865; 654.
444. Turnbull A, Tindall VR, Beard RW. *Report on Confidential Enquiry into Maternal Deaths in England and Wales 1982-1984.* London: HMSO, 1989; 28–36.
445. Turpie AGG, Gent M, Doyle DJ, *et al.* An evaluation of suloctidil in the prevention of deep vein thrombosis in neurosurgical patients. *Thromb Res* 1985; **39:** 173–81.
446. Vandenbroucke JP, Koster T, Briet E, Reitsma PH, Bertina RM, Rosendaal FR. Increased risk of venous thrombosis in oral-contraceptive users who are carriers of factor V Leiden mutation. *Lancet* 1994; **344:** 1453–7.
447. Vessey MP, Doll R. Investigation of relation between use of oral contraceptives and thromboembolic disease: a further report. *Br Med J* 1968; **2:** 199.
448. Vessey MP, Doll R, Fairburn AS. Post-operative thromboembolism and the use of oral contraceptives. *Br Med J* 1970; **3:** 123.
449. Vessey MP, Mann JI. Female sex hormones and thrombosis. Epidemiological aspects. *Br Med Bull* 1978; **34:** 157.
450. Vessey M, Mant D, Smith A, Yeates D. Oral contraceptives and venous thromboembolism: findings in a large prospective study. *Br Med J* 1986; **292:** 526.
451. Vianna JL, Khamashta MA, Ordi-Ros J, *et al.* Comparison of the primary and secondary antiphospholipid syndrome: a European multicenter study of 114 patients. *Am J Med* 1994; **36:** 3–9.
452. Villa P, Aznar J, Mira Y, Angeles F, Vaya A. Third generation oral contraceptives and low free protein S as a risk for venous thrombosis. *Lancet* 1996; **347:** 397.
453. Vinnicombe J, Shuttleworth KED. Aminocaproic acid in the control of haemorrhage after prostatectomy. Safety of aminocaproic acid – a controlled trial. *Lancet* 1966; **1:** 232.
454. Virchow R. Die Verstopfung den Lungenarteries und ihre Folgen. *Beitr Exp Pathol Physiol* 1846; 21.
455. Von Kaulla E, Von Kaulla KM. Oral contraceptives and low antithrombin III activity. *Lancet* 1970; **1:** 36.
456. Von Kaulla E, Von Kaulla KN. Antithrombin III and diseases. *Am J Clin Pathol* 1967; **48:** 69.
457. Von Kaulla E, Von Kaulla KN. Deficiency of antithrombin III activity associated with hereditary thrombosis tendency. *J Med* 1972; **3:** 349.
458. Von Recklinghausen F. Handbuch der allgemeinen Pathologie des Kreislaufs und der Ernäbrung. *Dtsche Chir* 1883; **2:** 52.
459. Voorberg J, Roelse J, Koopman R, *et al.* Association of idiopathic venous thromboembolism with a single point mutation at Arg506 of factor V. *Lancet* 1994; **343:** 1535–6.
460. Walsh JJ, Bonnar J, Wright FM. A study of pulmonary embolism after deep leg vein thrombosis after major gynaecological surgery using labelled fibrinogen, phlebography and lung scanning. *J Obstet Gynaecol Br Commonw* 1974; **81:** 311.
461. Warlow C, Ogston D. The ^{125}I-fibrinogen technique in the diagnosis of venous thrombosis. *Clin Haematol* 1973; **2:** 199.
462. Warlow C, Ogston D, Douglas AS. Deep venous thrombosis of the legs after strokes. Part 1. Incidence and predisposing factors. *Br Med J* 1976; **1:** 1178.
463. Warren R, Lauridsen J, Belko J. Alteration in numbers of circulating platelets following surgical operation and administration of adrenocorticotrophic hormone. *Circulation* 1953; **7:** 481.
464. Waugh TR, Ruddick DW. Studies on increased coagulability of the blood. *Can Med Assoc J* 1944; **51:** 11.
465. Welch CE, Fexon HH. Thrombophlebitis and pulmonary embolism. *JAMA* 1941; **117:** 1502.
466. Wells RE. Rheological aspects of stasis in thrombus formation. In: Sherry S, Brinkhous KM, Genton E, Stengle JM, eds. *Thrombosis*. Washington, DC: National Academy of Sciences USA, 1969.
467. Welsh WH. The structure of white thrombi. *Trans Pathol Soc Phil* 1887; **13:** 281.
468. Wessler S. Studies in intravascular coagulation. I. Coagulation changes in isolated venous segments. *J Clin Invest* 1952; **31:** 1011.
469. Wessler S. Studies in intravascular coagulation. III. The pathogenesis of serum induced venous thrombosis. *J Clin Invest* 1955; **34:** 647.
470. Wessler S. Thrombosis in the presence of vascular stasis. *Am J Med* 1962; **33:** 648.
471. Wessler S, Yin ET. Experimental hypercoagulable state induced by factor X: comparison of the nonactivated and activated forms. *J Lab Clin Med* 1968; **72:** 256.
472. Wessler S, Yin ET. On the mechanism of thrombosis. *Prog Hematol* 1969; **6:** 201.
473. Wheeler HB, Anderson FA, Cardullo PA, Patwarden NA, Jian-Ming L, Cutler BS. Suspected deep vein thrombosis: management by impedance plethysmography. *Arch Surg* 1982; **117:** 1206.

474. Wigton DH, Kociba GJ, Hoover EA. Infectious canine hepatitis: animal model for viral induced disseminated intravascular coagulation. *Blood* 1976; **47:** 287.

475. Wilkins RW, Mixter G, Stanton JR, Litter J. Elastic stockings in the prevention of pulmonary embolism: a preliminary report. *N Engl J Med* 1952; **246:** 360.

476. Wilkins RW, Stanton JR. Elastic stockings in the prevention of pulmonary embolism. II. A progress report. *N Engl J Med* 1953; **248:** 1087.

477. Willms-Kretschumer K, Flax MH, Cotran RS. The fine structure of the vascular response in hapten-specific delayed hypersensitivity and contact dermatitis. *J Lab Invest* 1967; **13:** 334–49.

478. Wills AL, Kuhn DC. A new potential mediator of arterial thrombosis whose biosynthesis is inhibited by aspirin. *Prostaglandins* 1973; **4:** 127.

479. Winter JH, Fenech A, Bennett B, Douglas AS. Thrombosis after venography and familial antithrombin III deficiency. *Br Med J* 1981; **283:** 1436.

480. Wiseman R. *Several Surgical Treatises.* London: Norton & Macock, 1676.

481. Wolfe JHN, Morland M, Browse NL. The fibrinolytic activity of varicose veins. *Br J Surg* 1979; **66:** 185.

482. Wright G Payling. *An Introduction to Pathology.* London: Longmans Green, 1958.

483. Wright H Payling, Osborn SB, Edmonds DG. Effects of post-operative bedrest and early ambulation on the rate of venous blood flow. *Lancet* 1956; **1:** 222.

484. Wright H Payling. Changes in the adhesiveness of blood platelets following parturition and surgical operations. *J Pathol Bacteriol* 1942; **54:** 461.

485. Wu AVO, Mansfield A. The relationship between the blood and vein wall fibrinolytic activity in response to surgical trauma. *Acta Haematol* 1980; **63:** 191.

486. Yeager RA, Moneta GL, Edwards JM, Taylor LM Jr, McConnell DB, Porter JM. Deep vein thrombosis associated with lower extremity amputation. *J Vasc Surg* 1995; **22(5):** 612.

487. Ygge J. Studies on blood coagulation and fibrinolysis in conditions associated with an increased incidence of thrombosis. Methodological and clinical investigations. *Scand J Haematol Suppl* 1970; **11:** 1–45.

488. Yin ET, Wessler S, Stoll PJ. Identity of plasma activated factor X inhibitor with antithrombin III and heparin co-factor. *J Biol Chem* 1971; **246:** 712.

489. Zahn W. Untersuchungen über Thrombose. *Zentralbl Med Wissenschaften* 1872; **10:** 129.

490. Zucker MB. Platelet agglutination and vasoconstriction as factors in spontaneous hemostasis in normal, thrombocytopenic, heparinized and hypoprothrombinemic rats. *Am J Physiol* 1947; **148:** 275.

491. Zucker MB, Borelli J. Platelet clumping produced by connective tissue suspensions and by collagen. *Proc Soc Exp Biol Med* 1962; **109:** 779.

CHAPTER 9

Deep vein thrombosis: diagnosis

Practical significance of the symptoms and signs   299
Investigations   301
Clinical application of tests for deep vein
   thrombosis   308

Conclusions   310
References   311

The clinical diagnosis of deep vein thrombosis can be extremely difficult because many patients have no symptoms or signs in the affected limb.

Symptoms

The symptoms that are commonly produced by deep vein thrombosis are pain, swelling, and a faint blue–red discoloration of the skin (Figure 9.1). Profound cyanotic discoloration (phlegmasia cerulea dolens), or pallor (phlegmasia alba dolens) and frank venous gangrene (Figure 9.3) are much less common.

The more proximal and occlusive the thrombus, the more marked are the symptoms and physical signs. Postoperative calf thrombi often do not cause any symptoms,[73] and the clinical significance of small symptomless calf thrombi has been questioned;[22,61,150] there is, however, no doubt that calf thrombi can progress to extensive life-threatening proportions if they are left untreated.[143]

Deep vein thrombosis may also present as a pyrexia of unknown origin or with the symptoms of pulmonary embolism without any leg symptoms.

A paradoxical embolus (seen only a few times during a surgeon's career) occurs when a venous thromboembolus passes from the right to the left side of the heart through a congenital defect and then impacts in the arterial side of the circulation.[23,37,42] The cardiac abnormality is usually an atrial or ventricular septal defect but a patent ductus arteriosus can also be responsible. A patent foramen ovale seems to be a common predisposing cause. A paradoxical embolus should be suspected if no cause can be found for an arterial embolus in a patient with a cardiac murmur, pulmonary hypertension and a swollen limb. Transthoracic echocardiography or, better still, transoesophageal echocardiography[144] demonstrates the cardiac abnormality and can also confirm the right-to-left shunt.

Many patients who present with the clinical signs of a post-thrombotic limb, confirmed by phlebography, have no previous history of a clinical deep vein thrombosis or pulmonary embolism, the whole process having been completely silent. This finding fits with the fact that half the patients who have a positive fibrinogen uptake test have no symptoms.[73]

Signs

The physical signs of a deep vein thrombosis may be as ephemeral as the symptoms, and often there are none.

Tenderness

The most common but most inaccurate physical sign is tenderness on compressing the calf muscles, or tenderness over the course of the main veins of the thigh. Tenderness should be elicited carefully with firm but gentle manual pressure along the course of the veins and over both bellies of the gastrocnemius muscle with the knee flexed to 150°.

Only half the patients with calf muscle tenderness have a thrombosis.[73] Tenderness at other sites (e.g. the lateral part of the thigh) rarely indicates a thrombosis. The aetiology of the tenderness remains obscure, as it does not appear to be related to either the extent or adherence of the thrombus.[27]

Oedema

Deep vein thrombosis often causes mild pitting oedema of the ankle. This is a significant clinical sign and is a true indicator of thrombosis in 70% of cases, especially if it is unilateral.[154] Oedema of the foot and calf indicates that the thrombus has probably extended into the popliteal vein and above (Figure 9.1). Swelling of the whole leg is associated with ilio-femoral or vena caval thrombosis (Figure 9.2).

Muscle induration

The calf muscles may feel 'woody' hard if there is extensive intramuscular thrombosis but it may be possible to palpate small tender patches before this happens; these small areas are presumably related to localized areas of intramuscular thrombosis. As the muscles become stiff, there may be a detectable difference in the mobility (floppiness) of one calf which can be observed by gently shaking the calves with the hand or by flexing the knees to 150° and gently knocking them together.

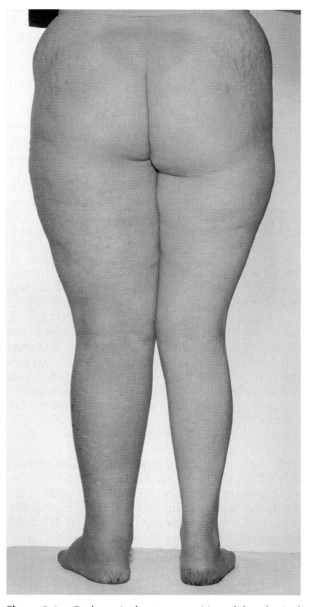

Figure 9.1 Oedema is the most sensitive of the physical signs of deep vein thrombosis; it correctly indicates the diagnosis in approximately 70% of cases. This patient complained of swelling of the left ankle but the photograph reveals that there was swelling of the whole leg. The left calf was firm but not tender. The skin had a bluish tinge. Phlebography revealed a complete popliteal–femoral–iliac thrombosis.

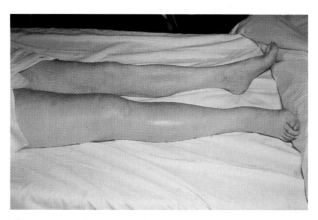

Figure 9.2 This patient had a right ilio-femoral thrombosis causing swelling pain, tenderness and discoloration of the whole leg.

Warm and distended superficial veins

The skin of the leg may feel warm and the superficial veins may be distended and fail to collapse when the limb is elevated if there is significant venous outflow obstruction. Veins may become distended in the affected groin of a limb with an ilio-femoral thrombosis indicating a major degree of venous obstruction.

Homans' dorsiflexion test

Homans' dorsiflexion sign is another method of testing calf tenderness but even Homans recognized that it was unreliable.[29] In 1944 Homans made the following statement.[100]

'Homans' sign. I prefer to call it the dorsiflexion sign. Actually the dorsiflexion of the feet is intended to bring out, on the side of the venous thrombosis, some degree of irritability of the posterior muscles, the soleus and gastrocnemius. *Discomfort need have no part in this reaction.* Dorsiflexion may be less complete in response to an equal degree of upward pressure on the affected side as compared with the normal, or the patient may involuntarily flex the knee, as the forefoot is forced upwards, to release the tension on the posterior muscles. If one looks at the dorsiflexion sign as evidence of even the faintest irritability of the posterior muscles (the early stage of the thrombosis occurring within and about them), the sign will be found more frequently than either tenderness or swelling.'

Archer[9] chided Sandler and Martin[197] with this direct quote from Homans when they had defined the sign as 'pain in the calf on passive dorsiflexion of the foot'. Sandler's riposte[196] was to quote four medical textbooks in which pain was included in the definition of Homans' sign, and to carry out a small survey amongst junior doctors in Sheffield, all of whom understood Homans' sign to be pain in the calf on dorsiflexion of the foot (but he did not state if he had himself been teaching these students!). A review of three surgical textbooks before the last edition of this book confirmed[5,99,183] that Homans' sign is commonly defined as 'pain' on dorsiflexion of the foot, though Hobsley,[99] like Browse,[31] went on to point out that Homans tried to disown the sign.

We suspect that pain has crept into the definition of 'Homans' sign' because 'increased resistance' is imprecise. We neither use nor recommend the test, irrespective of its definition, because it is inaccurate, and we would happily relegate it to obscurity.

The Loewenberg test

This was an attempt to quantify Homans' sign; it elicited 'tenderness' by inflating a pneumatic tourniquet placed around the calf muscles to different pressures to determine the pressure that caused pain. It has proved as unreliable as the dorsiflexion test.[149]

Skin discoloration

A white, swollen, and often painful leg (phlegmasia alba dolens) is a common and significant abnormality. It is more often observed by the clinician than complained of by the patient. The pallor is probably caused by extensive oedema which obscures the capillary circulation of the skin,[10] though some have suggested that it is the result of arterial spasm.[170] A 'white leg' is usually caused by an ilio-femoral thrombosis.

A blue leg (phlegmasia cerulea dolens)[81] is usually associated with a degree of pain and swelling which often initially overshadows the cyanosis. The 'blue' appearance is caused by venous congestion secondary to a thrombosis in both the external and common iliac veins (and often the internal iliac veins). The skin may be covered with small petechiae, and areas of skin may become gangrenous if the outflow obstruction is not relieved.

Venous gangrene

When the venous outflow of a limb is severely reduced, as in phlegmasia cerulea dolens, the arterial inflow may become obstructed. The tips of the toes become deep blue and then black, or the skin blisters (Figure 9.3). These changes usually affect all the toes, unlike arterial gangrene where only one or two toes may be affected, and may spread onto the dorsal and ventral surfaces of the forefoot. The general swelling and blueness of the limb, even when elevated, distinguishes it from the pale, cold, shrivelled limb of acute arterial ischemia.

Loss of peripheral arterial pulses

It is often difficult to palpate the foot pulses in a limb with phlegmasia cerulea dolens or venous gangrene. This observation led Oschner and DeBakey to suggest that an extensive venous thrombosis causes arterial spasm.[170]

Doppler ultrasound examination of the distal pulses usually shows them to be present and if so, and the patient is able to tolerate a tourniquet being inflated around the limb, the pressure index is normal.

The arterial inflow to the limb is usually reduced by the massive obstruction to venous outflow, but Lea Thomas and Carty[134] suggested that in some limbs obstruction to arterial inflow might be the prime abnormality, precipitating a secondary venous thrombosis.

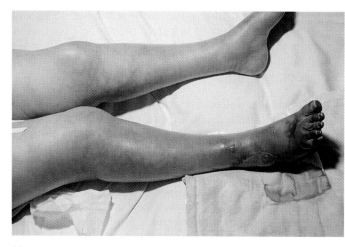

(a)

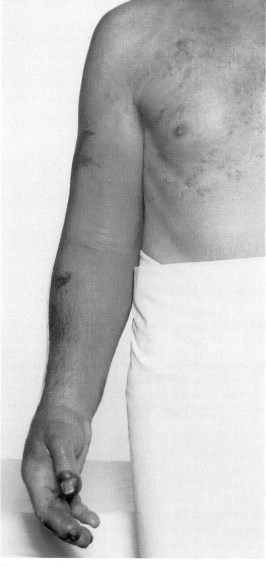

(b)

Figure 9.3 Two examples of venous gangrene. (a) Extensive gangrene of the forefoot with blistering around the ankle. (b) Venous gangrene of the fingertips following an extensive axillary/subclavian vein and superior vena cava thrombosis caused by malignant disease in the mediastural lymphnodes.

We have performed arteriograms on a few of these patients and found evidence of arterial emboli, possibly arising from the artery adjacent to the primary site of the venous thrombosis. Venous obstruction, arterial spasm and arterial emboli all probably play a part in different circumstances.

Very occasionally, a paradoxical embolus may be the cause of a blue swollen limb in which the pulses are absent.

Emboli may pass through a patent foramen ovale and lodge in the cerebral, arm or leg arteries. Duplex ultrasound and echocardiography have increased the recognition of this condition.[23,37,42]

Superficial thrombophlebitis

Any patient who presents with a superficial thrombophlebitis may have a deep vein thrombosis (see Chapter 23).[19]

Pyrexia

Patients with a deep vein thrombosis often have a low persistent fever. A patient who is found to have this type of fever in the postoperative period should be carefully screened to exclude a silent deep vein thrombosis. A similar fever is often found in patients who have repeated small pulmonary emboli.

Table 9.1 A method for estimating the probability of the presence of deep vein thrombosis based upon risk factors, clinical history and signs; devised by Wells *et al.*[222]

Checklist	Clinical probability of deep vein thrombosis
Major points Active cancer (treatment ongoing or within previous 6 months or palliative) Paralysis, paresis, or recent plaster immobilization of the lower extremities Recently bedridden >3 days and/or major surgery within 4 weeks Localized tenderness along the distribution of the deep venous system Thigh and calf swollen (should be measured) Calf swelling 3 cm > symptomless side (measured 10 cm below tibial tuberosity) Strong family history of DVT (≥2 first-degree relatives with history of DVT)	**High** ≥3 major points and no alternative diagnosis ≥2 major points and (2 minor points + no alternative diagnosis **Low** 1 major point + ≥2 minor points + has an alternative diagnosis 1 major point + ≥1 minor point + no alternative diagnosis 0 major points + ≥3 minor points + has an alternative diagnosis 0 major points + ≥2 minor points + no alternative diagnosis
Minor points History of trauma within the past 60 days to the symptomatic leg Pitting oedema; symptomatic leg only Dilated superficial veins (non-varicose) in symptomatic leg only Hospitalization within previous 6 months Erythema	**Moderate** All other conditions

Signs of pulmonary embolism

The clinical features of pulmonary embolism are discussed in detail in Chapter 21. Many patients with a silent deep vein thrombosis present with chest pain, haemoptysis or shortness of breath.

The discriminant value of the symptoms and signs

In a prospective study of deep vein thrombosis diagnosed with the fibrinogen uptake test and confirmed by phlebography, Flanc *et al.*[73] found that 11% of the patients with a proven thrombosis had a marked increase in ankle size, 25% had calf tenderness, 34% had a distinguishable difference in limb temperature, 52% had mild unilateral ankle oedema, and 68% showed some induration of the calf muscles. In a similar study, Howe[104] reported that the presenting symptoms of thrombosis were pain and tenderness in 66% of patients, swelling in 10%, and pulmonary embolism in 10%. The remaining 15% of patients presented with massive axial vein occlusion (white or blue legs).

McLachlin *et al.*[154] reported that unilateral leg swelling gave a correct indication of the diagnosis of deep vein thrombosis in 80% of patients, local tenderness and a positive Homans' sign correctly diagnosed thrombosis in only 50% and 8%, respectively.

Gibbs[79] also found that ankle oedema was a reliable clinical sign of deep vein thrombosis.

Differential diagnosis

As the history and physical signs of deep vein thrombosis are so imprecise,[73,127,184,202] a firm diagnosis depends upon the use of special tests but a recent study[222] has shown that patients can be divided into high, intermediate and low probability groups on the basis of symptom and signs, risk factors and potential alternative diagnoses (see Table 9.1).

The definitive investigation is probably still bipedal ascending phlebography although many clinicians have now abandoned this in favour of duplex Doppler ultrasound (see Chapter 4). It is essential always to confirm a clinical diagnosis of deep vein thrombosis with an objective investigation because treatment is not without risk.[16,74,127,146,150] However clinical assessment may be stratified and semiquantified,[222] it will always be wrong in 20–50% of cases.

The place of the alternative tests that can be used to diagnose thrombosis is discussed in the final section of this chapter.

The many conditions that mimic a deep vein thrombosis and must be excluded are listed in Table 9.2.

Table 9.2 Conditions that mimic deep vein thrombosis

Torn gastrocnemius muscle
Ruptured Baker's cyst
Calf haematomata
Lymphoedema with cellulitis
Acute arterial ischaemia
Extrinsic obstruction of veins and lymphatics in pelvis
Pathological fracture of femur
Superficial thrombophlebitis
Acute arthritis of the knee
Haemarthrosis of the knee
Torn meniscus
Achilles tendonitis
Oedema from congestive cardiac failure or the
    nephrotic syndrome
Rapidly growing sarcoma
Myositis ossificans
Munchausen's syndrome

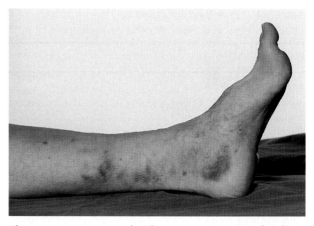

Figure 9.4 A ruptured Baker's cyst. A ruptured Baker's cyst is an important differential diagnosis of deep vein thrombosis. The bruising and discoloration of the skin in the groove behind and above the medial malleolus, shown here, is diagnostic of the condition.

Ruptured Baker's cyst

This is now recognized as one of the most important and most difficult conditions to distinguish from acute deep thrombosis.[118] Both conditions present with an acute onset of pain and swelling in the calf, and only a few patients give a prior history of arthritic pains in the knee joint.[202]

Once the cyst has ruptured, there may be few physical signs of arthritis in the knee joint, and there is usually no residual effusion or palpable cyst.[152] There is often some bruising but this commonly appears in the lower part of the leg, anterior to the Achilles tendon, days later and is of no help in making the diagnosis in the acute stage (Figure 9.4).

Deep vein thrombosis and a ruptured Baker's cyst can occur simultaneously[16,202] or the latter may precipitate the former; these situations make the diagnosis extremely difficult.

Duplex ultrasound will often confirm the diagnosis[214] but radiographs of the knee, MRI arthrography and even phlebography may be required for complete certainty.[130]

Torn gastrocnemius or plantaris muscle

These conditions cause a pain of sudden onset, sometimes followed by swelling of the leg. The pain usually develops faster than the pain of a thrombosis, and the patient is often taking some form of strenuous exercise when the symptoms begin. Unlike a rupture of the Achilles tendon, partial tears of the fibres of gastrocnemius muscle have no physical signs other than some muscle tenderness and pain when the muscle is contracted against resistance.

Duplex ultrasound may demonstrate a spindle-shaped echo-free cystic structure within the calf[214] but it may be difficult to decide if this is caused by a muscle rupture or disruption of a Baker's cyst (see above).

Lymphoedema with cellulitis

A limb with mild lymphoedema may suddenly develop a severe cellulitis, causing pain, redness and swelling. In the early stages this may be quite difficult to differentiate from an acute deep vein thrombosis. The diagnosis usually becomes apparent when the red area of skin extends and the patient develops a high pyrexia with rigors; neither of these signs is really typical of a thrombosis. Nevertheless, every year we see several patients with lymphoedema whose attacks of cellulitis have been misdiagnosed as deep vein thrombosis, and who have been treated, some for many years, with anticoagulants. A normal phlebograph and an abnormal lymphogram (isotopic or x-ray)[121,207] differentiate between lymphoedema with cellulitis and deep vein thrombosis.

Lipodystrophy: with or without erythrocyanosis frigida

Some ladies have extensive deposition of fat in their legs and buttocks. This may on occasion be very

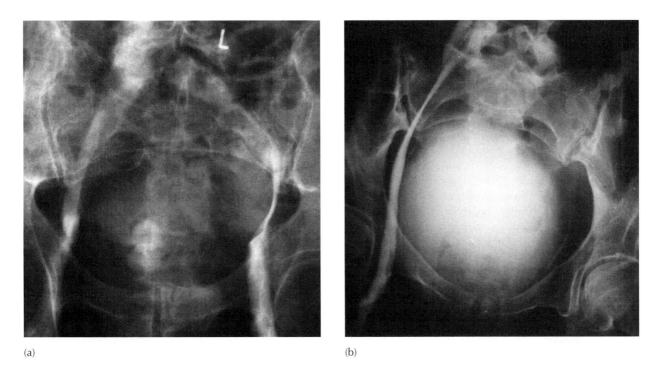

(a)   (b)

Figure 9.5 Compression of a deep vein causes the same symptoms as a deep vein thrombosis. (a) This patient's pain and leg swelling were caused by a large pelvic mass compressing the left external iliac vein. (b) This patient's swollen right leg was caused by a large bladder compressing the right iliac vein.

painful and, when confined to the lower leg, misdiagnosed as the oedema of a deep vein thrombosis. This is especially true if there is accompanying erythrocyanosis frigida – which can cause discoloration, pain and discomfort in the posterior and medial sides of the lower one-third of the leg.

Acute arterial ischaemia

This usually presents with severe pain but without swelling. Occasionally, arterial occlusion and venous thrombosis occur simultaneously;[16] the venous congestion and oedema are then often the dominant signs. The pallor of the limb and developing muscle weakness and paraesthesiae should quickly indicate the correct diagnosis. Pedal Doppler pressures are greatly reduced and provide useful confirmation that arteriography is required.

Haemorrhage into the limb

Patients on anticoagulants or patients with coagulation defects may suffer a sudden acute bleed into a joint or the soft tissues following minor trauma. Haemorrhage is often suspected if a coagulation defect has already been confirmed but may not be diagnosed correctly if the clinician is unaware of the condition. A painful immobile swollen joint or muscle, associated with abnormal coagulation tests makes this diagnosis highly likely, but ultrasound, CT or MR scans are usually necessary for complete certainty.

Pelvic or intra-abdominal tumours obstructing the veins

Patients with pelvic or intra-abdominal tumours are at increased risk of developing deep vein thrombosis, but sometimes a tumour obstructs the veins without causing a thrombosis. This can only be confirmed by phlebography, CT or MR scans and may be clinically important when planning the management of the tumour, especially if treatment may cause tumour regression (Figure 9.5a and b).

It is important to perform an abdominal, rectal and/or a vaginal examination on all patients who present with a spontaneous deep vein thrombosis to exclude an abdominal or pelvic malignancy.[50,60,188,205]

The value of routine pelvic ultrasound or CT in excluding abdominal or pelvic malignancy in patients with sporadic deep vein thrombosis is discussed later.

Pathological fractures

A history of injury is invariably present in patients with ordinary fractures. In patients with pathological fractures, however, a history of injury may be absent, and these patients often present with an unexplained and sudden onset of severe limb pain and swelling. Pathological fractures are usually correctly suspected if the patient is known to have had prior treatment for a malignant disease or has clinical evidence of malignant disease elsewhere. A careful clinical examination usually reveals localized tenderness, immobility and deformity but these signs may occasionally be minimal and easily missed. Radiographs of the bones confirm the diagnosis and obviate the need for phlebography. A radioactive isotope bone scan may provide evidence of other bony metastases.

Superficial thrombophlebitis

Superficial thrombophlebitis presents as a hot tender linear swelling of the skin and subcutaneous tissues. It is common in patients with varicose veins (see Figure 9.6 and Chapter 23).

Superficial thrombophlebitis and deep vein thrombosis often coexist,[19,114] and superficial thrombophlebitis is often mistaken for a deep vein thrombosis. As the association between the two types of thrombosis is so common (20–30%), duplex ultrasound or phlebography should be considered in all patients who do not have visible varicose veins.[19,114] Some patients who have recurrent superficial thrombophlebitis have an unsuspected malignant disease, particularly if their superficial thrombophlebitis is associated with a deep vein thrombosis (see Chapter 23).[65]

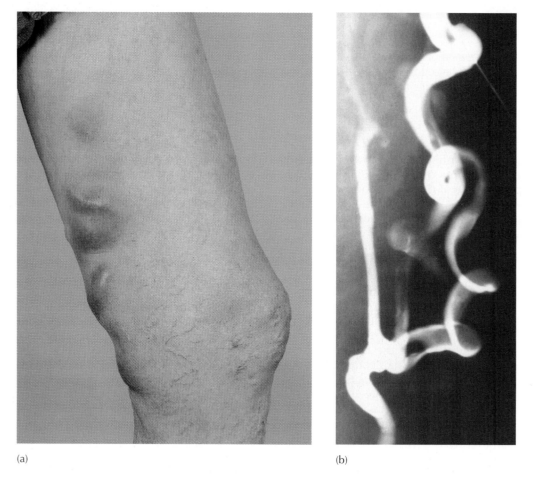

(a)   (b)

Figure 9.6 Superficial thrombophlebitis. (a) Large tender blue–red thrombosed varicose veins. This thrombus is adherent to the inflamed vein. (b) A phlebograph showing extensive adherent thrombus. Superficial thrombophlebitis is a common complication of varicose veins but when it occurs in a normal vein it is often associated with a deep vein thrombosis and is frequently caused by occult malignant disease (see Chapter 23).

Acute arthritis

Acute arthritis of the knee joint may cause pain, redness and swelling of the calf.[129] The pain is usually centred on the joint and is exacerbated by movement but it does occasionally spread throughout the leg. The diagnosis is easy to make if other joints are affected but even rheumatoid arthritis can be mono-articular. Clinical examination is usually diagnostic but plain radiographs and serological tests may be helpful.

Internal derangements of the knee

Many abnormalities of the knee joint (e.g. meniscal tears, meniscal cysts, loose bodies, effusions, chondromalacia patellae, recurrent dislocation of the patella, osteochondritis) can cause swelling and pain, both in and around the knee. These conditions should be distinguishable from deep vein thrombosis by the history and by physical signs related to knee movements. MR and arthroscopy confirm the diagnosis.

Achilles tendonitis

This causes pain which is localized to the Achilles tendon. It is usually the result of excessive and unaccustomed exercise but may be associated with Reiter's syndrome. There is usually pain on forcible dorsiflexion of the foot and tenderness over the tendon rather than over the calf. There may be a swelling palpable within the tendon.

Generalized oedema

Ankle oedema is common in patients with congestive cardiac failure, protein depletion, renal failure and fluid overload. The swelling is invariably bilateral, but deep vein thrombosis is also often bilateral and this may cause diagnostic difficulties, particularly during the postoperative period. The absence of calf tenderness or fever does not help because these features are often not present when there is a thrombosis. As there is a high incidence of thrombosis in patients with conditions that cause generalized oedema, it is often necessary to confirm or exclude the presence of thrombosis with duplex ultrasound or phlebography.

Soft-tissue sarcoma

A sarcoma of the muscles, fibrous tissue, or bone of the leg usually causes a localized swelling in the thigh or lower leg but may cause chronic pain, venous obstruction and generalized swelling of the limb. In the early stages the diagnosis may be very difficult to make. CT, MR scanning, arteriography and surgical exploration with biopsy should be considered if the phlebogram of a leg in which there is persistent pain and swelling is normal (see Chapter 27 and Figure 27.12).

Leiomyosarcoma of the femoral vein is a rare cause of leg swelling that can mimic a deep vein thrombosis.

Myositis ossificans

This condition rarely causes diagnostic difficulties, as it invariably follows a well-remembered major injury to the thigh. The swelling and pain may occasionally be mistaken for a thrombosis, especially if the patient has forgotten about the original injury. Plain radiographs always show extensive soft-tissue calcification.

Focal myositis has also been reported to have been mistaken for deep vein thrombosis.[92]

Arteriovenous fistula or fistulae

Arteriovenous (A-V) fistulae may cause swelling and pain in the limb. The swelling is invariably chronic and is confirmed by hearing a machinery murmur on auscultation and a positive Branham's test. Arteriography is usually diagnostic. Proximal fistulae between the aorta or iliac arteries and the vena cava or iliac veins may cause gross swelling of the leg and lead to a misdiagnosis of deep vein thrombosis.[212]

Popliteal vein entrapment

Three patients have recently been reported where the oedema associated with this condition was originally thought to be caused by a deep vein thrombosis.[41]

Munchausen's syndrome

Some patients deliberately induce swelling of the leg by applying a tourniquet; the swelling is then mistaken for lymphoedema or recurrent deep vein thrombosis.

Practical significance of the symptoms and signs

Deep vein thrombosis occurs in two groups of patients. In most instances the patient has a predisposing condition (e.g. medical illness or a surgical operation) and is in hospital. A few patients, however, present with the symptoms and signs of thrombosis or embolism as the first and only event, and do not have an obvious predisposing cause; most of these patients are seen in the doctor's office as out-patients and may require urgent admission to hospital for the investigation of their symptoms and subsequent treatment.

Patients in hospital known to be at risk

The diagnosis of deep vein thrombosis must be considered as a possibility at all times if it is not to be missed in patients who are in hospital. Prophylaxis is now universally employed in high-risk patients, but as no type of prophylaxis is infallible, a high degree of clinical vigilance must be maintained. All staff (junior and senior) should routinely inspect the temperature charts and examine the legs of patients for swelling and tenderness every day. Any symptoms or signs which are suggestive of deep vein thrombosis or pulmonary embolism should stimulate a detailed clinical examination followed by the appropriate tests to confirm or exclude the diagnosis. Every surgeon must remember that any patient may develop a deep vein thrombosis. The incidence in medical patients is somewhat less but occurs in a significant proportion of the total 'in-patient' population.

Patients who present with symptoms and signs that suggest thrombosis or embolism, de novo

Patients who suddenly develop symptoms in the legs or chest which suggest deep vein thrombosis or pulmonary embolism require a detailed clinical examination and basic investigations in order to answer the following questions.

- Is a deep vein thrombosis the most likely diagnosis?
- If not, what is the cause of the symptoms and signs?
- Is there any evidence of a pre-existing condition which could have caused the deep vein thrombosis?
- Has the patient had a pulmonary embolus?
- If not, what is the cause of the chest symptoms?

These questions are not difficult to answer when the symptoms and signs are typical. For example, a patient who has an aching pain in the calf that has developed over several hours and is associated with leg swelling and a predisposing factor (e.g. a past history of thrombosis, ingestion of the contraceptive pill, a family history of thrombosis, a known malignancy, an haematological disease, a recent illness, operation or an injury) almost certainly has

a deep vein thrombosis, especially if a pleuritic chest pain, haemoptysis or shortness of breath are also present.

In many patients, however, the story is less clear-cut, the symptoms and signs are vague, there is no obvious predisposing cause and in some cases the history is so 'atypical' that the diagnosis is merely considered within a long list of differential diagnoses. In this group of patients a meticulous systematic clinical examination may detect another cause of the symptoms.

When the history and examination have been completed it should be possible to place the patient in one of the following four categories and to obtain some indication of an underlying cause.

1. The patient almost certainly has deep vein thrombosis complicated by pulmonary embolism.
2. The patient almost certainly has a deep vein thrombosis.
3. The possibility of a deep vein thrombosis is sufficiently strong to justify its investigation before excluding other causes of the symptoms.
4. It is unlikely that the patient has a deep vein thrombosis, and other causes of the symptoms should be investigated first.

This degree of stratification is similar to that achieved by the clinical scoring system referred to earlier (page 295), which was originally developed to try to reduce the number of patients being sent for unnecessary investigation.[222]

Immediate management based upon the clinical assessment

The patient almost certainly has had a deep vein thrombosis complicated by pulmonary embolism
Treatment with heparin should begin at once, and the patient must be admitted to hospital immediately for confirmation of the diagnosis, to assess the risk of further embolism, and to plan further treatment.

The patient almost certainly has a deep vein thrombosis
The diagnosis must be confirmed so that appropriate treatment can be started to prevent extension of the thrombus and reduce the risk of embolism.

The patient may have had a deep vein thrombosis
When there is doubt but a genuine possibility that the patient has had a deep vein thrombosis, the diagnosis should be confirmed or excluded as soon as possible with duplex ultrasound as the first line

investigation. Two out of three patients will be given the wrong treatment if they are treated solely on clinical evidence as a clinical diagnosis has been shown repeatedly to be incorrect in 63% of patients,[184] and at best carries only a 50% chance of being correct.[73,202] Treatment with anticoagulants should not be commenced before objective evidence of thrombosis has been obtained.[27,73] The place of the various diagnostic tests in the management of deep vein thrombosis is discussed in the next section.

The patient is unlikely to have had a deep vein thrombosis

The investigations indicated for this group of patients are those which will help to confirm the cause of the symptoms (e.g. x-rays of the chest and lower limb to confirm a pathological fracture caused by a metastasis from a carcinoma of bronchus).

It is probably not necessary to carry out specific tests to exclude a deep vein thrombosis in these patients, except when all the other tests are negative and the symptoms and signs persist.

Is there a cause for the deep vein thrombosis?

Once the diagnosis of deep vein thrombosis has been confirmed by an objective test, every attempt should be made to detect or exclude an underlying cause. In the absence of obvious symptoms and signs, the major concern is to exclude occult malignant disease.[50,60,188,205] A careful history and physical examination may reveal a neoplasm of the rectum or prostate, or lymphadenopathy which suggests Hodgkin's disease. Examination of the male genitalia may reveal a testicular tumour. A chest radiograph, an ultrasound scan of the liver, kidneys and pelvis should be obtained if there is a history of weight loss, or a raised erythrocyte sedimentation rate (ESR), or the patient is elderly. An upper gastrointestinal endoscopy and a barium enema or colonoscopy should be arranged if there are appropriate indications from the history.

Abdominal CT scanning, MR imaging and endoscopic retrograde cholangiopancreatography (ERCP) are only indicated if there is a strong indication or intuition that there is an occult malignant lesion in the upper abdomen.

If the results of all these tests are within normal limits, the patient must be followed carefully with regular re-examinations and further specific tests as required. It is sometimes several years before the occult cause of a deep vein thrombosis becomes apparent.[14]

Recurrent deep vein thrombosis

There is a special group of patients who develop recurrent episodes of thrombosis, often despite adequate anticoagulation therapy. In these patients it is important to exclude malignant disease (as outlined above) and any cause of thrombophilia. The coagulation factors currently measured are: antithrombin III,[1,65,82,86,172,191,199,217,218,230] protein C,[20,82,103,174] protein S, lupus anticoagulant,[24,40] heparin cofactor II[215] and activated protein C resistance. Plasminogen, tissue plasminogen activator and its inhibitors[32,47,109,111,166,167,229] should also be measured. A platelet count and platelet function studies complete the assessment.

Investigations

The techniques used to investigate the venous system have already been described in detail in Chapter 4. This section discusses the accuracy, advantages and disadvantages of each of the methods used to diagnose deep vein thrombosis.

ASCENDING PHLEBOGRAPHY

For a full discussion of ascending plebography see Chapter 4, page 87.

Indications

Bipedal ascending phlebography provides adequate information in 95% of patients[30] thought to have a deep vein thrombosis, but it is an expensive and invasive investigation which is open to misinterpretation by the inexperienced. For example, one recent study on intra-observer variation had a kappa statistic of 0.63–0.74. This variability between radiologists significantly affected the interpretation of the results of a low molecular weight heparin prophylaxis study.[51]

Phlebographs can be obtained even when there are contraindications (e.g. sensitivity to iodine, the early stages of pregnancy and circulatory shock caused by a pulmonary embolism) provided special precautions are taken.[132]

Advantages

1. The diagnosis of deep vein thrombosis can be confirmed with certainty in 95% of limbs.[30,138]
2. The nature of the thrombus, its site, extent, degree of adherence and age can be determined (see Figures 4.22 and 4.23, pages 96 and 98).[34,138]

3. The risks of embolization can be estimated (see Figure 4.22).[34,138]
4. The clinical diagnosis may be firmly refuted if the phlebogram is normal.[52,73,87,106,107,171,179]
5. Thrombus within the calf veins can be detected satisfactorily.

Disadvantages

1. There may be disagreement over the interpretation of some phlebographic appearances,[51,59,153] but this decreases with the experience of the observer (see Figure 4.23).[59,135] The use of long-leg films appears to improve the accuracy of the procedure.[140]
2. Not all the veins of the limb can be filled with contrast medium.
   (a) The foot veins are not usually examined (Figure 9.7a).
   (b) Some calf veins are not regularly opacified (see Figure 4.15).[30,131,132]
   (c) The deep femoral vein is only displayed in 30% of patients (see Figure 4.16a and Figure 9.7b).[55]
   (d) The tributaries of the internal iliac vein are never shown with standard ascending phlebography (see Figure 4.16b and Figure 9.7c, d).[33,133]
   (e) The common iliac veins and inferior vena cava may be poorly opacified if the radiological technique is poor.[26,131,132,138]
3. The superficial veins may fill with contrast medium if the tourniquets are not correctly applied, making interpretation difficult.[131]
4. Phlebography only shows the state of the veins at the time of the examination. Progression or regresssion of thrombus can only be assessed by repeated examination.[30]
5. The procedure used to be unpleasant and painful but the new iso-osmolar contrast media have almost abolished these complaints (see Chapter 4).
6. Bilateral ascending phlebography takes 30 minutes and requires standard x-ray equipment and an experienced radiologist. It costs approximately the same as an intravenous excretory urogram (IVU).
7. Many hospitals do not have experience of this investigation and it is therefore poorly performed.[169]
8. The complications of the procedure have been discussed in Chapter 4.[137] The advent of iso-osmolar contrast media dramatically reduced the incidence of complications.[6,7] The risks of inducing thrombosis and producing tissue necrosis from extravasation have been virtually eliminated.[2] The risk of the injection and manipulation causing a pulmonary embolism is theoretical rather than real.

Accuracy

It is very difficult to obtain a precise estimate of the accuracy with which plebography detects deep vein thrombosis. Phlebography appears to detect more thrombi than duplex ultrasound but it detected fewer thrombi than the fibrinogen uptake test when this was available.[28,73,115,163,195,220] This could be because the fibrinogen uptake test is oversensitive or because phlebography is failing to reveal small thrombi. Phlebography can miss thrombi in the deep femoral vein[55] and internal iliac veins (Figure 9.7).[133] Thrombi are also easily missed in the foot veins (Figure 9.7)[139] because these veins are not usually examined during standard ascending phlebography. However, none of these blind areas is easily accessible to examination by any of the other techniques available.

There have been few reports in the literature of patients dying as a result of a proven pulmonary embolism after apparently normal phlebograms[105] but there have been no large planned comparisons between phlebography during life and autopsy examination.[160]

Hull *et al.*[105] reviewed a cohort of 150 patients who were referred for phlebography because of the suspicion of deep vein thrombosis who had normal studies. Only two developed problems after the study (at 5 days) and these may have been caused by the phlebogram.

Figure 9.7 (facing page)   The three segments of the veins of the lower limb not usually visualized by ascending phlebography are the foot veins, the deep femoral vein and the internal iliac vein and its tributaries but they may all contain thrombus. (a) A phlebograph showing thrombus in a foot vein (arrowed). (b) This large thrombus, which is extending up the common femoral vein, has its origin in the deep femoral vein. The superficial femoral vein is normal. The deep femoral vein is only visible in 30% of ascending phlebographs. (c) Fresh thrombus in the internal iliac vein. (d) The tributaries of the internal iliac vein are only fully visualized by intraosseous phlebography (see Chapter 4). In this example there is fresh thrombus in the left inferior gluteal vein.

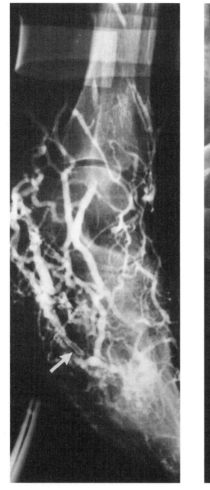

(a)

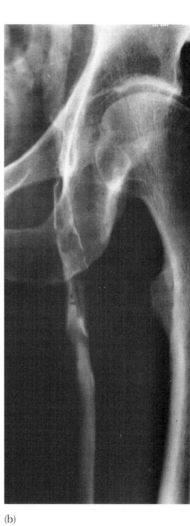

(b)

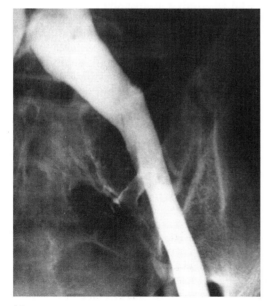

(c)

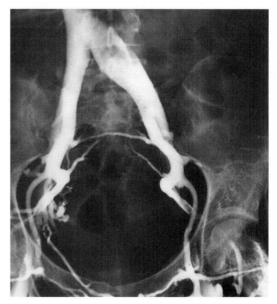

(d)

The overall accuracy and the positive and negative test accuracy is over 90%[30] and phlebography remains the standard against which other tests have always traditionally been compared. Phlebography still provides more information about the site, the extent and the age of the thrombus than its main rival, duplex ultrasound in the hard copy form available to the clinician.

The role of other phlebographic techniques

Cinephlebography

Cinephlebography[10,116] adds little to the standard screening and cut film techniques.[132] It is useful in the assessment of calf pump function but not in the diagnosis of deep vein thrombosis.

'No-tourniquet' technique

This technique, described by Nylander[8,26,88,168,169] is associated with a high incidence of false-positive interpretations caused by underfilling of the deep veins and 'knot-hole' effects in the superficial veins. We are not aware of any published comparison between this technique and our standard tourniquet technique.[136]

Perfemoral venography

Perfemoral venography[131,132] is carried out under local anaesthesia and is frequently used to provide better quality images of the iliac veins and vena cava. If there is a good flow of blood into the syringe before injection is made, there is no danger of disrupting a femoral vein thrombus and causing an embolus. The main indication for the use of this technique is the display of the upper limit of an ilio-femoral thrombosis that is not clearly visible on the ascending phlebogram or duplex ultrasound examination. Contrast CT scanning or MR venography are alternative means of assessing iliac thrombus.

Intraosseous phlebography

Intraosseous phlebography[131,132] has largely been abandoned, because of its complications, and the fact that patients have to be fully anaesthetized.

Spiral CT of leg veins

Baldt *et al.*[13] examined 52 patients suspected of having a deep vein thrombosis with spiral CT and conventional phlebography. Colour flow duplex ultrasound was used if the contrast phlebographs were inconclusive. The spiral CT examination covered a 100 cm section from the ankle to the inferior vena cava. Spiral CT was 100% sensitive, 90% specific and had a positive predictive value of 91% and a negative predictive value of 100%; 8% less contrast medium was used and the technique was especially valuable when the thrombus involved the pelvic veins or inferior vena cava.

Digital subtraction angiography of leg veins

One study[125] of this technique simply reports that it is possible to outline the leg veins following multiple intra-arterial injections of contrast medium. The advent of MR angiography and spiral CT phlebography has made this technique redundant.

Magnetic resonance angiography

This technique has the major advantage that it does not require the injection of a contrast medium into the veins. Preliminary studies to define the best application (spin echo, gradient echo or comparative gradient and spin echo) were followed by a number of trials comparing it with phlebography and duplex ultrasound (see Table 9.3). These all showed sensitivities between 80 and 100% and specificities between 92 and 100%. There is therefore little doubt that this is a valuable technique for diagnosing deep vein thrombosis. It is especially accurate at detecting thrombus in the iliac veins and vena cava where contrast phlebography and colour duplex ultrasonography are least reliable.[63] Because of its cost it will not replace colour-coded duplex ultrasound as the investigation of first choice but it is an alternative to bipedal ascending phlebography in patients where there is doubt about the diagnosis of deep vein thrombosis and confirmation of the diagnosis is essential. It is particularly indicated in preference to conventional phlebography during pregnancy, when the lower limbs are very swollen, when the foot veins are impossible to cannulate or when iliocaval thrombosis is suspected.[63]

Table 9.3 Some preliminary studies of the diagnostic sensitivity and specificity of MR venography when compared with various 'gold standards'[63]

MR venography study	Sensitivity (%)	Specificity (%)
Erdman *et al.*[68] 36 patients	90	100
Spritzer *et al.*[204] 66 patients	100	92.9
Arrivé *et al.*[12] ? patients	92	95
Dupas *et al.*[63] 25 patients	100	98.5
Carpenter *et al.*[39] 27 patients	100	96

ULTRASOUND

There are two methods of detecting venous thromboses with ultrasound – *indirectly* through the assessment of the venous blood flow and *directly* with greyscale ultrasound imaging (echo or sonography). Nowadays both are combined, hence the term duplex, with the blood flow colour-coded into the greyscale image – this is commonly described as duplex ultrasonography.

For a full discussion of ultrasound see Chapter 4, page 78.

Ultrasound blood flow detection

Many physicians[70,71,155,198,200,208,210] have studied the value of the ultrasound flow detector as a means of detecting deep vein thrombosis. They all found that the blood flow response in the deep axial veins to calf squeezing or the Valsalva manoeuvre is reduced in patients with extensive thrombus in the popliteal, femoral or iliac veins. Evans[70,71] also claimed that there was a reduction in the femoral vein blood flow response to squeezing the calf when there was calf vein thrombus present. Most of the subsequent published studies showed that the test was only useful in diagnosing thrombus in the large axial veins (i.e. the popliteal vein and above), and it has now been completely superseded, except as a bedside test, by duplex scanning.

Ultrasound imaging (colour flow duplex ultrasonography)

Although B-mode ultrasound imaging of the veins was originally described in 1976,[57] it was only when Strandness successfully combined the image with the Doppler assessment of blood flow that the value of ultrasound for detecting deep vein thrombosis became recognized. In many hospitals it is now the investigation of first choice for establishing or excluding a diagnosis of deep vein thrombosis.[157,225]

Indications

1. Confirmation of the clinical diagnosis of deep vein thrombosis.

Contraindications

There are no contraindications.

Advantages

1. It is truly non-invasive.
2. The addition of blood flow colour coding has made the technique easier to use with a Doppler flow detection facility, and more accurate.
3. It can give some indication of the precise extent and degree of adherence of the thrombus but is less accurate at defining thrombus age.[147]
4. It is safe to use during pregnancy.

Disadvantages

1. It is totally operator-dependent.
2. A full examination takes quite a long time (half an hour or more for both limbs) and requires considerable skill and anatomical knowledge.
3. The apparatus is expensive, and if the past 10 years are a guide, needs regular upgrading.

Accuracy

In 1976, the B-mode technique was shown to detect thrombi in 30 out of 32 limbs with phlebographically proven major vein thrombi,[57] and to confirm the presence of normal axial veins in 17 out of 18 limbs with normal phlebographs. The technical improvements that have been made in the probes and the combination of pulsed Doppler flow detection with real time B-mode imaging (duplex ultrasonography) have provided better information which has allowed the presence of venous thrombi to be detected even more accurately.[189,211] Cranley and his team[209] reported an overall accuracy of 94%, a positive test accuracy of 92%, and a negative test accuracy of 96%. These results are extremely good and still represent the best reported figures. Between 1990 and 1996, 17 publications reported specificities between 86% and 100% and sensitivities between 50% and 100%.

The limitations of the procedure have now clearly been defined.[46,113,128,190,223]

- It is only 50% sensitive as a screening test for calf thrombi in symptomless limbs.
- It is of limited value in detecting new thrombi in limbs that have already had previous thrombosis.
- Oversaturation of the colour image is a potential source of error.
- Many studies fail technically to demonstrate all the calf veins,[147,201] whereas thrombus in the popliteal vein and above is diagnosed with great accuracy (nearly 100%).[156]

- One patient is reported to have had a pulmonary embolus during compression.[177]

Comment

Although the capital outlay for this equipment is large, the ability to diagnose deep vein thrombosis by a non-invasive test which is both reproducible and repeatable, and does not expose the patient to the hazards of radiation, is a great advance. Because it has hardly any undesirable side-effects it is being overused, 75% of the studies being performed revealing normal deep veins.[75]

FIBRINOGEN UPTAKE TEST

Because of the risk of the fibrinogen transmitting infection (hepatitis and HIV) this test has been completely withdrawn from clinical use. This has left an unfortunate gap in our diagnostic armamentarium which has not been filled by duplex ultrasound.

This test was originally devised by Hobbs and Davies[98] but was developed for use as a screening test for deep vein thrombosis by Flanc et al.[73] and Negus et al.[163] It was designed to detect a thrombus as it developed (e.g. before or after an operation). It was much less accurate at detecting established thrombus.[28,176] It was used chiefly to assess different regimens of thrombosis prophylaxis. It was never taken up as a universal screening test on the grounds of expense.

For a discussion of the fibrinogen uptake test, see Chapter 4, page 76.[28,115,145,187,195]

Accuracy

Because so many of the studies upon which current prophylaxis regimens are based were established using the fibrinogen uptake test, it is important to remember its limitations.

Both the positive and the negative test accuracies for thrombus below the mid-thigh were between 95% and 100% when the test was used proleptically and compared with phlebography, provided all limbs with clinically detectable causes of false positives were excluded from testing.[28,73,115,117,145,163,195] The positive and negative test accuracies, under similar conditions, for established thrombus less then 7 days old were both 75%.[28,176] The incidence of pulmonary embolism after a negative scan was very low (0 out of 687).[117]

OTHER ISOTOPE UPTAKE TESTS

Technetium-99m (^{99m}Tc) plasmin uptake test

The technetium-99m plasmin uptake test[3,58,64,108,173] was developed to improve on the accuracy of 75% which was found when the ^{125}I-fibrinogen uptake test was used to examine patients with established thrombosis.[28,30,176] It was reported to be 97% sensitive, and 55% specific, with a predictive value of 79% in positive cases and 92% in negative cases.[108] The isotope has a short half-life and the injectate has to be specially prepared for each test. There is a high false-negative rate in patients with bilateral thrombosis.

There are few, if any, reports on this investigation in recent medical literature, but another paper in 1986 reported that the test was highly sensitive (increase of 90%) but not very specific (50–70%). It is perhaps because of this low specificity that the test has not become established.[123]

Technetium-99m (^{99m}Tc) streptokinase uptake test

The streptokinase uptake test[62,119] was also developed to try to provide faster results in diagnosing established thrombosis than the fibrinogen uptake test. The early results were encouraging but there have been problems involving sensitivity reactions to streptokinase and the short half-life of the isotope. It has largely been abandoned.

Technetium-99m (^{99m}Tc) labelled red cells

This test had a sensitivity of 100% and a specificity of 89% in one study.[21] It gives an anatomical picture of the whole venous tree which is imaged by a gamma camera. The quality of the image is markedly inferior to phlebography. This technique has not been widely adopted because of the time needed to label the red cells and the requirements for highly sophisticated imaging apparatus.

Radiolabelled plasminogen uptake test

This test is identical in principle and accuracy to the plasmin and streptokinase uptake tests described above.[91]

Indium-labelled platelets

This technique was also introduced to provide a quicker result than that given by the ^{125}I-fibrinogen uptake test.[72,122] Grimley *et al.*[83] reported that it was 60% accurate for calf thrombi and correctly detected 66% of thigh thrombi. There were 14% false positives in the calf and 19% false positives in the thigh. The test requires time and skill, and is expensive to prepare the platelets. These disadvantages have restricted its application.

Platelets labelled by 99mTc HMPAO

This is now preferred to indium as a means of labelling platelets. Blood pool and accumulation images show up 'hot-spots' indicative of thrombi. Patients on anticoagulation may be 'missed' by this technique and it has a poor sensitivity of 65%.[102]

Technetium-labelled macroaggregates of albumin

This technique is used to provide images which are similar to a phlebograph but their quality is far inferior to the images obtained from a standard x-ray contrast phlebograph.[96,192,193,221] The sensitivity for thigh thrombus has been claimed to be 80% with a specificity of 98%. Unfortunately, this test cannot detect calf vein thrombi.[165] It can be a useful axial vein screening test when performed as part of a perfusion lung scan.[120]

Technetium-99m (⁹⁹ᵐTc) labelled fibrinogen

The ⁹⁹ᵐTc-labelled fibrinogen test[112,198] provided a combination of static and dynamic scans of the leg veins following the injection of technetium-labelled fibrinogen into a foot vein. It was called 'the venoscan' by Sandler *et al.*[198] who claimed that it has an 80% accuracy with a sensitivity of 83% and a specificity of 76%. The nature of the equipment needed for this test has inhibited its study by other investigators, and fibrinogen can no longer be used.

Radiolabelled monoclonal antibodies

These have been produced against fibrin platelets, and tissue plasminogen activator.[123,194,219] As many are recombitant proteins, they are safe for human use, but at present none has proved clinically useful. Further studies and compounds are required.

Comment

False-positive scans will always occur in patients who have bruising, haematomata or inflammation in the legs. The loss of the fibrinogen uptake test has made the assessment of new methods of deep vein thrombosis prophylaxis much more difficult.

PLETHYSMOGRAPHY

Various forms of plethysmography have been used to diagnose deep vein thrombosis (see Chapter 4, pages 87–101). These include impedance plethysmography,[90,161,162,198,226,227] strain-gauge plethysmography,[35,89] segmental air plethysmography,[43,66,77] phleborheography[53,54] and light reflection rheography.[11,213]

All these techniques are based on the principle that thrombus interferes with venous blood flow.

Indications

1. Confirmation of the diagnosis of established deep vein thrombosis.
2. As a screening test.

Contraindications

There are no contraindications.

Advantages

1. It is non-invasive and moderately reproducible.
2. All the methods are relatively cheap and easy to learn.

Disadvantages

None can detect small calf vein thrombi or non-occlusive axial vein thrombi with certainty.

Accuracy

Strain-gauge plethysmography detects venous thrombosis by measuring the maximum venous outflow. It has a sensitivity for axial vein thrombosis of 90% but its sensitivity for calf vein thrombosis is only 60%.[35,89]

Phleborheography measures the changes in calf volume in response to upstream and downstream limb compression and the Valsalva manoeuvre. It has a sensitivity of 90% for axial vein thrombosis, but a sensitivity for calf vein thrombosis of only 70–80%.[53,54]

Impedance plethysmography detects thrombosis from the relationship between calf filling during venous congestion and the rate of emptying after congestion. Its sensitivity for detecting axial vein thrombus is 90%, but its sensitivity for calf vein thrombus is only 40%.[161,162,227]

Comment

All the plethysmographic techniques are good at detecting axial vein thrombosis that is causing a significant obstruction to blood flow, but they are relatively poor at detecting small haemodynamically insignificant calf vein thrombi. If it is accepted that axial vein thrombosis is the clinically significant form of deep vein thrombus, these tests should be classified as good but if the clinician wishes to detect all forms of thrombus, the plethysmographic techniques are far from ideal because their overall accuracy is only 60–70%.

THERMOGRAPHY

A number of publications have examined the value of thermography for the diagnosis of deep vein thrombosis.[17,18,25,36,48,49,95,110,142,175,180,186,197,206] When Bergqvist[18] compared the ^{125}I-fibrinogen uptake test with thermography, he found a sensitivity of only 62% but a specificity of 90%. Thermography detected developing thrombi slightly slower than the ^{125}I-fibrinogen uptake test. Bystrom *et al.*,[36] however, found a 94% agreement between phlebography and thermography. Sandler and Martin, using liquid crystal contact thermography,[197] showed a 97% sensitivity but a specificity of only 62%. This level of accuracy has been confirmed by others.[25,206]

For a full discussion of thermography, see Chapter 4, page 73.

Comment

Thermography is a non-specific and relatively insensitive test. False-positive results are a major problem and it is only of value in screening patients with established thrombosis.

BLOOD TESTS

A number of groups[36,84,97,228] originally measured the fibrin degradation products and felt they were of some value in diagnosing deep vein thrombosis. The development of the D-Dimer assay has provided

greater sophistication. There are a number of different techniques for measuring these products but all are insensitive (80–90%), not very specific (75%) and tend towards an accuracy of 70%. The ELISA assay is probably better than the later assay but is a slow test. There are now a huge number of studies on this assay and it is probably the best simple screening test but has the drawbacks mentioned above.

Other tests that have been used with variable success include fibrin peptide A estimation, thrombin–antithrombin complexes, soluble fibrin and fibrin monoclonal antibodies. These are all less satisfactory than the D-Dimer test.

SUMMARY

Despite the plethora of tests that have been described above, bipedal ascending phlebography has stood the test of time. Duplex ultrasound imaging is now favoured as the first line investigation by most physicians. Combinations of plethysmography with duplex ultrasound and D-Dimer assays may provide greater accuracy. No test can determine the extent, age and fixity of the thrombus as satisfactorily as phlebography, although duplex technology is continuing to improve.

Clinical application of tests for deep vein thrombosis

Although the physical signs of deep vein thrombosis and pulmonary embolism are variable and imprecise, they are the only clinical indication of the presence of thrombosis. Consequently, these signs must be sought by diligent daily examination, especially in the postoperative period when there is a high risk of deep vein thrombosis, and if any signs are detected they should be accepted as an important indication for further investigations to confirm or refute clinical suspicion. No suspicious physical sign should be ignored but *no treatment should be given without objective confirmation of the diagnosis.*

It is clearly impractical to use either duplex ultrasound or phlebography to investigate every patient who has suspicious physical signs. No hospital has the facilities to study phlebographs of every postoperative patient who has a tender calf and, as more than half these patients will not have a thrombosis, such an approach would be expensive and impractical. This is why clinical stratification is not only helpful but cost-effective.[222]

Patients fall into four distinct *clinical* categories; patients with

1. *Definite clinical evidence of pulmonary embolism*, which may or may not be life threatening (i.e. patients with the full clinical picture of pulmonary embolism described in Chapter 21 and in whom there is little doubt about the diagnosis).
2. *Symptoms or signs that could be caused by pulmonary embolism*, which are not life threatening (these patients often have one symptom, e.g. chest pain, which could be caused by embolism or could be caused by other conditions, for example, pneumonia, myocardial infarction or oesophageal spasm).
3. *Definite clinical evidence of deep vein thrombosis*, that is to say, symptoms and signs unlikely to be caused by anything other than deep vein thrombosis (e.g. phlegmasia cerulea dolens, a hard woody calf or a warm leg with mild ankle oedema and tenderness in the calf or along the femoral vein in the thigh).
4. *Symptoms or signs that could be caused by deep vein thrombosis* (e.g. minor calf tenderness).

Our methods of using the above investigations after categorizing the patients into one of these groups are described below. The reason for our preferences, which are italicized, are discussed in the subsequent section.

Definite clinical pulmonary embolism

The three objectives of investigation are to confirm the diagnosis of pulmonary embolism, assess its severity and exclude the possibility of further embolism. If the patient is collapsed and hypotensive we resuscitate him/her with oxygen, plasma volume expansion, vasoconstrictor drugs, intubation and ventilation, cardiac massage if indicated and give 12 500 units heparin intravenously. Once the patient has been resuscitated the next stage is to:

- assess the state of the major limb veins from the popliteal to the iliac veins with duplex;
- request *pulmonary angiography* if the clinical signs suggest severe pulmonary artery obstruction with continuing shock and if thrombolysis or embolectomy is contemplated;
- request *lung scans* if, or when, the patient's condition becomes more stable.

Pulmonary angiography may have to be performed on the operating table before an emergency embolectomy if the patient's condition is rapidly deteriorating. Embolectomy or thrombolysis should not be attempted without firm objective proof of the diagnosis. Treatment depends upon the severity of the pulmonary artery obstruction. If the obstruction is extensive and reducing the cardiac output, pulmonary embolectomy or thrombolysis may be indicated (see Chapter 21).

Anticoagulants should be given to the patient, if the embolus is not severe or life threatening. The leg veins should then be investigated to assess the likelihood of a further embolism, and a ventilation–perfusion (VQ) scan should be obtained to confirm the diagnosis of pulmonary embolism. Appropriate action can then be taken (see Chapter 10).

Possible, non-life-threatening pulmonary embolism

The first objective of treatment is the assessment of the possibility of a second, potentially fatal embolism. The second objective is to confirm the diagnosis.

- We first assess the patency of the major limb veins (popliteal to iliac) at the bedside with a duplex ultrasound scan, or hand-held Doppler flow detector.
- If this test is abnormal, we give the patient 10 000 units of heparin intravenously. If the thrombus cannot be accurately assessed by the duplex ultrasound scan or is seen to be extending into the iliac veins or IVC, phlebographs are obtained. If large amounts of loose thrombus are present, a filter is usually inserted to prevent massive pulmonary embolus. Ventilation–perfusion lung scans are obtained within 24 hours to confirm or refute the clinical diagnosis of pulmonary embolism.
- If the bedside tests are normal, we request an urgent *ventilation–perfusion lung scan* followed within 24 hours by *bipedal ascending phlebography* if the VQ scan is positive.

If the ventilation–perfusion lung scan is positive but duplex ultrasound scanning fails to show residual thrombus within the limbs, the risk of further embolism is small. Phlebography is usually arranged on the following day to be quite certain that the ultrasound scan has not missed a large, non-adherent potential embolus within the leg veins. The phlebograph also helps to decide upon the best form of treatment for the leg vein thrombosis.

Definite, clinical evidence of deep vein thrombosis without evidence of embolism

The objective of investigating these patients is to confirm the diagnosis and obtain information which may help the clinician to choose the best form of treatment. Duplex ultrasound assessment is usually the investigation of first choice. Equivocal results should be clarified by phlebography, to document the features of the thrombus, and to help with future management.

If the ultrasound scan shows that there is thrombus in the major axial veins (the popliteal vein or above), we still request urgent *bilateral ascending phlebography* in order to assess the possibility of using other forms of treatment (e.g. thrombolysis or thrombectomy) (see Chapter 10). The ultrasound scan is still not sufficiently accurate and does not give enough information about the features and nature of the thrombus for management decisions.

For a major vein thrombus we require information about its size, site, age and adherence. Our approach to patients who have definite deep vein thrombosis is therefore similar to our approach to those patients with pulmonary embolism that is not life threatening. We proceed to *phlebography* in all patients in whom the duplex ultrasound test suggests that the thrombosis extends into or above the popliteal vein.

Symptoms or signs that could be caused by deep vein thrombosis

This category contains the largest number of patients because non-specific physical signs (e.g. calf tenderness or minor ankle oedema) are very common.

Non-invasive tests are extremely useful in this group because they enable the clinician to exclude the possibility of an extensive calf or axial vein thrombosis in most patients and they can be used to screen the patients, daily if necessary, to confirm a negative diagnosis or the absence of thrombus extension. The best approach is to *combine two tests*, for example *duplex ultrasound* with D-Dimer assay or plethysmography.

Phlebography is only indicated if thrombus is found in the axial veins or if the patient develops symptoms that suggest a pulmonary embolism.

Conclusions

It can be seen from the management schemes presented above that before a deep vein thrombosis can be properly managed the following information is required.

1. Is a thrombus present below the knee?
2. Is a thrombus present above the knee?
3. What is the precise extent of the thrombus?
4. Is the thrombus adherent or non-adherent?
5. What is the age of the thrombus?
6. Is the thrombus likely to threaten the life of the patient?
7. Is the thrombus likely to threaten the limb?
8. Will the thrombus cause post-thrombotic symptoms?

The various non-invasive investigations discussed in this chapter and described in detail in Chapter 4 can answer questions 1, 2 and 3 with varying degrees of accuracy, depending upon the site of the thrombus. The relative accuracy of these tests is shown in Table 9.4. These tests provide sufficient information if the clinician is satisfied with approximate answers to questions 1 and 2. If the thrombus

Table 9.4 Accuracy of tests used to diagnose deep vein thrombosis

Question	Approximate degree of accuracy (%)				
	DUAK	DUBK	PRG	IPG	Phleb
1. Is there thrombus below the knee?	–	60	60	70	95
2. Is there thrombus above the knee?	95	–	90	90	99
3. What is the precise extent of the thrombus?	95	40	60	60	99
4. What is the size (length and width) of the thrombus?	90	40	–	–	99
5. Is the thrombus adherent or non-adherent?	85	40	–	–	95
6. What is the state of the upper (cephalad) end of the thrombus?	80	20	–	–	95

DUAK, duplex ultrasound above the knee; DUBK, duplex ultrasound below the knee, PRG, phleborheography; IPG, impedance plethysmography; Phleb, phlebography.

This table gives an indication of the ability of four tests to answer the clinicians' questions about deep vein thrombosis. A test which examines a whole segment of vein (e.g. the iliac and femoral veins) but which cannot give a precise indication of the exact extent of a thrombus site but can differentiate between above-knee and below-knee thrombosis is scored 60%. Similar estimates have been made to give an approximate score of the ability of each test to answer each question.

is in a major axial vein, we always want to know the answers to questions 3, 4, 5 and 6, and this information is often helpful even if the thrombus is confined to the calf; consequently, we still rely heavily upon phlebography, although duplex scanning has a major screening role.

There is no doubt that the information provided by phlebography is still superior to that provided by duplex ultrasound scanning. Now that non-ionic iso-osmolar contrast media are available, phlebography is an extremely safe procedure. It requires an x-ray suite and a radiologist's time but is far less expensive than many other radiological investigations. Although phlebography cannot be performed at the bedside or in the vascular laboratory by a technician, the information it provides still cannot be obtained from any of the other methods. This information is invaluable in determining management. In our opinion the use of the non-invasive tests should be restricted to screening. Phlebograms should be requested for any patient who has had a pulmonary embolism, for any patient who has thrombus above the knee and whenever thrombectomy, thrombolysis or caval interruption is contemplated. In our opinion it is acceptable to administer anticoagulants on the evidence of a non-invasive test if the thrombus is confined to the calf and to accept that no significant thrombosis is present on the basis of a negative non-invasive test, provided the test can moderately accurately (70–80%) detect thrombus both in the calf and in axial veins.

It is not acceptable to give anticoagulants solely on the basis of a clinical diagnosis, except to cover the period between making the clinical diagnosis and seeing the results of objective tests.

References

1. Aberg M, Nilsson I M, Hedner U. Antithrombin III after operation. *Lancet* 1973; **2:** 1337.
2. Aburahma AF, Powell M, Robinson PA. Prospective study of safety of lower extremity phlebography with nonionic contrast medium. *Am J Surg* 1996; **171:** 255–60.
3. Adolfsson L, Nordenfelt I, Olssen H, Torstensson I. Diagnosis of deep venous thrombosis with 99Tc plasmin. *Acta Med Scand* 1982; **211:** 365.
4. Agnelli G, Volpato R, Radicchia S, *et al.* Detection of asymptomatic deep vein thrombosis by real-time B-mode ultrasonography in hip surgery patients. *Thromb Haemost* 1992; **68:** 257–60.
5. Aird I. *A Companion in Surgical Studies.* London: Churchill Livingstone, 1957.
6. Albrechtsoon U, Olsson CG. Thrombosis after phlebography: a comparison of two contrast media. *Cardiovasc Radiol* 1979; **2:** 9.
7. Almen T, Hartel M, Nylander G, Olivercrona N. Effects of metrizamide on silver staining of the aortic endothelium. *Acta Radiol Suppl (Stockh)* 1973; **335:** 233.
8. Almen T, Nylander G. False signs of thrombosis in lower leg phlebography. *Acta Radiol* 1964; **2:** 345.
9. Archer GJ. Homans' sign. *Lancet* 1985; **1:** 816.
10. Arnoldi CC, Greitz T, Linderholm H. Variations in the cross sectional area and pressure in the veins of the normal human leg during rhythmic muscular exercise. *Acta Chir Scand* 1966; **132:** 507.
11. Arora S, Lam DJK, Kennedy C, Meier GH, Gusberg RJ, Negus D. Light reflection rheography: a simple noninvasive screening test for deep vein thrombosis. *J Vasc Surg* 1993; **18:** 767–72.
12. Arrivé L, Menu Y, Dessarts I, *et al.* Diagnosis of abdominal venous thrombosis by means of spin-echo and gradient-echo MR imaging: analysis with receiver operating characteristic curves. *Radiology* 1991; **181:** 661–8.
13. Baldt MM, Zontsich T, Stumpflen A, *et al.* Deep venous thrombosis of the lower extremity: efficacy of spiral CT venography compared with conventional venography in diagnosis. *Radiology* 1996; **200:** 423–8.
14. Bastounis EA, Karayianakis AJ, Makri EG, Alexiou D, Papalambros EL. The incidence of occult cancer in patients with deep venous thrombosis: a prospective study. *J Intern Med* 1996; **239:** 153–6.
15. Bautovich G, Angelides S, Lee FT, *et al.* Detection of deep venous thrombi and pulmonary embolus with technetium-99-m-DD-3B6/22 anti-fibrin monoclonal antibody Fab' fragment. *J Nucl Med* 1994; **35:** 195–202.
16. Belch JJF, McMillan NC, Fogelman I, Capell H, Forbes CD. Combined phlebography and arthrography in patients with painful swollen calf. *Br Med J* 1981; **282:** 949.
17. Bergqvist D, Dahleren S, Efsing HO, Hallbook T. Thermographic diagnosis of deep venous thrombosis. *Br Med J* 1975; **4:** 684–5.
18. Bergqvist D, Hallbook T. Thermography in screening post-operative deep vein thrombosis: a comparison with the ^{125}I-fibrinogen test. *Br J Surg* 1978; **65:** 443–5.
19. Bergqvist D, Jaroszewski H. Deep vein thrombosis in patients with superficial thrombophlebitis of the leg. *Br Med J* 1986; **292:** 658–9.
20. Bertina RM, Broekmans AW, Van Der Linden IK, Mertens K. Protein C deficiency in a Dutch family with thrombotic disease. *Thromb Haemost* 1982; **48:** 1.
21. Beswick W, Chmiel R, Booth R, Vellar I, Gilford E, Chesterman CN. Detection of deep venous thrombosis by scanning of ^{99m}Tc labelled red cell venous pool. *Br Med J* 1979; **1:** 82.
22. Blaisdell FW. Low dose heparin prophylaxis of venous thrombosis. *Am Heart J* 1979; **97:** 685.
23. Bochsner MA, Appleberg M. Paradoxical embolus. *Med J Aust* 1993; **158:** 127.
24. Boey LM, Cloaco CB, Gharavi AE, Elkon KB, Loizou S, Hughes GRV. Thrombosis in systemic

lupus erythematosis: striking association with the presence of circulating 'lupus anticoagulant'. *Br Med J* 1983; **287:** 1021.

25. Bounameaux H, Khabiri E, Huber O, *et al.* Value of liquid crystal contact thermography and plasma level of D-dimer for screening of deep venous thrombosis following general abdominal surgery. *Thromb Haemost* 1992; **67:** 603–6.

26. Brodelius A, Lorinc P, Nylander G. Phlebographic techniques in the diagnosis of acute deep venous thrombosis in the lower limb. *Am J Roentgenol Rad Ther Nucl Med* 1971; **111:** 794.

27. Browse NL. Diagnosis of deep vein thrombosis. *Br Med J* 1969; **4:** 676.

28. Browse NL. The ^{125}I-fibrinogen uptake test. *Arch Surg* 1972; **104:** 160.

29. Browse NL. The value of signs in the diagnosis of deep vein thrombosis. In: *Venous Disease: Medical and Surgical Management.* Montreux: Foundation International Cooperation in Medical Sciences, 1974.

30. Browse NL. Diagnosis of deep vein thrombosis. *Br Med Bull* 1978; **34:** 163.

31. Browse NL. *An Introduction to the Symptoms and Signs of Surgical Disease.* London: Edward Arnold, 1997.

32. Browse NL, Gray L, Morland M, Jarrett PEM. Blood and vein wall fibrinolytic activity in health and vascular disease. *Br Med J* 1977; **1:** 478.

33. Browse NL, Lea Thomas M. Source of non-lethal pulmonary emboli. *Lancet* 1974; **1:** 258.

34. Browse NL, Lea-Thomas M, Solan M, Young AE. Prevention of recurrent pulmonary-embolism. *Br Med J* 1969; **3:** 382.

35. Bygdeman S, Aschberg S, Hindmarsch T. Venous plethysmography in the diagnosis of chronic venous insufficiency. *Acta Chir Scand* 1971; **131:** 423.

36. Bystrom L-G, Larsson T, Lundell L, Abom P-E. The value of thermography and the determination of fibrin-fibrinogen degradation products in the diagnosis of deep venous thrombosis. *Acta Med Scand* 1977; **202:** 319.

37. Caes FL, Van Belleghem YV, Missault LH, Coenye KE, Van Nooten GJ. Surgical treatment of impending paradoxical embolism through patent foramen ovale. *Ann Thorac Surg* 1995; **59:** 1559–61.

38. Carpenter JP, Holland GA, Baum RA, Owen RS, Carpenter JT, Cope C. Magnetic resonance venography for the detection of deep venous thrombosis: comparison with contrast venography and duplex Doppler ultrasonography. *J Vasc Surg* 1993; **18:** 734–41.

39. Carpenter JP, Holland GA, Baum RA, Riley CA. Preliminary experience with magnetic resonance venography; comparison with findings at surgical exploration. *J Surg Res* 1994; **57:** 373–9.

40. Carreras LO, Vermylen JG. Lupus anticoagulant and thrombosis: possible role of inhibition of prostacyclin formation. *Thromb Haemost* 1982; **48:** 38.

41. Cerkin TM, Beebe HG, Williams DM, Bloom JR, Wakefield TW. Popliteal vein entrapment presenting as deep venous thrombosis and chronic venous insufficiency. *J Vasc Surg* 1993; **18:** 760–6.

42. Chaikof EL, Campbell BE, Smith RB. Paradoxical embolism and acute arterial occlusion: rare or unsuspected. *J Vasc Surg* 1994; **20:** 377–84.

43. Christopoulos D, Nicolaides AN, Malouf GM, Zukowski A, Szendro G, Christodoulou C. Absolute blood volume changes in the lower limb using air-plethysmography. In: Negus D, Jantet G, eds. *Phlebography '85.* London: Libbey, 1986.

44. Cogo A, Lensing A, Prandoni P, *et al.* Failure of thrombin–antithrombin III complexes in the diagnosis of deep vein thrombosis. *Angiology* 1992; **43:** 975–9.

45. Comerota AJ, Katz ML, Greenwald LL, Leefmans E, Czeredarczuk M, White JV. Venous duplex imaging: should it replace haemodynamic tests for deep vein thrombosis? *J Vasc Surg* 1990; **11:** 53–9.

46. Comerota AJ, Katz ML, Hashemi HA. Venous duplex imaging for the diagnosis of acute deep venous thrombosis. *Haemostasis* 1993; **23:** 61–71.

47. Conard J, Veuillet-Duval A, Horellou MH, Samama M. Etude de la coagulation et de la fibrinolyse dans 131 cas de thromboses veineuses récidivants. *Nouv Rev Fr Hematol* 1982; **24:** 205.

48. Cooke ED, Pilcher MF. Deep vein thrombosis: preclinical diagnosis by thermography. *Br J Surg* 1974; **61:** 971.

49. Cooke ED, Pilcher MF. Thermography in diagnosis of deep vein thrombosis. *Br Med J* 1973; **2:** 523.

50. Coon WW, Coller FA. Some epidemiological considerations of thrombophlebitis. *Surg Gynecol Obstet* 1959; **109:** 487.

51. Couson F, Bounameaux C, Didier D, *et al.* Influence of variability of interpretation of contrast venography for screening of postoperative deep venous thrombosis on the results of a thromboprophylactic study. *Thromb Haemost* 1993; **70:** 573–5.

52. Cranley JJ, Canos AJ, Sull WJ. The diagnosis of deep vein thrombosis. *Arch Surg* 1976; **111:** 34.

53. Cranley JJ, Canos AJ, Sull WJ, Grass AM. Phleborheographic technique for diagnosis of deep vein thrombosis of the lower extremities. *Surg Gynecol Obstet* 1975; **141:** 331.

54. Cranley JJ, Gay AY, Grass AM, Simeone FA. A plethysmographic technique for the diagnosis of deep venous thrombosis of the lower extremities. *Surg Gynecol Obstet* 1973; **58:** 111.

55. Culver D, Crawford JS, Gardiner JH, Wiley AM. Venous thrombosis after fractures of the upper end of the femur. A study of incidence and site. *J Bone Joint Surg (Br)* 1970; **52:** 61–9.

56. Davidson BL, Elliott CG, Lensing AW. Low accuracy of color Doppler ultrasound in the detection of proximal leg vein thrombosis in asymptomatic high-risk patients. The RD Heparin Arthroplasty Group. *Ann Intern Med* 1992; **117:** 735–8.

57. Day TK, Fish PJ, Kakkar VV. Detection of deep vein thrombosis by Doppler angiography. *Br Med J* 1976; **1:** 618–20.

58. Deacon JM, Ell PJ, Anderson P, Khan O. Technetium 99m plasmin: a new test for the detection of deep vein thrombosis. *Br J Radiol* 1980; **53:** 673–7.

59. DeWeese JA, Rogoff SM. Phlebographic patterns of acute deep venous thrombosis of the leg. *Surgery* 1963; **53:** 99.

60. Donati MB, Poggi A. Malignancy and haemostasis. *Br J Haematol* 1980; **44:** 173.

61. Douss TW. The clinical significance of venous thrombosis of the calf. *Br J Surg* 1976; **63:** 377.

62. Dugan MA, Kozar JJ, Ganse G. Localization of deep vein thrombosis using radioactive streptokinase. *J Nucl Med* 1973; **14:** 233.

63. Dupas B, El Kouri E, Curtet C, *et al.* Angiomagnetic resonance imaging of iliofemorocaval venous thrombosis. *Lancet* 1995; **346:** 17–19.

64. Edenbrandt CM, Nilsson J, Oulin P. Diagnosis of deep venous thrombosis by phlebography and ^{99}Tc plasmin. *Acta Med Scand* 1982; **211:** 59.

65. Egeberg O. Inherited antithrombin deficiency causing thrombophilia. *Thromb Diath Haemorrh* 1965; **13:** 516.

66. Eriksson E. Plethysmographic studies of venous disease of the legs. *Acta Chir Scand Suppl* 1973; **436:** 1.

67. Elliott CG, Suchyta M, Rose SC, *et al.* Duplex ultrasonography for the detection of deep vein thrombi after total hip or knee arthroplasty. *Angiology* 1993; **44:** 26–33.

68. Erdman WA, Jayson HT, Redman HC, Miller GL, Parkey RW, Peshock RW. Deep venous thrombosis of extremities: role of MR imaging in the diagnosis. *Radiology* 1990; **174:** 425–31.

69. Evans AJ, Sostman HD, Knelson MH, *et al.* 1992 ARRS Executive Council Award. Detection of deep venous thrombosis: prospective comparison of MR imaging with contrast venography. *Am J Roentgenol* 1993; **161:** 131–9.

70. Evans DS. The early diagnosis of venous thrombosis by ultrasound. *Br J Surg* 1970; **57:** 726.

71. Evans DS, Cockett FB. Diagnosis of deep venous thrombosis using an ultrasonic Doppler technique. *Br Med J* 1968; **2:** 802.

72. Fenech A, Dendy PP, Hussey JK, Bennett B, Douglas AS. Indium-111 labelled platelets in diagnosis of leg vein thrombosis: preliminary findings. *Br Med J* 1980; **280:** 1571.

73. Flanc C, Kakkar VV, Clark MB. The detection of venous thrombosis of the legs using ^{125}I labelled fibrinogen. *Br J Surg* 1968; **55:** 742.

74. Forfar JC. A seven year analysis of haemorrhage in patients on long-term anticoagulant treatment. *Br Heart J* 1979; **142:** 128.

75. Fowl RJ, Strothman GB, Blebea J, Rosenthal GJ, Kempczinski RF. Inappropriate use of venous duplex scans: an analysis of indications and results. *J Vasc Surg* 1996; **23:** 881–5 (discussion 885–6).

76. Francis CW, Totterman S. Magnetic resonance imaging of deep vein thrombi correlates with response to thrombolytic therapy. *Thromb Haemost* 1995; **73:** 386–91.

77. Gardner GP, Cordts PR, Gillespie DL, LaMorte W, Woodson J, Menzoian JO. Can air plethysmography accurately identify upper extremity deep venous thrombosis? *J Vasc Surg* 1993; **18:** 808–13.

78. Gerkin TM, Beebe HG, Williams DM, Bloom JR, Wakefield TW. Popliteal vein entrapment presenting as deep venous thrombosis and chronic venous insufficiency. *J Vasc Surg* 1993; **18:** 760–6.

79. Gibbs NM. Venous thrombosis of the lower limbs with particular reference to bed rest. *Br J Surg* 1957; **45:** 209.

80. Ginsberg JS, Siragusa S, Douketis J, *et al.* Evaluation of a soluble fibrin assay in patients with suspected deep vein thrombosis. *Thromb Haemost* 1995; **74:** 833–6.

81. Gregoire R. La phlébite bleue (phlegmasia cerulea dolens). *Presse Méd* 1938; **2:** 1313.

82. Griffin JH, Evatt B, Zimmerman TS, Kleiss AJ, Widemann C. Deficiency of protein C in congenital thrombotic disease. *J Clin Invest* 1981; **68:** 1370.

83. Grimley RP, Slaney G, Hawker RJ, Rafiqi E, Drolc Z. Diagnosis of deep vein thrombosis using indium[111] labelled platelets. *Br Med J* 1981; **282:** 1626.

84. Gurewich V, Hume M, Patrick M. The laboratory diagnosis of venous thromboembolic disease by measurement of fibrinogen/fibrin degradation product and fibrin monomer. *Chest* 1973; **64:** 585.

85. Gyde OHB, Littler WA, Stableforth DE. Familial antithrombin III deficiency. *Br Med J* 1978; **1:** 508.

86. Gyde OHB, Middleton MD, Vaughan GR, Fletcher DJ. Antithrombin III deficiency hypertriglyceridaemia and venous thromboses. *Br Med J* 1978; **1:** 621.

87. Haegar K. Den kliniska thrombusdiagnosens (o) tillforlitlighet. *Svenska Lak Sallsk Forhandl* 1965; **62:** 1067.

88. Haeger K, Nylander G. Acute phlebography. *Triangle* 1967; **8:** 18.

89. Hallbrook T, Gothlin J. Strain gauge plethysmography and phlebography in diagnosis of deep venous thrombosis. *Acta Chir Scand* 1971; **137:** 37.

90. Hanel KC, Abbott WM, Reidy NC, *et al.* The role of two noninvasive tests in deep venous thrombosis. *Ann Surg* 1981; **194:** 725.

91. Harwig SSL, Harwig JF, Sherman R, Coleman RE, Welch MJ. Radioiodinated plasminogen: an imaging agent for pre-existing thrombi. *J Nucl Med* 1977; **18:** 42.

92. Hassell AB, Planet MJ, Dawes PT. Focal myositis: another cause of pseudothrombophlebitis (letter). *Br J Rheumatol* 1994; **33:** 687.

93. Heijboer H, Cogo A, Buller HR, Prandoni P, ten Cate JW. Detection of deep vein thrombosis with impedance plethysmography and real-time compression ultrasonography in hospitalized patients. *Arch Intern Med* 1992; **152:** 1901–3.

94. Heijboer H, Jongbloets LM, Buller HR, Lensing AW, ten Cate JW. Clinical utility of real-time compression ultrasonography for diagnostic management of patients with recurrent venous thrombosis. *Acta Radiol* 1992; **33:** 297–300.

95. Henderson HP, Cooke ED, Bowcock SA, Hackett MEJ. After exercise thermography for predicting postoperative deep vein thrombosis. *Br Med J* 1978; **1:** 1020.

96. Highman J, O'Sullivan E. Isotope venography. *Br J Surg* 1973; **60:** 58.
97. Hirsch J, Gallus AS, Cade JF. Diagnosis of thrombosis. Evaluation of ^{125}I fibrinogen scanning and blood test. *Thromb Diath Haemorrh* 1974; **32:** 11.
98. Hobbs JT, Davies JWL. Detection of venous thrombosis with ^{131}I labelled fibrinogen in the rabbit. *Lancet* 1960; **2:** 134.
99. Hobsley M. *Pathways in Surgical Management.* London: Edward Arnold, 1979.
100. Homans J. Diseases of the veins. *N Engl J Med* 1944; **231:** 51.
101. Homans J. Thrombophlebitis of the lower extremities. *Ann Surg* 1928; **88:** 641.
102. Honkanen T, Jauhola S, Karppinen K, Paul R, Sakki S, Vorne M. Venous thrombosis: a controlled study on the performance of scintigraphy with 99TcM-HMPAO-labelled platelets versus venography. *Nucl Med Commun* 1992; **13:** 88–94.
103. Horellou MH, Conard J, Bertina RM, Samama M. Congenital protein C deficiency and thrombotic disease in nine French families. *Br Med J* 1984; **289:** 1285.
104. Howe CT. The management of deep vein thrombosis. *Br J Hosp Med* 1970; 348.
105. Hull R, Hirsch J, Sackett DL. Clinical validity of a negative venogram in patients with clinically suspected venous thrombosis. *Circulation* 1981; **64:** 622–5.
106. Hull R, Hirsch J, Sackett DL, Powers P, Turpie AGG, Walker I. Combined use of leg scanning and impedance plethysmography in suspected venous thrombosis. *N Engl J Med* 1977; **296:** 1497.
107. Hull R, Hirsch J, Sackett DL, Stoddart G. Cost effectiveness of clinical diagnosis, venography and non-invasive testing in patients with symptomatic deep vein thrombosis. *N Engl J Med* 1981; **304:** 1561.
108. Husted SE, Kraemmer Nielsen L, Krusell L, *et al.* Deep vein thrombosis detection by 99mTc-plasmin test and phlebography. *Br J Surg* 1984; **71:** 65–6.
109. Isacson S, Nilsson IM. Defective fibrinolysis in blood and vein walls in recurrent 'idiopathic' venous thrombosis. *Acta Chir Scand* 1972; **138:** 313.
110. Jensen C, Knudsen LL, Hecedus V. The role of contact thermography in the diagnosis of deep vein thrombosis. *Eur J Radiol* 1983; **3:** 99.
111. Johansson L, Hedner U, Nilsson IM. A family with thromboembolic disease associated with deficient fibrinolytic activity in vessel wall. *Acta Med Scand* 1978; **208:** 477.
112. Jonckheer MH, Abramovici J, Jeghers O, Derume JP, Goldstein M. The interpretation of phlebograms using fibrinogen labeled with 99mTc. *Eur J Nucl Med* 1978; **3:** 233–8.
113. Jongbloets LMM, Lensing AWA, Koopman MMW, Buller HR, ten Cate JW. Limitations of compression ultrasound for the detection of symptomless postoperative deep vein thrombosis. *Lancet* 1994; **343:** 1142–4.
114. Jorgensen JD, Hanel KC, Morgan AM, Hunt JM. The incidence of deep vein thrombosis in patients with superficial thrombophlebitis of the lower limbs. *J Vasc Surg* 1993; **18:** 70–3.
115. Kakkar VV. The diagnosis of deep vein thrombosis using fibrinogen test. *Arch Surg* 1972; **104:** 152.
116. Kakkar VV, Howe CT, Laws JW, Flanc C. Late results of treatment of deep vein thrombosis. *Br Med J* 1969; **1:** 810.
117. Kakkar VV, Sasahara AA. Diagnosis of venous thrombosis and pulmonary embolism. In: Bloom AL, Thomas DP, eds. *Haemostasis and Thrombosis.* Edinburgh: Churchill Livingstone, 1981.
118. Katz RS, Zizic TM, Arnold WP, Stevens MB. The pseudothrombophlebitis syndrome. *Medicine* 1977; **56:** 151.
119. Kempi V, Van der Linden W, Von Schéele C. Diagnosis of deep vein thrombosis with ^{99m}Tc-streptokinase: a clinical comparison with phlebography. *Br Med J* 1974; **4:** 748–9.
120. Kilpatrick TK, Lichenstein M, Andrews J, Gibson RN, Neerhut P, Hopper J. A comparative study of radionuclide venography and contast venography in the diagnosis of deep venous thrombosis. *Aust N Z J Med* 1993; **23:** 641–5.
121. Kinmonth JB. Lymphangiography in man. *Clin Sci* 1952; **11:** 13.
122. Knight LC, Primeau JL, Siegel BA, Welch MJ. Comparison of ^{111}In labelled platelets and iodinated fibrinogen for the detection of deep vein thrombosis. *J Nucl Med* 1978; **19:** 891.
123. Kohn H, Mostbeck A, Lofferer O, Konig B, Swetly C. Non-invasive screening for deep vein thrombosis: comparison between 99mTc labelled compounds, thermography I-131 fibrinogen uptake test and x-ray phlebography. *Phlebology* 1986; **1:** 65–72.
124. Kolecki RV, Sigel B, Jujstin J, *et al.* Determining the acuteness and stability of deep venous thrombosis by ultrasonic tissue characterization. *J Vasc Surg* 1995; **21:** 976–84.
125. Kudo S, Kishikawa T, Kuroiwa T, *et al.* Digital subtraction angiography for leg venography. *Radiat Med* 1992; **10:** 1–5.
126. Labropoulos N, Leon M, Kalodiki E, al Kutoubi A, Chan P, Nicolaides AN. Colour flow duplex scanning in suspected acute deep vein thrombosis; experience with routine use. *Eur J Vasc Endovasc Surg* 1995; **9:** 49–52.
127. Lambie JM, Mahaffey RG, Barber DC, Karmody AM, Scott MM, Matheson NA. Diagnostic accuracy in venous thrombosis. *Br Med J* 1970; **2:** 142.
128. Lausen I, Jensen R, Wille-Jorgensen P, *et al.* Colour Doppler flow imaging ultrasonography versus venography as screening method for asymptomatic postoperative deep venous thrombosis. *Eur J Radiol* 1995; **20:** 200–4.
129. Layfer LF, Jones JV. Calf pain in rheumatoid arthritis. *IMJ* 1979; **155:** 104.
130. Lazarus ML, Ray CE Jr, Manquis CG. MRI findings of concurrent acute DVT and dissecting popliteal cyst. *Magn Reson Imaging* 1994; **12:** 155–8.
131. Lea Thomas M. Deep vein thrombosis. *Proc R Soc Med* 1970; **63:** 123.
132. Lea Thomas M. *Phlebography of the Lower Limb.* Edinburgh: Churchill Livingstone, 1982.

133. Lea Thomas M, Browse NL. Internal iliac vein thrombosis. *Acta Radiol (Diagn) (Stockh)* 1972; **12:** 660.

134. Lea Thomas M, Carty H. Arteriographic changes in phlegmasia cerulia dolens. *Australas Radiol* 1975; **19:** 57.

135. Lea Thomas M, Carty H. The appearances of artefacts on lower limb phlebograms. *Clin Radiol* 1975; **26:** 527.

136. Lea Thomas M, McAllister V, Tonge K. The radiological appearances of deep vein thrombosis. *Clin Radiol* 1971; **22:** 295.

137. Lea Thomas M, McDonald LM. Complications of phlebography of the leg. *Br Med J* 1978; **2:** 307.

138. Lea Thomas M, McDonald LM. The accuracy of bolus ascending phlebography in demonstrating the ilio-femoral segment. *Clin Radiol* 1977; **28:** 165.

139. Lea Thomas M, O'Dwyer JA. A phlebographic study of the incidence and significance of venous thrombosis in the foot. *Am J Roentgenol* 1978; **130:** 751.

140. Lensing AW, Buller HR, Prandoni P, *et al.* Contrast venography, the gold standard for the diagnosis of deep-vein thrombosis: improvement in observer agreement. *Thromb Haemost* 1992; **67:** 8–12.

141. Lewis BD, James EM, Welch TJ, Joyce JW, Hallett JW, Weaver AL. Diagnosis of acute deep venous thrombosis of the lower extremities: prospective evaluation of color duplex flow imaging versus venography. *Radiology* 1994; **192:** 651–5.

142. Lindhagen A, Berquist D, Hallbook K, Lindroth B. After-exercise thermography and prevention of deep vein thrombosis. *Br Med J* 1982; **284:** 1825.

143. Lohr JM, James KV, Desmukh RM, Hasselfield KA, Alistair B. Kamody award. Calf vein thrombi are not a benign finding. *Am J Surg* 1995; **170:** 86–90.

144. Loscalo J. Paradoxical embolism: clinical presentation, diagnostic strategies and therapeutic options. *Am Heart J* 1986; **112:** 141–5.

145. Loudon JR. ^{125}I-fibrinogen uptake test. *Br Med J* 1976; **1:** 793.

146. Lowe GDO, McKillop JH, Prentice AG. Fatal retroperitoneal haemorrhage complicating anticoagulant treatment. *Postgrad Med J* 1979; **55:** 18.

147. Machi J, Sigel B, Roberts AB, Kahn MB. Oversaturation of color may obscure small intraluminal partial occlusions in color Doppler imaging. *J Ultrasound Med* 1994; **13:** 735–41.

148. Magnusson M, Eriksson BI, Kalebo P, Sivertsson R. Is colour Doppler ultrasound a sensitive screening method in diagnosing deep vein thrombosis after hip surgery? *Thromb Haemost* 1996; **75:** 242–5.

149. Makin GS. Assessment of a simple test to detect postoperative deep vein thrombosis. *Br J Surg* 1968; **55:** 822.

150. Mant MJ, O'Brien BD, Thong KL, Hammond GW, Birtwhistle RV, Grace MG. Haemorrhagic complications of heparin therapy. *Lancet* 1977; **1:** 1113.

151. Markel A, Weich Y, Gaitini D. Doppler ultrasound in the diagnosis of venous thrombosis. *Angiology* 1995; **46:** 65–73.

152. McFarlane DG, Bacon PA. Popliteal cyst rupture in normal knee joints. *Br Med J* 1980; **281:** 1203.

153. McLachlan MSF, Thomson JG, Taylor DW, Kelly M, Sackett DL. Observer variation in the interpretation of lower leg venograms. *Am J Roentgenol* 1979; **132:** 227.

154. McLachlin J, Richards T, Paterson JC. An evaluation of clinical signs in the diagnosis of venous thrombosis. *Arch Surg* 1962; **85:** 738.

155. Meadway J, Nicolaides AN, Walker CJ, O'Connell JD. Value of Doppler ultrasound in diagnosis of clinically suspected deep vein thrombosis. *Br Med J* 1975; **4:** 552.

156. Mitchell DC, Grasty MS, Stebbings WSL, *et al.* Comparison of duplex ultrasonography and venography in the diagnosis of deep venous thrombosis. *Br J Surg* 1991; **78:** 611–13.

157. Montefusco-Von Kleist CM, Bakal C, Sprayregen S, Rhodes BA, Veith FJ. Comparison of duplex ultrasonography and ascending contrast venography in the diagnosis of venous thrombosis. *Angiology* 1993; **44:** 169–75.

158. Montgomery KD, Potter HG, Helfet DL. Magnetic resonance venography to evaluate the deep venous system of the pelvis in patients who have an acetabular fracture. *J Bone Joint Surg (Am)* 1995; **77:** 1639–49.

159. Moreno-Cabral R, Kistner RL, Mordyka RA. Importance of calf-vein thrombophlebitis. *Surgery* 1976; **80:** 735.

160. Morris GK, Mitchell JR. Evaluation of ^{125}I fibrinogen test for venous thrombosis in patients with hip fractures: a comparison between isotope scanning and autopsy. *Br Med J* 1977; **1:** 254.

161. Moser KM, Brach BB, Dolan GF. Clinically suspected deep venous thrombosis of the lower extremities: a comparison of venography, impedance plethysmography and radiolabelled fibrinogen. *JAMA* 1977; **237:** 2195.

162. Mullick SC, Wheeler HB, Songster GP. Diagnosis of deep venous thrombosis by electrical impedance. *Am J Surg* 1970; **119:** 417.

163. Negus D, Pinto DH, LeQuesne LP, Brown N, Chapman M. [125]I labelled fibrinogen in the diagnosis of deep vein thrombosis and its correlation with phlebography. *Br J Surg* 1968; **55:** 835.

164. Nicolaides A, Kalodiki E. Duplex scanning in postoperative surgical patients. *Haemostasis* 1993; **23:** 72–9.

165. Nillius AS, Lindvall R, Nylander G. Dynamic radionucleotide phlebography. A clinical study in patients after total hip replacement. *Eur J Nucl Med* 1978; **3:** 161.

166. Nilsson IM, Krook H, Sternby N-H, Soderberg E, Soderstrom N. Severe thrombotic disease in a young man with bone marrow and skeletal changes and with a high content of an inhibitor in the fibrinolytic system. *Acta Med Scand* 1961; **169:** 323.

167. Nilsson IM, Ljungner H, Tengborn L. Two different mechanisms in patients with venous thrombosis and defective fibrinolysis: low concentration of plasminogen activator or increased concentration of plasminogen activator inhibitor. *Br Med J* 1985; **290:** 1453.

168. Nylander G. Phlebographic diagnosis of acute deep leg thrombosis. *Acta Chir Scand Suppl* 1968; **397:** 30.

169. Nylander G. Comments on reason for conflicting results of venography. *Haemostasis* 1993; **23 (Suppl):** 85–8.

170. Ochsner A, DeBakey ME. Thrombophlebitis: role of venospasm in the production of the clinical manifestations. *JAMA* 1940; **114:** 117.

171. O'Donnell TF, Abbott WM, Athanasoulis CA, Milan VG, Callow AD. Diagnosis of deep vein thrombosis in the outpatient by venography. *Surg Gynecol Obstet* 1980; **150:** 69.

172. Ollson P. Variations in antithrombin activity in plasma after major surgery. *Acta Chir Scand* 1963; **126:** 24.

173. Olsson CG, Albrechtsson U, Darte L, Persson RBR. Tc99m plasmin for rapid detection of deep venous thrombosis. *Nucl Med Commun* 1982; **3:** 41–52.

174. Pabinger-Fasching I, Bertina RM, Lechner K, Niessner H, Korininger CH. Protein C deficiency in two Austrian families. *Thromb Haemost* 1983; **50:** 180.

175. Partsch H, Kahn P, Roser-Maass E, Tham B. Teletthermography for screening ambulatory patients with leg vein thrombosis. *Vasa* 1981; **10:** 242.

176. Partsch H, Loefferer O, Mostbeck A. Diagnosis of established deep-vein thrombosis in the leg using ^{131}I fibrinogen. *Angiology* 1974; **25:** 719.

177. Perlin SJ. Pulmonary embolism during compression US of the lower extremity. *Radiology* 1992; **184:** 165–6.

178. Peters AM, Lavender JP, Needham SG, *et al.* Imaging thrombus with radiolabelled monoclonal antibody to platelets. *Br Med J* 1986; **293:** 1525–7.

179. Phillips RS. Prognosis in deep venous thrombosis. *Arch Surg* 1963; **87:** 732.

180. Pochaczevsky R, Pillari G, Feldman F. Liquid crystal contact thermography of deep vein thrombosis. *Am J Roentgenol* 1981; **738:** 717.

181. Poulose K, Kapcar A, Reba R. False positive ^{125}I fibrinogen test. *Angiology* 1976; **27:** 258.

182. Provan JL. Raised skin temperature in the early diagnosis of deep vein thrombosis. *Br Med J* 1965; **3:** 334.

183. Quist G. *Surgical Diagnosis.* London: HK Lewis, 1977.

184. Ramsay LE. Impact of venography on the diagnosis and management of deep vein thrombosis. *Br Med J* 1983; **286:** 698.

185. Riambau V, Carrio I, Berna L, Estorch M, Torres G, Viver E. Evaluation of indium-111 antifibrin monoclonal antibody imaging in deep venous thrombosis diagnosis. *Phlebology* 1992; **7:** 7–11.

186. Ritchie WGM, Lapayowker MS, Soulen RL. Thermographic diagnosis of deep venous thrombosis: anatomically based diagnostic criteria. *Radiology* 1979; **132:** 321.

187. Roberts VC. Fibrinogen uptake scanning for diagnosis of deep vein thrombosis: a plea for standardization. *Br Med J* 1975; **3:** 455.

188. Roberts VC, Cotton LT. Prevention of postoperative deep vein thrombosis in patients with malignant disease. *Br Med J* 1974; **1:** 358.

189. Rollins D, Ryan TJ, Semrow C, Buchbinder D. Diagnosis of deep venous thrombosis using real time ultrasound imaging. In: Negus D, Jantet G, eds. *Phlebology '85.* London: Libbey, 1986.

190. Rosen MP, Sheiman RG, Weintraub J, McArdle C. Compression sonography in patients with indeterminate or low-probability lung scans: lack of usefulness in the absence of both symptoms of deep-vein thrombosis and thromboembolic risk factors. *Am J Roentgenol* 1996; **166:** 285.

191. Rosenberg RD. Actions and interactions of antithrombin and heparin. *N Engl J Med* 1975; **292:** 146.

192. Rosenthall L. Radionucleotide venography using ^{99m}Tc pertechnetate and the gamma ray scintillation camera. *Am J Roentgenol* 1966; **97:** 874.

193. Rosenthall L. Combined inferior vena cavography, iliac venography and lung imaging with ^{99m}Tc albumin macroaggregates. *Radiology* 1971; **98:** 623.

194. Rosenthall L, Leclerc J. A new thrombus imaging agent. Human recombinant fibrin binding domain labeled with In-111. *Clin Nucl Med* 1995; **20:** 398–402.

195. Ruckley CV. [125]I fibrinogen test in the diagnosis of deep vein thrombosis. *Br Med J* 1975; **2:** 498.

196. Sandler DA. Homans' sign and medical education. *Lancet* 1985; **1:** 1130.

197. Sandler DA, Martin JF. Liquid crystal thermography as a screening test for deep vein thrombosis. *Lancet* 1985; **1:** 665.

198. Sandler D, Martin JF, Duncan JS, *et al.* Diagnosis of deep vein thrombosis. Comparison of clinical evaluation, ultrasound, plethysmography and venoscan with xray venogram. *Lancet* 1984; **2:** 716.

199. Sas G, Blasko G, Bankegyi D, Jako J, Palos A. Abnormal antithrombin III (antithrombin III 'Budapest') as a cause of a familial thrombophilia. *Thromb Diath Haemorrh* 1974; **32:** 105.

200. Sigel B, Popky GL, Boland JP, Wagner DK, Mapp EMcD. Diagnosis of venous disease by ultrasonic flow detection. *Surg Forum* 1967; **18:** 185.

201. Simons GR, Skibo LK, Polak JF, Creager MA, Klapec-Fay JM, Goldhaber SZ. Utility of leg ultrasonography in suspected symptomatic isolated calf deep venous thrombosis. *Am J Med* 1995; **99:** 43–7.

202. Simpson FG, Robinson PJ, Bark M, Losowsky MS. Prospective study of thrombophlebitis and 'pseudothrombophlebitis'. *Lancet* 1980; **1:** 331.

203. Spritzer CE, Evans AC, Kay HH. Magnetic resonance imaging of deep venous thrombosis in pregnant women with lower extremity edema. *Obstet Gynecol* 1995; **85:** 603–7.

204. Spritzer CE, Norconk JJ, Sostman HD, Coleman RE. Detection of deep venous thrombosis by magnetic resonance imaging. *Chest* 1993; **104:** 54–60.

205. Sproull EE. Carcinoma and venous thrombosis: the frequency of association of carcinoma in the body or tail of the pancreas with multiple venous thrombosis. *Am J Cancer* 1938; **34:** 566.

206. Stevenson AJM, Moss JG, Kirkpatrick AE. Comparison of temperature profiles (Devetherm) and conventional venography in suspected lower limb thrombosis. *Clin Radiol* 1990; **42:** 37–9.

207. Stewart G, Gaunt JI, Croft DN, Browse NL. Isotope lymphography: a new method of investigating the role of the lymphatics in chronic limb oedema. *Br J Surg* 1985; **72:** 906–9.

208. Strandness DE, Sumner DS. Ultrasonic velocity detector in the diagnosis of thrombophlebitis. *Arch Surg* 1972; **104:** 180.

209. Sullivan ED, David JP, Cranley JJ. Real time B mode venous ultrasound. *J Vasc Surg* 1984; **1:** 465–71.

210. Sumner DS, Baker DW, Strandness DE. The ultrasonic velocity detector in a clinical study of venous disease. *Arch Surg* 1968; **97:** 75.

211. Szendro G, Nicolaides AN, Zukowski AJ, *et al.* Duplex scanning in the assessment of deep venous incompetence. *J Vasc Surg* 1986; **4:** 237.

212. Teh A, Jeyamalar R, Habib ZA. Arteriovenous fistula simulating deep vein thrombosis as a complication of lumbar disc surgery. *Med J Malaysia* 1993; **48:** 440–2.

213. Thomas PRS, Butler CM, Bowman J, *et al.* Light reflection rheography: an effective non-invasive technique for screening patients with suspected deep venous thrombosis. *Br J Surg* 1991; **78:** 207–9.

214. Thulesius O, Thun A. Extravascular masses masquerading as deep venous thrombosis. *Phlebology* 1993; **8:** 158–61.

215. Tran TH, Marbet GA, Duckert F. Association of heriditary heparin co-factor 2 deficiency with thrombosis. *Lancet* 1985; **2:** 413.

216. Vanninen R, Maninen H, Soimakallio S, Katila T, Suomalainen O. Asymptomatic deep venous thrombosis in the calf: accuracy and limitations of ultrasonography as a screening test after total knee arthroplasty. *Br J Radiol* 1993; **66:** 199–202.

217. Von Kaulla E, Von Kaulla KN. Antithrombin III and diseases. *Am J Clin Pathol* 1967; **48:** 69.

218. Von Kaulla E, Von Kaulla KN. Deficiency of antithrombin III activity associated with hereditary thrombosis tendency. *J Med* 1972; **3:** 349.

219. Vorne MS, Honkanen TT, Lantto TJ, Laitinen RO, Karppinen KJ, Jauhola SV. Thrombus imaging with ^{99m}Tc-HMPAO-labelled platelets and ^{111}In-labelled monoclonal antifibrin antibodies. *Acta Radiol* 1993; **34:** 59–63.

220. Warlow C, Ogston D. The ^{125}I-fibrinogen technique in the diagnosis of venous thrombosis. *Clin Haematol* 1973; **2:** 199.

221. Webber M, Bennet L, Craig M. Thrombophlebitis: demonstration by scintiscanning. *Radiology* 1969; **92:** 620.

222. Wells PS, Hirsh J, Anderson DR, *et al.* Accuracy of clinical assessment of deep vein thrombosis. *Lancet* 1995; **345:** 1326–30.

223. Wells PS, Hirsh J, Anderson DR, *et al.* Comparison of the accuracy of impedance plethysmography and compression ultrasonography in outpatients with clinically suspected deep vein thrombosis. A two centre paired-design prospective trial. *Thromb Haemost* 1995; **74:** 1423–7.

224. Wells PS, Lensing AW, Davidson BL, Prins MH, Hirsh J. Accuracy of ultrasound for the diagnosis of deep venous thrombosis in asymptomatic patients after orthopedic surgery. A meta-analysis. *Ann Intern Med* 1995; **122:** 47–53.

225. Wester JP, Holtkamp M, Linnebank ER, *et al.* Non-invasive detection of deep venous thrombosis: ultrasonography versus duplex scanning. *Eur J Vasc Surg* 1994; **8:** 357–61.

226. Wheeler HB, Anderson FA, Cardullo PA, Patwardhan NA, Jian-Ming L, Cutler BS. Suspected deep vein thrombosis. Management by impedance plethysmography. *Arch Surg* 1982; **117:** 1206.

227. Wheeler HB, Mullick SC, Anderson JN, Pearson D. Diagnosis of occult deep vein thrombosis by a non-invasive bedside technique. *Surgery* 1971; **70:** 20.

228. Wood EH, Prentice ER, McNicol GP. Association of fibrinogen-fibrin related antigen (FR antigen) with postoperative deep-vein thrombosis and systemic complications. *Lancet* 1972; **1:** 166.

229. Ygge J. Studies on blood coagulation and fibrinolysis in conditions associated with an increased incidence of thrombosis. Methodological and clinical investigations. *Scand J Haematol Suppl* 1970; **11:** 1–45.

230. Yin ET, Wessler S, Stoll PJ. Identity of plasma associated factor X inhibitor with antithrombin III and heparin co-factor. *J Biol Chem* 1971; **246:** 712.

CHAPTER 10

Deep vein thrombosis: treatment

Thrombolysis	320	Defibrogenation	351
Thrombectomy	329	Summary	352
Anticoagulation	340	References	353

Thrombosis in a deep vein often occludes its lumen and invariably destroys its valves.[42] If by the term 'treatment' we imply restoration to complete normality, then the treatment of deep vein thrombosis requires either the removal of the thrombus before it has destroyed the valves, or the manipulation of the natural history of the thrombus with measures that will encourage reopening of the lumen and recovery of the valves. The latter approach is not yet possible and therefore the only available treatment is thrombus removal.

When a thrombus cannot be removed, its ultimate effect is, at present, beyond our control. All we can do is prevent further thrombosis or propagation, by giving anticoagulants, or stop complications (e.g. pulmonary embolism) by performing surgical venous blockade.

As a result of the inadequacies of the available forms of treatment, other clinical objectives are sought – often just the relief of symptoms. These efforts are called 'treatment', even though they do not cure. They are for the most part palliation.

The main clinical objectives are:

- Waiting for natural lysis or organization of the thrombus to occur while ensuring the patient does not develop thrombus propagation or fatal pulmonary embolus by providing adequate anticoagulation.
- The prevention of fatal pulmonary embolism. This can be achieved by thrombus removal, venous blockade or the prevention of new or propagated thrombosis with anticoagulants.
- To reduce the severity of the post-thrombotic syndrome. This may be achieved by thrombus removal or by preventing new or propagated thrombosis with anticoagulants but it may be made worse by venous blockade.
- Reduction of the severity of the presenting symptoms. This is usually achieved by measures such as pain relief which have no effect on the thrombus.

The first two of these four objectives – which entail saving the patient's life – override all others, and therefore when the ideal treatment (i.e. the complete removal of a thrombus leaving the veins and the valves intact) is unattainable, the patient may have to accept the post-thrombotic syndrome as the cost of being alive.

There are still only two methods for removing thrombus, surgical thrombectomy and pharmacological thrombolysis, although the latter may now be combined with endovascular techniques for breaking up or compressing the thrombus. Both methods are most effective when the thrombus is fresh and non-adherent, when it is often symptomless. By the time symptoms appear, the thrombus is often old and adherent, two features which make its removal or dissolution difficult. Both methods of removal have their contraindications. Whenever possible, pharmacological lysis of thrombus is preferred to surgical thrombectomy because it attempts to clear all the thrombus from the limb, some of which is inaccessible to the surgeon, and it avoids the risks and complications of surgery (although of course it has risks of its own).

Intravenous unfractionated heparin given by continuous infusion followed by a 3–6 months course of oral warfarin is the most common regimen used to treat extensive deep venous thrombosis even when it is associated with a small or moderate sized pulmonary embolism.[146] This form of treatment is aimed at avoiding further pulmonary embolism and preventing propagation of thrombus, which it may achieve although the evidence is mostly slight and indirect. It does nothing to prevent the subsequent development of the post-thrombotic limb syndrome (see Chapter 15) because it does not actively remove the thrombus which is progressively organized by the body's own defence mechanisms. Most patients who develop a sporadic deep vein thrombosis, or those who present with shortness of breath, haemoptysis or chest pain associated with a pulmonary embolism, are now admitted under the care of physicians who are content to treat these problems with heparin and warfarin. Increasing numbers are now treating deep vein thrombosis with subcutaneously administered low molecular weight heparin which appears to be equally efficacious to the intravenously administered unfractionated compound. Although we recognize the simplicity and limited effectiveness of these regimens, we continue to champion the concept of tailored treatment for each patient based on the extent, age, feasibility and the lethal potential of their venous thrombus. This means that the best approach is to consider thrombolytic therapy or surgical thrombectomy in every patient after a full assessment by contrast phlebography.

Thrombolysis

The body's fibrinolytic system can be activated to a state in which it will lyse thrombi by two exogenous plasminogen 'activators' – streptokinase (derived from the streptococcus) and urokinase (derived from human urine).[111,171] The body's own plasminogen activator, tissue plasminogen activator, has now been isolated and cloned and is available as a recombinant protein. All three activators work by activating plasminogen. Streptokinase acts directly by complexing with plasminogen; this exposes the active site on the plasminogen which catalyses the cleavage of plasminogen to plasmin. Urokinase and tissue plasminogen activator act directly on plas-

minogen, coverting it to plasmin. The plasmin produced by these two enzymes breaks fibrin down into a number of soluble products.

Streptokinase is neutralized in the blood by antibodies that have been produced in response to previous streptococcal infections. These antibodies must be blocked before the streptokinase can begin to complex with plasminogen. Streptokinase is itself highly antigenic, and the level of antistreptococcal antibodies rises and remains very high for 6 months after treatment, making the continuation of treatment beyond 3 weeks ineffective. Tissue plasminogen activator and urokinase are human proteins and are therefore not antigenic.

Streptokinase

This substance has been more widely used in Europe than urokinase or tissue plasminogen activator (mainly because it is considerably less expensive), though its antigenicity causes more side-effects. Perhaps for this reason urokinase remains more popular in the USA. It is tending to be replaced by the natural compound and tissue plasminogen activator but the lessons learnt from the use of streptokinase are still applicable because tissue plasminogen activator still works through the conversion of plasminogen to plasmin.

Dose

The blood of the majority of European and American patients has an antistreptokinase titre that can be neutralized by a loading dose of 250 000 units of streptokinase.[5,7,69,70] Most clinicians do not measure the antibody titre before beginning treatment, unless the patient has a history of a recent streptococcal infection or has had a recent course of streptokinase. The loading dose is given intravenously over 30–60 minutes and is followed by a standard maintenance dose of 100 000 units/hour which is continued for 3–5 days. Other dose regimens have been described but their benefits do not appear to be any greater than those of the regimen described above.[57,85,148]

Control

The clinical and haematological effects of streptokinase are monitored in the following ways.

1. Careful clinical observations to detect any sign of haemorrhage (i.e. blood pressure and pulse rate) and microscopic haematuria (i.e. urinalysis by dipstick).
2. Daily or twice daily measurement of the haematocrit.

3. The administration of streptokinase should be stopped if bleeding occurs from wounds, the urinary tract, or the gastrointestinal tract and, if necessary, the effect of streptokinase should be reversed by giving a fibrinolytic inhibitor (e.g. tranexamic acid). Administration of fresh plasma may be given if there is an urgent need to prevent bleeding, but this is not always effective, as the circulating streptokinase may lyse the infused fibrinogen, producing more fibrinogen degradation products which themselves interfere with the coagulation cascade.

4. Measurements of fibrin degradation products, plasma fibrinogen, plasmin, antiplasmin, and the bleeding time do not really assist the clinical control of treatment.

Urokinase

Urokinase is extremely expensive when produced by extraction from human urine. Newer methods of production may reduce the cost but both streptokinase and urokinase are being replaced by genetically engineered tissue plasminogen activator.

Dose

The standard treatment regimen for urokinase is a loading dose of 4000 units/kg given intravenously over 30 minutes followed by 4000 units/kg/h.[49,69,161]

Control

The clinical and haematological effects of urokinase are monitored in the following ways.

1. Careful clinical observations of blood pressure and pulse rate and dipstick urinalysis to detect microscopic haematuria.
2. Twice daily haematocrit estimations may reveal occult haemorrhage.
3. Bleeding is reversed by stopping the administration of urokinase and giving plasma, cryoprecipitates, and fibrinolytic inhibitors.
4. Measurement of plasma fibrinogen, fibrin degradation products, plasmin, antiplasmin and the bleeding time do not really assist the clinical control of treatment.

Streptokinase analogues

Streptokinase analogues consist of a streptokinase–plasminogen complex with a chemical bond across the active site that is released when the complex is warmed within the bloodstream. A number of these substances have been manufactured. They have a thrombolytic effect which is similar to that of streptokinase,[23] but as the effect lasts longer it was hoped that they would reduce the risks of haemorrhage. These analogues can be given by once or twice daily intravenous injections. These drugs have not been shown to be any more effective than streptokinase and the risk of causing bleeding has not been reduced. Research should continue with the aim of developing a safe thrombolytic drug which can be given by a single daily injection.

Tissue plasminogen activator

It was hoped that tissue plasminogen activator would only activate the plasminogen that was bound to fibrin and would not activate the plasminogen which was free in the circulation. If this was the case, thrombolysis would be achieved with fewer bleeding complications.

The tissue plasminogen activator glycoprotein was originally isolated from a cell line of human malignant melanoma cells.[169] It was shown experimentally in animals to have a higher specific thrombolytic activity than urokinase and to produce thrombolysis without systemic fibrinolytic activation. It does not, however, appear to be any more thrombolytically active than streptokinase in humans and still carries considerable risks of haemorrhage.

The structure of tissue plasminogen activator has now been identified by gene probes and the pure compound has been genetically engineered. This has the major advantage that the compound has no species antigen problems and it may be safely given on more than one occasion. Although it remains expensive, lower doses are more effective than similar doses of streptokinase and local delivery directly into the thrombus through a catheter may increase its efficacy.[152] This early report, however, needs confirmation by other studies.

COMPLICATIONS OF THROMBOLYSIS: PREVENTION AND TREATMENT

Haemorrhage

The incidence of haemorrhagic complications varies in different publications. Minor bruising at venepuncture sites and pressure areas (e.g. the elbows and buttocks) are common (i.e. they occur in up to 50% of patients). Serious bleeding occurs in 6–30% of patients.[101]

Fresh wounds, arterial puncture sites and gastrointestinal ulcers are common sites of serious bleeding, and patients with these abnormalities

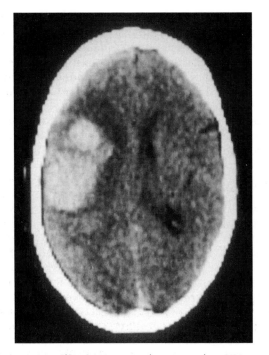

Figure 10.1   The computerized tomography (CT) scan of a patient treated with a streptokinase analogue showing a large intracerebral haemorrhage which caused a massive stroke and death.

should not be treated with thrombolytic drugs. Spontaneous urinary tract, gastrointestinal and, occasionally, intracerebral bleeding can occur (Figure 10.1). This latter devastating complication can occur in 1 or 2% of all those receiving treatment. Elderly, hypertensive patients who have had a previous stroke are particularly at risk.

The treatment of haemorrhage is the same irrespective of the type of thrombolytic drug being used. There are no specific antidotes to the thrombolytic drugs themselves, only measures which reverse their effect.

Local pressure on bleeding wounds and vascular puncture sites is important and usually effective. Surgical intervention to stop bleeding should be delayed until the blood fibrinolytic activity returns to normal.

The systemic treatment of haemorrhage includes:

- Stopping the thrombolytic drug
- Restoring the blood volume with a transfusion
- Restoring the plasma fibrinogen, fresh plasma or cryoprecipitates
- Reversing the fibrinolysis by giving intravenous tranexamic acid, 1 g immediately and then if necessary 8-hourly, until the bleeding stops.

Allergic reactions

These are only a problem with streptokinase; they are the body's response to the injection of a foreign protein.

Fever occurs in about a third of patients receiving streptokinase, and the more serious reactions (e.g. shivering, rigors, itching, urticarial rashes and loin pain) occur in less than 10% of patients.

Treatment should be withdrawn from patients who have rigors, hypotension and loin pain to avoid serious renal damage.

Minor reactions are not an indication to stop treatment, and they can often be prevented by administering antihistamines or hydrocortisone. We give 20 mg chlorpheniramine (Piriton) and 25 mg prednisolone intramuscularly one hour before giving streptokinase to reduce the incidence of fever, itching and urticaria. Additional corticosteroids can be given during treatment if minor reactions continue.

Major reactions should be treated with intravenous hydrocortisone (100 mg), Piriton (50 mg) and, if necessary, subcutaneous adrenaline (0.5 ml, 1 in 1000).

CONTRAINDICATIONS TO THROMBOLYSIS

The principal contraindication to all forms of thrombolytic therapy is the presence of a site of potential bleeding; the common sites are discussed below.

Fresh surgical wounds

Some clinicians have administered thrombolytic therapy within 4 days of surgery but we never give thrombolytic drugs within 7 days of any form of surgical operation. Even more caution should be used after ophthalmic, vascular and neurosurgical operations.

Recent arterial puncture wounds

It is unlikely that a patient with a deep vein thrombosis will have had a recent arteriogram but it must be remembered that arterial puncture wounds are sealed by thrombus and thrombolytic therapy may lyse the sealing plug of thrombus up to 7 days after the puncture.

Liver and kidney biopsies

Lytic therapy is contraindicated for 7–10 days after a liver or kidney biopsy has been taken.

Known gastrointestinal ulceration

A history of peptic ulceration or the presence of an alimentary tract carcinoma are contraindications to thrombolysis because both conditions can bleed spontaneously and heavily, even when they have caused no previous bleeding problems. A gastrointestinal haemorrhage which begins during thrombolytic therapy may be the first indication of gastrointestinal disease. The first line of treatment is to stop the bleeding by reversing the activation of fibrinolysis; surgical treatment should not be attempted until this has been achieved.

Haemorrhagic diatheses (e.g. thrombocytopenia and haemophilia)

These are absolute contraindications to thrombolysis. The effect of any previously administered anti-coagulant should be reversed before giving a thrombolytic drug because the combination of anti-coagulation with plasminogen activation is difficult to control and even more difficult to reverse if bleeding occurs. Heparin should be administered if thrombolysis is being considered because its action can be rapidly reversed by protamine.

Intracardiac thrombus

Thrombolysis softens thrombus before turning it into soluble split products and therefore makes the thrombus more likely to fragment. Emboli from peripheral venous thrombi during thrombolytic therapy are uncommon because these thrombi are not subjected to repeated local trauma, but thrombi in the heart may fragment. A history of a myocardial infarction or the presence of atrial fibrillation should alert the physician to the possibility that thrombolysis could cause an intracardiac thrombus to embolize into the brain or the peripheral vessels. In these patients cardiac thrombus should be excluded by transoesophageal echocardiography before giving thrombolytic drugs.

Hypertension

Elderly, hypertensive patients have a high risk of stroke, and may have already had a minor stroke. Fibrinolytic treatment should be avoided in this group because it may precipitate intracerebral bleeding.

DURATION AND TERMINATION OF TREATMENT

The dissolution of a thrombus by plasmin depends upon the age and accessibility of its contained fibrin.[19] Old fibrin is less susceptible to lysis[27] because of the polymerization and cross-linking between its molecules.

Thrombolysis occurs at the surface of a thrombus and throughout its substance (depending upon the presence of plasminogen trapped within the thrombus). The effect of a thrombolytic agent partly depends upon its ability to penetrate into the thrombus and this in turn depends upon the surface area of thrombus exposed to the bloodstream. The penetration of thrombolysis may now be enhanced by local delivery combined with mechanical damage to the thrombus by a pulse spray technique.[152]

A fresh non-adherent thrombus (i.e. one with young loose-knit fibrin and the majority of its surface exposed to flowing blood) is much more likely to lyse than an old adherent thrombus containing well polymerized fibrin with only 5% of its surface exposed to the blood. It may seem surprising that thrombolytic agents can diffuse into old adherent thrombi, but it must be remembered that thrombi are not inert 'backwaters' of the circulation. Fibrinogen and plasminogen can diffuse into thrombi, even when they are 7 or 10 days old.

The symptoms and signs of deep vein thrombosis give little indication of the true age of the thrombus; the phlebograph provides a crude estimate, but only in terms of weeks not days (see Chapters 4 and 9). It is rarely worth giving thrombolytic drugs when the thrombus is more than 7–10 days old. We attempt to estimate the age of the thrombus from the phlebographic appearance and the history, and only treat patients who have radiologically fresh (less than 7 days old), non-adherent thrombi, or patients who have adherent thrombus but a definite, short clinical history.

The response to thrombolytic therapy is unpredictable. Fresh non-adherent thrombus can be expected to lyse more readily than old non-adherent thrombus but the only way to achieve maximum thrombolysis is to monitor the process closely with *repeated phlebography or duplex scanning*,[29] although the latter does not provide equivalent visual resolution. Repeated phlebography is easier if the thrombolysis is being delivered through a local catheter. When systemic lysis is being given, most clinicians treat their patients for 3 days before performing a check phlebogram and deciding whether to continue treatment. This is a reasonable approach because there is usually little change in the thrombus during the first 24 or 48 hours of treatment. Comerota *et al.*[29] recommend repeat duplex scanning every 12–24 hours to determine response.

Treatment should be continued for another 48 hours if there has been worthwhile but incomplete lysis at 72 hours. When there has been no evidence of thrombus dissolution after 72 hours, but there is haematological evidence of adequate activation of the fibrinolytic system, treatment should be abandoned as it is unlikely to have any further effect on the thrombus. After 5 days the level of antistreptokinase antibodies begins to rise and the patient becomes resistant to treatment with streptokinase.

Treatment can be stopped abruptly because there is no evidence of any rebound phenomenon but the effect of thrombolytic drugs takes at least 4 hours to wear off. Intravenous heparin can be started 4 hours after stopping treatment providing there are no bleeding problems. Heparin, 20 000–40 000 units per 24 hours is given; the dose depends upon the coagulation tests used (usually the accelerated partial thromboplastin time). When there have been bleeding complications, the thrombin clotting time should be measured 4 hours after stopping treatment and, if necessary, repeated every 2 hours. Heparin should not be given until the thrombin clotting time is less than twice the pretreatment control value. It may be 12 hours before the test indicates that it is safe to give heparin.

Anticoagulation after thrombolytic therapy is important because any new thrombi that form contain little plasminogen and are less susceptible to further attempts at thrombolysis.

RESULTS

The results of thrombolysis can be divided into two categories – the lysis of the thrombi and the long-term clinical results. Lysis of the thrombi has been studied in detail over the past 15 years but the long-term clinical results, which are far more important, have still not been fully evaluated by good prospective trials.

Factors affecting the success of thrombolysis

Age of thrombus

After the early studies of streptokinase, between 1965 and 1970, it became apparent that young thrombus was more susceptible to lysis than old thrombus.[19,27,142] All the subsequent studies have confirmed this but also stress the difficulty of determining the age of a thrombus (Figures 10.2–10.4).

Most patients have thrombi of different ages throughout their lower limbs. A patient may develop a calf pain, indicative of a calf vein thrombosis, 3 weeks before their leg swells, a symptom that indicates that the thrombosis has extended into the popliteal or femoral vein. At that moment

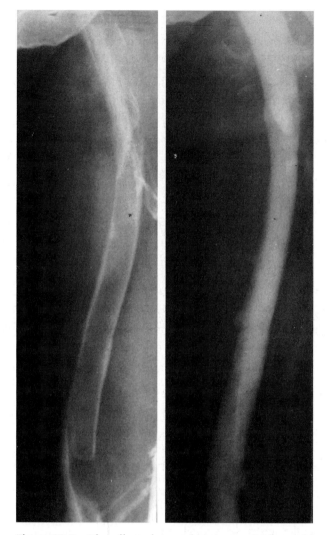

Figure 10.2   The effect of streptokinase on a 24-hour old thrombus. This patient was being screened daily with a Doppler flow detector. Twenty-four hours before the left-hand phlebogram was performed the superficial femoral vein was patent. On the day of the phlebogram the Doppler flow detector indicated that the vein was occluded, and the x-ray revealed fresh non-adherent thrombus. After 48 hours of streptokinase therapy (right-hand panel) the thrombus was completely lysed.

the calf thrombus is 3 weeks old and the propagated thrombus in the thigh is a few days old. Thrombolytic therapy may lyse the young thrombus in the thigh but not the old thrombus in the calf. Nevertheless, it may be better to try treatment than to withhold it, even when the age of the thrombus is in doubt, provided treatment can be given safely.

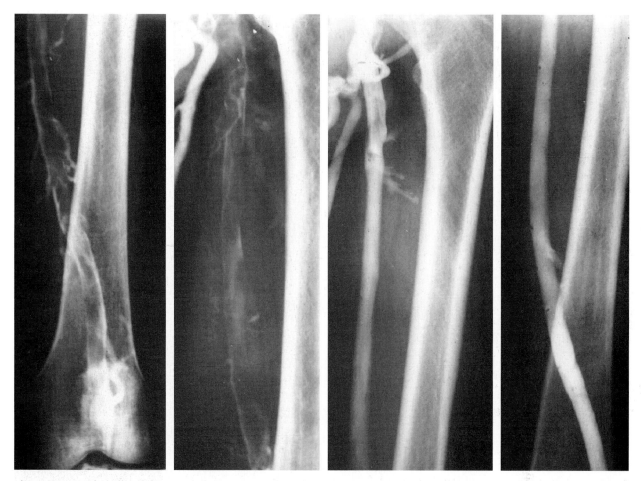

Figure 10.3   The effect of streptokinase on a 3–4-day old thrombus. This patient had experienced swelling of the leg for 3 days before admission to hospital. The phlebograph (left-hand panels) showed a fresh non-adherent thrombus. After 3 days of streptokinase therapy (right-hand panels) the thrombus was completely lysed but no valves were visible in the superficial femoral vein.

Adherence of thrombus

In our early studies[19] we were impressed by the failure of streptokinase to lyse thrombi that were totally adherent to the vein wall and completely occluding the lumen (Figure 10.5). This observation has subsequently been confirmed by some workers and refuted by others[41,62,82,113,114,121,140,160] This lack of agreement has been caused by two problems. First, the quality of the phlebography or duplex scan examination affects the number of times that complete occlusion is correctly diagnosed. A poor phlebogram often shows an unfilled segment of the venous tree which suggests a complete venous occlusion where an investigation of better quality may show a thin streak of contrast medium outlining the thrombus, indicating partial adhesion. This applies equally to duplex scanning (see Chapter 4). Secondly, it is impossible to give a 'phlebographic' or duplex ultrasound age to a thrombus that completely occludes a vein. A completely occluded vein may contain very old thrombus, or a young thrombus that has just blocked the vein. Complete occlusion and apparent radiological adherence should therefore not be a contraindication to treatment if the clinical history is distinct and short. Successful lysis is, however, less likely when there is occlusive thrombosis than when there is a 'free-floating' thrombus, and until we have a precise method for determining the age of thrombus, the published results of thrombolysis will continue to vary, although local intrathrombus delivery may improve lysis when combined with mechanical dissolution (Figure 10.6).

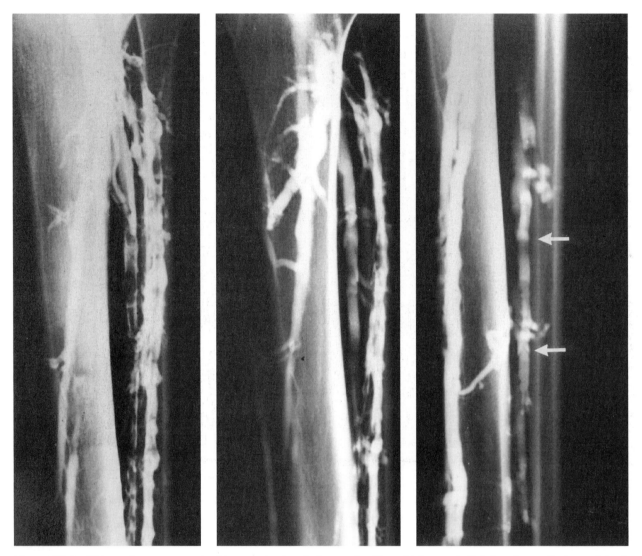

Figure 10.4 This patient presented with an episode of chest pain. The phlebograph (left-hand panel) showed fresh thrombus in the calf. After 3 days of streptokinase therapy most of the calf thrombus had been lysed (centre panel). Eighteen months later the calf veins were patent and the veins that had contained thrombus had normal functioning valves (right-hand panel, arrowed).

Site of thrombosis

Most published studies have reported better thrombolysis of axial than of calf vein thrombosis.[41,172] When all the published results are combined, however, there seems to be little difference between the rate of successful lysis of ilio-femoral thrombi when compared with lysis of thrombus in the superficial femoral vein. Between 60 and 80% of fresh thrombi in the major outflow tract veins can be completely or partially lysed, with preservation of valves in less than a third. A fresh non-adherent thrombus in an axial vein is particularly susceptible to lysis but occasionally this type of

thrombus may detach or fragment and become a pulmonary embolus.

Thrombus in the calf is less susceptible to thrombolytic therapy (Figure 10.7), but neither duplex ultrasound nor phlebography is ideal for assessing calf thrombosis because neither can display every calf vein. Studies with the now abandoned ^{125}I-fibrinogen uptake test demonstrated that radioactivity fell rapidly during the administration of streptokinase[81] but in other instances it rose, indicating that the thrombi extended despite lytic therapy. This observation suggested that local thrombogenic factors occasionally overrode a systemically induced thrombolytic state.

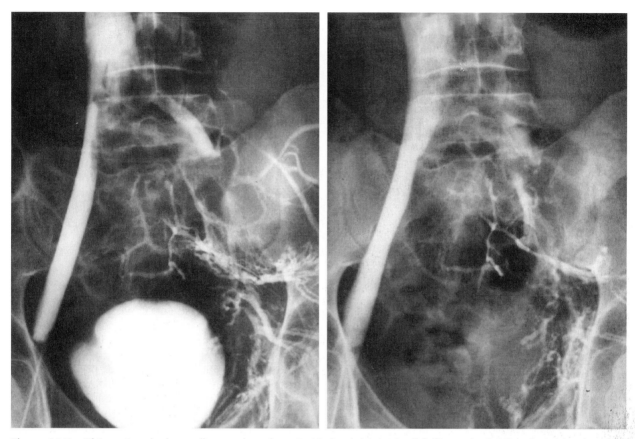

Figure 10.5 This patient had an adherent thrombus, 7–10 days old, in the left iliac vein (left-hand panel). The phlebograph also showed thrombus jutting into the vena cava. After 3 days of streptokinase therapy the vena caval thrombus was lysed but the adherent iliac thrombus was unaltered (right-hand panel). Streptokinase is not effective on ageing adherent thrombus.

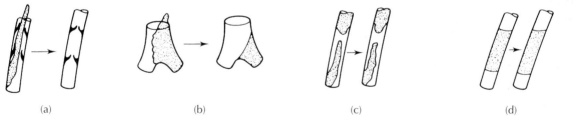

Figure 10.6 The circumstances in which thrombolysis can be expected to be effective. (a) Fresh non-adherent thrombus will lyse. (b) Thrombus jutting into flowing blood will lyse. (c) Non-adherent thrombus below an occlusion may fail to lyse. (d) Adherent thrombus which is more than 3 days old is unlikely to lyse.

The number of segments of the venous tree that contain thrombus does not seem to affect the response in individual segments. The iliac and calf thrombi of a combined ilio-femoral calf thrombosis lyse at the same rate as isolated iliac or calf thrombi.

Prevention of pulmonary embolism

There are few published data on the effect of thrombolysis on recurrent pulmonary embolism. Emboli may occur as the result of thrombolytic therapy but when they reach the lungs they are

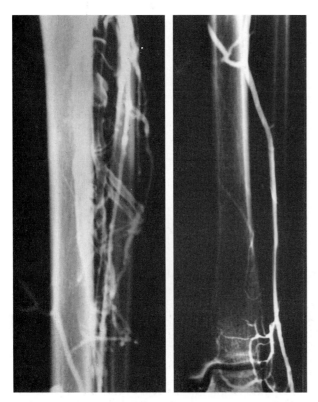

Figure 10.7   An example of the failure of streptokinase to lyse calf thrombi. The left-hand panel shows the calf veins filled with fresh non-adherent thrombus. After 3 days of streptokinase therapy (right-hand panel) all the calf veins were totally occluded (an os calcis intraosseous phlebogram was needed to confirm this). Nevertheless, the patient's pain and swelling had gone, and she was 'clinically' cured. This highlights the inadequacy of physical signs as indicators of the extent of deep vein thrombosis or the success of treatment.

usually lysed by the circulating lytic agent and the lungs' own very efficient natural thrombolytic system. In view of this potential complication, however, thrombolysis cannot be recommended when embolus prevention is the prime objective of treatment.

Long-term value of thrombolysis

The main purpose of giving a thrombolytic drug is to prevent the development of the calf pump failure syndrome. This is only going to be achieved if valve function, as well as vein patency, is restored (Figure 10.4),[19,141] though it is possible that communicating vein valve preservation is more important than axial vein valve preservation (see Chapter 15).

There are few long-term controlled comparisons of the effect of thrombolysis and routine anticoagulation on the post-thrombotic syndrome. Arnesen *et al.*[6] reviewed 35 patients 6 years and 6 months after treatment. Seventeen patients had been treated with streptokinase and 18 had been given heparin.[5] Thirty-four per cent of the group treated with streptokinase and 66% of the group treated with heparin had post-thrombotic symptoms and signs. Three patients in the group treated with heparin developed venous ulcers.

Elliot *et al.*[45] followed 51 patients for a mean of 18 months and they found 32% of the group treated with streptokinase had post-thrombotic symptoms compared with 76% of the group treated with heparin.

By contrast, Kakkar and Lawrence studied a much larger group (153 patients) for 2 years using clinical and physiological (foot volumetry) assessment; they found no difference in the late results between streptokinase and heparin treatment.[84]

It is difficult to compare these three studies. Almost all the patients in the first two studies had axial vein thrombosis, whereas the third study included patients with calf and popliteal vein thrombosis from a number of different trials. It seems logical that the removal of a large thrombus (destined to cause serious obstruction) from an axial vein should reduce the incidence of post-thrombotic sequelae,[123] whereas the partial removal of an extensive thrombosis from the calf is unlikely to restore calf pump function to normal. Ultimately, the risk of developing the post-thrombotic syndrome depends upon the relative long-term significance of axial vein obstruction and incompetence and communicating vein incompetence. Failure to relieve obstruction might cause early symptoms but these may regress as collateral veins develop. The extent of this collateral development, which may vary considerably in different individuals, may well also have a considerable impact on the eventual outcome. Communicating vein incompetence takes much longer to appear and, as most patients with deep vein thrombosis have some degree of calf vein thrombosis, the short-term improvements derived from the lysis of axial vein thrombus may disappear in the long term as the problems related to the calf vein damage develop. The majority of the long-term haemodynamic studies following thrombolysis report an incidence of moderate or severe dysfunction in half the patients, only a quarter having returned to normal. *These results suggest that thrombolysis has not yet significantly reduced the incidence of the post-thrombotic syndrome.*[2,25,30,79,83,122,148,170] There are no recent studies which have provided a more optimistic picture.

INDICATIONS FOR THROMBOLYSIS

It is customary to state the indications for a treatment before describing either the technique or the results. The proceeding paragraphs reveal that there is considerable doubt about the clinical value of thrombolysis. Furthermore, new dose regimens and substances are continually being introduced. When the results of a treatment are uncertain, the indications are also in doubt.

Our opinions on the present status and expectations of thrombolytic therapy, based on the conflicting evidence presented above, are given below (see also Figure 10.6).

Main axial vein thrombosis, which is either adherent or non-adherent, less than 7 days old, in the absence of contraindications

This should be treated with a thrombolytic drug which should be locally delivered through a catheter placed directly in the thrombus and regularly advanced on the basis of repeated phlebographic assessments.[152] The clinical significance of the contraindications increases with the age and adherence of the thrombus because these factors reduce the chance of successful lysis. For example, we rarely attempt thrombolysis of an adherent 7-day-old femoral vein thrombosis in a patient with only moderate symptoms, 14 days after an operation. By contrast, we consider that thrombolysis is the treatment of choice for a young patient who has not had an operation with a fresh, non-adherent, ilio-femoral thrombosis, or a similar but symptomless thrombus discovered on duplex ultrasound screening after a small pulmonary embolism. We make one exception to this approach. When the phlebogram suggests that the risk of another major pulmonary embolism is very high, we prefer to prevent further embolism as quickly as possible by removing the thrombus surgically (thrombectomy) or locking it into the limb (vena caval filter insertion) rather than rely on thrombolysis.

We expect the lysis of axial vein thrombi to relieve the obstruction to blood flow and perhaps save femoral vein valves and, if there is little or no calf vein thrombus, reduce the late sequelae (although we have no evidence that this is the case).

Combined axial and calf vein thrombosis, adherent or nor-adherent, less than 7 days old, in the absence of contraindications

We treat this in a similar manner but have less expectation (almost none) of preventing late sequelae. We consider that limb-threatening phlegmasia cerulea dolens should still be treated urgently by thrombectomy,[128] although high rates of rethrombosis have been reported after thrombectomy for this condition[88] and poor long-term results are common, with many limbs still remaining swollen and painful.[137] Thrombolysis is therefore a more attractive option in these patients if the limb is not immediately threatened,[46] especially if it is delivered directly into the thrombus[143] or into the femoral artery of the affected limb.[174]

Isolated calf vein thrombi

These thrombi should not be treated with thrombolytic drugs. They are not a threat to life or limb, whereas thrombolytic drugs can kill. There is a considerable chance that calf thrombi will lyse spontaneously, and there is no evidence that their lysis reduces the incidence of post-thrombotic sequelae. There is, however, good evidence that these thrombi should be treated with anticoagulants as they can extend[104] and can be the source of pulmonary emboli.[91]

The newer techniques for administering lytic therapy directly into the thrombus, e.g. via a catheter passed via the internal jugular or the popliteal vein (ultrasound guided), have rekindled interest in thrombolysis. Some have even advocated intra-arterial delivery (femoral artery) of the lytic agents. Endovascular technology with stents and clot-breaking devices are also developing and these ideas are encouraging a new assessment of concomitant thrombolysis. New studies must be carefully controlled and patients must be followed up for many years before justifiable claims can be made. It must be remembered that all invasive techniques have a down side and one death from an iatrogenic pulmonary embolus or intracerebral haemorrhage during thrombolysis may quickly dampen a clinician's enthusiasm. There is already some evidence that local delivery has no benefit over systemic therapy in achieving successful recanalization.[151]

Thrombectomy

The surgical removal of deep vein thrombi, mainly from the large axial veins, was first practised in the 1920s but was not widely adopted until phlebography improved in the 1940s and 1950s[40,54,66,71,100,105,107] and Fogarty introduced the balloon catheter in 1963.[51–53]

Technically and radiologically, controlled thrombectomy has therefore been practised for as long as thrombolysis, and a similar amount of information is available about its early and late results. Much of this information is anecdotal and almost none of it has been scientifically controlled or prospectively planned. Thrombectomy is used by individual surgeons, in the light of their own interpretation of the significance of the published results, and the indications for its use will therefore be discussed after a description of the technique and a summary of the published results.

Preoperative preparation

Patients with a deep vein thrombosis should be given the *anticoagulant* heparin if a firm clinical diagnosis has been made. The administration of heparin can always be stopped. If subsequent investigations show that the clinical diagnosis is wrong, its effect will wear off in 4 hours and no harm will have been done. Failure to give anticoagulants once the clinical diagnosis has been made may allow extension of the thrombus while the patient is awaiting special investigations. A standard loading dose of 5000–10 000 units of heparin followed by a continuous infusion that will provide 20 000–40 000 units/24 hours is sufficient.

Initial assessment by duplex scanning should be followed by complete *bilateral* phlebography to display fully the lower and upper limits of the thrombus, and the intervening partially occluded veins, and the state of the collateral veins before a thrombectomy can be considered. The decision to perform a thrombectomy is based upon the nature and extent of the thrombus seen on the phlebograph and the severity of the clinical symptoms and signs. At present this cannot be made on the basis of a duplex scan although magnetic resonance venography may give adequate information in the near future.

Ascending phlebography usually provides all the information required but it may have to be supplemented with percutaneous femoral vein injections to display the upper limits of the thrombus. A lung scan or pulmonary angiogram may be required to confirm the diagnosis of pulmonary embolism and determine the extent of the pulmonary artery obstruction (see Chapter 21). The bladder should be catheterized so that it does not obscure the intra-operative phlebographs when it fills with radio-opaque urine. As venous thrombectomy is often accompanied by a significant blood loss, 4 units (2 litres) of blood should be cross-matched.

Anaesthesia

General inhalation anaesthesia with muscle relaxation, endotracheal intubation, and positive pressure ventilation is preferable. This ensures a positive pressure gradient between the thorax and the groin so that blood flows down the vena cava and iliac veins and out of the femoral venotomy – once the venotomy has been made – thus preventing any loose thrombi moving centrally into the lungs. Controlled positive pressure ventilation plus a steep foot-down position (reversed Trendelenburg) produces a sustained pressure in the inferior vena cava of 20–30 mmHg and ensures retrograde flow.

Some surgeons prefer to carry out the operation under local, spinal or epidural anaesthesia so that the patient can perform a Valsalva manoeuvre during the passage of the thrombectomy catheter but if the operation takes a long time, such patients may find it difficult to cooperate.

The manoeuvres undertaken to ensure retrograde blood flow in the vena cava are extremely important because they prevent intraoperative pulmonary embolism and obviate the need for vena caval balloon blockade.[44]

Operating room preparation

The patient is placed supine on a radiographic operating table. The table is tipped 30° head-up and the patient's legs are abducted to 30°.

The skin of the whole chest, abdomen and both legs is painted with antiseptic. Towels are placed to cover the upper chest, the head and arms, the genitalia and the feet. The abdomen must be prepared in case it is necessary to explore the iliac veins or the vena cava, and the chest is prepared in case an emergency pulmonary embolectomy is necessary.

Good intravenous access should be available, and the central venous pressure should be monitored. The anaesthetist should insert an intra-arterial pressure line and place a Swan–Ganz catheter in the pulmonary artery to monitor pulmonary capillary wedge pressure if the patient has had a pulmonary embolism or has evidence of right-sided cardiac embarrassment.

Thrombectomy for ilio-femoral thrombosis[21,22,84]

The common femoral vein below the groin provides access to both the iliac and the superficial femoral veins. An incision is made in the skin of the thigh along the line of the vein, from the inguinal ligament downwards for about 6 inches (15 cm). Subcutaneous oedema may make identification and dissection of the veins difficult. The common femoral vein and its main tributaries (the superficial and deep femoral veins) must be exposed and snared. Minor tributaries should be ligated. The patient should already have been given heparin but, if this has been omitted, 5000 units heparin are administered before any clamps are applied or a venotomy made.

It is essential to handle the veins with great care. They should never be compressed with clamps which could break the thrombus and cause an embolus.

The venotomy should be made before placing clamps on any of the vessels. If the veins are found not to contain thrombus they may then be occluded with soft cushioned clamps of the Fogarty type.

The venotomy must be large enough to allow access to the iliac and superficial femoral vein and the mouths of the deep femoral veins. It should be confined to the common femoral vein and not extended down into the superficial femoral vein where the blood flow is less and the risk of postoperative thrombosis is more likely. Thrombus in the common femoral vein immediately bulges through the venotomy under the influence of the hydrostatic pressure and *the additional positive pressure that the anaesthetist must apply as the venotomy is made.* A non-adherent 'floating' thrombus in the iliac veins may be completely extruded by the positive pressure alone. There is always some bleeding but this can usually be controlled by gentle manipulation of the snares, taking care not to break the thrombus.

A balloon catheter which has a diameter large enough to obstruct the vena cava is then inserted into the venotomy, passed up into the vena cava, inflated and withdrawn until it jams against the end of the common iliac vein to prevent any thrombus in the iliac vein becoming dislodged as an embolus. This technique has replaced prior insertion of a caval blocking balloon through a tributary of the long saphenous vein in the opposite groin. Some surgeons rely solely on the positive pressure ventilation and head-up tilt and use no form of proximal blockade. The only way of ensuring that the balloon catheter is in the vena cava is by watching its passage with an x-ray image intensifier having filled the balloon with a radioopaque contrast medium instead of saline. A catheter can pass to its full extent but be in the ascending lumbar vein, rather than the vena cava. A plain radiograph may be taken if an image intensifier is not available. This confirms the position of the catheter in relation to the spine and gives some indication of the likelihood of misdirection.

A second balloon catheter is then passed up the iliac vein until it reaches the first balloon, before being inflated and withdrawn; the pressure in the second balloon is carefully controlled by light pressure on the barrel of the syringe to provide a gentle resistance between the balloon and the vein wall during the removal of the balloon. Overenthusiastic inflation of the balloon can rupture the vein. The procedure is repeated until no further thrombus is obtained. The blockading balloon is then slowly deflated until it can be withdrawn, bringing with it any small loose pieces of thrombus that have been trapped below it.

The iliac segment is then flushed with heparinized saline and an *operative phlebogram* is performed to display the iliac vein and vena cava (Figure 10.8). The ballooning is repeated if this investigation demonstrates residual mural thrombosis or if the upper end of the iliac vein is still occluded.

The presence of good back-bleeding from the external iliac vein does not mean that the whole iliac system is patent, because the blood can come from the internal iliac vein. Without radiographic control it is not possible to be certain that the veins are clear of thrombus.[109,116]

If the balloon will not pass into the inferior vena cava or the terminal portion of the common iliac vein cannot be opened, a decision must be made about whether to explore the iliocaval segment through a transperitoneal or retroperitoneal abdominal incision. Exploration of the termination of the common iliac vein in the presence of acute thrombosis is unfruitful unless there is a small spur (see Chapter 13) which can be divided. Dissection and exposure of the vessels and the liberation of any venous compression by the right common iliac artery is theoretically attractive but rarely helps when there is extensive oedema and inflammation in the vein wall. Occasionally, a retroperitoneal exposure of the iliac vein makes it possible to guide the catheter into the cava in those patients where the catheter persists in entering the ascending lumbar vein. Forcible blind passage of a catheter is extremely dangerous because balloon catheters can pierce the vein wall.[112] Insertion of a metallic stent is now an alternative method of holding the vessel open.[77]

Thrombi are subsequently removed from the distal veins of the leg by elevation, gentle compression with an Esmarch bandage applied from the toes upwards, and the retrograde passage of a balloon catheter. The last option can be difficult because the catheter often impacts in a valve cusp. Partial inflation of the balloon just above a valve sometimes centralizes the tip of the catheter and helps it to pass between the cusps but catheters rarely pass beyond the popliteal vein. The venotomy is closed with a fine monofilament suture.

Thrombus which cannot be removed by these manoeuvres can be attacked in two further ways. Some surgeons expose the upper part of the popliteal vein through an incision on the medial

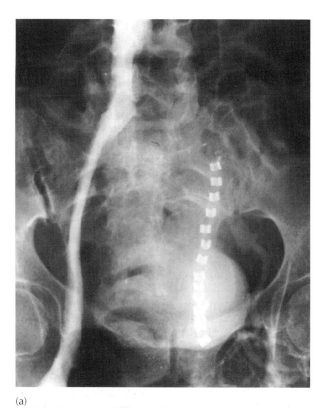

(a)

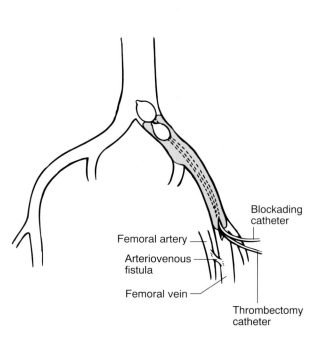

(b)

Blockading catheter

Femoral artery

Arteriovenous fistula

Femoral vein

Thrombectomy catheter

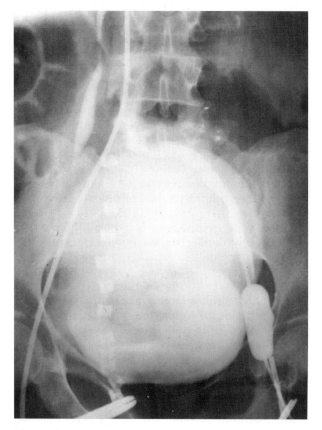

(c)

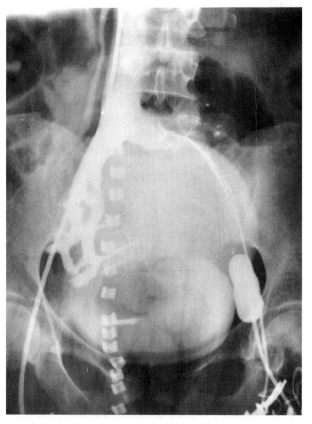

(d)

aspect of the lower thigh and make another venotomy for the passage of a balloon catheter in both directions. A few surgeons attempt a more vigorous removal of thrombus from the distal veins with long forceps which are similar to Desjardin's gallstone forceps.

An alternative approach is to pass a guide wire from the posterior tibial vein at the ankle up to the groin with the open end of a balloon catheter attached to the guide wire. This end of the catheter is then pulled up to the groin in an orthograde direction. The balloon is inflated as it enters the vein at the ankle. A special modification to the open end of the catheter is required for this technique.[90]

Although these ingenious techniques sound attractive, no evidence has been published to show that they improve either the immediate or the long-term results.

Full anticoagulation, compression stockings, passive and active exercises in bed and early activity out of bed encourage venous blood flow and help to reduce the chances of a postoperative thrombosis.

Adjuvant arteriovenous fistulae

There is good experimental evidence which proves that the addition of an arteriovenous fistula below a venous anastomosis improves its chance of staying patent.[44,65] It may also increase the size of the collateral vessels if the thrombectomy is only partially

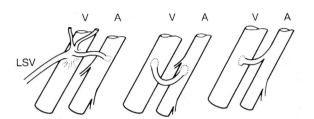

Figure 10.9 Three simple methods of fashioning an arteriovenous fistula to enhance blood flow after a thrombectomy. (a) A tributary of the long saphenous vein (LSV) anastomosed to the artery (A). (b) A segment of superficial vein (a tributary of the long saphenous vein not the main trunk) sewn between the common femoral artery (A) and the vein (V). (c) A branch of the femoral artery anastomosed to the vein (V).

successful. When non-adherent thrombus can be extracted from the iliac vein with ease, the vein wall is probably not inflamed and there is no need to form an arteriovenous fistula. The blood flow from the limb combined with anticoagulation should ensure that the vein remains patent. Conversely, an arteriovenous fistula is probably helpful if the vein wall is inflamed, the lumen narrowed, or thrombus has been left on the vein wall. This situation is encountered after an attempt has been made to remove an adherent thrombus when the chance of rethrombosis is high.

The simplest method of making an arteriovenous fistula is to sew a tributary of the long saphenous vein end-to-side to the femoral artery (Figure 10.9). A loop of ligature material should be left lying loosely around the fistula to help identify it when the decision to ligate it is taken 2–3 months later.

An alternative technique is to divide a branch of the superficial femoral artery in the thigh and sew it end-to-side to the superficial femoral vein. This type of fistula is harder to find and to close and does not usually provide such a high blood flow. Fistulae can now be closed by covering their origin with a covered stent or blocking them with a metal coil.

Postoperative phlebography

It is important to assess the results of all deep vein operations by confirming vein patency with phlebography. Clinical improvement does not mean that the vein is patent (Figure 10.10). The symptoms of most legs with extensive axial vein thrombosis improve spontaneously without any form of treatment as collateral vessels enlarge and the thrombus retracts. Although the object of thrombectomy is the relief of symptoms, objective evidence must be obtained when claiming that any

Figure 10.8 Ilio-femoral thrombectomy. (Operative phlebography is an essential part of thrombectomy.) (a) The preoperative phlebograph of a patient with a complete left iliac vein thrombosis following a hysterectomy. (b) A diagrammatic representation of the positioning of the occluding and thrombectomy balloon catheters. (c) The thrombectomy has been completed and radio-opaque contrast is being injected into the iliac vein above a balloon catheter which is occluding the common femoral vein. The vena cava is still occluded with a balloon catheter passed via a tributary of the right long saphenous vein. The thrombectomized segment is smooth and patent. There is no residual thrombus. (d) A second film showing contrast medium in the vena cava confirming the patency of the right iliac vein and vena cava and the clearance of that part of the thrombus that can be seen in (a) spreading up the side wall of the vena cava, from the left iliac vein.

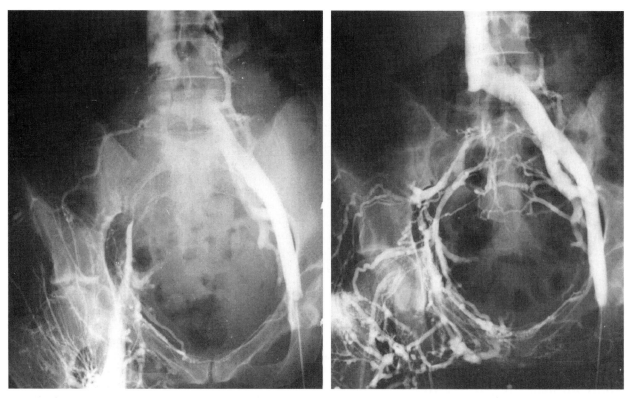

Figure 10.10 An example of the failure of thrombectomy. The left-hand panel shows an extensive but localized right iliac vein thrombosis with thrombus in the vena cava. A thrombectomy was performed and the operative phlebograph showed complete clearance of thrombus. Heparin was given to the patient postoperatively. Five days later the patient's leg was not painful and the swelling had subsided, this was considered a 'clinical' success but the phlebograph (right-hand panel) showed a total rethrombosis. This case (and Figure 10.7) emphasizes the inadequacy of using physical signs for the assessment of the results of treatment.

improvement is the direct result of the operation and not simply the result of the natural changes in the thrombus and the collateral vessels.

COMPLICATIONS

Haemorrhage

The main intraoperative complication is blood loss during the passages of the balloon catheter. Rapid loss of blood and a reduction of venous return may precipitate a cardiac arrest if the patient is hypotensive or on the edge of cardiac failure as a result of previous pulmonary embolism.

Pulmonary embolism

Pulmonary embolism is uncommon if positive pressure ventilation and head-up tilting are used during the passage of the balloon. Postoperative pulmonary

embolism from residual axial vein mural thrombus or calf vein thrombus occurs in 20% of patients if anticoagulants are not given.[84,133,173] Anticoagulants must be given postoperatively and, though thrombectomy is an alternative to thrombolysis when the risk of haemorrhage is high, it should not be considered as an alternative to the administration of anticoagulants, except in the most exceptional circumstances.

Rethrombosis

Rethrombosis is the most common postoperative complication. It may occur silently and can only be detected by follow-up phlebography, or it may be associated with the return of physical signs. Recurrent thrombus is invariably firmly adherent to the vein wall and a repeat thrombectomy is not worthwhile unless the new thrombosis has occurred within 24 hours of the first operation and the repeat operation can be done immediately. Unfortunately, the reappearance of physical signs indicating a rethrombosis tends to occur only when the vein has totally occluded, even though mural thrombus has been building up from the moment of the operation. Such thrombus is fixed firmly to the vein wall and is difficult to remove. The best way to avoid recurrent thrombosis is to avoid operating on adherent thrombus.

Rethrombosis is common when the precipitating cause is disseminated malignant disease, or one of the other hypercoagulable states (see Chapter 8). It is prudent to avoid thrombectomy in these circumstances.

RESULTS

There are three objectives of thrombectomy:

- Prevention of pulmonary embolism
- Relief of symptoms in the leg
- Reduction of the incidence of late post-thrombotic sequelae.

Prevention of embolism

It is assumed that the removal of a large floating thrombus reduces the risk of pulmonary embolism though there have been no controlled trials to test this hypothesis. Pulmonary emboli do occur after thrombectomy but in the many large series few cases of fatal emboli occurred either during or after the operation.

Mavor analysed the incidence of pulmonary embolism (based upon a clinical diagnosis) after thrombectomy in a large series of 260 patients,[115] 127 of whom had had an embolus before operation. Thirty (25%) had postoperative emboli, seven of which (6%) were fatal. One hundred and thirty-three patients had no clinical evidence of embolism before operation but six (5%) of these had postoperative emboli, one (1%) of which was fatal.

In this study only half the thrombectomies were performed with radiological control. When the incidence of embolism was analysed according to the degree of clearance of the thrombus from the peripheral veins (in those patients who had intraoperative phlebography), fatal emboli occurred only when there was incomplete clearance or a failed operation.

These rates of postoperative embolism seem to be high but many of the patients were elderly and 20% had concurrent serious medical illness or malignant disease. Other series have reported a lower incidence of postoperative embolism. Mansfield[108] recorded no fatal emboli and five non-fatal emboli after thrombectomy in 62 patients.

Eklof studied the incidence of emboli after thrombectomy by performing repeat lung scans. Fifty-six per cent of the 63 patients in a controlled prospective trial had perfusion defects before operation. One week later, 23% of those patients who had been treated surgically had additional defects compared with 15% in the group who had been treated conservatively.[44]

All these studies confirm that thrombectomy does not provide complete protection against subsequent pulmonary embolism. Consequently, it is probably safer to combine thrombectomy with, or replace it by, the insertion of a caval filter (see later and Chapter 22) if the intraoperative phlebogram shows residual thrombus or when another embolus might be expected to be fatal. Using a similar approach some years ago we were able to show in a retrospective case-controlled study that we could reduce the incidence of 14% fatal and 26% non-fatal recurrent emboli to 0% fatal and 12% non-fatal emboli.[18] This was, however, not just a comparison of thrombectomy with and without venous blockade but included patients who were given anticoagulants alone if the phlebogram showed no loose thrombus. Van de Berg[163] examined the incidence of preoperative and postoperative embolism associated with four forms of treatment (Figure 10.11). Two of the 23 patients who had a thrombectomy alone had fatal postoperative emboli, whereas only two of 56 patients who had a thrombectomy and vena caval interruption had a non-fatal embolus. In this study the results

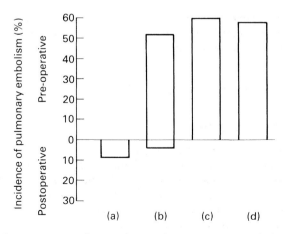

Figure 10.11 The incidence of postoperative embolism after three types of treatment (after Van de Berg[163]). (a) After thrombectomy (23 patients). (b) After thrombectomy plus vena cava filter or clip (56 patients). (c) After thrombectomy plus vena cava clip plus arteriovenous fistula (15 patients). (d) After vena cava clip alone (31 patients).

were weighted against the second (caval interruption) group as 29 of these patients had had preoperative emboli whereas none of the first group had had previous emboli.

The results of these studies have been presented in detail to emphasize the paucity of good controlled evidence about thrombectomy and embolism and this remains true since the first edition of this book. The results appear to support what would seem obvious, namely that if fresh non-adherent thrombus is completely removed and the patient is given anticoagulants, fatal embolism is eliminated and minor embolism rarely occurs. When the operation fails or is only partially successful (leaving either non-adherent thrombus in the calf or mural adherent thrombus in the axial veins), recurrent embolism is not only common but more common than when patients are given anticoagulants alone.

Except when it is thought to be the only way to save the life of the limb, thrombectomy should only be performed when the phlebogram indicates that all the thrombus can be removed. When the thrombus cannot be completely removed, a caval filter procedure should be added or thrombectomy should be avoided.

Relief of symptoms

The massive swelling that may accompany an ilio-femoral thrombosis often disappears as soon as axial vein patency is restored. Pain and immobility are also relieved and the patient notices the improvement on waking from the anaesthetic. Areas of blue discoloration, which if left untreated may become patches of venous gangrene, often improve in colour and become less painful.[55,63,67,94,106] This relief persists if the vein does not rethrombose.

Phlebographic clearance, axial vein patency

It must be stressed again that the relief of symptoms must not be interpreted as an indicator of axial vein patency because symptoms are also relieved by the development of collaterals. The only way to confirm patency is by phlebography. Our interpretation of the many published studies is that approximately 60% of iliac veins can be expected to stay permanently patent after thrombectomy of the ilio-femoral segment. The success rate is probably 40% and 80%, respectively, if the patients are divided into those with adherent and those with non-adherent thrombus. In Mavor's series of 75 operations in which he used radiological control,[115,116] 27% had either a partial or a complete rethrombosis at 14

days. Five years after operation, 66% of his smaller series, treated without radiological screening, had evidence of rethrombosis. The state of the vein 14 days after operation is not necessarily its final condition.

Mansfield found that 76% of the veins that had a thrombectomy appeared 'normal' by 6 months.[108] Andriopoulos *et al.*[4] had a 60% patency rate when the operation was performed for floating thrombus or phlegmasia cerulea dolens, and Brunner and Wirth[20] reported that 69% of their patients had a complete or partial clearance at 2 years. Ecklof studied 70 patients who had a temporary arteriovenous fistula added to the thrombectomy for 6 months.[44] He found that 38% of iliac veins were normal, 23% had post-thrombotic stenosis and 39% were occluded. In a second study[133] in which 31 patients who had been treated surgically were compared with 32 who had been given anticoagulants, 76% of the surgical group had normal iliac veins at 6 months compared with 35% of the controls. This last observation is very important because iliac veins often recanalize spontaneously and do not have valves. Nevertheless, the difference between the two forms of treatment is highly significant ($P = 0.005$). Unfortunately, none of the published studies has described or analysed the results according to the nature of the thrombus and its exact distribution, few studies have a control series for comparison, and the results differ widely between studies.[37,78,92]

It appears that thrombectomy has a 60% chance of restoring ilio-femoral vein patency – sometimes to normal, sometimes with some degree of stenosis. Whether this benefits the patient with respect to the relief of swelling and the development of late post-thrombotic sequelae is not clear. As the ilio-femoral segment has few valves, its main function is that of a conduit; maintaining its patency should therefore be beneficial.

None of the publications quoted report much about superficial femoral vein patency or valve competency. It is therefore impossible to decide whether or not thrombectomy of the superficial femoral vein is worthwhile; in our view it depends upon the presence of popliteal vein thrombosis. It is probably worth removing discontinuous superficial femoral vein thrombus above a normal popliteal vein but a femoral vein thrombus that is continuous, through the popliteal vein, with calf vein thrombus, is almost impossible to remove, and we doubt if thrombectomy is then going to be clinically beneficial, except in the rare circumstance when all the thrombus is fresh and non-adherent and can be extruded easily through the venotomy, without the need for a balloon catheter.

Calf pump failure syndrome

The evidence that thrombectomy affects subsequent calf pump failure is extremely poor and mostly anecdotal. Mavor[115] found a relationship between the state of the ilio-femoral segment and symptoms 6 years after operation. Only two of his 13 patients with normal iliac veins had symptoms, whereas seven of the nine patients who had recanalized veins, and 13 of the 14 patients with collaterals across the floor of the pelvis had symptoms. The incidence of leg symptoms was lower in the group in which the operation was carried out under radiological control. Overall, 34 (58%) of Mavor's 59 patients who were studied clinically and venographically between 3 and 6 years after operation had some problem with their legs.

We suspect that these results are not significantly different from the natural history of venous thrombus resolution, and this view is supported by the results of non-invasive testing of calf pump function in Ecklof's study. Only 23% of Ecklof's first series of patients[44] had normal calf pump function 6 months after operation; 60% had poor ejection, 17% had reflux, and only 7.5% had a normal venous outflow when measured with a strain-gauge plethysmography. In Ecklof's second controlled study,[44,131,132] there were no statistically significant differences in the calf function tests between the group treated with thrombectomy and the group given only anticoagulants, though the phlebographic patency and the absence of ilio-femoral vein obstruction correlated well with femoral vein pressure. Unfortunately, patency was usually associated with reflux. At 6 months all symptoms occurred less frequently in the surgical group, and the difference between the percentage of patients in the control and the percentage of patients in the thrombectomy group that were 'symptom free' (7% vs 42%) was significant; this was also true for ilio-femoral patency (36% vs 76%) and the presence of competent valves (26% vs 52%). Once again the anatomical appearances and the physiological tests failed to correlate. When these patients were reviewed after 5 years, 37% of the operated patients were free of symptoms compared with 18% of those treated conservatively, and their foot vein pressures were significantly better. The clinical improvement did not, however, reach statistical significance.[131]

INDICATIONS FOR OPERATION

The indications for thrombectomy are presented at the end of this section, as for thrombolysis, because they depend upon the reader's interpretation of the significance of the results described above.

It is self-evident that the only circumstance in which thrombectomy can prevent embolism and abolish the incidence of late sequelae is when all the thrombus is removed. This can only be achieved when the thrombus is fresh, non-adherent (floating) and limited in extent (i.e. with a clear-cut top and bottom in a large axial vein) (Figures 10.12, 10.13). In these circumstances the balloon catheter can be passed beyond either end of the thrombus and the whole thrombus can be extracted. Thrombus which is adherent cannot be completely removed, and thrombectomy in these circumstances is associated with a significant incidence of minor embolism. This risk would be acceptable if the reopening of the axial vein was definitely going to be permanent and beneficial to calf pump function. A proportion of the veins that are successfully opened by thrombectomy, perhaps as many as half, stenose or even occlude during the subsequent 2 years in spite of a course of anticoagulants, and there is little evidence that normal calf pump function can be restored in any patient who has extensive calf vein thrombosis.

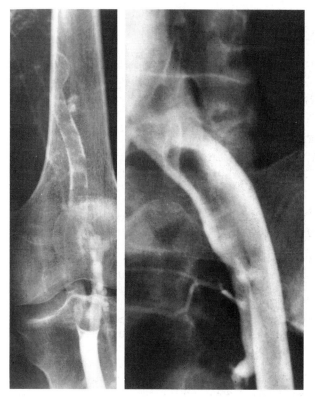

Figure 10.12 A fresh non-adherent thrombus with clearly defined proximal and distal limits. Thrombectomy is the most suitable method of treatment for this type of thrombus.

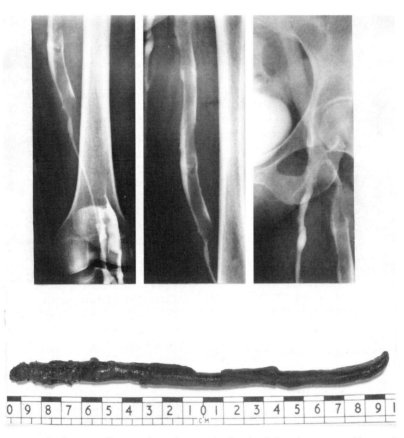

Figure 10.13 A fresh non-adherent thrombus with clearly defined upper and lower limits that was completely removed with one passage of a balloon catheter. The patient had had two pulmonary emboli in spite of adequate anticoagulation with heparin, and the thrombus shown was removed from the clinically normal leg.

We therefore believe that there is little justification for performing a thrombectomy on an occluded superficial femoral vein. We would only advise surgery on the ilio-femoral segment when the thrombus is localized to this segment, the clinical history suggests that the thrombus is less than 5 days old, and the clinical signs confirm a significant functional obstruction. In these circumstances we would prefer to use a thrombolytic drug but would operate if these drugs are contraindicated.

Our attitude to surgical thrombectomy for ilio-femoral thrombosis can be summarized as follows (Figure 10.14).

- Thrombectomy is only indicated when thrombolysis is contraindicated.
- Thrombectomy should be used to remove non-adherent thrombus localized to the ilio-femoral or superficial femoral vein, young (less than 3 days old) adherent thrombus localized to the

ilio-femoral segment (the iliac and common femoral vein), and recent thrombus in an axial vein threatening the viability of the limb (severe phlegmasia cerulea dolens).
- There is no evidence that the partial removal of floating or adherent superficial femoral vein thrombus which is continuous with calf vein thrombus reduces the late sequelae, and there is considerable evidence that the risk of pulmonary embolism is increased if the thrombus is not completely removed. Under these circumstances the placement of an inferior vena caval filter must be considered.
- All patients must be given adequate anticoagulants for 6 months after the operation.
- An arteriovenous fistula improves patency after thrombectomy but probably only in patients with adherent thrombus. We would fashion an arteriovenous fistula after removing an adherent limited ilio-femoral thrombus, but not if we have removed a floating non-adherent thrombus.

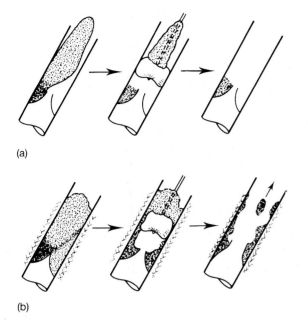

(a)

(b)

Figure 10.14 The type of thrombus which is removable by surgical thrombectomy. (a) Fresh non-adherent thrombus with clearly defined proximal and distal limits can be completely removed. (b) Adherent thrombus cannot be completely removed, and the residual mural thrombus gives rise to recurrent pulmonary emboli and causes rethrombosis.

THROMBECTOMY FOR PHLEGMASIA CERULEA DOLENS

A total obstruction of the venous outflow from a limb causes ischaemia of the distal tissues. Even when the majority of the limb veins are blocked, the blood usually finds some small vessels to act as collaterals and the limb survives. The worse the obstruction, however, the greater the swelling and discoloration and the greater the chance of tissue necrosis.

Phlegmasia cerulea dolens is a swollen, blue painful limb caused by venous obstruction. Its clinical features are described in Chapter 9.

The skin may blister and become gangrenous (venous gangrene). Treatment in these circumstances is aimed at saving the limb, the risks of minor embolism and late post-thrombotic sequelae become secondary considerations.

- The initial treatment should be full anticoagulation with heparin to try to stop extension of the thrombosis.
- Swelling should be reduced by steep elevation of the leg.

- Analgesics are invariably required to alleviate the associated pain.
- Phlebography is essential to define the limits of the thrombosis. It is likely that the deep femoral veins and the internal iliac veins will have become occluded as well as the axial veins.
- A general examination is essential to determine a hidden cause of the thrombosis, especially malignant disease, because this may influence the management decisions.
- If the skin is ischaemic, blistering, and likely to die, an urgent attempt must be made to relieve the outflow tract obstruction. This can only be done surgically. Fibrinolysis has been used but in our experience it may take too long to work and sometimes causes interstitial bleeding from the congested veins within the limb. Recently both the local delivery of the thrombolytic agent by the 'pulse-spray' technique[167] and intra-arterial administration of lytic agents have been described,[174] but the speed of thrombus dissolution may still be too slow to avoid tissue loss.[128]
- A thrombectomy of the ilio-femoral segment and the superficial and deep femoral veins should be performed to restore some venous drainage from the limb.
- If thrombectomy fails, some surgeons have tried an emergency vein bypass operation to the other limb or the vena cava. These operations are, however, unlikely to work because the veins carrying the blood to the root of the limb are usually blocked and the bypass has an inadequate inflow.
- Do not be in a hurry to amputate tissues which look ischaemic. It is remarkable how dark blue–black, apparently dead skin can recover with time, particularly the skin underneath blisters which always looks purple and dead but often recovers. Two series of patients with this condition have reported good results from conservative management with heparin, elevation, and fluid replacement;[72,126] however, four of 12 patients died in the first series[72] and two of six died in the second,[126] most of widespread malignancy. Some patients will still proceed to amputation despite valiant attempts at restoring venous damage.[128]

INFERIOR VENA CAVA THROMBECTOMY

The technique of thrombectomy described on pages 329–333 is only applicable to ilio-femoral thrombosis. Thrombus may propagate into the vena cava, and if it is not adherent, it may be a source of potentially lethal emboli (Figure 10.15). The risk of embolism can be prevented by inserting a vena

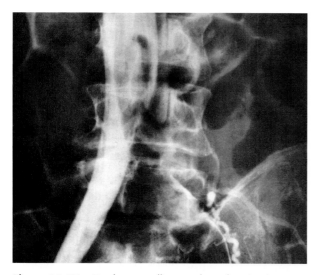

Figure 10.15 Fresh non-adherent thrombus in the vena cava that might fragment and become a pulmonary embolism if it was treated with streptokinase. We prefer to remove this type of thrombus surgically or confine it to the vena cava with vena caval blockade.

caval filter (see Chapter 22) but while this saves life it does nothing to improve gross limb swelling or prevent the subsequent development of post-thrombotic limb. A thrombolytic drug can be used but there is a significant risk of it causing a major embolism.

Inferior vena caval thrombus can be removed by balloon catheters passed via the femoral veins, but there is a considerable risk that the passage of the catheter will dislodge thrombus and cause emboli. Most surgeons prefer a direct approach to the vena cava but many would insert a temporary filter from above before beginning the exposure.

The vena cava is best exposed through an abdominal transperitoneal incision. A retroperitoneal exposure gives only limited access and cannot be extended. If a temporary filter has not been inserted, the first manoeuvre should be to place a clamp on the vena cava well above the thrombus to prevent embolism during the subsequent dissection of the cava. The vena cava and common iliac veins are best exposed by reflecting the caecum, ascending colon and duodenum to the left (see Figure 26.6, page 718). A venotomy is then made in the lower part of the vena cava and thrombus is then extracted with forceps or a balloon. Once the thrombus has been extracted, bleeding from the lumbar veins can be controlled with direct finger pressure (see Figure 26.6, page 718) and the venotomy held closed by a partially occluding Satinsky clamp. Inferior vena cava thrombosis is often the extension of an iliac vein thrombosis and therefore vena cava thrombectomy

may have to be followed by an ilio-femoral thrombectomy. Further embolism can be prevented by plicating or clipping the vena cava just below the renal veins, if the thrombectomy is incomplete, but this is now usually avoided by the early placement of a temporary filter.

COMBINED THROMBECTOMY AND THROMBOLYSIS

Attempts have been made to improve the results of thrombectomy by infusing fibrinolytic agents into the thrombectomized segment of vein after the operation.[117,120] A fine catheter is passed into an iliac vein via a small tributary of the long saphenous vein, and a low dose of streptokinase or tissue plasminogen activator is given in an attempt to produce local thrombolysis without causing a generalized systemic activation of the fibrinolytic system. There is little published evidence to show that this addition produces better results than thrombectomy alone, and the incidence of complications (e.g. wound haematoma) is increased.

It is only necessary to use thrombolytic drugs in this way if the thrombectomy is incomplete. This usually occurs when the operation has been performed on an ageing adherent thrombus, i.e. in the wrong circumstances. When a thrombectomy is performed in the correct circumstances, postoperative thrombolysis should be unnecessary.

Anticoagulation

Effective anticoagulation should prevent the propagation of existing thrombus by stopping the formation of new thrombus but it has no effect on the behaviour of existing thrombus. Thrombus fragmentation, retraction or adhesion still occurs, and therefore anticoagulants do not prevent embolism or deep vein damage. The most effective anticoagulant is heparin. Heparin should always be given as the initial treatment and should only be replaced by an oral anticoagulant when the circumstances causing the precipitating hypercoagulable state begin to recede. The value of long-term oral anticoagulation is now clearly established as a means of preventing delayed embolism and rethrombosis.[35,58,102,129,139,149]

HEPARIN

Heparin is a mucopolysaccharide glycosaminoglycan with a molecular weight of about 16 000, which inhibits the action of thrombin. It is produced by mast cells and contains a high content of esterified sulphuric acid. It has a strong negative charge. Small doses of heparin accelerate the inhibitory effect of antithrombin III on the activation of factor X and it can prevent thrombosis if given *before* thrombosis develops. Much larger doses are, however, required to stop existing thrombus propagating because in these circumstances the heparin has to inhibit thrombin in both the plasma and the thrombus, where it is combined with fibrin. The doses required for the treatment of existing thrombus are therefore 20 times greater than those needed for prophylaxis.

Dose

The precise blood level of standard heparin that prevents an existing thrombus growing has not been determined. Studies in animals in which a thrombus has been induced by physical means have shown that thrombosis does not occur if the plasma heparin level is more than 0.3 units/ml or if the accelerated partial thromboplastin time (APPT) is one and one-half times longer than the normal.[26]

Animal studies do not equate to clinical practice where the patient has a systemic hypercoagulable state, an existing thrombus and possibly some local vein wall damage and a reduced venous blood flow.

It is generally accepted that thrombus growth will only be prevented in humans when the plasma heparin is greater than 0.3 units/ml, the accelerated partial thromboplastin time (APTT) is more than twice normal, or the whole blood clotting time two to three times normal.[69,87] These blood levels are obtained by giving an intravenous loading dose of heparin of 5000 units followed by 20 000–40 000 units/24 hours; the dose should be controlled by a coagulation test. Patients whose APTT level is high before starting treatment develop an APTT which is twice the laboratory standard plasma normal level with a low level of plasma heparin. Patients with a low APTT level before starting treatment need more heparin, and therefore have a high blood level, by the time their APTT is doubled (Figure 10.16).[69] This explains why a small proportion of patients are inadequately anticoagulated and some are overtreated when the dose of heparin is compared with the APTT or other coagulation tests on laboratory control plasma. The correct plasma heparin levels are obtained when the patient's own pretreatment APTT (not a laboratory plasma APTT) is doubled (see Figure 10.17). However, the value of using the APTT to monitor heparin

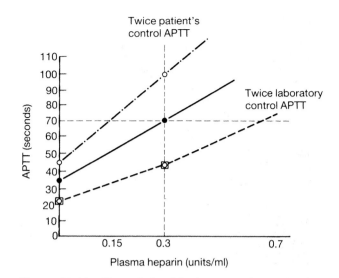

Figure 10.16 The relationship between the patient's pretreatment APTT (accelerated partial thromboplastin time) and the plasma heparin level during treatment. A patient with an APTT similar to that of the laboratory control plasma (●–●) will have a plasma heparin of 0.3 units/ml when his APTT is doubled. A patient with an APTT which is lower than that of the laboratory control plasma (□–□) will have a plasma heparin of 0.7 units/ml when his APTT is prolonged to twice that of the laboratory control plasma, but a plasma heparin level of 0.3 units/ml when his APTT is prolonged to twice that of his own pretreatment level. Similarly, a patient with an APTT which is higher than that of the laboratory control plasma (○–·–·○) will have a plasma heparin level of 0.15 units/ml when his APTT is prolonged to twice that of the laboratory control plasma, but a plasma heparin level to 0.3 units/ml when his APTT is prolonged to twice that of his own pretreatment level. This graph explains why some patients are inadequately anticoagulated and other patients are over-anticoagulated if the APTT ratio is based upon a standard laboratory control plasma. The APTT ratio must be based upon the patient's own pretreatment plasma. If the APTT ratio is based on the patient's pretreatment plasma, doubling the ratio will give a plasma heparin level of 0.3 units/ml. (Redrawn from Hirsh *et al.*[69])

therapy is not universally accepted. In a wide-ranging review of the relationship between the laboratory tests of coagulation blood heparin levels and clinical effectiveness, Blaisdell[17] concluded that there was little correlation between laboratory measurements and clinical response and that effectiveness and complications were more closely related to risk factors and individual idiosyncracies than blood levels. If this conclusion is correct, then complex laboratory studies could

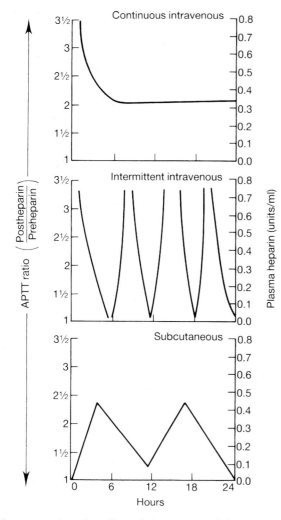

Figure 10.17   The effect of the route and frequency of administration on the pretreatment and post-treatment APTT ratio and plasma heparin levels. If the pretreatment APTT is doubled, the plasma heparin should be between 0.3 units/ml and 0.4 units/ml – the ideal therapeutic range. It can be seen that neither 6-hourly intravenous injections nor 12-hourly subcutaneous injections produce a sustained therapeutic level of plasma heparin. After 6 hours the effect of an intravenous bolus of heparin has worn off. Four-hourly injections provide a sustained effect but also result in frequent periods of excessive anticoagulation. (Redrawn from Hirsh *et al.*[69])

be replaced by careful clinical monitoring. Unfortunately, clinical monitoring only detects overtreatment (bleeding) not inadequate treatment. Much needs to be learnt about heparin and its control – especially the dosage and control of the newer low molecular weight heparins.

Administration

Standard heparin can be administered *intravenously* and *continuously*[60,146] or by subcutaneous injections.[3] Administration by the subcutaneous route is not so easily controlled or reversed but the use of fixed doses of the heparin fragments based on the patient's weight have made this a much more feasible route.[8,56,155]

A number of studies have compared intermittent with continuous administration of standard heparin. Figure 10.17 shows the blood levels obtained as a result of 6-hourly injections. The half-life of heparin is approximately 1 hour. The anticoagulant effect of a single injection has almost disappeared within 4 hours. *Patients who are given 6-hourly injections are therefore not anticoagulated for 2 of the 6 hours.* If, for logistic or clinical reasons, it is decided to give standard heparin intermittently, it must be given 4-hourly.

Studies of the incidence of bleeding complications have shown that a continuous infusion causes fewer bleeding complications than intermittent dosage.[60,110,146] This is not surprising in view of the high level of anticoagulation which occurs in the few minutes following each dose. A mathematical compilation of five controlled studies[69] reveals that the incidence of major bleeds was 5% when standard heparin was administered continuously compared with 12% after intermittent administration.

Comparative trials of low molecular weight heparin given subcutaneously against intravenous unfractionated heparin have shown that the former gives a more constant blood level and is just as effective in preventing recurrent thromboembolism. Low molecular weight heparins have now become the treatment of choice.[103,155] This is confirmed by the meta-analyses of Leizarovitz *et al.* who found by an analysis of 16 and 19 randomized control trials that subcutaneous low molecular weight heparins appeared to be better at reducing thrombus extension and recurrent thromboembolism than unfractionated heparin.[97,98]

Laboratory control

If a continuous infusion of standard heparin is used it should be monitored by measuring the accelerated partial thromboplastin time (APTT) or the clotting time.[12,59,134]

A pretreatment test should be performed and control studies should be repeated 4 hours and 8 hours after beginning treatment. Thereafter the frequency of testing depends upon the variability of the results but a coagulation test should be performed at least once a day.[48,125]

The preceding paragraph is the counsel of perfection. Many surgeons rely on a standard dose of 40 000 units/24 hours; they reduce this dose if bleeding complications occur, and they measure nothing. This regimen usually succeeds in providing adequate anticoagulation and stops further thrombosis without causing a high incidence of bleeding problems because the relationship between high doses and bleeding is not nearly as clear as that between low doses and recurrent thrombosis. Most authorities have now switched to subcutaneous low molecular heparin given in a fixed dose dependent upon the patient's weight. The dose varies according to the variety of unfractionated heparin and so it is important to follow the manufacturer's instructions with care. Monitoring is then unnecessary. This route of administration reduces laboratory and nursing costs.

Duration of treatment

There is no scientific evidence on which to base a decision concerning the duration of heparin therapy. Heparin is given initially because of its instant effect. Oral anticoagulants take 3–5 days to work but the actual anticoagulant effectiveness of these two types of drug has not been compared.

There is a large amount of anecdotal clinical evidence which suggests that heparin prevents new thrombosis and relieves symptoms more effectively than warfarin or phenindione. Most clinicians have seen the sudden return of symptoms with apparent extension of thrombosis when heparin is replaced by an oral anticoagulant (even when the prothrombin time is within the therapeutic range), followed by the rapid abatement of symptoms and, presumably, the cessation of thrombus growth on reinstituting heparin therapy. This experience is so common that many clinicians give heparin for 7 days before giving the loading dose of an oral anticoagulant although the Gallus study[58] suggested that warfarin started after 3 days is more effective in reducing further episodes of embolism and thrombosis than delaying its introduction for 7 days. The 7 days of heparin therapy covers the time when it is thought that the hypercoagulable state is maximal and the thrombus is most likely to extend. It allows the thrombus to retract, polymerize, and become adherent to the vein wall. After this period the risk of recurrent embolism and thrombosis is less and oral anticoagulants are more likely to be effective. Heparin therapy (standard or fragment) should probably be given for 7–10 days with a loading dose of an oral anticoagulant being given on the third day, followed by 3–6 months of warfarin to prevent rethromboses, especially in patients with sporadic rather than postoperative deep vein

thromboses. _Heparin must not be withdrawn until the prothrombin time is within the therapeutic range._ This means that the heparin should be stopped on the 6th or 7th day, and 4 hours later, when its effect has worn off, blood samples should be taken for a prothrombin time estimation. The heparin must then be resumed until the result of the laboratory test is available. The heparin can be stopped if the prothrombin time is two to three times the normal. The heparin must be continued for another 24 hours and the testing process must be repeated if it is less than twice the normal.

It is very important to ensure that the patient is not unprotected at any stage. This will happen if the heparin is just stopped on the assumption that the oral anticoagulant is working. Heparin should only be withdrawn after a satisfactory prothrombin time has been achieved.

Complications and their treatment
Bleeding

Bleeding is the most serious complication of heparin treatment.[33] The relationship between overdose and bleeding is unclear. Some studies have shown an increased rate of bleeding when the coagulation time is longer than 60 minutes, some show no relation between APTT and bleeding, and other studies show an increased rate of bleeding with doses greater than 40 000 units/24 hours. Some of the variations in these observations are probably caused by the effect of heparin on platelet function.[147] Some are almost certainly the result of heparin sensitivity.[144]

Bleeding occurs either spontaneously or from wounds. Spontaneous bleeding usually occurs in the subcutaneous tissues beneath pressure areas, or in the retroperitoneum, and it is more common in patients with severe hypertension. Surgical wounds, peptic ulcers and neoplastic ulcers of the gastrointestinal and renal tract may also bleed during heparin therapy.

Bleeding is reduced by the following measures:

- Stopping the heparin.
- Reversing the effect of the heparin by administering protamine sulphate.[127] Protamine sulphate combines directly with heparin and inactivates it. If a bolus of heparin has just been given, every 100 units of heparin will require 1 mg protamine to neutralize it. If the patient has been having a continuous infusion of heparin it is wise to give 25 mg protamine over 10 minutes and then measure the clotting time or the APTT. Further doses of protamine can be given until the anticoagulation is reversed. During vascular surgery we have found that 25 mg of protamine always

reverses the effect of 5000 units heparin given 30–60 minutes previously. *If protamine is given quickly it can cause hypotension; it should therefore be given slowly and carefully.*
- Restoring the blood volume with blood.
- Applying local measures as necessary, including surgery to bleeding vessels or ulcers if the blood loss continues after the anticoagulant effect of the heparin has been reversed. There is quite a lot of evidence that bleeding complications are less common when using subcutaneous low molecular weight heparins[97] as is heparin-induced thrombocytopaenia.

Thrombocytopenia

Standard unfractionated heparin will induce antiplatelet antibodies in approximately 2% of patients.[168] This can cause a thrombocytopenia which may become apparent after 2–3 days of treatment or can be delayed.[1] The development of this complication may cause serious bleeding complications and, paradoxically, may also cause thromboembolic complications as a result of platelet aggregation.[86,159] These patients have heparin specific antibodies.[1]

If arterial platelet emboli occur, the temptation is to continue or increase the heparin but instead heparin administration must be stopped and any problem of tissue ischaemia should be treated surgically. Thrombocytopenic complications (e.g. arterial emboli) are associated with a high morbidity and mortality, but fortunately, they are rare. The platelets return to normal when the standard heparin is stopped. The condition has a high morbidity and mortality unless actively treated.[93]

All patients who have been given therapeutic doses of standard heparin for more than 5 days should have a platelet count at the same time as their daily APTT. A rising demand for heparin (i.e. a falling APTT) and a falling platelet count should raise suspicion of heparin-induced thrombocytopenia. The platelet count should be repeated and platelet aggregation studies obtained and, if the number of platelets continues to fall, the heparin must be stopped and replaced with an oral anticoagulant. Low molecular weight heparin rarely causes thrombocytopenia[73] and patients can be converted to treatment with a heparin fragment if anticoagulation must be continued.

Sensitivity reactions

Heparin occasionally causes an itchy red maculopapular rash. This rash settles quickly when the heparin is stopped, and the itching can be controlled with an antihistamine. Anaphylactic reactions are very rare.

Alopecia

Loss of hair is a rare but distressing complication of prolonged heparin therapy. The precise incidence is not known but is likely to be small (<1%).

Osteoporosis

Patients who are given heparin for more than 6 months may become osteoporotic and present with pathological fractures of their vertebrae, ribs and metatarsals.[64,150] This complication is seldom seen, and is said not to occur if the dose of heparin is kept below 10 000 units/day.

In recent years it has become popular to use long-term subcutaneous heparin for the prevention of recurrent deep vein thrombosis and pulmonary embolism when oral anticoagulation is difficult to control or the risks of bleeding are high (e.g. during pregnancy). It is important to restrict the dose of heparin to 5000 units 12-hourly to avoid osteoporosis. Nowadays the use of low molecular weight heparin, delivered subcutaneously, is replacing standard heparin because it is easier to deliver – once a day, fixed dose based on weight, no monitoring, fewer side-effects.

Results

The efficacy of heparin must be judged against the three objectives of its administration:
- Prevention of pulmonary embolism
- Prevention of recurrent deep vein thrombosis
- Prevention of post-thrombotic sequelae.

In 1979, Bentley *et al.*[15] suggested that the subcutaneous route might be appropriate to treat established venous thrombosis. They found that this route of administration was as efficacious as the intravenous route in preventing further thromboembolic complications without any obvious increase in the risk of bleeding complications. This was not widely accepted for a number of years because clinicians were concerned that reversal of heparin's action when it was associated with major bleeding might be more difficult. A large multicentre study published in 1987, however, confirmed the value of subcutaneous administration[167] and in fact suggested that the subcutaneous route was more efficacious in preventing extension of thrombus.

When the low molecular weight heparins became available, around the same time, the subcutaneous route of administration became very attractive.[145] These heparins had a longer plasma half-life, had a clearer dose response and a reduced risk of causing unwanted haemorrhage. In 1992, two large controlled trials were published,[76,136] which showed that

Table 10.1 Incidence of pulmonary embolism during anticoagulation with heparin*

Reference	No. cases studied	No. fatal emboli	No. non-fatal emboli	Total no. emboli
119	149	0	4	4
35	107	1	3	4
80	346	0	28	28
124	60	7	?	7
36	124	2	12	14
31	152	9	12	21
11	54	0	3	3
24	118	22	?	22
158	20	0	3	3
89	26	0	4	4
Totals	1156	41 (3.5%)	69 (11%)	110 (9.5%)

*Ten studies performed between 1947 and 1966.

low molecular weight heparin given in fixed doses based purely on the patient's weight was as efficacious and safe as a comparable intravenous administration of adjusted dose standard heparin. In addition, it had the advantage that it is easy to administer and patients may leave hospital earlier. These studies have stimulated most physicians to use this treatment for all patients with deep vein thrombosis and few now make any assessment of the thrombus (other than its presence), but simply start all patients on subcutaneous low molecular weight heparin without any knowledge of the problem they are treating. Such an approach assumes that embolism, further thrombosis and late sequelae will be adequately treated. Low molecular weight heparin will certainly do as well and perhaps better than standard heparin but will it achieve the three principal therapeutic objectives? The evidence derived from the existing studies on unfractionated heparin suggest that it will not.

Prevention of recurrent embolism

Heparin (standard or low molecular weight) is given to patients with a deep vein thrombosis in the hope that it will prevent existing thrombus fragmenting and embolizing. Evidence that thrombus repeatedly fragments comes from the natural history study of Barker and Priestley[9,10] who showed that 30% of patients who have had one embolus have a further embolus and that 20% of these second emboli are fatal.

The value of heparin in preventing death after the first embolus is based on the study by Barritt and Jordan[11] which is discussed in detail in Chapter 11. By modern standards this study has many defects but heparin is now established as the accepted initial treatment for pulmonary embolism.[34]

Table 10.1 gives the incidence of recurrent embolism during heparin therapy in 10 studies on 1157 patients, published between 1947 and 1966. It could be argued that knowledge and control of heparin treatment was not as good 20 years ago as it is now, but nevertheless the incidence of both fatal and non-fatal recurrent emboli (3.5% and 11% respectively) is significant and has not fallen over the years. Since then, however, monitoring has improved and low molecular weight heparin has been developed. Nevertheless, new modern studies are still required. Some years ago[13] we reviewed 50 of our patients who had been treated with heparin alone and found that seven (14%) had had recurrent fatal emboli and 13 (26%) had had recurrent non-fatal emboli. This showed that heparin did not stop the fragmentation and embolization of existing thrombus, which in 40% of our trial patients was non-adherent (Figure 10.18).

More recent studies have confirmed that pulmonary emboli still occur in fully heparinized patients, though the incidence is lower than in untreated patients; for example, 21% of the patients with deep vein thrombosis who were given heparin in the control arm of a thrombectomy study had new ventilation–perfusion defects after 7 days of treatment.[133]

The incidence of recurrent embolism is dependent upon the degree of anticoagulation; Basu *et al.*[12] found a recurrence rate of 25% when the APTT was below 50 seconds but found no recurrences when it was above 50 seconds.

We conclude that *heparin therapy, fractionated or unfractionated, does not completely abolish recurrent embolism.* A definitive comparison of the

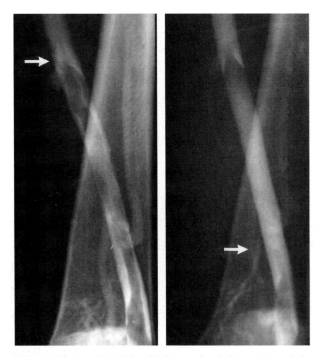

Figure 10.18   The first phlebograph of this patient (left-hand panel) revealed a non-adherent thrombus showing some signs of ageing, retraction and irregularity. The patient was fully anticoagulated with heparin. Two days later he experienced a severe pleuritic chest pain. A second phlebograph (right-hand panel) showed that part of the thrombus had broken off at a narrow segment to become an embolus.

effect of heparin against no treatment on the mortality and recurrence rate following pulmonary embolism has yet to be performed. As it is logical to prevent new thrombosis in the legs and new thrombus developing around the embolus in the pulmonary artery, a controlled trial with an untreated group will probably never be performed, for ethical and so-called logical reasons.

Prevention of recurrent deep vein thrombosis

The concept that heparin can induce the resorption of thrombus and thus reduce post-thrombotic late sequelae is based upon the belief that it is thrombolytic. This idea was supported by Bauer's claim[13] that 10 years after a thrombosis only 1.3% of a group of patients who had been given anticoagulants had the post-thrombotic syndrome compared with 58% of those patients who had not been given anticoagulants. It was assumed that this difference was caused by thrombolysis but it is unacceptable

to make deductions about the effect of heparin from clinical evidence as the physical signs are affected by many different factors. The only way to prove that a drug is thrombolytic is by demonstrating thrombolysis with phlebography. Recently, Vairel et al.[162] have suggested that low molecular weight heparin may enhance thrombolysis. This was also suggested by the multicentre study of Walker et al.[167]

The majority of the phlebographic studies of heparin and deep vein thrombosis are the control arms of studies of thrombolysis. There are no studies comparing the effect of heparin against no treatment. Nevertheless, these studies of thrombolysis do describe a small thrombolytic effect of heparin, even though the methods of administration, dosage and control vary considerably from study to study.

In 1968, Robertson et al.[141] compared heparin with streptokinase. They reported that half the 23 patients who were given heparin had poor results but unfortunately they did not say whether 'poor' was a worsening or unchanging phlebographic appearance.

In 1969,[19] we compared five patients treated with heparin for 5 days against five patients who were given streptokinase for 3 days and found no change in the phlebographic appearance of the thrombus in those patients given heparin.

In 1969, Kakkar[81] compared heparin with streptokinase and ancrod (Arvin). One of the 10 patients who were given heparin had a fatal pulmonary embolism. Two of the remaining nine patients showed clearance of the thrombus; in two patients the size of the thrombus was slightly reduced and in five patients it was unchanged. Fibrinogen uptake tests were also performed. In the two legs in which the thrombus cleared, the radioactivity fell quickly, but these legs contained only calf vein thrombi which are known to lyse spontaneously without treatment; it is therefore not known whether the disappearance of the thrombus was the result of spontaneous lysis or fragmentation and embolization. In two patients the radioactivity of the thrombus rose, suggesting further deposition of thrombosis in spite of adequate anticoagulation.

In 1969, we began a study, based on phlebography, designed to compare the effects of intermittent heparin with those of continuous heparin on deep vein thrombosis. In the pilot study 10 patients with deep vein thrombosis were given 5000 units of heparin 4-hourly for 7 days. When the phlebograms were repeated 5 days later the thrombi of four patients had progressed from being non-adherent to adherent thrombus, the thrombi of four patients were unchanged and two patients showed retraction and shrinkage (Figures 10.19–10.21). The progression to

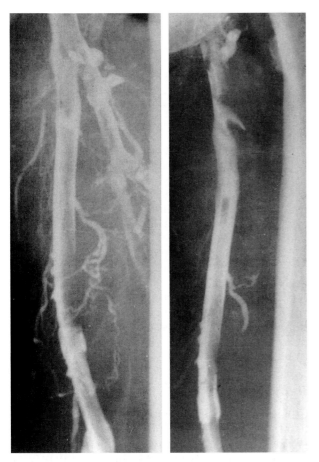

Figure 10.19 Retraction of thrombus during anticoagulation with heparin. These phlebographs were obtained before and after 5 days of treatment. The thrombus has retracted to half its original width.

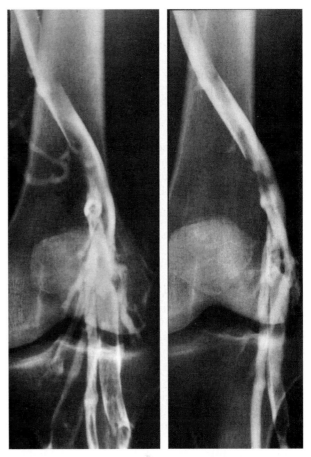

Figure 10.20 A phlebograph showing moderate retraction of the thrombus in the upper popliteal vein before and after 5 days of anticoagulation treatment with heparin, and considerable retraction of the thrombus in the lower half of the popliteal vein.

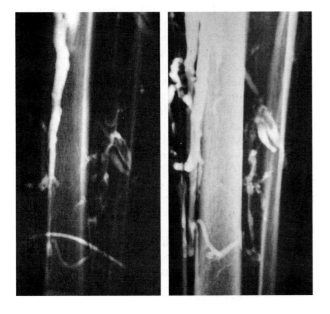

Figure 10.21 These phlebographs were obtained before and after 5 days of anticoagulation treatment with heparin. They show retraction of the thrombus in a communicating vein but no change in the thrombus in the deep axial vein. The changes in calf vein thrombus during anticoagulation are usually less pronounced than the changes of non-adherent axial vein thrombus.

thrombus adhesion and total obliteration of the lumen was most marked in the calf veins. Two patients had pulmonary emboli during treatment; the source of these emboli was clearly visible on the second phlebograph as a square cut end to a previously long loose thrombus. In the light of these results and the four studies described above, the trial was stopped and we were convinced that heparin was not thrombolytic, that it was unethical to treat patients who had non-adherent thrombus with anticoagulants alone, and that though an adequate dose of heparin might stop new thrombus forming, it failed to stop emboli or prevent partially occluded vessels becoming totally occluded.

Other studies have also emphasized the failure of heparin to do anything other than maintain the 'status quo'. Elliot[45] has reported that two patients of 25 who were given heparin developed extension of their thrombosis in spite of a clotting time which was 2.5–3 times the normal. Widmer[171] also found no lytic effect with heparin. The phlebographs of 89% of Widmer's 132 patients were unchanged by treatment, 6% had thrombus retraction, 3% got worse, developing more thromboses, and only 2% showed a significant reduction in the size of the thrombus.

In our opinion there is little clinical evidence that heparin causes or accelerates thrombolysis, to a degree that is clinically beneficial. Natural thrombolysis is common in small calf vein thrombi but uncommon in the axial veins. The chance of new thrombus forming during adequate anticoagulant therapy is between 5 and 10% and the chance of non-adherent thrombus becoming adherent and totally occluding its containing vein, rather than retracting to one side and leaving the lumen open, is probably 50%. It does, however, appear that low molecular weight heparin given subcutaneously is the most effective method of preventing thrombus progression and allowing natural lysis to occur. New controlled trials of this treatment against lytic therapy are required.

Prevention of the calf pump failure syndrome

The possibility that heparin might stop the progression of thrombosis raised the hope that it might reduce the incidence of the post-thrombotic syndrome. There are, however, no good long-term controlled trials comparing no treatment against a course of heparin. Controls are essential because of the variability of the natural history of thrombosis. Bauer[13] observed that half of his patients had a post-thrombotic syndrome 5 years after a deep vein thrombosis. Many of these patients had been given heparin.

Our own study,[175] comparing anticoagulants alone with anticoagulants combined with embolus-preventing operations (when indicated), showed that 58% of those patients who were given heparin alone had post-thrombotic symptoms at 3 years. The incidence of post-thrombotic symptoms in patients who had had surgical procedures and anticoagulants was similar. We also found that 20% of the legs without phlebographic evidence of thrombosis at the time of presentation had post-thrombotic symptoms.

Widmer studied 34 patients who had been given heparin as part of the control arm of a streptokinase trial 4 years and 7 months after the acute event, and he found that only 35% were normal.[170–172] The remaining 65% of patients had symptoms and signs of venous insufficiency; 12% had venous ulcers.

These studies do not give any indication that anticoagulants reduce the incidence of the post-thrombotic syndrome, and they confirm the view, repeatedly expressed throughout this book, that all you can expect from anticoagulants is the prevention of further thrombosis. This will save a life or prevent late sequelae in a limb on only a few occasions.

Indications

From the above section the reader might conclude that there is little justification for the use of heparin. A scientific evidence-based argument supporting this view could be produced, and we still believe that it would be ethical to restudy the value of heparin in all aspects of the treatment of thromboembolism. Nevertheless, low molecular weight heparin usually stops new thrombosis, and its use is justified in the light of our present knowledge.

We give unmonitored subcutaneous low molecular weight heparin by fixed dose based on weight, to *all patients with deep vein thrombosis* provided that there are no contraindications. This treatment is started as soon as the diagnosis is made on clinical grounds, but the heparin *is never continued without obtaining objective proof that there is a deep vein thrombosis.* Phlebography still provides the most complete information about the thrombus. Many of the non-invasive tests can provide proof of the diagnosis but none gives the additional information that we need to help us decide which is the best method of protecting the 5% of patients that the phlebographs reveal need other measures to protect them from recurrent embolism.

ORAL ANTICOAGULANTS

The oral anticoagulants, the coumarins (dicoumarol, nicoumalone and warfarin) and the indanediones (anisindione, diphenadione and phenindione) are easily absorbed by the gastrointestinal tract, and when absorbed they become bound to plasma albumin. The bound drug is inactive; only the small proportion (1–10%) that is unbound is active. These drugs inhibit the action of vitamin K in the synthesis of factors VII, IX and X so that inactive coagulation factors are produced. Only the coumarins are now used as they have fewer side-effects.

The effect of the coumarins is assessed by measuring the prothrombin time. This is usually expressed as the International Normalized Ratio (INR), the ratio between the patient's prothrombin time and the control time obtained with a standardized animal-derived thromboplastin; the thromboplastin is calibrated against an international reference preparation. A therapeutic level of anticoagulation is achieved when the INR is 2.5–3.5. This is a method of calculating the prothrombin time, and was brought about by the withdrawal of the standard human brain thromboplastin because it may contain human immunodeficiency viruses (HIV).

Dose

Warfarin is given as a loading dose of 10 mg followed by 6–10 mg/day, depending upon the prothrombin time. The loading dose of phenindione is 200 mg and the average maintenance dose is 100 mg/day.

Most physicians use warfarin in the first instance because its effect is more predictable, but if the effect of warfarin is difficult to control, it may be necessary to change to phenindione, nicoumalone or dicoumarol.

The half-life of warfarin is 35 hours and a full anticoagulant effect may take 3 or 4 days to develop.

Control

The anticoagulant effect is monitored with the prothrombin time, using the standardized thromboplastin described above. It must be measured daily until the maintenance dose and the test results are stable. The first measurement should be made 48 hours after the loading dose. Subsequently, the dose is varied by 2 mg amounts until the prothrombin time is between two and three times the normal value.

The prothrombin time cannot be measured accurately in heparinized blood; heparin administration should therefore be stopped 4 hours before taking blood for a prothrombin time test. The heparin should then be resumed until the result of the test is known.

Complications and their treatment

Haemorrhage

Bleeding may occur in up to 20% of patients.[69] Haematuria, spontaneous bruising and gastrointestinal bleeding are the common forms of bleeding.

Death as a result of bleeding occurs in less than 0.1% of patients.

Bleeding is stopped by the following measures:

- Administration of vitamin K_1 to reverse the effect on the coagulation factors. Vitamin K_1 can be given orally or intravenously. Intravenous administration is usually required when there are bleeding complications. If 5 mg vitamin K_1 are given intravenously (slowly to avoid hypotension and tachycardia), the prothrombin time should return to normal within 4–8 hours.[28]
- Infusion of plasma concentrates of factors II, VII, IX and X; this may be required if severe bleeding demands rapid reversal of anticoagulation.
- Replacement of blood lost with fresh blood or plasma.
- Application of local measures, including surgery, if the bleeding is severe.

Interaction with other drugs

Many drugs affect the way in which anticoagulants change the action of vitamin K; they are summarized in Table 10.2.

The modes of interaction of these drug vary. Some drugs affect the absorption of vitamin K or the anticoagulant, others affect metabolic processes in the liver, some alter the plasma albumin binding and some interfere with the metabolism of vitamin K itself. It is important to warn the patient of these interactions and to ask about any drugs they may have taken if a previously stable prothrombin time goes awry. The drugs which most commonly cause problems are the barbiturates, phenylbutazone, aspirin, sulphonamides, steroids and antibiotics.

Sensitivity reactions

The indanediones may cause rashes and fever. Fatal renal and liver failure have been reported but these complications are extremely rare. Warfarin produces very few sensitivity reactions but occasionally causes skin necrosis.[47] Skin necrosis is more common in females and affects areas which are well covered with fat (e.g. the breasts, buttocks and thighs). The skin turns red and oedematous, blisters and then turns blue–black. A necrotic area of skin may need to be excised and skin grafts may have to be applied.

Table 10.2 Some of the drugs which affect the effect of oral anticoagulants

Drugs which *increase* anticoagulant effect	Drugs which *decrease* anticoagulant effect
Allopurinol	Alcohol
Alcohol	(regular/heavy intake)
(occasional intake)	Antacids
Anabolic steroids	Antihistamines
Aspirin	Barbiturates
Cephalosporins	Carbamazepine
Chloramphenicol	Cholestyramine
Cholestyramine	Corticosteroids
Cimetidine	Dichloralphenazone
Clofibrate	Diuretics
Chlorpromazine	Glutethimide
Chloral	Griseofulvin
Co-trimoxazole	Oral contraceptives
Disulfiram	Phenytoin
Glucagon	Rifampicin
Metronidazole	
Naproxen	
Neomycin	
Oxyphenbutazone	
Phenylbutazone	
Quinine	
Quinidine	
Salicylates	
Sulphonamides	
Sulphonylureas	
Tamoxifen	
Tetracyclines	
Thyroxine	
Tricyclics (imipramine, amitriptyline, nortriptyline)	

Pregnancy

As warfarin can cross the placental barrier it may cause fetal abnormalities.[157] Chondrodysplasia punctata (skeletal deformities, nasal dysplasia and optic atrophy), mental retardation and blindness have been reported. Oral anticoagulants should not be given in the first trimester of pregnancy and should be given only after careful thought in the second trimester. Fetal abnormalities are unlikely to occur after the first trimester but fetal death may follow placental or maternal haemorrhage. Oral anticoagulants should be avoided in the last 2 months of pregnancy because the trauma of delivery may cause both internal haemorrhage in an anticoagulated fetus and in the mother.

The simplest solution is to avoid the use of oral anticoagulants at any time during pregnancy or when a woman thinks she might be pregnant. It is safe to give anticoagulants after pregnancy, and breast fed babies do not become anticoagulated because only a small quantity of the drug is excreted in the milk.

The anticoagulant of choice during pregnancy is heparin because it does not cross the placental barrier. This can be self-administered as a subcutaneous injection. The low molecular weight heparins are now usually used.

Results

Oral anticoagulants are given to prevent recurrent embolism and recurrent thrombosis and to reduce the incidence of post-thrombotic sequelae.

Prevention of recurrent embolism

There are now a number of controlled studies on the value of long-term oral anticoagulation in preventing recurrent embolism.[38,58,75,91,102,129,139,149]

Coon and Willis[33] found a 12.5% incidence of recurrent embolism in patients who had been given a short course of treatment as an in-patient, a 7.2% incidence in patients who had received a full course of treatment as an in-patient, and a 4.6% incidence in patients who had had proper in-patient treatment followed by 3 months of treatment as an out-patient.

The rationale for continuing anticoagulant therapy for 3–6 months is the phlebographic evidence that thrombus continues to show changes of retraction, vessels recanalize, and collaterals enlarge throughout this time. Furthermore, as we are not usually able to discover the cause of a thrombosis, it is not unreasonable to assume that whatever the cause was, it may take 3–6 months to disappear (i.e. until the patient is fully recovered and active)[18]. Our own study showed a reducing incidence of recurrent embolism over several months and few emboli after 6 months, except in those patients who were later found to have had a chronic recurrent thrombotic problem.

Hull *et al.*[75] performed a prospective study of 14 days of heparin therapy followed by the administration of low-dose subcutaneous heparin (5000 units 6-hourly) or full oral anticoagulation therapy for 6 weeks (for calf thrombosis) or 3 months (for axial vein thrombosis). Forty-seven per cent of the patients with axial vein thrombosis (27% of the whole group) who were given uncontrolled long-term heparin developed further thrombosis; there were no recurrences in the group of patients given oral anticoagulants. The incidence of embolism was 3% for the group treated with heparin and no patients had further embolism the group given oral anticoagulants. When this study was repeated[74] using a variable dose of heparin, adjusted weekly to prolong the APTT to one and one-half times the normal, the recurrent emboli stopped but bleeding complications increased.

The study by Gallus *et al.*[58] showed that warfarin started at 3 days was more efficacious than continuing heparin for 10 days before beginning anticoagulation as a means of preventing recurrent thromboembolism. The Research Council of the British Thoracic Society[139] found that there were significantly fewer episodes of recurrent thromboembolism in patients treated for 3 months with warfarin than those treated for 4 weeks [14 (4%) vs 27 (7.8%); $P = 0.04$]. A similar multicentre trial by Schulman *et al.*[149] in 1995 showed 80 recurrences (18.1%) in a group of patients treated for 6 weeks with warfarin compared with 43 (9.5%) in a group treated for 6 months. Similar results were found by Levine *et al.*[102]

The evidence therefore now clearly confirms that continuous anticoagulation therapy with warfarin for 6 months after giving heparin for 3 days does reduce the incidence of recurrent embolism.

Prevention of recurrent thrombosis

The study by Hull[75] provides objective evidence that oral anticoagulants reduce the incidence of new thrombosis. No conclusions can be made about the heparin group as some of these patients were not fully anticoagulated. This is supported by the other studies quoted above. Lagerstedt *et al.*[91] compared two groups of 23 and 28 patients with symptomatic calf vein thrombosis. One group was given heparin for 5 days, the other group was given heparin for 5 days and warfarin for 3 months. Both groups wore elastic stockings. The recurrence rate after 3 months was zero in the group that had been given warfarin and 29% in the group that had not received warfarin ($P = 0.01$). At 1 year the recurrence rates were 4% and 68%, respectively.

There is no reason to believe that oral anticoagulants increase the possibility of spontaneous thrombolysis or reduce the likelihood that non-adherent thrombi will become adherent.[39]

Prevention of calf pump failure syndrome

There are no published data on the incidence of post-thrombotic sequelae in patients given long-term anticoagulants compared to patients treated with only a 10-day course of heparin. Although warfarin may reduce the incidence of recurrent axial vein thrombosis, the incidence of post-thrombotic sequelae probably depends upon the extent of the initial calf vein thrombosis. There is some evidence from the longitudinal duplex ultrasound studies of

Meissner *et al.* that recurrent thrombosis does equate with increasing valvular incompetence.[118]

Indications

There appears to be enough evidence to support the belief that oral anticoagulants reduce the incidence of recurrent embolism during the 6 months following a thrombosis. There is also some evidence to suggest that oral anticoagulants reduce the development of new axial vein thrombosis, and thus may reduce the chance of post-thrombotic calf pump failure but the evidence for this last supposition is extremely weak.

On the basis of these beliefs (not facts) our practice is *to treat all deep vein thrombosis, in the absence of any strong contraindication, with heparin for 3–7 days followed by full anticoagulation with warfarin for 6 months.* Some workers argue that calf vein thrombosis is not a serious problem and treat this for only 6 weeks or 3 months. We think that calf vein thrombosis is a serious problem; it is a major cause of the post-thrombotic syndrome, and calf thrombi can become emboli. There is published support for this hypothesis.[104] We therefore draw no distinction between the site or the age of the thrombus, or the initial form of treatment (i.e. anticoagulants, surgery or thrombolysis) but prescribe 6 months of anticoagulation therapy for *all* patients after thrombosis.

If the patient remains well during this 6-month treatment period we 'tail-off' the warfarin over a 2-week period (even though there is no evidence of a 'rebound' phenomenon), but ask the patient to return immediately if they experience any leg or chest symptoms. Low molecular weight heparin is restarted and a phlebogram and ventilation–perfusion scan are performed if the patient returns with recurrent symptoms. The patient is given warfarin for another 6 months if we find any evidence of new thrombosis or embolism. Recurrence after 1 year of treatment is rare and usually means that the patient has thrombophilia (see Chapter 8). Blood coagulation factors (e.g. antithrombin III and protein C) and tissue fibrinolysis should be measured and the possibility of life-long anticoagulation or long-term enhancement of fibrinolysis should be considered. Recurrent thromboembolic disease of this nature occurs in less than 0.5% of patients.

Defibrinogenation

The treatment of venous thromboembolism by defibrinogenation has not developed into a useful form of therapy because it is difficult to control and is of limited value, as antibodies to the defibrinogenating agent develop after 2–3 weeks of administration.[14,130,138]

Summary

Our approach to treatment of deep vein thrombosis based upon phlebography

The treatment options described in this chapter can be used in many ways; the choice of method often depends upon individual preferences and contraindications rather than on hard scientific evidence of suitability or superiority.

Our approach is as follows (see Figure 10.22). The pretreatment investigations used must provide sufficient information for management. They must:

1. Confirm the presence of thrombosis
2. Establish the site of the thrombosis
3. Establish whether the thrombus, particularly its upper limit, is adherent or non-adherent, and indicate its age
4. Confirm the presence or absence of pulmonary embolism (time and circumstances may only allow this to be done by clinical examination).

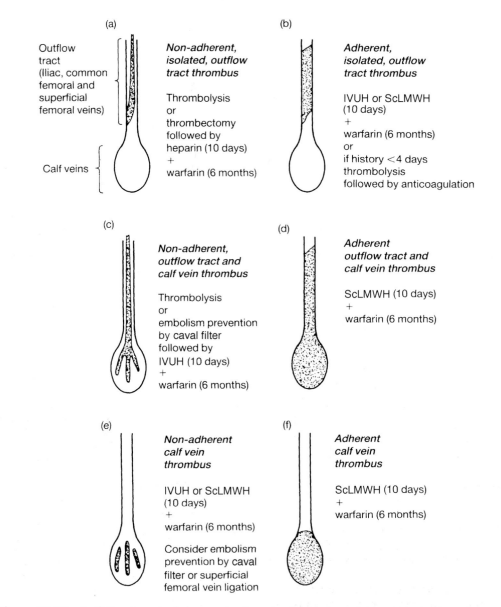

Figure 10.22 (a–f) Treatment of deep vein thrombosis. A plan of management based upon the phlebographic appearances of the thrombus. ScLMWH, subcutaneous low molecular weight heparin; IVUH, intravenous unfractionated heparin.

When the patient has had a pulmonary embolus, the principal object of treatment is the prevention of a second embolus. The ways in which this can be done are described in Chapter 22.

When the patient has not had a pulmonary embolism, the aims of treatment are to abolish the risk of embolism and to minimize the damage to the deep veins.

Fresh (less than 5 days old) non-adherent isolated thrombus in the outflow tract (popliteal and above)

This should be removed (Figure 10.22a). Our preference, in the absence of the risk of bleeding complications, is to use thrombolysis with tissue plasminogen activator delivered locally or systemically.

When there is a risk of bleeding (e.g. postoperatively) and when the thrombus is limited to the ilio-femoral segment we use thrombectomy. If neither thrombolysis nor thrombectomy can be used, we prevent embolism by placing a filter in the inferior vena cava.

All patients are given intravenous heparin before and after their initial treatment for 7–10 days followed by warfarin for 6 months.

Adherent isolated thrombus in the outflow tract (popliteal and above)

This should be removed if possible (Figure 10.22b). The problem is the unknown age of the thrombus. Some clinicians would try a course of lysis if the clinical picture suggests that the thrombus is less than 4 days old, in spite of its phlebographic adherence.

We give heparin to prevent further thromboses if there are contraindications to thrombolysis and if the history is longer than 3 days. We do not use thrombectomy in these circumstances because it usually fails and embolism is not a risk.

Heparin is continued for 10 days, followed by warfarin for 6 months.

Non-adherent continuous calf and outflow tract thrombus

This should be removed by thrombolysis (Figure 10.22c). Thrombectomy is not very effective in these circumstances because it cannot remove the calf vein thrombus.

When thrombolysis is not possible, prevention of embolism should be considered, e.g. a combination of ilio-femoral thrombectomy and vein ligation or vena caval interruption).

Adherent continuous calf and outflow tract thrombus

This should be treated with anticoagulants unless there is good evidence (a rare circumstance) that the thrombus is less than 3 days old in which case thrombolysis may be tried (Figure 10.22d).

Non-adherent calf thrombus

This should be treated with anticoagulants (Figure 10.22e). If the patient has already had a pulmonary embolus which has embarrassed cardiac function, prevention of embolism, a vena cava filter or superficial femoral vein ligation should be considered. A few clinicians would consider thrombolysis.

Adherent calf vein thrombus

This should be treated with anticoagulants (Figure 10.22f).

References

1. Adams JG, Humphrey LJ, Zhang Xinchao, Silver D. Do patients with the heparin-induced thrombocytopenia syndrome have heparin-specific antibodies? *J Vasc Surg* 1995; **21(2):** 247–54.
2. Albrechtsson U, Anderson J, Einarsson E, Eklof B, Norgren L. Streptokinase treatment of deep vein thrombosis and the postthrombotic syndrome. Follow-up evaluation of venous function. *Arch Surg* 1981; **116:** 33–7.
3. Anderson G, Fagrell B, Holmgren K, *et al.* Subcutaneous administration of heparin. *Thromb Res* 1982; **27:** 631–9.
4. Andriopoulos A, Wirsing P, Botticher R. Results of iliofemoral venous thrombectomy after acute thrombosis. Report on 165 cases. *J Cardiovasc Surg* 1982; **23:** 123–4.
5. Arnesen H, Heilo A, Jakobsen E, Ly B, Skaga E. A prospective study of streptokinase and heparin in the treatment of deep vein thrombosis. *Acta Med Scand* 1978; **203:** 457–63.
6. Arnesen H, Hoiseth A, Ly B. Streptokinase or heparin in the treatment of deep vein thrombosis. *Acta Med Scand* 1982; **211:** 65–8.
7. Astedt B, Robertson B, Haeger K. Experience with standardized streptokinase therapy of deep vein thrombosis. *Surgery* 1974; **139:** 387–8.
8. Barber ND, Hoffmeyer UK. Comparison of the cost-effectiveness of administering heparin subcutaneously or intravenously for the treatment of deep vein thrombosis. *Ann R Coll Surg Engl* 1993; **75:** 430–3.
9. Barker NW, Nygaard KK, Walters W, Priestley JT. A statistical study of postoperative venous thrombosis and pulmonary embolism. III. Time of

occurrence during the postoperative period. *Proc Staff Meet Mayo Clin* 1941; **16:** 17.

10. Barker NW, Priestley JT. Postoperative thrombophlebitis and embolism. *Surgery* 1942; **12:** 411.

11. Barritt DW, Jordan SC. Anticoagulant drugs in treatment of pulmonary embolism: controlled trial. *Lancet* 1960; **1:** 1309–12.

12. Basu D, Gallus A, Hirsh J, Code J. A prospective study of the value of monitoring heparin treatment with the activated partial thromboplastin time. *N Engl J Med* 1972; **287:** 324–7.

13. Bauer G. A roentgenological and clinical study of the sequels of thrombosis. *Acta Chir Scand* 1942; **86:** Suppl 74.

14. Bell WR, Pitney WR, Goodwin JF. Therapeutic defibrination in the treatment of thrombotic disease. *Lancet* 1968; **1:** 490–3.

15. Bentley PG, Kakkar VV, Scully F, *et al.* An objective study of alternative methods of heparin administration. *Thromb Res* 1980; **18:** 177–87.

16. Bird RL. Treatment options for phlegmasia caerulea dolens. *J Vasc Surg* 1994; **21:** 998.

17. Blaisdell FW. Heparin – controversies and misconceptions. *J Cardiovasc Surg* 1996; **4:** 691–7.

18. Browse NL, Lea Thomas M, Solan MJ, Young AK. Prevention of recurrent pulmonary embolism. *Br Med J* 1969; **3:** 382–6.

19. Browse NL, Thomas ML, Pim HP. Streptokinase and deep vein thrombosis. *Br Med J* 1968; **3:** 717–20.

20. Brunner U, Wirth W. Spatresultate nach Thrombecktomie bei Iliofemoralvenenthrombose in klinisch-radiologischen vergleich. *Schweiz Med Wochenschr* 1971; **101:** 1327–34.

21. Brunner V. Surgery of acute femoro-iliac phlebothrombosis. In: May R, ed. *Surgery of the Veins of the Leg and Pelvis.* Stuttgart: G Thieme, 1979.

22. Brunner V. Thrombektomie bei iliofemoral venenthrombose. *Helv Chir Acta* 1971; **38:** 57.

23. Burnand KG, Sheen J, Lea Thomas M, Browse NL, Feers R, Standing R. Treatment of deep vein thrombosis by slow deacylating streptokinase plasminogen complex (BRL 33575). In: Negus D, Jantet G, eds. *Phlebology '85.* London: John Libbey, 1986; 476.

24. Byrne JJ. Phlebitis. A study of 979 cases at the Boston City Hospital. *JAMA* 1960; **174:** 113.

25. Cairols MA, Marco-Luque MA, Caralt MT, Ballon H, Aced S, Capdevila JM. A phlebographic and ultrasonic evaluation of fibrinolytic therapy. *Vasc Diagn Ther* 1983; **3:** 37–40.

26. Carey LC, Williams RD. Comparative effects of dicoumarol, tromexan and heparin on thrombus propagation. *Ann Surg* 1960; **152:** 919.

27. Chavatzas D, Martin P. A study of streptokinase in deep vein thrombosis of the lower extremities. *Vasa* 1975; **4:** 68–72.

28. Clagett GP, Salzman E. Prevention of venous thromboembolism. *Prog Cardiovasc Dis* 1975; **17:** 345–66.

29. Comerota AJ, Katz ML, White JV. Thrombolytic therapy for acute deep venous thrombosis: how much is enough? *Cardiovasc Surg* 1996; **4(1):** 101–4.

30. Common HH, Seaman AJ, Rosch J, Porter JM, Dotter C. Deep vein thrombosis treated with streptokinase or heparin – follow up of a randomized study. *Angiology* 1976; **27:** 645–54.

31. Coon W, MacKenzie JW, Hodgson PK. A critical evaluation of anticoagulant therapy in peripheral venous thrombosis and pulmonary embolism. *Surg Gynecol Obstet* 1958; **106:** 129.

32. Coon WW, Willis PW. Haemorrhagic complications of anticoagulant therapy. *Arch Intern Med* 1974; **133:** 386–92.

33. Coon WW, Willis PW. Thromboembolic complications during anticoagulant therapy. *Arch Surg* 1972; **105:** 209–12.

34. Coon WW, Willis PW, Symons MJ. Assessment of anticoagulant treatment of venous thromboembolism. *Ann Surg* 1969; **170:** 559–68.

35. Cosgriff SW, Cross RJ, Habif DV. Management of venous thrombosis and pulmonary embolism. *Surg Clin North Am* 1948; **28:** 324.

36. Crane C. Deep venous thrombosis and pulmonary embolism. *N Engl J Med* 1957; **257:** 147.

37. Cranley JJ, Krause RJ, Stasser ES, Hafner CD. Femoroiliac thrombophlebitis. Immediate and late results after thrombectomy, caval ligation and conservative management. *J Cardiovasc Surg* 1969; **10:** 463–7.

38. Das SK, Cohen AT, Edmondson RA, Melissari E, Kakkar VV. Low-molecular weight heparin versus warfarin for prevention of recurrent venous thromboembolism: a randomized trial. *World J Surg* 1996; **20:** 521–7.

39. Davies JA, Merrick MV, Sharp AA, Holt JM. Controlled trial of ancrod and heparin in treatment of deep vein thrombosis of lower limb. *Lancet* 1971; **1:** 113–15.

40. DeWeese JA, Jones TI, Lyon J, Dale W. Evaluation of thrombectomy in the management of iliofemoral venous thrombosis. *Surgery* 1960; **47:** 140–59.

41. Duckert F, Muller G, Nyman D, *et al.* Treatment of deep vein thrombosis with streptokinase. *Br Med J* 1975; **1:** 479–81.

42. Edwards EA, Edwards JE. Effect of thrombophlebitis on venous valves. *Surg Gynecol Obstet* 1937; **65:** 310.

43. Eichinger S, Kyrle PA, Brenner B, *et al.* Thrombocytopenia associated with low molecular-weight heparin. *Lancet* 1991; **337:** 1425–6.

44. Eklof B, Einarsson E, Plate G. Role of thrombectomy and temporary arteriovenous fistula in acute venous thrombosis. In: Bergan JJ, Yao JST, eds. *Surgery of the Veins.* Orlando, FL: Grune & Stratton, 1985.

45. Elliot MS, Immelman EJ, Jeffrey P, *et al.* A comparative randomized trial of heparin versus streptokinase in the treatment of acute proximal venous thrombosis. *Br J Surg* 1979; **66:** 838–43.

46. Elliot MS, Immelman EJ, Jeffrey P, *et al.* The role of thrombolytic therapy in the management of phlegmasia caerulea dolens. *Br J Surg* 1979; **66:** 422–4.

47. Faraci PA, Deterling R, Stein A, Rheinlander H, Cleveland R. Warfarin induced necrosis of the skin. *Surg Gynecol Obstet* 1978; **146:** 695–700.

48. Fennerty AG, Thomas P, Backhouse G, Bentley P, Campbell IA, Routledge PA. Audit control of heparin treatment. *Br Med J* 1985; **290:** 27–8.

49. Fletcher AP, Alkjaersig N, Sherry S. The development of urokinase as a thrombolytic agent. Maintenance of a sustained thrombolytic state in man by its intravenous infusion. *J Lab Clin Med* 1965; **65:** 713.

50. Fogarty TJ, Dennis D, Krippaehen WW. Surgical management of ilio-femoral venous thrombosis. *Am J Surg* 1966; **112:** 211–17.

51. Fogarty TJ, Cranley JJ, Krause RJ, Strasser ES, Hafner CD. A method for extraction of arterial emboli and thrombi. *Surg Gynecol Obstet* 1963; **116:** 241.

52. Fogarty TJ, Cranley JJ, Krause RJ, Strasser ES, Hafner CD. Surgical management of phlegmasia cerulea dolens. *Arch Surg* 1963; **86:** 256–63.

53. Fogarty TJ, Krippaehue WW. Catheter technique for venous thrombectomy. *Surg Gynecol Obstet* 1965; **121:** 362–4.

54. Fontaine R. Remarks concerning venous thrombosis and its sequelae. *Surgery* 1957; **41:** 6.

55. Fontaine R, Tuchmann L. The role of thrombectomy in deep venous thrombosis. *J Cardiovasc Surg* 1964; **5:** 298–313.

56. Friedel HA, Balfour JA. Tinzaparin. A review of its pharmacology and clinical potential in the prevention and treatment of thromboembolic disorders. *Drugs* 1994; **48(4):** 638–60.

57. Gallus AS, Hirsh J, Cade JF, Turpie AGG, Walker IR, Gent M. Thrombolysis with a combination of small doses of streptokinase and full doses of heparin. *Semin Thromb Hemost* 1975; **2:** 14–32.

58. Gallus A, Jackaman J, Tillett J, Mills W, Wycherley A. Safety and efficacy of warfarin started early after submassive venous thrombosis or pulmonary embolism. *Lancet* 1986; **2:** 1293–6.

59. Genton E. Guidelines for heparin therapy. *Ann Intern Med* 1974; **80:** 77–82.

60. Glazier RL, Crowell EB. Randomized prospective trial of continuous or intermittent heparin therapy. *JAMA* 1976; **236:** 1365–7.

61. Gmelin E, Theiss W. Repeated phlebographic examination during and after fibrinolytic therapy with streptokinase and urokinase. *Cardiovasc Radiol* 1978; **1:** 157–64.

62. Gormsen J, Laursen B. Treatment of acute phlebothrombosis with streptase. *Acta Med Scand* 1967; **181:** 373–83.

63. Goto H, Wada T, Matsumoto A, Matsummoto A, Souna T. Iliofemoral venous thrombectomy. *J Cardiovasc Surg* 1980; **21:** 341–6.

64. Griffiths GC, Nichols G, Aster JD. Heparin osteoporosis. *JAMA* 1965; **193:** 85.

65. Gruss JD, Lanbach K. Modifikation der operations technik bei teifer Becken- und Oberschenkel-Venen thrombose. *Thoraxchirurgie* 1971; **19:** 509–14.

66. Haller JA. *Deep Thrombophlebitis.* Philadelphia, PA: WB Saunders, 1967.

67. Haller JA, Abrams BL. Use of thrombectomy in the treatment of acute iliofemoral venous thrombosis in forty five patients. *Ann Surg* 1963; **158:** 561–9.

68. Hirsh J. Long term treatment of venous thromboembolism with oral anticoagulants. *Pract Cardiol* 1984; **10:** 235.

69. Hirsh J, Genton E, Hull R. *Venous Thromboembolism.* New York: Grune & Stratton, 1981.

70. Hirsh J, O'Sullivan E F, Martin M. Evaluation of a standard dosage schedule with streptokinase. *Blood* 1970; **35:** 341–9.

71. Homans J. Exploration and division of femoral and iliac veins in treatment of thrombophlebitis of leg. *N Engl J Med* 1941; **224:** 179.

72. Hood DB, Weaver FA, Modrall JG, Yellin AE. Advances in the treatment of phlegmasia cerulea dolens. *Am J Surg* 1993; **166(2):** 206–10.

73. Huisse MG, Guillin MC, Bezeaud A, Toulemonde F, Kitsis M, Andreassian B. Heparin associated thrombocytopenia. *In vitro* effects of different molecular weight heparin fractions. *Thromb Res* 1982; **27:** 485–90.

74. Hull R, Delmore T, Carter C, *et al.* Adjusted subcutaneous heparin versus warfarin sodium in the long term treatment of venous thrombosis. *N Engl J Med* 1982; **306:** 189–94.

75. Hull R, Delmore T, Genton E, *et al.* Warfarin sodium versus low dose heparin in the long term treatment of venous thrombosis. *N Engl J Med* 1979; **301:** 855–8.

76. Hull RD, Raskob GE, Pineo GF, *et al.* Subcutaneous low-molecular weight heparins compared with continuous intravenous heparin in the treatment of proximal vein thrombosis. *N Engl J Med* 1992; **326:** 975–82.

77. Jakob H, Maass D, Schmiedt W, Schild H, Oelert H. Treatment of major venous obstruction with an expandable endoluminal spiral prosthesis. *J Cardiovasc Surg* 1989; **30:** 112–17.

78. Johansson E, Nordlander S, Zetterquist S. Venous thrombectomy in the lower extremity. Clinical phlebographic and plethysmographic evaluation of early and late results. *Acta Chir Scand* 1973; **139:** 511–16.

79. Johansson L, Nylander G, Hedner U, Nilsson IM. Comparison of streptokinase with heparin. Late results in the treatment of deep vein thrombosis. *Acta Med Scand* 1979; **206:** 93–8.

80. Jorpes JE. On the dosage of the anticoagulants, heparin and dicoumarol in the treatment of thrombosis. *Acta Chir Scand Suppl* 1950; **149.**

81. Kakkar VV, Flanc C, Howe CT, O'Shea M, Flute PT. Treatment of deep vein thrombosis. A trial of heparin, streptokinase and arvin. *Br Med J* 1969; **1:** 806–10.

82. Kakkar VV, Flanc C, O'Shea MJ, Flute PT, Howe CT, Clarke MB. Treatment of deep vein thrombosis with streptokinase. *Br J Surg* 1969; **56:** 178–83.

83. Kakkar VV, Howe CT, Laws JW, Flanc C. Late results of treatment of deep vein thrombosis. *Br Med J* 1969; **1:** 810–11.

84. Kakkar VV, Lawrence D. Hemodynamic and clinical assessment after therapy for acute deep vein thrombosis: a prospective study. *Am J Surg* 1985; **150 (Suppl 4A):** 54–63.

85. Kakkar VV, Sagar S, Lewis M. Treatment of deep vein thrombosis with intermittent streptokinase and plasminogen infusion. *Lancet* 1975; **2**: 674–6.

86. Kapsch D, Adelstein E, Rhodes G, Silver D. Heparin induced thrombocytopenia, thrombosis and haemorrhage. *Surgery* 1979; **86**: 148–55.

87. Kapsch DN, Kasulke RJ, Silver D. Anticoagulant therapy. *Vasc Diagn Ther* 1981; **19:**.

88. Karp RB, Wylie EJ. Recurrent thrombosis after iliofemoral venous thrombectomy. *Surg Forum* 1966; **17:** 147.

89. Kernohan RJ, Todd C. Heparin therapy in thromboembolic disease. *Lancet* 1966; **1**: 621–3.

90. Kiely PK. A new venous thrombectomy technique. *Br J Surg* 1973; **60**: 850–2.

91. Lagerstedt CI, Olsson CG, Fagher BO, Oqvist BW, Albrechtsson V. Need for long term anticoagulant treatment in symptomatic calf vein thrombosis. *Lancet* 1985; **2**: 515–18.

92. Lansing AM, Davis WM. Five year follow up study of iliofemoral venous thrombectomy. *Ann Surg* 1968; **168**: 620–8.

93. Laster J, Cikrit I, Walker N, Silver D. The heparin-induced thrombocythaemia syndrome – an update. *Surgery* 1987; **102**: 763–70.

94. Lawen A. Weitere Erfahrungen Über operative thromben-entfernung bei Venenthrombose. *Arch Klin Chir* 1938; **193**: 723.

95. Lawen A. Ueber Thombektomie bei venen thrombose und Arteriospasmus. *Zentralb Chir* 1937; **64**: 961–8.

96. Le Compte T, Luo SK, Stieltjes N, LeCrubier C, Samama MM. Thrombocytopenia associated with low-molecular-weight heparin. *Lancet* 1991; **338**: 1217.

97. Leizorovitz A, Simmoneau G, Decousus H, Boissel JP. Comparison of efficacy and safety of low molecular weight heparins and unfractionated heparin in initial treatment of deep venous thrombosis: a meta-analysis. *Br Med J* 1994; **309**: 299–304.

98. Lensing AW, Prins MH, Davidson BL, Hirsh J. Treatment of deep venous thrombosis with low-molecular-weight heparins. A meta-analysis. *Arch Intern Med* 1995; **155(6)**: 601–7.

99. Leriche R. Traitement chirurgical des suites éloignées des phlébites des grandes oedemes non-médicaux des membres inférieures. *Bull Med Soc Nat Chir* 1927; **53**: 187–95.

100. Leriche R, Geisendorf W. Résultats d'une thrombectomie précoce avec resection veineuse dans une phlébite grave des deux membres inférieurs. *Presse Méd* 1939; **47**: 1239.

101. Levine MN, Goldhaber SZ, Califf RM, Gore JM, Hirsh J. Hemorrhagic complications of thrombolytic therapy in the treatment of myocardial infarction and venous thromboembolism. *Chest* 1992; **102(4)**: 364–73.

102. Levine MN, Hirsh J, Gent M, *et al.* Optimal duration of oral anticoagulant therapy: a randomized trial comparing four weeks with three months of warfarin in patients with proximal deep vein thrombosis. *Thromb Haemost* 1995; **74(2)**: 606–11.

103. Lindmarker P, Holmstrom M, Granqvist S, Johnsson H, Lockner D. Comparison of once-daily subcutaneous Fragmin with continuous intravenous unfractionated heparin in the treatment of deep vein thrombosis. *Thromb Haemost* 1994; **72(2)**: 186–90.

104. Lohr JM, James KV, Deshmukh RM, Hasselfeld KA. Allastair B Karmody Award. Calf vein thrombi are not a benign finding. *Am J Surg* 1995; **170(2)**: 86–90.

105. Mahorner H. A new method of management for thrombosis of deep veins of the extremities. *Am Surg* 1954; **20**: 487.

106. Mahorner H. Results of surgical operations for venous thrombosis. *Surg Gynecol Obstet* 1969; **129**: 66–70.

107. Mahorner H, Castleberry JW, Coleman WC. Attempts to restore function in major veins which are the site of massive thrombosis. *Ann Surg* 1957; **146**: 510–22.

108. Mansfield AO. Control of pulmonary embolism. *Ann R Coll Surg Engl* 1972; **51**: 373–88.

109. Mansfield AO, Carmichael JHE, Parry EW. Thrombectomy employing continuous radiographic control. *Br J Surg* 1971; **58**: 119–23.

110. Mant MJ, O'Brien BD, Thong KL, Hammond GW, Birtwhistle RJ, Grace MG. Haemorrhagic complications of heparin therapy. *Lancet* 1977; **1**: 1133–5.

111. Marder VJ. Guidelines for thrombolytic therapy of deep vein thrombosis. *Prog Cardiovasc Dis* 1979; **21**: 327–32.

112. Masuoka S, Shinomura T, Audo T, Goto K. Complications associated with the use of the Fogarty balloon catheter. *J Cardiovasc Surg* 1980; **21**: 67–74.

113. Mavor GE, Bennett B, Galloway M, Karmody AM. Streptokinase in iliofemoral venous thrombosis. *Br J Surg* 1969; **56**: 564–7.

114. Mavor GE, Dhall DP, Dawson AA, *et al.* Streptokinase therapy in deep vein thrombosis. *Br J Surg* 1973; **60**: 468–74.

115. Mavor GE, Galloway JMD. Iliofemoral venous thrombosis. *Br J Surg* 1969; **56**: 45–58.

116. Mavor GE, Galloway JMD. Radiographic control of iliofemoral venous thrombectomy. *Br J Surg* 1967; **54**: 1019–22.

117. Mavor GE, Ogston D, Galloway JMD, Karmody AM. Urokinase in iliofemoral venous thrombosis. *Br J Surg* 1969; **56**: 571–4.

118. Meissner MH, Caps MT, Bergelin RO, Manzo RA, Strandness DE. Propagation, rethrombosis and new thrombus formation after acute deep venous thrombosis. *J Vasc Surg* 1995; **22(5)**: 558–67.

119. Murray G. Anticoagulants in venous thrombosis and the prevention of pulmonary embolism. *Surg Gynecol Obstet* 1947; **84**: 665.

120. Nachbur BB, Beck EA, Senn A. Can the results of treatment of deep venous thrombosis be improved by combining surgical thrombectomy with regional fibrinolysis. *J Cardiovasc Surg* 1980; **21**: 347–52.

121. Nilsson IM, Olow B. Fibrinolysis induced by streptokinase. *Acta Chir Scand* 1962; **123**: 247–66.

122. Norgren L, Gjores JE. Venous function in previously thrombosed legs. *Acta Chir Scand* 1977; **143:** 421–4.

123. Norgren L, Widmer LK. Venous function evaluated by foot volumetry in patients with a previous deep vein thrombosis treated with streptokinase. *Vasa* 1978; **7:** 412–14.

124. Oschner A, DeBakey ME, De Camp PT, De Rocha E. Thrombo-embolism. An analysis of cases at the Charity Hospital in New Orleans over a 12 year period. *Ann Surg* 1951; **134:** 405.

125. O'Shea MJ, Flute PT, Pannell GM. Laboratory control of heparin therapy. *J Clin Pathol* 1971; **24:** 542–6.

126. Patel KR, Paidas CN. Phlegmasia cerulea dolens: the role of non-operative therapy. *Cardiovasc Surg* 1993; **1(5):** 518–23.

127. Perkins HA, Osborn JJ, Hurt R, Gerbode F. Neutralization of heparin *in vivo* with protamine. A simple method of estimating the required dose. *J Lab Clin Med* 1956; **48:** 223.

128. Perkins JMT, Magee TR, Galland RB. Phlegmasia cerulea dolens and venous gangrene. *Br J Surg* 1996; **83:** 19–23.

129. Pini M, Aiello S, Manotti C, *et al.* Low molecular weight heparin versus warfarin in the prevention of recurrences after deep vein thrombosis. *Thromb Haemost* 1994; **72(2):** 191–7.

130. Pitney WR, Raphael MJ, Webb Peploe MM, Olsen EGJ. Treatment of experimental venous thrombosis with streptokinase and ancrod. *Br J Surg* 1971; **58:** 442–7.

131. Plate G, Akesson H, Einarsson E, Ohlin P, Eklof B. Long term results of venous thrombectomy combined with a temporary arterio-venous fistula. *Eur J Vasc Surg* 1990; **4:** 483–9.

132. Plate G, Einarsson E, Ohlin P, Jensen R, Clvarfordt P, Eklof B. Thrombectomy with temporary arterio-ovenous fistula. The treatment of choice in acute iliofemoral venous thrombosis. *J Vasc Surg* 1984; **1:** 867–76.

133. Plate G, Ohlin P, Eklof B. Pulmonary embolism in acute iliofemoral venous thrombosis. *Br J Surg* 1985; **72:** 912–15.

134. Poller L, Thomson JM, Yee KF. Heparin and partial thromboplastin time – an international survey. *Br J Haematol* 1980; **44:** 161–5.

135. Porter JM, Seamen AJ, Common HH, Rosch J, Eidemiller LR, Calhoun AD. Comparison of heparin and streptokinase in the treatment of venous thrombosis. *Am Surg* 1975; **41:** 511–19.

136. Prandoni P, Lensing AWA, Buller HR, *et al.* Comparison of subcutaneous low-molecular-weight heparin with intravenous standard heparin in proximal deep vein thrombosis. *Lancet* 1992; **339:** 441–5.

137. Quafordt P, Ecklof B, Ohlin P. Intramuscular pressure in the lower leg in deep vein thrombosis and phlegmasis cerulea doleus. *Ann Surg* 1983; **197:** 450–3.

138. Rahintoola SH, Raphael MJ, Pitney WR, Olsen EJG, Webb Peploe MM. Therapeutic defibrination and heparin therapy in the prevention and resolution of experimental venous thrombosis. *Circulation* 1970; **42:** 729.

139. Research Committee of the British Thoracic Society. Optimum duration of anticoagulation for deep vein thrombosis and pulmonary embolism. *Lancet* 1992; **340:** 873–6.

140. Robertson BR, Nilsson IM, Nylander G. Thrombolytic effect of streptokinase as evaluated by phlebography of deep venous thrombi of the leg. *Acta Chir Scand* 1970; **136:** 173–80.

141. Robertson BR, Nilsson IM, Nylander G. Value of streptokinase and heparin in treatment of acute deep vein thrombosis. *Acta Chir Scand* 1968; **134:** 203–8.

142. Robertson BR, Nilsson IM, Nylander G, Olow B. Effect of streptokinase and heparin on patients with deep venous thrombosis. *Acta Chir Scand* 1967; **133:** 205–15.

143. Robinson DL, Teitelbaum GP. Phlegmasia cerulea doleus, treatment by pulse spray and infusion thrombolysis. *Am J Roentgenol* 1993; **160:** 1258–90.

144. Rhodes GR, Dixon RH, Silver D. Heparin induced thrombocytopaenia with thrombotic and haemorrhagic complications. *Surg Gynecol Obstet* 1973; **136:** 409–16.

145. Salzman EW. Low-molecular-weight heparin: is small beautiful? *N Engl J Med* 1986; **315:** 957–9.

146. Salzman EW, Deykin D, Shapiro RM, Rosenberg R. Management of heparin therapy: controlled prospective trial. *N Engl J Med* 1976; **292:** 1046–50.

147. Salzman EW, Rosenberg RD, Smith MH, Lindon JN, Favreau L. Effect of heparin and heparin fractions on platelet aggregation. *J Clin Invest* 1980; **65:** 64–73.

148. Schulman S, Lockner D, Granqvist S, Bratt G, Paul C, Nyman D. A comparative randomized trial of low dose versus high dose streptokinase in deep vein thrombosis of the thigh. *Thromb Haemost* 1984; **51:** 261–5.

149. Schulman S, Rhedin AS, Lindmarker P, *et al.* A comparison of six weeks with six months of oral anticoagulant therapy after a first episode of venous thromboembolism. Duration of Anticoagulation Trial Study Group. *N Engl J Med* 1995; **332(25):** 1661–5.

150. Schuster J, Meier-Ruge W, Elgi F. Zur Pathologie der Osteopathie nach Heparinbehandlung. *Dtsch Med Wochenschr* 1969; **94:** 2334–8.

151. Schwieder G, Grimm W, Siemens HJ, *et al.* Intermittent regional therapy with rt-PA is not superior to systemic thrombolysis in deep vein thrombosis (DVT) – a German multicenter trial. *Thromb Haemost* 1995; **74(5):** 1240–3.

152. Semba CP, Dake MD. Iliofemoral deep vein thrombosis: aggressive therapy with catheter-directed thrombolysis. *Radiology* 1994; **191:** 487–94.

153. Sherry S. Tissue plasminogen activator. Will it fulfil its promise? *N Engl J Med* 1985; **313:** 1014–17.

154. Silver D, Kapsh DN, Tsoi EK. Heparin induced thrombocytopenia, thrombosis and haemorrhage. *Ann Surg* 1983; **198:** 301–6.

155. Simonneau G, Charbonnier B, Decousus H, *et al.* Subcutaneous low-molecular-weight heparin compared with continuous intravenous unfractionated

heparin in the treatment of proximal deep vein thrombosis. *Arch Intern Med* 1993; **153(13):** 1541–6.

156. Standing Advisory Committee for Haematology. Drug interaction with coumarin derived anticoagulants. *Br Med J* 1982; **285:** 274–5.

157. Stevenson R, Burton M, Ferlauto G, Taylor H. Hazards of oral anticoagulants during pregnancy. *JAMA* 1980; **243:** 1549–51.

158. Thompson EN, Hamilton M. Pulmonary embolic disease. *Lancet* 1962; **1:** 1369.

159. Towne JB, Berhard VM, Hussey C, Garancis JC. White clot syndrome peripheral vascular complications of heparin therapy. *Arch Surg* 1979; **114:** 372–7.

160. Tsapogas MJ, Peabody RA, Wis TK, Karmody AM, Devaraj KT, Eckert C. Controlled study of fibrinolytic therapy in deep vein thrombosis. *Surgery* 1973; **74:** 973–84.

161. Urokinase pulmonary embolism trial: phase I results: a cooperative study. *JAMA* 1970; **214:** 2163–72.

162. Vairel EG, Bonty-Boye H, Toulemonde F, Dontremepuich C, Marsh NA, Gaffney PJ. Heparin and low molecular weight fraction enhances thrombolysis and by this pathway exercises a protective effect against thrombosis. *Thromb Res* 1983; **30:** 219–24.

163. Van de Berg L. Venous thrombectomies and partial interruption of the vena cava in 125 cases of thrombophlebitis. *J Cardiovasc Surg* 1978; **19:** 143–50.

164. Verstraete M, Bernand R, Bory M, *et al.* Randomized trial of intravenous recombinant tissue-type plasminogen activator versus intravenous streptokinase in acute myocardial infarction. *Lancet* 1985; **1:** 842–7.

165. Verstraete M, Bleifeld W, Brower RW, *et al.* Double blind randomized trial of intravenous tissue-type plasminogen activator versus placebo in acute myocardial infarction. *Lancet* 1985; **2:** 965–69.

166. Verstraete M, Vermylen J, Amery A, Vermylen C. Thrombolytic therapy with streptokinase using a standard dosage scheme. *Br Med J* 1966; **1:** 454–6.

167. Walker MG, Shaw JW, Thomson GJL, Cumming JGR, Lea Thomas M. Subcutaneous calcium heparin versus intravenous sodium heparin in treatment of established acute deep vein thrombosis of the legs: a multicentre prospective randomised trial. *Br Med J* 1987; **294:** 1189–92.

168. Warken T, Kelton JG. Heparin induced thrombocytopenia. *Prog Haemost Thromb* 1991; **10:** 1–34.

169. Weimar W, Stibbe J, Van Seyen AJ, Billan A, de Somer P, Collen D. Specific lysis of an iliofemoral thrombus by administration of extrinsic plasminogen activator. *Lancet* 1981; **2:** 1018–20.

170. Widmer LK, Brandenberg E, Schmitt HE, *et al.* Zum Schicksal des Patienten mit tiefer Venenthrombose. *Dtsch Med Wochenschr* 1985; **110:** 993–7.

171. Widmer LK. The treatment of venous thrombosis. Angiological aspects. *Triangle* 1977; **16:** 47–61.

172. Widmer LK, Madar G, Duckert F, Müller G, Schmitt HE. Acute deep thrombophlebitis: thrombolytic versus anticoagulant therapy. *Acta Univ Carol (Mea Monogr) (Praha)* 1972; **52:** 137–42.

173. Wilson H, Britt LG. Surgical treatment of iliofemoral thrombosis. *Ann Surg* 1967; **165:** 855–9.

174. Wlodarczyk ZK, Gibson M, Dick R, Hamilton G. Low-dose intra-arterial thrombolysis in the treatment of phlegmasia caerulea dolens. *Br J Surg* 1994; **81(3):** 370–2.

175. Young AE, Lea Thomas M, Browse NL. Comparison between sequelae of surgical and medical treatment of venous thromboembolism. *Br Med J* 1974; **4:** 127–30.

CHAPTER 11

Deep vein thrombosis: prevention

Pharmacological methods of prevention	360	Commentary	371
Mechanical methods of prevention	368	References	373

Deep vein thrombosis in the lower limb causes three clinical problems:

- *symptoms* – e.g. pain, swelling and difficulty with walking
- *the post-thrombotic calf pump failure syndrome* – pain, swelling, pigmentation, dermatitis, lipo-dermatosclerosis and ulceration
- *pulmonary embolism.*

The ideal method of prophylaxis would abolish all these clinical problems by completely eliminating deep vein thrombosis. This objective cannot yet be achieved; our current methods of prophylaxis therefore fall into two categories – those that reduce the incidence of deep vein thrombosis by administering prophylaxis before the causal event and those that prevent pulmonary embolism in the presence of established thrombosis. The first approach (primary prophylaxis) should reduce the incidence of all three clinical problems caused by the thrombosis. The second approach (secondary prophylaxis) is unlikely to affect the initial symptoms or the late sequelae, but may save the patient's life.

It is often assumed that any form of prophylaxis that reduces the incidence of deep vein thrombosis will *pari passu* reduce the incidence of pulmonary embolism. This assumption is true if deep vein thrombosis is totally abolished but not necessarily true if the incidence is only reduced. As the evidence concerning the effectiveness of prophylactic regimens at preventing deep vein thrombosis is far better

than that concerning pulmonary embolism,[220] these aspects of prevention are discussed separately – deep vein thrombosis prophylaxis in this chapter and pulmonary embolism prophylaxis in Chapter 22.

The 10 years since the first edition of this book was published has witnessed the introduction of the low molecular weight heparins (which have virtually supplanted the use of unfractionated heparin for deep vein thrombosis prophylaxis), many more clinical trials especially in orthopaedic surgery, the development of the statistical techniques of meta-analysis and overview, and the prohibition of the use of the fibrinogen uptake test. Overall, these changes have not altered our basic understanding and use of prophylactic techniques but the loss of the fibrinogen uptake test has made it more difficult to conduct good quality objective clinical trials.

Because of the vast number of books and articles published on the prevention of deep vein thrombosis in the past 10 years, this chapter can only present a summary of their conclusions. Those seeking far more detailed information should refer to the many excellent reviews and monographs currently available.[27,43]

The aetiology of deep vein thrombosis was summarized by Virchow in 1856 as changes in the coagulability of the blood, changes in the blood flow and changes in the vessel wall (see Chapter 8). The two forms of prophylaxis most studied modify the first two of these factors. No method has been devised to change the vessel wall, though attempts to stimulate fibrinolysis might be construed to act in this way, and it is also claimed that the effect of dihydroergotamine may be through its direct effect on the vein wall. The pharmacological methods mainly alter blood coagulability; the mechanical methods alter blood flow.

Pharmacological methods of prevention

Many pharmacological methods of prevention have been studied but there is no doubt that anticoagulants, particularly heparin, are the most effective agents for reducing the incidence of deep vein thrombosis.

ORAL ANTICOAGULANTS

In 1959 Sevitt and Gallagher clearly established[293] that oral anticoagulation (they used phenindione) reduces the incidence of deep vein thrombosis and pulmonary embolism.

The two main groups of oral anticoagulants are the coumarins and the indanediones. Both groups work by inhibiting the role of vitamin K in the synthesis of coagulation factors II, III, IX and X, so that biologically inactive factors are produced.

The effect of oral anticoagulants is monitored by measuring the activated partial thromboplastin time or the prothrombin time. The prothrombin time is a reliable test provided standardized tissue thromboplastins are used. For effective anticoagulation, the prothrombin time (using British Standard Thromboplastin) must be between two and four times the control value. Therapeutic prothrombin times measured with Simplastin (a rabbit brain/lung thromboplastin) should be one and one-half to two times the control value.

Fractured hips

Sevitt and Gallagher studied patients with fractures of the neck of femur and showed, at autopsy, a reduction of deep vein thrombosis from 83 to 14%. Other workers[40,101,141,281] have confirmed these findings (Table 11.1). The value of oral anticoagulants in the management of hip fractures has also been confirmed with the fibrinogen uptake test by Morris and Mitchell[225,227] who found a reduction in the incidence of thrombosis from 68% to 31%.

Overall, seven studies[40,102,141,226,258,281,293] show that oral anticoagulants will reduce the incidence of deep vein thrombosis after hip fracture from an average of 36% to 12% and, incidentally the incidence of fatal pulmonary embolism from 10% almost to zero.

Hip replacement surgery

A number of studies[115,147,251] have shown that oral anticoagulants are equally valuable in preventing deep vein thrombosis after hip replacement surgery – the overall effect being a reduction of deep vein thrombosis from approximately 50% to 19%. The use of smaller doses of warfarin,[110] over a longer period pre- and postoperatively failed to reduce the incidence of thrombosis, whereas an adjusted normal dose was slightly more effective.[331] A comparison[331] of a regular dose of 2 mg warfarin daily against a higher adjusted daily dose, taken for 1 month after discharge from hospital, showed that the adjusted dose was far more effective in preventing late post-discharge thrombosis.

Knee replacement surgery

The value of warfarin during knee replacement has not been studied.

General surgery and gynaecology

There are only a few studies of the value of oral anticoagulants in gynaecological[161,305] and general surgery but almost all show a beneficial effect.[64,256]

Table 11.1   The effect of oral anticoagulants on the incidence of deep vein thrombosis and pulmonary embolism after hip fractures

	Deep vein thrombosis	Fatal embolism	Death
Sevitt and Gallagher[293] (autopsy study)			
No treatment (150 patients)	83%	10%	28%
Phenindione (150 patients)	14%	0	17%
Morris and Mitchell[225,227] (autopsy plus isotope scanning)			
No treatment (74 patients)	100%	8.5%	31%
Warfarin (74 patients)	31%	0	22%

Medical patients

There are few studies of the use of prophylactic warfarin in medical patients. Those most often studied, patients with myocardial infarction or stroke, often need full anticoagulation for other reasons. One study[241] showed warfarin to reduce the incidence of thrombosis from 38% to 5%.

Disadvantages of oral anticoagulants

The four main disadvantages of oral anticoagulants are:

- The time taken to produce an effect (2–4 days)
- The need to perform frequent measurements of the prothrombin time
- The sensitivity of the anticoagulant effect to many other drugs
- The risks of haemorrhage.

The risks of haemorrhage involve not only per-operative bleeding and wound haematomata but spontaneous retroperitoneal and intestinal intramural haemorrhage, and bleeding from gastrointestinal ulceration. It is these problems that have inhibited surgeons from using oral anticoagulation for routine prophylaxis in both general and orthopaedic surgery.[226] Nevertheless, it is important to emphasize that an effective form of prophylaxis has been available since 1959, a method proven by a variety of tests, including autopsy, to be effective against venous thrombosis and pulmonary embolism. These drugs have also been shown to reduce the overall mortality rate following hip fractures, an important fact which is discussed in Chapter 22 (page 632).

UNFRACTIONATED LOW-DOSE SUBCUTANEOUS HEPARIN (UFH)

Heparin is a sulphated polysaccharide that accelerates the serine protease neutralizing effects of antithrombin III. Antithrombin III will inhibit those activated clotting factors that have a serine residue at their enzymatically active centre – factors XII, XI, IX, X and thrombin. As the coagulation process is a mutiplying cascade, the amount of heparin required to inhibit one of the factors at the beginning of the cascade (e.g. Xa) is far less than that needed to inhibit thrombin because far less Xa is produced than thrombin. Thus it has been calculated that the inhibition of 32 units of Xa will prevent the formation of 1600 NIH units of thrombin.[336] As inactivation is on a one-to-one basis this means that only one-fiftieth of the amount of heparin required to inactivate thrombin is needed to achieve the same effect if it is given at the beginning of the cascade (at the factor Xa stage) *before* the thrombin has formed. This is the rationale for giving small doses of heparin before the coagulation process that causes a deep vein thrombosis begins. The critical word in the previous sentence is *before*. Prophylactic heparin is most effective when given before the operation, before the illness or before the accident; only the first situation is practical.

Low molecular weight heparin and heparin analogues are said to have a greater inhibitory effect on factor Xa than on thrombin.[8]

In 1950 de Takats[91] suggested that a low dose of heparin given before an operation might prevent thrombosis. Sharnoff[294–296] treated a large number of patients in this way, and claimed a reduction in the incidence of fatal pulmonary embolism. Unfortunately he had no control patients and used no objective evaluation of the incidence of thrombosis in the limbs.

Scientific assessment of the value of low doses of heparin given subcutaneously quickly followed the introduction and validation of the fibrinogen uptake test in 1968. Many studies on the value of low-dose heparin have since been published.[25,27]

General surgery

Heparin started at least 2 hours before an operation, and continued in doses of 5000 units 12-hourly or 8-hourly, significantly reduces the incidence of postoperative radioactive fibrinogen detectable calf vein thrombi in general surgical patients. An arithmetical compilation of 24 studies (published between 1971 and 1980) on 4932 patients undergoing general surgical operations who were each given 5000 units heparin 12-hourly or 8-hourly and three major overviews published in 1988[61,76,202] all show that heparin reduces the incidence of deep vein thrombosis from around 30% to 9% (Table 11.2).

Table 11.2 The effect of subcutaneous unfractionated heparin on the incidence of deep vein thrombosis following general surgical operations – a compilation of 24 studies* on 4932 patients

No heparin	30%
Heparin (5000 units, subcutaneous, 8- or 12-hourly)	9%

*References 9–11,32,52,57,65,79,122,123,132,136,138,166,171, 176,181,184,192,237,255,264,269,270,275,300,307,309,329,334

There is little difference between the clinical effects of sodium and calcium heparin or between the effects of 8-hourly and 12-hourly administration; most surgeons therefore prefer a 12-hourly regimen.

It is important to note that these regimens do not *abolish* thrombosis. In all studies of all forms of prophylaxis there remains a stubborn 5–8% of patients whose thrombi cannot be prevented.

Urology

At least nine trials[32,72,183,239,275,283,292,319,329] have shown that UFH reduces, in the region of 40% to 20%, the incidence of deep vein thrombosis after general urological operations. The incidence of thrombosis after transurethral resection is much lower[239] than that following open prostatectomy but UFH still has a worthwhile effect.

Gynaecology

Six controlled trials[14,41,66,68,154,305] have shown that UFH can reduce the incidence of deep vein thrombosis after gynaecological surgery from 19% to 8%.

Prophylaxis with any from of anticoagulant is rarely used in obstetric practice. Warfarin is contranidicated in pregnancy so when necessary most obstetricians use a low dose of unfractionated or low molecular weight heparin.

Hip fracture

A number of studies[30,60,119,123,171,222,225,228,273,304,335] have shown that UFH will reduce the incidence of deep vein thrombosis after hip fracture but because the incidence when not prevented is so high – 50%+ – and the reduction only to 30%, the patient is still at considerable risk. Even this effect is only achieved when the heparin is begun soon after the fracture, something that is often difficult to achieve. Most orthopaedic surgeons therefore consider that UFH gives an inadequate level of protection.

Hip replacement surgery

A similar or sometimes better reduction of the incidence of deep vein thrombosis by UFH has been observed after hip replacement surgery[22,187] and this effect can be improved by adjusting the dose of the heparin[200,306] but the incidence of thrombosis in those receiving heparin is still high (29%) (Table 11.3). The reasons for the failure of UFH to work effectively in hip fracture and hip replacement are not clear but may be related to the severity of the trauma and to local vein wall damage. Attempts to adjust the dose of UFH[107] reduced the incidence of thrombosis but increased the incidence of bleeding.

Table 11.3 The effect of subcutaneous unfractionated heparin on the incidence of deep vein thrombosis following elective hip operations – a compilation of 11 studies* on 979 patients

No heparin	50%
Heparin (5000 units, subcutaneous, 8- or 12-hourly)	19%

*References 30,87,89,90,142,207,209,224,228,280,320

Medical patients

A few studies have examined the value of low-dose subcutaneous UFH in patients with myocardial infarction.[97,143,324] One study[143] showed no effect but two others[97,324] showed a reduction of the incidence of deep vein thrombosis from around 20% to 5%.

Similarly, three studies of general medical patients[24,54,140] showed an overall reduction of thrombosis from 25% to 9% and one study of 81 patients with stroke[82] showed that heparin reduced the incidence of thrombosis from 48% to 24%. The effect of UFH on the mortality rate of medical patients is not known. Gardland[125] compared 5776 patients given 12-hourly subcutaneous UFH until discharged from hospital or for 3 weeks with 5917 untreated patients. There were eight autopsy-proven fatal emboli at 30 days in the treated group and 13 in the untreated group. At 60 days fatal emboli had occurred in 15 and 16, respectively. Though not a blind trial with possibly an inadequate dose of UFH, this study highlights the need for more research on the effect of heparin on embolism.

Comment

Phlebographic evidence suggests that heparin is less effective at preventing axial vein than calf vein thrombosis.[32] Unfortunately, some of the studies supporting the opposite view, that heparin has a better effect on proximal thrombi, have been based upon the fibrinogen uptake test which is not accurate above mid-thigh level and are consequently misleading.

Low-dose subcutaneous UFH prophylaxis should be continued while the patient is still at risk of developing a thrombosis (i.e. during continuing bedrest and any debilitating postoperative complications). Once the patient is eating and walking normally, most surgeons stop the heparin, although there is a well documented incidence of late, even post-discharge thrombosis.[328]

There is no doubt that low-dose subcutaneous heparin increases the incidence of bleeding complications.[250] The most common complications are bruising and wound haematomata. It is generally assumed that these are unimportant but if they cause an increase in the incidence of wound infection and incisional hernia, then they should be taken into account. Some studies have shown an increase in blood transfusion requirements and operative blood loss but these increases have not always been statistically significant.

The clinical problems caused by bleeding are also related to the nature of the operation. Orthopaedic surgery and open prostatectomy are operations which are bound to cause bleeding but the blood loss rarely causes problems. On the other hand, minor blood loss in ophthalmic or spinal surgery, or bleeding beneath a skin graft can destroy the effect of the operation; any prophylactic regimen that increases the bleeding tendency should therefore be avoided with operations where a small amount of bleeding can cause serious harm. The 8-hourly regimen is generally reported to cause more bleeding than the 12-hourly regimen.[310]

Thrombocytopenia is a well-known complication of intravenous heparin administration[130,288] but it may occasionally occur with low-dose subcutaneous prophylaxis if the initial platelet count is low or if the prophylaxis is continued for a long period. It is advisable to request a platelet count and test platelet function if heparin is given for more than 10 days.

Heparin and dihydroergotamine (DHE)

Dihydroergotamine (DHE) increases the tone of the peripheral veins by stimulating the α-adrenergic receptors and the smooth muscle cells directly. It therefore increases the velocity of venous blood flow by reducing the diameter of the veins but in some patients it also reduces the arterial blood flow. The effect on venous blood flow might be antithrombotic in itself and might increase the effect of the heparin or reduce the dose requirement.

Studies of the effect of dihydroergotamine alone have shown no effect on postoperative calf vein thrombosis but when it was combined with heparin the prophylactic effect of the heparin was enhanced. An arithmetical compilation of four studies[175,180,182,299] on 728 general surgical patients comparing heparin alone (5000 units, 12-hourly) with heparin plus dihydroergotamine (5000 units + 0.5 mg, 12-hourly) showed an incidence of thrombosis of 10% and 6%, respectively. As the number of patients in these trials is relatively small, this difference is not statistically significant; all the studies do, however, show the same trend.

A multicentre study[230] of the effect of heparin alone, two doses of heparin plus DHE, DHE alone, and a placebo suggest that 5000 units heparin plus 0.5 mg DHE given subcutaneously 2 hours preoperatively, and 12-hourly for 5–7 days, was superior to the other combinations, but the incidence of deep vein thrombosis in the 'DHE 5000 heparin' was no less than the 9% incidence seen in the majority of the other published studies of subcutaneous alone.

In three series[175,280,289] of 390 patients undergoing elective hip surgery, the overall incidence of thrombosis in the control and treated groups was 23% and 10%, respectively; this difference approaches statistical significance. It is possible that the greater effect in orthopaedic patients was related to the higher incidence of axial vein thrombosis in these patients and the possibility that dihydroergotamine increases blood flow more effectively in the axial veins than the calf veins.

Unfortunately, this promising combination of a thrombotic agent and a venomotor agent has had to be withdrawn from the market because of complications such as angina,[262] vasospasm and renal failure.[211] Cases of peripheral gangrene have been reported, the presentation being similar to ergotism.[96,318] *DHE should no longer be used.*

Intravenous unfractionated heparin

Negus[236] has shown that the administration of a minute quantity of heparin intravenously (1 unit/kg/hour) can reduce the incidence of deep vein thrombosis to the same extent as subcutaneous heparin. In a controlled study of 100 patients, the incidence of isotopically diagnosed thrombi in the control group was 22% whereas the incidence in the test group was 4.3%. There was no difference between the effect of intravenous heparin given for 5–7 days and the effect of intravenous heparin given for 2 days followed by 5 days of subcutaneous heparin, but the incidence of wound haematomata in the patients given only intravenous heparin was 2% whereas the incidence of thrombosis in patients given subcutaneous heparin for 5 days after receiving 2 days of intravenous heparin was 7.5%. These studies are interesting because the dose of heparin is so small that the blood levels are not measurable. It is not known whether the mechanism of action is through the inhibition of factor Xa.

SUBCUTANEOUS LOW MOLECULAR WEIGHT HEPARIN (LMWH)

Although low molecular weight heparin (LMWH) has almost replaced standard unfractionated heparin (UFH) as the drug of choice for the prevention of deep vein thrombosis, the previous section on unfractionaed heparin has been retained in this edition because it is this research that proved that heparin given subcutaneously in low doses was an effective prophylactic agent. Chapter 22 highlights the difficulties that exist in wholeheartedly accepting that low doses of unfractionated heparin really do reduce the incidence of postoperative pulmonary embolism but most clinicians are sufficiently convinced to the extent that they do not believe trials of any new variety of heparin against an untreated control group would be ethical. Consequently, all the studies of the new LMWHs compare their effect against another form of prophylaxis, usually UFH, and concentrate on the incidence of deep vein thrombosis, because this reduces the size of the trial to manageable proportions. *There are therefore no trials of the effect of LMWHs against no treatment to enable us to say unequivocally that they do reduce the incidence of pulmonary embolism.* Our belief that they reduce the incidence of deep vein thrombosis is based on the knowledge that they are as effective as UFH and we know UFH works. All current studies show that LMWHs have the same effect as UFH, and so much of the preference for LMWH resides in the convenience of its daily, as opposed to UFH's thrice daily, rate of administration.

What are low molecular weight heparins?

Heparin is a simple but long chain of disaccharide units, all of which contain glucosamine and uronic acid. It exerts its main anticoagulant activity via the plasma protein – antithrombin III. In the mid 1970s,[8,167] it was noticed that low molecular weight fractions made from standard heparin by gel filtration had an anticoagulant profile different from that of unfractionated heparin. Further studies showed that these fractions of heparin might have a similar effect on deep vein thrombosis as standard heparin with the possible added benefit of a reduced risk of bleeding complications.[15,106] As long as the molecular weight distributions are similar (4000–6500 Da), the method of production appears to have little significance[249] and so there are a number of different preparations available, each with confusingly different trade names. The activity of LMWHs is measured in anti-xa and anti-Xa units. The ratio of these

two activities for UFH is 1:1, the ratio for LMWHs varies from 4:1 to 2:1, i.e. LMWHs have a reduced ability to catalyse the inactivation of thrombin relative to their ability to inhibit factor Xa. This ratio is now usual compared to an international reference standard with a specific activity of 168 anti-Xa units/mg and 68 anti-IIa units/mg.[17,21,185,210,322]

In addition to these anticoagulant properties, LMWHs have three valuable pharmacodynamic advantages over UFH:

- Almost 100% of the active substance is absorbed following subcutaneous injection
- Their biological half-life is longer than that of UFH
- The anticoagulant response to weight adjusted doses is less variable.[33,195,212,321]

The actual doses recommended by the manufacturers depend upon the anti-Xa and anti-IIa activity of each specific product. Some recommend different doses for moderate and high risk patients. For example, the dose of enoxaparin recommended for medium-risk patients is 20 mg (providing 2000 anti-Xa units) daily but for high-risk patients such as those undergoing hip replacement the recommended dose is 40 mg.[321] It is essential, therefore, to take particular note of the manufacturer's instructions.[284]

General surgery

In one placebo controlled trial,[247] Dalteparin significantly reduced the incidence of deep vein thrombosis in general surgical patients from 15.9% to 4.2%. The unusual feature of this trial in the low incidence of thrombosis is the untreated group.

All the other reliable trials of the LMWHs compare them with other forms of prophylaxis – principally unfractionated heparin. A selection of these trials is listed.[1,14,16,18,26–28,31,35,36,41,55,56,63,83,84,118,149,174,179,188,195,246,284] The effect of LMWHs on deep vein thrombosis following general surgical operations is summed up in Table 11.4. These figures are based upon the trials mentioned above and the meta-analysis published by Nurmohamed and colleagues in 1992.[245] Almost every trial obtained similar results. The incidence of deep vein thrombosis in

Table 11.4 The effect of LMWHs on the incidence of postoperative deep vein thrombosis following major general surgical operations based on a meta-analysis by Nurmohamed *et al.*[245] of 17 trials on 6878 patients

	Deep vein thrombosis	Major bleeding
Unfractionated heparin s.c. 5000 IU 8- or 12-hourly starting preoperatively	6.7%	2.6%
Low molecular weight heparin manufacturer's recommended dose	5.3%	2.6%

patients given 5000 IU UFH, 8- or 12-hourly, beginning preoperatively was 6–7%. This incidence is similar to that found in the older trials of the 1960s and 1970s, shown in Table 11.2, of 9%. The effect of the LMWHs was identical, a thrombosis incidence between 5 and 6% (Table 11.4).

Although there are variations between the many trials that have been performed, it is noticeable that the higher the scientific quality of the trial the more likely it is to find UFH and LMWH having the same effect.

All the studies included in Nurmohamed's meta-analysis used the fibrinogen uptake test for diagnosis. This may not reveal the full picture. Bounameaux[44] performed an ascending phlebogram 8 days after operation, having given half his patients a low dose (2500 anti-Xa units of Dalteparin) and half a high dose (3075 anti-Xa units Nadroparin) of LMWH and found a 31% and 18% incidence of thrombosis, respectively. He concluded that both regimens failed. Studies such as this are reminiscent of the occasional older studies that failed to show the expected effect of UFH.

It is quite clear that neither UFH or LMWH completely abolishes the incidence of postoperative deep vein thrombosis. They will not therefore completely abolish pulmonary embolism and there is no reason to believe that the relative reduction of embolism will be of the same magnitude as the reduction of deep vein thrombosis. More research and better drugs are needed. There is no cause for complacency.

Urological and gynaecological surgery

The effect of subcutaneous LMWHs on the incidence of deep vein thrombosis following gynaecological operations has not been extensively studied but appears to be similar to that of UFH.[164,317] Many of the studies referred to in the general surgery section above deal with abdominal surgery and consequently include procedures such as hysterectomy.

The same comment applies to major urological surgery such as nephrectomy and prostatectomy. Specialists in these subjects, having established the efficacy of UFH and accepting the many studies

that show LMWHs are as effective as UFH in general surgery, are content to extrapolate those results to their own specialties without performing new specific speciality trials. This is a justifiable and acceptable approach.

Comments
The last 10 years have seen the introduction of many less invasive techniques into surgical practice such as laparoscopic cholesystectomy, laparoscopic vaginal hysterectomy, percutaneous nephrolithotomy and the endovascular grafting of aortic aneurysms. The reduction of trauma tends to outweigh the extended length of these procedures but most are likely to be associated with a lower incidence of deep vein thrombosis. Nevertheless, the risk persists and the majority of surgeons still give full prophylaxis patients being treated by these new methods.

Orthopaedic surgery

The incidence of deep vein thrombosis after major orthopaedic surgery on the hip or knee is higher than that following abdominal surgery. Estimates range for hip surgery from 54 to 45%[22,121,163,189,316] and for knee surgery from 80 to 40%.[208,243,301–303]

These thrombi develop not only in the calf veins but in the superficial and common femoral veins and it is thrombi from these latter sites that become fatal emboli. Unfortunately, UFH does not cause the same reduction of calf vein thrombosis in orthopaedic patients as it does in general surgical patients and has still less effect on axial vein thrombi.

The advent of LMWHs raised the hope that they would be more effective in orthopaedic patients and many studies have been performed. A selection is included in the references.[88,99,103,153,169,193,197,198,200,248,254]

Hip surgery
Nurmohamed's[245] meta-analysis of the best six of these orthopaedic hip surgery trials which include both elective and traumatic hip operations[16,88,99,103,200,254] shows (Table 11.5) that LMWHs are a little more effective than UFH but still leave the patient with a 14% risk of developing a thrombosis. This is clearly better than an untreated risk

Table 11.5 The effect of LMWHs on the incidence of postoperative deep vein thrombosis following elective or traumatic hip surgery, based upon a meta-analysis by Nurmohamed *et al.*[245] of 6 trials on 1294 patients

	Deep vein thrombosis	Major bleeding
Unfractionated heparin s.c. 5000 IU 8- or 12-hourly starting preoperatively	21%	1.3%
Low molecular weight heparin manufacturer's recommended dose	14%	0.9%

of 50% but nowhere near the 5% that can be achieved in general surgical patients.

Although some of these studies include both traumatic and elective cases, it appears that the effect of LMWHs is the same in both groups provided it is started before the operation. The trauma, followed by an operation, for a fractured neck of femur, is clearly greater and more thrombogenic than the trauma of the fracture itself. One study[197] has shown that when the heparins are started after the operation, they have little effect. Some of these studies[127,248] have shown LMWHs to have some effect on the axial vein thrombosis associated with hip replacement. Planes[254] showed that within an overall reduction of deep vein thrombosis (comparing LMWHs with UFH) of 25% to 12.5%, the incidence of axial vein thrombosis fell from 18.5% to 7.5%. But this degree of major vein thrombosis still leaves a significant risk and patients are still dying from pulmonary embolism in spite of receiving adequate prophylactic doses of LMWHs. When the same investigators[253] looked at the rate of thrombosis after discharge from hospital in two groups of patients, one given placebo and the other a LMWH, they found that amongst the 179 patients who had no phlebographic evidence of thrombosis at the time of discharge, 23 had phlebographically proven thrombi in their legs 21 days later, 17 (19%) in the placebo group and six (7%) in the LMWH group. The incidence of distal thrombi was 11% and 1%, respectively, but the incidence of axial vein thrombi was equal (8% and 6%). Thus, the risk of axial vein thrombosis continues for at least 3 weeks after operating and this risk is not reduced by the normal in-hospital administration of LMWH, whereas distal thrombosis is. This difference is probably related to damage in the axial veins the effect of which may well last longer than the simple post-surgical hypercoagulability which causes thrombosis in the distal veins.

Because LMWHs are more effective than UFH in preventing deep vein thrombosis after elective hip surgery, it has been calculated[95] that their use, though expensive in themselves, would save approximately £20 per patient – a saving brought about by the reduced frequency of injections and the fewer thromboembolic complications needing treatment.

Knee replacement surgery
There are very few studies of the effect of LMWHs on the incidence of deep vein thrombosis after knee surgery. As this area of surgery is rapidly expanding, this deficiency needs to be addressed. The reported incidence of deep vein thrombosis after knee replacement as assessed in five studies by phlebography between the fourth and eleventh day varied from 25% to 70%, four studies being in the 60–70% range.[157,177,301,303,332]

This thrombosis usually begins in the calf vein but extends into the popliteal and femoral veins in 10–20%.[115,157,208] Isolated femoral vein thrombosis is rare.

Thrombus propagating out of the calf into the axial veins is a potential lethal embolus. McKenna[216] found positive lung scans in 12 patients who had had knee replacements and positive scans in six of 10 patients with thrombus that had propagated into the popliteal vein. The risk of pulmonary embolism after knee replacement surgery is high, and the reported low incidence[223,301] of fatal embolism must be viewed with caution – there may be few deaths but there are probably many unrecognized non-fatal emboli.

Leclerc[193] compared 41 patients given LMWH with 54 patients given placebo. The incidence of deep vein thrombosis was 19.5% and 64.8%, respectively. No patient died. One patient in the placebo group had a pulmonary embolism and the incidence of major bleeding was 6% and 7%, respectively. Thus LMWHs have a significant effect but 20% of patients remain unprotected.

Trauma

Thromboembolism is a common complication of major trauma. Geerts[126] showed that 70% of 349 patients developed deep vein thrombosis after major injuries. Injuries to the chest and abdomen are associated with a incidence of deep vein thrombosis of 50–60%, this increases to 60–70% with injuries of the spine, pelvis and lower limbs.[186] Proximal deep vein thrombosis in these two categories of patients is approximately 15% and 25%, respectively.

The reduction of deep vein thrombosis after hip fractures is discussed above. There are few studies of the value of LMWHs after other forms of trauma but studies of acute spinal cord injury[133,135] have shown that LMWHs reduce the incidence of deep vein thrombosis from 60–70% to very low levels. The studies are small and need repeating and expanding.

Many cases of trauma are associated with haemorrhage and the clinician will always be faced with a choice between using an effective thrombophylactic agent which might cause further bleeding, such as a LMWH, and a mechanical method of thrombophylaxis which does not cause bleeding.

Medical patients and children

The incidence of deep vein thrombosis in patients in medical wards is extremely variable because these patients have many variable risk factors and multiple diseases. Without prophylaxis the incidence ranges between 15% and 35% – a similar range to that seen in general surgical patients – and many studies have shown that LMWHs reduce this incidence to 7–10%.[24,83,120,145]

The incidence of deep vein thrombosis after a major stroke is higher than that seen in general medical patients – between 50 and 70%. UFH reduces this incidence to 15–20%[82,214,215] and LMWHs have a similar effect.[260,286,314,315] This still leaves stroke patients at significant risk,[323,324] presumably mainly because of their immobility.

Deep vein thrombosis in children is rare[274] and prophylaxis is not indicated.

NEW THROMBOPHYLACTIC DRUGS

Drugs other than heparin and its subfractions affect the coagulation cascade and some may prove useful for deep vein thrombosis prophylaxis. Hirudin derivatives and dermatan sulphate have both been shown to reduce the incidence of postoperative deep vein thrombosis to a similar degree as that achieved by UFH and LMWH. They have not replaced heparin but their effect is encouraging researchers to seek similar but more effective agents.[99,129,259]

DEXTRAN

Dextran 70 or dextran 40, dissolved in 5% dextrose and given intravenously, has an antithrombotic effect by expanding blood volume, coating the formed elements of the blood so preventing their interaction with any damaged areas of vessel wall, inactivating factor VIII and polymerizing with fibrin to make a soft degradable thrombus.[234]

The dose of dextran is usually 500 ml given during the operation, 500 ml given during the next 24 hours and a further 500 ml given the following day.

General surgery

In most controlled studies of deep vein thrombosis after general surgery using the fibrinogen uptake test[3,168] for diagnosis, dextran has had little or no effect.[25]

Bergqvist[25,32] reviewed 16 trials on a total of 1707 patients in which the fibrinogen uptake test was used to diagnose deep vein thrombosis and found an incidence of 26% in the control group and 20% in the treated group. However, some of these and other studies indicated a possible reduction in the

incidence of pulmonary embolism.[205] The reasons for this finding are discussed in Chapter 22. As there are no controlled studies of the effect of dextran on fatal embolism in general surgical patients, and as subcutaneous heparin administration has become so much easier with the introduction of low molecular weight heparin, dextran is rarely used in general surgical patients.

Gynaecology

A similar situation applies to gynaecological surgery. There are studies[39,41,154,213] which have demonstrated the effectiveness of dextran after gynaecological surgery but its use has been superseded by LMWHs.

Orthopaedic surgery

The situation concerning the value of dextran following elective or emergency hip surgery is a little less clear because of the possible worthwhile effect on pulmonary embolism. Nevertheless, all trials[3,30,86,87,105,116,168,190,232,244,298,325] show a persistent high incidence of thrombosis in spite of the administration of dextran and it has been superseded by the LMWHs.

Dextran has three adverse side-effects. It may overload the circulation and precipitate heart failure; it should therefore be used with caution in the elderly and is contraindicated in many patients with medical cardiac conditions. It prolongs the bleeding time[81] but none of the clinical studies of its use reports an increase of bleeding complications. It causes anaphylactoid reactions;[261] this is its most serious complication because these reactions can be fatal. However, a fatal reaction probably occurs in less than 0.008% of infusions and in less than 0.01% of patients.[267,290] This problem can be overcome by the preliminary infusion of dextran 1 (molecular weight = 1000) which acts as a hapten and blocks the formation of immune complex.[137,266] In a review of 30 000 patients who were given hapten (dextran 1) before dextran 70, serious immune reactions occurred in 0.0001%.[218]

Anaphylaxis should be treated by intravenous hydrocortisone (100 mg), subcutaneous adrenaline (0.5 ml; 1:1000) and antihistamines.

ASPIRIN

Aspirin prolongs the bleeding time by inhibiting the ability of platelets to adhere to collagen and to each other. Acetylsalicylic acid inhibits the synthesis of endoperoxides and thromboxane A2 from the arachidonic acid in platelet membranes by acetylating the platelet enzyme cyclo-oxygenase which catalyses the oxidation of the arachidonic acid to endoperoxide PGG_2.

The principal effect of aspirin is on the platelets but there is also an effect on prostacyclin production by the vein wall. These two effects are dose dependent, and there is still controversy over the correct therapeutic dose of aspirin. A low dose reduces platelet aggregation by reducing thromboxane A2 production from the platelets; a high dose inhibits the endothelial cell production of PGI_2 which inhibits platelet aggregation, thus its effect may be thrombogenic.

The doses in the published studies of the value of aspirin as a prophylactic agent vary from 450 mg/day to 4000 mg/day. This makes comparisons difficult. In an attempt to decide whether aspirin was of value the Antiplatelet Trialists Collaboration Group performed an overview of 53 trials (8400 patients) on general surgical or orthopaedic patients, nine trials (600 patients) on other categories of immobility and 18 trials (1000 patients) which compared two different antiplatelet regimens.[12] They concluded that aspirin seems to reduce the average risk of deep vein thrombosis from 34% to 25% and the incidence of pulmonary embolism from 2.7% to 1%. However, the authors themselves point out the tremendous variations of dose and duration of administration. There appeared to be a marginally greater risk of bleeding in those receiving aspirin.

Our view of these studies is that the value of aspirin remains unproven. It causes gastrointestinal complications, might affect bleeding and must be begun well before any surgical intervention. On the other hand, it is easy to take, particularly in the long term after an operation. It may find a place as an adjunct to the more effective prophylactic agents such as LMWHs.

OTHER PLATELET INHIBITING DRUGS

Dipyridamole, sulphinpyrazone, hydroxychloroquine, flurbiprofen and ticlopidine have been studied, and none has had a worthwhile effect on deep vein thrombosis.

There are a few studies of the combination of aspirin with dipyridamole which show a significant effect but an equal number of studies that do not. If the conclusions of the overview of the effect of aspirin on deep vein thrombosis are correct then other antiplatelet drugs may be more effective than we think but, as with aspirin, they will not replace LMWHs.

STIMULATION OF FIBRINOLYSIS

Venous thrombosis is often associated with a reduction of blood and vein wall fibrinolytic activity.[19,162] Attempts to reduce the incidence of thrombosis by stimulating fibrinolysis have failed,[13,47,112] probably for two reasons. First, the few active drugs which will do this take 2–3 weeks to have an effect. Secondly, though resting blood fibrinolytic activity is increased, the fibrinolytic shutdown in response to surgery is not prevented.

Mechanical methods of prevention

Surgeons have long believed that early ambulation after an operation prevents venous thrombosis. Unfortunately, early ambulation often means sitting out of bed in a chair, a state which would better be described as 'early stagnation'.

There have been no controlled studies of early ambulation but a number of uncontrolled studies suggest that it is beneficial.[108,194,235,312] Early ambulation is a worthwhile form of physiotherapy for many other reasons and should therefore always be encouraged.

LEG ELEVATION

Elevating the legs during an operation increases the velocity of venous blood flow but does not decrease the incidence of fibrinogen detectable thrombi.[50,276] Nevertheless, it is still a common, and probably sensible, practice to increase venous velocity by elevating the foot of the bed of patients with venous disease and swelling of the lower limb.

ELASTIC COMPRESSION

One of the earliest studies of elastic stockings, based upon clinical diagnosis in a large group of patients, indicated that elastic compression might have a worthwhile effect on the incidence of thrombosis and embolism,[327] but when the fibrinogen uptake test became available the studies of the stockings and bandages then available failed to show that they had a beneficial effect.[50,277] However, better stockings were developed which produced a compression of 20 mmHg at the ankle, gradually reducing along the length of the leg. This pressure is sufficient to produce venous compression and an increased velocity of blood flow *when the patient is supine*, without affecting arterial inflow. These stockings have also been carefully designed so that their tops do not become constriction bands around the thighs.

General surgery and gynaecology

A number of studies of modern anti-thromboembolism stockings have shown that they have a significant effect. An arithmetical compilation of nine studies on 1505 patients shows that stockings reduce the incidence of thrombosis from 19% to 8% (Table 11.6). The untreated incidence in this group of patients is low; nevertheless, even when it is higher, e.g. 31%, stockings can still reduce the incidence to 11%.[165] When the untreated incidence is low, as in gynaecological surgery, stockings seem to be even more effective with thrombosis rates being reduced from 5% to 0.[313] The length of the stocking does not alter its effect on the incidence of thrombosis. A comparison of below-knee and thigh-length stockings[257] has shown no difference in their effect on either calf or thigh vein thrombosis.

Table 11.6 The effect of graduated compression stockings on the incidence of deep vein thrombosis following general abdominal operations based upon a compilation of 9 studies* on 1505 patients

No compression	19%
Graduated compression stockings	8%

*References 4,37,155,163,217,291,313,326,330

Similar reductions in thrombosis rates have been reported for neurosurgery[315] and urology.[144] Although the compresssion profiles of different makes of stocking are not identical, this does not seem to alter their effectiveness significantly.[330]

A meta-analysis by Wells[326] concludes that when graduated compression stockings are used in surgical patients they reduce the risk of thrombosis by 68%.

Orthopaedic surgery

The majority of the studies of the value of graduated compression stockings in orthopaedic patients are comparisons between stockings and other mechanical methods. Overall, they tend to show that stockings are less effective in these patients with incidences reduced from 54% to 20% and 46% to 30%,[116,163] with little effect on the above-knee

axial vein thrombosis that causes so much concern with hip surgery.

Medical patients

Graduated compression stockings are often prescribed for patients with medical illnesses but evidence of their effect on thrombosis is lacking.

The modern stocking is comfortable to wear and can be used throughout the patient's stay in hospital. It has no adverse effects other than when a tight stocking is applied to a leg with a poor circulation[242] and therefore can and should be used as a routine part of the prophylaxis regimen of all patients over the age of 40 years, and in all patients (whatever their age) who have a history of previous deep vein thrombosis.

PNEUMATIC COMPRESSION

The logical extension of the elastic stocking is a pneumatic compression device that squeezes the leg intermittently, preferably in a graduated, sequential manner, from ankle to groin. The first devices were simple single chamber leggings; the most modern devices have many chambers which can be inflated sequentially to different pressures.

The obvious effect of pneumatic compression is to accelerate venous blood flow.[297] This effect is closely related to the rapidity and duration of the compression.[271,278] Those devices which do not produce a large increase in venous velocity but still reduce the incidence of thrombosis may work by emptying the blood from the valve cusps (the site of origin of thrombi), or by stimulating the release of fibrinolytic activator from the endothelium.[4,178,268] We could not confirm this last suggestion in an unpublished study on 50 patients, and another more recent detailed investigation also suggests that it does not occur.[204]

Two forms of compression have been developed – a rapid short (square wave) compression for 10 seconds at 50 mmHg followed by a rest for 60 seconds,[279] and a slowly applied (sine wave) compression taking 30 seconds to reach a pressure of 50 mmHg followed by a slow reduction with no pressure applied for 60 seconds.[152] There have been a number of studies of the effect of these different forms of compression on both venous and capillary blood flow. The rapid compression devices have the greatest effect on the velocity of femoral vein blood flow but there is little difference in the clinical effect on calf vein thrombosis of the two types of compression. Some devices have many chambers and produce sequential compression.[238] The slowly compressing single chamber device is the cheapest.

Table 11.7 The effect of intermittent pneumatic compression on the incidence of deep vein thrombosis following general surgical operations – a compilation of 12 studies* on 1900 patients

No pneumatic compression	26%
Intermittent pneumatic compression	10%

*References 49,52,57,65,72,152,165,178,269,270,279,307

General surgery

An arithmetical compilation of 12 trials which studied 1900 patients (Table 11.7) showed that intermittent pneumatic compression reduces the incidence of deep vein thrombosis in general surgical patients from the region of 26% to approximately 10%. This effect has been confirmed by an overview.[74] Although this is clearly a worthwhile reduction, the residual incidence is still higher than that associated with LMWH's unprotected residue of 5–7%.

Urology

Two studies[72,144,283] have shown that pneumatic compression has a similar effect on patients undergoing urological operations with the incidence of thrombosis being reduced to 6–7%.

Gynaecological surgery

Results similar to those above have been reported in patients undergoing gynaecological surgery,[41,67,69] together with evidence that the effect is appreciably greater if the pneumatic compression is continued for 5 days after operation, not just for 24 hours.

Orthopaedic surgery

Hip operations
There are surprisingly few data about the value of pneumatic compression in preventing deep vein thrombosis after hip operations for trauma but there are many publications on its value in elective hip surgery. Four good studies[124,148,160,251] of more than 300 patients record an overall incidence of deep vein thrombosis in untreated patients in the region of 45% against an incidence of 23% in the treated group. It has also been shown that pneumatic compression reduces the incidence of axial vein as well as calf vein thrombosis.[333]

Knee replacement
Studies which have used mixtures of mechanical methods of prophylaxis, but include pneumatic compression,[139,157,216,252] have shown that pneumatic compression can reduce the high incidence of thrombosis after knee replacement from >60% to the region of 20%.

Medical patients

We have not found any studies of the use of this form of prophylaxis in medical patients.

Comment

A plastic pneumatic legging, even with an absorbant stocking between it and the skin, can be uncomfortable to wear. This may account for the low compliance and improper use reported in some studies.[77] Nevertheless, it is a simple and relatively cheap device and easily combined with graduated compression stockings and/or heparin or warfarin.[251]

There are other forms of compression. Two studies[45,111] of foot compression, which only increases the velocity of venous blood flow, have shown this technique to be of value.

ELECTRICAL STIMULATION OF THE CALF MUSCLES

Contractions of the calf muscle not only eject venous blood from the calf but also increase venous blood flow indirectly because they cause an exercise hyperaemia.[93]

A number of studies have been performed to test the effect of electrically induced calf muscle contractions on fibrinogen detectable thrombi in the calf.[20,51,94,240] The variations of method, especially the frequency and strength of the muscle contractions induced, make it unacceptable to consider the results as a single group but the largest studies with similar protocols show a significant reduction of thrombosis from approximately 25% to 12%.

The disadvantage of electrical stimulation is that it can only be applied to the anaesthetized patient because the stimulus, even when applied gradually rather than as a square wave, is uncomfortable and sometimes painful. In the studies mentioned above, the stimulus was applied only during anaesthesia and there was a significant effect. It is, however, well established that many postoperative thrombi begin 2 or 3 days after the operation and therefore electrical stimulation is unlikely to be as effective as methods which can be used after an operation when the patient is conscious.

Other methods

The incidence of thrombosis has been shown to be reduced by, for example, the use of a mechanical foot pedal[272] and by a patient-driven pedalling machine[219] – perhaps the best way of getting the patient to exercise after an operation.

Commentary

This chapter has been limited to a discussion of methods for preventing deep vein thrombosis. In surgical patients the main objective of preventing deep vein thrombosis is the prevention of pulmonary embolism, any reduction of the incidence of late thrombotic sequelae being an extra benefit.

There are, however, many patients in whom the prevention of deep vein thrombosis is especially a worthwhile end in its own right. These are the patients who are put to bed for long periods to help cure the complications of their venous disease. Patients with venous ulcers often need long periods of bedrest. If the ulcer is the result of previous deep vein thrombosis, the risk of a further thrombosis during the period of bedrest is high. Another thrombosis will add to the calf pump dysfunction and greatly increase the likelihood of recurrent ulceration. These patients should be given an effective form of prophylaxis from the moment they enter hospital. There is no doubt that subcutaneous low molecular weight heparin is the most efficient and safe method for preventing deep vein thrombosis in patients not having an operation. None of the other pharmacological methods approaches its effectiveness, and mechanical methods, even elastic stockings, are often unsuitable for limbs with venous disease and ulcers.

Mechanical methods are suitable for all other categories of patient. As a result of the logistic problems of giving injections of subcutaneous heparin to all patients in hospital, the simplest solution is to use the modern graduated anti-thromboembolism stocking. Although stockings will not have as great an effect on the incidence of thrombosis as subcutaneous heparin, their effect will be worthwhile. Stockings may also help to prevent those thrombi that begin as a result of admission to hospital, before operation.[151]

A note of caution

Whether any of these methods reduces the incidence of pulmonary embolism or the post-thrombotic syndrome is a question discussed in Chapters 15 and 22.

When these methods of prophylaxis are being used to prevent pulmonary embolism, the arguments for and against them must be based on the published evidence of their effect on the incidence of embolism, not on their effect on deep vein thrombosis. It is also important to consider the use of prophylactic agents in the light of current knowledge of the incidence of thromboembolism. The incidence of thromboembolism appears to have diminished over the past 20 years,[92] not because of the use of prophylaxis but because of other unknown factors.[5,156,203] Does this reduced incidence mean that prophylactic methods will be more effective or that those thrombi that do occur are those that are more resistant to our current methods of prevention?

With the increasing use of prophylaxis our knowledge of the natural incidence of thrombosis and its natural history will gradually diminish as will our knowledge of whether we are using prophylaxis necessarily or unnecessarily. It is essential to keep the situation under constant review using the most accurate diagnostic methods available.

Prediction of risk (Table 11.8)

A number of workers have measured every conceivable coagulation factor preoperatively in an attempt to predict those patients at risk and thus avoid giving a prophylactic drug to those not at risk[263] (see Chapter 8). Crandon et al. produced a complex risk index which has been shown in a prospective study to be accurate.[53,70,80] Lowe produced a simplified index.[206] Both these studies showed that the levels of fibrinogen and fibrinolysis are the most useful blood tests for predicting thrombosis (not the coagulation factors), and other investigators have confirmed this. The laboratory tests required to calculate these indices are, however, complex and time consuming, and this approach has not been generally adopted. Nevertheless, it is the logical way to approach the problem and, if simpler tests can be devised,[150] it may become generally applicable.

Table 11.8 Two methods for calculating the risk of developing a postoperative deep vein thrombosis

---

Crandon et al. 1980[70,71,80]
Index = $-11.3 + 0.009 \times$ (ELT) + 0.22 × (FRAs) + 0.085 × (Age) + 0.043 × (% overweight) + 2.19 × (VVs)
Lowe et al. 1982[206]
Index = Age + 1.3 × (% weight)

ELT, Euglobulin lysis time; FRA, fibrin related antigen; Age, years; % overweight, % overweight for height; VVs, varicose veins (present = 1, absent = 0); Weight, as % mean population weight for age, sex and height

In recent years our knowledge of the coagulation cascade has grown. Many abnormalities which produce an hypercoagulable state such as antithrombin III, protein C and protein S deficiencies, dysfibrinogenaemia, disorders of plasminogen and plasminogen activation, antiphospholipid antibodies and lupus anticoagulant and hyperviscosity syndromes have been described.[287] In a small number of patients these abnormalities undoubtedly predispose towards the development of deep vein thrombosis and embolism. They are rarely sought for or detected by routine screening tests but tend to be detected when investigating the problem of a recurrent thromboembolism. A careful record of the family history is an important simple way of detecting these high risk patients.[7]

The current use of prophylactic regimens

Knowledge of the value of oral anticoagulants has existed for 40 years. The effectiveness of subcutaneous heparin was established over 20 years ago, at the same time as the value of elastic and pneumatic compression was described, yet the use of these methods varies from surgeon to surgeon, country to country and between specialties.[6,23,58,109,191] Most surveys reveal that 30–40% of surgeons do not routinely use some form of prophylaxis. Often this non-usage occurs when there is a heavy workload of surgical emergencies, sometimes when surgeons become disillusioned when they see fatal emboli occurring in patients who have been given theoretically adequate prophylaxis.[128]

The scientific evidence that deep vein thrombosis can be significantly reduced is overwhelming. All doctors, physicians as well as surgeons, should take one of two approaches: the blanket approach – give all patients some form of prophylaxis; or the individual approach – consider each patient separately before deciding what to do. That may mean no prophylaxis for the 30-year-old having a hernia repaired under local anaesthesia as a day case,[265] but will mean that a clear decision is made for each patient and recorded in the patient's records. This approach should apply as much to medical patients as surgical patients.[308] One decision that has previously not received much attention is the duration of the prophylaxis. The standard practice is to give the prophylaxis whilst the patient is confined to bed or partly immobile, yet a number of studies have described thrombosis and embolism many days after discharge from hospital and return to full mobility.[2,328] Careful long-term follow-up studies are needed to determine which patients should be given long-term rather than short-term prophylaxis.

SUMMARY

This chapter has attempted to give an overview of the many publications which describe the prevention of deep vein thrombosis. Those with a special

Table 11.9 The clinical application of pharmacological and mechanical methods for preventing deep vein thrombosis

Type of patient	Risk of thrombosis (%)	Recommended prophylaxis
Minor general surgery (<30 min)	Low (0–5%)	GCS
Patients under 40 years old General surgery (>30 min)	Moderate (10–30%)	sLMWHs or IPC ± GCS

Patients over 40 years old
Patients less than 40 years old on contraceptive pill
General surgery in patients with
    Malignant disease
 	
    History of thromboembolism
	High (40–60%)	sLMWHs + GCS or oral anticoagulants

Orthopaedic surgery on hip, knee and spine	High (50–60%)	sLMWHs + IPC or oral anticoagulants
Multiple trauma	High (50%)	sLMWHs
Stroke	High (40%)	sLMWHs
Myocardial infarction	Moderate (25%)	sLMWHs
Immobile patients with active medical disease	Low (0–5%)	GCS

GCS, Graduated compression stockings; IPC, intermittent pneumatic compression; sLMWHs, subcutaneous low molecular weight heparin interest in this subject must read the many overviews and analyses that have been published,[59,62,63,73,76,78,131,158,197,221,245,282] taking particular note of those that assess the risks,[26,27,43] and form their own opinion.

In the first edition we classified patients into those at risk from thromboembolism and those at risk from bleeding.[48] This approach remains valid, although the risk of bleeding from subcutaneous low molecular weight heparin is sufficiently small that it is only of concern in particular patients undergoing delicate neurosurgical or plastic surgical procedures.

Fortunately, intermittent pneumatic compression (whose effect is almost equal to that of LMWH) can always be used when bleeding might jeopodize the result of an operation.

Table 11.9 summarizes the information currently available. The data has been rounded up to simple numbers; the recommendations are very similar to those of the first edition[48] and those of the 1991 European Consensus meeting.[104] A choice is always given between a heparin derivative and a mechanical method to allow the bleeding risk to be considered. Oral anticoagulation with warfarin, i.e. full anticoagulation, must always remain as the fall-back prophylaxis for those in whom the risk is life threatening.

References

1. Adolf J, Knee H, Roder JD, van de Fierdt E, Siewert JR. Thromboembolieprophylaxe mit niedermolekularem Heparin in der Abdominalchirurgie. *Dtsch Med Wochenschr* 1989; **114:** 48–53.
2. Agnelli G, Ranucci V, Verchi F, Rinonapoli E, Lupathlelli P, Nenci GG. Clinical outcome of orthopaedic patients with negative lower limb venography at discharge. *Thromb Haemost* 1995; **74:** 1042–4.
3. Ahlberg A, Nylander G, Robertson B, Cronberg S, Nilsson IM. Dextran in prophylaxis of thrombosis in fractures of the hip. *Acta Chir Scand Suppl* 1968; **387:** 83.
4. Allenby F, Boardman L, Pflug JJ, Calnan JS. Effects of external pneumatic intermittent compression on fibrinolysis in man. *Lancet* 1973; **2:** 412.
5. Anderson FA, Wheeler HB, Goldberg RJ, *et al.* A population-based perspective of the hospital incidence and case-fatality rates of deep vein thrombosis and pulmonary embolism. *Arch Intern Med* 1991; **151:** 933–8.
6. Anderson FA, Wheeler HB, Goldberg RJ, Gent M. Physician practices in the prevention of venous thromboembolism. *Ann Intern Med* 1991; **115:** 591–5.
7. Anderson FA, Wheeler HB, Goldberg R, Hosmer D, Forcier A. The prevalence or risk factors for venous thromboembolism among hospital patients. *Ann Intern Med* 1992; **152:** 1660–4.
8. Anderson LO, Barrowcliffe TW, Holmer E, Johnson EA, Sims GEC. Anticoagulant properties of heparin fractionated by affinity chromatography on matrix bound antithrombin III and by gel filtration. *Thromb Res* 1976; **9:** 573.
9. Anon. Heparin versus dextran in the prevention of deep-vein thrombosis. A multi-unit controlled trial. *Lancet* 1974; **2:** 118–20.
10. Anon. Prevention of fatal postoperative pulmonary embolism by low doses of heparin. An international multicentre trial. *Lancet* 1975; **2:** 45–51.
11. Ansay J, Fastres R, Kutnowski M, Kraytman M. Prevention des thromboses veineuses profondes post-opératoires par l'héparine souscutanée a faible doses. *Ann Chir* 1977; **31:** 263.
12. Antiplatelet Trialists' Collaboration. Collaborative overview of randomized trials of antiplatelet therapy III. Reduction in venous thrombosis and pulmonary embolism by antiplatelet prophylaxis among surgical and medical patients. *Br Med J* 1994; **308:** 235–46.
13. Atkins P, Brown IK, Downie RJ, *et al.* The value of phenformin and ethyloestrenol in the prevention of deep venous thrombosis in patients undergoing surgery. *Thromb Haemost* 1978; **39:** 89.
14. Ballard M, Bradley-Watson PJ, Johnstone ED, *et al.* Low doses of subcutaneous heparin in the prevention of deep venous thrombosis after gynaecologic surgery. *J Obstet Gynaecol Br Commonw* 1973; **80:** 469.
15. Bang CJ, Berstad A, Talstad I. Haemorrhagic effects of unfractionated and two low molecular weight heparins, enoxaparin and Fragmin in rats. *Haemostasis* 1991; **21:** 30–6
16. Barre J, Pfister G, Potron G, *et al.* Efficacité et tolérance comparées du Kabi 2165 et de l'héparine standard dans la prévention des thromboses veineuses profondes au cours de prothèses totale de hanche. *J Mal Vasc* 1987; **12:** 90–5.
17. Barrowcliffe TW, Curtis AD, Johnson EA, Thomas DP. An international standard for low molecular weight heparin. *Thromb Haemost* 1988; **60:** 1–7.
18. Baumgartner A, Jacot N, Moser G, Krähenbühl B. Prevention of postoperative deep vein thrombosis by one daily injection of low molecular weight heparin and dihydroergotamine. *Vasa* 1989; **18:** 152–6.
19. Becker J. Fibrinolytic activity of the blood and its relation to postoperative venous thrombosis of the lower limbs. A clinical study. *Acta Chir Scand* 1972; **138:** 787.
20. Becker J, Schampi B. The incidence of postoperative venous thrombosis of the legs. A comparative study on the prophylactic effect of dextran 70 and electrical calf-muscle stimulation. *Acta Chir Scand* 1973; **139:** 357.
21. Beguin S, Lindhout T, Hemker HC. The mode of action of heparin in plasma. *Thromb Haemost* 1989; **60:** 457–62.

22. Beisaw NE, Comerota A, Groth HE, *et al.* Dihydroergotamine/heparin in the prevention of deep vein thrombosis after total hip replacement. *J Bone Joint Surg (Am)* 1988; **70:** 2.

23. Belcaro G, Laurora G, D'Alterio A, *et al.* An Italian survery on the prophylaxis of venous thromboembolism. *Phlebology* 1992; **7:** 71–4.

24. Belch JJ, Lowe GDO, Ward AG. Prevention of deep vein thrombosis in medical patients by low dose heparin. *Scott Med J* 1981; **26:** 115.

25. Bergqvist D. *Postoperative Thromboembolism.* Berlin: Springer-Verlag, 1983; 98.

26. Bergqvist D. Review of clinical trials of low molecular weight heparins. *Acta Chir Scand* 1992; **158:** 67.

27. Bergqvist D, ed. *Prevention of Venous Thromboembolism.* London: Med Orion, 1994.

28. Bergqvist D, Burmark US, Flordal PA, *et al.* Low molecular weight heparin started before surgery as prophylaxis against deep vein thrombosis 2500 versus 5080 Xa units in 2070 patients. *Br J Surg* 1995; **82:** 496–501.

29. Bergqvist D, Burmark US, Frisell J, *et al.* Low molecular weight heparin once daily compared with conventional low dose heparin twice daily. *Br J Surg* 1986; **73:** 204.

30. Bergqvist D, Efsing HO, Hallbook T, Hedlund T. Thromboembolism after elective and posttraumatic hip surgery – a controlled prophylactic trial with dextran and low-dose heparin. *Acta Chir Scand* 1979; **145:** 213.

31. Bergqvist D, Flordal PA, Friberg B, Frisell J, Hedberg M, Ljungstrom KG. Thromboprophylaxis with a low molecular weight heparin (tinzaparin) in emergency abdominal surgery. *Vasa* 1996; **25:** 156–60.

32. Bergqvist D, Hallbook T. Prophylaxis of postoperative venous thrombosis in a controlled trial comparing dextran 70 and low-dose heparin. A study with the ^{125}I-fibrinogen test. *World J Surg* 1980; **4:** 239.

33. Bergqvist D, Hedner U, Sjorin E, Holmer E. Anticoagulant effects of two types of low molecular weight heparin administered subcutaneously. *Thromb Res* 1983; **381:** 91.

34. Bergqvist D, Lindblad B, Matzsch T. Low molecular weight heparin for thromboprophylaxis and epidural/spinal anaesthesia – is there a risk? *Acta Anaesth Scand* 1992; **36:** 605–9.

35. Bergqvist D, Lowe GD, Berstad A, *et al.* Prevention of venous thromboembolism after surgery: a review of enoxaparin. *Br J Surg* 1992; **79:** 495–8.

36. Blum A, Desruennes E, Elias A, Lagrange G, Loriferne JF. DVT prophylaxis for digestive tract cancer comparing the LMW heparinoid oRG 10172 (Lomoparan) with calcium heparin (abstr). *Thromb Haemost* 1989; **62:** 126.

37. Bolton FJ. The prevention of post-operative deep venous thrombosis by graduated compression stockings. *Scott Med J* 1978; **23:** 333.

38. Boneu B. An international multicentre study: Clivarin ® in the prevention of venous thromboembolism in patients undergoing general surgery. Report of the International Clivarin ® Assessment Group. *Blood Coag Fibrinolysis* 1993; **4(Suppl 1):** S21–2.

39. Bonnar J, Walsh JJ, Haddon M, *et al.* Coagulation system changes induced by pelvic surgery and the effect of dextran 70. *Bibl Anat* 1973; **12:** 351.

40. Borgstrom S, Greitz T, van der Linden W, Molin J, Rudics I. Anticoagulant prophylaxis of venous thrombosis in patients with fractured neck of the femur. A controlled clinical trial using venous phlebography. *Acta Chir Scand* 1965; **129:** 500.

41. Borow M, Goldson H. Postoperative venous thrombosis: evaluation of five methods of treatment. *Am J Surg* 1981; **141:** 245.

42. Borris LC, Lasseu MR. Orthopaedic surgery. In: Hull R, Raskob G, Pineo G, eds. *Venous Thromboembolism: an Evidence-based Atlas.* Armonk, NY: Futura Publishing Co, 1996; 53–62.

43. Bounameaux H. Low molecular weight heparin in prophylaxis and therapy of thromboembolic disease. New York: Marcel Dekker, 1994.

44. Bounameaux H, Huber O, Khabiri E, Schneider PA, Didier D, Rohner A. Unexpected high rate of phlebographic deep vein thrombosis following elective abdominal surgery among patients given prophylaxis with low molecular weight heparin. *Arch Surg* 1993; **128:** 326–8.

45. Bradley JG, Krugener GH, Jager HJ. The effectiveness of intermittent plantar venous compression in prevention of deep venous thrombosis after total hip arthroplasty. *J Arthroplasty* 1993; **8:** 57–61.

46. Briel RC. Low dose heparin prophylaxis and post operative wound haematoma. *Int Surg* 1983; **68:** 241.

47. Brown IK, Downie RJ, Haggart B, *et al.* Pharmacological stimulation of fibrinolytic activity in the surgical patient. *Lancet* 1971; **1:** 774.

48. Browse NL. Personal views on published facts. *Ann R Coll Surg Engl* 1977; **59:** 138.

49. Browse NL, Clemenson G, Bateman NT, Gaunt JI, Croft DN. Effect of intravenous dextran 70 and pneumatic leg compression on incidence of postoperative pulmonary embolism. *Br Med J* 1976; **2:** 1281.

50. Browse NL, Jackson BT, Mayo ME, Negus D. The value of mechanical methods of preventing postoperative calf vein thrombosis. *Br J Surg* 1974; **61:** 219.

51. Browse NL, Negus D. Prevention of postoperative leg vein thrombosis by electrical muscle stimulation. An evaluation with ^{125}I-labelled fibrinogen. *Br Med J* 1970; **3:** 615.

52. Butson R. Intermittent pneumatic calf compression for prevention of deep venous thrombosis in general abdominal surgery. *Am J Surg* 1981; **142:** 525.

53. Butterman G, Haluszcynski I, Theisenger W, Pabst HW. Postoperative thromboembolie-prophylaxe mit reduziertem low-doseHeparin-Anteil und Dihydroergotamin in fixer Kombination. *MMW* 1981; **123:** 1213.

54. Cade JH. High risk of the critically ill for venous thromboembolism. *Crit Care Med* 1982; **10:** 448.

55. Cade J, Gallus A, Ockelford P, Magnani H. Org 10172 or heparin for preventing venous thrombosis

(VT) after surgery for malignant disease? A double blind multi-centre comparison (abstr). *Thromb Haemost* 1989; **62:** 42.

56. Caen JP. A randomized double-blind study between a low molecular weight heparin Kabi 2165 and standard heparin in the prevention of deep vein thrombosis in general surgery. *Thromb Haemost* 1988; **59:** 216–19.

57. Calnan JS, Allenby F. The prevention of deep vein thrombosis after surgery. *Br J Anaesth* 1975; **47:** 151.

58. Campbell WB, Ridler BMF. Varicose vein surgery and deep vein thrombosis. *Br J Surg* 1995; **82:** 1494–7.

59. Carter C, Gent M, Leclerc JR. The epidemiology of venous thrombosis. In: Coleman RW, Hirsh J, Marder VJ, *et al.*, eds. *Hemostasis and Thrombosis.* Philadelphia, PA: JB Lippincott, 1987; 1185–98.

60. Checketts RG, Bradley JG. Low dose heparin in femoral neck fractures. *Injury* 1974; **6:** 42.

61. Clagett GP. Overview of prevention of venous thromboembolism. In: Hull R, Raskob G, Pineo G, eds. *Venous Thromboembolism: an Evidence-based Atlas.* Armonk, NY: Futura Publishing Co, 1996; 37–43.

62. Clagett GP, Anderson FA, Levine MN, Salxman EW, Wheeler HB. Prevention of venous thromboembolism. *Chest* 1992; **102:** 319S–407S.

63. Clagett GP, Reisch JS. Prevention of venous thromboembolism in general surgical patients. Results of a meta analysis. *Ann Surg* 1988; **208:** 227.

64. Clagett GP, Salzman E. Prevention of venous thromboembolism. *Prog Cardiovasc Dis* 1975; **17:** 345.

65. Clark WB, MacGregor ILB, Prescott RJ, Ruckley CV. Pneumatic compression of the calf and postoperative deep vein thrombosis. *Lancet* 1974; **2:** 5.

66. Clarke-Pearson DL, Coleman RE, Synan IS, *et al.* Venous thromboembolism prophylaxis in gynecologic oncology: a prospective controlled trial of low dose heparin. *Am J Obstet Gynecol* 1983; **145:** 606.

67. Clarke-Pearson DL, Creasman WT, Coleman RE, *et al.* Perioperative external pneumatic calf compression as thromboembolism prophylaxis in gynecologic oncology: report of a randomised controlled trial. *Gynecol Oncol* 1984; **18:** 226.

68. Clarke-Pearson DL, DeLong ER, Synan IS, *et al.* A controlled trial of two low dose heparin regimens for the prevention of deep vein thrombosis. *Obstet Gynecol* 1990; **75:** 684.

69. Clarke-Pearson DL, Synan IS, Hinshaw WM, Coleman RE, Creasman WT. Prevention of postoperative venous thromboembolism by external pneumatic calf compression in patients with gynaecologic malignancy. *Surg Gynecol Obstet* 1984; **63:** 92.

70. Clayton JK, Anderson JA, McNicol GP. Preoperative prediction of postoperative deep vein thrombosis. *Br Med J* 1976; **2:** 910.

71. Clayton JK, Crandon AJ, Peel KR, McNicol GP. Postoperative deep vein thrombosis prophylaxis in high risk patients. *Thromb Haemost* 1979; **42:** 260.

72. Coe N, Collins R, Klein L, *et al.* Prevention of deep vein thrombosis in urological patients. A controlled, randomized trial of low-dose heparin and external pneumatic compression boots. *Surgery* 1978; **83:** 230.

73. Cohen AT, Skinner JA, Kakkar VV. Antiplatelet treatment for thromboprophylaxis: a step forward or backwards. *Br Med J* 1994; **309:** 1213–17.

74. Colditz GA, Tuden RL, Oster G. Rates of venous thrombosis after general surgery: combined results of randomised clinical trials. *Lancet* 1986; **2:** 143.

75. Coleridge-Smith PD. European workshop on the prevention of thromboembolism. *Phlebology* 1992; **7:** 45–6.

76. Collins R, Scrimgeour A, Yusuf S, *et al.* Reduction in fatal pulmonary embolism and venous thrombosis by perioperative administration of subcutaneous heparin. *N Engl J Med* 1988; **318:** 1162.

77. Comerota AJ, Katz ML, White JV. Why does prophylaxis with external pneumatic compression for deep vein thrombosis fail? *Am J Surg* 1992; **164:** 265–8.

78. Coon WW. Epidemiology of venous thromboembolism. *Ann Surg* 1977; **186:** 149–64.

79. Covey TH, Sherman L, Baue AK. Low-dose heparin in postoperative patients. A prospective coded study. *Arch Surg* 1975; **110:** 1021.

80. Cranden AJ, Peel KR, Anderson JA, Thompson V, McNicol GP. Prophylaxis of postoperative deep vein thrombosis. Selective use of low dose heparin in high risk patients. *Br Med J* 1980; **2:** 345.

81. Cronberg S, Robertson B, Nilsson IM, Nilehn J-E. Suppressive effect of dextran on platelet adhesiveness. *Thromb Diath Haemorrh* 1966; **16:** 384.

82. Czechanowski B, Heinrich F. Prophylaxe venöser Thrombosen bei frischem ischaemischem zerebrovaskulariën Indult. *Dtsch Med Wochenschr* 1981; **106:** 1254.

83. Dahan R, Houlbert D, Caulin C, *et al.* Prevention of deep vein thrombosis in elderly medical inpatients by a low-molecular weight heparin: a randomised double-blind trial. *Haemostasis* 1986; **16:** 159–60.

84. Dahan M, Levasseur PH, Bogaty J, Boneu B, Samama M. Prevention of post-operative deep vein thrombosis (DVT) in malignant patients by Fraxiparine (a low molecular weight heparin). A cooperative trial (abstr). *Thromb Haemost* 1989; **62:** 519.

85. Daniel WJ, Moore AR, Flanc C. Prophylaxis of deep vein thrombosis (DVT) with dextran 70 in patients with a fractured neck of the femur. *Aust N Z J Surg* 1972; **41:** 289.

86. Darke SG. Ilio-femoral venous thrombosis after operations of the hip – a prospective controlled trial using dextran 70. *J Bone Joint Surg (Br)* 1972; **54:** 615.

87. Dechavanne M, Saudin F, Viala J-J, Kher A, Bertrix L, de Mourgues G. Prevention des thromboses veineuses. Succes de l'heparine a fortes doses lors des coxerthroses. *Nouv Presse Med* 1974; **3:** 1317.

88. Dechavanne M, Ville D, Berruyer M, *et al.* Randomized trial of a low molecular weight heparin (Kabi 2165) versus adjusted dose subcutaneous standard heparin in the prophylaxis of deep vein thrombosis after elective hip surgery. *Haemostasis* 1989; **1:** 5–12.

89. Dechavanne M, Ville D, Viala J-J, Kher A, Fairre J, Pousset MB, Dejour H. Controlled trial of platelet anti-aggregating agents and subcutaneous heparin in prevention of postoperative deep vein thrombosis in high risk patients. *Haemostasis* 1975; **4:** 94.

90. De Mourgues F, Pagnier F, Clermont N, Yille D, Moyen B. Etude de l'efficacité de l'héparine sous-cutanée utilisée selon deux protocoles dans la prévention de la thromboge veineuse post-opérative après prothise totale de hanche. *Rev Chir Orthop* 1979; **65(Suppl 2):** 74–6.

91. de Takats G. Anticoagulants in surgery. *JAMA* 1950; **142:** 527.

92. Dismuke SE, Wagner EH. Pulmonary embolism as a cause of death: the changing mortality in hospitalized patients. *JAMA* 1986; **255:** 2039–42.

93. Doran FSA, Drury M, Sivyer A. A simple way to combat the venous stasis which occurs in the lower limb during surgical operations. *Br J Surg* 1964; **51:** 486.

94. Doran FSA, White HM. A demonstration that the risk of postoperative deep vein thrombosis is reduced by stimulating the calf muscles electrically during operation. *Br J Surg* 1967; **54:** 686.

95. Drummond A, Amitides M, Davies L, Forbes C. Economic evaluation of standard heparin and enoxaparin for prophylaxis against deep vein thrombosis in elective hip surgery. *Br J Surg* 1994; **81:** 1742–6.

96. Echterhoff HM, Kottmann UR, O'Koye XR, Rohner HG. Ergotismus: Eine wichtige Komplikation in der medikamentosen Thromboembolieprophylaxe. *Dtsch Med Wochenschr* 1981; **106:** 1717.

97. Emmerson PA, Marks P. Preventing thromboembolism after myocardial infarction: effect of low dose heparin or smoking. *Br Med J* 1977; **1:** 18.

98. Encke A, Breddin K. Comparison of a low molecular weight and unfractionated heparin for the prevention of deep vein thrombosis in patients undergoing abdominal surgery. *Br J Surg* 1988; **75:** 1058–63.

99. Eriksson B, Ekman S, Kalebo P, Zachrisson B, Bach D, Close P. Prevention of deep vein thrombosis after total hip replacement, direct thrombin inhibition with recombinant hirudin. CGP 39393. *Lancet* 1996; **347:** 635–9.

100. Eriksson BI, Eriksson E, Wadenvik H, Tengborn L, Risberg B. Comparison of low molecular weight heparin and unfractionated heparin in prophylaxis of deep vein thrombosis and pulmonary embolism in total hip replacement (abstr). *Thromb Haemost* 1989; **62:** 470.

101. Eskeland G. Prevention of venous thrombosis and pulmonary embolism in injured patients. *Lancet* 1962; **1:** 1035.

102. Eskeland G, Solheim K, Skjörten F. Anticoagulant prophylaxis, thromboembolism and mortality in elderly patients with hip fractures. A controlled clinical trial. *Acta Chir Scand* 1966; **131:** 16–29.

103. Estoppey D, Hochreiter J, Breyer HG, *et al.* Org 10172 (Lomparan) versus heparin-DHE in prevention of thromboembolism in total hip replacement – a multicentre trial (abstr). *Thromb Haemost* 1989; **62:** 356.

104. European Consensus Statement. Prevention of venous thromboembolism. *Int Angiol* 1992; **11(3):** 151–9.

105. Evarts CM, Feil EJ. Prevention of thromboembolic disease after elective surgery of the hip. *J Bone Joint Surg (Am)* 1971; **53:** 1271–80.

106. Fareed J, Walenga JM, Hoppensteadt D, Huan X, Racanelli A. Comparative study on the in vitro and the in vivo activities of seven low-molecular weight heparins. *Haemostasis* 1988; **18 (Suppl 3):** 3–15.

107. Feller JA, Parkin JD, Phillips GW, Hannon PJ, Hennessy O, Higgins RM. Prophylaxis against venous thrombosis after hip arthroplasty. *Aust N Z J Surg* 1992; **62;** 606–10.

108. Flanc C, Kakkar VV, Clarke M. Postoperative deep vein thrombosis. Effect of intensive prophylaxis. *Lancet* 1969; **1:** 75.

109. Fletcher JP, Koatts J, Ockelford PA. Deep vein thrombosis prophylaxis: a survey of current practice in Australia and New Zealand. *Aust N Z J Surg* 1992; **62:** 601–5.

110. Fordyce MJ, Baker AS, Stadden G. Efficacy of fixed minidose warfarin prophylaxis in total hip replacement. *Br Med J* 1991; **303:** 219–20.

111. Fordyce MJ, Ling RSM. A venous foot pump reduced thrombosis after total hip replacement. *J Bone Joint Surg (Br)* 1992; **74:** 45–9.

112. Fossard DP, Field ES, Kakkar VV, Friend JR, Corrigan TP, Flute PT. Fibrinolytic activity and postoperative deep-vein thrombosis. *Lancet* 1974; **1:** 9.

113. Francis CW, Marder VJ, Evarts CM, *et al.* Two-step warfarin therapy. *JAMA* 1983; **249:** 374.

114. Francis CW, Marder VJ, McCollister E, Yaukoolbodi S. Two step warfarin therapy. Prevention of postoperative venous thrombosis without excessive bleeding. *JAMA* 1983; **249:** 374.

115. Francis CW, Pellegrini VD, Marder VJ, *et al.* Prevention of venous thrombosis after total hip replacement. *J Bone Joint Surg (Am)* 1989; **71:** 327.

116. Fredin H, Bergqvist D, Cerderholm C, Lindblad B, Nyman U. Thrombopraphylaxis in hip arthroplasty, dextran with graded compression or perioperative dextran compared in 150 patients. *Acta Orthop Scand* 1989; **60:** 678–81.

117. Fredin HO, Rosverg B, Arborelius Jr M, Nylander G. On thromboembolism after total hip replacement in epidural analgesia: a controlled study of dextran 70 and low-dose heparin combined with dihydroergotamine. *Br J Surg* 1984; **71:** 58–60.

118. Fricker JP, Vergnes Y, Schach R, *et al.* Low dose heparin versus low molecular weight heparin (Kabi 2165, Fragmin) in the prophylaxis of thromboembolic complications of abdominal oncological surgery. *Eur J Clin Invest* 1988; **18:** 561–7.

119. Galasko CSB, Edwards DH, Fearn CBD'A, Barber HM. The value of low dosage heparin for the prophylaxis of thromboembolism in patients with transcervical and intertrochanteric femoral fractures. *Acta Orthop Scand* 1976; **47:** 276.

120. Gallus AS. Medical patients. In: Hull R, Raskob G, Pineo G, eds. *Venous Thromboembolism: an Evidence-based Atlas.* Armonk, NY: Futura Publishing, 1996; Chapter 8.

121. Gallus A, Cade J, Ockelford P, *et al.* (ANZ-Organon Investigators' Group). Orgaran (Org 10172) or heparin for preventing venous thromboembolism after elective surgery for malignant disease? A double-blind, randomised multicentre comparison. *Thromb Haemost* 1993; **70(4):** 562–7.

122. Gallus AS, Hirsh J, O'Brien S, McBride J, Tuttle R, Gent M. Prevention of venous thrombosis with small, subcutaneous doses of heparin. *JAMA* 1976; **235:** 1980.

123. Gallus AS, Hirsh J, Tuttle R, *et al.* Small subcutaneous doses of heparin in prevention of venous thrombosis. *N Engl J Med* 1973; **288:** 545.

124. Gallus A, Raman K, Darby T. Venous thrombosis after elective hip replacement – the influence of preventive intermittent calf compression and of surgical technique. *Br J Surg* 1983; **70:** 17–19.

125. Gardlund B. Randomised controlled trial of low dose heparin for prevention of fatal pulmonary embolism in patients with infectious disease. *Lancet* 1996; **347:** 1357–61.

126. Geerts WH, Code KJ, Jay RM, *et al.* A prospective study of venous thromboembolism after major trauma. *N Engl J Med* 1994; **331:** 1601–6.

127. German Hip Arthroplasty Trial Group. Prevention of deep vein thrombosis with low molecular weight heparin in patients undergoing total hip replacement. *Arch Orthop Trauma Surg* 1992; **111:** 110–20.

128. Gilliei TE, Ruckley CV, Nixon SJ. Still missing the boat with fatal pulmonary embolism. *Br J Surg* 1996; **83:** 1394–5.

129. Ginsberg JS, Nurmohamed MT, Gent M, *et al.* Use of Hirulog in the prevention of venous thrombosis after major hip or knee surgery. *Circulation* 1994; **90:** 2385–9.

130. Godal HC. Report of the international committee on thrombosis and haemostasis. Thrombocytopenia and heparin. *Thromb Haemost* 1980; **43:** 222.

131. Goldhaber SZ, Savage DD, Garrison RJ, *et al.* Risk factors for pulmonary embolism: the Framlington study. *Am J Med* 1983; **74:** 1023–8.

132. Gordon-Smith IC, Grundy DJ, Le Quesne LP, Newcombe JF, Bramble FJ. Controlled trial of two regimens of subcutaneous heparin in prevention of postoperative deep-vein thrombosis. *Lancet* 1972; **1:** 1134.

133. Green D. Prophylaxis of thromboembolism in spinal cord-injured patients. *Chest* 1992; **102:** 649S–51S.

134. Green D, Hirsh J, Heit J, Prins M, Davidson B, Lensing AWA. Low molecular weight heparin: a critical; analysis of clinical trials. *Pharmacol Rev* 1994; **46:** 89–109.

135. Green D, Lee MY, Lim AC, *et al.* Prevention of thromboembolism after spinal cord injury using low-molecular-weight heparin. *Ann Intern Med* 1990; **113:** 571–4.

136. Groote Schunr Hospital Thromboembolus Study Group. Failure of low-dose heparin to prevent significant thromboembolic complications in high-risk surgical patients. Interim report of a prospective trial. *Br Med J* 1979; **1:** 1447.

137. Gruber UF, Allemann U, Gerber H, Wettler H. Erster direkter Vergleich der allergischen Nebenwirkungen des Dextrans mit und ohne Hapten. *Schweiz Med Wochenschr* 1982; **112:** 605.

138. Gruber UF, Fridrich R, Duckert F, Torhorst J, Rem J. Prevention of postoperative thromboembolism by dextran 40, low-doses of heparin, or xantinol nicotinate. *Lancet* 1977; **1:** 207.

139. Haas SB, Insall JN, Scuderi GR, Windsor RE, Ghelman B. Pneumatic sequential-compression boots compared with aspirin prophylaxis of deep-vein thrombosis after total knee arthroplasty. *J Bone Joint Surg (Am)* 1990; **72:** 27–31.

140. Halkin H, Goldberg J, Nodan M, *et al.* Reduction of mortality in general medical inpatients by low dose heparin prophylaxis. *Ann Intern Med* 1982; **96:** 561.

141. Hamilton HW, Crawford JS, Gardiner JH, Wiley AM. Venous thrombosis in patients with fracture of the upper end of the femur – a phlebographic study of the effect of prophylactic anticoagulation. *J Bone Joint Surg (Br)* 1970; **52:** 268–89.

142. Hampson WG, Harris FC, Lucas HK, *et al.* Failure of low-dose heparin to prevent deep-vein thrombosis after hip replacement arthroplasty. *Lancet* 1974; **2:** 795.

143. Handley AJ. Low dose heparin after myocardial infarction. *Lancet* 1972; **2:** 623.

144. Hansberry KL, Thompson IM, Bauman J, Deppe S, Rodriguez FR. A prospective comparison of thromboembolic stockings, external sequential pneumatic compression stockings and heparin sodium/dihydroergotamine mesylate for the prevention of thromboembolic complications in urological surgery. *J Urol* 1991; **145(6):** 1205–8.

145. Harenberg J, Kallenbach B, Martin U, *et al.* Randomized controlled study of heparin and low molecular weight heparin for prevention of deep-vein thrombosis in medical patients. *Thromb Res* 1990; **59:** 639–50.

146. Harris WH, Athanasoulis C, Waltman AC, *et al.* High and low dose aspirin prophylaxis against venous thromboembolic disease in total hip replacement. *J Bone Joint Surg (Am)* 1982; **64:** 63.

147. Harris WH, Salzman EW, Athanasoulis C, *et al.* Comparison of warfarin, low-molecular-weight dextran, aspirin, and subcutaneous heparin in prevention of venous thromboembolism following total hip replacement. *J Bone Joint Surg (Am)* 1974; **56:** 1552–62.

148. Harris WH, Salzman EW, Athanasoulis C, *et al.* Aspirin prophylaxis of venous thromboembolism after total hip replacement. *N Engl J Med* 1977; **297:** 1246.

149. Hartl P, Brücke P, Dienstl E, Vinazzer H. Prophylaxis of thromboembolism in general surgery: comparison between standard heparin and Fragmin. *Thromb Res* 1990; **57:** 577–84.

150. Heather B, Jennings S, Greenhalgh R. The saline dilution test – a preoperative predictor of DVT. *Br J Surg* 1980; **67:** 63.

151. Heatley RV, Hughes LE, Morgan A. Pre- or post-operative deep vein thrombosis. *Lancet* 1976; **1:** 437.

152. Hills NH, Pflug JJ, Jeyasingh K, Boardman L, Calnan JS. Prevention of deep vein thrombosis by intermittent pneumatic compression of calf. *Br Med J* 1972; **1:** 131.

153. Hoek J, Nurmohamed MT, Flamelynck KJ, *et al.* Prevention of deep-vein thrombosis following total hip replacement by a low-molecular-weight heparinoid. *Thromb Haemost* 1992; **67:** 28–32.

154. Hohl MK, Luscher KJP, Tichy J, *et al.* Prevention of postoperative thromboembolism by dextran-70 or low dose heparin. *Obstet Gynecol* 1980; **55:** 497.

155. Holford CP. Graded compression for preventing deep venous thrombosis. *Br Med J* 1976; **2:** 969.

156. Huisman MV, Buller H, Jan W, *et al.* Unexpected high prevalence of silent pulmonary embolism in patients with DVT. *Chest* 1989; **95:** 498–502.

157. Hull R, Delmore TJ, Hirsh J, *et al.* Effectiveness of intermittent pulsatile elastic stockings for the prevention of calf and thigh vein thrombosis in patients undergoing elective knee surgery. *Thromb Res* 1979; **16:** 37.

158. Hull RD, Pineo GF. Therapeutic use of low molecular weight heparin. *Haemostasis* 1993; **23(Suppl 1):** 2–9.

159. Hull RD, Raskob GE. Prophylaxis of venous thromboembolic disease following hip and knee surgery. *J Bone Joint Surg (Am)* 1986; **68:** 146.

160. Hull RD, Raskob GE, Gent M, *et al.* Effectiveness of intermittent pneumatic leg compression for preventing deep vein thrombosis after total hip replacement. *JAMA* 1990; **263:** 2313.

161. Hunter GR, Barney MF, Crapo RO, Broadbent TR, Reilly WF, Jensen RL. Perioperative warfarin therapy in combined abdominal lipectomy and intra-abdominal gynecological surgical procedures. *Ann Plast Surg* 1990; **25:** 37.

162. Isacson S. Low-fibrinolytic activity of blood and vein wall in venous thrombosis. *Scand J Haematol Suppl* 1971; **16:** 1–29.

163. Ishak M, Morley K. Deep venous thrombosis after total hip arthroplasty: a prospective controlled study to determine the prophylactic effect of graded pressure stockings. *Br J Surg* 1981; **68:** 429.

164. Jeffcoate TNA, Tindall VR. Venous thrombosis and embolism in obstetrics and gynaecology. *Aust N Z J Obstet Gynaecol* 1965; **5:** 119–30.

165. Jeffrey PC, Nicolaides AN. Graduated compression stockings in the prevention of post operative deep vein thrombosis. *Br J Surg* 1990; **77:** 380.

166. Joffe SN. Drug prevention of postoperative deep vein thrombosis. A comparative study of calcium heparinate and sodium pentosan polysulphate. *Arch Surg* 1976; **111:** 37.

167. Johnson EA, Kirkwood TBL, Stirling Y, Perez-Requejo JL. Four heparin preparations: anti-Xa potentiating effect of heparin after subcutaneous injection. *Thromb Haemost* 1976; **35:** 586–91.

168. Johnson SR, Bygdeman S, Eliasson R. Effect of dextran on postoperative thrombosis. *Acta Chir Scand Suppl* 1968; **387:** 80.

169. Jørgensen PS, Knudsen JB, Broeng L, *et al.* The thromb-prophylactic effect of a low molecular weight heparin (Fragmin) in hip fracture surgery. A placebo controlled study. *Clin Orthop* 1992; **278:** 95–100.

170. Kakkar VV, Cohen AT, Edmondson RA, *et al.* Low molecular weight versus standard heparin for the prevention of venous thromboembolism after major abdominal surgery. *Lancet* 1993; **341:** 259–65.

171. Kakkar VV, Corrigan T, Spindler J, *et al.* Efficacy of low doses of heparin in prevention of deep-vein thrombosis after major surgery. *Lancet* 1972; **1:** 101.

172. Kakkar VV, Djazari B, Fok J, Fletcher M, Sailly MF, Westwick J. Low-molecular weight heparin and prevention of post-operative deep vein thrombosis. *Br Med J* 1982; **284:** 375.

173. Kakkar VV, Lawrence D, Bentley PG, Detlas HA, Ward VP, Scully MF. A comparative study of low doses of heparin and a heparin analogue in the prevention of post-operative deep vein thrombosis. *Thromb Res* 1918; **13:** 111.

174. Kakkar VV, Murray WJG. Efficacy and safety of low molecular weight heparin (CY216) in preventing postoperative thrombo-embolism: a cooperative study. *Br J Surg* 1985; **72:** 786–91.

175. Kakkar VV, Stamatakis J, Bentley P, Lawrence D, de Haas H, Ward V. Prophylaxis for postoperative deep-vein thrombosis. Synergistic effect of heparin and dihydroergotamine. *JAMA* 1979; **241:** 39.

176. Kettunen K, Poikolainep E, Karjalainen P, *et al.* Low-dose heparin as prophylaxis against postoperative deep vein thrombosis (In Finnish). *Duodecim* 1974; **90:** 834.

177. Kim YH. The incidence of deep vein thrombosis after cementless and cemented knee replacement. *J Bone Joint Surg (Br)* 1990; **72:** 779.

178. Knight MTN, Dawson R. Effect of intermittent compression of the arms on deep venous thrombosis in the legs. *Lancet* 1976; **2:** 1265.

179. Koller M, Schoch UK, Buchmann P, Largiadèr F, von Felten A, Frick PG. Low molecular weight heparin (Kabi 2165) as thromboprophylaxis in elective visceral surgery. *Thromb Haemost* 1986; **56:** 243–6.

180. Koppenhagen K, Wiechmann A, Zuhlke H-V, Wenig HG, Haring R. Leistungsfahigkeit und Risiko der Thromboembolieprophylaxe in der Chirurgie. Eine vergleichende Untersuchung von Heparin-Dibydergot und 'low-dose' Heparin. *Therapiewoche* 1979; **29:** 5920.

181. Kraytman M, Kutnowski M, Ansay J, Fastrez R. Prophylaxie par heparine sous-cutanée a faibles doses des thromboses veineuses postopératoires. *Acta Chir Belg* 1976; **5:** 519.

182. Kunz S, Drahne A, Briel RC. Prophylaxe der postoperativen Thromboembolie. Erfahrungen mit Heparin-Dihydergot in der Gynakologie. In: Pabst HW, Maurer G, eds. *Postoperative Thromboembolieprophylaxe.* Stuttgart, New York: Schattauer, 1977; 133.

183. Kutnowski M, Vandendris M, Steinberger R, Kraytman M. Prevention of deep vein thrombosis by low-dose heparin in urological surgery. *Urol Res* 1977; **5:** 123.

184. Lahnborg G, Bergstrom K, Friman L, Lagergren H. Effect of low-dose heparin on incidence of postoperative pulmonary embolism detected by photoscanning. *Lancet* 1974; **1:** 329.

185. Lane DA, Pejler G, Flynn AM, Thompson EA, Lindahl U. Neutralization of heparin-related saccharides by histidine-rich glycoprotein and platelet factor 4. *Biol Chem* 1986; **262:** 3980–6.

186. Lassen MR, Borris LC. Trauma. In: Hull R, Raskob G, Pineo G, eds. *Venous Thromboembolism: an Evidence-based Atlas.* Armonk NY: Futura Publishing Co, 1996; Chapter 9.

187. Lassen MR, Borris LC, Christiansen HM, *et al.* Heparin/dihydroergotamine for venous thrombosis prophylaxis: comparison of low dose heparin and low molecular weight heparin in hip surgery. *Br J Surg* 1988; **75:** 686.

188. Lassen MR, Borris LC, Christiansen HM, *et al.* Clinical trials with low molecular weight heparins in the prevention of postoperative thromboembolic complications: a meta-analysis. *Semin Thromb Hemost* 1991; **17(Suppl 3):** 284–90.

189. Lassen MR, Borris LC, Christiansen HM, *et al.* Prevention of thromboembolism in 190 hip arthroplasties. Comparison of LMW heparin and placebo. *Acta Orthop Scand* 1991; **62:** 33–8.

190. Lassen MR, Borris LC, Hauch O, *et al.* Enoxaparin versus dextran 70 in the prevention of postoperative deep vein thrombosis after total hip replacement. A Danish multicentre study. *Proceedings of the Danish Enoxaparin Symposium, February 3, 1990.*

191. Laverick MD, Croal SA, Mollan RAB. Orthopaedic surgeons and thromboprophylaxis. *Br Med J* 1991; **303:** 549–50.

192. Lawrence JC, Xabregas A, Gray L, Ham JM. Seasonal variation in the incidence of deep vein thrombosis. *Br J Surg* 1977; **64:** 777.

193. Leclerc JR, Geerts WH, Desjardins L, *et al.* Prevention of deep vein thrombosis after major knee surgery – a randomized, double-blind trial comparing a low molecular weight heparin fragment (enoxaparin) to placebo. *Thromb Haemost* 1992; **67:** 417–23.

194. Leithauser PH, Saraf L, Smyka S, Sheridan M. Prevention of embolic complications from venous thrombosis after surgery; standardized regimen of early ambulation. *JAMA* 1951; **147:** 300.

195. Leizorovicz A, Bara L, Samama MM, Haugh MC. Factor Xa inhibition. Correlation between the plasma levels of anti-Xa activity and occurrence of thrombosis and haemorrhage. *Haemostasis* 1993; **23(Suppl 1):** 89–98.

196. Leizorovicz A, Haugh MC, Chapuis FR, Samama MM, Boissel JP. Low molecular weight heparin in prevention of perioperative thrombosis. *Br Med J* 1992; **305:** 913–20.

197. Levine MN, Hirsh J, Gent M, *et al.* Prevention of deep vein thrombosis after elective hip surgery: a randomized trial comparing low molecular weight heparin with standard unfractionated heparin. *Ann Intern Med* 1991; **114:** 545–51.

198. Leyvraz P, Bachmann F, Bohnet J, *et al.* Thromboembolic prophylaxis in total hip replacement: a comparison between the low molecular weight heparinoid Lomoparan and heparin-dihydroergotamine. *Br J Surg* 1992; **79:** 911–14.

199. Leyvraz PF, Bachmann F, Hoek J, *et al.* Prevention of deep vein thrombosis after hip replacement: randomized comparison between unfractionated heparin and low-molecular-weight heparin. *Br Med J* 1991; **303:** 531–2.

200. Leyvraz PF, Postel M, Bachmann F, Hoeck JA, Samama M, Vandenbroek D. Prevention of deep vein thrombosis after total hip replacement: randomized comparison between adjusted dose unfractionated heparin and low molecular weight heparin (CY216). In: Hoek JA, ed. *Deep Vein Thrombosis following Total Hip Replacement.* PhD thesis, University of Amsterdam, 1990; 105–17.

201. Leyvraz PF, Richard J, Bachmann F, *et al.* Adjusted versus fixed-dose subcutaneous heparin in the prevention of deep-vein thrombosis after total hip replacement. *N Engl J Med* 1983; **309:** 954–8.

202. Lindblad B. Prophylaxis of post operative thrombo embolism with low dose heparin alone or in combination with dihydroergotamine. A review. *Acta Chir Scand Suppl* 1988; **543:** 31–42.

203. Lindblad B, Eriksson A, Bergqvist D. Autopsy-verified pulmonary embolism in a surgical department: analysis of the period from 1951 to 1988. *Br J Surg* 1991; **78:** 849–52.

204. Ljungner H, Bergqvist D, Nilsson IM. Effect of intermittent pneumatic and graded static compression on factor VIII and the fibrinolytic system. *Acta Chir Scand* 1981; **147:** 657.

205. Ljunström K-G. Dextran prophylaxis of fatal pulmonary embolism. *World J Surg* 1983; **7:** 767–72.

206. Lowe GDO, Osborne DH, McArdle BM, *et al.* Prediction and selective prophylaxis of venous thrombosis in elective gastrointestinal surgery. *Lancet* 1982; **1:** 409.

207. Lowe L. Venous thrombosis and embolism. *J Bone Joint Surg (Br)* 1981; **63:** 155.

208. Lynch JA, Baker PL, Polly RE, *et al.* Mechanical measures in the prophylaxis of postoperative thromboembolism in total knee arthroplasty. *Clin Orthop* 1990; **260:** 24–9.

209. Mannucci PM, Citterio L, Panajotopoulos N. Low-dose heparin and deep-vein thrombosis after total hip replacement. *Thromb Haemost* 1976; **36:** 157.

210. Marciniak E. Factor X, inactivation by antithrombin III: evidence for biological stabilization of factor X_2 by factor V–phospholipid complex. *Br J Haematol* 1973; **24:** 391–400.

211. Mattson E, Ohlin A, Balkfors B, *et al.* Lower-limb vasospasm and renal failure during postoperative thromboprophylaxis. *Eur J Surg* 1991; **157:** 289–92.

212. Mätzsch T, Bergqvist D, Fredin H, Hedner U. Low molecular weight heparin compared with dextran as prophylaxis against thrombosis after total hip replacement. *Acta Chir Scand* 1990; **156:** 445–50.

213. McCarthy TG, McQueen J, Johnstone FD, *et al.* A comparison of low dose subcutaneous heparin and intravenous dextran-70 in the prophylaxis of deep venous thrombosis after gynaecologic surgery. *J Obstet Gynaecol Br Commonw* 1974; **81(6):** 486–91.

214. McCarthy ST, Robertson D, Turner JJ, Hawkey CJ. Low-dose heparin as a prophylaxis against deep vein thrombosis after acute stroke. *Lancet* 1977; **2:** 800–1.

215. McCarthy ST, Turner J. Low-dose subcutaneous heparin in the prevention of deep vein thrombosis and pulmonary emboli following acute stroke. *Age Ageing* 1986; **15:** 84–8.

216. McKenna R, Galante J, Bachmann F, Wallace DL, Kaushal S, Meredith P. Prevention of venous thromboembolism after total knee replacement by high-dose aspirin and intermittent calf and thigh compression. *Br Med J* 1980; **280:** 514.

217. Mellbring G, Dahlgren S, Winan B. Prediction of deep vein thrombosis after extensive abdominal operations by the quotient between plasmin and α2-antiplasmin complex and fibrinogen concentration in plasma. *Surg Gynecol Obstet* 1985; **161:** 339.

218. Messmer K, Ljunstroom K-G, Gruber U, Richter W, Hedin H. Prevention of dextran-induced anaphylactoid reactions by hapten inhibition. *Lancet* 1980; **1:** 975.

219. Milhe E. Physikalische Moglichkeiten der Thromboseprophylaxe. *Langenbecks Arch Chir* 1977; **345:** Kongressbericht.

220. Mitchell JRA. Can we really prevent postoperative pulmonary emboli? *Br Med J* 1979; **1:** 1523.

221. Mohr DN, Silverstein MD, Mutaugh PA, Harrison JM. Prophylactic agents for venous thrombosis in elective hip surgery. Meta analysis of studies using venographic assessment. *Arch Intern Med* 1993; **153:** 2221–8.

222. Montrey JS, Kistner RL, Kong AYT, *et al.* Thromboembolism following hip fracture. *J Trauma* 1985; **25:** 534.

223. Morrey BF, Adams RA, Ilstrup DM, Bryan RS. Complications and mortality associated with bilateral or unilateral total knee arthroplasty. *J Bone Joint Surg (Am)* 1987; **69:** 484.

224. Morris GK, Henry APJ, Preston BJ. Prevention of deep-vein thrombosis by low-dose heparin in patients undergoing total hip replacement. *Lancet* 1974; **2:** 797.

225. Morris GK, Mitchell JR. Evaluation of ^{125}I-fibrinogen test for venous thrombosis in patients with hip fractures: comparison between isotope scanning and necropsy findings. *Br Med J* 1977; **1:** 254.

226. Morris GK, Mitchell JR. Prevention and diagnosis of venous thrombosis in patients with hip fractures. A survey of current practice. *Lancet* 1976; **2:** 867.

227. Morris GK, Mitchell JR. Warfarin sodium in prevention of deep venous thrombosis and pulmonary embolism in patients with fractured neck of femur. *Lancet* 1976; **2:** 869.

228. Moskovitz PA, Ellenberg SS, Feffer HL, *et al.* Low-dose heparin for prevention of venous thromboembolism in total hip arthroplasty and surgical repair of hip fractures. *J Bone Joint Surg (Am)* 1978; **60:** 1065.

229. Mottier D. Prophylaxis of deep vein thrombosis in medical geriatric patients. *Thromb Haemost* 1996; **9(Suppl):** 1115.

230. Multicentre Trial Committee. Prophylactic efficacy of low-dose dihydroergotamine and heparin in post-operative deep venous thrombosis following intra abdominal operation. *J Vasc Surg* 1984; **1:** 608.

231. Murray WJG. MS Thesis, 1986. University of London.

232. Myhre H, Holen A. Thrombosis prophylaxis. Dextran or sodium warfarin? A controlled clinical study. *Nord Med* 1969; **82:** 1534.

233. Myhre HO, Storen EJ, Ausen CA. Pre or post-operative start of anticoagulation prophylaxis in patients with fractured hips? *Oslo City Hosp* 1973; **23:** 15.

234. Nair CH, Shah GA, Dhall DP. Operation, dextran and fibrin network structure. *Clin Invest Med* 1985; **8:** A125.

235. Nanson E. Useful measures in the prevention of deep vein thrombosis of the legs. *Can Med Assoc J* 1963; **195:** 88.

236. Negus D. Prevention and treatment of venous ulceration. *Ann R Coll Surg Engl* 1985; **67:** 144.

237. Nicolaides AN, Desai S, Douglas JN, *et al.* Small doses of subcutaneous sodium heparin in preventing deep venous thrombosis after major surgery. *Lancet* 1972; **2:** 890.

238. Nicolaides AN, Fernandes F, Pollack AV. Intermittent sequential pneumatic compression of the legs in the prevention of venous stasis and postoperative deep venous thrombosis. *Surgery* 1980; **87:** 69.

239. Nicolaides AN, Field ES, Kakkar VV. Prostatectomy and deep vein thrombosis. *Br J Surg* 1972; **50:** 487.

240. Nicolaides AN, Kakkar VV, Field ES, Fish P. Optimal electrical stimulus for prevention of deep vein thrombosis. *Br Med J* 1972; **4:** 756.

241. Nicolaides AN, Kakkar VV, Renney TJG, *et al.* Myocardial infarction and deep vein thrombosis. *Br Med J* 1971; **1:** 432.

242. Nicolaides AN, Miles C, Hoare M, *et al.* Intermittent sequential pneumatic compression of the legs and thromboembolism-deterrent stockings in the prevention of postoperative deep venous thrombosis. *Surgery* 1983; **94:** 21–5.

243. Nielson PT, Jorgensen LN, Albrecht-Beste E, Leffers M, Rasmussen LS. Lower thrombosis risk with epidural blockade in knee arthoplasty. *Acta Orthop Scand* 1990; **61:** 29.

244. Nillius A, Nylander G. Deep vein thrombosis after total hip replacement: a clinical and phlebographic study. *Br J Surg* 1979; **66:** 324.

245. Nurmohamed MT, Rosendaal FR, Buller HR, *et al.* Low molecular weight heparin versus standard heparin in general and orthopaedic surgery: a meta-analysis. *Lancet* 1992; **340:** 152–6.

246. Nurmohamed MT, Verhaeghe R, Irarte JA, Vogel G, vanRij AM, Prentice CR. A comparative trial of a low molecular weight heparin (enoxaparin) versus standard heparin for the prophylaxis of deep vein

thrombosis in general surgery. *Am J Surg* 1995; **196:** 567–71.

247. Ockelford PA, Patterson J, Johns AS. A double blind randomised placebo controlled trial of thrombo-prophylaxis in major elective general surgery using once daily injections of a low molecular weight heparin fragment (Fragmin). *Thromb Haemost* 1989; **62:** 1046.

248. Oertli D, Hess P, Dung M, *et al.* Prevention of deep vein thrombosis in patients with hip fracture. Low molecular weight heparin versus dextran. *World J Surg* 1992; **16;** 980–4.

249. Østergaard PB, Nilsson B, Bergqvist D, Hedner U, Pederson PC. The effect of low molecular weight heparin on experimental thrombosis and haemostasis. The influence of production method. *Thromb Res* 1987; **45:** 739–49.

250. Pachter L, Riles T. Low dose heparin: bleeding and wound complications in the surgical patient. A prospective randomized study. *Ann Surg* 1977; **186:** 669.

251. Paiement G, Weissinger SJ, Waltman AC, *et al.* Low dose warfarin versus external pneumatic compression for prophylaxis against venous thromboembolism following total hip replacement. *J Arthroplasty* 1987; **2:** 23.

252. Pidala MJ, Donovan DL, Kepley RF. A prospective study on intermittent pneumatic compression in the prevention of deep vein thrombosis in patients undergoing total hip or total knee replacement. *Surg Gynecol Obstet* 1992; **175:** 47–51.

253. Planes A, Vochelle N, Darmon JY, Fagola M, Belland M, Huet Y. Risk of deep vein thrombosis after hospital discharge in patients having undergone total hip replacement. Double blind randomized trial of enoxaparin versus placebo. *Lancet* 1996; **348:** 224–8.

254. Planes A, Vochelle N, Mazas F, *et al.* Prevention of postoperative venous thrombosis: a randomized trial comparing unfractionated heparin with low molecular weight heparin in patients undergoing total hip replacement. *Thromb Haemost* 1988; **60:** 407–10.

255. Plante J, Boneu B, Vaysse C, Barret A, Gouzi M, Bierme R. Dipyridamole–aspirin versus low doses of heparin in the prophylaxis of deep venous thrombosis in abdominal surgery. *Thromb Res* 1979; **14:** 399.

256. Poller L, McKernan A, Thomson JM, Elstein M, Hirsh PJ, Jones JB. Mixed mini-dose warfarin: a new approach to prophylaxis against venous thrombosis after major surgery. *Br Med J* 1987; **295:** 1309–12.

257. Porteous MJ, Nicholson EA, Morris LT, James R, Nejus D. Thigh length versus knee length stockings in the prevention of deep vein thrombosis. *Br J Surg* 1989; **76:** 296–7.

258. Powers PJ, Gent M, Jay RM, *et al.* A randomized trial of less intensive postoperative warfarin or aspirin therapy in the prevention of venous thromboembolism after surgery for fractured hip. *Arch Intern Med* 1989; **149:** 771.

259. Prandoni P, Meduri F, Cuppini S, *et al.* Dermatan sulphate, a safe approach to prevention of post operative deep vein thrombosis. *Br J Surg* 1992; **79:** 505–9.

260. Prins MH, Gelsema R, Sing AK, *et al.* Prophylaxis of deep venous thrombosis with a low-molecular weight heparin (Kabi 2165/Fragmin) in stroke patients. *Haemostasis* 1989; **19:** 245–50.

261. Pulsaki EJ. Present status of plasma volume expanders in the treatment of shock. *Arch Surg* 1951; **63:** 745.

262. Raberger G, Schwarz M, Benke T, Kraupp O. Die Wirkung von Dihydroergotamin auf den grosser und kleinen Kreislauf. In: Tscherne H, Deutsch E, eds. *Postoperative Thromboembolei-Prophylaxe aus aktueller Sicht.* Stuttgart, New York: Thieme, 1981.

263. Rakoczi I, Chamone D, Collen D, Verstraete M. Prediction of postoperative leg-vein thrombosis in gynaecological patients. *Lancet* 1978; **1:** 509.

264. Rem J, Duckert F, Fridrich R, Gruber UF. Subkutane kleine Heparindosen zur Thrombosprophylaxe in der allgemeinen Chirurgie und Urologie. *Schweiz Med Wochenschr* 1975; **105:** 827.

265. Riber C, Alstrup N, Nymann T, Bogstad JW, Wille-Jorgensen P, Tonnesen H. Postoperative thromboembolism after day case herniorrhaphy. *Br J Surg* 1996; **83:** 420–1.

266. Richter W. Hapten inhibition of passive antidextran anaphylaxis in guinea pigs. [Role of molecular size in anaphylactogenicity and precipitability of dextran fraction.] *Int Arch Allergy Appl Immunol* 1971; **41:** 826.

267. Ring J, Messmer K. Incidence and severity of anaphylactoid reactions to colloid volume substitutes. *Lancet* 1977; **1:** 466.

268. Risberg B. Fibrinolysis and tourniquets. *Lancet* 1977; **2:** 360.

269. Roberts VC, Cotton LT. Failure of low-dose heparin to improve efficacy of peroperative intermittent calf compression in preventing postoperative deep vein thrombosis. *Br Med J* 1975; **3:** 458.

270. Roberts VC, Cotton LT. Prevention of postoperative deep vein thrombosis in patients with malignant disease. *Br Med J* 1974; **1:** 358.

271. Roberts VC, Sabri S, Beeley AH, Cotton LT. The effect of intermittently applied external pressure on the haemodynamics of the lower limb in man. *Br J Surg* 1972; **59:** 223.

272. Roberts VC, Sabri S, Pietroni MC, Gurewich V, Cotton LT. Passive flexion and femoral vein flow; a study using a motorized foot mover. *Br Med J* 1971; **3:** 78.

273. Rogers PH, Walsh PN, Marder VJ, *et al.* Controlled trial of low dose heparin and sulfinpyrazone to prevent venous thromboembolism after operation on the hip. *J Bone Joint Surg (Am)* 1978; **60:** 758.

274. Rohrer MJ, Cutler BS, MacDougall E, Herrman JB, Anderson FA, Wheeler HP. A prospective study of the incidence of deep venous thrombosis in hospitalized children. *J Vasc Surg* 1996; **24:** 46–50.

275. Rosenberg IL, Evans M, Pollock AV. Prophylaxis of postoperative leg vein thrombosis by low dose subcutaneous heparin or peroperative calf muscle stimulation: a controlled clinical trial. *Br Med J* 1975; **1:** 649.

276. Rosengarten DS, Laird J. The effect of leg elevation on the incidence of deep vein thrombosis after operation. *Br J Surg* 1971; **58:** 182.

277. Rosengarten DS, Laird J, Jeyasingh K, Martin P. The failure of compression stockings (Tubi-grip) to prevent deep venous thrombosis after operation. *Br J Surg* 1970; **57:** 296.

278. Sabri S, Roberts VC, Cotton LT. Effects of externally applied pressure on the haemodynamics of the lower limb. *Br Med J* 1971; **3:** 503.

279. Sabri S, Roberts VC, Cotton LT. Prevention of early postoperative deep vein thrombosis by intermittent compression of the leg during surgery. *Br Med J* 1971; **4:** 394.

280. Sagar S, Stamatakis JD, Higgins AF, *et al.* Efficacy of low dose heparin in prevention of extensive deep-vein thrombosis in patients undergoing total-hip replacement. *Lancet* 1976; **1:** 151.

281. Salzman EW, Harris WH, DeSanctis RW. Anticoagulation for prevention of thromboembolism following fractures of the hip. *N Engl J Med* 1966; **275:** 122–30.

282. Salzman EW, Hirsh J. Prevention of venous thromboembolism. In: Colman RW, Hirsh J, Marder VJ, Salzman EW, eds. *Hemostasis and Thrombosis: Basic Principles and Clinical Practice.* Philadelphia, PA: JP Lippincott Co, 1987; 1253.

283. Salzman EW, Ploetz J, Bettman M, Skillman J, Klein L. Intraoperative external pneumatic calf compression to afford long-term prophylaxis against deep vein thrombosis in urological patients. *Surgery* 1980; **87:** 239.

284. Samama H. Low molecular weight heparins: moded action and dosage. In: Bergqvist D, ed. *Prevention of Venous Thromboembolism.* London: Med Orion, 1994; Chapter 13.

285. Samama M, Boissel JP, Combe-Tamzali S, Leizorovicz A. Clinical studies with low molecular weight heparins in the prevention and treatment of venous thromboembolism. *Ann N Y Acad Sci* 1989; **556:** 386–405.

286. Sandset PM, Dahl T, Stiris M, *et al.* A double-blind and randomized placebo-controlled trial of low molecular weight heparin once daily to prevent deep vein thrombosis in acute ischemic stroke. *Semin Thromb Hemost* 1990; **16:** 25–33.

287. Schafer AI. The hypercoagulable states. *Ann Intern Med* 1985; **102:** 814–28.

288. Schmitt BP, Adelman B. Heparin-associated thrombocytopenia: a critical review and pooled analysis. *Am J Med Sci* 1993; **305:** 208–15.

289. Schondorf T, Weber U. Prevention of deep vein thrombosis in orthopaedic surgery with the combination of low dose heparin plus either dihydroergotamine or dextran. *Scand J Haematol Suppl* 1980; **36:** 126.

290. Schoning B, Koch H. Pathergiequote verschiedener Plasmasubstitute an Haut und Respirationstractus orthopadischer Patienten. *Anaesthesist* 1975; **24:** 507.

291. Scurr JH, Ibrahim SZ, Faber RG, Le Quesne LP. The efficacy of graduated compression stockings in the prevention of deep vein thrombosis. *Br J Surg* 1977; **64:** 371.

292. Sebeseri O, Kummer H, Zingg E. Controlled prevention of post-operative thrombosis in urological diseases with depot heparin. *Eur Urol* 1975; **1(5):** 229–30.

293. Sevitt S, Gallagher NG. Prevention of venous thrombosis and pulmonary embolism in injured patients. *Lancet* 1959; **2:** 981.

294. Sharnoff JG, De Blazio G. Prevention of fatal postoperative thromboembolism by heparin prophylaxis. *Lancet* 1970; **2:** 1006.

295. Sharnoff JG, Kass HH, Mistica BA. A plan of heparinization of the surgical patient to prevent postoperative thromboembolism. *Surg Gynecol Obstet* 1962; **115:** 75.

296. Sharnoff JG. Results in the prophylaxis of postoperative thromboembolism. *Surg Gynecol Obstet* 1966; **123:** 303.

297. Sigel B, Edelstein A, Felix R, Memhardt C. Compression of the deep venous system of the lower leg during inactive recumbency. *Arch Surg* 1973; **106:** 38.

298. Stadil F. Prophylaxis of postoperative venous thrombosis with dextran-70. *Ugeskr Laeger* 1970; **132:** 1817.

299. Stamatakis JD, Sagar S, Lawrence D, Kakkar VV. Dihydroergotamine in the prevention of postoperative deep venous thrombosis. *Br J Surg* 1977; **64:** 294.

300. Strand L, Bank-Mikkelsen OK, Lindewald H. Small heparin doses as prophylaxis against deep-vein thrombosis in the major surgery. *Acta Chir Scand* 1975; **141:** 624.

301. Stringer MD, Steadman CA, Hedges AR, Thomas EM, Morley TR, Kakkar VV. Deep vein thrombosis after elective knee surgery: an incidence study in 312 patients. *J Bone Joint Surg (Br)* 1989; **71:** 492.

302. Stulberg GN, Francis CW, Pellegrinin VD, *et al.* Antithrombin III/low dose heparin in the prevention of deep vein thrombosis after total knee arthroplasty. *Clin Orthop* 1989; **248:** 152.

303. Stulberg GN, Insall JN, Williams GW, Ghelman B. Deep vein thrombosis following total knee replacement. An analysis of six hundred and thirty-eight arthroplasties. *J Bone Joint Surg (Am)* 1984; **66:** 194.

304. Svend-Hansen H, Bremerskov V, Gøtrok J, Ostri P. Low dose heparin in proximal femoral fractures – failure to prevent deep vein thrombosis. *Acta Orthop Scand* 1981; **52:** 77.

305. Taberner DA, Poller L, Burslem RW, Jones JB. Oral anticoagulants controlled by the British comparative thromboplastin versus low-dose heparin in prophylaxis of deep vein thrombosis. *Br Med J* 1978; **1:** 272.

306. Taberner DA, Poller L, Thomson JM, *et al.* Randomised study of adjusted versus fixed low dose heparin prophylaxis of deep vein thrombosis in hip surgery. *Br J Surg* 1989; **736:** 933.

307. Takkunen O. The effect of different modes of artificial ventilation and of some prophylactic means on the incidence of postoperative deep vein thrombosis. *Ann Chir Gynaecol Fenn (Suppl)* 1975; **191:** 3–43.

308. Thromboembolic Risk Factors (THRIFT) Consensus Group. Risk of and prophylaxis for venous thromboembolism in hospital patients. *Br Med J* 1992; **305:** 567–74.

309. Torngren S, Forsberg K. Concentrated or diluted heparin prophylaxis of postoperative deep venous thrombosis. *Acta Chir Scand* 1978; **144:** 283.

310. Torngren S. Optimal regimen of low-dose heparin prophylaxis in gastrointestinal surgery. *Acta Chir Scand* 1979; **145:** 87.

311. Torngren S, Kettunen K, Lahtinen J, *et al.* A randomized study of a semisynthetic heparin analogue and heparin in prophylaxis of deep vein thrombosis. *Br J Surg* 1984; **71:** 817.

312. Tsapogas MJ, Gousous H, Peadbody RA, Karmody AM, Eckert C. Postoperative venous thrombosis and the effectiveness of prophylactic measures. *Arch Surg* 1971; **103:** 561.

313. Turner GM, Cole SE, Brooks JH. The efficacy of graduated compression stockings in the prevention of deep vein thrombosis after major surgery. *Br J Obstet Gynaecol* 1984; **91(6):** 588–91.

314. Turpie AGG, Gent M, Cote R, *et al.* A low-molecular weight heparinoid compared with unfractionated heparin in the prevention of deep vein thrombosis in patients with acute ischemic stroke. *Ann Intern Med* 1992; **117(5):** 353–7.

315. Turpie AGG, Hirsh J, Gent M, Julian D, Johnson J. Prevention of deep vein thrombosis in potential neurosurgical patients: a randomized trial comparing graduated compression stockings alone or graduated compression stockings plus intermittent pneumatic compression with control. *Arch Intern Med* 1989; **149:** 679–81.

316. Turpie AGG, Levine MN, Hirsh J, *et al.* A randomized-controlled trial of a low-molecular-weight heparin (Enoxaparin) to prevent deep-vein thrombosis in patients undergoing elective hip surgery. *N Engl J Med* 1986; **315:** 925–7.

317. UrlepSalinovic V, Jelatancev B, Gorisek B. Low doses of heparin and heparin dihydergot in postoperative thromboprophylaxis in gynaecological patients. *Thromb Haemost* 1994; **72(1):** 16–20.

318. Van den Berg E, Walterbusch G, Gotzen L, Rumpf K-D, Otten B, Frohlich H. Ergotism leading to threatened limb amputation or to death in two patients given heparin-dihydroergotamine prophylaxis. *Lancet* 1982; **1:** 955.

319. Vandendris M, Kutnowski M, Futeral B, Giannakopoulos X, Krayman M, Gregoir W. Prevention of postoperative deep vein thrombosis by low dose heparin in open prostatectomy. *Urol Res* 1980; **8:** 219.

320. Venous Thrombosis Clinical Study Group. Small doses of subcutaneous sodium heparin in the prevention of deep vein thrombosis after elective hip operations. *Br J Surg* 1975; **62:** 348.

321. Verstraete M. Pharmacotherapeutic aspects of unfractionated and low molecular weight heparins. *Drugs* 1990; **40:** 498–530.

322. Wallenga JM, Fareed J. Relative contribution of factor Xa and factor IIa. Inhibition in the mediation of the antithrombotic actions of LMWHs and synthetic heparin pentasaccharides. *Thromb Haemorrh Dis* 1991; **3:** 53–9.

323. Warlow C, Ogston D, Douglas AS. Venous thrombosis following strokes. *Lancet* 1972; **1:** 1305–6.

324. Warlow C, Terry G, Kenmere AC, *et al.* A double blind trial of low dose subcutaneous heparin in the prevention of deep vein thrombosis after myocardial infarction. *Lancet* 1973; **2:** 934.

325. Welin-Berger T, Bygdeman S, Mebium C. Deep vein thrombosis following hip surgery. Relation to activated factor X inhibitor activity: effect of heparin and dextran. *Acta Orthop Scand* 1982; **53:** 937.

326. Wells PS, Lensing AWA, Hirsh J. Graduated compression stockings in the prevention of postoperative venous thromboembolism. A meta analysis. *Arch Intern Med* 1994; **154:** 67–72.

327. Wilkins RW, Stanton JR. Elastic stockings in the prevention of pulmonary embolism. *N Engl J Med* 1953; **248:** 1087.

328. Wille-Jorgensen P, Lansen I, Jorgensen L. Is there a need for long term thrombo-prophylaxis following general surgery. *Haemostasis* 1993; **23(Suppl 1):** 10–14.

329. Williams HT. Prevention of postoperative deep vein thrombosis with perioperative subcutaneous heparin. *Lancet* 1971; **2:** 950.

330. Williamson M, Thomas S, Edward A, Johnson R, Riggs J, Lewis M. Graduated compression stockings in the prevention of postoperative deep vein thrombosis a comparative study of pressure profiles and patient complications. *Phlebology* 1990; **5:** 135–9.

331. Wilson MG, Pei LF, Malone KM, Polak JF, Creager MA, Goldhaber SZ. Fixed low-dose versus adjusted higher-dose warfarin following orthopaedic surgery. *J Arthroplasty* 1994; **2:** 127–30.

332. Wilson NV, Das SK, Maurice H, Smibert G, Thomas EM, Kakkar VV. Thrombosis prophylaxis in total knee replacement. A new mechanical device. *Thromb Haemost* 1991; **65:** 1131.

333. Woolson ST, Watt M. Intermittent pneumatic compression to prevent proximal deep venous thrombosis during and after hip replacement. *J Bone Joint Surg (Am)* 1991; **73:** 507.

334. Wu T, Tsapogas M, Jordan R. Prophylaxis of deep venous thrombosis by hydroxychloroquine sulfate and heparin. *Surg Gynecol Obstet* 1977; **145:** 714.

335. Xabregas A, Gray L, Ham JM. Heparin prophylaxis of deep vein thrombosis in patients with a fractured neck of the femur. *Med J Aust* 1978; **1:** 620.

336. Yin ET, Wessler S. Heparin accelerated inhibition of activated factor X by a natural plasma inhibitor. *Biochim Biophys Acta* 1970; **201:** 387.

CHAPTER 12

Chronic deep vein incompetence

Normal valves	385	Treatment	394
Pathology	387	Commentary	404
Pathophysiology	389	References	405
Diagnosis	389		

The demonstration that the valves in the veins ensured a unidirectional flow of blood was the key-stone experiment in Harvey's investigations which proved that the blood circulated from the heart through the arteries and capillaries and returned through the veins.

The valves in the veins of the lower limbs are particularly important because hydrostatic forces encourage retrograde flow in the erect posture.

Although the structure of venous valves has been well described, their function is understood at only the most basic level. They prevent blood refluxing within and between the venous systems of the leg and are important in preventing sudden changes of venous pressure and volume. Beyond this, little is known of their static and dynamic properties or of factors that coordinate and modulate their action. Attempts to reproduce the structure and function of venous valves are still in their infancy.

Normal valves

MORPHOLOGY

Valves may be termed parietal and ostial, depending on their position.[29,105] Parietal valves are commonest and are found at any site in the length of a vein, often just distal to the entry site of tributaries. Valves unrelated to tributaries are termed free pari-etal valves. The vast majority of human parietal valves are bicuspid, although unicuspid, tricuspid and quadricuspid valves have rarely been found.[24] Two cusps dividing a circumferential sinus are the fundamental elements. Parietal valve anatomy is depicted in Figure 12.1. Ostial valves occur at the

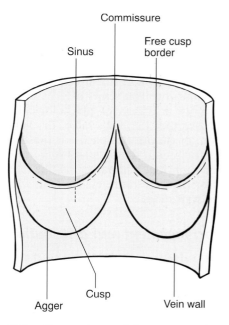

Figure 12.1 The anatomy of the venous valve as seen when a valve-bearing length of vein is split longitudinally through a commissure.

entry site of a small vein into a larger vein. Two types of bicuspid ostial valves have been noted by von Kügelgen and Greinemann[105] and their original classification has been amended by Gottlob and May[29] who describe marginal ostial valves and recessed ostial valves.

Light microscopy shows a unicellular layer of endothelium covering the luminal and parietal faces of the valve cusp and the sinus wall. A thin, undulating elastic lamina extending from the vein wall is found under the endothelium of the luminal cusp face from which thin fibrils extend into the underlying collagenous layer.[86] A collagenous stroma is found between the two layers of cusp endothelium. Smooth muscle cells are found in the region of the agger. Few connective tissue cells are present and the collagen fibres run between the aggers, parallel to the free cusp border.[105] Fibres also run from the cornu to the opposite side of the agger, in a cruciate configuration.

Electron microscopy has confirmed that smooth muscle cells are found in the region of the agger but indicates that the numbers are so small that functionally they are probably insignificant.[8] Smooth muscle cells are, however, found in greater numbers in the region of the commissures and may have some role to play in the 'tuning' of the valve.

Physical properties

Ackroyd *et al.*[3] have investigated the mechanical properties of parietal valve cusps, sinuses and vein wall. They found that strips of valve cusp cut parallel to the free border exhibited great physical strength compared with the vein wall in spite of their apparently delicate structure. The mean ultimate tensile strength of valve leaflets was 9 N/mm^2 compared with 5 N/mm^2 for circumferential strips and 2.5 N/mm^2 for axial strips of vein wall. These figures are far in excess of physiological venous pressures exerted on the valve or vein wall. Calculation of strain for each of these regions showed that circumferential strips of vein wall are less elastic than longitudinal strips but circumferential sinus strips are more elastic than circumferential vein wall strips.

Spatial arrangement and distribution

In general, valves are found distal to the point of entry of major tributaries.[101] The lower the vein in the limb the greater is the frequency of valves within it with the exception of the soleal venous sinuses which are devoid of valves.[56] Valve cusp edges lie in the long axis of the elliptical cross-section of the partially compressed vein and consequently lie parallel to the skin or deep fascia.[18,85]

The inferior vena cava is devoid of valves whilst valves in the common iliac veins are rare.[52] Most normal subjects have one valve in the external iliac or common femoral vein above the sapheno-femoral junction,[56] although 20–25% of subjects have no valve in this site.[78] Valves are found just distal to the junction of the superficial and deep femoral veins in 90% of legs and in the upper region of the popliteal vein just distal to the adductor hiatus in 96% of legs. Most of the other deep vein valves are variable in position.

FUNCTION

Unlike cardiac valves, the activity of venous valves is frequently random. When venous blood flow is steady during standing or sitting, the valve cusps are open and the venous pressure is the resultant of the hydraulic, hydrostatic and central venous pressures. Only following contraction of one of the muscle pumps, after which the intramuscular vein pressure falls to zero, do the valves maintain the reduction of venous pressure by preventing reflux. This effect is most pronounced during rhythmical activity such as walking.[35]

Hydrostatic function

In the venous system, flow is rarely static even when the muscle pumps are inactive. When the venous pressure changes rapidly during a change in posture or coughing, the valves shut and dampen the distal transmission of the sudden rise in pressure. Similarly, when the calf pump stops contracting at the end of a period of exercise, the valves remain shut for some time, preventing sudden exposure of the limb to the hydrostatic pressure. The gradual rise in venous pressure is a reflection of the shielding effect of the valves from the hydrostatic pressure and the gradual refilling of the venous circulation from the capillary bed. In addition to these pressure damping effects, the valves also prevent sudden volume changes so that blood does not suddenly pool in the legs on rapid standing.

The hydrostatic properties of valves, including the leak rates under varying pressure gradients and the pressure gradients generated by valves at different flow rates, are largely unknown, in contrast to the extensive literature available on the hydrostatic and hydrodynamic behaviour of cardiac valves.[115] Rosenbloom *et al.*[80] have examined the hydrostatic properties of an autogenous valve mechanism constructed from the external jugular vein of dogs for implantation in the femoral vein. They infused saline against closed valves at a known hydrostatic pressure and found that four valves remained competent to a pressure of 55 cmH$_2$O and two valves remained competent to a pressure of 300 mmHg. Two valves were viewed through an endoscope placed in a small side branch and found to close at pressures in the range 3–5 cmH$_2$O.

Hydrodynamic function

The deep vein valves perform their anti-reflux role at different phases of the calf pump cycle.[55] The valves of the communicating veins and the veins downstream to the pump close during calf pump systole in an analogous fashion to the mitral valve. The axial deep vein valves of the popliteal and femoral segments are arranged in series and open during calf pump systole, mimicking the aortic valve. In calf pump diastole the action is reversed.

The study of hydrodynamic properties of the valves themselves has largely been neglected. The opening and closing pressures, pressure gradients across valves, and closing and regurgitation fractions under varying conditions are unknown. The relationship of valve function to calf pump function and venous insufficiency is understood at only the most basic level.

In-vivo function

In-vivo assessment may involve an individual valve or a whole system of valve-bearing veins. Modified techniques of ascending and descending phlebography have been used to investigate valve competence,[4,17,58] but duplex ultrasonography is now used increasingly to demonstrate valve function[6] and reflux and attempts are underway to quantify these parameters.[102,104]

Calf pump function is determined by the force of muscle pump contraction, outflow resistance and valve competence. A global indication of valve function is given by foot vein pressure or plethysmographic methods in the recovery time to resting venous pressure[64] or volume after calf pump exercise.

Miscellaneous properties of the valve sinus

Because the valve sinus is wider than the adjacent vein,[13] the valve cusps do not lie flat against the sinus wall but float in the long axis of the vein. This leads to the presence of a relatively static pool of blood in the valve sinus. Paired vortices occur between the sinus and the valve cusps during conditions of steady flow.[29] The haematocrit is higher and the oxygen tension lower in the blood contained in the vortex at the bottom of the valve sinus.[32]

Fibrinolytic activity in the cusp sinuses appears minimal compared with other parts of the vein wall[53] and this may explain why thrombus is initiated in the valve sinus.

Pathology

Retrograde flow in the deep veins may be permitted by one of the following abnormalities.

Age-related valve changes

Histological changes occur within the valves from the age of 30 years onwards. There is a replacement of areolar tissue by collagen fibres and flattening of the crypts on the luminal cusp face where the elastic membrane extends, thickens and becomes tortuous.[87] There is a generalized hypertrophy of the subendothelial elements just distal to the valve that appears from the age of 40 onwards. The cause of this 'endophlebohypertrophy' is unclear, although repeated buffeting of the vein wall by eddy currents has been proposed.

Advancing age is accompanied by the appearance of polynuclear cells in the endothelium of the human vein wall.[29] Endothelial giant cells are found in the left common iliac vein secondary to the trauma inflicted on the left common iliac vein by the right iliac artery.[84] In the valves, giant cells are rare, although binucleate cells are found.

Congenital absence of valves

Congenital absence of deep vein valves is very rare and was first reported by Luke.[57] Lodin et al.,[54] Basmajian[7] and Plate et al.[70] have all reported the condition which characteristically causes bilateral leg ulcers from the early teens onwards. Varying degrees of impaired valve development occur and other associated vascular anomalies including haemangiomas and naevi have been described[33] (see Figure 24.7). Lindvall and Lodin[54] demonstrated heredity of valve agenesis over several generations of their patients and autosomal dominant inheritance seems most likely.[70]

Trauma

Mechanical trauma to the vein wall causes desquamation of endothelial cells and a similar response is seen in the valve cusps.[29] Highly acidic, alkaline, hypertonic and hypotonic solutions and protein-denaturing substances produce similar changes.

Valve inflammation

Saphir and Lev[86] described venous valvulitis in five patients suffering from endocarditis. Polymorph and lymphocyte infiltration was found in these valves together with leucocyte and red cell aggregations on the cusps which resembled vegetations. In some cases the cusps were damaged by adherent thrombus. It is unclear whether a bacteraemia from other sources affects the valves.

Primary non-thrombotic valve incompetence (floppy valve cusps)

The length of the free edge of a valve cusp is critical to its competence. When closed, the edge should be taut and straight and abut against its fellow across the whole width of the vein, with the valve sinus full and tense. If the valve edge is too long, it can evert in an upstream direction and render the valve incompetent. The incompetence, but not the valve eversion, can be demonstrated by descending phlebography.

Kistner[43] identified a group of patients in Hawaii who apparently have a primary non-thrombotic valvular incompetence ('floppy valve cusps') and suggested that this defect may be congenital, traumatic or age-related. Other authors have also recognized this condition.[36,75,88] There is some evidence that post-thrombotic disease at a distant site may somehow cause valvular incompetence without direct thrombotic valve damage.[9,102] Indeed, Kistner[43] states that most patients with primary femoral vein valve incompetence have post-thrombotic changes in the popliteal and tibial veins. The possibility that deep vein valves may be rendered incompetent by indirect and distant post-thrombotic damage requires further investigation. This abnormality is much less common than post-thrombotic deep vein valve incompetence.

Valve ring dilatation

Normal valve cusps will not meet across the lumen of the vein, if the valve ring (the cross-section of the vein at the level of the commissures) dilates. The most common example of this form of incompetence is seen in varicose superficial veins when either an underlying defect in the strength of the vein wall or prolonged high pressure dilates not only the valve ring but the whole vein, making the valves incompetent and the vein large and tortuous (see Chapter 5).

This type of valvular incompetence is rare in the deep veins, perhaps because they are supported by the surrounding muscles and the connective tissues of the neurovascular bundle. The phlebographic diameter of the deep veins is remarkably uniform from patient to patient and is only slightly increased even when there is gross reflux.

A few cases of patients with very large deep veins have been reported in association with arteriomegaly but there is no equivalent condition that can be called 'phlebomegaly'.[50]

There are publications which describe varicose veins of the deep compartment. These veins may have incompetent valves secondary to valve ring dilatation but this abnormality is rare and usually localized to one or two veins in the calf, the other veins being of normal size.[49]

The vein walls relax during pregnancy under the influence of raised hormone levels. This certainly makes the superficial veins dilate and become incompetent and sometimes the deep veins follow suit but the incidence and degree of the deep vein change has not been documented. Most of the vein changes of pregnancy reverse after delivery.

Valves and thrombosis

Thrombosis (see Chapter 15) invariably causes irrecoverable damage to the valve cusps and causes secondary deep vein incompetence. It is an important cause of deep vein reflux.

Paterson and McLachlin[65] examined the femoral veins of 165 cadavers and found 21 cases of early thrombosis. Careful examination of serial sections revealed that in 17 of the 21 cases the valve sinus was the origin of the thrombosis. Gibbs,[27] Sevitt and Gallagher[90] and Sevitt[89] also detected isolated valve sinus thrombosis, especially in elderly patients who were confined to bed. Sevitt[89] considers the valve sinus to be the origin of deep vein thrombosis. He has identified red cell/fibrin and platelet/fibrin foci in otherwise healthy valve sinuses and postulated that these act as a nidus for thrombus formation. McLachlin et al.[60] studied the rate of clearance of contrast medium from the leg veins of supine patients. They found that contrast remained in the valve sinuses for as long as 27 minutes after injection. They proposed that these low velocities and attendant eddy currents predispose to thrombus formation, particularly in the face of endothelial damage, possibly caused by hypoxaemia. In support of Sevitt's theory, Gottlob and May[29] have cited evidence that the frequency of thrombosis in any given vein is proportional to the density of valves within it. Valvular incompetence in the popliteal vein appears to predispose towards postoperative deep vein thrombosis.[45] Although valves appear important in the pathogenesis of deep vein thrombosis, the avalvular soleal sinuses are also a common site for thrombus formation.

Thrombosis destroys valve cusps by fragmentation, fibrosis and capillary infiltration as organization of the thrombus advances.[19] Where thrombosis occurs in the region of a valve whose cusps are open, these cusps fuse to the vein wall. Recanalization leaves a fibrotic, valveless conduit. Incomplete thrombosis causes patchy valve damage, with partial adherence of cusps to the sinus wall, shortening and fibrosis of the cusps leading to stenosis of the vein.

Whether the thrombosis is partial or complete, the affected valves, if still present, frequently become incompetent. There appears to be a 40–60% chance of deep vein valve incompetence occurring in veins affected by a thrombosis.[61] Serial duplex studies indicate that this process takes many years to develop fully.[103]

Pathophysiology

Reflux is the single most important abnormality of the venous system contributing to the pressure changes and clinical features of venous insufficiency. Patterns of reflux in the deep, communicating and superficial venous system have become clearer since the advent of colour-flow duplex ultrasound scanning, but the best way to quantify reflux has yet to be defined. The anatomical demonstration of reflux by descending phlebography has been largely superseded by duplex ultrasound and plethysmography. A number of variables including reflux flow velocity, reflux flow volume, valve closure time (duplex ultrasound) and venous filling index (air plethysmography) have been described but there is poor correlation between them and none seems to quantify reflux accurately.[79,109]

Some degree of reflux is found in most normal veins but reflux persisting for longer than 0.5 seconds at ultrasound scanning in any venous system is now regarded as pathological. The presence of segmental reflux has been identified where one venous segment is affected while its neighbouring veins function normally. The physiological significance of this is gradually becoming apparent with multisegmental reflux and reflux affecting the common femoral, popliteal and posterior tibial veins having the greatest significance in the development of calf pump failure.[66,81] Deep vein reflux appears commoner in limbs with severe venous disease than in those with mild or moderate skin changes.[110] From our own studies, deep vein reflux appears to be the principal cause of venous ulceration in approximately 30% of patients affected. Frequently it is difficult to incriminate one segment or system specifically with reflux occurring globally in the superficial, deep and communicating venous systems. The significance of communicating vein reflux remains unclear, however.[82] It should be remembered that deep vein reflux does not always induce venous insufficiency with 6–7% of apparently normal legs demonstrating marked deep vein reflux.[47] Deep vein reflux impairs calf pump function, although the ability of the calf pump to eject venous blood does not seem to be impaired.[48]

Diagnosis

Clinical presentation

Swelling

This is the principal complaint and has usually been present for many years. Swelling begins at the ankle and slowly extends to involve the lower leg and sometimes the thigh. It is rarely so great that it impedes the movements of the limb but it does restrict activity because it makes the leg feel tight. Swelling increases as the day passes and goes down a little after a night in bed.

Swelling is caused by the lack of venous hypotension during exercise; its presence therefore implies that there is poor calf pump function. Some patients with severe reflux have no swelling because they are able to reduce their superficial vein pressure by exercise. This makes it likely that the swelling associated with deep vein reflux is not caused by the axial vein reflux alone but by the secondary effects of this reflux on the veins of the calf, particularly the lower leg communicating veins.

Pain

Pain is not a common complaint. The leg becomes tight and aches as the day passes but the patient rarely says that the ache is severe enough to merit calling it a pain.

Venous claudication

A few patients develop muscle pain on exercise similar to the venous claudication caused by severe outflow tract obstruction. This is difficult to explain when there is no mechanical obstruction to venous outflow from the limb and indicates that the reflux is so great that it is producing the same effect as a severe outflow tract obstruction.

Night cramps are common.

Skin changes

Skin changes such as eczema, pigmentation, lipo-dermatosclerosis and ulceration rarely appear while the calf pump is efficient, even when there is grade 4 reflux, but as soon as the communicating veins become incompetent as a result of the prolonged strain on the pump caused by the reflux, the sub-cutaneous tissues and the skin rapidly deteriorate.

The skin changes in the 'gaiter' area of the leg are identical to those seen following severe calf vein thrombosis.

Clinical examination reveals the swelling and the skin changes and may also detect superficial vari-cose veins. Varicosities are not invariably present but, like the skin changes, they indicate calf pump insufficiency and communicating vein incompe-tence.

INVESTIGATIONS

Doppler insonation

Retrograde flow in the deep veins can be detected using a bidirectional Doppler flow probe (see also Chapter 4, page 123). The transducer is placed over the common or superficial femoral vein to observe the direction of blood flow during and after a Valsalva manoeuvre, and a thigh squeeze. In a normal person venous blood flow stops when the intrathoracic pressure is raised by a Valsalva manoeuvre. If the valves are incompetent, the flow stops and then reverses to flow retrogradely down the vein. A similar biphasic signal (forward and reversed flow) will be heard during and after squeezing the thigh (Figure 12.2).

The common and superficial femoral veins are easy to insonate with the Doppler probe. It is not easy to find the popliteal vein. When popliteal vein blood flow is being studied it must be done with the short saphenous vein occluded because incompe-tence of this vein allows retrograde flow in the segment of the popliteal vein above its termination. In fact there are a number of anatomical variations and pathological abnormalities which can allow ret-rograde flow in a segment of the popliteal vein between competent valves (Figure 12.3); this vein must therefore be examined very carefully and the results interpreted with caution. The combined use of venous imaging with flow observations will make flow studies much more reliable as the point of flow measurement will be visible on the grey-scale image.

When the popliteal vein is examined, the patient must be standing with the knee slightly flexed and the weight on the opposite leg. The transducer is placed over the centre of the popliteal fossa at an angle of 45–60°. The vein usually lies over or to one side of the arterial signal. Blood flow in the vein can be heard if it is accelerated by squeezing the calf. If retrograde flow follows squeezing the calf, the test should be repeated with a finger compressing the short saphenous vein. If the retrograde flow per-sists, the popliteal vein is incompetent.

Figure 12.4 shows the various situations in which retrograde flow can occur in a segment of popliteal vein, even when its valves are competent, and indi-cates that this test should be interpreted with caution.

Duplex ultrasound

This technique has become a mainstay of investi-gation in the venous system over the past decade. The combination of Doppler and real time B-mode imaging gives flow velocity information and anatomical/morphological detail. The addition of colour flow demonstrates flow direction and turbu-lence, visually simplifying and shortening most examinations. Duplex ultrasound is most useful in demonstrating venous occlusion or stenosis and reflux. The B-mode element allows anatomical localization of flow abnormalities, unlike pure Doppler ultrasound. Antegrade venous flow can be produced in the leg veins by manual calf compres-sion in the standing or lying positions. Reflux can be induced in the standing position by manual calf compression and relaxation or by deflation of a thigh cuff. Significant reflux is defined as reversed

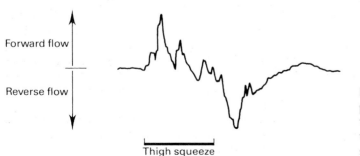

Figure 12.2 The Doppler signal from an incom-petent superficial femoral vein. Forward blood flow occurs when the lower thigh is squeezed, but the direction of blood flow reverses when the pres-sure on the lower thigh is released.

flow lasting at least 0.5 seconds. Duplex ultrasound has superseded descending phlebography as the method of choice for demonstrating venous reflux[6] but ascending phlebography is preferred for the demonstration of fine morphological detail such as post-thrombotic damage. The technique and colour coded examples are described in Chapter 4, pages 125–6.

Ambulatory venous pressure and plethysmography

Failure to reduce pressure in the veins of the lower leg with exercise defines venous insufficiency and direct pressure measurements can be made by cannulating a dorsal foot vein. Venous pressure can be measured using a water manometer or with a pressure transducer (see Chapter 4). The veins are emptied by exercise or compression and the time taken to return to the resting pressure indicates valve function. Normally the venous pressure should fall to less than 20 mmHg and return to its resting level not less than 20 seconds after cessation of exercise. Shorter times than this indicate venous reflux. Although the technique does not give information about individual valves, the use of tourniquets to occlude the long or short saphenous veins can localize reflux to an individual venous system.

Plethysmographic methods correlate well with ambulatory venous pressure measurements and their use has become widespread in preference to dorsal foot vein cannulation. Foot volumetry, photo-, strain-gauge, air and isotope plethysmography detect volume changes in the foot and/or calf as blood is expelled during exercise and refills at rest (see Chapter 4). Air plethysmography has assumed popularity in recent years, but there are concerns about its reproducibility.

The refilling rate can be expressed in various ways – the complete refilling time, the 90% or the 50% refilling time, or the maximum rate of refilling. None of these expressions is particularly superior to any other. All are acceptable provided each laboratory establishes its own normal range and adheres to a standardized method.

Normal refilling of the veins of the leg when the superficial veins are occluded is a slow process depending solely upon the arterial inflow. The normal rate of refilling determined by foot volumetry is between 2.0 and 2.5 ml/100 ml of calf per minute. When there is gross deep or superficial reflux this rate can increase to 10–15 ml/100 ml/min.[100] When measured with isotope plethysmography,[111] the normal refilling rate is 5%/min, deep vein incompetence alone can increase this to 10%/min, and a combination of deep and superficial vein incompetence increases it to 15%/min (Figure 12.5).

Figure 12.6 shows a foot volume trace of a normal limb and the tracing of a patient with deep vein incompetence, with and without the superficial

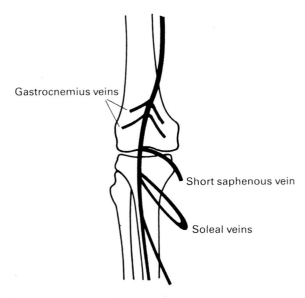

Figure 12.3 The tributaries of the popliteal vein join it above and below the knee joint. Many of the muscle veins do not have valves so blood can flow retrogradely into them from the main vein.

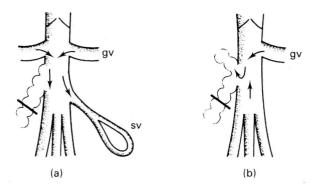

Figure 12.4 The situations in which retrograde blood flow can occur in the popliteal vein even when the short saphenous vein is occluded. (a) Blood flowing into the popliteal vein from a gastrocnemius vein (gv) and out into a valveless soleal sinusoid (sv). (b) Blood flowing out into incompetent tributaries deep to the popliteal fascia and above the point of short saphenous vein obstruction. In both these circumstances blood may be flowing forwards in the lower half of the popliteal vein and backwards in the upper half, even when the popliteal vein contains a competent valve.

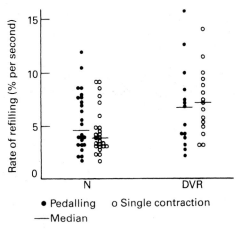

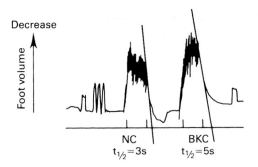

Figure 12.5 The rate of venous refilling of the calf measured with isotope plethysmography after pedalling and a sustained calf muscle contraction in 25 normal subjects (N) and 15 patients with phlebographically proven deep vein reflux (DVR). The increased rate of refilling in the patients was statistically significant. (Redrawn from Whitehead *et al.*[111])

Figure 12.6 The foot volume trace of a limb with deep vein incompetence (NC, no superficial vein occluding cuff; BKC, below-knee cuff). The $t_{1/2}$ (refilling time) without a cuff was 3 seconds. The $t_{1/2}$ was 5 seconds when the superficial veins were occluded below the knee. If the rapid refilling had been caused by superficial vein reflux, the below-knee cuff would have restored the refilling time to normal (i.e. 15–25 seconds).

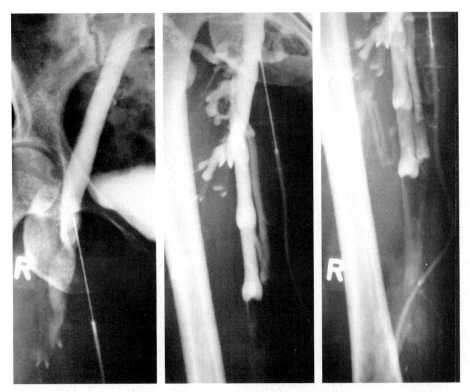

Figure 12.7 A descending phlebograph showing reflux down to a valve in the mid-thigh during a Valsalva manoeuvre (middle panel) with a small amount of contrast medium trickling through down to a point just above the knee. We would classify the mid-thigh valve as normal and call this grade 2, not grade 3, reflux.

veins occluded by a tourniquet. The rapid refilling caused by the deep vein reflux is quite obvious.

Phlebography

Despite advances in duplex ultrasound technology over recent years, ascending phlebography currently remains the investigation of choice for demonstrating the fine detail of post-thrombotic change (wall irregularity, recanalization, collaterals and absent valves) and incompetent communicating veins in patients with deep vein incompetence. We perform ascending phlebography routinely in the investigation of patients with severe venous insufficiency.

Because descending phlebography fails to demonstrate distal and segmental reflux and correlates poorly with plethysmographic refilling-time assessment of reflux, it has largely been abandoned in favour of duplex ultrasound.[6] The technique is still useful for studying the behaviour of individual valves, however, and has been used extensively in the development and evaluation of techniques for correction of deep vein incompetence.

The technique of descending phlebography is fully described in Chapter 4. Provided the position of the patient is kept constant (we prefer the patient to be supine, other investigators favour a 65° head-up tilt) and the stimulus to reflux is controlled (a Valsalva manoeuvre at 40 mmHg for 30 seconds), the distance the x-ray contrast medium refluxes down the leg is reproducible and measurable.[23] Five grades of reflux are recognized[13] (see Chapter 4 and Figures 12.7 and 12.8):

- grade 0 – none
- grade 1 – reflux down to the first valve below the site of injection
- grade 2 – reflux down to the upper third of the thigh
- grade 3 – reflux down to, but not below the knee joint
- grade 4 – reflux below the knee joint.

An examination of the correlation between the presence of symptoms and signs and the degree of reflux strongly suggests that grades 0, 1 and 2 reflux are normal, whereas the reflux of grades 3 and 4 is abnormal and usually, but not always,[2,35] associated with calf pump failure.

An *arm phlebogram* should be performed if a valve transplant is being considered for avalvular or congenitally absent abnormal lower limb valves. In one of our patients valves were absent from both the arms and the legs.

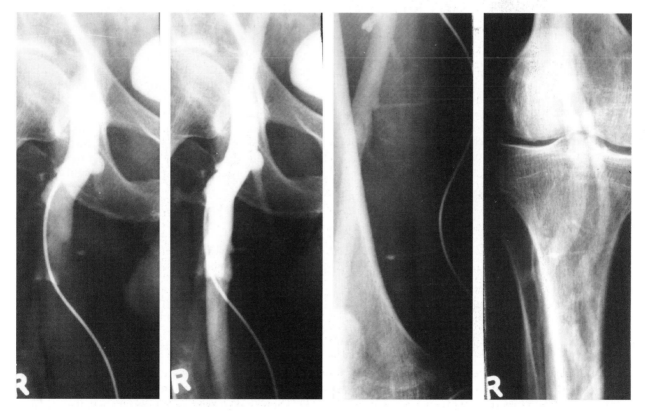

Figure 12.8 A descending phlebograph showing reflux of contrast medium down to the mid-calf. This is grade 4 reflux.

Treatment

All varieties of deep axial vein incompetence should, initially, be treated conservatively. The most important objective is the reduction and control of the swelling with good quality compression stockings and elevation of the leg whenever possible.

Below-knee stockings are usually sufficient as most of the swelling is usually below the knee. Effective stockings should compress the limb with a pressure of 30–40 mmHg at the ankle. The patient must be told to avoid standing still, to put his/her legs up on a leg rest when sitting and, if possible, to spend 10–15 minutes each day lying on the floor with legs propped up vertically against a wall. At night the patient should raise the foot of the bed by 12 inches (30 cm) and elevate the affected limb or limbs still further by resting them upon a wedge of pillows.

Regular support and elevation of the limb, assisted by gentle massage of the whole limb, with special attention to areas of skin or subcutaneous thickening, will often relieve the aching and keep the limb to an acceptable size.

A distinct group of patients exists who suffer persistent ulceration despite the above measures and many of these patients have post-thrombotic deep vein damage. Significant deep reflux is a common finding together with grossly abnormal pump function after conventional superficial vein surgery. It is this group that is most likely to benefit from deep vein valve surgery.

Various studies have indicated that correction of one abnormality in isolation is likely to be overstressed and fail.[22,23] Where communicating, deep and superficial vein incompetence coexist, all abnormalities should be corrected.[112]

SURGICAL CORRECTION OF DEEP VEIN INCOMPETENCE

History

In 1953, Eiseman and Malette[20] reported the first technique of valve construction. This technique, performed in the inferior vena cava of the dog, produced a valve by intussuscepting the vessel wall. In 1960, De Weese and Niguidula[16] performed venous valve autotransplantation in the dog, but it was not until 1968 that Kistner[41] first described a technique of venous valve repair in man. In 1979, Kistner and Sparkuhl[44] described the technique of valve transposition and in 1982, Taheri *et al.*[96] reported the first vein valve autotransplant in man. Since 1985, interest in venous valve surgery has increased and a number of reports have appeared describing new valve repair methods and valve replacement techniques using homografts, xenografts and prosthetic materials.

The valve abnormality: valve repair or replacement?

Valves may be made incompetent by thrombosis, stretching of the valve cusps and/or the valve sinus, or may be congenitally absent.

Valve repair (valvuloplasty) and replacement are quite distinct techniques and are suitable for different groups of patients. To achieve effective valve repair, the basic structure of the valve must be intact. The abnormality most suited to this kind of procedure is non-thrombotic valve incompetence. This may be caused by valve cusp prolapse ('floppy valve cusps') as described by Kistner,[43] or valve ring dilatation,[31,75] or a combination of the two. Whether these are two distinct conditions remains unclear. They may represent a primary defect, or be secondary to, or associated with post-thrombotic damage in the more distal calf veins.[43,102] Raju[75] has suggested that such deep vein thrombosis may be a secondary event to venous reflux consequent on a primary valve abnormality. Whatever its aetiology, non-thrombotic valve incompetence appears less common than post-thrombotic incompetence, although it has been recognized and treated by a number of groups.[39,42,76]

Direct post-thrombotic valve damage usually destroys the valve cusps beyond repair, making them unsuitable for valvuloplasty. In this situation and valve agenesis, valve replacement techniques are the only suitable procedures.

The ideal number and site of valves to be repaired or replaced remains unclear, but abolition of reflux in the popliteal vein seems to confer the greatest improvement in calf pump function.

Principles and aims of venous valve surgery

The requirements for effective deep vein valve surgery in the treatment of venous insufficiency are as follows:

1. Demonstration of significant deep vein reflux with impaired calf pump function refractory to conservative measures and conventional superficial/communicating vein surgery.
2. Adequate definition and proof of correction of significant coexisting venous abnormalities contributing to the venous insufficiency.
3. The use of a valve with physiological static and dynamic properties.

4. Avoidance of thrombosis.
5. Maintenance of long-term competence.
6. Ease of valve procurement of construction.

Valve repair techniques

Valve repair techniques aim to prevent reflux by producing secure cusp apposition without cusp prolapse. Direct valvuloplasty achieves this by shortening the redundant floppy valve cusp edges, whilst the indirect methods narrow the dilated valve sinus to produce greater cusp contact.

Direct valvuloplasty: valve cusp procedures

Direct valvuloplasty was first described by Kistner[41] in 1968. The vein containing the valve to be repaired is exposed through a longitudinal incision. Valve incompetence is confirmed by Harvey's test, the patient is anticoagulated with heparin and the vein occluded with soft atraumatic vascular clamps. A longitudinal venotomy is made passing between the valve cusps through the commissure so that the cusps are not damaged. The redundant cusp edges are tightened by fine prolene sutures that reef its free edge into the two commissures, restoring competence to the valve unit (Figure 12.9). The venotomy is then closed and the competence tested by Harvey's test. Descending phlebography or duplex ultrasonography may be employed to further confirm competence.

Kistner advocates perioperative anticoagulation with heparin and continuation of this for 2 weeks postoperatively, followed by oral anticoagulation for 2 months. In 1982, Ferris and Kistner[23] reported the late results of 31 valvuloplasty procedures and showed that competency was restored to the majority of these valves and was sustained for up to 13 years when assessed by descending phlebography (Figure 12.10). Calf pump function was improved (Figure 12.11), but the effect on clinical venous disease is more difficult to interpret since most of these patient also underwent communicating vein surgery. Indeed, Kistner[43] states that the best results were seen in patients undergoing total correction of the various refluxing systems. Raju,[75] Raju and Fredericks[76] and Eriksson[21] have also shown long-term improvement of reflux and symptoms in the majority of their patients undergoing Kistner's procedure. Cheatle and Perrin[12] have reported freedom from reflux in 85% and correction of venous refilling time in 68% in 52 limbs one year after superficial femoral vein direct valvuloplasty.

Modifications of Kistner's technique have been described, Raju and Fredericks[76] advocating a

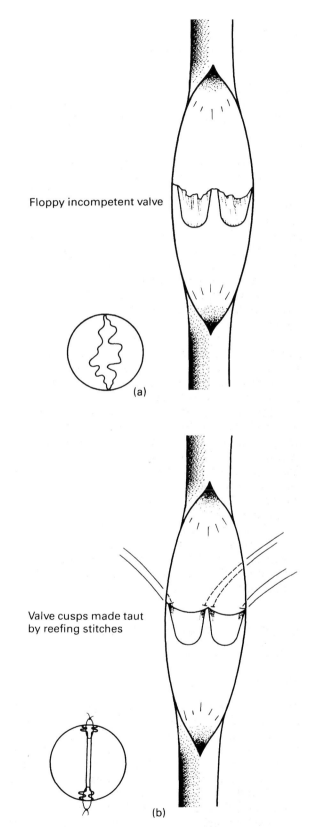

Floppy incompetent valve

(a)

Valve cusps made taut by reefing stitches

(b)

Figure 12.9 Primary floppy valve incompetence corrected by Kistner's technique of direct valvuloplasty.

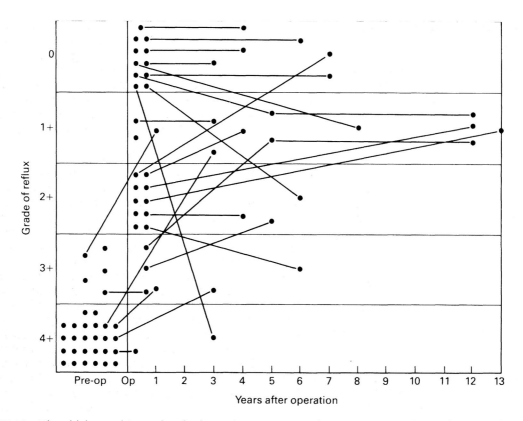

Figure 12.10 The phlebographic results of valve repair 3–13 years after operation. (Redrawn from Ferris and Kistner.[23])

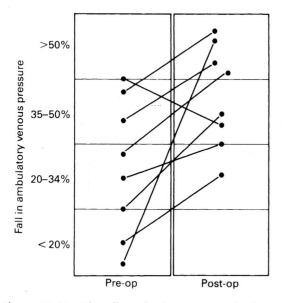

Figure 12.11 The effect of valve repair on the foot vein pressure during exercise. Seven of the eight patients studied had improved calf pump function. (Redrawn from Ferris and Kistner.[23])

transverse venotomy to gain access to the redundant cusps in preference to the original vertical incision, and Sottiurai[92] employing a combination of the two, using a T-shaped incision. Angioscopy has been used to assess competence of valves repaired at direct and indirect valvuloplasty.[51,109] Gloviczki *et al.*[28] have recently described a technique for the direct repair of floppy valve cusps using angioscopy to guide the placement of the cusp-reefing sutures, thus eliminating the need to perform a venotomy in the region of the valve. A prosthetic cuff was also used to provide external support to the valve sinus, a technique described below.

Kistner's long-term results[62] in 51 limbs over a mean period of 10.6 years indicate that the performance of repaired valves can deteriorate for up to 6 years after surgery, but thereafter the repairs remain durable. Freedom from severe symptoms and ulceration was achieved in 73% of limbs undergoing valvuloplasty for correction of primary valve incompetence. Calf pump function was universally improved but did return to normal in all cases. The importance of correcting communicating vein incompetence was once again demonstrated.

Indirect valvuloplasty: valve sinus procedures

In 1972, Hallberg[31] reported a technique to reduce sinus dilatation by wrapping a Dacron cuff around the valve (Figure 12.12). The diameter of the cuff was adjusted to restore valve competence. One patient with chronic venous ulceration (despite superficial and communicating vein surgery and bandaging) was treated in this way and patency and competence were demonstrated phlebographically 2 months after procedure. Clinical improvement apparently occurred during this short period, although details of long-term follow-up are not available.

Jessup and Lane[37] have investigated a similar technique in the external jugular vein of the sheep, where a Dacron-reinforced silicone cuff (Venocuff) was used to resolve natural or induced valve incompetence. The cuff restored competence in most valves, but was surrounded by a fibrous capsule and induced a mild fibrosis of the vein wall, although the endothelium remained intact.

Axial plication of the valve sinus has also been employed to reduce excessive dilatation and restore valve competence (Figure 12.13). The valve ring is reduced in circumference by a longitudinal series of plication sutures at right angles to the valve ring and midway between the commissures. This does not shorten the cusps but may stop them prolapsing. Jones *et al.*[39] performed this procedure in five patients with chronic venous disease and achieved resolution of oedema and ulceration up to one year.

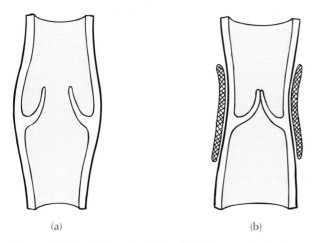

(a) (b)

Figure 12.12 The principle of indirect valvuloplasty using an external cuff. (a) An incompetent valve with healthy valve cusps. (b) Competence restored by an encircling slightly constricting Dacron mesh.

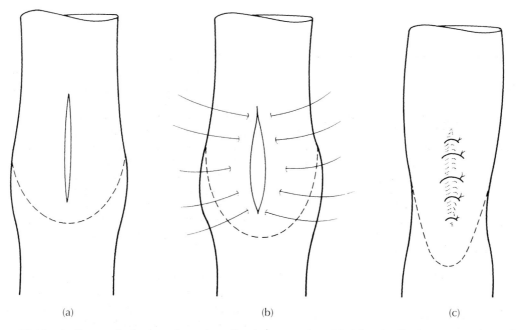

(a) (b) (c)

Figure 12.13 Indirect valvuloplasty by valve plication operation. (a) A longitudinal venotomy is made level with the edge of the valve cusp, midway between the commissures. It is then enlarged towards the centre of the attached border of the cusp. (b) Sutures are placed to close the venotomy but at an increasing distance from the edge of the venotomy at its centre. (c) When the sutures are tied the circumference of the valve ring is reduced.

Comment

Direct valvuloplasty apparently confers lasting competence in the majority of valves, together with long-term improvement of calf pump function and resolution of clinical disease when combined with other appropriate procedures. Meticulous technique is required and considerable measures are necessary to avoid thrombosis. The great advantage of indirect valvuloplasty techniques is that they do not require a venotomy and leave no foreign material within the lumen. Clamping of the vein is avoided, and heparinization and other antithrombotic measures are unnecessary. The long-term effects of a cuff on the valve wall are not yet clear.

The use of both direct and indirect valvuloplasty techniques is limited to the correction of non-thrombotic valve incompetence, but they may be of use in valve transposition or transplantation procedures in maintaining or restoring competence.

Our interpretation of all the studies published to date is that valve repair is not in itself sufficient to relieve the swelling and skin changes of deep axial vein incompetence. We think that these studies suggest that symptoms do not appear until the communicating veins become incompetent and that axial vein valve repair will have only a temporary effect if the communicating vein abnormality is not corrected.

Valve replacement techniques

These techniques are used in the aftermath of deep vein thrombosis (where valve cusps are damaged beyond repair or no longer present) or, in the much rarer condition of congenital avalvulosis. A considerable number of valve mechanism replacement techniques have been described in animal studies, but apart from transposition and transplantation, few have been attempted in man.

Valve transposition operations

The valves of the three major veins that meet below the inguinal ligament – the superficial and deep femoral veins and the long saphenous vein – are not usually afflicted with the same abnormality. In 1979, Kistner and Sparkuhl[44] described a technique for restoring competence to a refluxing superficial femoral vein. This involves transposing a competent valve-bearing segment of long saphenous vein (end-to-end anastomosis), or profunda femoris vein (end-to-side anastomosis) onto the incompetent superficial femoral vein (Figure 12.14). The best operation is probably the anastomosis of the superficial femoral vein to a competent deep femoral vein. The saphenous vein is often unsuitable because it is incompetent in most forms of chronic venous insufficiency.

The anastomosis must be made with care using fine monofilament materials. A-V fistulae are not usually employed but the patient should be given anticoagulants for 3–6 months.

This technique was performed in 14 patients, all of whom had grade 3 or 4 reflux.[23] Reflux and foot vein pressures were improved in all patients initially, but by 3 years several had recurrence of their reflux and many had recurrent symptoms. One of the criticisms of this study has been that most of the patients underwent communicating vein surgery which may have masked the effect of the transposition.[33]

Queral *et al.*[74] performed a similar study in 12 patients but performed only the transposition procedure. Three months postoperatively, the mean post-exercise foot vein pressure recovery time had returned to normal and all ulcers had healed. At one year, however, the mean recovery time had become abnormal and nine patients had developed recurrent ulceration.[38] All these patients had gross communicating vein reflux. Unfortunately, only two patients underwent late descending phlebography, and thus, the performance of the transposed valves is impossible to assess.

Kistner's study failed to demonstrate the value of valve transposition in the restoration of calf pump function, and suggests that subsequent deterioration is largely due to failure of the transposed valve. Queral's study, however, shows that valve transposition alone can restore calf pump function to normal, thus suggesting that deep reflux is of major importance in determining calf pump function, but fails to demonstrate whether the recurrence of calf pump failure in this study was caused solely by deteriorating communicating vein reflux or failure of the transposed valve.

The evidence published to date suggests that the insertion of a functioning valve in the femoral vein by transposition improves calf pump function initially, but fails to confer long-term deep axial vein competence. Addition of an external valvuloplasty technique to the transposed valve may promote long-term competence. Long-term competence and calf pump function are also dependent on correction of superficial and communicating vein reflux.

Valve transplantation

Although Carrel and Guthrie[10] transplanted valve-bearing vein segments in the dog in 1906, it was not until 1960 that De Weese and Niguidula[16] specifically studied the fate of autotransplanted valves. They transplanted femoral vein valves from the contralateral leg in 20 dogs, achieving primary

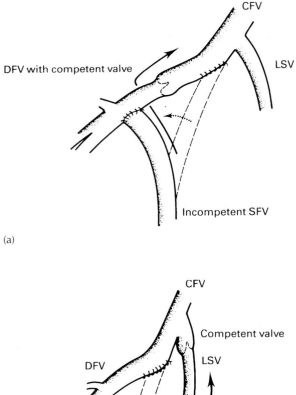

(a)

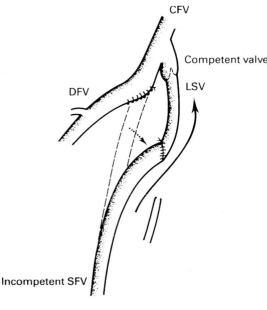

(c)

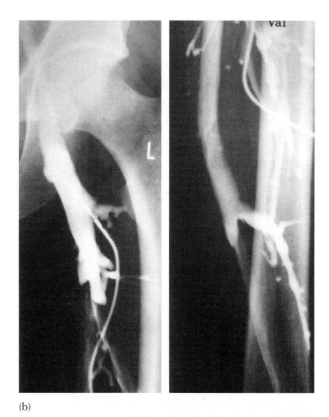

(b)

Figure 12.14 Valve transposition. (a) An incompetent superficial femoral vein (SFV) anastomosed to the deep femoral vein (DFV) below a competent valve. CFV, common femoral vein; LSV, long saphenous vein. (b) A phlebograph showing a competent deep femoral vein (left hand panel) and an incompetent superficial femoral vein (right hand panel). This patient could be treated with the operation shown in Figure 12.14(a). (c) An incompetent superficial femoral vein anastomosed to the long saphenous vein below a competent valve. This operation is rarely performed as the long saphenous vein is usually incompetent in patients with long-standing post-thrombotic deep vein damage.

patency 14–21 days after implantation in 11, with competence in nine, as assessed by Harvey's strip test. They demonstrated that early thrombosis followed by recanalization could give a false impression of patency but that where this occurred the valve was always incompetent.

During the 1960s, further animal studies followed, particularly evaluating the role of autotransplanted valves in healthy and experimentally thrombosed veins.[5,11,46,59,106] These studies demonstrated that valve autotransplantation was a practical proposition, and in 1982, Taheri _et al._[96] reported the first human procedures involving transplantation of a brachial vein valve into the superficial

femoral vein of patients with post-thrombotic reflux.

The method used by Taheri to assess incompetence was retrograde injection through a catheter introduced via an arm vein. Taheri stated that even when a competent valve was found in the common femoral vein the catheter could be passed through the valve cusps so that valves below this level could be assessed. Taheri therefore advocates valve transplants for patients with segmental valvular incompetence as well as complete axial vein valve incompetence when there is reflux to the knee and below (grades 3 and 4), and when there has been no response to conservative treatment, providing the phlebographic abnormality is confirmed by foot vein pressure studies and atrophic changes in a calf muscle biopsy.[95]

Technique of valve transplantation

An incision is made on the medial aspect of the thigh centred on the adductor tubercle so that the upper part of the popliteal vein can be exposed. Division of the long head of adductor magnus greatly enhances this exposure. If the popliteal vein wall is healthy, the brachial vein is exposed through a 4 cm incision, beginning just below the axilla. The valves are tested with Harvey's manoeuvre, and a 2 cm segment of vein with a healthy valve is removed.

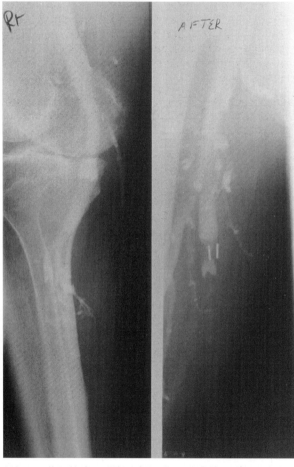

(a)   (b)

Figure 12.15   Autogenous valve transplantation. A pre-operative descending phlebograph (a) showing reflux to the calf, and a postoperative phlebograph showing a competent transplanted valve in the middle of the superficial femoral vein (b). The metal clips indicate the level of the upper anastomosis of the transplanted segment of brachial vein. (Reproduced by kind permission of Dr Syde Taheri.)

The popliteal vein is divided, approximately 1 cm is excised and the transplant is sewn in, end to end, with fine (7/0) monofilament sutures. An A-V fistula is not fashioned. Figure 12.15 shows pre- and postoperative phlebographs of one of these patients, demonstrating the restoration of valvular competence.

Full systemic heparinization followed by oral anticoagulation for 3–6 months were employed initially, but latterly Taheri has used pneumatic compression to prevent thrombosis and abandoned postoperative anticoagulation. Since 1983, he has placed the transplanted valve in the popliteal vein rather than the femoral vein.[94]

In 1985, Taheri *et al.*[97] reported the results of 71 valve transplants performed over a 5-year period in patients with severe symptoms refractory to conservative measures, grade 3 or 4 reflux, elevated venous pressures, and muscle changes. Follow-up was conducted by consultation, postal survey, and telephone enquiry. Forty-eight of the patients responded. Thirty-six patients reported improvement or complete relief of symptoms and 17 of the 18 respondents with leg ulceration reported healing (Figure 12.16).

Foot vein pressure measurements were performed before and after operation in only 20 patients. The average improvement of pressure reduction during exercise was 13%, i.e. all the patients still had abnormal calf pump function, and the exercising venous pressures for two patients were increased (Figure 12.17). Postoperative descending phlebography was performed in 31

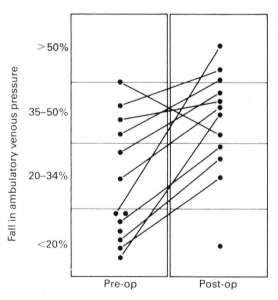

Figure 12.16   The results of a postal and telephone survey of 67 valve transplants performed on 62 patients. (Reproduced by kind permission of Dr Syde Taheri.)

patients. Twenty-eight valves were judged patent and competent, one was occluded and two were incompetent. How long after transplantation these studies were performed is unclear. It is also unclear how many patients had previously undergone superficial and communicating vein surgery.

Nash[36] has reported the results of 25 valve autotransplants, from the brachial to the popliteal vein in 23 patients with post-thrombotic reflux. All patients had persistent ulceration or skin changes despite previous superficial and communicating vein surgery. Of 17 patients, 15 healed their ulcers and six patients with skin changes showed rapid healing with resolution of symptoms. Ambulant venous pressure fell by an average of 18% postoperatively and this improvement was sustained in most patients 18 months later when all 18 valve transplants were patent, although five showed phlebographic evidence of reflux.

Venous valve transplantation is undoubtedly successful in correcting reflux and improving calf pump function and is associated with the resolution of ulceration and symptoms in some patients. However, the symptoms, signs and impairment of venous function tend to recur as time passes.[21] It seems that correction of deep reflux alone is inadequate and that correction of all refluxing systems should be undertaken.

Obtaining a suitable valve for transplantation can be difficult. Many harvested valves are incompetent once transplanted, despite being competent at preoperative descending phlebography. Such valves require an adjunct valvuloplasty.

In an attempt to overcome the limitations of valve supply inherent in autotransplantation, interposition of glutaraldehyde-preserved homografts and xenografts has been attempted.[1,40] Low patency and competence rates have so far precluded the use of these techniques in man. Brachial and axillary valve autotransplants tend to fail with the passage of time.[75] Possible reasons for this are:

- Size mismatch between the transplanted valve and recipient vein resulting in valve dilatation and incompetence – even in the popliteal position[63]
- Shedding of valvular endothelium during the first 4 months following transplantation, resulting in thrombosis and/or incompetence[77]
- Late fibrosis and degeneration, possibly caused by ischaemia.[99]

Such problems make valve autotransplantation unsuitable for universal use in the correction of deep venous reflux.

Psthakis' substitute valve

Psthakis[72] first performed the substitute valve technique in 1963, employing a sling fashioned from the gracilis muscle to compress the popliteal vein externally during walking. Fibrosis and adhesion formation prompted him to modify the technique, and he subsequently employed a silastic strip sutured to the gracilis tendon. He has claimed excellent late phlebographic, functional, and clinical results in 145 patients.[73] This technique has been evaluated in a few other centres, and their early results do not match those of Psthakis.

Experimental valve replacement techniques

Interest in alternative valve replacement techniques has developed over the past 10 years. This has been provoked by increasing awareness of the prominent role of deep reflux in venous insufficiency and failure of the currently available techniques to provide long-term patency and competence, particularly in post-thrombotic reflux. Most of these techniques have been described in single case reports or animal studies.

Case reports

Garcia-Rinaldi *et al.*[25] have implanted a xenograft monocusp valve mechanism in the superficial

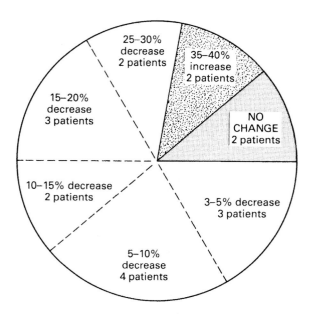

Average change = 13% decrease

Figure 12.17 The changes in foot vein pressure during exercise 1 month to 4 years after valve transplantation in 18 patients. The average decrease in foot vein pressure was 13%. (Reproduced by kind permission of Dr Syde Taheri.)

femoral and long saphenous veins of a patient with chronic venous ulceration refractory to conservative treatment in whom descending phlebography and Doppler examination had revealed gross deep and superficial reflux. The monocusp valves were constructed using preserved bovine pericardium and incorporated into the vein wall. Descending phlebography 4 weeks postoperatively demonstrated full competence, as did Doppler examination at intervals up to 14 months. Photoplethysmography performed 14 months postoperatively suggested normal calf pump function. Ulceration and symptoms resolved without the use of compression stockings. The patient was anticoagulated for 6 months.

Simpkin et al.[91] have described the construction of a choke mechanism in the femoral and popliteal veins by the creation of a stenosis. Although not strictly a valve, this was said to impede deep reflux, but no evidence is presented to confirm the claim. The clinical results in the four patients concerned are obscure. The mechanism seems just as likely to produce outflow obstruction as reduce reflux.

Sloan (personal communication, 1989) has employed a cryopreserved infant pulmonary valve homograft. This was placed in the common femoral vein of a patient with post-thrombotic ulceration. Symptoms and ulceration had resolved 6 months later but no details of late patency, competence or calf pump function are available. This technique depends on a supply of infant cardiac valves and cryopreservation techniques, neither of which is yet widely available in the United Kingdom.

Animal studies

Autografts

In 1953, Eiseman and Malette[20] used the principle of wall intussusception to produce an autogenous caval valve in 14 dogs. No anticoagulation was used and no gross thrombosis was found between 24 hours and 6 months later. Descending phlebography via the right renal vein was used to demonstrate competence of the valves, but no results were presented. In 1987, Rosenbloom et al.[80] described a method of valve construction using autologous external jugular vein in the dog. A segment of external jugular vein was harvested and the media and adventitia partially stripped from the intima which was then invaginated and secured to produce a cusp mechanism. The resultant valve was then interposed in the canine femoral vein. Fifteen such valves were constructed. The pressure gradient required to open the valve (opening pressure) was less than 3 cm H_2O in the three valves that were studied, and the closing pressures of two valves 3–5 cm H_2O. Four valves remained competent at pressure gradients of 55 cm H_2O. After implantation in six dogs not treated with

anticoagulants, thrombus formation prevented cusp closure, leading to incompetence in four, whereas the valves implanted in three anticoagulated dogs stayed patent and competent for 13 days after implantation. This is one of the few studies to give an account of the hydrostatic properties of a constructed valve, showing that it will function within the physiological range.

We have developed a technique of in-situ venous valve construction employing vein wall intussusception to produce a bicuspid valve (Figure 12.18).[113] The vein is lengthened using an interposition vein graft prior to valve construction to compensate for the shortening that intussusception creates. The technique avoids devascularization of the valve segment and avoids problems of incorrect size matching of valve to its adjacent vein segments, problems which may cause the long-term failure of transplanted valves. Forty-one valves were constructed in the femoral vein of the dog and all were patent and competent by Harvey's test immediately after construction. Descending phlebography confirmed competence in 38 valves (Figure 12.19).

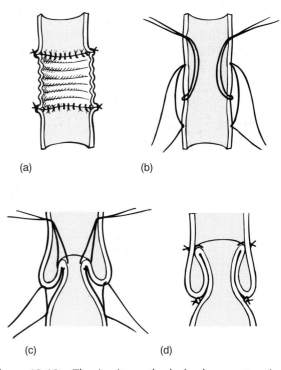

(a)   (b)

(c)   (d)

Figure 12.18   The *in-situ* method of valve construction. (a) Interposition graft. The vein is first lengthened by inserting a segment of transplanted autogenous vein or PTFE graft. (b) Intussuscepting sutures. Prolene sutures are placed through the lumen and on the outer surface of the vein to effect the intussusception. (c) When these sutures are tightened the vein intussuscepts. (d) When the sutures are tight the intussuscipiens forms a bicuspid valve.

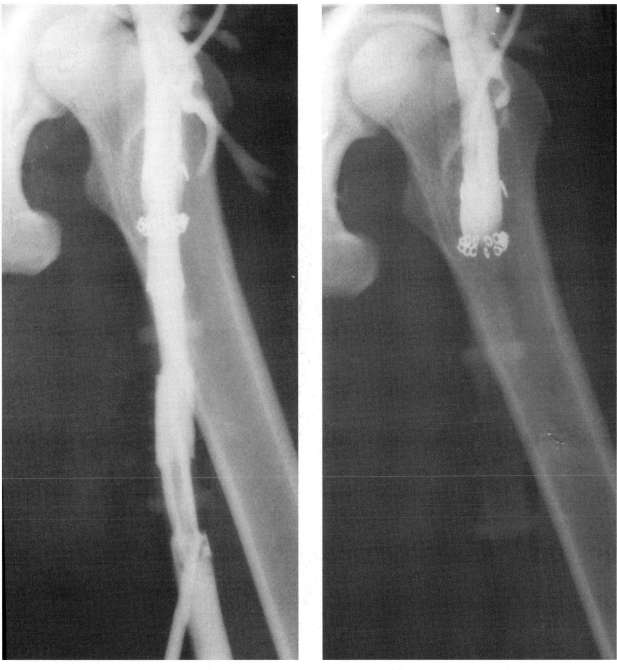

(a)   (b)

Figure 12.19   (a) An ascending phlebograph of an *in-situ* valve. (b) A descending phlebograph showing complete competence. Apart from the sutures which produced the intussusception and which were marked with small Ligaclips, all the other anastomoses and sutures were made with microclips.

Static pressure testing indicated full competence between 0.5 and 250 cm H_2O in 24 of 27 valves tested. Five of six valves constructed in surviving animals remained competent up to 112 days after construction.

Homografts

The first valved venous homograft was implanted by Waddell *et al.*[106] in the dog. They achieved patency in 40% but competence in only 10% at 2–3 weeks post-implantation, at which time marked inflammatory changes were present in all valves. McLachlin *et al.*[59] had no patent grafts in a series of 14 fresh homografts. Wright *et al.*[114] found little difference in the patency rates of fresh or frozen irradiated homografts. Perloff *et al.*[68] demonstrated in rats that venous grafts provoke a cellular immune response emphasized by the subsequent rejection of donor skin grafts. Although this response was attenuated by immunosuppressive agents and thrombosis delayed by peroperative heparinization (seven dogs), defibrinogenation (three dogs), and the construction of an arteriovenous fistula (eight dogs), all preserved valves had thrombosed by 6 weeks. In a similar study, Kaya *et al.*[40] found that glutaraldehyde-preserved valve autografts had superior patency and competence than preserved homografts 7 weeks after implantation.

Xenografts

Xenografts require preservation and neutralization of antigenic determinants. Glutaraldehyde has been used extensively for treatment of xenograft valves in the cardiac and arterial circulations,[15] but is associated with an unacceptable degree of thrombosis in the venous system.

Phifer *et al.*[69] have implanted glutaraldehyde-preserved cardiac bioprosthetic xenograft valves in the inferior vena cava of 22 dogs. Despite promising early results, 10 valves had thrombosed by 28 months and nine had caused pulmonary emboli.[26]

Prosthetic valves

The limitations of autogenous vein valve autotransplantation, including inadequate donor valves and late cusp degeneration,[99] have prompted various attempts to produce a readily available valve prosthesis that is convenient to use. Unfortunately, prosthetic materials have suffered from low patency rates when used as venous conduits,[14,30] although results recently obtained using expanded polytetrafluoroethylene (ePTFE) have been more favourable.[71,93]

Hill *et al.*[34] have designed a bicuspid flutter valve mechanism which has been produced in both pellethane polymer and tanned human umbilical vein. Ten pellethane and ten umbilical vein valves were implanted into the external jugular veins of 20 dogs. The umbilical vein valves were all occluded by 48 hours, and all the pellethane valves were thrombosed by 8 days, in spite of full anticoagulation.

Warmenhoven *et al.*[108] have implanted valve-shaped silastic mandrels in dogs to excite the production of a corresponding collagen sheath. After 5–13 weeks, the mandrel was removed and the collagen valve removed for implantation into the femoral or external jugular vein. Fifteen valves

were produced in this way and inserted without anticoagulation. All valves had thrombosed 16 weeks after implantation.

Taheri *et al.*[98] have developed a centre-hinged bileaflet valve which they have constructed in platinum or pyrolite carbon-covered titanium. These valves were initially tested for fatigue and wear characteristics over a 5-month period. One valve showed cracking adjacent to a cusp hinge. Hydrodynamic pressure and flow studies showed regurgitation of approximately 48% of the ejected stroke volume per cycle in the first few valves, although this improved subsequently. Ten valves (five of each material) were then implanted into nine dogs, seven in the inferior vena cava and three in the femoral vein. All five titanium valves showed evidence of thrombosis with complete occlusion of four between 14 and 18 months after implantation. Two of these valves also became grossly displaced. The four platinum valves studied plebographically were patent and competent 14–18 months after implantation.[99]

Problems such as displacement, regurgitation and thrombosis seem to preclude any human trial at present.

Commentary

Venous reflux appears central to the development of calf pump failure. How best to define and measure pathological reflux remains unclear and this is illustrated by the poor correlation between measurements of calf pump function, venous reflux and the clinical expression of calf pump failure. Improvements in ultrasound technology have facilitated the increasingly accurate study of deep vein reflux and rendered the duration and velocity of reflux measurable as well as revealing phenomena such as segmental reflux. Deep vein reflux is clearly important in the pathogenesis of calf pump failure, but is inextricably linked with superficial and communicating vein reflux. Attempts to correct reflux in one isolated system tend to fail and the early studies in valvuloplasty, transposition and transplantation have demonstrated the close interdependence of the deep, superficial and communicating veins of the leg. There are indications that correction of reflux in one system may improve reflux in other systems with various reports demonstrating resolution of deep vein reflux following abolition of long saphenous vein reflux.[83,107] The concept of global reflux has developed and attempts have been made to define a level of total reflux in the leg which will lead to calf pump failure.[104]

Deep vein reflux has generally been attributed to post-thrombotic valve damage, or to non-thrombotic floppy valves. The prevalence of the latter condition remains unclear, but our own studies suggest that non-thrombotic reflux accounts for 10–15% of the whole. Increasingly it appears that the two lesions are not so clearly defined, with subtle post-thrombotic changes being detected in the veins adjacent to apparently non-thrombotic floppy valves. It may well be that floppy valve reflux predisposes to deep vein thrombosis. We suspect that the detection of post-thrombotic deep vein reflux is dependent on how hard it is sought. Venous valves are sensitive to injury and appear central to the process of venous thrombosis.

The development, morphology and function of venous valves are complex and incompletely understood with research in the fields of static and dynamic valve function being virtually non-existent.

Attempts to repair and replace human venous valves have met with mixed success and none of the available techniques is widely used. Currently, direct valvuloplasty to restore competence in non-thrombotic deep vein reflux with correction of coexisting superficial and communicating vein reflux offers the best long-term relief from calf pump failure. Unfortunately, a readily available 'off-the-shelf' valve replacement is far away with problems relating to thrombosis and long-term competence appearing insurmountable. There is a need for a valve construction technique which can overcome these problems and an autogenous mechanism seems most promising. Further studies are required to establish the optimum type, number and position of valves to restore and maintain normal venous physiology.

Techniques for abolishing reflux in the deep venous system remain the province of the specialist clinical researcher. Treatment of coexisting superficial and communicating vein reflux, where appropriate, with the provision of good quality graduated compression hosiery remains central to the management of most patients with calf pump failure associated with deep vein reflux.

References

1. Ackroyd JS. *Venous Valve Homografts.* MChir Thesis, University of Cambridge, 1985.
2. Ackroyd JS, Browse NL. The investigation and surgery of the post-thrombotic syndrome. *J Cardiovasc Surg* 1985; **27:** 5–16.
3. Ackroyd JS, Pattison M, Browse NL. A study of the mechanical properties of fresh and preserved human femoral vein wall and valve cusps. *Br J Surg* 1985; **72:** 117–19.
4. Ackroyd JS, Thomas ML, Browse NL. Deep vein reflux: an assessment by descending phlebography. *Br J Surg* 1986; **73:** 31–3.
5. Baird RJ, Lipton IH, Miyagishima RT, Labrosse CJ. Replaclement of deep veins of the leg. *Arch Surg* 1964; **89:** 797–805.
6. Baker SR, Burnand KG, Sommeville KM, Thomas ML, Wilson NM, Browse NL. Comparison of venous reflux assessed by duplex scanning and descending phlebography in chronic venous disease. *Lancet* 1993; **341:** 400–3.
7. Basmajian JV. The distribution of valves in the femoral, iliac and common iliac veins and their relationship to varicose veins. *Surg Gynecol Obstet* 1952; **95:** 537–42.
8. Böck P. Vergleich der morphologie von arterien – und venenklappen. *Verh Anat Ges* 1975; **69:** 145–9.
9. Caps MT, Manzo RA, Bergelin RO, Meissner MH, Strandness DE. Venous valvular reflux in veins not involved at the time of acute deep vein thrombosis. *J Vasc Surg* 1995; **22:** 524–31.
10. Carrel A, Guthrie CC. Uniterminal and biterminal venus transplantations. *Surg Gynecol Obstet* 1906; **2:** 266–86.
11. Cerino M, McGraw JY, Luke JC. Autogenous vein graft replacement of thrombosed deep veins. Experimental approach to the postphlebitic syndrome. *Surgery* 1964; **55:** 123–34.
12. Cheatle TR, Perrin M. Venous valve repair: early results in fifty-two cases. *J Vasc Surg* 1994; **19:** 404–13.
13. Cotton LT. Varicose veins. Gross anatomy and development. *Br J Surg* 1961; **48:** 589–98.
14. Dale WA, Scott HW. Grafts of the venous system. *Surgery* 1963; **53:** 52–71.
15. Dardik H, Ibrahim IM, Sprayregen S, Dardik II. Clinical experience with modified human umbilical cord vein for arterial bypass. *Surgery* 1976; **79:** 618–24.
16. De Weese JA, Niguidula F. The replacement of short segments of veins with functional autogenous venous grafts. *Surg Gynecol Obstet* 1960; **110:** 303–8.
17. Dohn K. Tilt phlebography. *Acta Radiol* 1958; **50:** 293–309.
18. Edwards EA. The orientation of venous valves in relation to body surfaces. *Anat Rec* 1936; **64:** 369–81.
19. Edwards EA, Edwards JE. The effect of thrombophlebitis on the venous valves. *Surg Gynecol Obstet* 1937; **65:** 310–20.
20. Eiseman B, Malette W. An operative technique for the construction of venous valves. *Surg Gynecol Obstet* 1953; **97:** 731–4.
21. Eriksson I. Vein valve surgery for deep valvular incompetence . In: Eklöf B, Gjöres JE, Thulesius O, Berqvist D, eds. *Controversies in the Management of Venous Disorders.* London: Butterworth, 1989.
22. Eriksson I, Almgren B. Influence of the profunda femoris vein on venous hemodynamics of the limb. *J Vasc Surg* 1986; **4:** 390–5.
23. Ferris EB, Kistner RL. Femoral vein reconstruction in the management of chronic venous insufficiency. *Arch Surg* 1982; **117:** 1571–9.

24. Franklin KJ. Valves in veins: an historical survey. *Proc R Soc Med* 1927; **2:** 1–33.

25. Garcia-Rinaldi R, Revuelta JM, Martinez MJ, Granada E, De Santos L. Femoral vein incompetence: treatment with a xenograft monocusp patch. *J Vasc Surg* 1986; **3:** 932–5.

26. Gerlock AJ, Phifer TJ, McDonald JC. Venous prosthetic valves. The first step towards an investigation in the canine model. *Invest Radiol* 1985; **20:** 42–4.

27. Gibbs NM. Venous thrombosis of the lower limbs with particular reference to bed rest. *Br J Surg* 1957; **45:** 209–36.

28. Gloviczki P, Merrell SW, Bower TC. Femoral vein valve repair under direct vision without venotomy: a modified technique with use of angioscopy. *J Vasc Surg* 1991; **14:** 645–8.

29. Gottlob R, May R. *Venous Valves.* Vienna: Springer-Verlag, 1986.

30. Haimovici H, Hoffert PW, Zinicola M, Steinman C. An experimental and clinical evaluation of grafts in the venous system. *Surg Gynecol Obstet* 1970; **131:** 1173–86.

31. Hallberg D. A method for repairing incompetent valves in deep veins. *Acta Chir Scand* 1972; **138:** 143–5.

32. Hamer JD, Malone PO, Silver JA. The pO2 in venous valve pockets: its possible bearing on thrombogenesis. *Br J Surg* 1981; **68:** 166–70.

33. Hepp W. Zur kongenitalen aplasie und avalvulie der beinvenen. *Vasa* 1980; **9:** 316–20.

34. Hill R, Schmidt S, Evancho M, Hunler T, Hillegass D, Sharp W. Development of a prosthetic venous valve. *J Biomed Mater Res* 1985; **19:** 827–32.

35. Högensgård IC, Stürup H. Static and dynamic pressures in superficial and deep veins of the lower extremity in man. *Acta Phys Scand* 1953; **27:** 49–67.

36. Huse JB, Nabseth DC, Bush HL, Widrich WC, Johnson WC. Direct venous surgery for venous valvular insufficiency of the lower extremity. *Arch Surg* 1983; **118:** 719–23.

37. Jessup G, Lane RJ. Repair of incompetent venous valves: a new technique. *J Vasc Surg* 1988; **8:** 569–75.

38. Johnson ND, Queral LA, Flinn WR, Yao JST, Bergan JJ. Late objective assessment of venous valve surgery. *Arch Surg* 1981; **116:** 1461–5.

39. Jones JW, Elliot F, Kerstein MD. Triangular venous valvuloplasty. *Arch Surg* 1982; **117:** 1250–1.

40. Kaya M, Grogan JB, Lentz D, Tew W, Taju S. Glutaraldehyde-preserved venous valve transplantation in the dog. *J Surg Res* 1988; **45:** 294–7.

41. Kistner R. Surgical repair of a venous valve. *Straub Clin Proc* 1968; **34:** 41–3.

42. Kistner RL. Surgical repair of the incompetent femoral vein valve. *Arch Surg* 1975; **110:** 1336–42.

43. Kistner RL. Primary venous valve incompetence of the leg. *Am J Surg* 1980; **140:** 218–24.

44. Kistner RL, Sparkuhl MD. Surgery in acute and chronic venous disease. *Surgery* 1979; **85:** 31–41.

45. Konradsen L, Jorgensen LN, Albrecht-Best E, Nielsen SP. Popliteal valve incompetence and postoperative deep vein thrombosis. *Acta Chir Scand* 1990; **156:** 441–3.

46. Kunlin J, Lengua F, Richard S, Tregouet T, Mourton A. Grafting of valvulated veins: an experimental study. *J Cardiovasc Surg* 1966; **7:** 520–3.

47. Labropoulos N, Delis KT, Nicolaides AN. Venous reflux in symptom-free vascular surgeons. *J Vasc Surg* 1995; **22:** 150–4.

48. Labropoulos N, Delis KT, Nicolaides AN, Leon M, Ramaswami G. The role of the distribution and anatomic extent of reflux in the development of signs and symptoms in chronic venous insufficiency. *J Vasc Surg* 1996; **23:** 504–10.

49. Lea Thomas M. *Phlebography of the Lower Limb.* Edinburgh: Churchill Livingstone, 1982; 164.

50. Lea Thomas M, Andress MR. Phlebographic changes in arteriomegaly. *Acta Radiol Diagn (Stockh)* 1970; **10:** 427–32.

51. Lermusiaux P, De Forges MR. Angioscopy-assisted valvuloplasty for primary deep venous valvular insufficiency. *Ann Vasc Surg* 1996; **10:** 233–8.

52. Lindvall N, Lodin A. Congenital absence of valves in the deep veins of the leg. *Acta Derm Venereol Scand* 1961; **41:** Suppl 45.

53. Ljungnér H, Bergqvist D. Decreased fibrinolytic activity in the bottom of human vein valve pockets. *Vasa* 1983; **12:** 333–6.

54. Lodin A, Lindvall A, Gentele H. Congenital absence of venous valves as a cause of leg ulcers. *Acta Chir Scand* 1958; **116:** 265–71.

55. Ludbrook J. Functional aspects of the veins of the leg. *Am Heart J* 1962; **64:** 706–13.

56. Ludbrook J. *Aspects of Venous Function in the Lower Limbs.* Springfield, IL: Thomas, 1966.

57. Luke JC. The diagnosis of chronic enlargement of the leg, with the description of a new syndrome. *Surg Gynecol Obstet* 1941; **73:** 472–80.

58. Mathieson FR. Tilt phlebography. A reliable method for diagnosing incompetent communicating veins. *Acta Radiol* 1958; **50:** 430–43.

59. McLachlin AD, Carroll SE, Meads GE, Amacher AL. Valve replacement in the recanalized incompetent superficial femoral vein in dogs. *Ann Surg* 1965; **162:** 446–51.

60. McLachlin AD, McLachlin JA, Jory YA, Rawling EG. Venous statis in the lower extremities. *Ann Surg* 1960; **152:** 678–85.

61. Markel A, Manzo RA, Bergelin RO, Strandness DE. Valvular reflux after deep vein thrombosis; incidence and time of occurrence. *J Vasc Surg* 1992; **15:** 377–82.

62. Masuda M, Kistner RL. Long-term results of venous valve reconstruction: a four- to twenty-one-year follow-up. *J Vasc Surg* 1994; **19:** 391–403.

63. Nash T. Long-term results of vein valve transplants placed in the popliteal vein for intractable postphlebetic venous ulcers and pre-ulcer skin changes. *J Cardiovasc Surg* 1988; **29:** 712–16.

64. Nicolaides AN, Zukowski AJ. The value of dynamic venous pressure measurements. *World J Surg* 1986; **19:** 919–24.

65. Paterson JC, McLachlin J. Precipitating factors in venous thrombosis. *Surg Gynecol Obstet* 1954; **98:** 96–102.

66. Payne SP, London NJ, Jagger C, Newland CJ, Barrie WW, Bell PRF. The clinical significance of venous reflux detected by duplex scanning. *Br J Surg* 1994; **81:** 39–41.

67. Perloff LJ, Reckard CR, Barker CF. Studies of the venous homograft. *Surg Forum* 1972; **23:** 245–6.

68. Perloff LJ, Reckard CR, Rowlands DT, Barker CF. The venous homograft: an immunological question. *Surgery* 1972; **72:** 961–70.

69. Phifer TJ, Gerlock AJ, Grafton WD, McDonald JC. Valvular xenografts in the inferior vena cava. *Am J Surg* 1989; **157:** 588–92.

70. Plate G, Brudin L, Eklöf B, Jensen R, Ohlin P. Physiologic and therapeutic aspects in congenital vein valve aplasia of the lower limb. *Ann Surg* 1983; **198:** 229–33.

71. Plate G, Hollier LH, Gloviczki P, Dewanji MK, Kaye MP. Overcoming failure of venous vascular prostheses. *Surgery* 1984; **96:** 503–10.

72. Psthakis N. Has the substitute valve at the popliteal vein solved the problem of venous insufficiency of the lower extremity? *J Cardiovasc Surg* 1968; **9:** 64–70.

73. Psthakis ND, Psthakis DN. Surgical treatment of deep venous insufficiency of the lower limb. *Surg Gynecol Obstet* 1988; **166:** 131–41.

74. Queral LA, Whitehouse WM, Flinn WR, Neiman HL, Yao JST, Bergan JJ. Surgical correction of chronic deep venous insufficiency by valvular transposition. *Surgery* 1980; **87:** 688–95.

75. Raju S. Venous ulceration of the lower limb and stasis ulceration. *Ann Surg* 1983; **197:** 688–97.

76. Raju S, Fredericks R. Valve reconstruction procedures for nonobstructive venous insufficiency: rationale, technique and results in 107 procedures with two- to eight-year follow-up. *J Vasc Surg* 1988; **7:** 301–10.

77. Raju S, Perry JT. The response of venous valvular endothelium to autotransplantation and in vitro preservation. *Surgery* 1983; **94:** 770–5.

78. Reagan B, Folse R. Lower limb venous dynamics in normal persons and children of patients with varicose veins. *Surg Gynecol Obstet* 1971; **132:** 15–18.

79. Rodriguez AA, Whitehead CM, McLaughlin RL, Umphrey R, Welch HJ, O'Donnell TF. Duplex-derived valve closure times fail to correlate with reflux flow volumes in patients with chronic venous insufficiency. *J Vasc Surg* 1996; **23:** 606–10.

80. Rosenbloom MS, Schuler JJ, Bishara RA, Ronan SG, Flanigan DP. Early experimental experience with a surgically created totally autogenous venous valve: a preliminary report. *J Vasc Surg* 1988; **7:** 642–6.

81. Rosfors S, Lamke LO, Nordstrom E, Bygdeman S. Severity and location of venous valvular insufficiency: the importance of distal valve function. *Acta Chir Scand* 1990; **156:** 689–94.

82. Ruckley CV, Makhdoomi KR. The venous perforator. *Br J Surg* 1966; **83:** 1492–4.

83. Sales CM, Bilof ML, Petrillo KA, Luka NL. Correction of lower extremity deep venous incompetence by ablation of superficial venous reflux. *Ann Vasc Surg* 1966; **10:** 186–9.

84. Salomonowitz E, Gottlob R. Untersuchungen am endothel der vena iliaca communis sinistra als beitrag zur pathogenese des venensporna. *Vasa* 1981; **10:** 194–8.

85. Samuels PB, Plested WG, Haberfelde GC, Cincotti JJ, Brown CE. In situ saphenous vein arterial bypass: a study of the anatomy pertinent to its use in situ as a bypass graft with a description of a new valvulotome. *Am Surg* 1968; **34:** 122–30.

86. Saphir O, Lev M. Venous valvulitis. *Arch Pathol* 1952; **53:** 456–69.

87. Saphir O, Lev M. The venous valve in the aged. *Am Heart J* 1952; **44:** 843–50.

88. Schanzer H, Pierce EC. A rational approach to surgery of the chronic venous stasis syndrome. *Ann Surg* 1982; **195:** 25–9.

89. Sevitt S. The structure and growth of valve-pocket thrombi in femoral veins. *J Clin Pathol* 1974; **27:** 517–28.

90. Sevitt S, Gallagher NG. Prevention of venous thrombosis and pulmonary embolism in injured patients. *Lancet* 1959; **2:** 981–9.

91. Simpkin R, Esteban JC, Bulloj R. By pass venovenosus y valvuloplastias en el tratamiento quirúrgico del síndrome postrombótico. *Angiologia* 1988; **40:** 30–5.

92. Sottiurai VS. Technique in direct venous valvuloplasty. *J Vasc Surg* 1988; **8:** 646–8.

93. Soyer T, Lempineu M, Cooper P, Norton L, Eisman B. A new venous prosthesis. *Surgery* 1972; **72:** 864–72.

94. Taheri SA, Elias SM, Yacobucci GN, Heffnner R, Lazar L. Indications and results of vein valve transplant. *J Cardiovasc Surg* 1986; **27:** 163–8.

95. Taheri SA, Heffner R, Williams J, Lazar L, Elias S. Muscle changes in venous insufficiency. *Arch Surg* 1984; **119:** 929–31.

96. Taheri SA, Lazar L, Elias S, Marchand P, Heffner R. Surgical treatment of postphlebitic syndrome with vein valve transplant. *Am J Surg* 1982; **144:** 221–4.

97. Taheri SA, Prendergast D, Lazar E, *et al.* Vein valve transplantation. *Am J Surg* 1985; **150:** 203–6.

98. Taheri SA, Rigan D, Wels P, Mentzer R, Shores RM. Experimental prosthetic vein valve. *Am J Surg* 1988; **156:** 111–14.

99. Taheri SA, Shores R. Successful use of prosthetic vein valves in dog. In: Davy A, Stemmer R, eds. *Phlébologie '89.* London: Libbey, 1989; 1035–7.

100. Thulesius O, Norgren L, Gjores JE. Foot volumetry: a new method for objective assessment of edema and venous function. *Vasa* 1973; **2:** 325–9.

101. Turner Warwick W. Valvular defects in relation to varicosis. *Lancet* 1930; **2:** 1278–86.

102. Van Bemmelen PS, Bedford G, Beach K, Strandness DE. Quantitative segmental evaluation of venous valvular reflux with duplex ultrasound scanning. *J Vasc Surg* 1989; **10:** 425–31.

103. Van Haarst EP, Liasis N, van Romshorst B, Moll FL. The development of valvular incompetence after deep vein thrombosis: a seven year follow-up study with duplex scanning. *Eur J Vasc Endovasc Surg* 1996; **12:** 295–9.

104. Vasdekis SN, Clarke GH, Nicolaides AN. Quantification of venous reflux by means of duplex scanning. *J Vasc Surg* 1989; **10:** 670–7.

105. Von Kügelen A, Greinemann H. Die Klappen in den menschlichen nierenvenen, besonders in der mündung der nierenbeckenvenen. *Z Zellforsch* 1959; **47:** 648–73.

106. Waddell WG, Vogelfanger IJ, Prudhomme P, Ram JD, Beattie WG, Ewing JB. Venous valve transplantation. *Arch Surg* 1964; **88:** 5–15.

107. Walsh JC, Bergan JJ, Beeman S, Comer TP. Femoral venous reflux abolished by greater saphenous vein stripping. *Ann Vasc Surg* 1994; **8:** 566–70.

108. Warmenhoven PG, Klopper PJ, Keeman JN. Construction of valves in the venous system. A preliminary report of an experimental study in dogs. *Eur Surg Res* 1985; **17(Suppl 1):** 105.

109. Welch HJ, McLaughlin RL, O'Donnell TF. Femoral vein valvuloplasty: intraoperative angioscopic evaluation and haemodynamic improvement. *J Vasc Surg* 1992; **16:** 694–700.

110. Welch HJ, Young CM, Semegran AB, Iafrati MD, Mackey WC, O'Donnell TF. Duplex assessment of venous reflux and chronic venous insufficiency: the significance of deep venous reflux. *J Vasc Surg* 1996; **24:** 755–62.

111. Whitehead S, Clemenson G, Browse NL. The assessment of calf pump function by isotope plethysmography. *Br J Surg* 1983; **70:** 675.

112. Wilson NM, Rutt DL, Browse NL. Repair and replacement of deep vein valves in the treatment of venous insufficiency. *Br J Surg* 1991; **78:** 388–94.

113. Wilson NM, Rutt DL, Browse NL. In situ venous valve construction. *Br J Surg* 1991; **78:** 595–600.

114. Wright CB, Hobson RW, Giordano JM, de Witt PL, Rich NM. Acute femoral venous occlusion (management by segmental venous replacement in the dog). *J Cardiovasc Surg* 1977; **18:** 523–9.

115. Wright JTM. Hydrodynamic evaluation of tissue valves. In: Ionescu MI, ed. *Tissue Heart Valves.* London: Butterworth, 1979.

CHAPTER 13

Chronic deep vein obstruction

Pathology	409	Treatment	419
Clinical presentation	415	References	425
Investigations	416		

The commonest cause of deep vein obstruction, acute or chronic, is deep vein thrombosis. The pathology, diagnosis and treatment of acute deep vein thrombosis are described in Chapters 8, 9 and 10. This chapter deals with one of the late sequelae of deep vein thrombosis, namely chronic deep vein obstruction; the other serious sequel, deep vein incompetence is described in Chapter 12.

Deep vein obstruction is not caused solely by deep vein thrombosis. Consequently the first part of this chapter describes the pathology of the non-thrombotic causes of obstruction. The treatments available are applicable to all varieties of obstruction whatever their pathology, but in non-thrombotic cases should be used to supplement the treatment of the prime cause.

Non-thrombotic occlusion of the deep axial veins of the lower limbs is uncommon. Minor degrees of compression by external structures, such as compression of the left common iliac vein by the right common iliac artery, are found in the majority of the population, making it difficult to define what is normal and what is abnormal. The ultimate test of an obstruction must be the physiological demonstration of an increased resistance to blood flow, not the demonstration of an anatomical abnormality or even the presence of collateral vessels. It is function, not appearance, that matters.

Pathology

Non-thrombotic deep vein obstruction may be caused by abnormalities outside, in the wall, or within the lumen of a vein.

EXTERNAL CAUSES

Right common iliac artery compression of the left common iliac vein

The left common iliac vein is crossed by the right common iliac artery in the midline, in front of the body of the fifth lumbar vertebra, just before it unites with the right common iliac vein to form the vena cava (Figure 13.1).

It is not surprising that this part of the vein is always flatter and wider than the vein upstream because it is compressed by the taut pulsating artery in front and the vertebral body behind. This compression is visible on a phlebograph as a segment with reduced opacification or an area of non-filling (Figure 13.2a–d) and is a normal appearance. If the lumbar lordosis increases or the intra-abdominal pressure rises (e.g. in pregnancy), the venous compression increases. When this happens blood flow is obstructed and a normal anatomical variant becomes a pathological entity.[1,8,11,63] This is an uncommon event and is termed Cockett's syndrome or May–Thurner syndrome. The clinical significance of iliac vein compression lies in its predisposing effect on deep vein thrombosis.[63] Compression of the vein and any small effect it has on blood flow does not matter under normal circumstances but if the patient is ill or has an operation, events which are thrombogenic, a minor degree of compression may increase the chances of the patient developing a left ilio-femoral thrombosis. Compression and webs in the left common iliac vein are thought to be the prime cause of the high incidence of left-sided deep vein thrombosis.

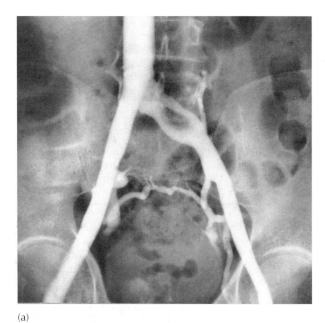

(a)

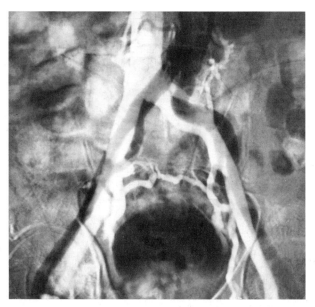

(b)

Figure 13.1   A phlebograph (a) and superimposed arteriogram (b) showing the right common iliac artery crossing and compressing the termination of the left common iliac vein. A kink in the left common iliac artery is causing a filling defect in the left common iliac vein.

Malignant disease

Malignant disease around the iliac veins can compress and obstruct them. The tumours most likely to do this are carcinoma of the cervix, ovary, colon and rectum, all of which may spread directly across the floor of the pelvis and encircle the vein. Secondary thrombosis in a vein constricted by tumour is common (see Figure 14.3, page 434).

Malignant enlargement of the iliac lymph nodes can also compress or occlude the iliac veins. The secondary tumours which commonly spread to the iliac lymph glands are neoplasms of the uterus, cervix, rectum and the anal canal. Testicular tumours which have spread outside the tunica albuginea and tumours of the leg and scrotal skin (e.g. malignant melanoma and squamous cell carcinoma) also metastasize to the iliac lymph nodes.

Retroperitoneal fibrosis

This condition is mainly found in front of and lateral to the aorta and vena cava, but it can spread across the posterior wall of the true pelvis and involve the iliac veins before it affects the vena cava (see Figure 14.4, page 435).

Internal iliac artery compression of the external iliac vein

The internal iliac artery crosses the termination of the external iliac vein on both sides to run down into the pelvis with its companion vein. It sometimes compresses the external iliac vein in a manner similar to that in which the right common iliac artery compresses the left common iliac vein. This rarely causes symptoms but may increase the risk of an external iliac vein thrombosis.

Tortuous or dilated arteries in any site may cause compression of an adjacent vein.

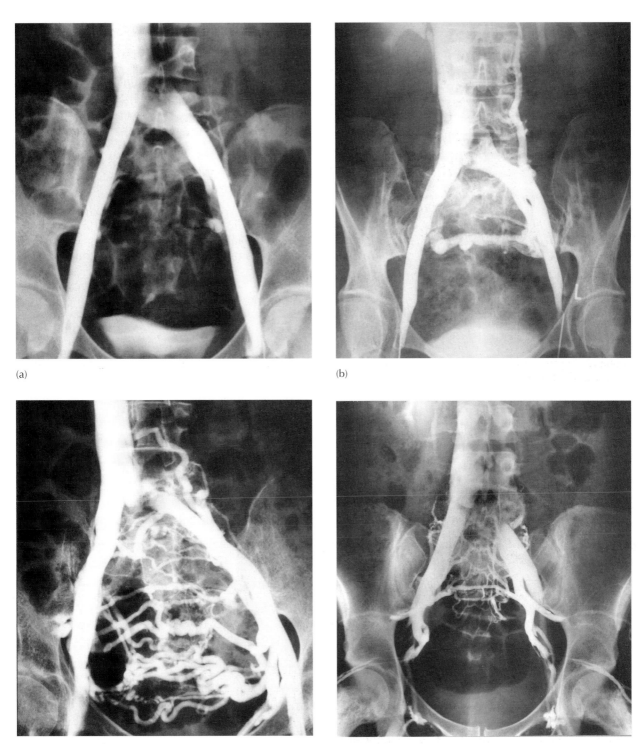

(a)

(b)

(c)

(d)

Figure 13.2 Three examples of compression of the left common iliac vein by the right common iliac artery varying from minor compression to complete occlusion. None of these patients had any symptoms from his/her abnormality. (a) A minor degree of arterial compression with no collateral vessels. (b) Arterial compression occluding half the width of the iliac vein with dilated ascending lumbar and presacral veins. (c) Arterial compression causing an almost complete band-like occlusion of the iliac vein with many dilated presacral veins. (d) Arterial compression causing a wide and almost complete occlusion of the whole common iliac vein with a few small presacral collateral veins.

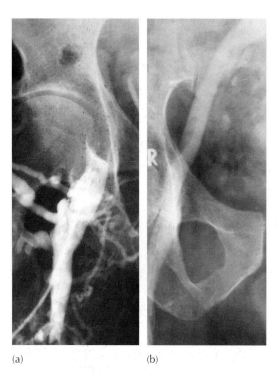

(a)   (b)

Figure 13.3   Gullmo's phenomenon. (a) During a Valsalva manoeuvre the common femoral vein was completely occluded. (b) When the raised intra-abdominal pressure was released the vein opened out to a normal size.

Pelvic masses

Masses arising from the hip joint may compress the iliac veins, including synovial cysts,[36] and cement following arthroplasty.[58] Bladder distension secondary to prostatic hypertrophy may compress the iliac veins causing ankle oedema.[44] Aortic and iliac artery aneurysms[13, 81] can cause similar effects.

Compression of the femoral vein (Gullmo's phenomenon)

Phlebographs of the femoral veins sometimes show an indentation on the medial side of the vein at the level of the inguinal ligament. There is much argument about the cause of this compression which can produce a total occlusion.

Gullmo[31] considers that it occurs when a weakness in the region of the femoral canal – a latent femoral hernia – allows the extraperitoneal fat to herniate downwards and laterally to compress the vein when the intra-abdominal pressure rises (Figure 13.3). Nylander[65] believes that it is the

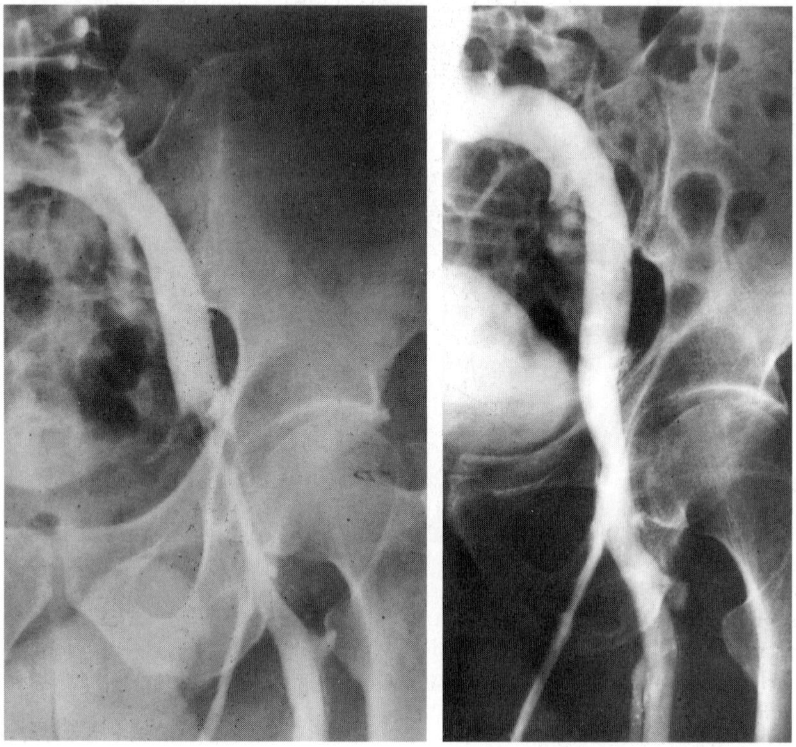

Figure 13.4 Compression of the common femoral vein by the inguinal ligament (a) which disappeared when the hip joint was slightly flexed (b).

(a)   (b)

combination of compression of the vein by abdominal pressure and retrograde flow, permitted by incompetent or absent common femoral vein valves, that allows the vein to empty. An indentation which is visible in the absence of a raised intra-abdominal pressure is probably caused by direct compression by the lacunar part of the inguinal ligament. This appearance is often exacerbated by hyperextension of the hip joint (Figure 13.4).

Gullmo's phenomenon and inguinal ligament compression are phlebographic abnormalities. They probably never cause symptoms. They are therefore of some anatomical interest but physiologically irrelevant.

Masses in the thigh

Large tumours or aneurysms in the thigh may compress the deep femoral vein and may stretch and compress the common and superficial femoral veins. The tumours are usually liposarcomata and fibrosarcomata, the aneurysms (true or false) in the common, superficial or deep femoral arteries.

The superficial femoral vein may also be compressed by the tendon forming the adductor canal (Figure 13.5).

Popliteal masses

A popliteal aneurysm, a large Baker's cyst or distended bursae or bone tumour can compress the popliteal vein. They may not be discovered until the patient presents with a popliteal or calf vein thrombosis caused by the venous obstruction. An abnormal band of muscle may cause popliteal vein entrapment (see Chapter 24, page 686).

VEIN WALL ABNORMALITIES

Aplasia

Aplasia of the pelvic veins is uncommon. When it occurs it is often part of a congenital venous abnormality such as the Klippel–Trenaunay syndrome (see Chapter 24).

Tumours

Primary tumours of the vein wall are rare but are found more often in the lower limb than in the upper limb. They are usually leiomyosarcomata (see Chapter 27). Cystic degeneration producing a lesion which is similar to the common subcutaneous ganglion and the cystic mucoid degeneration of the popliteal artery has been reported as a rare cause of femoral vein obstruction (see Chapter 27).

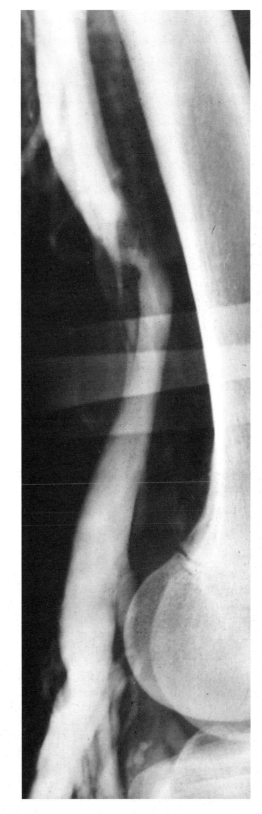

Figure 13.5 Compression of the superficial femoral vein as it passes through the adductor canal.

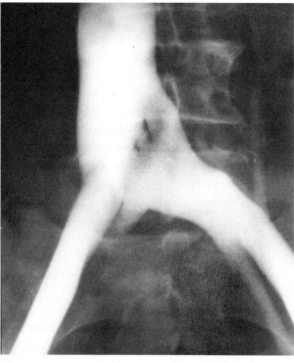

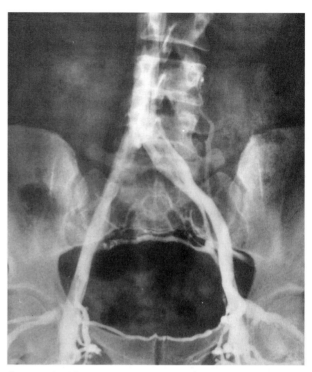

(a)   (b)

Figure 13.6 (a) Two left common iliac vein webs (central spurs). The two filling defects correspond to two bands of connective tissue connecting the anterior to the posterior wall of the iliac vein. Note that they lie within the area of vein compressed by the right common iliac artery but they are not post-thrombotic. (b) Multiple synechiae between the anterior and posterior wall of the left common iliac vein. These are the remnants of an iliac vein thrombosis. There is also a similar synechia in the inferior vena cava.

INTRALUMINAL CAUSES

Spurs/webs

The most important intraluminal cause of venous obstruction is the venous web or septum. Webs (spurs) occur at the termination of the left common iliac vein in 20% of the population at the point where the vein is compressed by the common iliac artery.[55,57,70] May has described three varieties – the lateral spur, the central spur and the perforated septum (Figure 13.6a).[55]

Histological studies have shown these spurs to consist of connective tissue and endothelium but they do not contain elastic tissue, muscle or haemosiderin. These observations suggest that they are not congenital remnants of the vein wall or the remnant of a thrombus. May believes they are caused by the combination of an inflammatory response and endothelial proliferation in response to repeated minor trauma to the two adjacent surfaces of the vein by the overlying compressing iliac artery.[55]

Only when obstruction of the veins is almost complete do these spurs cause symptoms, and then only when the collateral vessels are inadequate. Similar webs have been observed in the femoral vein.[75]

Post-thrombosis webs

Although this section of this chapter is concerned with non-thrombotic abnormalities, this condition is mentioned here to remind the reader that post-thrombotic lesions are by far the most common cause of chronic intraluminal obstruction of the deep veins of the lower limbs (Figure 13.6b).

IATROGENIC CAUSES

Ligation of the deep veins is sometimes unavoidable when dealing with the damage caused by local trauma but ligation of the femoral or popliteal veins during varicose vein surgery, though clearly negligent, is sadly not uncommon (Figure 13.7).

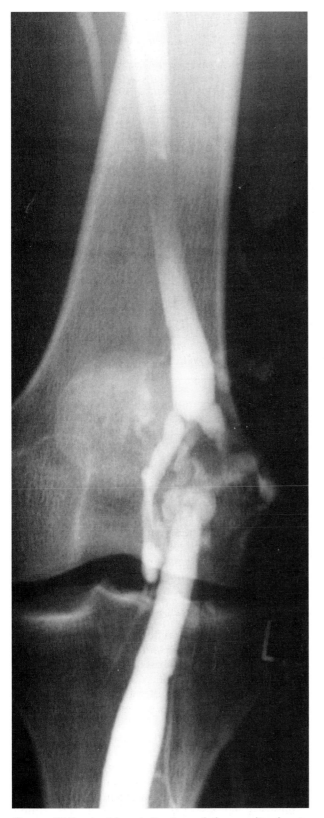

Clinical presentation

Many of the conditions described above are symptomless and only present when they precipitate a deep vein thrombosis. Their symptoms and treatment in such circumstances are described in Chapters 9 and 10.

The symptoms that occur when an extraluminal or intraluminal abnormality causes a chronic impediment to blood flow fall into two categories, those of the venous obstruction and those of the underlying abnormality.

VENOUS OBSTRUCTION

Distended veins

Collateral veins enlarge as the obstruction to blood flow increases. Common iliac vein obstruction is mainly bypassed by collateral veins in the pelvis and posterior abdominal wall, which cannot be seen, and by subcutaneous veins running across the lower abdominal wall just above the pubis and inguinal ligament which may become very large (Figure 13.8).

If there is some obstruction of the inferior vena cava, the collateral vessels may extend across the

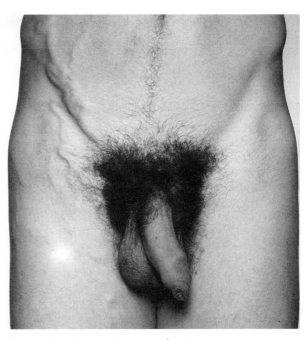

Figure 13.7   Accidental ligation of the popliteal vein during short saphenous vein surgery.

Figure 13.8   Large tortuous subcutaneous veins crossing the groin carrying blood around an occluded iliac vein.

abdominal wall towards the axilla. Proof that these veins are collaterals is obtained by confirming the retrograde flow of blood within them by Harvey's test (see Figure 1.6, page 7).

Oedema

Iliac vein obstruction usually causes swelling of the whole leg and sometimes causes swelling of the buttock and lower abdominal wall.

Obstruction of the superficial femoral vein below the termination of the deep femoral vein may cause swelling of the lower leg and ankle but may be symptomless.

Pain

If there is only a minor obstruction to blood flow, the patient will complain of an aching pain in the leg that is made worse by standing and is relieved by rest and elevation.

Severe obstruction may cause venous claudication, a deep (muscle) pain within the leg which is induced by the rise in venous and interstitial pressures within the muscle compartments during exercise (see Chapters 16 and 17).[71]

Skin changes

Prolonged severe obstruction will eventually damage the skin. This damage may be visible as pigmentation 'atrophie blanche', lipodermatosclerosis and ulceration (see Chapter 15). These symptoms are unusual in non-thrombotic obstruction except when it has not been complicated by secondary thrombosis.

EVIDENCE OF THE UNDERLYING PATHOLOGY

Iliac compression and webs only cause the symptoms and signs described above. Patients with obstruction caused by disease outside the veins may have other local or distant evidence of their underlying disease. For example, debility, loss of weight, lower abdominal pain and vaginal bleeding would suggest the presence of pelvic malignancy. Testicular enlargement, palpable inguinal lymph nodes, and lesions on the skin of the leg would suggest the possible presence of iliac lymphadenopathy.

It is absolutely essential to conduct a complete clinical examination to exclude such abnormalities in a patient who presents with recent symptoms or signs of venous obstruction.

SECONDARY THROMBOSIS

Patients with a primary non-thrombotic venous compression or obstruction may develop an acute thrombosis and present with acute pain in the iliac fossa and groin and rapid swelling of the leg. The leg may be white (phlegmasia alba dolens) or blue (phlegmasia cerulea dolens), depending upon the degree of venous obstruction. Although the initial clinical management should be directed towards treating the thrombosis, it is important to remember that there may be an underlying local abnormality which requires treatment. This must be excluded by a careful clinical assessment and investigation. Local or distant malignant disease is the underlying cause of half the cases of phlegmasia cerulea dolens.

Pulmonary embolism is not a common complication of thrombosis secondary to obstruction because the obstruction prevents the downstream propagation of the thrombus and the upstream thrombosis is 'locked in' by the obstruction.

Investigations

The initial investigations should define the state of the veins and the cause of the obstruction.

PHLEBOGRAPHY

Phlebography is an essential, primary investigation because it will confirm or refute the clinical diagnosis of a venous obstruction. All forms of phlebography may be required but bilateral ascending and percutaneous direct femoral vein phlebograms are sufficient in most patients.

Common iliac compression causes a variety of phlebographic appearances (see Figure 13.2) – mildly reduced opacification, a lateral defect, or a full width complete filling defect. Collateral vessels may be visible across the floor of the pelvis (Figure 13.9) and the ascending lumbar and ovarian veins may be enlarged. The presence of large collateral veins must not be interpreted as indicating a major degree of obstruction; in fact, the larger the collaterals the less the obstruction. Large collaterals indicate that there has been a significant obstruction, not that it still exists. Obstruction can only be diagnosed by a physiological test (see page 417).

A series of films taken after a femoral vein injection of radio-opaque contrast medium will show the direction of blood flow in the collaterals.

Tumour compression causes irregular filling defects on the vein wall (Figure 13.10a), usually the result of external compression but sometimes

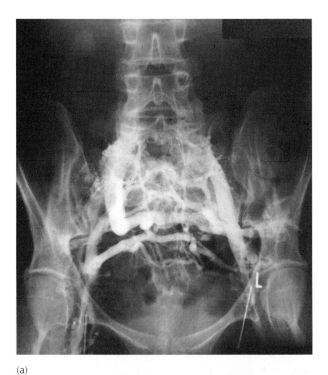

(a)

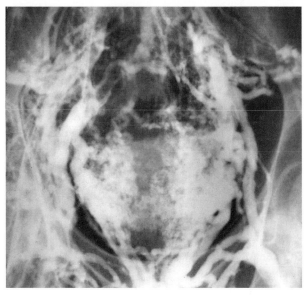

(b)

Figure 13.9   The vessels that bypass an iliac vein occlusion. (a) The presacral veins. (b) The vesical and rectal plexi and the subcutaneous pubic veins.

caused by mural thrombosis developing in response to tumour infiltrating the vein wall.

When enlarged lymph glands surrounding a vein are irradiated the subsequent fibrosis may cause a long stricture (Figure 13.10b).

Arterial impressions are common but can only be confirmed by the superimposition of an arteriogram on a phlebograph (see Figure 13.1). Indentations of the common and external iliac veins by their accompanying arteries are common, especially as the arteries dilate and elongate with age.

Femoral vein compression is best seen if the patient performs a Valsalva manoeuvre during the phlebogram as this accentuates the size of the impression (see Figure 13.3). Primary vein wall tumours produce filling defects which are usually indistinguishable from defects caused by external compression (see Chapter 27).

ULTRASOUND

Ultrasound can provide morphological information about extrinsic sources of compression and colour flow Duplex ultrasound can demonstrate changes in flow velocity or direction induced by stenoses or obstruction. Unfortunately, ultrasound imaging of the pelvic veins is often suboptimal because of their inaccessibility and overlying bowel gas. Ultrasound techniques do not yet provide the fine detail of the shape of the veins and the number and size of the collateral veins that can be obtained from high quality phlebograms.

GENERAL INVESTIGATIONS

General investigations such as a chest radiograph and blood studies (haematological and biochemical) are important screening tests to exclude distant primary abnormalities. Coagulation studies may be necessary.

Special techniques such as lymphography, ultrasound imaging, computerized tomography (CT) scanning and magnetic resonance imaging (MRI) may help to detect and define masses compressing the veins.

PHYSIOLOGICAL TESTS OF VENOUS OBSTRUCTION

Quite major anatomical abnormalities may not obstruct blood flow when the limb is at rest, but will cause obstruction during exercise when the limb blood flow and consequently the deep vein blood flow increases 10- or 20-fold. The non-invasive techniques for detecting venous outflow obstruction are extremely insensitive because they are usually performed with the leg at rest.

Phleborheography is usually normal in the presence of long-standing femoral or popliteal occlusion.

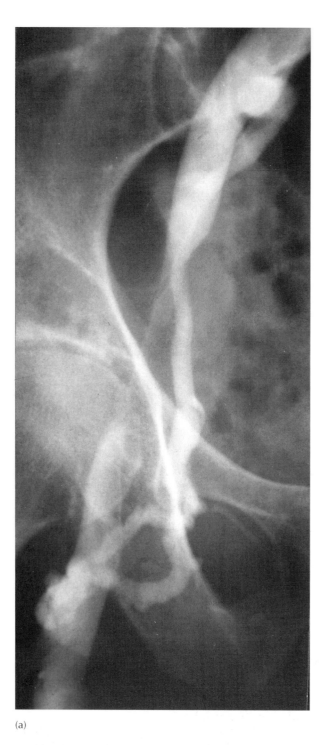

(a)

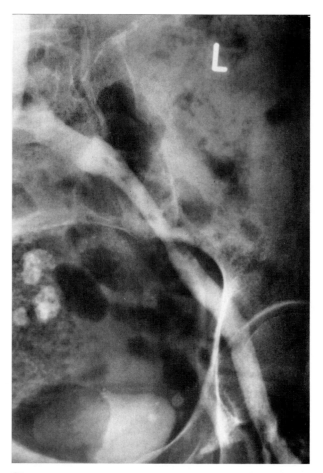

(b)

Figure 13.10   (a) A phlebograph showing indentation and compression of the common femoral and external iliac veins by enlarged lymph glands. (b) A phlebograph showing a long stenosis of the external iliac vein caused by fibrosis and contraction in a mass of iliac lymph glands treated with radiotherapy.

Venous outflow strain-gauge plethysmography may help. It has been claimed[64] that a maximum venous outflow of less than 65 ml/100 ml/min is diagnostic of outflow obstruction and that a decrease in calf volume during exercise of less than 0.75 ml/100 ml indicates calf pump insufficiency secondary to outflow obstruction and communicating vein incompetence. In our own laboratory we find the measurements of maximum venous outflow are extremely variable and no help with diagnosis.

Isotope plethysmography, which can measure the amount of blood expelled by both exercise and compression, detects only severe obstruction (Figure 13.11).

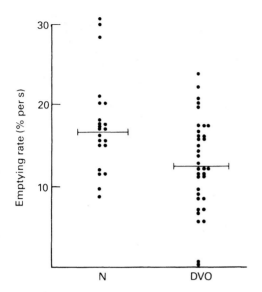

Figure 13.11 The rate of emptying of the calf veins of 22 normal limbs (N) and 35 limbs with deep vein obstruction (DVO) in response to a single calf contraction, measured with isotope plethysmography. There is no significant difference between the mean rate of emptying of the two groups. Only two patients' calves did not empty at the normal rate. This type of test does not reveal even moderate outflow obstruction.

Comment

We do not find any of the non-invasive tests helpful in the diagnosis of venous outflow obstruction. The few patients who do have grossly abnormal test results usually have venous claudication, a symptom which makes the tests almost superfluous.

Femoral vein pressure

Measurement of this pressure before and during exercise will indicate the severity of an iliac vein obstruction.[62] The technique is simple. A fine needle or cannula is inserted into the femoral vein with the patient lying supine. The patient is then asked to forcibly plantar flex the foot against a resistance, once every second.

Under normal circumstances the femoral vein pressure will rise by only 1 or 2 mmHg. When there is an iliac obstruction it will increase by 5–10 mmHg. An increase of more than 5 mmHg is significant but the best test of significance is the comparison of the pressure rise in the abnormal limb with that in the normal limb (Figure 13.12).

The ability of the clinician to diagnose superficial femoral vein obstruction would be improved if popliteal vein pressure could be measured during exercise.

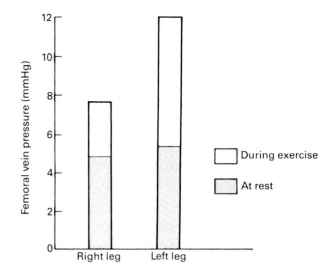

Figure 13.12 The effect of leg exercise on the femoral vein pressures in a patient with a left iliac vein occlusion. In the normal leg pressure rose by only 2.2 mmHg. In the abnormal leg the pressure rose by 6.7 mmHg, indicating a physiologically significant obstruction. (Modified from May _et al._[53])

Treatment

Operations should only be considered when conservative treatment has failed.

ELASTIC COMPRESSION

The symptoms of pain and swelling can usually be relieved by the external compression provided by elastic stockings. Below-knee stockings are usually sufficient, but full-length stockings can be used if there are many large veins in the thigh and the thigh is swollen. In most patients the swelling and discomfort are mainly in the calf and a below-knee stocking is adequate.

If the patient wears a stocking regularly, the dilatation of the peripheral subcutaneous veins will slow down, and the development of skin changes and ulceration will be delayed.

If lipodermatosclerosis is present, its resolution may be accelerated by the use of drugs which stimulate interstitial fibrinolysis (see Chapter 17).

SURGICAL TREATMENT

There are two surgical methods for relieving deep vein obstruction – a bypass operation or a local disobliteration.

Iliac vein bypass operations

Iliac occlusion or compression causing symptoms can be bypassed by the simple, extra-anatomic, extra-abdominal, femoro-femoral saphenous vein bypass operation, described by Palma in 1959 and 1960 (Figure 13.13a and b).[68,69]

The Palma operation

This operation is indicated when there are severe symptoms in the leg which are unrelieved by elastic compression.[14,15,19] The most important symptom is venous claudication. Operations for mild swelling ‘and moderate aching are unlikely to be successful.

The Palma operation should only be considered when there is physiological evidence of venous obstruction during exercise as shown by an *abnormal rise in femoral vein pressure during exercise* (Figure 13.12)[51,53] Only under these circumstances can the surgeon be certain of an adequate perfusion pressure to maintain graft patency.

The femoral vein in the groin of the abnormal leg is explored through a vertical incision, and its tributaries are dissected until a healthy patent segment is found, usually in the deep femoral vein. The results are better if the femoral vein does not have post-thrombotic changes.

The long saphenous vein of the normal leg is exposed through either a single or multiple incisions. After ligating its tributaries, the vein is divided between ligatures at a point well down the thigh where it will be long enough to stretch, still attached to the femoral vein, across the abdomen to the opposite groin.

A subcutaneous tunnel is made across the lower abdomen by blunt dissection or with a tunneller, above the crest of the pubis to the opposite groin, and the saphenous vein is threaded through it.

An end-to-side anastomosis is made between the saphenous vein and the healthiest segment of femoral vein that can be found, sometimes the common or superficial femoral vein but often the deep femoral vein.

Most surgeons fashion an arteriovenous fistula just below the anastomosis to help maintain patency, using a segment of the saphenous vein or one of its tributaries.[24,26,48]

The patient is given anticoagulants for 36 months. If a fistula is fashioned, it should be closed 3 months after operation. This can be a difficult operation, and it is facilitated by leaving a loose, non-absorbable suture around the fistula to help to identify it within the scar tissue. Alternatively, the fistula may be closed by the insertion of a small detachable balloon by an interventional vascular radiologist.

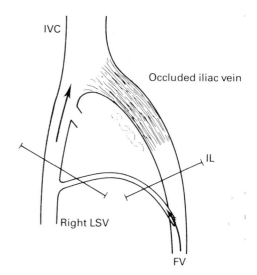

(a)

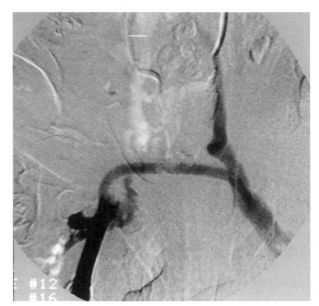

(b)

Figure 13.13   The Palma operation. (a) A diagrammatic representation showing the right long saphenous vein (LSV) swung across the pubis and anastomosed to the left femoral vein (FV). IL, inguinal ligaments. (b) A digital subtraction phlebograph of a successful Palma operation performed to bypass an occluded right iliac vein.

Results

The results of this operation may be judged by clinical or phlebographic criteria; the clinical results are usually better than the phlebographic results for reasons that are not entirely clear. Clinical improvement in the presence of an occluded graft may be related to an increase in the number of collaterals,

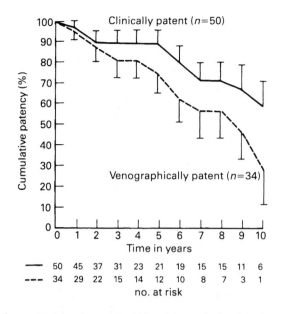

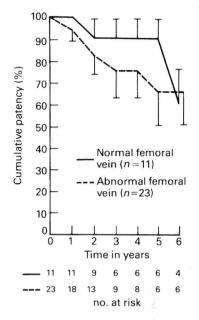

Figure 13.14 A modified life table analysis of the cumulative patency of femoro-femoral vein crossover grafts as determined by clinical examination and phlebography. (Modified from Halliday *et al.*[34])

Figure 13.15 A modified life table analysis of the cumulative phlebographic patency of 34 femoro-femoral vein crossover grafts subdivided according to the preoperative state of the superficial femoral vein - normal,[12] or post-thrombotic damage.[25] (Modified from Halliday *et al.*[34])

or the proper use of better quality elastic stockings, factors which may also be responsible for clinical improvement in patients with patent grafts.

The results of 50 operations performed by Halliday are shown in Figure 13.14.[34] Unfortunately, preoperative femoral vein pressure studies had not been carried out on any of these patients. None had arteriovenous fistulae. All had patency judged on clinical grounds (patency = relief of symptoms). Postoperative phlebograms were performed on only 34 patients.

It can be seen that at 5 years when 21 patients were available for assessment, 90% had clinical relief, and 75% had patent grafts. Beyond 5 years the number of patients available for study was too small for detailed analysis but there were clearly a considerable number of patients whose graft was patent 10 years after the operation.

The majority of Halliday's series of Palma operations were for post-thrombotic occlusion and, consequently, some patients had post-thrombotic changes in the femoral vein at and below the site of the anastomosis. In Figure 13.15 the results are subdivided according to the state of the superficial femoral vein. At 5 years those patients with normal femoral veins had better patency rates but this was not the case with the 10 patients studied 6 years after operation.

Other surgeons have reported similar long-term patency rates of 75%.[18,40] Few surgeons have

measured femoral vein pressures after this operation.[47] It has been suggested that some bypasses thrombose and then recanalize so that the clinical benefit does not appear for 3–6 months.[17]

The development of better vascular prostheses has tempted some surgeons to use these artificial materials for femoro-femoral bypass when the long saphenous vein is inadequate. Only small numbers have been reported[16,65] but the results with prostheses made of PTFE (polytetrafluoroethylene) are encouraging, particularly if the prostheses are strengthened with external ring supports.[4] An arteriovenous fistula is essential when using a prosthesis. External support of the anastomosis with rings[46,47] and anticoagulation by defibrinogenation[6,37,42,67] appear to be of value in maintaining the patency of venous anastomoses in experimental animals but there are no clinical studies to confirm the value of these techniques in man.

Other bypass operations

Kunlin inserted a saphenous vein between the left external iliac vein and the right common iliac vein to bypass a terminal common iliac vein occlusion.[45] Hardin used the ipsilateral saphenous vein as a bypass between the femoral vein and the vena cava.[35]

These operations have not been widely practised because entering the abdomen adds a morbidity to the procedure which can be avoided by using the Palma operation which is entirely subcutaneous.

Reports of femoral-caval and femoro-femoral bypasses of iliac blocks using externally supported PTFE[4,9,20,61,66] indicate promising results in small numbers of patients but there are no large series yet reported.

Iliac vein disobliteration

A localized obstruction at the termination of the common iliac vein can be treated by a direct operation on this vein.[12]

The vein is best approached through an abdominal incision. The right common iliac artery is mobilized and the underlying common iliac vein is exposed. After the vena cava and both iliac veins have been controlled with soft clamps, the iliac vein can be opened and any spurs or membranes carefully excised. It is sometimes necessary to enlarge the vein with a patch of autogenous superficial vein, as a long-standing occlusion often narrows the vein.

This type of procedure is only applicable to short localized stenoses. The iliac artery should be freed so that it does not compress the site of the operation; if necessary it can be held to one side with a peritoneal sling.

Some authors have suggested placing a plastic bridge beneath the artery to protect the vein.[78] No long-term results of this procedure have been published. We have not used this technique because of the potential risk of arterial erosion and late aneurysm formation.

Iliac vein decompression

If the left common iliac vein is compressed between the fifth lumbar vertebra and the right common iliac artery, the compression can be relieved by dividing and elongating the artery or removing the bony prominence of the vertebra. Both these operations have been proposed by Dick[23] but no long-term results have been published.

Endovascular iliac vein dilatation and stenting

Endovascular techniques including venous angioplasty and stent placement are being used successfully to treat caval and iliac vein stenosis secondary to post-thrombotic stenosis, malignant infiltration, retroperitoneal fibrosis and iliac artery compression.[3,80] No large or comparative series have yet been published and it remains unclear whether these techniques will provide long-term patency but early results (Figures 13.16, 13.17) are extremely encouraging.

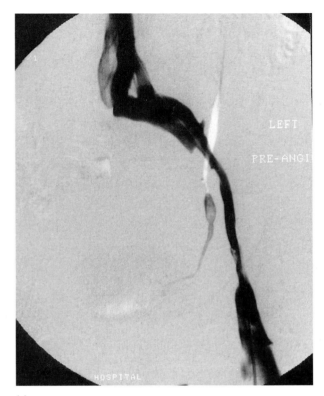

(a)

Figure 13.16 Angioplasty and stenting for a radiation stricture of the left iliac vein following the treatment of a carcinoma of the prostate. (a) This phlebograph shows the extent and severity of the stricture.

Figure 13.17 Dilatation and stenting of a malignant obstruction of the common femoral vein. (a) A digital unsubtracted phlebograph showing a complete occlusion of the femoral vein (caused by enlarged lymph nodes containing metastatic carcinoma from the vulva) which has been traversed by a guide wire. (b) A wall stent with an angioplasty balloon *in situ*. The stent was deployed from the left groin. (c) Phlebograph showing satisfactory flow through the stent.

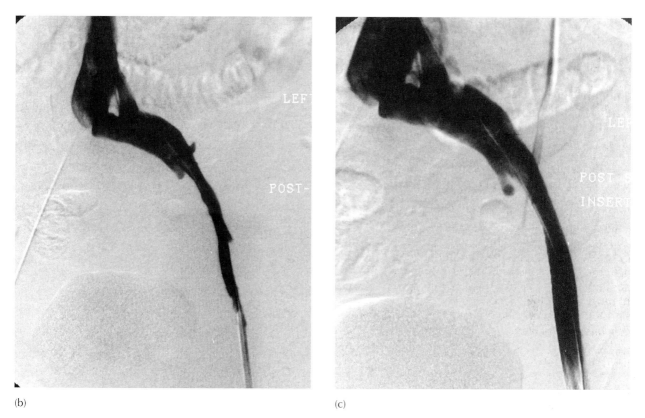

(b)   (c)

Figure 13.16   (b) A phlebograph after balloon angioplasty. The stricture is just as tight. (c) A phlebograph after the insertion of a stent shows that the stricture is being held open and that there is now an adequate venous outflow tract for the limb.

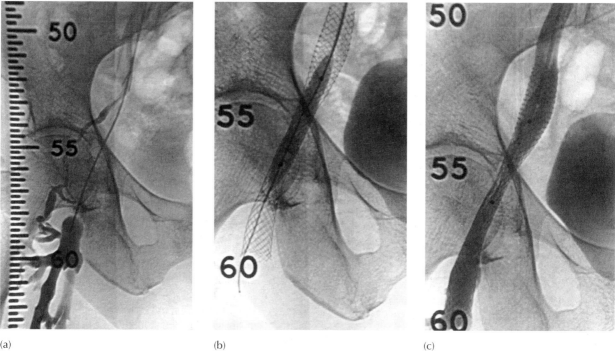

(a)   (b)   (c)

Femoral vein bypass operations (Warren–May–Husni operation)[41,50,82]

Non-thrombotic obstruction of the superficial femoral vein is rare. Post-thrombotic obstruction is common, and most of the published series of femoral vein bypass operations have been for post-thrombotic problems.[39]

Popliteal to common femoral vein bypass using the *in-situ* long saphenous vein was first described by Warren in 1954,[82] and a few surgeons have used it occasionally since the early 1970s (Figure 13.18).

This bypass is indicated when there is severe pain and swelling below the knee caused by a superficial femoral vein occlusion without adequate collaterals. Although maximum venous outflow rates may be prolonged in this situation, there is no good test of femoral vein obstruction during calf exercise and so the indications for this operation are entirely clinical. The long saphenous vein must be patent, and the popliteal and common femoral veins must be healthy.

The most valuable investigations are phlebography (Figure 13.19) and a foot vein pressure study confirming a severe degree of obstructive calf pump insufficiency.

The saphenous vein is exposed at the level of the knee, divided and anastomosed end-to-side to the popliteal vein. Provided its valves are competent, its tributaries do not have to be ligated. Gruss[29,30] adds

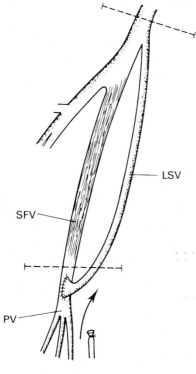

Figure 13.18 A diagrammatic representation of the Warren popliteal-to-common femoral vein saphenous vein bypass operation. The long saphenous vein (LSV) has been divided and anastomosed to a patent popliteal vein (PV) to bypass an occluded superficial femoral vein (SFV). The broken lines indicate the level of the hip and knee joints.

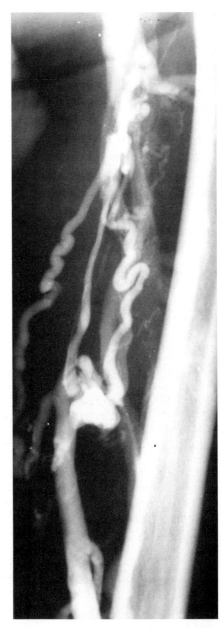

Figure 13.19 This superficial femoral vein occlusion is suitable for a saphenous vein bypass operation because the popliteal vein is healthy. This patient's symptoms were, however, mild, and surgical interference was not justified.

an arteriovenous fistula, not just below the anastomosis, but well down the leg, just above the medial malleolus between the posterior tibial artery and saphenous vein. As the saphenous vein has been divided at the knee level, it is assumed that the additional arterial blood flowing through the fistula travels up the long saphenous vein, into the deep veins via the communicating veins, up the deep veins and then through the venous anastomosis into the bypass. Whether it actually does this is debatable.

Results

Gruss[28] has described the results of 12 popliteal to femoral vein bypass operations, four without and eight with arteriovenous fistulae. The late follow-up studies (6–10 years later) revealed that three bypasses had occluded and eight were patent, but the calf pump function (assessed by foot vein pressure measurements) of four of the eight that were patent had deteriorated. Two of the bypasses in the four patients whose calf pump function had improved had become dilated and varicose. May[54] described the initial results in 16 patients and the late results of seven; four had improved, three had deteriorated. Husni has reported a 60% late patency rate. Frileux[27] has described a series of 20 patients with similar results.

An alternative bypass has been suggested by Annous and Queral.[1] They anastomosed the lower end of a divided femoral vein, at the level of the adductor hiatus end-to-side to the saphenous vein. No long-term results are available.

Comment

It seems that only half of these bypasses remain patent and in a smaller proportion of patients there is worthwhile improvement in calf pump function. The results are not encouraging, and this operation should not be carried out unless it is part of a careful clinical research trial. It may be that functioning valves are required as well as a patent conduit. If the long saphenous vein is already acting as a collateral, there seems little point in dividing and anastomosing it to a deep vein. Perhaps the operation should be restricted to those patients in whom the application of a mid-thigh superficial vein occluding tourniquet does not adversely affect calf pump function (i.e. those patients in whom the long saphenous vein is not already acting as a collateral vessel).

Other measures

When venous obstruction is caused by an external mass, it may be relieved by removing the mass or reducing its size.

Popliteal aneurysms can be bypassed or resected. Enlarged lymph nodes can be excised or reduced in size by radiotherapy, which may also be used to relieve the effect of infiltrating tumours.

Compression of the femoral vein by the inguinal ligament can be relieved by dividing the ligament.

It is important to relieve any functionally significant persistent compression of a major axial vein to reduce the risk of secondary thrombosis.

Experimental studies

The relatively few clinical reports of vein grafts and vein replacement belie the intense interest in this problem. Over the past 30 years there have been many laboratory studies which have aimed to produce a satisfactory method of replacing occluded veins. Autografts,[22,25,72,83] heterografts,[38] inverted small bowel and many types of prosthesis have been studied.[2,5,7–9,21,32,33,43,59,60,73,74,77] The results have been disappointing. The only consistent finding has been the increased patency rate conferred by the use of a temporary arteriovenous fistula. It is likely that endovascular techniques, particularly endoluminal stents, will prove increasingly useful for the treatment of venous stenoses, but as for all treatments of venous problems, the value of each technique must be properly established by large, long-term controlled clinical trials.

Direct venous surgery remains in its infancy because of the unsolved technical problems and the small number of patients whose symptoms justify direct surgical interference.

References

1. Annous MO, Queral LA. Venous claudication successfully treated by distal superficial femoral-to-greater saphenous vein bypass. *J Vasc Surg* 1985; **2(6):** 870–3.
2. Baird RJ, Lipton IH, Miyagishima RT. Replacement of the deep veins of the legs. *Arch Surg* 1964; **89:** 797.
3. Berger A, Jaffe JW, York TN. Iliac compression syndrome treated with stent placement. *J Vasc Surg* 1995; **21:** 510–14.
4. Bernstein EF, Chan EL, Bardin JA. Externally supported grafts for inferior vena cava bypass. In: Bergan JJ, Yao JST, eds. *Surgery of the Veins.* New York: Grune & Stratton, 1985; 33.
5. Bower R, Fredericci V, Howard JM. Continuing studies of replacement of segments of the venous system. *Surgery* 1960; **47:** 132.
6. Browse NL, Clemenson G. Vein surgery during defibrinogenation. *Br J Surg* 1978; **65:** 452.
7. Bryant MF, Lazenby WD, Howard JM. Experimental replacement of short segments of vein. *Arch Surg* 1958; **76:** 289.

8. Ceriso M, McGraw JY, Luke JC. Autogenous vein graft replacement of thrombosed deep veins. Experimental approach to the treatment of the post-phlebitic syndrome. *Surgery* 1964; **55**: 123.

9. Chan EL, Bardin JA, Bernstein EF. Inferior vena cava bypass. Experimental evaluation of externally supported grafts and initial clinical application. *J Vasc Surg* 1984; **1**: 675.

10. Chermet J. Left common iliac vein syndrome. *Anat Clin* 1979; **1**: 347.

11. Cockett FB, Thomas ML, Negus D. Iliac vein compression, its relation to iliofemoral thrombosis and the post thrombotic syndrome. *Br Med J* 1967; **2**: 14.

12. Cockett FB, Thomas Lea M. The iliac compression syndrome. *Br J Surg* 1965; **52**: 816.

13. Combe J, Besancenot J, Milleret P, Camelot G. Iliocaval venous compression due to aneurysm of the abdominal aorta: report of ten cases. *Ann Vasc Surg* 1990; **4**: 20–5.

14. Dale WA. Crossover grafts for iliofemoral venous occlusion. In: Bergan JJ, Yao JST, eds. *Venous Problems*. Chicago & London: Year Book Medical Publisher, 1978.

15. Dale WA. Crossover vein grafts for relief of iliofemoral venous block. *Surgery* 1965; **57**: 608.

16. Dale WA. Synthetic grafts in venous reconstruction. In Bergan JJ, Yao JST, eds. *Surgery of the Veins*. New York, Grune & Stratton, 1985; 233.

17. Dale WA. Thrombosis and recanalization of veins used as venous grafts. *Angiology* 1961; **12**: 603.

18. Dale WA. Venous bypass surgery. *Surg Clin North Am* 1982; **62**: 391.

19. Dale WA, Harris J. Crossover vein grafts for iliac and femoral venous occlusion. *J Cardiovasc Surg* 1969; **10**: 458.

20. Dale WA, Harris J, Terry RB. Polytetrafluor-ethylene reconstruction of inferior vena cava. *Surgery* 1984; **95**: 625.

21. Dale WA, Scott HW. Grafts of the venous system. *Surgery* 1963; **53**: 52.

22. De Weese JA, Niguidula F. The replacement of short segments of veins with functional autogenous venous grafts. *Surg Gynecol Obstet* 1960; **110**: 303.

23. Dick W. Klinik und therapie der venensperre am confluens der beiden gemeinsamen iliacalvenen. *Langenbecks Arch Chir* 1962; **301**: 573.

24. Dumanian AV, Santschi DR, Park K, Walker AP, Frahm CJ. Cross-over saphenous vein graft combined with a temporary femoral arteriovenous fistula. A case report. *Vasc Surg* 1968; **2**: 116.

25. Eadie DG, de Takats G. The fate of autogenous grafts in the canine femoral vein. *J Cardiovasc Surg* 1966; **7**: 148.

26. Ecklof B, Albrechtson V, Einarsson E, Plate G. The temporary arteriovenous fistula in venous reconstructive surgery. *Int Angiol* 1985; **4**: 455.

27. Frileux C, Pillot-Bienayme P, Gillot C. Bypass of segmental obliterations of ilio-femoral venous axis by transposition of saphenous vein. *J Cardiovasc Surg* 1972; **13**: 409.

28. Gruss JD. The saphenopopliteal bypass for chronic venous insufficiency (May-Husni Operation). In:

Bergan JJ, Yao JST, eds. *Surgery of the Veins*. New York: Grune & Stratton, 1985; 255.

29. Gruss JD. Zur Modifikation des Femoral bypass nach May. *Vasa* 1975; **4**: 59.

30. Gruss JD, Vargas-Mantano H, Bartels D, Hanschke D, Fietze-Fischer B. Direct reconstructive venous surgery. *Int Angiol* 1985; **4**: 441.

31. Gullmo A. The strain obstruction syndrome of the femoral vein. *Acta Radiol Scand* 1957; **47**: 119.

32. Haimovici H, Hoffert PW, Zinicola N, Steinman C. An experimental and clinical evaluation of the grafts in the venous system. *Surg Gynecol Obstet* 1970; **131**: 1173.

33. Haimovici H, Zinicola N, Noorani M, Hoffert PW. Vein grafts in the venous system. *Arch Surg* 1963; **87**: 542.

34. Halliday P, Harris J, May J. Femoro-femoral crossover grafts (Palma operation). A long term follow up study. In: Bergan JJ, Yao JST, eds. *Surgery of the Veins*. New York: Grune & Stratton, 1985; 241.

35. Hardin C. Bypass saphenous grafts for the relief of venous obstruction of the extremity. *Surg Gynecol Obstet* 1962; **115**: 709.

36. Harris RW, Andros G, Dulawa LB, Oblath RW, Horowitz R. Iliofemoral venous obstruction without thrombosis. *J Vasc Surg* 1987; **6**: 594–9.

37. Hobson RW, Croom RD. Influence of heparin and low molecular weight dextran on the patency of autogenous vein grafts in the venous system. *Ann Surg* 1973; **178**: 773.

38. Horsch S, Pichlmaier H, Walter P, Landes TH. Replacement of the inferior vena cave and iliac veins with heterologous grafts in animal tests. *Surgery* 1978; **84**: 644.

39. Husni EA. Clinical experience with femoropopliteal venous reconstruction. In: Bergan JJ, Yao JST, eds. *Venous Problems*. Chicago: Year Book Medical Publishers, 1978; 485.

40. Husni EA. Reconstruction of veins, the need for objectivity. *J Cardiovasc Surg* 1983; **24**: 525.

41. Husni EA. *In situ* saphenopopliteal bypass graft for incompetence of the femoral and popliteal veins. *Surg Gynecol Obstet* 1970; **130**: 279.

42. Ishimaru S, Fujiwara Y, Domeki D, Horiguchi Y, Furukawa K, Takahashi M. Defibrinogenation therapy in venous reconstructive surgery with PTFE Graft. *J Jpn Coll Angiol* 1977; **17**: 515.

43. Katy NM, Spence IJ, Wallace RB. Reconstruction of the inferior vena cava with a PTFE tube graft after resection for hypernephroma of the right kidney. *J Thorac Cardiovasc Surg* 1984; **87**: 791.

44. Kopesky K, Schwartz R, Silver D. Lower extremity edema from bladder compression of the iliac veins. *J Vasc Surg* 1988; **7**: 778–80.

45. Kunlin J. Le rétablissement de la circulation veineuse par greffe en cas d'obliteration trauma-tique ou thrombophlétique. Greffe de 18 cm entre la veine saphene interne et la veine iliaque externe. Thrombose après trois semaines de perméabilité. *Mem Acad Chir* 1953; **79**: 109.

46. Kunlin J, Benitte AM, Richard S. La suspension de la suture veineuse. Etude experimentale. *Bull Soc Int Chir* 1960; **19**: 336.

47. Kunlin J, Kunlin A, Richard S, Tregovet T. Le remplacement et l'anastomose latéro-latérale des veines par greffon avec suture suspendue a anneau. *J Chir (Paris)* 1963; **85:** 305.

48. Levin PM, Rich NM, Hutton JE Jr, Barker WF, Zeller JA. Role of arteriovenous shunts in venous reconstruction. *Am J Surg* 1971; **122:** 183.

49. Matsumoto T, Homes RH, Burdick CO, Hersterkamp CA, O'Connell TJ. The fate of the inverted segment of small bowel used for the replacement of major veins. *Surgery* 1966; **60:** 739.

50. May R. Femoralis bypass beim posthrombotischen Zustandsbild. *Vasa* 1972; **1:** 267.

51. May R. The femoral bypass. *Int Angiol* 1985; **4:** 435.

52. May R. Veins of the pelvis. In: May R, ed. *Surgery of the Veins of the Leg and Pelvis.* Stuttgart: Georg Thieme, 1974; 25.

53. May R, DeWeese JA. Surgery of the pelvic veins. In: May R, ed. *Surgery of the Veins of the Leg and Pelvis.* Stuttgart: Georg Thieme, 1974; 171.

54. May R, Nissl R. The post-thrombotic syndrome. In: May R, ed. *Surgery of the Veins of the Leg and Pelvis.* Stuttgart: Georg Thieme, 1974; 153.

55. May R, Thurner J. Ein gefasseporn in der V. iliaca comm. sin. als wahrscheinliche Ursache der uberwiegend linksseifigen Beckenvenenthrombose. *Z Kreislaufforsch* 1956; **45:** 912.

56. May R, Thurner J. The cause of the predominantly sinistral occurrence of thrombosis of the pelvic vein. *Angiology* 1957; **8:** 419.

57. McMurrich JP. The occurrence of congenital adhesions in the common iliac veins and their relation to the thrombosis of the femoral and iliac veins. *Am J Med Sci* 1908; **135:** 342.

58. Middleton RG, Reilly DT, Jessop J. Occlusion of the external iliac vein by cement. *J Arthroplasty* 1996; **11:** 346–7.

59. Mitsuoka H, Howard JM. Experimental grafting of the vena cava. *J Cardiovasc Surg* 1968; **9:** 190.

60. Moore TC, Young NK. Experimental replacement and bypass of large veins. *Bull Soc Int Chir* 1964; **23:** 274.

61. Murchan P, Sugrue ME, O'Malley MK, Feely TM, Shanik DG, Moore DJ. A new technique for bilateral iliac vein and inferior vena cava reconstruction using reinforced polytetrafluoroethylene. *Ann Vasc Surg* 1990; **4:** 302–4.

62. Negus D, Cockett FB. Femoral vein pressures in postphlebitic iliac vein obstruction. *Br J Surg* 1967; **54:** 522.

63. Negus D, Fletcher EWL, Cockett FB, Lea Thomas M. Compression and band formation at the mouth of the left common iliac vein. *Br J Surg* 1968; **55:** 369.

64. Nicolaides AN, Fernandes JF, Schull K, Miles C. Calf volume plethysmography. In: Nicolaides AN, Yao JST, eds. *Investigation of Vascular Disorders.* New York: Churchill Livingstone, 1981; 495.

65. Nylander G. Haemodynamics of the pelvic veins in incompetence of the femoral vein. *Acta Radiol (Stockh)* 1961; **56:** 369.

66. Okadome K, Muto Y, Eguchi H, Kusaba A, Sugimachi K. Venous reconstruction for iliofemoral venous occlusion facilitated by temporary arteriovenous fistula. Long term results in nine patients. *Arch Surg* 1989; **124:** 957–60.

67. Olsson P, Ljungqvist A, Goransson L. Vein graft surgery in Defibrase defibrinogenated dogs. *Thromb Res* 1973; **3:** 161.

68. Palma EC, Esperon R. Tratamiento del sindrome posttrombo-flebitico mediante transplante de safena interna. *Angiologica* 1959; **11:** 87.

69. Palma EC, Esperon R. Vein transplants and grafts in the surgical treatment of the post-phlebitic syndrome. *J Cardiovasc Surg* 1960; **1:** 94.

70. Pinsolle J, Videau J. Anomalies du carrefour iliocave. *Chirurgie* 1982; **108:** 451.

71. Qvarfordt P, Eklof B, Ohlin P, Plate G, Saltin B. Intramuscular pressure blood flow and skeletal muscle metabolism in patients with venous claudication. *Surgery* 1984; **95:** 191.

72. Scobie AH, Scobie TK, Vogelfeueger LJ. Venous autografts. *Can J Surg* 1962; **5:** 471.

73. Silver D, Anlyan WG. Peripheral vein grafts in dogs. *Surg Forum* 1961; **12:** 259.

74. Sitzmann JV, Imbembo AI, Ricotta JJ, McManama GP, Hutchins GM. Dimethylsulfoxide treated cryopreserved venous allografts in the arterial and venous system. *Surgery* 1984; **95:** 154.

75. Stirling GA, Tsapogas MJ. Extrapulmonary vascular bands and webs. *Ann Surg* 1969; **169:** 308.

76. Sztankasy G, Szabo Z. Ilio-caval dysplasia. Studies on the pathogenesis of venous diseases in the lower extremities. *J Cardiovasc Surg* 1969; **10:** 16.

77. Takaro T, Smith DE, Peasley ED, Kim JS. Experimental vena caval anastomoses and grafts. *Surg Gynecol Obstet* 1962; **115:** 49.

78. Trimble C, Bernstein EF, Pomerantz M. A prosthetic bridge device to relieve iliac venous compression. *Surg Forum* 1972; **23:** 249.

79. Vollmar J. Reconstruction of the iliac vein and inferior vena cava. In: Hobbs JT, ed. *The Treatment of Venous Disorders.* Philadelphia, PA: Lippincott, 1977; 308.

80. Vorwerk D, Guenther RW, Wendt G, Neuerberg J, Schurmann K. Iliocaval stenosis and iliac venous thrombosis in retroperitoneal fibrosis: percutaneous treatment by use of hydrodynamic thrombectomy and stenting. *Cardiovasc Int Radiol* 1996; **19:** 40–2.

81. Walsh JJ, Williams LR, Driscoll JL, Lee JF. Vein compression by arterial aneurysms. *J Vasc Surg* 1988; **8:** 465–9.

82. Warren R, Thayer T. Transplantation of the saphenous vein for postphlebitic stasis. *Surgery* 1954; **35:** 867.

83. Zinicola N, Hoffert PW, Haimovici H. Autogenous vein bypass grafts in the venous system. *Bull Soc Int Chir* 1962; **21:** 265.

CHAPTER 14

Acquired obstruction of the inferior vena cava (IVC)

Pathology	429	Treatment	437
Clinical presentation	430	Prognosis	440
Investigations	431	References	441

Most congenital anomalies of the inferior vena cava (IVC) cause no symptoms because they either provide additional pathways for blood flow, as in the double vena cava, or are well compensated by collateral vessels. Aplasia and other congenital abnormalities of the IVC are discussed in Chapter 24.

Acquired obstruction of the vena cava is a distinct clinical entity commonly caused by spontaneous thrombosis in a normal vessel, thrombosis secondary to external compression or thrombosis upon pathological changes in the vein wall.

Pathology

The causes of obstruction of the vena cava are as follows.

THROMBOSIS

Spontaneous thrombosis

Spontaneous thrombosis usually follows a *surgical operation* or major systemic trauma, and is commonly an extension of an ilio-femoral vein thrombosis into the vena cava but may occur in isolation or in association with deep vein thrombosis elsewhere in the lower limbs. A small proportion of patients have pro-thrombotic coagulation abnormalities such as antithrombin III deficiency, protein C and protein S deficiency.

Thrombosis secondary to local trauma

Direct trauma, caused by blunt and penetrating injuries, iatrogenic injuries inflicted during arterial operations, and indirect trauma such as tears and bruising from spinal fractures are the injuries that commonly cause secondary thrombosis.

Thrombosis secondary to malignant tumour invasion

Primary and secondary malignant disease in the lymph nodes, and carcinoma of the pancreas, stomach and pelvic organs may infiltrate into the wall of the vena cava and, by damaging the endothelium, initiate thrombosis.

Renal carcinoma can spread via the lumen of the renal vein into the vena cava where it may cause an occluding thrombosis, or spread along the lumen without blocking it and give rise to tumour emboli. Adrenal tumours can cause similar effects.

Thrombosis secondary to external compression (see below)

Iatrogenic

Caval ligation or partitioning with stitches, clips, or filters (all procedures performed to prevent pulmonary embolism) may cause a partial or total obstruction or initiate an occlusive thrombosis.

EXTERNAL COMPRESSION

External compression may in itself occlude the vena cava but it commonly causes a secondary thrombosis once the compression significantly reduces the rate of blood flow. The common causes of external compression are given below.

Lymph glands

The pre-aortic and para-aortic lymph nodes are often enlarged by lymphomatous change and secondary carcinoma.

Retroperitoneal fibrosis

This begins as a plaque of fibrous tissue across the front of the vena cava and aorta and may totally occlude it as the fibrosis thickens and contracts.

Aortic aneurysms

These commonly stretch and partly compress the IVC but rarely cause a complete occlusion or a thrombosis. Rupture of an aneurysm into the IVC to produce an aorto-caval fistula raises the pressure in the distal IVC and causes symptoms similar to those caused by an IVC block. The increased venous return gives rise to a high central venous pressure and congestive cardiac failure. Inflammatory aneurysms with retroperitoneal fibrosis may occlude the vena cava.

Large abdominal malignant tumours

Tumours such as carcinoma of the kidney and tumours of the ovary may compress the IVC.

Ascites

This may become so tense that it compresses the IVC, obstructs venous return and causes oedema of the legs.

VEIN WALL PATHOLOGY

Vein wall membranes such as those causing the Budd–Chiari syndrome may give rise to caval thrombosis. Leiomyosarcoma of the caval wall narrows the lumen and, more rarely, leads to thrombosis (Chapter 27).

Clinical presentation

The symptoms of occlusion of the vena cava which were first described in 1644[21] may appear suddenly or slowly.[12,17,26] A rapid onset is almost always caused by an acute thrombosis. The gradual development of symptoms may be caused by a slowly increasing compression that causes symptoms as it develops or, some time after the occlusion, the slow decompensation of collateral vessels and the slow development of peripheral valve incompetence.

ACUTE THROMBOSIS

The symptoms of an acute IVC thrombosis may appear spontaneously or following a recent unrelated operation or injury. They may also follow a chronic debilitating illness or as an addition to the symptoms of a chronic IVC obstruction.

The patient often complains of low back or buttock pain which is frequently misdiagnosed as lumbago and treated by putting the patient to bed – an action which exacerbates the thrombotic process. If a renal vein becomes involved, the patient will develop loin pain and haematuria. Abdominal pain is uncommon and the abdomen is rarely tender.

The legs become oedematous within 6–12 hours of the IVC becoming totally blocked. The whole of both limbs, buttocks and sometimes the lower abdominal wall become oedematous. The swelling is soft and pits but is not tender.

The abdomen may become swollen with ascitic fluid or may already be swollen before the onset of the leg swelling if the caval obstruction is caused by an intra-abdominal abnormality.

The skin of the legs may develop a bluish tinge. If there is extensive thrombosis in the pelvic and femoral veins as well as in the IVC, the skin may turn a deep blue (phlegmasia cerulea dolens) and develop areas of skin blistering and gangrene.

Renal vein thrombosis will cause haematuria and, if bilateral, oliguria, anuria and the symptoms of uraemia.[12]

The patient may complain of chest pain and breathlessness if there is an associated pulmonary embolus.

There may be other physical signs indicating the cause of the thrombosis, such as a large abdominal mass.

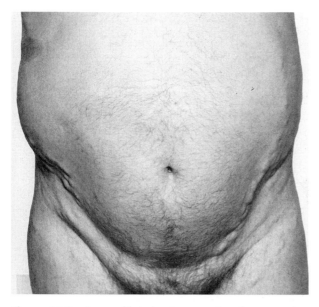

Figure 14.1 Large dilated veins crossing the anterolateral aspect of the abdominal wall in a patient with occlusion of the inferior vena cava.

Dilated veins appear on the abdominal wall between the groins and the axillae within days of the thrombosis (Figure 14.1).

CHRONIC OCCLUSION (PLUS THROMBOSIS)

The symptoms and signs of a slowly progressive occlusion are similar to those of an acute thrombosis but their time course is different.[10]

There may be a history of a serious illness, accident or operation years before, often in the teenage years, which produced no symptoms or minimal leg swelling which regressed rapidly and spontaneously. Some patients will give a history of symptoms relevant to the cause of the IVC compression whilst others will complain of no symptoms other than those caused by the venous obstruction.

A few patients have no symptoms, the IVC occlusion being discovered during a routine examination when collateral veins are found on the abdominal wall.

The principal symptoms of a chronic IVC occlusion are swelling and dull aching pains in the legs and the appearance of varicose veins on the abdomen and the legs. The swelling often becomes gross and may extend into the buttocks and lower abdominal wall.

The large varicosities on the abdominal wall follow the course of the superficial inferior epigastric

and superficial external iliac veins (Figure 14.1). Normally, blood flows down these veins to the sapheno-femoral junction. Compression and stroking the veins (Harvey's test) will reveal that the blood flow is upwards towards the tributaries of the superior vena cava.

The longer the history of leg swelling and varicose veins, the more likely is there to be skin pigmentation, eczema, lipodermatosclerosis and ulceration. If these changes develop, they are invariably extensive, often affecting the whole of the lower legs, not just the gaiter areas, with multiple areas of ulceration.

The patient may complain of bursting pain on exercise which is relieved by rest and elevation (venous claudication) and notice that the leg swelling increases with exercise.

General examination may reveal evidence of the cause of the IVC obstruction, such as an abdominal mass or generalized lymph node enlargement.[6] Albuminuria in patients with chronic renal vein occlusion is rare.[10]

Investigations

Two questions need to be answered. Is the IVC obstructed? What is the cause of the obstruction?

The state of the IVC is best determined by cavography which was first performed by Dos Santos in 1938.[4]

IVC PHLEBOGRAPHY[5,7,11,16,25]

Bilateral simultaneous foot injections of a radio-opaque contrast medium, combined with the application of thigh tourniquets during the injection which are suddenly released to allow a bolus of contrast to enter the pelvic veins, usually gives good quality images of the IVC, but they are not as good as those obtained with bilateral femoral vein injections.

Thrombotic IVC occlusion is often associated with iliac and femoral vein thrombosis; it is therefore worthwhile performing bilateral ascending phlebograms first to determine both the state of the veins in the legs and the patency of the femoral veins. A recanalized or fully patent femoral vein can then be punctured for a femoral injection using the ascending phlebogram to identify the position of the patent vein at the groin. Twenty millilitres of contrast medium should be injected into both veins by hand.

On the rare occasion when both femoral veins are occluded, the IVC can be opacified with bilateral intratrochanteric injections,[22] or with a retrograde

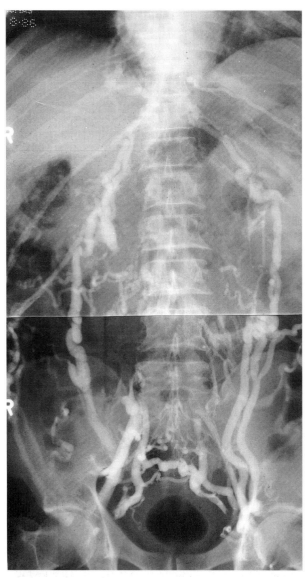
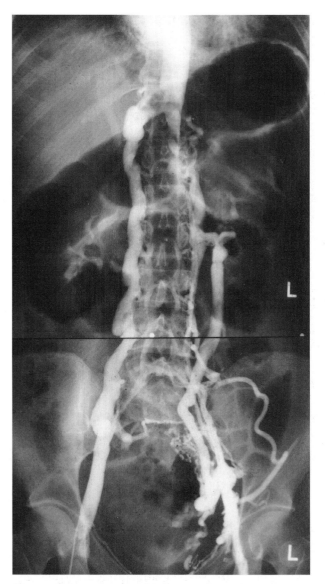

(a)   (b)

Figure 14.2   The phlebographic appearances of inferior vena cava obstruction. (a) Total occlusion of the inferior vena cava from its origin to the entry of the renal veins. This phlebograph shows large inferior epigastric, deep circumflex iliac and ascending lumbar veins draining into the lower intercostal and azygos veins just below the diaphragm. This is the preoperative phlebograph of the patient illustrated in Figure 14.9. (b) The phlebograph of a patient with a total occlusion of the inferior vena cava. The two collateral vessels are a large azygos vein on the patient's right and a large ascending lumbar vein on the left. (c) A montage of the phlebographs of a patient with a total occlusion of the inferior vena cava showing collateral vessels carrying blood from the internal iliac veins into the perirectal venous plexus and from there into the inferior mesenteric vein and the portal vein.[11] (d) An excretory urograph showing multiple external indentations into both ureters caused by dilated peri-ureteric veins acting as collaterals for a totally occluded vena cava.

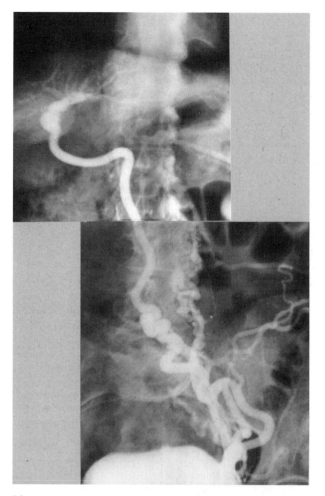

(c)

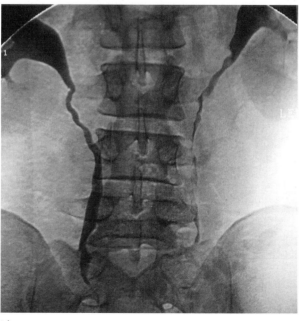

(d)

injection from a catheter passed down into the IVC from an arm vein, or by digital subtraction enhancement of the venous phase of an aortogram.

The typical appearances of IVC obstruction and the common collaterals (the inferior epigastric, deep external iliac, ascending lumbar and azygos veins) are shown in Figure 14.2.

If the IVC is not completely blocked, phlebography may reveal external compression by enlarged lymph glands (Figure 14.3a, b), retroperitoneal fibrosis (Figure 14.4a, b), a caval clip (Figure 14.5) or the intraluminal spread of a tumour (Figure 14.6a, b). A chest radiograph may reveal an enlarged azygos vein (Figure 14.7).

The cause of an IVC obstruction can usually be determined by the combination of clinical examination, phlebography and other radiological investigations.

Unless there is a definite history of a previous venous thrombosis, it is wise to exclude all other reasons for a thrombosis before accepting that it is spontaneous.

Physical examination may reveal an abdominal mass, generalized lymphadenopathy or signs of a distant neoplasm.

DUPLEX ULTRASOUND SCANNING

Duplex scanning can demonstrate caval stenosis or occlusion, but overlying bowel gas frequently causes technical difficulties.

COMPUTERIZED TOMOGRAPHY

The CT scan is the most useful investigation for detecting retroperitoneal abdominal masses as it reveals both the lumen of the great abdominal vessels and the anatomy of any masses compressing them.[20] Ultrasound will detect masses but does not give as much information about the vessels as a CT scan.

Retroperitoneal fibrosis is not always visible on a CT scan and may only be diagnosed when an intravenous excretory urogram shows the ureters to be drawn medially and perhaps partially obstructed.

MAGNETIC RESONANCE IMAGING

MRI is accurate in demonstrating the location and extent of IVC thrombosis and provides useful information about the heterogeneity and morphology (hence age) of the thrombus.[23] MRI also provides detailed information about caval wall abnormalities and retroperitoneal masses.[13]

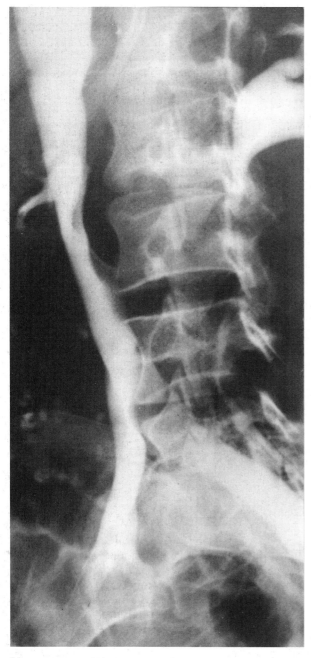

(a)

(b)

Figure 14.3   (a) Compression of the inferior vena cava by a large mass of lymphomatous preaortic lymph nodes. (b) Two phlebographs taken 2 months apart. The upper panel shows an irregular filling defect at the termination of the left common iliac vein and the beginning of the vena cava. This is too lateral and too irregular to be confused with a physiological iliac vein compression. CT scanning confirmed a mass of enlarged lymph nodes in this region. Two months later the patient developed oedema of both legs. A new phlebograph (lower panel) showed total occlusion of the vena cava and both iliac veins.

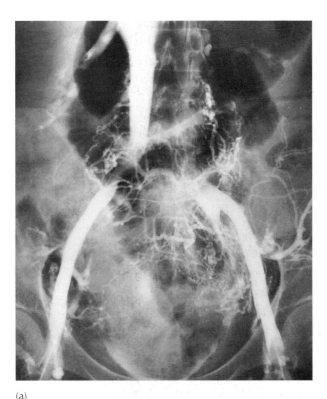

(a)

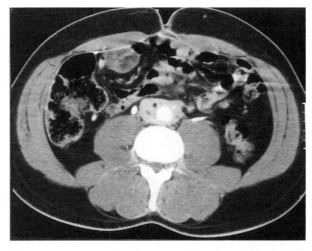

(b)

Figure 14.4 (a) A phlebograph showing stenoses of the iliac vein and the first part of the inferior vena cava caused by retroperitoneal fibrosis. (b) An enhanced CT scan showing retroperitoneal fibrosis, especially around the aorta, completely occluding the vena cava. The ureters have been released by a previous ureterolysis.

BLOOD INVESTIGATIONS

These are rarely helpful. A raised erythrocyte sedimentation rate should raise the suspicion of a generalized disease or retroperitoneal fibrosis. Coagulation factors are usually normal in patients with venous thrombosis, though the rare conditions of antithrombin III, protein C and protein S deficiency must not be forgotten. The haemoglobin concentration and white cell count should be measured as they will be abnormal in patients with generalized debilitating disease, infections and retroperitoneal fibrosis. Biochemical tests of renal function may suggest the presence of ureteric obstruction by retroperitoneal fibrosis or renal vein thrombosis.

OTHER INVESTIGATIONS

A surgical biopsy of an enlarged peripheral lymph node may be required to define the histology of lymph node disease.

Bipedal lymphangiography is occasionally helpful in defining the extent of an abdominal lymph node mass but has been largely superseded by CT scanning.

Arteriography is rarely required.

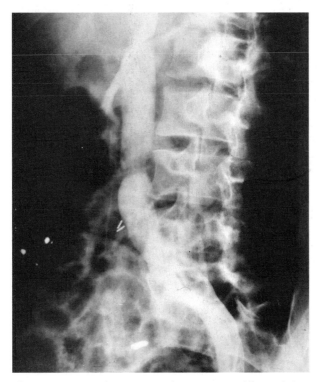

Figure 14.5 A linear partial transverse filling defect caused by a Miles clip (see Chapter 22, page 640).

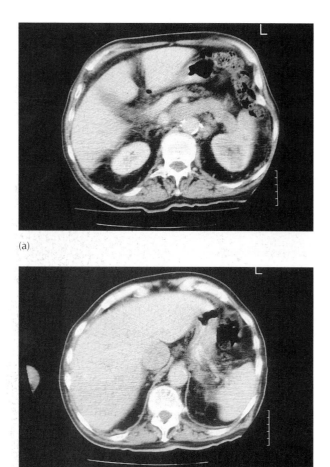

(a)

(b)

Figure 14.6   (a) A CT scan showing a carcinoma of the left kidney spreading into the inferior vena cava via the left renal vein. (b) A CT scan showing a vena cava full of tumour and thrombus from a renal carcinoma. This thrombus extended into the right atrium.

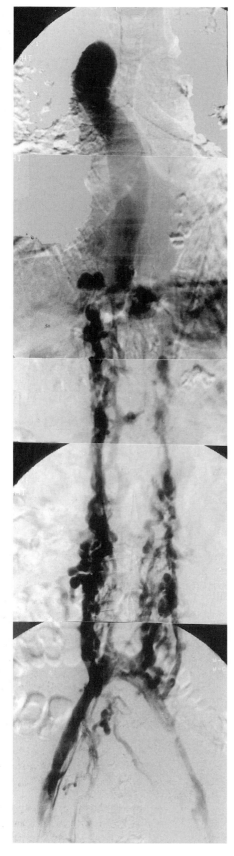

Figure 14.7   A subtraction film showing a dilated azygos vein carrying blood past an occluded inferior vena cava. The distortion of the mediastinal shadow at the point where the azygos vein turns forwards to join the superior vena cava may be the first indication that a patient has a vena cava occlusion. Ligation of an azygos vein such as this which is carrying the whole of the visceral and lower limb venous return can cause renal vein thrombosis and death.

The decision to investigate the cause of an IVC occlusion depends upon the degree of suspicion raised by the history and clinical findings that an extravascular abnormality might exist.

Treatment

The treatment of an acute thrombosis of the IVC is similar to the treatment of any other type of venous thrombosis, fully discussed in Chapter 10. Removal of the thrombus, if possible, and by whatever means, will not, however, result in long lasting patency if the cause of the thrombosis (e.g. external compression) is not corrected.

It is, therefore, essential to decide before beginning treatment whether the thrombosis is spontaneous (idiopathic) or secondary to compression. The investigations required may take some time to carry out and so the immediate treatment, the administration of heparin to prevent further thrombosis, must be based upon a clinical diagnosis. A loading dose of 10 000 units of heparin intravenously should be followed by 40 000 units/24 hours, with the dose controlled and monitored by a laboratory test (the clotting time or the activated partial thromboplastin time) until a definite diagnosis is made and plan of treatment formulated.

ACUTE 'IDIOPATHIC' THROMBOSIS

If no abnormality is detected other than the caval thrombosis, the clinician has three choices – prevent further thrombosis by giving heparin, remove the thrombus surgically or pharmacologically, or confine the thrombus to the vena cava to prevent embolism. The second and third approaches should be considered when the thrombus is fresh and non-adherent or only partially adherent to the vein wall. The first approach is only safe when the whole thrombus is fixed to the vein wall. Radomski *et al.*[18] found that pulmonary embolism occurred in 27% of patients with free-floating caval thrombi and 17% with adherent thrombi despite adequate anticoagulation.

Thrombolysis of fresh non-adherent thrombus

This may be achieved with urokinase, streptokinase or tissue plasminogen activators which are all described in Chapter 10.

The worry about dissolving a large IVC thrombus is that it might fragment and become a large pulmonary embolus. Emboli do occur during throm-

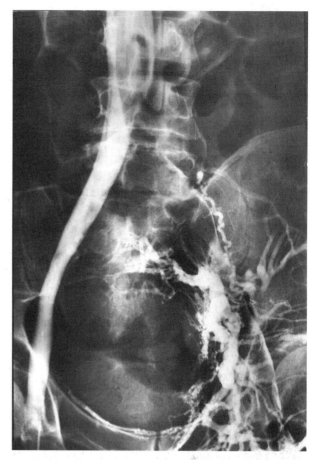

Figure 14.8 A large loose coiled non-adherent thrombus floating in the inferior vena cava. We prefer to treat such a threat to the patient's life by thrombectomy rather than thrombolysis. The left iliac and common femoral veins also contain fresh partially adherent thrombus. The vena caval thrombus is an extension of the iliac vein thrombosis.

bolysis, and the larger the thrombus being lysed the greater this concern. A decision about the use of thrombolysis will depend upon the general state of the patient, evidence of previous emboli and any contraindications to lytic therapy. Our preference is to remove large non-adherent thrombi surgically (Figure 14.8) and to reserve thrombolysis for the relatively small caval thrombus which is usually just an extension of an iliac vein thrombus.

Thrombectomy

Thrombectomy of fresh IVC thrombus is performed through a long midline abdominal incision. The IVC is exposed by reflecting the caecum, ascending colon and duodenum to the left and controlled with a clamp above the upper limit of the thrombus as displayed by the phlebogram. The thrombus is then extracted with a Fogarty balloon catheter passed directly through a venotomy in the lower half of the IVC. Bleeding from the IVC below the venotomy and the lumbar veins is controlled by direct digital pressure or by a balloon catheter.

Renal vein thrombectomy can be performed but is a considerable surgical 'tour de force'.

There is little point in removing thrombus from the IVC if both iliac veins are irretrievably occluded. If one iliac vein is patent, it is worthwhile clearing the IVC, even if the occluded iliac vein cannot be cleared, because a patent IVC will benefit the leg with the blocked iliac vein as well as the leg with the normal iliac vein by increasing the outflow routes of its potential collaterals.

If both iliac veins and the IVC are cleared of thrombus, which implies bilateral groin incisions as well as the abdominal incision, then patency should be maintained with bilateral A-V fistulae fashioned between the femoral arteries and veins.

Neglen *et al.*[14] studied 52 patients with iliofemoral thromboses extending into the IVC. Of these, 27 underwent successful thrombectomy combined with the construction of an arteriovenous fistula and anticoagulation. None of these patients developed venous ulceration or other features of calf pump failure on long-term follow-up, whereas 20% of non-thrombectomized patients developed ulceration. Thrombectomy was performed with low morbidity and mortality but was only successful in patients with a short history and fresh thrombus.

Caval blockade

Patients who are not fit enough to withstand a major abdominal operation and who have contraindications to thrombolysis should be considered for caval blockade (see Chapter 22). It is not possible to predict whether a fresh thrombus will fragment and embolize; it must therefore be assumed that it will. A history of chest pain, haemoptysis or a positive lung scan suggests that the risk of further embolism is high.

Caval blockade can be performed under local anaesthesia by inserting a filter into the upper part of the IVC, usually below the entry of the renal veins, through a venotomy in the right internal jugular vein.

Most forms of filter or external clip effectively prevent further emboli, and in these circumstances we are not concerned with IVC patency. Indeed if there is a large fresh thrombus in the IVC, it is highly likely that the IVC will become totally occluded after inserting a filter. Heparin must be given to reduce further thrombosis, and placing the filter below but as close to the entry of the renal

veins as possible will also reduce the chances of thrombosis above the filter.

Heparin

Patients who have a complete vena cava occlusion by the time they present, with no propagating tail of thrombus and no symptoms or signs of embolism, should be treated with a 7-day course of heparin followed by oral anticoagulation for at least 6 months. Thrombectomy or thrombolysis when the phlebograph shows a completely occluded IVC and well developed collateral channels usually fails because the thrombus is frequently more than 6 days old.

ACUTE SECONDARY THROMBOSIS

Most of the conditions that compress the vena cava and precipitate thrombosis are unsuitable for surgical treatment. In such cases anticoagulants to prevent further thrombosis and caval blockade to prevent embolism are the main forms of treatment.

Even surgically correctable conditions such as aortic aneurysms are not easy to treat at the same time as IVC thrombectomy, though a combined operation is technically feasible. It is safer to allow the acute thrombosis to settle before treating the aneurysm, or opt for embolus prevention by inserting a caval filter before proceeding to repair the aneurysm.

Thrombus in a compressed or infiltrated IVC is usually adherent and without a propagating tail, so controllable with anticoagulants. Direct venous surgery is rarely indicated.

CHRONIC OCCLUSION

When the initial cause of the IVC occlusion is compression the compression should, if possible, be treated first. Many of the patients in this group have advanced malignant disease. The cause of their IVC obstruction is often beyond treatment and their venous symptoms are often clinically insignificant.

The symptoms of the patients with a long-standing IVC occlusion following thrombosis fall into two groups: swelling and post-thrombotic changes in the skin of the legs, and venous claudication.

Swelling and skin changes can usually be controlled by conservative measures. Venous claudication is uncommon and can only be relieved by some form of direct vascular surgery.

Conservative treatment

Conservative treatment of the leg swelling, varicose veins and skin changes caused by a long-standing

IVC obstruction aims to reverse the effect of the high peripheral venous pressure by counteracting it with external compression.

Patients must wear high quality, high compression (40 mmHg), full-length, bilateral, elastic compression stockings at all times (see Chapter 16). Patients should elevate their legs whenever possible. At night the foot of their beds should be raised 12 inches (30 cm). During the day they should avoid standing and sitting. When sitting, they should raise their legs on a foot stool so the legs are horizontal. Patients should lie on the floor and raise their legs vertically against a wall for 15 minutes at least once each day. If the swelling is severe, they may have to spend 1 or 2 days in bed each week.

Once lipodermatosclerosis and ulceration have developed, elastic compression alone has little effect. Long periods of bed rest are required to heal chronic ulcers, and areas of severe tissue damage may have to be excised and replaced with skin grafts. Patients who have reached this state and those with venous claudication can only be helped by bypass surgery.

Vena cava bypass operations

Venous bypass operations have not been widely practised because of their high failure rate.[24,27] However, a number of animal studies have shown that prostheses made of expanded polytetrafluoroethylene (PTFE) will stay patent in the venous system if venous blood flow is enhanced by a distal A-V fistula.[2,3,8] Sporadic case reports and small series indicate that the large bore, externally supported expanded polytetrafluoroethylene (ePTFE) graft is the preferred conduit for caval repair or replacement and that long-term patency rates are acceptable,[15] although no large trials have been reported.

Some isolated clinical reports of bypasses of the iliac veins remaining patent for 2 years are encouraging.[1,3]

For the bypass procedure to be successful there must be a relatively healthy vein at both ends of the bypass for the anastomoses. Unfortunately, many patients with an IVC occlusion have extensive postthrombotic damage of the iliac and femoral veins as well as of the IVC, and a bypass is therefore not possible.

If, however, a patient has disabling symptoms of claudication or extensive skin damage in the lower limb and patent, moderately healthy femoral veins, it is worthwhile attempting a bifemoral caval bypass with an externally supported PTFE prothesis with A-V fistulae below the lower anastomoses (Figure 14.9).

The patient who is to have a bypass operation must be well past the thrombotic state of his original

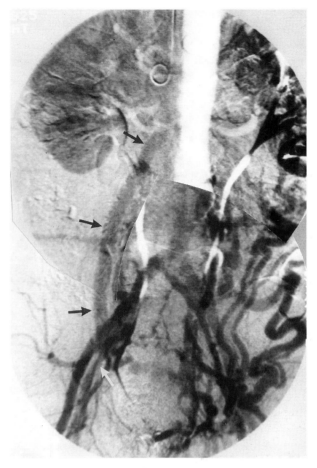

Figure 14.9 A montage of two films from a digital subtraction angiogram showing an externally supported PTFE graft between the right external iliac vein and the inferior vena cava, just below the entry of the right renal vein. In the upper part the aorta is white but in the lower part arteries are black. In the lower part the ureters are white. The black arrows indicate the bypass. The white arrow indicates the external iliac vein just below the anastomosis. This is the patient illustrated in Figure 14.2(a).

illness and have severe symptoms. Anticoagulants must be given postoperatively, and the fistulae must be closed 3–6 months later.

While the fistulae are open, swelling of the patient's leg may increase because the venous pressure in the legs will be increased.

When a Budd–Chiari syndrome is associated with a vena caval thrombosis a cavo-atrial bypass may relieve the symptoms in the legs.[9]

Much careful clinical experimentation needs to be done before these procedures become generally adopted. Venous claudication should improve following a bypass operation but improvement in the state of the skin of the lower leg depends mainly on

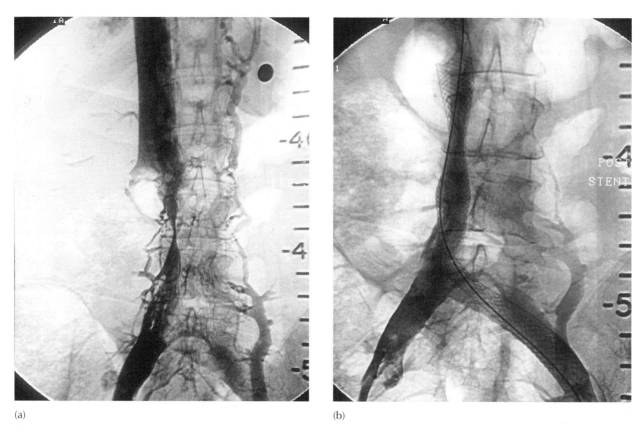

(a)

(b)

Figure 14.10 (a) Obstruction of the inferior vena cava and termination of the left common iliac vein caused by tumour infiltration from an adjacent carcinoma of the ureter. (b) Treatment by dilatation and the insertion of a Wall stent into the left common iliac vein and vena cava.

the degree of post-thrombotic damage in the calf. Additional surgery may be needed to ablate secondarily incompetent communicating veins.

Excisional operations

When the vena caval occlusion is caused by tumour infiltration, or intraluminal spread of the tumour, a wide excision of the tumour and the vena cava may produce worthwhile palliation of symptoms and an occasional cure.[19]

Stenting

When external compression of the vena cava is causing symptoms, an alternative approach is transvenous dilatation and stenting. This form of treatment is especially valuable when seeking to palliate the symptom of venous compression caused by malignant disease (Figure 14.10a, b). Its role in relieving post-thrombotic stenoses has not yet been assessed by long-term studies. Provided the stent maintains the dilatation and does not thrombose,

stenting will become an extremely valuable form of therapy, but will only be of value when obstruction rather than incompetence is the principal physiological problem.

Prognosis

The prognosis for patients with IVC obstruction depends upon their ability to form collateral channels, the likelihood of further episodes of thrombosis, and the presence of post-thrombotic damage in the deep veins of the lower limb.

The younger the patient the better the collaterals. Many of the cases of spontaneous IVC thrombosis seen in our clinic occurred during the teenage years but did not present until the patient was 30 or 40 years old, presentation being related to the slow progression of symptoms or to a new episode of thrombosis. Once symptoms have appeared, their progression is inexorable unless the patient is exceptionally diligent with the use of elastic stockings.

Direct venous surgery will be applicable to only a small proportion of these patients, even when the techniques are fully developed; the clinical emphasis must therefore be on the prevention of thrombosis or its effective treatment when it first occurs. Progressive destruction of the skin of the lower leg following bilateral femoral and iliac thrombosis plus an IVC thrombosis sometimes ends with the patient requesting an amputation.

References

1. Chan EL, Bardin JA, Bernstein EF. Inferior vena cava bypass. Experimental evaluation of externally supported grafts and initial clinical experience. *J Vasc Surg* 1984; **1:** 675.
2. Dale WA. Synthetic grafts for venous reconstruction. In: Bergan JJ, Yao JST, eds. *Surgery of the Veins.* New York: Grune & Stratton, 1985; 233.
3. Dale WA, Harris J, Terry RB. Polytetrafluoroethylene reconstruction of the inferior vena cava. *Surgery* 1984; **95:** 625.
4. Dos Santos JC. La phlébographie directe. *J Int Chir* 1938; **3:** 625.
5. Filler RM, Edwards EA. Collaterals of the lower inferior vena cava in man as revealed by venography. *Arch Surg* 1962; **84:** 10.
6. Filler RM, Harris SH, Edwards EA. Characteristics of inferior vena cava venogram in retroperitoneal cancer. *N Engl J Med* 1962; **266:** 1194.
7. Fletcher EWL, Lea Thomas M. Chronic post thrombotic obstruction of the inferior vena cava investigated by cavography. *Am J Roentgenol* 1968; **102:** 363.
8. Gloviczki P, Hollier LH, Dewanjee MK, Trastek VF, Hoffman EA, Kaye MP. Experimental replacment of the inferior vena cava. Factors affecting patency. *Surgery* 1984; **95:** 657.
9. Huguet C, Deliere T, Ollivier JM, Levy VG. Budd–Chiari syndrome with thrombosis of the inferior vena cava: long term patency of meso-caval and cavo-atrial prosthetic bypass. *Surgery* 1984; **95:** 108.
10. Jackson BT, Thomas ML. Post-thrombotic inferior vena caval obstruction. A review of 24 patients. *Br Med J* 1970; **1:** 18.
11. Kendall B. Collateral flow to portal system in obstruction of iliac veins and inferior vena cava. *Br J Radiol* 1965; **38:** 798.
12. Missal ME, Robinson JA, Tatum RW. Inferior vena cava obstruction. Clinical manifestations, diagnostic methods and related problems. *Ann Intern Med* 1965; **62:** 133.
13. Monig SP, Gawenda M, Erasmi H, Zieren J, Pichlmaier H. Diagnosis, treatment and prognosis of the leiomyosarcoma of the inferior vena cava. Three cases and summary of published reports. *Eur J Surg* 1995; **161:** 231–5.
14. Neglen P, Nazzal MM, al-Hassan HK, Christenson JT, Eklof B. Surgical removal of an inferior vena cava thrombus. *Eur J Vasc Surg* 1992; **6:** 78–82.
15. Okada Y, Kumada K, Terachi T, Nishimura K, Tomoyoshi T, Yoshida O. Long-term follow up of patients with tumour thrombi form renal cell carcinoma and total replacement of the inferior vena cava using an expanded polytetrafluoroethylene tubular graft. *J Urol* 1996; **155:** 444–6.
16. O'Loughlin BJ. Roentgen visualisation of inferior vena cava. *Am J Roentgenol* 1947; **58:** 617.
17. Pleasants JH. Obstruction of the inferior vena cava with a report of eighteen cases. *Johns Hopkins Hosp Rep* 1911; **15:** 363.
18. Radomski JS, Jarrell BE, Carabasi RA, Yang SL, Koolpe H. Risk of pulmonary embolus with inferior vena cava thrombosis. *Am Surg* 1987; **53:** 97–101.
19. Schechter DC. Cardiovascular surgery in the management of exogenous tumours involving the vena cava. In: Bergan JJ, Yao JST, eds. *Venous Surgery.* New York: Grune & Stratton, 1985; 393.
20. Schechter DC, Vogel JM. The challenge of venous extension in malignant renal neoplasms. *N Y State J Med* 1983; **83:** 55.
21. Schenk. *Observationum Medicarum Rariorum.* Lugduni, 1644; 339.
22. Schobinger RA. *Intra-osseus Phlebography.* New York: Grune & Stratton, 1960.
23. Soler R, Rodriguez E, Lopez MF, Marini M. MR imaging of inferior vena cava thrombosis. *Eur J Radiol* 1995; **19:** 101–7.
24. Stansel HC. Synthetic inferior vena cava grafts. *Arch Surg* 1964; **89:** 1096.
25. Stein S, Blumsohn D. Clinical and radiological observations of inferior vena caval obstruction. *Br J Radiol* 1962; **35:** 159.
26. Welch WH. In: Allbutt TC, Rollerton HD, ed. *A System of Medicine,* Vol. 6. London: Macmillan, 1899; 217.
27. Wilson SE, Jabour H, Stone R, Stanley TM. Patency of biological and prosthetic inferior vena cava grafts with distal limb fistula. *Arch Surg* 1978; **113:** 1174.

CHAPTER 15

The calf pump failure syndrome: pathology

The effect of deep vein thrombosis on vein function	444	The effect of calf pump failure on the microcirculation of the lower limb	458
The effect of thrombosis on calf pump function	454	Prevalence	466
		References	467

The changes in the veins, subcutaneous tissues and skin of the lower limb that follow a deep vein thrombosis have for many years been called the post-phlebitic syndrome. The terms thrombophlebitis and phlebothrombosis are misleading[29,41,56] because they imply a dominance of one form of pathological change and furthermore suggest that it is possible to identify the dominant abnormality, namely the thrombosis or the vein wall inflammation.

Most clinicians and pathologists now prefer to use the all embracing and non-committal term 'deep vein thrombosis' for all forms of venous thrombosis except for the variety in the superficial veins which is called 'superficial thrombophlebitis' (see Chapter 23) because it is invariably associated with an inflammation of the vein wall. Conversely, as the principal cause of the late sequelae of deep vein thrombosis is the thrombosis rather than the vein wall inflammation, it is preferable to use the term 'post-thrombotic syndrome' rather than post-phlebitic syndrome.

This chapter is, however, entitled 'The calf pump failure syndrome', not the post-thrombotic syndrome, because the clinical features of this condition can develop in the absence of any evidence of a previous deep vein thrombosis. Patients with the calf pump failure syndrome fall into three distinct groups: those with a definite history of proven deep vein thrombosis, those with no history of thrombosis but phlebographic evidence of a previous thrombosis, and those with no history of a thrombosis and a normal phlebograph. The syndrome in the latter group is not the result of thrombosis but primary deep or superficial valve incompetence. The resulting symptoms and signs are caused by failure of the calf pump; hence the name 'calf pump failure syndrome' covers all possibilities and can be preceded by the adjective post-thrombotic if there is definite evidence of thrombosis.

The anatomy and physiology of the calf pump are described in Chapter 3. The calf pump is in essence a set of valved tubes surrounded by muscle with a series of inflow and outflow tracts. The pump receives blood from the superficial and deep tissues of the lower half of the leg and propels it back towards the heart. To function properly the veins within and outside the pump must be patent, their valves competent and the muscle strong. The commonest cause of calf pump vein obstruction and valve incompetence is deep vein thrombosis and it is important to consider how, when and where thrombosis damages the calf pump. The ways in which other conditions affect vein patency and valve competence – such as external compression and primary valve abnormalities – are more obvious even though their aetiology may not be fully understood and are described in Chapters 12–14.

The effect of deep vein thrombosis on vein function

Most venous thrombi seem to begin within valve cusps and muscle sinusoids[29,44,59,65,110,124,125,130,132] (see Chapter 8). As the thrombus grows it gets thicker, changing from a thin non-adherent non-obstructing thrombus to one that completely obstructs the vein. The obstruction becomes haemodynamically significant when the thrombus occupies more than 75% of the cross-sectional area of the vein. When this occurs collateral vessels begin to open, the main stimulus to collateral vein dilatation being the pressure gradient between the occluded vein's tributaries on either side of the obstruction.

As the thrombus grows it either surrounds the valve cusps or pushes them flat against the wall of the vein. These are the most serious effects of thrombosis because they destroy the valves. At first the valves become stiffened by a covering of fibrin and thrombus, soon they adhere to the vein wall and eventually they fragment. These changes destroy the valve's ability to function and leave the vein incompetent if it recanalizes.[48] Valves can only be saved from destruction by thrombosis if the thrombus is dissolved or removed during the first few hours of its life, before it has engulfed the valve. The period of time which is necessary for a valve to be completely destroyed has not been established.

Once established a thrombus may retract, adhere or recanalize.

Retraction

As a thrombus ages, its fibrin matures and contracts, causing the whole thrombus to shrink.[11,77,85] This is a slow process which takes many months to complete. As the thrombus gets smaller it usually becomes adherent to the vein wall, fixing and destroying any remaining valves which were not incorporated within it when it first formed. Sometimes the thrombus adheres to opposite sides of the vein and then, as it retracts, turns the vein into a double channelled vessel (see Figure 8.12).[93,115]

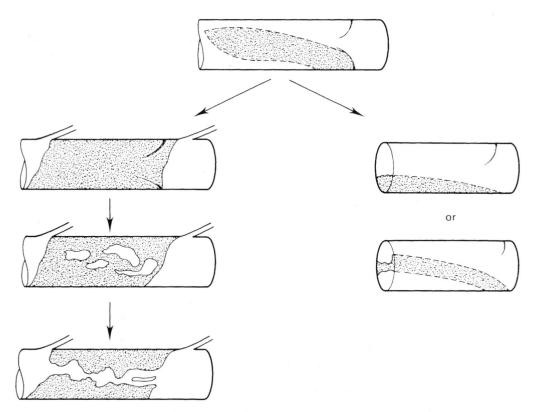

Figure 15.1   The changes in a venous thrombus that lead to recanalization (left-hand pathway) and reopening (right-hand pathway). The former is true recanalization (i.e. intrinsic thrombolysis producing a channel through the thrombus). The latter is simply retraction and adherence of the thrombus to one or both sides of the vessel wall.

Adhesion

Most thrombi grow steadily until they fill the whole vein and either engulf or completely flatten the valves against the vein wall. In the process of adhering to the vein wall the thrombus initiates an inflammatory response in the wall.[48] The thrombus may then retract but more often it totally occludes the vein which either remains permanently occluded or recanalizes.

The inflammatory response in the vein wall is the first step in the organization of the thrombus. The thrombus is infiltrated by chronic inflammatory cells and new capillary loops. The whole process leads to the conversion of the thrombus into an organized scar consisting of fibrin, fibrous tissue, and a few capillaries. The end result is a solid cord of tissue consisting of the original vein containing a thin totally organized thrombus.

Recanalization

The term recanalization is often used loosely to describe the new channels that can be seen to replace the original vein on a phlebograph. The reopening of most veins results from the retraction and adhesion of the thrombus to one side of the vein, leaving part of the original lumen open. True recanalization is rare.

True recanalization is the development of a new channel through the thrombus.[123] As time passes, areas within the thrombus soften and liquify, just as a haematoma liquifies, by spontaneous proteolysis. The role of the venous endothelium and the fibrinolytic activator it produces in this process of recanalization is not known.[32,81] Cystic spaces develop throughout the thrombus and if they join together and reach to both ends of the thrombus a new channel is formed (Figure 15.1). The chances of this process producing a good-sized channel are few, and the new channel is valveless. Strictly speaking, the development of large patent channels at the site of a previously thrombosed major vein should not be called recanalization. If the channel is large and in direct continuity with anatomically recognizable vessels above and below, the original vein has *reopened* as a result of thrombus *retraction* (Figures 15.1 and 15.3a).

If there are one or two large vessels, almost but not precisely in the anatomical course of the thrombosed vein, they are probably dilated vena venorum acting as collaterals (Figure 15.2). If there is a narrow and irregular channel bridging the gap between two anatomically definable veins, the thrombus may have recanalized. If there is a plexus of small tortuous vessels they are probably dilated vena venora (Figure 15.3b).

Whatever the form of channel that develops, it will probably be valveless, certainly incompetent, but not necessarily an obstruction to blood flow. The lumen of a reopened iliac or femoral vein can be as large as the normal vein if the thrombus retracts down to a thin cord on one side of the vein but most reopened veins are rarely as big as the original vessel and usually cause some obstruction to blood flow.

THROMBOSIS AND VEIN PATENCY

The reopening of veins after thrombosis has been observed frequently on serial phlebographs[85] but the development of duplex ultrasound scanning which allows frequent non-invasive assessments has enabled the rate and frequency of reopening to be assessed more accurately.

Over the past 5 years a number of workers[78,102,117] have shown that at least 50% of occluded vein segments reopen within 1 to 3 months but most of these studies have examined and recorded changes

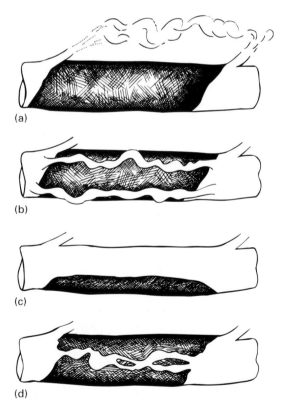

(a)

(b)

(c)

(d)

Figure 15.2 The four ways in which blood can bypass or pass through an obstruction caused by thrombosis. (a) Via true collateral vessels. (b) Via dilated vena venora. (c) Alongside retracted thrombus. (d) Through true recanalization.

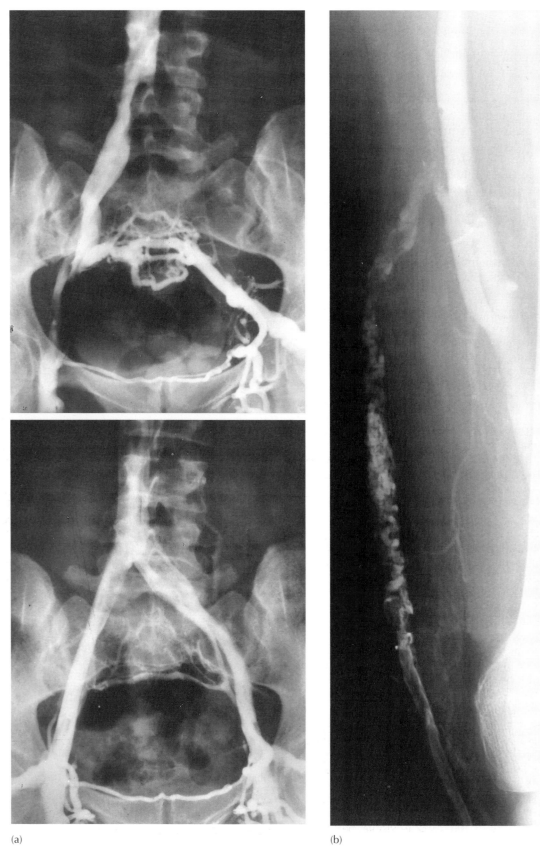

(a)

(b)

Table 15.1 Percentage reopening of veins after an occlusive thrombosis

	Common femoral vein	Superficial femoral vein	Popliteal vein	Calf vein
After 4 weeks				
Fully open	20	25	26	30
Improved	56	45	52	52
No change/worse	23	30	22	18
After 12 weeks				
Fully open	54	38	50	48
Improved	42	50	41	42
No change/worse	4	4	9	10
After 24 weeks				
Fully open	78	70	75	70
Improved	15	22	19	24
No change/worse	8	8	6	6

After Caprini _et al._[31]

in segments of the venous system (Table 15.1),[31] not the whole limb. Although there does not appear to be a significant difference in the incidence of reopening between different segments (except that the reopening of the smaller calf veins may be a little faster than that of the larger thigh veins), not every segment will reopen in a leg, and the degree of reopening and subsequent obstruction to flow as well as incompetence varies. Johnson _et al._[76] found only 12% of the limbs that they followed up after a deep vein thrombosis to have completely normal veins by their duplex scan criteria. Furthermore, as will be seen later, neither the extent of the initial thrombosis nor subsequent reopening correlates well with the incidence of calf pump failure.

Although a high proportion of veins reopen, mostly as a result of thrombus retraction not thrombus recanalization, and are reported by the duplex scan as patent, these veins are not normal. They

almost all show, on phlebography, the stigmata of the previous thrombosis described in Chapter 4 and it should not be assumed that reopening is necessarily an advantage and aid to the calf pump. A patent but stiff slightly narrow vessel without valves – the commonest sequel of deep vein thrombosis – presents an obstruction to flow during calf muscle contraction and reflux during calf muscle relaxation, both impeding proper calf pump function.

The rate of reopening is extremely variable. Meissner _et al._[97] measured the time taken for segments of thrombosed veins to reopen fully in a follow-up which involved regular re-examinations at 1 day, 7 days, 1 month, 3 monthly for 1 year and then annually. Segments that partially reopened were not analysed. Their results are summarized in Table 15.2. Full reopening of a segment may take from 15 to 500 days. They observed that the segments that reopened quickly were less likely to show evidence

Figure 15.3 (a) An example of complete reopening of a major vein probably caused by retraction of the thrombus rather than true recanalization. The lower phlebograph was obtained 2 years after the upper film. (b) A fine plexus of collateral vessels derived from the vena venora. In this case they are circumventing a thrombosis of the saphenous vein and connecting it with a Hunterian communicating vein. Retracted thrombus is visible below the totally occluded segment.

Table 15.2 Time taken (days) for a vein to open after an acute thrombosis

	Approx. median opening time	Range
Common femoral avein	155	37–577
Superficial femoral vein	198	95–736
Popliteal vein	148	29–388
Posterior tibial vein	78	28–182

NB. Initial thrombosis was completely occlusive in 2/3 of the segments and partially occlusive in 1/3.
After Meissner _et al._[97]

of reflux but the significance of these observations was not recorded. It is not possible to calculate the exact median complete reopening time for the whole group of patients they studied but it is clearly somewhere between 3 and 6 months.

Collateral vessel formation

The previous section describes the effect of thrombosis on vein patency. However, functional obstruction does not depend solely upon the degree of obstruction in the previously thrombosed vein but on the balance between that obstruction and the naturally developing compensating collaterals. Collateral vessels bypassing an occluded vein can develop very quickly. They are often visible on a phlebograph within 24 hours of an acute occlusion.

The peripheral veins are multiple, variable and frequently interconnect. Potential collateral channels are therefore immediately available. New vessels do not have to grow as they do in the arterial circulation.

The main sites for collateral vessel development are discussed in Chapter 2. The deep femoral vein provides an escape route for blood from the calf to the outflow tract at the root of the limb. The gluteal veins and their tributaries deep in the thigh help bypass an ilio-femoral occlusion by conducting blood into the internal iliac system, across the floor of the pelvis, to the contralateral internal iliac vein. The epigastric veins can conduct blood up the abdominal walls in cases of iliac and vena caval obstruction. Within the abdomen, vena caval obstruction is bypassed by the ascending lumbar, ovarian and azygos veins.

Collateral vessels on a phlebograph often appear to have a larger total cross-sectional area than the original blocked vessel. This gives a false impression. Collateral vessels are rarely adequate and nearly always obstruct blood flow and then make an additional contribution to calf pump dysfunction when their valves become incompetent as a result of their dilatation.

It must always be remembered that the superficial subcutaneous veins of the lower limb may also act as a collateral system when the deep veins are blocked but, in order to drain blood from the calf pump, they must receive blood via the communicating veins. They can only do this if the communicating vein valves are incompetent. Communicating vein incompetence is a common sequel to the high pressure that develops within the calf when there is pump outflow obstruction. This can occur with isolated pelvic vein obstruction but more often follows combined popliteal and femoral vein obstruction. Under these circumstances the communicating veins are acting more as a safety valve to reduce the

intrapump pressure than as vessels conducting a significant volume of blood flow, but the effect remains the same whether they are safety vents or blood conductors – superficial venous hypertension – which leads to the tissue damage we recognize as the calf pump failure syndrome.

THROMBOSIS AND VALVE FUNCTION

Valve incompetence is described in detail in Chapter 12. Incompetence was originally assessed with descending phlebography but this technique is invasive and only adequately assesses the main femoral and popliteal veins.

Duplex ultrasound scanning with its ability to detect and measure the direction of blood flow and provide an image of the veins has provided much new information about venous valve function – especially after deep vein thrombosis.

Meisner et al.[97] studied the incidence of reflux in vein segments that had completely reopened (Table 15.3) and found reflux present in less than half. In particular, only 17% of posterior tibial veins showed reflux. This study cannot be interpreted as indicating that the valves survive in half of the veins that reopened because the valves were not specifically investigated. Reflux in a damaged segment of vein may be prevented if there are healthy valves in an undamaged segment above or below that part which was damaged. Not all the valves in a limb are damaged by thrombosis. In a similar follow-up study, Ramshort et al.[116] found no patient with incompetence at all levels of the leg but they also found reflux in only 45% of the reopened veins, in contrast to an incidence of reflux of 7% in segments that had not been thrombosed. The average duration of reflux in normal veins following release of a pneumatic tourniquet, in the standing non-weight-bearing position, was less than 0.5 seconds whereas reflux durations up to 2 seconds were observed in the post-thrombotic segments. Other studies[76,82] whose main purpose was to relate symptoms and signs to the initial deep vein thrombosis record

Table 15.3 Incidence of reflux in reopened segments of vein following thrombosis

Vein	% Showing reflux
Common femoral vein	42
Superficial femoral vein	40
Popliteal vein	33
Posterior tibial vein	17

After Meissner et al.[97]

similar (45–50%) incidences of post-thrombotic deep vein reflex.

The overall picture of the progression and effect of deep vein thrombosis on patency and valve competence revealed by these ultrasound studies is as follows.

- 50–60% of occluded segments will reopen. This is a patchy event and not all venous segments reopen to the same extent or the same rate.
- The remaining 40% will stay occluded or show minor degrees of reopening or recanalization.
- Half of the reopened segments will be incompetent. Whether the other half have functioning valves, even though they do not show reflux is not known, but in our opinion, doubtful.
- The changes described refer to segments of the venous system. It is uncommon to find the whole venous system of a limb which was been the site of a previous deep thrombosis completely normal.
- The variable outcome of venous thrombosis, in both nature and site, explains the lack of correlation between the extent of the thrombosis and calf pump function and calf pump failure symptoms.
- In summary: six months after a segment of a deep vein has been occluded by thrombus there is a 40% chance that it will still be occluded or poorly recanalized; a 60% chance that it will be fully open and, if open, a 50% chance (30% overall) that it will be incompetent.

THROMBOSIS AND THE CLINICAL SEQUELAE

Deep vein thrombosis can vary from a single short (5 cm) thrombus in one calf vein following a surgical operation to a totally thrombotic occlusion of all the veins in legs. Such extremes clearly cause different physical signs at the time of the thrombosis and might be expected to cause very different late sequelae. The extremes mentioned are usually followed by very different sequelae so it is not unreasonable to assume that the severity of the late sequelae and the extent of the thrombosis are closely related for all circumstances between the extremes.

This is not the case. Almost all studies have shown a variable, indeterminate and therefore unpredicatable relationship between the site and extent of a thrombosis and the late sequelae. Unfortunately, many clinicians are prepared to diagnose the post-thrombotic syndrome in the absence of clinical evidence of a previous thrombosis, justifying this approach with the argument that at least 50% of episodes of deep vein thrombosis are symptomless. There are, however, two important facts which belie this approach.

First, 30% of general surgical patients over the age of 40 years have a deep vein thrombosis but only a small proportion subsequently develop the post-thrombotic syndrome.

Secondly, in the Basle survey of patients with varicose veins and the skin changes of chronic venous insufficiency, which would be called by many clinicians 'post-thrombotic', only 6% of men and 14% of women had any knowledge of a predisposing venous thrombosis (see Chapter 5).

Two questions therefore need to be answered. To what extent is the severity of the syndrome related to the site of the thrombosis? Is the syndrome always, and only caused by thrombosis?

Thrombosis in the calf

The most minor form of deep vein thrombosis is the asymptomatic calf vein thrombosis that occurs in 20–30% of patients after a major operation.[57,107] However, one-third of all patients who have had a major operation do not develop a post-thrombotic syndrome: the significance of these minor postoperative thrombi is therefore not clear.

Calf thrombosis alone may or may nor alter calf pump function, depending upon its effect on the communicating veins. It is almost impossible for a deep vein thrombosis to obliterate all the deep veins of the calf. Most of the thrombosed veins recanalize, collaterals always develop and the pump may return to normal if the outflow tract is undamaged and the communicating veins remain competent.

In 1974 we reviewed 44 patients between 3 and 4 years after they had had a positive postoperative fibrinogen uptake test.[21] Their mean age was 60 years. Three and a half years after operation 20% of the limbs that had contained a thrombus ached, 20% were slightly swollen and 50% had varicose veins. Of particular interest was the finding that 10% of the legs without thrombus (negative fibrinogen uptake tests) ached, 10% had some ankle swelling, and 50% had visible varicose veins. If the combination of aching, swelling and varicose veins is thought to be the beginning of the post-thrombotic syndrome, 20% of the legs that had a postoperative thrombosis and 10% of legs that did not have a thrombosis were developing the syndrome 3 years after an operation. However, although 50% of the legs studied had mild varicose veins before the operation, only 10% of the legs without varicose veins before operation developed new varicose veins.

When the legs without preoperative venous abnormalities were analysed, we found that six of the 34 legs known to have a thrombosis had developed an ankle flare and two of these had developed pigmentation and mild lipodermatosclerosis. At the same time, two of the 15 legs without a pre-existing venous abnormality that did not develop a thrombosis (negative fibrinogen uptake test) had also developed an ankle flare and one of these had developed lipodermatosclerosis. We cannot be absolutely certain that a thrombosis did not develop in these limbs as a late event, after the fibrinogen scanning, but this is unlikely.

Thus in the 49 legs without any evidence of preoperative venous abnormality, eight (16%) had developed signs suggestive of calf pump failure and the incidence of this change was similar in those legs with, and in those legs without thrombosis (18% and 14%, respectively).

A similar study was performed by Mudge and Hughes in 1978[101] on patients who 3 years previously had entered a trial of postoperative dextran prophylaxis. They found that 26 patients (out of 564) had clinical evidence of the post-thrombotic syndrome. This was present before the operation (3 years earlier) in 14 patients but was a new event in 12 patients, all of whom had had a postoperative deep vein thrombosis. This result (24%) is similar to ours (18%). Three-quarters of these patients developed their skin changes within 1 year of operation. The incidence of the post-thrombotic syndrome in the patients who did not develop a postoperative thrombosis was not studied as not all patients had a fibrinogen uptake test.

Widmer studied the incidence of the post-thrombotic syndrome 5 years after the initial thrombosis in 37 patients who had had localized calf thrombosis.[144] Although some patients had minor symptoms, none had developed a post-thrombotic syndrome. These results are difficult to interpret as some patients had been treated with streptokinase and others with heparin. Also, Widmer's symptom score differs from ours in placing far more weight on ulceration; for example, in Widmer's study a patient with an ankle flare, oedema and skin changes would not be classified as having a post-thrombotic syndrome, whereas in both the other studies they would. Such differences highlight the problems of definition and comparability in long-term follow-up studies.

Lindhagen *et al.*[92] found no difference in the incidence of the post-thrombotic syndrome between patients who had a positive or negative postoperative fibrinogen uptake test (23% and 21% respectively) but found a foot vein pressure fall during exercise of less than 30 mmHg more often in those who had had a positive test (18% compared with 7%).

Saarinen *et al.*[119] have recently studied the incidence of calf pump failure symptoms, 5 and 10 years

after a deep vein thrombosis, in patients with calf vein thrombosis and patients with more proximal vein thrombosis (popliteal, femoral or iliac). They found no difference in the incidence of symptoms between the two groups but a significantly greater incidence of severe symptoms in both groups at 10 years when compared to 5 years, severe symptoms increasing from 22% to 50% over the 5-year interval.

We must conclude that the sequelae of calf vein thrombosis are unpredictable and that *not all derangements of the calf pump are caused by thrombosis.*

Thrombosis in the outflow tract

Thrombosis that affects the venous outflow tract of the limb alone will obstruct the blood flow from the calf pump until the thrombosed vessels recanalize and collaterals develop. The obstruction will then become less but the valves in the recanalized segment are likely to be incompetent, making reflux an additional burden on the pump. At first the pump may be able to deal with the combined stress of outflow obstruction and reflux but it will become inefficient if progressive dilatation of the veins in the pump causes communicating vein incompetence. A thrombosis which is localized to the superficial femoral or the iliac vein will cause less of an obstruction than a thrombosis involving both these veins because, though both have potentially good collateral circulations, two sets of collaterals in series are rarely adequate. Thrombosis involving the whole of the deep venous system, from the calf veins to the vena cava, has an even greater chance of causing a post-thrombotic syndrome.

We examined 130 legs of 67 patients, 5–10 years after they had suffered a thrombosis, to see if there was any relationship between the site of the initial thrombosis and the subsequent development of the post-thrombotic syndrome.[22] All the patients had been treated with anticoagulants. Forty-seven of the legs were clinically and phlebographically normal and therefore acted as controls. The site and severity of the thrombosis was graded from the phlebograph and the current signs and symptoms assigned a symptom score. There was a higher incidence of post-thrombotic sequelae in the patients who had had a severe thrombosis when compared with those who had had a minor thrombosis (Figure 15.4).

Thirteen per cent of the legs with no thrombosis, 20% of the legs with small localized thrombosis (regardless of site), and 40% of the legs with an extensive thrombosis had developed the post-thrombotic syndrome. Many of these patients wore elastic stockings which may have retarded the

No or minor initial thrombosis (87 legs)

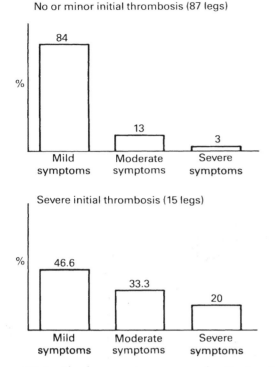

Severe initial thrombosis (15 legs)

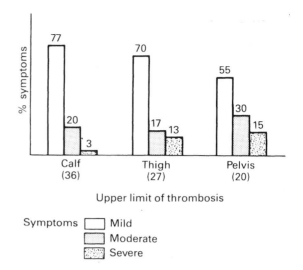

Upper limit of thrombosis

Symptoms ☐ Mild
☐ Moderate
☐ Severe

Figure 15.5 The leg symptom scores of patients 5–10 years after a deep vein thrombosis related to the site of the thrombosis. The symptom score was higher the more extensive the thrombosis but the differences were not statistically significant.

Figure 15.4 The leg symptom scores of patients with minor and major degrees of deep vein thrombosis (phlebographically determined) 5–10 years after the thrombosis. Only 16% of patients with a minor thrombosis had moderate or severe symptoms compared with a 53% incidence of moderate or severe symptoms amongst those who had a severe thrombosis.

development of the syndrome but the incidence of 40% with post-thrombotic symptoms 6 years after an extensive thrombosis is close to Bauer's finding of an incidence of 45% with induration 5 years after a thrombosis.

It is important to note that 16% of limbs developed significant symptoms in the absence of evidence of a thrombosis. As there was no evidence to suggest that these patients had had a late thrombosis, 6 months or more after the initial episode when their anticoagulants were stopped, we assume that their calf pump failure was not post-thrombotic.

A more detailed analysis of the effect of the site of the thrombosis was unexpectedly inconclusive (Figure 15.5). Legs with an axial vein thrombosis did not have a significantly higher incidence of problems (calf thrombus, 20%; thigh thrombus, 30%; and pelvic thrombus, 45%), though there was a definite trend which might have reached significance in a larger study. Almost half (42%) the 12 legs that had had a total calf-femoral-iliac thrombosis had no symptoms at 6½ years.

Widmer's 5-year follow-up of 415 patients with deep vein thrombosis,[144] some of whom had been treated with streptokinase, found a 21% incidence of post-thrombotic syndrome and a 6.5% incidence of ulceration. When the limbs were subdivided according to the extent of the initial thrombosis, the incidence of the post-thrombotic syndrome following calf and popliteal vein thrombosis was 17% (5% with ulcers); for calf, popliteal, and superficial femoral vein thrombosis it was 23% (7% with ulcers), and for calf, popliteal, femoral and iliac vein thrombosis it was 34% (8% with ulcers) (Figure 15.6). There may be two reasons for the lower incidence of post-thrombotic syndrome found by Widmer. First, his definition of the post-thrombotic syndrome placed more weight on ulceration and less on pre-ulcer skin changes. Secondly, the selection for treatment and the method of treatment were different. Despite these differences, the results of all the studies quoted follow the same trend and emphasize the high chance of late sequelae after a deep vein thrombosis.

We also found a positive correlation between the age of the thrombus – assessed radiographically at the time of presentation – and subsequent symptoms.[22] Fresh thrombi (which were also an indication of earlier diagnosis and subsequently early treatment with anticoagulants) were associated with a 9% incidence of symptoms, whereas thrombi more than 7 days old at presentation (which was usually an indication of occluding thrombi and late

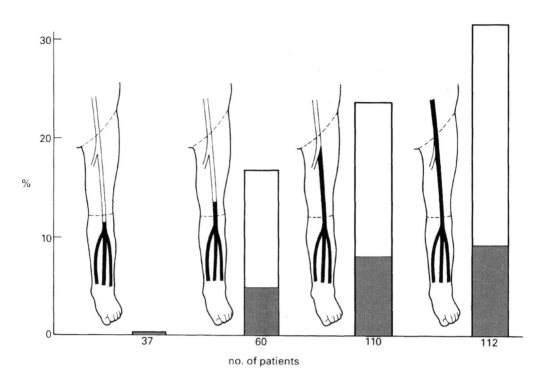

Figure 15.6 The incidence of the post-thrombotic syndrome and ulceration (shaded area) related to the site of thrombosis (black shading) in 341 patients 5 years after the thrombosis. This study showed a close correlation between the extent of the thrombosis and the incidence of symptoms. (Modified from Widmer.[144])

treatment) had a 46% incidence of symptoms (Figure 15.7). Perhaps some of the differences between the results of our study and those of Bauer are related to the time of diagnosis and the early use of heparin.

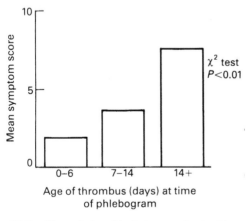

Figure 15.7 The relationship between the incidence of post-thrombotic symptoms 5–10 years after the thrombosis and the age of the thrombosis (judged phlebographically) at the time of clinical presentation. The older the thrombosis at presentation the greater the severity of the symptoms 5 years later.

The duplex ultrasound studies of the early 1990s show similar results. Araki *et al.*[2] found no correlation between the site of venous reflux, an indicator of the site of the original thrombosis, and the severity of clinical signs (Table 15.4). These workers also measured many other aspects of calf pump function and, although they found a relationship between ejection fractions and residual volume fractions and clinical severity, there was no significant relation between these test results and the extent of ultrasound detected valve incompetence.

Ramshorst *et al.*,[116] in a similar study of 252 vein segments 3 years after the thombosis, whilst finding a significant correlation between the extent of the initial thrombosis and the number of refluxing segments found no correlation between the extent of the initial thrombosis and the late clinical symptoms.

The effect and significance of outflow tract incompetence is further confused by the presence or absence of incompetent valves in the superficial and communicating veins. Labropoulos *et al.*[82] found that severe symptoms are more common where there is combined superficial and deep vein incompetence. Deep vein incompetence is most often post-thrombotic but superficial vein incompetence may be a primary abnormality or sec-

The effect of deep vein thrombosis on vein function

Table 15.4 Relationship between the rate of valve incompetence and severity of calf pump failure syndrome

Severity of symptoms	% Incidence of valve incompetence		
	All deep veins	Superficial femoral vein	Calf veins
Never ulcerated	59	67	43
Healed ulcer	74	72	54
Active ulcer	71	50	47

After Araki *et al.*[2]

ondary to any obstruction or incompetence in the deep system caused by the thrombosis. In such a complex system it is not surprising that tests of one part of the system fail to correlate with the overall clinical picture. The same workers expressed the view that in many patients superficial vein incompetence may be a more important cause of symptoms than the post-thrombotic deep vein reflux but if the superficial reflux is itself secondary to the original deep vein thrombosis then treatment of the initial effects of thrombosis (if we had any) might prevent the secondary damage to the superficial system and so reduce the risk of serious clinical sequelae.

Whereas duplex ultrasound can measure deep vein reflux, it is not very good at detecting deep vein obstruction. Nevertheless, Johnson *et al.*[76] tried to assess obstruction – using the effect on flow of distal compression and the release of proximal compression, as well as reflux, in 83 legs, 1–6 years (median 3 years) after a deep vein thrombosis.

Table 15.5 shows the incidence of reflux and obstruction, alone and combined, in legs with and legs without symptoms. Obstruction, alone or combined with reflux, occurred in 47% of the limbs without symptoms, and 80% of the limbs with symptoms. Reflux alone or combined with obstruction occurred in 70% of asymptomatic legs and

83% of legs with symptoms. This study suggests that a physiological obstruction occurs in at least half the limbs previously damaged by deep vein thrombosis. Manual compression tests fall far short of the haemodynamic stress caused by exercise. It seems most likely that outflow tract obstruction is as common and significant a cause of post-thrombotic calf pump failure as reflux, a conclusion obvious to the phlebographers of the past but until now difficult to prove.

It can be deduced from these studies that a patient with a thrombosis that extends into the popliteal vein or above has a 35% chance of getting a mild post-thrombotic syndrome and a 40% chance of getting a severe post-thrombotic syndrome within 6 years. Without doubt, 75% of all these patients will get some symptoms.[45]

It must also be remembered that 20% of patients with minor calf or small non-adherent axial vein thrombi and 13% of patients with no evidence of postoperative thrombosis will get symptoms. This later figure is almost identical to the 14% incidence of post-thrombotic syndrome that we found in patients who had had a negative fibrinogen uptake test after operation, a fact not detected by Bauer because he only studied legs with thrombosis. The symptoms in this group are caused by a combination of post-thrombotic venous obstruction and reflux, exacerbated by primary or secondary superficial vein reflux.

THE ROLE OF SUPERFICIAL VEIN INCOMPETENCE

Many of the patients in the studies discussed above had or developed varicose veins, and this raises the question of the role of superficial vein incompetence in the aetiology of the post-thrombotic syndrome.[134,146]

Mudge and Hughes[101] observed that 24% of their patients had varicose veins preoperatively but that new varicose veins had appeared 1 year later in

Table 15.5 The incidence of reflux and obstruction, alone or combined in 83 limbs 1–6 (median 3) years after thrombosis

	Legs without symptoms (49)	Legs with symptoms (34)
No abnormality	9 (18%)	1 (3%)
Reflux alone	17 (35%)	6 (18%)
Obstruction alone	6 (12%)	5 (15%)
Reflux and obstruction	17 (35%)	22 (65%)

After Johnson *et al.*[76]

16% of the patients who did not have a postoperative thrombosis, and in 35% of the patients who had had a thrombosis. We found a similar incidence of new varicose veins in previously normal legs (14%) but a lower incidence (18%) in the legs that had had a thrombosis.[22]

Superficial vein incompetence reduces calf pump efficiency by allowing superficial vein reflux during pump diastole; it is therefore possible that the calf pump failure symptoms that developed in the patients without evidence of thrombosis were related to the development of superficial vein reflux and its effect on the calf pump.

Phlebographic studies of the deep veins of patients with venous ulceration show that a significant proportion have normal looking deep veins.[104,118] Unless it is postulated that these veins, or the communicating veins, have been the site of minor thrombosis not detectable by phlebography, it is difficult to postulate that the ulceration, and the pre-ulcer calf pump failure was caused by a thrombosis.

The arguments set out above do not explain how a surgical operation can induce the appearance of varicose veins other than through the mechanism of thrombotic valve destruction. We have no alternative hypothesis to advance.

Superficial vein incompetence in the presence of normal deep veins can produce skin changes and ulceration,[70,122] but we suspect that this only happens when the communicating veins are involved in the 'varicose' process and dilate, thus making their valves incompetent. This is normally a very slow process. We would not expect it to occur in 1 year and so can see no mechanism that would rapidly affect the veins except minor thrombosis that is undetectable, confined to the communicating veins, and destroys their valves.

The problem remains unsolved. The 'post-thrombotic syndrome' may occur in patients with superficial vein incompetence and in patients with no firm evidence of a past thrombosis, yet we know of no mechanism by which a surgical operation can cause the development of varicose veins other than through valve destruction in the deep and communicating veins by thrombosis. There is still much to investigate and unravel.

THE ROLE OF TISSUE FIBRINOLYSIS

One of the predisposing causes of deep vein thrombosis is a deficiency of fibrinolysis.[68,111] A number of studies have suggested that patients who have had a thrombosis have a reduced level of blood fibrinolytic activity. Of all the haematological factors that have been studied before and after surgical operation,[74] the level of plasma fibrinogen and tests of blood fibrinolytic activity are the most reliable predictors of the likelihood of thrombosis.[36,61,75,112]

Varicose veins also have a reduced tissue fibrinolytic activity. This is mentioned here because if tissue fibrinolytic activity mirrors blood fibrinolytic activity, this may be the reason why varicose veins are a risk factor for thrombosis, and a major risk in the development of the post-thrombotic syndrome. The relationship between blood and vein wall fibrinolytic activator levels and the development of the post-thrombotic syndrome requires further study.

Comment

The interaction of factors such as interstitial fibrosis, valve ring dilatation and fibrinolysis may explain why a simple correlation between the degree of thrombosis and the post-thrombotic syndrome has not yet been found. Until an incontrovertible connection between thrombosis and all cases of the post-thrombotic syndrome can be established we shall continue to use the term 'calf pump failure syndrome'.

The effect of thrombosis on calf pump function

Because the effect of thrombosis on vein patency and valve function is so variable and unpredictable, the effect of thrombosis on calf pump function is equally variable, more so because in some patients the peripheral veins and calf pump seem able to compensate for significant degrees of obstruction and reflux whereas in others a minor thrombosis may cause serious sequelae, presumably because the thrombosis, though small, has damaged a critical part of the pump mechanism.

The aetiology of deep vein thrombosis is discussed in detail in Chapter 8. The initiating factor is usually systemic trauma (e.g. an accident or a surgical operation), a severe medical illness, or pregnancy and childbirth.

The risk of a thrombosis complicating these conditions is exacerbated by increasing age, a previous episode of deep vein thrombosis, the presence of malignant disease, the presence of varicose veins, obesity, and abnormalities in the blood such as polycythaemia, thrombocytosis, abnormal coagulation factors, a raised plasma fibrinogen or defective fibrinolysis.

In many patients these risk factors play a very small part; the ultimate trigger of the coagulation cascade is the undefined 'hypercoagulability' induced by the operation or injury, in association with the reduced venous blood flow that accompanies the prohibition of exercise enforced by the initial trauma or illness.

Nevertheless, all the conditions which predispose to thrombosis must be considered as risk factors of the post-thrombotic calf pump failure syndrome.

Chapter 3 describes the function of a normal calf pump by dividing it into two compartments: the *deep (pump) compartment* (the veins within the deep fascia, within and between the muscles) and the *superficial (pump) compartment* (all the veins in the subcutaneous tissues and skin). In addition there are the *communicating veins* connecting the two compartments and the *outflow tract* from the pump (the popliteal, femoral and iliac veins).

Thrombosis can occur in one, or any, combination of the four parts of this system with varying effects.

SUPERFICIAL VEIN INCOMPETENCE

This is mentioned first because superficial thrombophlebitis in superficial varicose veins is probably the most common form of thrombosis. In the Basle study,[143] 16% of women with varicose veins claimed to have had an episode of 'thrombosis'.

Occlusive thrombosis in a superficial vein may improve calf pump failure by stopping superficial reflux. This is the rationale of sclerotherapy and excision surgery although in the former form of treatment the benefit is often short-lived because the vein often recanalizes.

Superficial thrombophlebitis does not cause the 'calf pump failure syndrome' unless it extends into the communicating veins (Figure 15.8). It is not known how often this happens but phlebographic evidence suggests that it occurs in 20–40% of patients without varicose veins but in only 2–4% of patients with varicose veins.[10]

It is unusual to see the radiological features of recanalization in either the superficial veins or the communicating veins. Nevertheless, some authorities have suggested that it must be the cause of communicating vein incompetence even when there is no evidence of deep vein thrombosis.[38] Extension of thrombosis into the communicating veins certainly occurs if an intravenous infusion is given into the long saphenous vein at the ankle. This site of superficial thrombophlebitis has long been recognized as

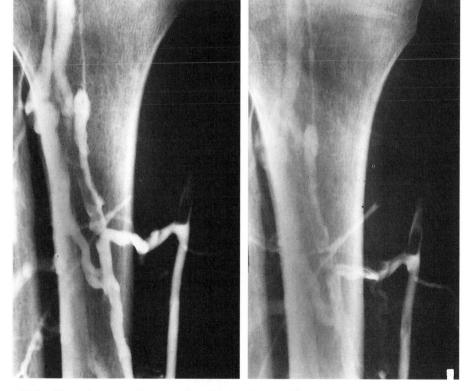

Figure 15.8 Thrombosis in the posterior tibial vein extending into a communicating vein (seen best in the right-hand panel) associated with a fresh thrombus in a superficial vein.

a cause of the calf pump failure syndrome and ulceration, and is the reason why intravenous infusions should always be given into arm veins. In most cases superficial thrombophlebitis in varicose veins does little harm to calf pump function and may improve it if it occludes a major pathway of superficial reflux.

The superficial venous network is so extensive that it never becomes totally occluded. Obstruction in superficial veins never seriously interferes with calf pump function.

CALF AND COMMUNICATING VEIN INCOMPETENCE

Communicating vein incompetence makes the pump 'leaky'[43,55,84] but the volume of blood that flows retrogradely through these veins is probably not the important factor. If the patient is upright, the superficial veins are full and at the top their stress–strain curve (see Figure 3.3, page 51). The veins cannot dilate further and so the addition of even a small amount of blood from the contracting calf pump produces a significant increase in pressure, and it is this increase in pressure rather than the volume of retrograde blood flow that causes the microvascular damage.[59,79,125]

It is unusual for all the communicating veins to be incompetent; the superficial vein pressure during exercise therefore depends upon the balance between those communications that are working normally and helping to decompress the superficial veins and those that are incompetent and allow blood to reflux and distend the superficial system. The blood may literally be going round in circles – in through one communicating vein and out through another. It is not the blood flow or its disordered direction that matters, it is the failure of the pump to produce superficial venous hypotension during exercise (i.e. the venous hypertension) that leads to the tissue changes described later.

The communicating veins have a relatively small cross-sectional area when compared with the large axial and muscle veins of the calf which combine to form the popliteal vein. A normal outflow tract presents less resistance to flow than three or four incompetent communicating veins.

It is therefore not surprising that the pump still works quite well when the only abnormality is communicating vein incompetence with the superficial venous pressure falling during exercise to a moderate level (40–50 mmHg).[26,83,94] Communicating vein incompetence alone therefore takes a long time to cause the microcirculatory changes of the calf pump failure syndrome; this explains why the majority of

patients have forgotten the symptoms of their initiating thrombosis (if they ever had any) by the time their skin changes develop. Isolated thrombosis within the calf veins that does not involve the communicating veins has little effect on the calf pump. Two long-term follow-up studies have failed to find an increased incidence of post-thrombotic symptoms in patients with minor calf vein thrombosis detected with radioactive fibrinogen.[21,101]

Calf vein thrombosis that propagates into the popliteal vein often leads to a severe post-thrombotic syndrome because it invariably causes a severe obstruction to the outflow of blood from the calf[144] or severe reflux if it recanalizes.[128] The muscle and stem veins of the calf all drain into the popliteal vein and are not connected with other veins which can become collaterals. If the communicating veins were involved in the initial thrombosis, the pump rapidly becomes inadequate. If the communicating veins were not involved in the initial thrombosis, they gradually dilate, become incompetent and act as collateral outflow channels from the pump. In these circumstances superficial venous pressure falls by only 10 or 20 mmHg during exercise and the calf pump failure syndrome quickly develops.

ISOLATED OUTFLOW TRACT OBSTRUCTION OR INCOMPETENCE

Isolated thrombosis and subsequent obstruction and/or incompetence in the outflow tract usually follows one of four common patterns: ilio-femoral vein thrombosis, superficial femoral vein thrombosis, superficial femoral and popliteal vein thrombosis, and ilio-femoro-popliteal vein thrombosis (i.e. thrombosis of the upper third, the middle third, the lower two thirds or the whole tract) (Figure 15.9). Solitary popliteal vein thrombosis is uncommon.

Isolated iliac vein obstruction and/or incompetence

This increases the resistance to the outflow of blood from the whole leg but is sufficiently distant from the calf pump and often so well compensated by collateral pathways that it may cause few or no symptoms. The veins below the obstruction dilate and connect with many vessels on the floor of the pelvis and posterior abdominal wall which act as collateral pathways.[39,96] Provided the valves in the superficial femoral vein remain competent, the calf pump can function normally, even though it has an increased load; the skin of the lower leg remains normal. In some patients the pump cannot push enough blood past the obstruction during exercise

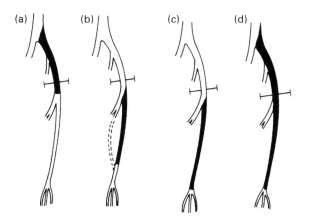

Figure 15.9 The four common varieties of calf pump outflow tract thrombosis. (a) Ilio-femoral thrombosis. (b) Superficial femoral vein thrombosis. (c) Superficial femoral and popliteal vein thrombosis. (d) Complete popliteal, femoral and iliac vein thrombosis.

and the veins become distended and painful – a symptom called venous claudication[103,137] (see Chapter 13).

If the veins upstream to the obstruction (i.e. in the femoral and popliteal veins) dilate, two complications may develop. At first, the valves of the outflow tract become progressively incompetent down to, and including, those in the popliteal vein[128] so the pump becomes overloaded with blood refluxing into it during diastole. The response of the calf pump is similar to that of the heart. The capacity of the pump and the ejection fraction increases but usually neither change is sufficient and so pump efficiency falls and less blood is drawn from the superficial into the deep compartment during diastole. Although the superficial vein pressure during exercise does not fall to the normal range, the resulting venous hypertension is often not sufficient to cause post-thrombotic changes in the skin. In other words, minimal outflow tract obstruction plus secondary outflow tract reflux, in the presence of a good pump with normal calf and communicating vein valves, may not cause severe symptoms or serious skin changes,[76] but eventually, the higher pressures and volumes within the pump caused by the minimal outflow tract obstruction and reflux will probably cause communicating vein incompetence. As soon as this occurs the calf pump failure syndrome rapidly appears because the combination of outflow obstruction and reflux with a leaky pump makes the pump extremely inefficient. Superficial venous pressure is reduced during exercise by only 10–20 mmHg and the persistent venous hypertension quickly causes the microcirculatory changes that lead to eczema, pigmentation, lipodermatosclerosis and ulceration.

Isolated superficial femoral vein obstruction and/or incompetence

This can cause the same sequence of events as isolated iliac vein disease but in many patients the collateral circulation from the upper popliteal vein to the deep femoral vein becomes an adequate and competent outflow tract and the patient has no symptoms. This explains the low incidence of calf pump failure after excision of the superficial femoral veins.[42] If, however, the collateral veins are inadequate, the pump begins to fail, the soleal sinusoids and the communicating veins dilate and the calf pump begins to fail.

The reopened superficial femoral vein is usually incompetent and an obstruction to pump outflow. The pump has to cope with obstruction during systole and reflux during diastole. This combination overloads the pump much more than either obstruction or reflux alone and leads to communicating vein incompetence. Patients affected in this way may occasionally complain of venous claudication as well as the calf pump failure syndrome but this is uncommon if the popliteal vein is patent.

Isolated popliteal vein occlusion or thrombosis

This is extremely rare. It is usually the result of the extension of a thrombus in a calf vein tributary. When it results from retrograde spread of a low superficial femoral vein thrombosis and the calf veins are normal, the symptoms are similar to those described above but appear sooner and are more severe because the element of obstruction is greater. A completely obstructed popliteal vein is a severe embarrassment to the calf pump and pump failure develops rapidly.

Combined iliac and superficial femoral vein obstruction and/or incompetence

This rapidly disturbs calf pump physiology in a way similar to that described above, because the collateral channels are seldom adequate.[148]

Reopening and recanalization does occur but is rarely sufficient to relieve the outflow obstruction. Reflux is almost always present. It is uncommon for extensive axial vein thrombosis to occur without the calf veins being involved, but if they are spared the pump may be able to cope, hence the enigma of patients with a normal leg years after an extensive thrombosis.[22,144] Even when the calf veins are spared, the obstruction and reflux may rapidly overload the pump, cause communicating vein incompetence, and the appearance of pump failure changes in the skin.

Once this occurs, the superficial veins become incompetent and superficial vein reflux is added to the load of the pump. These patients often present with a combination of venous claudication and severe skin changes.

COMBINED CALF AND OUTFLOW TRACT OBSTRUCTION AND/OR INCOMPETENCE

The calf pump fails in 80–90% of patients with extensive thrombosis but it is quite extraordinary that some patients can have an extensive mixture of obstruction and incompetence in their calf, popliteal, femoral, and iliac veins and yet be free of symptoms 10 years later. We were surprised to find that half our patients who had this degree of venous dysfunction were without symptoms 5 years after their thrombosis.[22] These results may, however, have been influenced by the length of follow-up and the relatively small numbers that we were able to study.[5,60,144]

When both the outflow tract and the communicating veins are damaged, pump failure is almost inevitable. As the calf muscles contract, the blood flow meets a massive resistance. The principal communicating veins cannot act as collaterals because they are occluded by thrombus; every other small unnamed vein therefore dilates to fill this role. Later the communicating veins reopen or recanalize and act as collateral outflows to the pump during exercise and at rest. By this stage some of the axial veins may have reopened but they are usually narrow and incompetent. There is no way in which such a damaged system can propel sufficient blood towards the heart to reduce the superficial venous pressure during exercise. There is constant superficial venous hypertension which is often exacerbated by exercise. The leg swells, becomes painful and the skin steadily deteriorates. Venous claudication and venous ulceration often appear within 2–3 years of a severe thrombosis.

Comment

The above descriptions of the haemodynamic effects of the various sites of deep vein thrombosis explain why the pathophysiological sequelae are unpredictable and variable.

The damaged outflow tract may obstruct blood flow or permit reflux; in many patients it does both. As a result of these abnormalities the communicating veins become incompetent. It is impossible with our current methods of investigation to isolate and quantify each of these abnormalities, and so we are usually unable to determine which of them is the cause of a patient's symptoms.

Obstruction, even with a healthy pump, may cause venous claudication, but it is debatable whether reflux alone can do the same. Skin changes appear once the valves in the communicating veins fail, and when this occurs the skin problems tend to overshadow the claudication. It is not known whether outflow obstruction or reflux is more likely to lead to communicating vein failure. Consequently, when a patient has a combination of outflow tract obstruction and incompetence we do not know which to correct. The problem is not academic because surgical repair of secondarily incompetent communicating veins will provide only a temporary improvement if the primary problem is obstruction and is not corrected. We will not be able to answer these questions and treat our patients rationally until we can measure the size of each abnormality individually and accurately, and discover each one's role in the production of symptoms and signs.

The effect of calf pump failure on the microcirculation of the lower limb

Inefficiency of the calf pump, whether it be the result of overloading from superficial venous incompetence, communicating vein leakage or outflow tract obstruction or incompetence or, as is most often the case, combinations of all these abnormalities, causes a persistent rise in the mean superficial venous pressure throughout the patient's daily life. The first effect of this venous hypertension appears in the subcutaneous veins and skin capillaries.

SUBCUTANEOUS VEINS

The raised venous pressure eventually causes the subcutaneous veins to dilate and their valves to become incompetent. The resulting retrograde blood flow exacerbates the venous hypertension at rest and during exercise and the veins become varicose. Very large dilated veins may appear over the point where incompetent communicating veins pierce the deep fascia. These localized varicosities have been called 'blow-out' veins by Cockett[38] and 'blow-down' veins by Gottleb.[62] We prefer the term 'blow-out' because it reminds us of the underlying and more important calf pump abnormality.

CAPILLARIES AND VENULES

Elongation and dilatation

The venules and venular capillaries dilate and become tortuous.[49,51,67,99] A cross-section of dermis from an area of the leg showing the skin changes of the calf pump failure syndrome reveals many more capillaries cut in cross-section than a cross-section of normal skin (Figure 15.10).[27,142]

In our early publications we called this 'capillary proliferation' but it is caused by elongation and tortuosity of existing capillaries, not new additional capillaries.[50] In many cases there are fewer capillary loops than normal.[58]

The number of venular capillaries seen in cross-section histological preparations of the skin is directly related to the efficiency of the calf pump as assessed by the reduction of foot vein pressure during exercise (Figure 15.11),[27] a confirmation that the dilatation elongation and tortuosity is a direct result of the raised venous pressure caused by the calf pump failure.

This change can be seen clinically as the leash of small intradermal venules that appears over the medial aspect of the ankle in patients with calf pump failure, known as the *ankle flare* or the *corona phlebectatica* (see Chapter 6, Figure 6.9). The degree of capillary elongation and tortuosity is closely related to the clinical classification of the calf pump failure (Figure 15.12).

PERMEABILITY

The dilated elongated dermal capillaries have an increased permeability to large molecules because the raised venous pressure enlarges the inter-epithelial pores, the pathway through which large

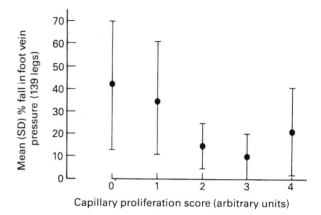

Figure 15.11 The relationship between the percentage reduction of foot vein pressure during exercise and the number of skin capillaries seen in cross-section in the skin of patients with calf pump failure (arbitary units). The less efficient the calf pump the greater the elongation and tortuosity of the capillaries.

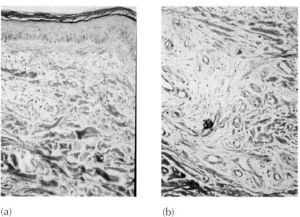

(a)   (b)

Figure 15.10 Photomicrographs of (a) normal skin and (b) skin stained with phosphotungstic acid haematoxylin (PTAH) showing the changes of lipodermatosclerosis. The magnification is slightly different but the increased number of capillaries seen in the cross-section of the abnormal skin is clearly apparent. This is the result of elongation and tortuosity. There may actually be fewer capillary loops. Fibrin stains blue with PTAH. The capillaries in the right-hand panel are surrounded with blue staining.

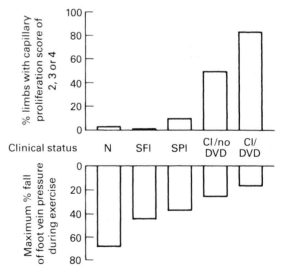

Figure 15.12 The relationship between the clinical state of the limb and the elongation and tortuosity of the skin capillaries in biopsies removed from an area 7 cm above the medial malleolus. N, normal; SFI, sapheno-femoral incompetence; SPI, sapheno-popliteal incompetence; CI/no DVD, communicating vein incompetence with phlebographically normal deep veins; CI/DVD, communicating vein incompetence with phlebographic evidence of post-thrombotic deep vein damage.

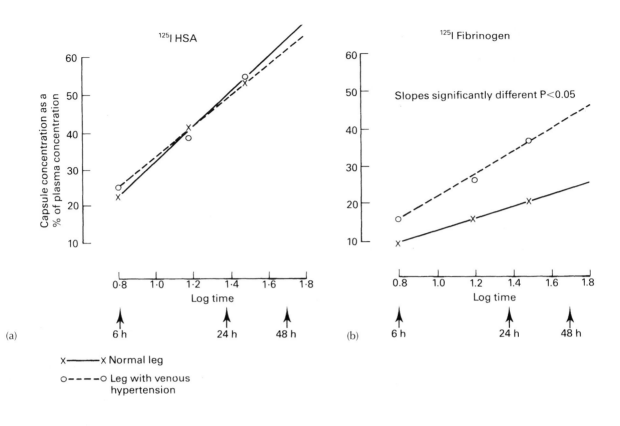

Figure 15.13 The rate of accumulation of (a) albumin and (b) fibrinogen in Guyton capsules in the subcutaneous tissues of six canine hind limbs with and six limbs without venous hypertension (produced by an arteriovenous fistula). The accumulation of fibrinogen in the capsules in the limbs with venous hypertension was significantly increased.

molecules leave the capillaries. We sought proof of this by measuring the accumulation of radioactively labelled sodium chloride, albumin and fibrinogen in the fluid that collects in the centre of a Guyton capsule implanted into the subcutaneous tissues of a dog's hind limb with venous hypertension produced by fashioning an A-V fistula at the groin.[25] These experiments showed that the accumulation of fibrinogen in the capsule fluid was significantly greater in the limbs which had a high venous pressure (Figure 15.13). The increase in permeability caused by venous hypertension causes pericapillary oedema. The halos visible around the capillaries on videomicroscopy are enlarged to the extent that they touch each other.[49,51,67,89,91]

The transcapillary diffusion of sodium fluorescein is also increased in patients with moderate disease[129] but diminishes as the calf pump failure becomes severe perhaps as a result of the reduction of the number of perfused capillaries seen in severe disease.[17]

Further evidence of an increased permeability is the fact that venous hypertension, both acute and long-term, increases the concentration of fibrinogen in the lymph leaving the limb. In the canine hind limb an increase in the venous pressure from 2 mmHg to 20 mmHg trebles the lymph flow and doubles the lymph fibrinogen concentration (Table 15.6). As the only source of fibrinogen in lymph is the plasma fibrinogen, the venous hypertension must have made the capillaries more permeable.[14-16]

Skin capillary blood flow is difficult to measure. Laser Doppler fluximetry measures the concentration of moving blood cells multiplied by the magnitude of their median velocity. It can only give a relative indication of blood flow changes, not an absolute value, and cannot differentiate between the skin nutritional and thermoregulatory blood flow, although 90% of the signal is believed to come from the subpapillary nutritional capillaries.[52,53]

In the normal limbs the laser Doppler flux shows regular fluctuation and decreases on standing as a result of the venoarteriolar reflex. This reflex is believed to be one of the capillaries' natural protecting mechanisms – a rise in venular pressure on standing which could be transmitted to the capillaries and increase capillary permeability being partially prevented by reducing capillary blood flow through arteriolar constriction.

Table 15.6 The effect of venous hypertension on canine hind limb lymph flow and lymph fibrinogen concentration[86]

Venous pressure (mmHg)	Lymph flow (μl/min)	Lymph fibrinogen (g/l)
Acute venous hypertension		
2.4	14.0	0.07
18.0	40.5	0.14
(An increased interstitial fluid transport of fibrinogen of 623%)		
Chronic venous hypertension		
1.0	11.6	0.11
25.0	38.6	0.20
(An increased interstitial fluid transport of fibrinogen of 602%)		

Laser Doppler flux is increased in patients with venous disease,[90,91] perhaps mainly because of the capillary dilatation and elongation. Patients with mild or moderate disease show the normal reduction of flux on standing but some workers[1,7,8,33] have noticed a decreased response and change in the rate and size of the normal rhythmic fluctuations in the flux of patients with severe disease (Table 15.7).[34,126] Loss of the venoarteriolar reflex would increase transcapillary filtration whilst standing and exacerbate all the effects of venous hypertension. It is most unlikely that this local axon reflex neuropathy is a prime factor in the aetiology of venous disease as it is only present when the disease is severe. One of the features of the calf pump syndrome is the progressive death of tissues and their replacement by scar tissue – seen clinically as 'atrophie blanche'. The small nerves are not immune to the process. The neuropathy is therefore likely to be caused by the death of neurones whose death is the result, not the cause, of the calf pump failure and capillary hypotension.

Table 15.7 The changes in laser Doppler flux in lipodermatosclerotic skin

	Normal	LDS
Hyperaemic response (peak/basal flow)		
At rest	2.25	1.0
After venous hypertension	1.7	1.05
Vasomotion		
Amplitude at rest (arbitary units)	14.17	19.98
Frequency at rest (min)	2.66	3.3

After Shami *et al.*[126]

WHITE BLOOD CELL TRAPPING

In 1987, Moyses *et al.*[100] observed that when blood was held in the leg for a longer period than normal it became concentrated and the refluxing blood contained fewer white blood cells. They explained the haemoconcentration by postulating an increase of capillary filtration and the cell loss by postulating that the white blood cells were trapped and held within the capillaries as a result of endothelial and white cell activation.

These observations led Thomas *et al.*[133] to see whether the same changes occurred in legs with chronic venous insufficiency. Their observations are illustrated in Figure 15.14. Where the abnormal leg was dependent there was significant reduction in the number of white cells leaving the leg followed by an increase when the leg was elevated. These changes correlated with the degree of calf pump failure as assessed by the calf expelled volume ratio (Figure 15.15). From these observations came the hypothesis that the tissue ischaemia of chronic venous disease which leads to ulceration is caused by the obstruction of capillaries by trapped white cells.[40] Attempts by other workers[145] to detect capillaries blocked by leucocytes were unsuccessful as were attempts to show significant excess numbers of white cells in the tissues.[121,145] T-lymphocytes and macrophages have been found in the perivascular tissues but there is no correlation between their presence and any of the usual tests of calf pump function. Wilkinson *et al.*[145] concluded 'it is probable that capillary occlusion by white cells is not a major contributor to skin damage in venous disease, and the injury may be related more to the inflammatory response'. In other words, the white cells appear as a result of the damage. They do not cause it.

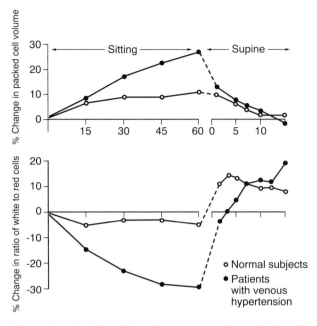

Figure 15.14 The effect of posture on the packed cell volume and ratio of white to red cells during 60 minutes of sitting and 15 minutes after resuming the supine position. (Redrawn from Thomas *et al.*[133])

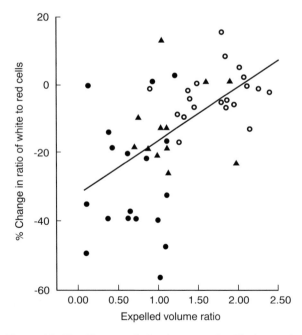

Figure 15.15 The correlation between the % change in the ratio of white to red cells leaving the lower limbs of patients after 60 minutes in the sitting position and the calf pump function expressed as the expelled volume ratio. (Redrawn from Thomas *et al.*[133]) ○, normal subjects; ▲, patients with varicose veins; ●, patients with deep vein insufficiency.

Endothelial and leucocyte activation

The search goes on to give a role to the trapped white cell. It is highly likely that a prolonged stay in a capillary will activate any contained white cells and cause changes in endothelial cell activity. Shields *et al.*[127] in a human experimental model have shown that an increase of venous pressure of 70 mmHg for 30 minutes when supine causes a significant rise in plasma lactoferrin. A similar response occurs when standing. Lactoferrin comes from the granules of neutrophils and its release is considered to be a reliable indicator of neutrophil activation. It is known that activated leucocytes, through the mechanism of oxygen-free radical liberation, damage the endothelium, increase capillary permeability[140] and stimulate an inflammatory response but whether the endothelial and possible interstitial damage followed by an inflammatory response is sufficient to cause tissue death is not known. Other substances in the interstitium, such as fibrin, may play a more important role.

If endothelial cell oedema and white cell trapping eventually cause capillary obstruction and focal ischaemia, red and white cell deformability may be decreased.[108] But it should be remembered that almost all of the evidence concerning white cells, endothelium and ischaemia comes from studies on the arterial side of the circulation. It is easy to understand how activated cells and noxious metabolites developing in the arterioles will affect the capillaries but difficult to understand how changes that require transmission by blood flow but which seem to occur primarily in the venules can affect capillaries which are upstream. As there is no evidence for capillary plugging by leucocytes and, in normal circumstances muscle activity will continually wash out any activated cells from the venules into the large veins, the theory that white cell activation causes the tissue changes of the calf pump failure must be considered 'not proven'.

Endothelial damage

The endothelial cells in limbs with calf pump failure certainly do show signs of damage. The cells may be irregular, oedematous, contain macro- and microcytotic vesicles, multivesicular bodies and widened interendothelial spaces.[88–91,141]

They also exhibit an increased production of intracellular adhesion molecules and factor VIII-related antigen.[19,139] There is an increase in the collagen IV layer of the basement membrane.

All this damage and all these reactions are just as likely to be the direct effect of the prolonged venular and capillary hypertension that we know exists. Whether the reperfusion injury situation required by the white cell plugging/activation theory exists and plays a real part in the production of the clinical signs of calf pump failure is still open to serious doubt.

FIBRINOLYTIC ACTIVITY

The amount of fibrinolytic activator produced by the endothelium can be measured by incubating thin slices of vein wall on a fibrin plate and measuring the areas of fibrinolysis.[135] Veins taken from limbs with the calf pump failure syndrome have a reduced level of tissue activator activity (Figure 15.16). Furthermore, in these patients plasma fibrinogen is raised, the dilute blood clot lysis time is prolonged and the fibrin plate lysis area is reduced.[23,75] Veins from their hands also have a reduced fibrinolytic activity (Figure 15.17).[24] Vanscheidt _et al._[138] also found a reduction in the release of tissue plasminogen activator inhibitor in response to venous congestion in the arms of patients with calf pump failure, but not to a statistically significant level.

These results imply that these patients have a systemic reduction of blood and tissue fibrinolytic activity. Whether this is a primary abnormality or is secondary to exhaustion of the activator stores in the legs caused by the chronic venous hypertension is not known. In favour of a primary systemic defect is the observation that patients with a history of deep vein thrombosis also have a reduced blood fibrinolytic activity.[24] Perhaps it is this abnormality which triggers the initial thrombosis and later exacerbates the interstitial changes caused by the damaged calf pump. This hypothesis would explain why only a proportion of a group of patients with similar calf pump dysfunction develop post-thrombotic syndrome skin changes.

Whatever the cause of the fibrinolytic deficiency, it definitely reduces the clearance of subcutaneous fibrin clots in limbs with lipodermatosclerosis (Table 15.8).

Table 15.8 The clearance of radioactive fibrin clots from the subcutaneous tissues of normal legs and legs with lipodermatosclerosis[87]

	Count rate (% of initial injection)			
	24 h	48 h	72 h	5 days
Normal legs	9 ± 1.8	4 ± 0.9	1 ± 0.5	0
Liposclerotic legs	17 ± 2.1*	12 ± 1.6*	8 ± 1.8*	9 ±2.7*

*$P<0.001$.
Subcutaneous clot = 0.05 ml ¹²⁵I-fibrinogen + 0.05 ml human thrombin)

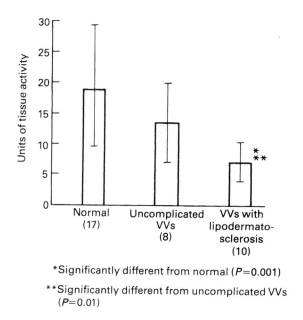

*Significantly different from normal (P=0.001)

**Significantly different from uncomplicated VVs (P=0.01)

Figure 15.16 The tissue fibrinolytic activity of veins removed from the feet of normal subjects, limbs with uncomplicated varicose veins and limbs with lipodermatosclerosis. The mean fibrinolytic activity of the veins from the limbs with skin changes was significantly less than the normal (means and standard deviations).

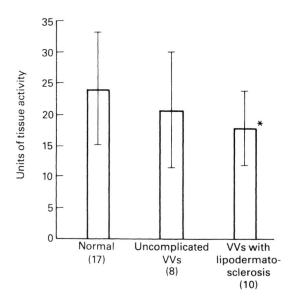

Figure 15.17 The tissue fibrinolytic activity of veins removed from the dorsum of the hands of normal subjects and patients with uncomplicated varicose veins and varicose veins (VVs) with lipodermatosclerosis. The mean fibrinolytic activity of the veins from the patients with lipodermatosclerosis was significantly less than the normal (means and standard deviations).

THE INTERSTITIAL SPACE

The raised venous pressure and increased capillary permeability increase the flow of capillary transudate through the interstitial spaces. Most of this transudate is cleared by the lymphatics but some remains, sometimes clinically apparent as oedema and always microscopically visible as enlarged pericapillary halos.[51] Venous hypertension increases the amount of fibrinogen crossing the interstitial spaces by 600% (see Table 15.6). Accompanying the fibrinogen are all the other components of plasma including clotting factors, fibrinolytic activators and inhibitors.[19] Our measurements of lymph composition in dogs' legs with venous hypertension showed only a slight reduction of fibrinolytic activity but revealed the appearance of an inhibitor of fibrinolysis, α2-antiplasmin. Thus not only is the amount of fibrinogen passing through the interstitial spaces increased,[86,87] but the interstitial fluid also contains a fibrinolytic inhibitor and less fibrinolytic activator. It may be that these changes explain the deposition of fibrinogen/fibrin around the capillaries.

Careful staining with specific dyes, fluorescent antibodies and immunohistochemistry has revealed layers of fibrinogen/fibrin around the dermal capillaries of lipodermatosclerotic skin[19,26,28,35,54,95,145] (Figure 15.18). Many other plasma proteins are also present. The presence of pericapillary fibrin is associated with calf pump inefficiency. We found the mean reduction in foot vein pressure during exercise in 26 legs with pericapillary fibrin in their skin biopsies to be 18 mmHg, whereas the mean reduction in foot vein pressure during exercise in 15 legs without pericapillary fibrin was 55 mmHg.[24,28] The presence of fibrin also correlates well with the degree of capillary elongation and dilatation, fibrin only being seen in limbs with an excessive number of dermal capillaries.

The presence of interstitial fibrin and other proteins may be the result of an increased deposition but could also be caused by a decreased rate of clearance as the changes in the skin associated with calf pump failure cause a progressive obliteration of the terminal lymphatics.[113,114]

The main lymphatic trunks of the limb are normal in patients with primary and post-thrombotic venous disease[105] but the small collecting lymphatics in the skin and subpapillary dermal plexus are abnormal in areas of lipodermatosclerosis. Bollinger has described a lymphatic microangiopathy causing an increase of permeability to fluorescent dextrans[14–16] and Fagrell has described a reduced lymphatic clearance from tissues showing post-thrombotic changes.[51]

A limb which has a chronically raised venous pressure has an increased lymph flow which can be shown by isotope lymphography to be two or three times higher than normal.[131]

Our assessment of the available evidence is that the lymphatics play no part in the initiation of the post-thrombotic syndrome but are affected by the changes in the capillaries and interstitial fluid and thereafter contribute as a secondary factor to the deterioration of the skin and subcutaneous tissues.

The pericapillary proteins can be found in skin showing the early stigmata of calf pump failure – thickening, tenderness and pigmentation – long before any ulceration, so it is not a phenomenon secondary to the inflammatory response caused by ulceration.

In the late stages of calf pump failure and especially when there is ulceration, the interstitial spaces contain all the elements of an inflammatory reaction – plasma proteins, white cells, red cells and haemosiderin.[69] In chronic long-standing cases, much of the normal tissue is replaced by scar tissue – collagen and fibroblasts.[145] The critical question remains – what causes the death of these tissues.

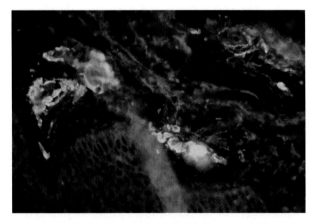

Figure 15.18 Pericapillary fibrin/fibrinogen. This section of skin taken from an area of lipodermatosclerosis and stained with fluorescent antibodies to fibrin shows each capillary surrounded by a layer of fibrin.

TISSUE OXYGENATION AND NUTRITION

Although many venous ulcers are started by a minor injury, none of the other changes of the calf pump failure syndrome is related to trauma. The skin and subcutaneous tissue fibrosis – which we have called 'lipodermatosclerosis' – and 'atrophie blanche' are the visible evidence of slow tissue death and replacement by scar tissue. Tissue death can only result from inadequate nutrition or anoxia if there is no trauma and no other detectable chemical or physical cause.

When we first described the presence of fibrin around the capillaries in tissues subjected to chronic venous hypertension, in man and in a canine experimental model, we suggested that this protein might impede the oxygenation and nutrition of nearby cells.[20,28]

Calculations by Michel, based upon the molecular structures of fibrin and oxygen and the space that the fibrin occupies within the pericapillary space, suggest that the quantity of fibrin we and others[19,35,54,95] have observed would not impede the movement of a small molecule such as oxygen.

Nevertheless, many investigators have shown that the transcutaneous oxygen tension of lipodermatosclerotic skin is reduced[37,58,95] and that the oxygen content of blood draining a limb with the calf pump failure syndrome is increased.[12,13] The only logical way to explain these findings is to postulate that oxygen transport through the capillary walls is reduced, the nutritional capillaries of the epidermis acting as physiological shunts.[98] The reflex reduction of blood flow caused by the increase of venous pressure cannot explain these two observations.[66]

Attempts to detect arteriovenous shunts by physiological methods have failed, though some workers claim, on the basis of arteriography and anatomical dissections, that they do exist.[63,64,120] If arteriovenous fistulae were present, there would be an increased tissue oxygen utilization. Studies with positron emission tomography[73] have shown that areas of lipodermatosclerosis have an increased blood flow but a reduced oxygen utilization; this finding is consistent with the interstitial barrier/physiological shunt hypothesis.

The permeability of the capillaries in the granulation tissue in the base of venous ulcers has also been shown to be directly related to the mean venous pressure; permeability reverts to normal when the patient is put to bed.[71] If anatomical A-V shunts were present, the venous pressure would remain high and the permeability would not fall during bed rest.

Unfortunately, the many publications describing the changes in skin blood using laser Doppler fluximetry have failed to clarify this problem because this technique cannot distinguish between the nutritive epidermal blood flow and the deeper dermal flow.[53]

Further support for the physiological shunt hypothesis comes from the observation that the venous hypertension seen in the hand after the formation of an arteriovenous shunt at the wrist causes lesions in the fingers similar to those seen in lipodermatosclerosis.[147]

If the physiological shunt is caused by the widening of the intercapillary spaces by the presence of excess proteins and possibly inflammatory cells, then it should be reduced and tissue oxygen tension improved by reducing the intercapillary space. This can be done very easily with external compression. Cheatle *et al.*[33] were unable to show a significant increase in $tcPO_2$ after 4 weeks of intermittent pneumatic compression or a change in percutaneous xenon clearance. Travers *et al.*,[136] however, showed a significant increase in the $tcPO_2$ measurements of lipodermatosclerotic skin following surgical treatment of the underlying incompetent veins, 19.6 mmHg rising to 40.6. They also observed an increase in the rate of increase of $tcPO_2$ following the inhalation of 100% oxygen for 5 minutes.

The reversal of abnormalities of tissue oxygen concentrations and laser Doppler flux[8] could not occur if there was a significant permanent obstruction to flow in capillaries and venules as suggested by those who postulated the white cell trapping hypothesis. However, the effect of the activators released by temporary trapping and activation on permeability and hence on the size and contents of the pericapillary space could be altered, thus bringing the two hypotheses together – the mechanical and the chemical elements both altering permeability, disrupting diffusion through the pericapillary tissues and so causing a physiological shunt.

The most valuable effect of our original 'fibrin barrier' hypothesis has been the stimulation of a considerable amount of new research into the effect on the microcirculation of venous hypertension. The older theories of venous stasis and anatomical A-V fistula have been discarded. Further work is needed to clarify the precise cause of the tissue death caused by venous hypertension because it does not occur in every patient and is associated with varying degrees of venous hypertension. This suggests a variable degree of tissue susceptibility and consequently gives the hope of not only more effective treatment but also pharmacological prophylaxis.

The current theories are illustrated in Figure 15.19; only time and more research will reveal which is correct.[6,72] The most important information we need is the pressure, blood flow, oxygen and cell content of the blood at the arterial and venous end of the capillaries.

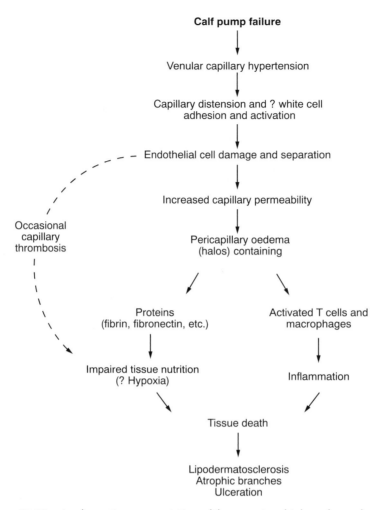

Calf pump failure

↓

Venular capillary hypertension

↓

Capillary distension and ? white cell
adhesion and activation

↓

Endothelial cell damage and separation

↓

Increased capillary permeability

↓

Pericapillary oedema
(halos) containing

Occasional
capillary
thrombosis

Proteins
(fibrin, fibronectin, etc.)

Activated T cells and
macrophages

↓

Impaired tissue nutrition
(? Hypoxia)

↓

Inflammation

Tissue death

↓

Lipodermatosclerosis
Atrophic branches
Ulceration

Figure 15.19   A schematic representation of the ways in which prolonged venous
hypertension may cause changes and damage in the microcirculation and interstitial spaces that lead to tissue death manifest by fibrosis or ulceration.

Prevalence

It is extremely difficult to determine the prevalence
of the calf pump failure syndrome. It certainly does
not occur in every patient who has had a venous
thrombosis. Indeed, if clinical history, fibrinogen
uptake tests and phlebographic studies are accepted,
it would appear to affect some patients who have
never had a thrombosis. Most workers, however,
believe that it is always caused by a thrombosis and
refuse to entertain other possibilities.

We think that 'calf pump failure syndrome' is a
better name than post-thrombotic syndrome as this
encompasses pump failure associated with hereditary varicose veins or a fibrinolytic deficiency
without evidence of an initiating thrombosis.

As there is no clear definition of the calf pump
failure syndrome, estimation of its incidence is
extremely difficult. The symptoms and signs may
vary from mild pain to severe venous claudication
and from an ankle flare with a little pigmentation
to a large ulcer.

Estimates of the prevalence of venous ulcers lie
between 0.1% and 0.25% (see Chapter 18). If we
knew the proportion of patients with the post-
thrombotic syndrome that had ulcers, we could
deduce the prevalence of the post-thrombotic syndrome.

The incidence of varicose veins, chronic venous
insufficiency and ulcers in the 4529 people (3744
men, 785 women) examined in the Basle survey was
45%, 15% and 1%, respectively.[47,144] 'Chronic
venous insufficiency' occurred in 16% of the men

and 13% of the women. 'Chronic venous insufficiency without ulceration' was also divided into mild, medium and severe, medium being hyperpigmentation or hypopigmentation with or without a 'corona phlebectatica'. If it is accepted that these changes are the early signs of calf pump failure, the Basle study suggests that calf pump failure was present in 6% of men and 5% of women.

This means that the prevalence of calf pump failure is five times that of ulceration. If we accept a figure of 0.1–0.2% as the prevalence of ulceration in the western hemisphere (one-tenth of that of the Basle III study), between 5 and 10 of every 1000 adults over the age of 25 years have an inadequate calf pump.

All the epidemiological studies have shown an increasing incidence with age, approximately 10-fold in men and 20-fold in women between the ages of 25 years and 65 years. As many as 100–200 of every 1000 women (10–20%) over the age of 65 years have some signs of chronic venous insufficiency which are compatible with a diagnosis of calf pump failure syndrome.[18] The prevalence in men is half this figure.[30]

The obvious difference in a woman's life compared to a man's life is pregnancy and childbirth. Both events are known to be complicated by venous dilatation and deep vein thrombosis.

Mudge and Hughes[101] reviewed the limbs that developed a deep vein thrombosis during a study of dextran prophylaxis, 5 and 10 years later. They found 26 of 564 (4.5%) patients had a post-thrombotic syndrome but this was present before the operation in 14 (2.5%). Their preoperative incidence matches the prevalence figures discussed above, and the postoperative incidence of 4.5% suggests that a major traumatic event in a person's life, such as a surgical operation, doubles the chances of developing a post-thrombotic syndrome.

The problem is massive. In a country with a population of 50 million, between 250 000 and 500 000 people will have a post-thrombotic syndrome. This figure will increase steadily as the mean age of the population rises. There are more than 8.0 million people over 65 years old in the United Kingdom – 3.2 million men and 4.8 million women. At least 0.65 million (160 000 men and 480 000 women) probably have clinical evidence of calf pump failure.

References

1. Allen AJ, Wright D, McCollum CN, Tooke JE. Impaired postural vasoconstriction, a contributory cause of oedema in patients with chronic venous disease. *Phlebology* 1988; **3:** 163–8.
2. Araki CT, Back TL, Padberg FT, *et al.* The significance of calf muscle pump function in venous ulceration. *J Vasc Surg* 1994; **20:** 872–9.
3. Arnoldi CC, Linderholm H. On the pathogenesis of venous leg ulcer. *Acta Chir Scand* 1968; **134:** 427.
4. Barnes MD, Marni K, Barrett DF, White JE. Changes in skin microcirculation at periulcerous sites in patients with chronic venous ulcers during leg elevation. *Phlebology* 1992; **7:** 36–9.
5. Bauer G. A roentgenological and clinical study of the sequels of thrombosis. *Acta Chir Scand* 1942; **86(Suppl 74):** 1.
6. Banersachs J, Fleming I, Busse R. Pathophysiology of chronic venous insufficiency. *Phlebology* 1996; **11:** 16–22.
7. Belcaro G, Christopoulos D, Nicolaides AN. Skin flow and swelling of the postphlebitic limbs. *Vasa* 1989; **18:** 136–9.
8. Belcaro G, Grigg M, Rulo A, Nicolaides AN. Blood flow in the perimalleolar skin in relation to posture in patients with venous hypotension. *AnnVasc Surg* 1989; **3:** 5–7.
9. Belcaro GV, Nicolaides AN. Effects of intermittent sequential compression in venous hypertensive microangiopathy. *Phlebology* 1994; **9:** 99–103.
10. Bergqvist D, Jaroszewski H. Deep vein thrombosis in patients with superficial thrombophlebitis of the leg. *Br Med J* 1986; **292:** 658.
11. Bergvall U, Hjelmstedt A. Recanalization of deep venous thrombosis of the lower leg and thigh. A phlebographic study of fracture cases. *Acta Chir Scand* 1968; **134:** 219.
12. Blalock A. Oxygen content of blood in patients with varicose veins. *Arch Surg* 1929; **19:** 898.
13. Blumoff RL, Johnson G. Saphenous vein pO_2 in patients with varicose veins. *J Surg Res* 1977; **23:** 35.
14. Bollinger A, Jager K. Trans and pericapillary diffusion of Na-fluorescein in scleroderma and venous insufficiency. *Bibl Anat* 1981; **20:** 679.
15. Bollinger A, Jager K, Geser A, Sgier F, Seglias J. Transcapillary and interstitial diffusion of Na fluorescein in chronic venous insufficiency with white atrophy. *Int J Microcirc Clin Exp* 1982; **1:** 5.
16. Bollinger A, Jager K, Roten A, Timeus C, Mahler F. Diffusion, pericapillary distribution and clearance of Na-fluorescein in the human nailfold. *Pflugers Arch Ges Physiol* 1979; **382:** 137.
17. Bollinger A, Leu AJ. Evidence for microvascular thrombosis obtained by intravital fluorescence videomicroscopy. *Vasa* 1991; **20:** 252–5.
18. Borschberg E. *The Prevalence of Varicose Veins in the Lower Extremities.* Basel: Karger, 1967.
19. Brakman M, Faber WR, Kerckhaedt JAM, Kraaijenhagen RJ, Hart H. Immunofluorescence studies of atrophie blanche with antibodies against fibrinogen, fibrin, plasminogen activator inhibitor, factor VIII related antigen and collagen type IV. *Vasa* 1992; **21:** 143–8.
20. Browse NL, Burnand KG. The cause of venous ulceration. *Lancet* 1982; **2:** 243.
21. Browse NL, Clemenson G. Sequelae of a ^{125}I-fibrinogen detected thrombosis. *Br Med J* 1974; **2:** 468.

22. Browse NL, Clemenson G, Lea Thomas M. Is the postphlebitic leg always postphlebitic? Relation between phlebographic appearance of deep vein thrombosis and late sequelae. *Br Med J* 1980; **282:** 1167.

23. Browse NL, Gray L, Jarrett PEM. Blood and vein wall fibrinolytic activity in health and vascular disease. *Br Med J* 1977; **1:** 478.

24. Burnand KG, Browse NL. The post-phlebitic leg and venous ulceration. In: Russell RCG, ed. *Recent Advances in Surgery 11.* Edinburgh: Churchill Livingstone, 1982.

25. Burnand KG, Clemenson G, Whimster I, Gaunt J, Browse NL. The effect of sustained venous hypertension on the skin capillaries of the canine hind limb. *Br J Surg* 1982; **69:** 41.

26. Burnand KG, O'Donnell TF, Lea Thomas M, Browse NL. The relative importance of incompetent communicating veins in the production of varicose veins and venous ulcers. *Surgery* 1977; **82:** 9.

27. Burnand KG, Whimster I, Clemenson G, Lea Thomas M, Browse NL. The relationship between the number of capillaries in the skin of the venous ulcer bearing area of the lower leg and the fall in foot vein pressure during exercise. *Br J Surg* 1981; **68:** 297.

28. Burnand KG, Whimster I, Naidoo A, Browse NL. Pericapillary fibrin in the ulcer bearing skin of the leg. *Br Med J* 1982; **285:** 1071.

29. Byrne JJ. Phlebitis. A study of 748 cases at the Boston City Hospital. *N Engl J Med* 1955; **253:** 579.

30. Callam MJ, Ruckley CV, Harper DR, Dale JJ. Chronic ulceration of the leg: extent of the problem and provision of care. *Br Med J* 1985; **290:** 1855.

31. Caprini JA, Arcelus JI, Hoffman KN, *et al.* Venous duplex imaging follow-up of acute symptomatic deep vein thrombosis of the leg. *J Vasc Surg* 1995; **21:** 472–6.

32. Chakrabarti R, Birks PM, Fearnley GR. Origin of blood fibrinolytic activity from veins and its bearing on the fate of venous thrombi. *Lancet* 1963; **1:** 1288.

33. Cheatle TR, McMullin GM, Farrah J, Coleridge-Smith PD, Scurr JM. Three tests of microcirculatory function in the evaluation of treatment of chronic venous insufficiency. *Phlebology* 1990; **5:** 165–72.

34. Chittenden SJ, Shami SK, Cheatle TR, Scurr JH, Coleridge Smith PD. Vasomotion in the leg skin of patients with chronic venous insufficiency. *Vasa* 1992; **21:** 138–42.

35. Claudy AI, Mirshahi S, Soria J. Detection of undergraded fibrin and tumour necrosis factor-α in leg ulcers. *J Am Acad Dermatol* 1991; **25:** 623–7.

36. Clayton JK, Anderson JA, McNicol GP. Preoperative prediction of post operative deep vein thrombosis. *Br Med J* 1976; **2:** 910.

37. Clyne CAC, Ramsden WH, Chant ADB, Webster JHH. Oxygen tension in the skin of the gaiter area of limbs with venous disease. *Br J Surg* 1985; **72:** 644.

38. Cockett FB, Elgan Jones DE. The ankle blow-out syndrome. *Lancet* 1953; **1:** 17.

39. Cockett FB, Thomas ML. The iliac compression syndrome. *Br J Surg* 1965; **52:** 816.

40. Coleridge Smith PD, Thomas P, Scurr JH, Dormandy JA. Causes of venous ulceration, a new hypothesis. *Br Med J* 1988; **296:** 1726–7.

41. Coon WW. Problems in thromboembolism. *Surg Clin North Am* 1961; **41:** 1343.

42. Corburn M, Ashworth C, Francis W, Morin C, Bronkhim M, Carney WI. Venous stasis complications of the use of the superficial femoral and popliteal veins for lower extremity bypass. *J Vasc Surg* 1993; **17:** 1005–9.

43. Corrigan TP, Kakkar VV. Early changes in the post-phlebitic limb: their clinical significance. *Br J Surg* 1973; **60:** 808.

44. Cotton LT, Clark C. Anatomical localization of venous thrombosis. *Ann R Coll Surg Engl* 1965; **36:** 214.

45. Cranley JJ, Krause RJ, Strasser ES. Chronic venous insufficiency of the lower extremity. *Surgery* 1961; **49:** 48.

46. Creutzig A, Caspary L, Alexander K. Changes in the microcirculation in patients with chronic venous insufficiency assessed by laser Doppler fluximetry and transcutaneous oxymetry. *Phlebology* 1994; **9:** 158–63.

47. Da Silva A, Widmer LK, Martin H, Mall TH, Claus L, Schneider M. Varicose veins and chronic venous insufficiency. *Vasa* 1974; **3:** 118.

48. Edwards EA, Edwards JE. Effects of thrombophlebitis on venous valves. *Surg Gynecol Obstet* 1937; **65:** 310.

49. Fagrell B. Local microcirculation in chronic venous incompetence and leg ulcers. *Vasc Surg* 1979; **13:** 217.

50. Fagrell B. Microcirculatory changes of the skin in venous disorders of the leg; studied by vital capillaroscopy. In: Schneider KW, ed. *Die Venose Insuffizienz.* Baden-Baden: Witztrock, 1972; 202.

51. Fagrell B. Microcirculatory disturbances – the final cause for venous ulcers. *Vasa* 1982; **11:** 101–3.

52. Fagrell B. How best to evaluate skin viability and the effect of therapy in patients with peripheral obliterative arterial disease. *Vasc Med Rev* 1990; **1:** 59–68.

53. Fagrell B. Laser Doppler flowmetry. In: Shepherd AP, Oberg A, eds. *Peripheral Vascular Diseases.* Boston: Kluwer, 1990.

54. Falanga V, Moosa HH, Nemeth AJ, Alstadt SP, Eaglestein WF. Dermal pericapillary fibrin in venous disease and venous ulceration. *Arch Dermatol* 1987; **123:** 620–3.

55. Fell SC, McIntosh HD, Hornsby AT, Horton CE, Warren JV, Pickrell K. The syndrome of the chronic leg ulcer. The phlebodynamics of the lower extremity: physiology of the venous valves. *Surgery* 1955; **38:** 771.

56. Fine J, Starr A. The surgical therapy of thrombosis of the deep veins of the lower extremity. *Surgery* 1945; **17:** 232.

57. Flanc C, Kakkar VV, Clarke MB. The detection of venous thrombosis of the legs using ^{125}I-labelled fibrinogen. *Br J Surg* 1968; **55:** 742.

58. Franzek UK, Bollinger A, Huch R, Huch A. Transcutaneous oxygen tension and capillary

morphologic characteristics and density in patients with chronic venous incompetence. *Circulation* 1984; **70:** 806–11.

59. Gibbs NM. Venous thrombosis of the lower limbs with particular reference to bed rest. *Br J Surg* 1957; **45:** 209.

60. Gjores JF. The incidence of venous thrombosis and its sequelae in certain districts of Sweden. *Acta Chir Scand Suppl* 1956; **206**.

61. Gordon-Smith IC, Hickman JA, LeQuesne LP. Postoperative fibrinolytic activity and deep vein thrombosis. *Br J Surg* 1974; **61:** 213.

62. Gottleb R. The clinical insignificance of the rami perforantes or communicantes in primary varicoses. In: May R, Partsch H, Staubesand J, eds. *Perforating Veins*. Munich: Urban & Schwarzenberg, 1981.

63. Guis JA. Arteriovenous anastomoses and varicose veins. *Arch Surg* 1960; **81:** 299.

64. Haimovici H. Arteriovenous shunting in varicose veins. *J Vasc Surg* 1985; **2:** 684.

65. Hamer JD, Malone PC, Silver IA. The pO2 in venous valve pockets. Its possible bearing on thrombogenesis. *Br J Surg* 1981; **68:** 166.

66. Hanna GB, Newton DJ, Harrison DK, Belch JJ, McCollum PT. Use of light guide spectrophotometry to quantify skin oxygenation in a variable model of venous hypertension. *Br J Surg* 1995; **82:** 1352–6.

67. Haselbach P, Vollenweider U, Moneta G, Bollinger A. Microangiopathy in severe chronic venous insufficiency evaluated by fluorescence videomicroscopy. *Phlebology* 1986; **1:** 159–69.

68. Hedner U, Nilsson IM, Isaacson S. Effect of ethyloestranol on fibrinolysis in the vessel wall. *Br Med J* 1976; **2:** 729.

69. Herrick SE, Sloan P, McGurk M, Freak L, McCollum CN, Ferguson N. Sequential changes in the histologic pattern and extra cellular matrix deposition during the healing of chronic venous ulcers. *Am J Pathol* 1992; **141:** 1085–95.

70. Hoare MC, Nicolaides AN, Miles CR, *et al.* The role of primary varicose veins in venous ulceration. *Br J Radiol* 1971; **44:** 653.

71. Hopkins NFG, Jamieson CW. Antibiotic concentration in the exudate of venous ulcers. A measure of local arterial insufficiency. *Br J Surg* 1982; **69(Suppl):** 676.

72. Hopkins NFG, Jamieson CW. Diffusion barriers in venous ulceration. *J R Soc Med* 1985; **78:** 355.

73. Hopkins NFG, Spinks TJ, Rhodes CG, Ranicar ASO, Jamieson CW. Positron emission tomography in venous ulceration and liposclerosis, study of regional tissue function. *Br Med J* 1983; **286:** 333.

74. Hume M, Chan YK. Examination of the blood in the presence of venous thrombosis. *JAMA* 1967; **200:** 747.

75. Isaacson S, Nilson IM. Defective fibrinolysis in blood and vein walls in recurrent idopathic venous thrombosis. *Acta Chir Scand* 1972; **138:** 313.

76. Johnson B, Manzo RA, Bergelin MS, Strandness MD. Relationship between changes in the deep venous system and the development of the postthrombotic syndrome after an acute episode of lower limb deep vein thrombosis. A one to six year follow up. *J Vasc Surg* 1995; **21:** 307–13.

77. Kakkar VV, Howe CT, Flanc C, Clarke MB. Natural history of postoperative deep vein thrombosis. *Lancet* 1969; **2:** 230.

78. Killewich LA, Bedford GR, Beach KW, Strandness DE. Spontaneous lysis of deep venous thrombosis. *J Vasc Surg* 1989; **9:** 89–97.

79. Killewich LA, Martin R, Cramer M, Beach KW, Strandness DE. An objective assessment of the physiologic changes in the post-thrombotic syndrome. *Arch Surg* 1985; **120:** 424.

80. Krupski WC, Bass A, Dilley RB, Bernstein EF, Otis SM. Propogation of deep venous thrombosis identified by duplex ultrasonography. *J Vasc Surg* 1990; **12:** 467–75.

81. Kwaan HC, Astrup T. Fibrinolytic activity in thrombosed veins. *Circ Res* 1965; **17:** 477.

82. Labropoulos N, Leon M, Nicolaides AN, *et al.* Venous reflux in patients with previous deep venous thrombosis. Correlation with ulceration and other symptoms. *J Vasc Surg* 1994; **20:** 20–6.

83. Lawrence D. *Haemodynamic Studies Relating to the Postphlebitic Syndrome.* MS Thesis, London University, 1982.

84. Lawrence D, Kakkar VV. Post phlebitic syndrome – a functional assessment. *Br J Surg* 1980; **67:** 686.

85. Lea Thomas M, McAllister V. The radiological progression of deep vein thrombosis. *Radiology* 1971; **99:** 37–49.

86. Leach RD. Venous ulceration, fibrinogen and fibrinolysis. *Ann R Coll Surg Engl* 1984; **66:** 258.

87. Leach RD, Browse NL. Effects of venous hypertension on canine hind limb lymph. *Br J Surg* 1985; **72:** 275.

88. Leu HJ. Morphology of chronic venous insufficiency – light and electron microscopic examination. *Vasa* 1991; **20:** 330–42.

89. Leu HJ, Wenner A, Spycher M, Brunner U. Veranderungen der transsendothelialen Permeabilitat als Ursache des Oedems bei der chronich-venosen Insuffizienz. *Phlebol Proktol* 1980; **9:** 67–73.

90. Leu AJ, Yanar A, Pfister G, Geiger M, Franzeck UK, Bollinger A. Microangiopathy in chronic venous insufficiency. *Dtsch Med Wochenschr* 1991; **116:** 447–53.

91. Leu AJ, Yanar A, Pfister G, Geiger M, Franzeck UK, Bollinger A. Mikroangiopathic bei chronischer venoser insuffizienz. *Dtsch Med Wochenschr* 1991; **116:** 447–53.

92. Lindhagen A, Bergqvist D, Hallbook T. Deep venous insufficiency after post operative thrombosis diagnosed with[125]I labelled fibrinogen uptake test. *Br J Surg* 1984; **71:** 511.

93. Luke JC. The deep vein valves: a venographic study in normal and post-phlebitic limbs. *Surgery* 1951; **29:** 381.

94. McMullin GM, Scott HJ, Coleridge PD, *et al.* A reassessment of the role of perforating veins in chronic venous insufficiency. *Phlebology* 1990; **5:** 85–94.

95. Mani R, White JE, Barrett DF, Weaver PW. Tissue oxygenation, venous ulcers and fibrin cuffs. *J R Soc Med* 1989; **82:** 345–6.

96. May R, Thurner J. Ein Gefassporn in der V. iliaca communis sinistra als Ursache der vorwiegend links-seitigen Beckenvenenthrombosen. *Z Kreislauf-forsch* 1956; **45:** 912.

97. Meissner MH, Manzo RA, Bergelin RO, Markel A, Strandness E. Deep venous insufficiency: The relationship between lysis and subsequent reflux. *J Vasc Surg* 1993; **18:** 596–608.

98. Moosa HH, Falanga V, Steed DL, *et al.* Oxygen diffusion in chronic venous ulceration. *J Cardiovasc Surg* 1987; **28:** 464–7.

99. Mourad MM, Barton SP, Marks P. Changes in endothelial cell mass, luminal volume and capillary number in the gravitational syndrome. *Br J Dermatol* 1989; **121:** 447–61.

100. Moyses C, Cederholm-Williams SA, Michel CC. Haemoconcentration and accumulation of white cells in feet during venous stasis. *Int J Microcirc Clin Exp* 1987; **5:** 311–20.

101. Mudge M, Hughes LE. The long term sequelae of deep vein thrombosis. *Br J Surg* 1978; **65:** 692–4.

102. Murphy TP, Cronan JJ. Evolution of deep venous thrombosis, a prospective evaluation with ultrasound. *Radiology* 1990; **177:** 543–8.

103. Negus D. Calf pain in the post thrombotic syndrome. *Br Med J* 1968; **2:** 156.

104. Negus D. Prevention and treatment of venous ulceration. *Ann R Coll Surg Engl* 1985; **17:** 144.

105. Negus D. The iliac veins in relation to lymphoedema. *Br J Surg* 1969; **56:** 481.

106. Negus D, Cockett FB. Femoral vein pressures in postphlebitic iliac vein obstruction. *Br J Surg* 1967; **54:** 522.

107. Negus D, Pinto DJ, Le Quesne LP, Brown N, Chapman M. ^{125}I-labelled fibrinogen in the diagnosis of deep vein thrombosis and its correlation with phlebography. *Br J Surg* 1968; **55:** 835.

108. Neuman FJ, Waas W, Muller-Bulh U, *et al.* Activated stiffened leucocytes in the circulation of the ischaemic leg in peripheral vascular occlusive disease. *Circulation* 1988; **78(Suppl II):** 404.

109. Nicolaides AN, Clark CT, Thomas RD, Lewis JD. Soleal veins and local fibrinolytic activity. *Br J Surg* 1972; **59:** 914.

110. Nicolaides AN, Kakkar VV, Field ES, Renney JTG. The origin of deep vein thrombosis. *Br J Radiol* 1971; **44:** 653.

111. Nilsson IM, Isacson S. New aspects of the pathogenesis of thrombo-embolism. In: Allgower M, Bergentz SE, eds. *Progress in Surgery.* Basel: Karger, 1973.

112. Pandolfi M, Isacson S, Nilsson IM. Low fibrinolytic activity in the walls of veins of patients with thrombosis. *Acta Med Scand* 1969; **186:** 1.

113. Partsch H. Lymphangiopathei bei chronischr Veneninsuffizienz. *Phlebol Proktol* 1984; **13:** 85–9.

114. Partsch H. Investigations on the pathogenesis of venous leg ulcers. *Acta Chir Scand* 1988; **544:** 25–9.

115. Phillips RS. Prognosis in deep vein thrombosis. *Arch Surg* 1963; **87:** 44.

116. Ramhorst B, Bemmelen PS, Hoenveld H, Eikelboom BC. The development of valvular incompetence after deep vein thrombosis. A follow-up study with duplex scanning. *J Vasc Surg* 1994; **20:** 1059–66.

117. Ramhorst B, Bemmelen PS, Hoeneveld H, Faber JAJ, Eikelboom BC. Thrombus regression in deep venous thrombosis: quantification of spontaneous thrombolysis with duplex scanning. *Circulation* 1992; **86:** 414–19.

118. Recek E. A critical appraisal of the role of the ankle perforators for the genesis of venous ulcers in the lower leg. *J Cardiovasc Surg* 1971; **12:** 45.

119. Saarinen J, Sisto T, Laurikka J, Salerius J-P, Tarkka M. Late sequelae of acute deep vein thrombosis. Evaluation five and ten years after. *Phlebology* 1995; **10:** 106–9.

120. Schalin L. Arteriovenous communications to varicose veins in the lower extremities studied by dynamic angiography. *Acta Chir Scand* 1980; **146:** 397.

121. Scott HJ, Coleridge-Smith PD, Scurr JH. Histological study of white blood cells and their association with lipoerdermatosclerosis and venous ulceration. *Br J Surg* 1991; **78:** 210–11.

122. Sethia KK, Darke SG. Long saphenous incompetence as a cause of venous ulceration. *Br J Surg* 1984; **71:** 754.

123. Sevitt S. The mechanism of canalization of deep vein thrombosis. *J Pathol* 1973; **110:** 153.

124. Sevitt S. The structure and growth of valve-pocket thrombi in femoral veins. *J Clin Pathol* 1974; **27:** 517.

125. Sevitt S, Gallagher NG. Venous thrombosis and pulmonary embolism. A clinicopathological study in injured and burned patients. *Br J Surg* 1961; **48:** 475.

126. Shami SK, Cheatle TR, Chittenden SH, Scurr JH, Coleridge Smith PD. Hyperaemic response in the skin microcirculation of patients with chronic venous insufficiency. *Br J Surg* 1993; **80:** 433–5.

127. Shields DA, Andaz S, Abeyside RD, Porter JB, Scurr JH, Coleridge-Smith PD. Neutrophil activation in experimental venous hypertension. *Phlebology* 1994; **9:** 119–24.

128. Shull KC, Nicolaides AN, Fernandes E, *et al.* Significance of popliteal reflux in relationship to ambulatory venous pressure and ulceration. *Arch Surg* 1979; **114:** 1304.

129. Speiser DE, Bollinger A. Microangiopathy in mild chronic venous incompetence, morphological alterations and increased transcapillary diffusion detected by fluorescein videomicroscopy. *Int J Microcirc Clin Exp* 1991; **10:** 55–66.

130. Stamatakis JD, Kakkar VV, Lawrence D, Bentley PG. The origin of thrombi in the deep veins of the lower limb: a venographic study. *Br J Surg* 1978; **65:** 449.

131. Stewart G, Gaunt J, Croft DN, Browse NL. Isotope lymphography, a new method of investigating the role of the lymphatics in chronic limb oedema. *Br J Surg* 1985; **72:** 906.

132. Thomas ML, O'Dwyer JA. Site of origin of deep vein thrombosis in the calf. *Acta Radiol Diagn (Stockh)* 1977; **4:** 418.

133. Thomas PRS, Nash GB, Dormandy JA. White cell accumulation in dependent legs of patients with venous hypertension: a possible mechanism for trophic changes in the skin. *Br Med J* 1988; **296:** 1693–5.

134. Thulesius O, Gjores JE, Eriksson O, Berlin E. Mechanische und biochemische Voraussetzungen der chronisch-venosen insuffizienz. *Vasa* 1984; **13:** 195.

135. Todd AS. The histological localization of fibrinolysis activator. *J Pathol Bacteriol* 1959; **78:** 281.

136. Travers JP, Berridge DC, Makin GS. Surgical enhancement of skin oxygenation in patients with venous lipodermatosclerosis. *Phlebology* 1990; **5:** 129–33.

137. Tripolitis AJ, Milligan EB, Bodily KC, Strandness DE Jr. The physiology of venous claudication. *Am J Surg* 1980; **139:** 447.

138. Vanscheidt W, Kresse O, Hach-Wunderle V, *et al.* Leg ulcer patients: no decreased fibrinolytic response but white cell trapping after venous occlusion of the upper limb. *Phlebology* 1992; **7:** 92–6.

139. Veraart JCJM, Verhaegh MEJM, Neumann HAM, Hulsmans RFMS, Arends JW. Adhesion molecule expression in venous leg ulcer. *Vasa* 1993; **22:** 213–18.

140. Weissman G, Smolen JE, Korchak M. Release of inflammatory mediators from stimulated neutrophils. *N Engl J Med* 1980; **303:** 27–34.

141. Wenner A, Leu HJ, Spycher M, Brunner U. Ultrastructural changes of capillaries in chronic venous insufficiency. *Exp Cell Biol* 1980; **48:** 1–14.

142. Whimster I. In: Dodd H, Cockett FB, eds. *The Pathology and Surgery of Veins of the Lower Limb.* Edinburgh: Churchill Livingstone, 1953.

143. Widmer LK. *Peripheral Venous Disorders.* Bern: Hans Huber, 1978.

144. Widmer LK, Zemp E, Widmer MT, *et al.* Late results in deep vein thrombosis of the lower extremity. *Vasa* 1985; **14:** 264–8.

145. Wilkinson LS, Brewster C, Edwards JWW, Scurr JH, Coleridge-Smith PD. Leukocytes: their role in the aetiopathogenesis of skin damage in venous disease. *J Vasc Surg* 1993; **17:** 669–75.

146. Wolfe JHN, Morland M, Browse NL. The fibrinolytic activity of varicose veins. *Br J Surg* 1979; **66:** 185.

147. Wood ML, Reilly GD, Smith GT. Ulceration of the hand secondary to a radial arteriovenous fistula, a model for varicose ulceration. *Br Med J* 1983; **287:** 1167.

148. Young AK, Thomas ML, Browse NL. Comparison between sequelae of surgical and medical treatment of venous thromboembolism. *Br Med J* 1974; **4:** 127.

CHAPTER 16

The calf pump failure syndrome: diagnosis

Diagnosis	473	**References**	483
Investigations	479		

The development of symptoms after a deep vein thrombosis is not entirely predictable. Nevertheless, a considerable proportion of patients do develop problems in their legs after a deep vein thrombosis which are sufficiently distinctive to be recognizable as the clinical syndrome, commonly known as the post-thrombotic syndrome, but more easily understood as 'the calf pump failure syndrome'.

Diagnosis

CLINICAL PRESENTATION

History

Not every patient with calf pump failure gives a history of a deep vein thrombosis. Some patients have never been seriously ill, undergone surgery or had any previous leg symptoms. The phlebographs of a significant number of these patients are normal which makes one question whether their symptoms are post-thrombotic (see Chapter 15). In our experience, fewer than one-third of patients with calf pump failure give a definite history of a previous deep vein thrombosis. It is easy for patients to forget past events and they may not have been told

their diagnosis, so when taking a history it is important to ask directly about episodes of leg swelling or pain in relation to pregnancy, to the puerperium, to previous operations, or to accidents, especially leg fractures. A number of women will deny a history of 'thrombosis' but then inform you that they had a swollen or 'white leg' after the birth of a child!

Thromboembolic events are sometimes familial; it is therefore important to ask about a family history of varicose veins, venous thrombosis or pulmonary embolism.

Symptoms and signs

Pain and tenderness

The most common complaint is of *an aching pain* in the leg that is exacerbated by standing. The pain is felt in the muscles of the calf or thigh and is relieved by rest and elevation of the leg. The muscles are not particularly tender.

Localized *throbbing pain* may be felt over areas of acute lipodermatosclerosis and superficial thrombophlebitis.

Ischaemic skin about to break down and form into an ulcer often causes *persistent pain* which is not relieved by rest and is similar to the 'rest pain' of arterial ischaemia. The surrounding skin is often very tender but the centre may be numb.

Venous claudication is a *bursting pain* experienced during exercise. It occurs when there is severe outflow obstruction and venous hypertension during exercise. The bursting sensation is felt deep inside the leg, mainly below the knee, though a few patients complain that the thigh becomes painful before the calf. The amount of exercise needed to produce the pain is not so constant and reproducible as that needed to cause the pain of arterial claudication. When the muscles are tense and 'bursting', they are usually tender. The acute pain subsides quickly with rest and elevation but a residual dull ache and mild tenderness often persists for some time.

Swelling

Oedema caused by venous obstruction may vary from mild ankle swelling to gross oedema of the whole leg from the foot to the groin. If the inferior vena cava (IVC) has been thrombosed, the oedema may extend into the lower abdominal wall and over the buttocks. The oedema of venous obstruction varies from day to day, is soft, pits easily and is not tender. It subsides rapidly with bed rest and limb elevation.

Localized oedema occurs in areas of lipodermatosclerosis and thrombophlebitis. An oedematous patch of acute lipodermatosclerosis, found commonly in the gaiter area of the leg, is usually hot, red and tender with an easily palpable edge.

Varicose veins

The subcutaneous veins become dilated after a deep vein thrombosis for two reasons. First, they are distended by the high venous pressures in the leg that follow the outflow obstruction and the valvular incompetence of the communicating veins. Secondly, they enlarge to carry more blood as they become collateral channels bypassing the occluded deep veins.

Some patients with the calf pump failure syndrome have no visible varicose veins. It was their absence in some patients with venous ulcers that confused the early physicians and stopped them recognizing the 'venous' nature of many ulcers.

When varicose veins do appear they may be situated anywhere but are often most prominent on the lower medial third of the leg, close to the important communicating veins. A very large dilated vein over the site of an incompetent communicating vein is often called a 'blow-out'.[2]

The long and short saphenous veins and their tributaries may also be dilated and incompetent, particularly when they are acting as collateral veins. Dilatation is more common in patients who had varicose veins before their thrombosis or who have a family history of varicose veins.

Post-thrombotic communicating vein incompetence often causes lower leg varicosities but may take many years to make the whole subcutaneous venous system dilated and incompetent. Once incompetent, the communicating veins may act as *collateral vessels*, but the direction in which blood flows in lower leg varicose veins during exercise cannot be deduced from their size or site.

Varicose veins which appear in the upper thigh, groin and lower abdomen following an ilio-femoral thrombosis are usually acting as collaterals. Large dilated subcutaneous veins at the root of the limb and crossing the groin are diagnostic of an iliac vein obstruction.

Varicose veins that appear as a sequel to deep vein damage cause the same symptoms as primary varicose veins, namely aching pains, night cramps, mild oedema and cosmetic disfigurement. They are often the patient's *presenting complaint*, especially if the patient is unaware of the initial thrombotic episode.

It is important to remember the patient's principal symptoms and their cause when phlebograms and other minor symptoms are tempting you to perform deep rather than superficial vein surgery.

Intradermal venules

Chronic venous hypertension dilates the veins, the venules and the venular capillaries (see Chapter 15). This is manifest clinically by the appearance of fine dilated veins in the skin. They bulge up under the epidermis, making the skin bosselated and irregular. They are prone to localized thrombosis. This turns them into small black nodules which eventually peel off and may bleed profusely after minor trauma. Intradermal venules are commonly seen in a triangular area, whose apex begins just above the medial malleolus and whose base is at the edge of the sole of the foot. This patch of dilated venules has been called the *ankle flare*,[1] or the corona phlebectactica[4] (see Figure 16.1). This is an apt description and its presence indicates long-standing calf pump failure, usually caused by communicating vein incompetence.

Venous 'stars'

The valves begin in venules which are 1 mm in diameter. If the first few valves of a venule become incompetent, the fine venular capillaries become distended and are visible on the skin as fine thread-like red–purple vessels. Their draining vein is situated either at their centre – the vessels radiating from it like the spokes of a wheel (hence the name

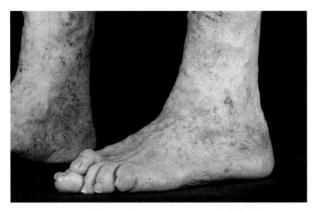

Figure 16.1 The 'ankle flare'. Chronic venous hypertension causes dilatation of the intradermal and subdermal venules around the ankle. This is usually seen as a triangle of dilated venules below the medial malleolus. The patient illustrated has medial and lateral ankle 'flares' on both legs.

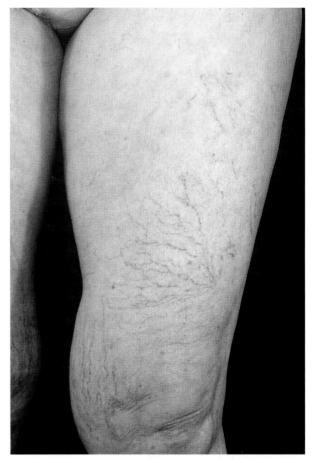

Figure 16.2 Venous telangiectases. These fine intradermal venules are also called venous stars and spider veins. They are commonly associated with calf pump failure. They can be treated by injection sclerotherapy but invariably recur if calf pump function is not improved.

'stars') – or at one corner with the vessels radiating out in a triangle (Figure 16.2). Extensive venous stars can give the skin of the whole leg an unsightly blue colour. Venous stars can occur in normal limbs without varicose veins and their aetiology and significance is therefore far from clear. They cause distress solely because of the cosmetic disfigurement. They do not cause pain or bleeding and are clinically and prognostically insignificant when compared with the larger intradermal venules discussed above.

Pigmentation

Prolonged venous hypertension causes venular dilatation and the extrusion of red blood cells through the inter-endothelial pores. The red cells are broken down and absorbed but the *haemosiderin* remains as a brown pigment staining the skin.

Pigmentation occurs mainly on the lower medial third of the lower leg but may slowly spread around the leg to involve the whole of the 'gaiter' area (Figure 16.3).

As the years pass, the pigmentation may get darker and eventually look almost black. The epidermis over such pigmented skin tends to become hypertrophic and scaly, probably as a result of the venous hypertension rather than as a response to the pigment.

Pigmentation may also occur in a linear form over the course of a subcutaneous vein and commonly occurs over a segment of superficial thrombophlebitis. The more vigorous the inflammatory response, the more likely it is that the inflammatory exudate will contain red cells.

Dermatitis

Dermatitis appears over prominent subcutaneous varicose veins and in areas of skin which have been subjected to chronic venous hypertension – usually the lower medial third of the leg (Figure 16.4). These changes are presumably a response to venous congestion, fibrin, and haemosiderin deposition and local oedema but the exact mechanism is not known.

Venous dermatitis (or 'varicose eczema') may be dry and scaly or vesicular, 'ulcerated' and weeping. Once the epidermis is lost there is a serious risk that

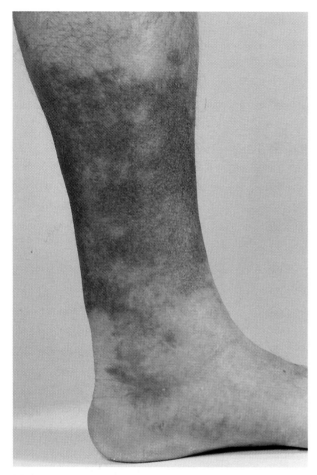

(a)

Figure 16.3   Two examples of pigmentation caused by calf pump failure. (a) The pigmentation is confined to the medial side of the gaiter area. (b) The pigmentation is beginning to spread all around the gaiter area and up the leg. In some patients the whole of the leg becomes deeply pigmented.

(b)

a venous ulcer may develop but as this is not an invariable sequence of events it is likely that the disorders of the microcirculation that cause the dermatitis are not always the same as those that cause ulcers. Ulcers are invariably started by minor local trauma, dermatitis is not. The difference between ulceration and dermatitis is particularly apparent in the patient with a linear patch of dermatitis over a large vein on the lateral aspect of the thigh, a site at which venous ulcers are never found.

The skin of patients with chronic venous disease appears to be more sensitive than normal. Contact dermatitis in response to any or all of the medica-

ments placed on ulcers, to the rubber in elastic bandages, and to the creams in impregnated bandages, is extremely common. This may be induced sensitization from repeated dressings but it is so common that it is conceivable that chronic venous hypertension, in some unknown way, increases skin sensitivity to chemical agents.

Lipodermatosclerosis

This is a rather unwieldy term which we coined to describe the progressive fibrosis of the skin and subcutaneous tissues induced by chronic venous

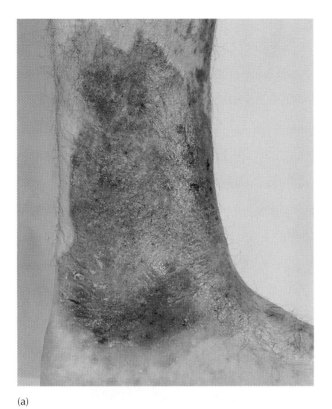

(a)

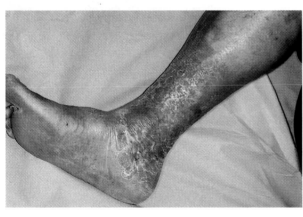

(a)

Figure 16.4 Two examples of venous dermatitis/eczema. (a) An area of dermatitis localized to the lower medial third of the leg with vesicles and exudate. (b) Dermatitis with scaling, fissures and weeping involving the whole of the lower leg.

hypertension.[1] Other investigators have called it fat necrosis, panniculitis and chronic cellulitis, but none of these names indicates the true pathology.

It appears in two forms – acute or chronic. It is usually found on the lower medial third of the leg but sometimes spreads around the whole of the lower third of the limb (the gaiter area) and occasionally higher up the calf. The acute variety eventually becomes chronic, but the chronic variety can develop without passing through an acute stage.

Acute lipodermatosclerosis is a painful disabling condition. It begins as a thickened, sometimes slightly raised red–brown, tender area in the skin of the lower leg (see Figure 16.5). The patient's main complaint is of pain and tenderness and a constant sensation of heat. The area gradually enlarges and has a distinct edge. The edge is not elevated like that of erysipelas but there is a palpable change between the hot, red, tense skin and subcutaneous tissue and the soft normal tissue. The redness, heat and tenderness frequently lead to a mistaken diagnosis of cellulitis or thrombophlebitis. The afflicted area may increase in size or the centre may suddenly break down and ulcerate.

The inguinal lymph nodes are not enlarged and the patient does not have a pyrexia or a leucocytosis. Acute lipodermatosclerosis occasionally resolves spontaneously but usually progresses to the chronic form, if an ulcer does not supervene.

Chronic lipodermatosclerosis may develop spontaneously or from burnt-out acute lipodermatosclerosis. The skin is stiff and shiny and fixed to the hard, indurated, contracting subcutaneous tissues. It has a palpable edge, and the dilated veins within it feel like deep pits. The skin is not red and hot but brown and shiny.

The progressive contraction of the skin and subcutaneous tissues make the gaiter area shrink and, with slight oedema of the calf above, gives the leg an inverted 'champagne bottle' shape (Figure 16.6).

The pigmented skin is often scarred from previous ulceration and the subcutaneous fat may become calcified, and feel rock hard.

Atrophie blanche

Skin can die and be replaced by scar tissue without ulcerating or sloughing. Atrophie blanche is the name given to small areas of skin scarring caused by chronic venous hypertension (and in other circumstances by arteritis).

The patches are grey–white and usually only a few millimetres in diameter. They form a slight depression on the skin surface and are covered with a thin transparent-looking epithelium which may be surrounded by a halo of fine dilated venules (see Figure 16.7).

Sometimes multiple small areas of atrophie blanche coalesce to form a large scar. These larger scars are fragile and may break down spontaneously or following minimal trauma to become an ulcer.

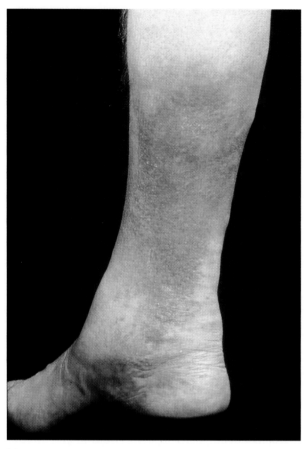

(a)

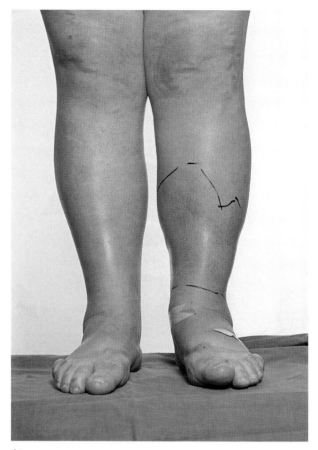

(b)

Figure 16.5 Two examples of acute lipodermatosclerosis. Chronic venous hypertension slowly destroys the skin and subcutaneous tissues so that they become replaced with scar tissue. In the early stages of this process the skin tissues become hot, red, thickened, painful and tender. We have called this condition acute lipodermatosclerosis. It is often misdiagnosed as cellulitis, thrombophlebitis or panniculitis. The edge of these changes can be palpated and marked out, as in one of these illustrations.

Stiffness of the ankle joint

The progressive subcutaneous thickening and scarring of lipodermatosclerosis may also extend into the subcutaneous tissue around the ankle joint. This restricts ankle movements, reduces calf pump efficiency and exacerbates the venous hypertension. The ankle joint may become completely fixed by scar tissue – a fibrous ankylosis.

Fixed plantar flexion

Chronic pain from lipodermatosclerosis or an ulcer makes patients avoid bearing weight on the sole of the foot. The patient limps on the toes of the affected leg to reduce ankle movements and gradually the ankle stiffens in plantar flexion and the Achilles tendon shortens. The calf muscles do not contract as the patient limps and calf pump efficiency diminishes. Painful callosities form on the ball of the foot and toes which also impede walking.

Walking with a plantar flexed ankle disturbs the whole leg, the knee, hip, and back, and can exacerbate any pre-existing symptoms of osteoarthritis.

Periostitis

Long-standing inflammation in the subcutaneous tissues may induce a hyperaemia in the underlying periosteum which then produces new subperiosteal bone. This can sometimes be felt as patchy thickening and roughening of the subcutaneous surface of the lower third of the tibia but is more often a coincidental finding observed on a plain radiograph (Figure 16.8).

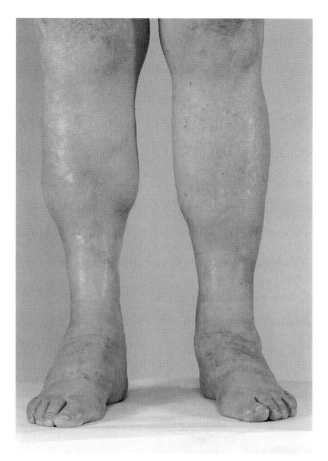

Figure 16.6 As lipodermatosclerosis dies out the tissues contract, narrowing the lower third of the lower leg to give the 'champagne bottle' shape and reducing the mobility of the ankle joint.

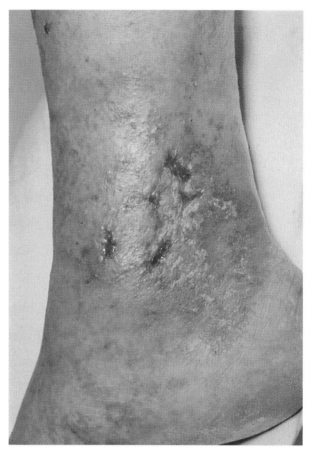

Figure 16.7 This figure illustrates all the different varieties of tissue damage caused by calf pump failure – dermatitis, healed and open ulceration and areas of white scarring (atrophie blanche) that have developed without passing through a period of ulceration.

Ulceration

All the conditions described above and collectively called the post-thrombotic syndrome are pre-ulcer changes. They are the signs of impaired tissue nutrition and oxygenation and slow tissue death which can be exacerbated in minutes by an injury and then progress rapidly to ulceration. Venous ulceration is discussed in detail in Chapters 18, 19 and 20.

Investigations

There are two main objectives in investigating a patient with symptoms and signs suggestive of the post-thrombotic syndrome. The first is to confirm the diagnosis, the second is to assess the severity of the

venous disease and the possible forms of treatment. The investigations comprise a general physical examination, blood studies and special radiological tests.

INVESTIGATIONS TO EXCLUDE OTHER DIAGNOSES

Other conditions which cause symptoms and signs which can be confused with the calf pump failure syndrome are given below.

Peripheral arterial disease

Arterial insufficiency can cause muscle pain on exercise, pain in the leg when at rest and skin ulceration. In each of these circumstances there will be

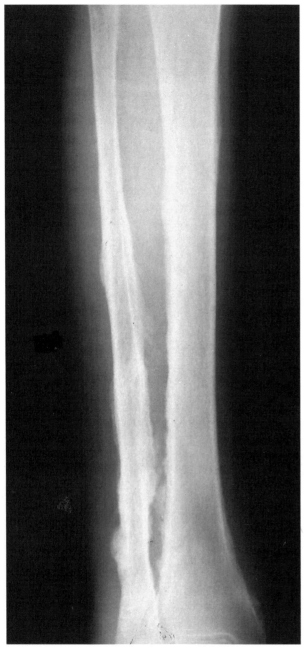

Figure 16.8 A plain radiograph showing periosteal new bone formation on the surface of the fibula underneath an area of chronic lipodermatosclerosis and recurrent ulceration.

some detectable abnormality of the arterial circulation such as pallor of the limb, absent peripheral pulses or arterial bruits. Many elderly patients have both peripheral arterial and venous disease, and it is sometimes difficult to decide which system is the cause of the symptoms. Special tests such as ankle arterial pressure measurements using Doppler ultrasound after treadmill exercise may be needed before arterial insufficiency can be excluded as a cause of symptoms.

Myositis and arteritis

These both cause muscle pains which are exacerbated by exercise and relieved by rest. Clinical examination may reveal persistent tenderness in the muscles after exercise and tenderness of the upper limb muscles. The erythrocyte sedimentation rate (ESR) is usually raised and there may be abnormal levels of immunoglobulins in the blood. A biopsy of the muscles or arteries may be needed to confirm the diagnosis.

Deep vein thrombosis

An acute thrombosis will not cause skin changes but may occur in a limb which is already the site of post-thrombotic damage and exacerbate the existing pain and swelling. Sudden onset of pain, calf tenderness and mild oedema should arouse suspicion of this diagnosis. Duplex ultrasound or phlebography are the quickest and most accurate methods for excluding fresh thrombus.

Arteriovenous fistulae

These can cause pain, varicose veins and skin ulceration – which are all symptoms of the calf pump failure syndrome. This diagnosis should be suspected if the patient is young, the limb is hot and enlarged and if there are flow murmurs over the main limb arteries. Arteriography and measurements of peripheral blood flow will confirm or exclude this diagnosis.

Lymphoedema

Lymphoedema is a possible diagnosis if the swelling is marked, the skin healthy and the varicose veins sparse. Lymphoedema can be distinguished from venous oedema by isotope lymphangiography. Venous oedema causes an increase of lymph flow, while in lymphoedema the lymph flow is reduced.

Other causes of pigmentation and dermatitis

The whole of the patient's skin should be carefully examined. Abnormalities in skin not subjected to chronic venous hypertension should raise the possibility of a primary skin disease such as pemphigoid, erythema nodosum and Bazin's disease. Biopsy of lesions on the legs and elsewhere may be necessary to determine whether pigmentation or dermatitis is venous in origin.

Locally applied medicaments may make the skin pigmented. A careful history should be taken of all previous local and systemic treatment.

Atrophie blanche

This can be caused by cutaneous vasculitis. The clue is often found in the site of the scarring. If the white patches are on the toes or feet and the other signs of venous insufficiency are unconvincing, the efficiency of the calf pump should be measured and, if it is normal, the blood should be examined for evidence of abnormal immunoglobulins and rheumatoid factors. These tests are often unhelpful, and non-venous atrophie blanche is often diagnosed by exclusion after finding that the calf pump function tests and the phlebograms are normal.

Rheumatoid arthritis

This may present with acute pain and redness of the subcutaneous tissues. Joint pain and immobility are usually severe. Serological tests and radiographs will help confirm this diagnosis.

Cellulitis

Acute lipodermatosclerosis is red, hot and tender, as is cellulitis, but the former has a long history and does not cause a pyrexia, lymphangitis, a leucocytosis or inguinal lymphadenopathy. A diagnostic course of antibiotics may, however, be the only way to prove that an area of lipodermatosclerosis is not a subcutaneous infection.

Superfical thrombophlebitis

If the inflammation in the vein is severe and spreads into the surrounding tissues, it may be difficult to confirm the diagnosis of superficial thrombophlebitis by feeling the underlying 'cord-like' thrombosed vein. Superficial thrombophlebitis is rarely confined to the lower third of the leg and settles quickly with bed rest. Phlebography is not helpful unless it shows thrombus in other veins.

Neurological disease

Peripheral neuropathy, ankle deformities, ulcers and oedema can all complicate neurological disease. A full neurological examination of the limb is essential.

Periostitis

This may be noticed by chance on a radiograph. Other causes of periostitis (e.g. ulcerative colitis) must be excluded.

Comment

The differential diagnoses of the calf pump failure syndrome can be excluded in most patients by a careful clinical history and examination. Simple blood tests, the occasional skin biopsy, phlebograms and arteriograms will help sort out the confusing clinical situation where the patient has post-thrombotic type symptoms and signs but normal calf pump function test results. The differential diagnoses of leg ulcers are discussed in Chapter 19.

INVESTIGATIONS TO CONFIRM AND ASSESS THE SEVERITY OF THE VENOUS DISEASE

Clinical examination

The severity of the pain and the extent of the swelling, pigmentation and lipodermatosclerosis indicate the severity of the damage to the microcirculation, but are poorly related to the crude measurements of calf pump function that are available and often have little correlation with the phlebographic abnormalities. It is therefore important to remember while performing special investigations on the veins that the main object is to treat the symptoms, not just the anatomical or physiological abnormalities demonstrated by the investigations; this objective can often be achieved with an elastic stocking. Surgery should be the last form of treatment.

Whatever treatment is prescribed, it is important to know which aspect of calf pump physiology is abnormal. The tourniquet tests should be used during clinical examination to see if the long or short saphenous systems or the communicating veins are incompetent. The latter assessment is difficult if the veins are not prominent and the tissues are thickened. Laboratory tests are more informative.

Tests of calf pump efficiency

The simple methods of assessing calf pump function are useful for confirming the presence of a venous abnormality and obtaining an estimate of its severity.

The best assessment of pump function is to measure venous emptying during exercise. This can be qualitatively assessed with photoplethysmography, which can be crudely calibrated to make it semi-quantitative. We find, however, that the simplest quantitative method is foot volumetry. This method gives a measure of venous emptying and refilling in absolute terms and in relation to the initial foot volume. The normal values of these measurements are remarkably similar in different laboratories and so can be used to diagnose the presence or absence of pump inefficiency with confidence (see Chapter 4). Many vascular laboratories now use air plethysmography rather than foot volumetry because it is less cumbersome and measures the same features of calf pump function.

It is essential to watch the patient performing these tests. A painful, stiff ankle will reduce movements and the strength of the calf contractions and show that correction of the joint problem might have a greater effect on the calf pump than correction of the venous abnormality.

Saphenous reflux

Superficial vein reflux can add a large burden to the work of the calf pump. Reflux can be detected with the clinical tourniquet tests and heard with the Doppler flow detector but its contribution to the calf pump failure syndrome can only be measured by combining the tourniquet tests with some form of plethysmography (see Chapter 4).

The simplest test is to combine the tourniquet tests with photoplethysmography. This only gives a qualitative answer but if the refilling rate becomes normal when a tourniquet is applied, the superficial vein reflux probably needs to be corrected surgically.

We prefer to identify the role of superficial reflux with foot volumetry because it gives a quantitative measure of reflux; air plethysmography can also be used for this purpose.

Descending phlebography will often show the presence of long saphenous reflux but is not indicated for this purpose alone because the simpler methods such as Doppler flow detection and the tourniquet tests are probably just as accurate (see Chapter 4).

Communicating vein reflux

There is no way of measuring the amount of blood that refluxes through the communicating veins. If a tourniquet is placed just below the knee, it will prevent reflux down the saphenous veins but not through the communicating veins. An abnormally fast refilling with a below-knee tourniquet in place implies that the communicating veins are incompetent. A tourniquet at the ankle will only restore refilling to normal if it is below the lowest incompetent communicating vein, compresses all the subcutaneous veins and does not interfere with ankle movements. As the lowest communicating vein is behind and just below the medial malleolus, and the subcutaneous tissues are often hard and incompressible, an ankle tourniquet is frequently ineffective.

Only 50–60% of incompetent communicating veins can be detected with a simple Doppler flow detector. This test also produces a high rate of false-positives. We find that the most reliable techniques for the detection of incompetent communicating veins are ascending phlebography and duplex ultrasound, but it must be accepted that although both tests have a high positive test accuracy, both have a high false-negative rate, phlebography because the contrast will not necessarily flow through every incompetent communicator, duplex ultrasound because it is not practical to scan every aspect of the whole leg. Neither method measures the amount of reflux, and so it has to be assumed that any detectable reflux is clinically significant.

By a complex series of manoeuvres involving multiple cuffs, passive squeezing of the calf, and the use of isotope plethysmography it is possible to detect the reflux of blood into the superficial compartment and measure the resulting increase in superficial venous volume. The volume of the reflux is very small and poorly correlated to the pressure change because of the variable compliance of diseased veins, thus making knowledge of the volume of reflux of little clinical significance.

A decision that the communicating veins are playing a significant role in the symptomatology of a patient's calf pump failure syndrome is based primarily on finding that these veins are incompetent by clinical, ultrasonic, or radiological means, and from the site and distribution of the skin changes.

The role of the deep veins

The deep veins may be contributing to calf pump inefficiency by obstructing forward blood flow or allowing blood to reflux. Maximum venous outflow measured with a plethysmograph around the calf gives a crude measure of femoral vein obstruction but is not very accurate. Wheeler[3] devised a measurement called the 'venous diameter index' derived from an impedance plethysmograph tracing but this test has been replaced by measurements derived from duplex ultrasound studies.

Iliac vein obstruction can be assessed from femoral vein pressures measured during exercise.

The presence of deep vein reflux can be detected and estimated using the photoplethysmograph or the foot volumeter if an increased rate of refilling persists after all the superficial reflux has been prevented with tourniquets, but the site and extent of the reflux can only be assessed by duplex ultrasound or descending phlebography (see Chapters 4 and 12).

The anatomy of the venous abnormalities

None of the tests of function indicates the precise site of the post-thrombotic abnormalities. This can only be done with ascending and femoral phlebography, or a very extensive ultrasound study. Phlebography can reveal calf, axial and communicating vein damage. Perfemoral or intraosseus phlebography may be needed to show abnormalities in the ilio-femoral segment (see Chapter 4).

Ultrasound in the hands of a skilled technician is an excellent method for detecting major vein (femoral and popliteal) abnormalities but not good for detecting post-thrombotic damage in the small axial veins of the lower leg or the intramuscular veins of the gastrocnemius and soleus muscles.

Biopsy

It may be necessary to take a biopsy of an area of post-thrombotic lipodermatosclerotic change to assess the effect of the venous hypertension on the skin and confirm the diagnosis. Very occasional patches of abnormal skin showing the clinical features of chronic calf pump failure dermatitis will be found to be basal or squamous cell carcinoma.

Blood studies

Part of the calf pump failure syndrome, and not just those cases that follow a deep vein thrombosis, is related to a deficiency of fibrinolysis. The fibrinolytic system of a patient with surgically incurable or recurrent post-thrombotic disease or unexplained symptoms suggestive of calf pump failure should be studied by measuring the plasma fibrinogen, euglobulin clot lysis time and plasminogen activity. Sometimes vein wall fibrinolytic activator production should be assessed on a vein biopsy from the dorsum of the foot.

Comment

Whereas most patients with simple varicose veins can be treated on the basis of clinical examination alone, patients with post-thrombotic calf pump failure need careful evaluation before advising treatment.

In our opinion the minimum investigations should be the following:

- A careful clinical examination supplemented with tourniquet tests and a Doppler flow detector analysis of saphenous reflux.
- A water, air or photoplethysmographic assessment, with and without tourniquets, of overall calf pump function, saphenous and deep vein reflux.
- A full duplex ultrasound and/or phlebographic study to detect incompetent communicating veins, post-thrombotic calf vein damage, axial vein obstruction, collaterals and any deep vein reflux.
- Measurements of blood and vein wall fibrinolytic activity when surgical correction of the calf pump is not possible.

References

1. Browse NL. Venous ulceration. *Br Med J* 1983; **286:** 1920–3.
2. Cockett FB, Elgan Jones DE. The ankle blow-out syndrome. *Lancet* 1953; **1:** 17–20.
3. Wheeler HB, Anderson FA. The diagnosis of venous thrombosis by impedance plethymography. In: Bernstein EF, ed. *Non-invasive Diagnostic Techniques in Vascular Disease.* St Louis, MO: CV Mosby, 1985.
4. Widmer LK. *Peripheral Venous Disorders.* Bern: Hans Huber, 1978.

CHAPTER 17

The calf pump failure syndrome: treatment

Natural history	485	References	500
Treatment	486		

Natural history

What happens once the symptoms and signs of calf pump failure have appeared?

Although collectively and individually the skin changes of the calf pump failure syndrome can be called pre-ulcer changes, not every patient develops an ulcer. It is not known whether the rate of progression of tissue damage is mainly related to:

- a critical level of calf pump inefficiency
- a steadily deteriorating efficiency
- a critical level at which the circulatory changes affect capillary permeability, white blood cell behaviour and interstitial oedema and protein deposition
- the presence of a pre-existing deficiency of fibrinolysis and interstitial protein clearance
- age and repeated trauma.

Probably all these factors are involved, but much more information is needed about the day-to-day and year-to-year fluctuations of lower limb superficial vein pressures, changes in the microcirculation, blood and tissue fluid fibrinolysis, and their relation to the development of symptoms.

When a patient with a history of venous thrombosis, secondary varicose veins and early skin pigmentation asks if he/she will develop a venous ulcer, we are inclined to answer in the affirmative in order to encourage the patient to take preventative measures and wear an elastic stocking. In truth, we do not know what will happen. The calf pump function tests of a patient with mild symptoms are usually not grossly abnormal, and yet one such patient may develop an ulcer 1 year later whereas another will have no new changes in the leg 10 or 20 years later, partly because the ultimate cause of an ulcer is often an unrelated, unpredictable event such as a minor injury.

When symptoms get worse, the results of the function tests are usually found to have deteriorated. It has been suggested that patients with exercising foot vein pressures which are lower than 45 mmHg never develop ulcers.[83] This may be close to the truth but the converse is not true. Not all, or even the majority, of patients with high exercising foot vein pressures develop ulcers. The lack of a close correlation between the onset of symptoms and the ways in which we currently measure calf pump inefficiency suggests that the clinical natural history is significantly affected by other factors. Whereas skin deterioration, once the skin changes are present, coincides with the deterioration of the calf pump, the initiation of skin changes may depend upon independent abnormalities of the microcirculation and interstitial spaces.

What makes the pump deteriorate? This is another unanswered question. Valves not destroyed by the initial thrombosis probably become incompetent because of valve ring dilatation. Dilatation is caused by the high venous pressure, but must also be related to vein wall strength. Is there a vicious circle in which the patient with a familial tendency to varicose veins gets a thrombosis because of the varicose veins,[5] which in turn causes further incompetence because of vein wall weakness? And is this connected with another vicious circle in which fibrinolytic deficiency leading to thrombosis leads to calf pump failure, leaky capillaries and the failure to lyse fibrin in the interstitial space and a further deterioration of endothelial cell production of fibrinolytic activators?

There is much to be discovered about the factors which affect the progression of the symptoms of the calf pump failure syndrome. In general it can be said that pigmentation and dry eczema are early mild signs that may remain static. Lipodermatosclerosis indicates serious tissue damage which will advance either to overt skin necrosis, an ulcer, or to a latent fibrous replacement of the skin and subcutaneous tissue clinically visible as 'atrophie blanche' and the 'champagne bottle' leg. Lipodermatosclerosis rarely regresses if the calf pump inefficiency and the abnormalities in the interstitial space are not treated. Its rate of progression is variable but usually inevitable.

The clinician has a problem. Mild disease causes few symptoms but is easier to investigate and treat than advanced disease, whereas advanced disease is complex and difficult to investigate and treat. If we knew for certain that early treatment with external support, pharmacological correction of the abnormalities of the microcirculation, the stimulation of natural fibrinolysis, or surgery would definitely stop the progression of skin changes, we would not hesitate to advise treatment at an early stage, but there is no scientifically acceptable evidence to support such an approach. As we are considering a pathological process that may take 30 years or more to progress to a measureable end point, a good experimental study would outlast a surgeon's working life, making its conduct a considerable challenge. Short-term studies based on the results of non-invasive investigations may be possible when we have improved the quality, reproducibility, and sensitivity of our tests and defined their significance and relationship to the clinical problems.[97]

With so many uncertainties, most surgeons prefer to observe the symptoms and signs over a number of years before pronouncing on an individual's natural history or need for early treatment.

Treatment

The common presenting symptom – aching pain – is often relieved by wearing a good quality elastic stocking.[41,60,87] Stockings can be prescribed after the patient's first consultation and worn while the investigations are being arranged. Relief of pain by a stocking is not only gratifying to the patient but is also a good diagnostic test of the clinical impression that the symptoms are caused by venous hypertension.

Once the diagnosis has been made and the severity and type of the venous abnormality defined, treatment falls into two distinct categories:[2]

- 'Curative' treatment – surgical correction of the calf pump abnormality
- Palliation of symptoms – principally, reducing the venous transmural pressure.

The term 'cure' when applied to venous disease is an optimistic overstatement; it might be loosely applied to the treatment of some types of primary varicose vein but should never be used to describe the treatment of the post-thrombotic calf pump failure syndrome. All forms of surgical treatment throw added stress on the remaining veins unless the treatment achieves the impossible and restores every part of the pump to normal. When one incompetent communicating vein is ligated, another has to take over its function as a collateral vessel and will in time become incompetent. At best, surgery improves calf pump function for a limited time, it rarely restores it permanently to normal – which is what most patients would consider to be a 'cure'.

SURGICAL CORRECTION OF CALF PUMP ABNORMALITIES

The two abnormalities of the veins of the lower limb that can be corrected surgically are valvular incompetence and obstruction to blood flow. The former is corrected by restoring valve function or ligating the incompetent vessel, the latter by bypassing the obstruction.

All patients admitted to hospital for the investigation and treatment of the post-thrombotic calf pump failure syndrome should be given 5000 units of heparin subcutaneously 12-hourly or a daily dose of a low molecular weight heparin from the day of their admission until discharge to prevent further deep vein thrombosis (see Chapter 11).

Prevention of reflux

The veins which become incompetent and strain the pump are those in the saphenous system, the communicating veins and the deep outflow tract. All these veins will become incompetent if the thrombosis has been extensive. It is usually impractical to correct all three systems at once and so most surgeons prefer to correct the superficial and communicating vein incompetence first, and leave the deep vein incompetence to be treated, if necessary and if technically possible, at a later date.

Saphenous vein reflux

Saphenous vein reflux is treated by ligation of the saphenous vein at the sapheno-femoral junction. This operation is described in detail in Chapter 7 (page 195). The long saphenous vein above the level of the knee often connects with the superficial femoral vein in the middle of the thigh through the Hunter's canal communicating vein and so the saphenous vein should be stripped out from the knee to the groin to abolish this site of deep-to-superficial reflux and so prevent an early or late recurrence (see page 204).

The correction of long saphenous and communicating vein incompetence rarely returns the foot vein pressure during exercise to normal (Figure 17.1). In a study in which the long saphenous incompetence was treated first, followed by a second operation on the communicating veins at least 3 months later, with frequent serial studies of calf pump function, Akesson and his colleagues[3] showed that pressure during exercise, was reduced and refilling after exercise prolonged by the correction of the long saphenous incompetence but not by ligating the

incompetent communicating veins. Neither operation restored the measurements to the normal range. Nevertheless, both operations produced clinical improvement. Such studies emphasize the lack of correlation between our current tests and clinical status. Simply measuring pressure or volume, without knowing the rates of inflow and outflow, compliance, and the point on the venous system's compliance curve at which the measurements are made, will never give us anything more than a very crude indication of calf pump function.

The saphenous vein should not be ligated or stripped if it is acting as a major collateral around an occluded superficial femoral vein. It is difficult to be certain from a clinical examination when this situation is present. If phlebographs show no filling of the superficial and deep femoral veins with all the contrast medium ascending from the mid-calf to the groin in the saphenous vein, the wisdom of removing the long saphenous vein should be questioned. But phlebography is an anatomical, not a physiological, test. The only physiological way to assess the role of the long saphenous vein is to measure the change of foot volume, or foot vein pressure, during exercise, before and after occluding the superficial veins in the thigh with a tourniquet. If the long saphenous vein is acting as a significant collateral, calf pump function will deteriorate when the tourniquet is inflated (i.e. the venous volume and pressure during exercise will increase when the cuff is inflated) (Figure 17.2a). The pressure may even increase above the resting level.

Much more commonly, occlusion of a large incompetent saphenous vein that is allowing gross reflux to overload the pump will improve calf pump function (Figure 17.2.b). In these circumstances an

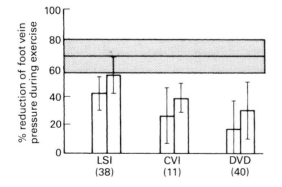

Figure 17.1   The effect of surgery on calf pump function in three groups of patients. The left-hand side of each histogram indicates the reduction of foot vein pressure during exercise before surgery. It can be seen that surgery almost returns the foot vein pressure to normal limits in patients with long saphenous vein incompetence (LSI), but does not return the pressure to normal in patients with incompetent calf communicating veins (CVI) or in patients with evidence of post-thrombotic damage on phlebography (DVD).

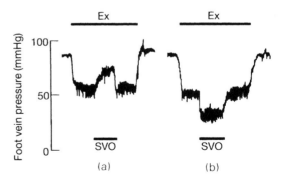

Figure 17.2   The effect of superficial vein occlusion (SVO) at mid-thigh level on the foot vein pressure during exercise (Ex). (a) If superficial vein occlusion during exercise causes an increase in foot vein pressure, the superficial veins must be acting as collateral outflow channels. (b) If superficial vein occlusion during exercise reduces foot vein pressure, the superficial veins must be incompetent and the reflux impeding calf pump function.

incompetent long saphenous vein can safely be ligated and stripped. The long saphenous vein functions as a significant collateral channel in only 5–10% of patients but this small group must be identified because ligation of their long saphenous veins will make their symptoms worse.

Communicating vein reflux

The presence of skin and subcutaneous tissue changes in the lower leg are usually sufficient to justify a diagnosis of communicating vein incompetence but an attempt should always be made to confirm the presence of the reflux within these veins with tourniquet and Doppler flow detection tests and the sites of reflux should be determined by duplex ultrasound or ascending phlebography.[24,85,97]

Whereas ligation of an incompetent long saphenous vein acting as a major collateral channel will do harm, ligation of communicating veins acting as collaterals does not appear to cause problems. The volume of blood that these veins conduct is small when compared to the presumed deleterious effect of their incompetence on the superficial venous pressure. This pressure abnormality must be abolished to stop the progression of the calf pump failure syndrome but the evidence is mounting that ligating incompetent communicating veins does not produce a major reduction of exercising pressure. Does the operation work in another so far unexplained way or are our tests of calf pump function too crude to detect the effect of abolishing communicating vein reflux? Alternatively, the clinical response might have nothing whatsoever to do with the communicating vein ligation!

The patient's symptoms seem only to be relieved until new incompetent communicating veins develop. It is not possible to predict how long this process will take but it is clearly related to the degree of deep vein damage. The rapid reappearance of symptoms plus new, dilated, incompetent communicating veins within 1–3 years usually indicates a severe degree of outflow tract obstruction. The usual phlebographic indication that this will occur is severe post-thrombotic changes in the calf veins and a totally occluded or very poorly recanalized popliteal vein.

Although the ligation of communicating veins which are acting as collaterals does no harm clinically because it reduces the superficial venous hypertension and so helps the subcutaneous tissues and skin to recover, it must embarrass the pump. Ligating these veins when the outflow tract is obstructed is the equivalent of introducing mitral stenosis in place of mitral incompetence in a patient with severe aortic stenosis. The incompetent communicating veins are the 'blow-out' safety vents for the pump. Ligating them increases the end systolic volume and the work that the pump must do during systole. If we could measure intra-pump volumes and pressures, with and without the incompetent communicating veins occluded, we could decide how their ligation would affect pump function in a way similar to the assessment of the role of an incompetent long saphenous vein that might be acting as a collateral or as a source of regurgitation. At present we cannot do this because although we can identify their position we cannot experimentally occlude each one and measure the pressure–volume relationships within the pump, with and without their occlusion. Perhaps this could now be done by measuring calf pump function between each communicating vein ligation if it were done under local anaesthesia with an 'endoscopic' technique.

The only means we have of predicting the long-term effect of communicating vein ligation is by examining the phlebograph for evidence of severe deep vein damage. In a series of our patients whose communicating veins were ligated following conservative treatment to heal a venous ulcer, the ulcer recurred within 5 years in all those with extensive deep vein damage. The ulcer did not recur in those patients with healthy deep veins. Neither group was provided with elastic stockings.[23]

How is deep vein damage best assessed? Occlusion, recanalization and stenosis of the main outflow tract is easy to see on phlebographs and with duplex ultrasound but post-thrombotic changes in the stem and muscle veins of the calf are much more difficult to see, describe and quantify with either technique. The deep vein changes that predict a poor result from communicating vein ligation (i.e. an early chance of recurrence) are narrowing and irregularity of clusters of veins, tortuous collateral vessels within the calf, occluded calf axial veins (there should always be three pairs of axial veins in the calf – posterior tibal, peroneal, and anterior tibial) and the absence of valves (Figure 17.3).

These abnormalities are rarely present in isolation, they are commonly all present. We try to avoid ligating the communicating veins when these changes are present because the results are often no better than those obtained with elastic compression but some patients prefer to have an operation even though they will experience a relapse in 3–5 years' time. It is important to discuss the prognosis in detail with the patient before proceeding to surgery.

Communicating vein ligation
This is described in detail in Chapter 7. If the deep veins are healthy, it is possible to cut through thick pigmented skin and obtain primary wound healing provided maximum care is taken to avoid skin

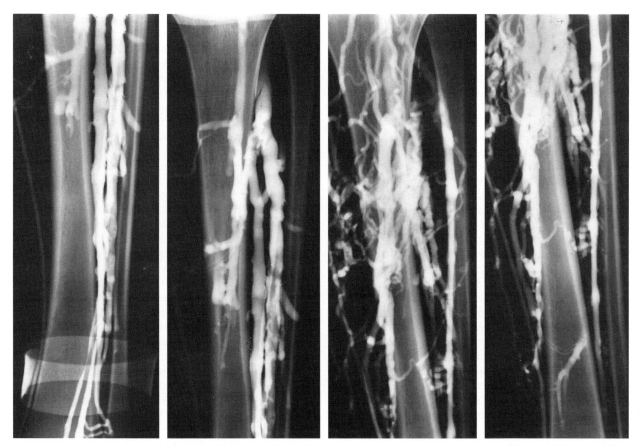

Figure 17.3 Phlebographs showing normal (left-hand panels) and damaged (right-hand panels) deep calf veins. The deep vein thrombosis has caused a mixture of partial and complete occlusion, tortuous collaterals and many thin irregular valveless vessels meandering in all directions.

damage, undercutting, and skin ischaemia as a result of tight stitches. 'Endoscopic' ligation through an incision in healthy skin is likely to replace the older direct approach. If there is an ulcer, the incision can be moved posteriorly to avoid cutting through unhealthy skin.[34,35,71,72]

When there are skin changes such as lipodermatosclerosis, exploration to find the communicating veins should *always be subfascial.* Undercutting the skin in the subcutaneous layer is likely to cause skin necrosis or delayed healing. The last thing a surgeon wants is to cause an ulcer when he is doing an operation to prevent ulceration. The skin should be closed with the minimum of stitches. It is often possible to hold the incision together with surface adhesive strips and thus avoid skin stitches altogether.

The leg should be firmly bandaged. If the patient has had an ulcer and is used to an impregnated bandage (e.g. Viscopaste or Calaband), this can be applied at the end of the operation and left in place for 2–3 weeks.

The patient should be kept in bed with the leg elevated for 2 or 3 days before being allowed to walk because ankle movements disturb the edges of the lower part of the incision. Patients are normally encouraged to walk as soon as possible after varicose vein operations but in these patients the main objective is to obtain healing by first intention and this requires a period of rest to give the wound a chance to knit together before being disturbed by weight bearing and walking.

A delayed healing rate of 10–15% is inevitable when operating through unhealthy tissues. If the wound is very painful, it must be inspected. Skin necrosis and haematomata are the common causes of postoperative pain and should be treated by excision and evacuation, respectively; the resulting defect may have to be closed with a skin graft.

Prophylaxis with subcutaneous heparin is essential in these patients, throughout their stay in hospital, as they are at risk of getting a further thrombosis – an event which could make their leg much worse. The heparin should not increase the incidence of wound haematomata if care is taken with haemostasis during the operation and the limb is firmly bandaged and elevated afterwards.

The clinical effect of communicating vein ligation on the pre-ulcer symptoms and signs of the calf pump failure syndrome has not been evaluated. The majority of surgeons have studied ulcer recurrence and claim a 5-year ulcer-free rate of 85% but few have assessed the state of the deep veins with phlebography preoperatively.[6,17,43,51,57,59,63,66,80,84,98] It is our experience that those legs that show progression of their lipodermatosclerosis or develop recurrent ulcers after operation are those with extensive deep vein damage.

Patients with incompetent communicating veins and scarred unhealthy skin often do better if the damaged skin is excised and replaced by a split skin graft. A few patients with extensive circumferential skin damage do best when all the skin of the lower leg is excised, from the ankle to the mid-calf, in a way similar to the Charles' reducing operation for lymphoedema. When there is extensive deep vein damage this may be the only treatment that can be offered. It should reduce the incidence of recurrence because the excision of all the communicating veins with the skin and subcutaneous fat leaves none to become incompetent. We have performed this operation on only four patients.

To avoid cutting through unhealthy skin many surgeons have adapted the instruments developed for laparoscopic abdominal surgery so that they can ligate incompetent communicating veins, subfascially, through a small incision placed high up the calf in healthy skin. This is no different from techniques described some years ago using long retractors and malleable lights.

No results of either the older indirect approaches to communicating vein ligation or the 'endoscopic' methods have yet been published. It must first be established that the new methods do successfully reveal and occlude all the incompetent communicators, and if they do, they should be used in a large study to identify the value of the technique. The 'endoscopic' methods significantly reduce the duration of postoperation hospitalization.

Communicating vein shearing

To avoid cutting through the unhealthy skin some surgeons push a blunt-ended shearing knife up and down the leg beneath the deep fascia, hoping to divide all the communicating veins.[37] This method can cause haematomata, bruising of the skin, and occasionally, skin necrosis. It cannot guarantee to divide all the communication veins and cannot be recommended.

Deep vein reflux

The treatment of non-thrombotic deep vein reflux has been discussed in Chapter 12. When reflux follows deep vein thrombosis the valves are totally destroyed, making attempts at valve repair inappropriate. The only two methods by which a valve can be inserted to prevent reflux in a previously thrombosed vein are valve transplantation[101] and valve segment transposition.[68] *Valve transplantation* has been described on page 398. It only works when a healthy valve can be transferred into a relatively healthy vein. In reflux without evidence of post-thrombotic damage (for which valve transplantation has been used by Taheri[102]), the popliteal or superficial femoral veins of the recipient legs have been healthy.[101] After popliteal or femoral vein thrombosis the segment of vein that recanalizes least well is the portion above and below the adductor canal – perhaps this is because of the stiff surrounding structures. Consequently, it is rarely possible to transplant a valve to this position after a thrombosis because of the poor quality of the recipient vein. It is unwise to sew a valve into a vein that is fibrosed, thickened and stenosed with endothelialized mural thrombus. Such a vein can be guaranteed to thrombose in spite of anticoagulants and the use of an adjuvant arteriovenous fistula.

Valve transplantation has little place in the treatment of the post-thrombotic syndrome and, because suitable patients are extremely hard to find, no large series describing its use has been published. For the same reasons the insertion of a preserved allograft valve will rarely be feasible.

Valve transposition

Deep vein thrombosis often affects the superficial femoral vein and spares the deep femoral vein. In such circumstances it may be possible to perform a transposition of the upper end of an incompetent superficial femoral vein into the side of a competent deep femoral vein, below a healthy valve (see Figure 12.14, page 399).[68]

A number of valve transpositions have been performed for post-thrombotic incompetence. Although many patients have a significant prolongation of deep vein refilling 3 months after operation, refilling often becomes abnormal again 9 months later, indicating that this simple and logical operation cannot stand the test of time.[65,91] This does not mean that it should be abandoned but that it should be studied when combined with additional procedures that might prevent valve ring dilatation and recurrent reflux.

During the time that an obstructed segment of vein takes to recanalize to allow sufficient reflux to cause symptoms, the original obstruction will have stimulated other collateral veins to dilate and thus made them incompetent. We do not know whether the restoration of deep vein competence will encourage superficial incompetent veins, which have dilated to act as collaterals, to constrict and become competent. Fegan has claimed that this phenomenon can occur in the long saphenous vein following occlusion of incompetent calf communicating veins,[40,92] but whether a similar change follows a successful valve transplant or transposition is not known. The evidence from Kistner's valve repair studies[42] suggests that the communicating veins do not recover as the majority of his patients still needed communicating vein surgery after a successful valve repair. This is not surprising because the pump still generates the same systolic pressure during exercise, and blood, taking the route of least resistance, will continue to flow retrogradely in the communicating veins even after the axial veins have been rendered competent. This means that incompetent communicating veins must be ligated at the same time as deep vein valve competence is restored.

A number of other anti-reflux procedures on the deep veins have been advocated over the years; none has stood the test of time.

Femoral vein and popliteal vein ligation

These methods have been tried and found to be unsatisfactory. The theories of Homans, Bauer and Linton[9–11] that femoral vein ligation would improve calf pump function were based on the belief that reflux down the recanalized femoral or popliteal vein was the main cause of the post-thrombotic syndrome and venous ulceration. Deep vein reflux cannot, however, be the only or even the main cause of post-thrombotic symptoms because many patients with incompetent communicating veins have normal popliteal and femoral veins.

Other investigators[29,96] have tried both these operations and have not found them to be of clinical benefit. Sometimes the bursting pain on walking is relieved for a few months but it soon returns. Oedema is unaffected, and the measurements of calf pump function deteriorate. The only explanation that can be advanced for Bauer's claim that two-thirds of his 136 patients were improved by deep vein ligation must lie in his simultaneous prescription of proper conservative treatment, particularly the use of elastic compression. Linton[71] frequently stated that femoral vein ligation must be followed by permanent elastic support otherwise the operation will fail. *Deep vein ligation should not be practised for the post-thrombotic syndrome.*

In 1964, Psathakis[89] devised an operation in which the tendon of the gracilis muscle was rerouted deep to the popliteal vein so that the vein was occluded when the muscle contracted, making it in effect an external compression valve. Psathakis[90] has also suggested using a plastic cord attached to the muscle in place of the tendon. This operation has not been widely practised as other investigators have reported poor results (e.g. four successes in 46 cases).[53,76] Unless the gracilis contracts and occludes the popliteal vein immediately the calf contraction stops – the time when the reflux begins – the operation cannot work. Such a course of events is most unlikely. Psathakis states that superficial vein and communicating vein incompetence should be treated at the same time as performing the sling operation. It seems likely that these additional procedures produce the clinical improvement.

The preceding paragraphs reveal the clinical importance of communicating vein incompetence even in the presence of extensive deep vein reflux. Although we do not understand the mechanism, far more benefit is achieved by preventing communicating vein reflux than by preventing deep vein reflux. Consequently, if it is thought that concomitant repair of the deep reflux might prevent the recurrence of communicating vein reflux, it should always be considered.

Deep vein obstruction

Any combination of lower limb venous outflow tract thrombosis can occur but there are four common varieties – ilio-femoral, superficial femoral, combined superficial femoral and popliteal and total ilio-femoro-popliteal thrombosis (see Figure 15.9, page 457).

If the diagram of these types of thrombosis is examined, it is apparent that the lesion most suited to treatment by a bypass operation is isolated iliac or ilio-femoral occlusion. Superficial femoral vein obstruction may be bypassed if the popliteal vein has been spared or has recanalized well. Total occlusion of the outflow tract is not amenable to surgical cure.

Iiliac vein obstruction

This can be treated by femoral–caval bypass or by an extra anatomic femoro-femoral bypass (the Palma operation). These operations are described on pages 420–5.

When an isolated ilio-femoral thrombosis occurs, the inferior vena cava and the opposite iliac vein are not affected. The femoral vein below the block is usually healthy but may contain some organized thrombus. Provided the contralateral long saphenous vein is healthy and of good calibre and there is a patent major vein in the groin of the affected side, a Palma operation is possible.[31] The operation should not, however, be performed without first showing that there is a significant rise in femoral vein pressure below the obstructions in response to leg exercise.

When the femoral vein below the obstruction at the site of the anastomosis is abnormal, it is wise to add an arteriovenous fistula because post-thrombotic damage at the site of anastomosis increases the risk of thrombosis. Some surgeons advocate the use of an arteriovenous fistula in all cases.

The long-term (5-year) patency rates for the Palma operation are approximately 75%, with a lower patency when there are post-thrombotic changes in the femoral vein (see Figures 13.13 and 13.14, pages 420 and 421).[58] If the graft remains patent, the patient can expect the symptoms of venous claudication to disappear and oedema to decrease. Skin changes in the leg should also improve but this will depend upon the degree of pre-existing damage in the other deep veins and the communicating veins. The main indication for a Palma operation is venous claudication. The addition of communicating vein ligation depends upon the symptoms, the state of the skin of the lower leg and the phlebographic appearance of the calf veins.

In a busy venous disease clinic the number of patients that might be seen who are suitable for this operation is small. Halliday[58] performed 50 operations between 1965 and 1984, less than three each year. Gruss[48] calculated that less than 2% of patients with the post-thrombotic syndrome are suitable for any type of bypass. Careful selection of patients is critically important, and the surgeon must be certain that it is the iliac obstruction that is the principal cause of the symptoms. The Palma operation is so simple that bypasses between the femoral vein and the vena cava with heterologous vein or prosthetic materials should only be considered when the long saphenous vein of the other leg is unsuitable or there is obstruction in both iliac veins.

Superficial femoral vein obstruction

This can be treated with a popliteal to femoral vein saphenous vein bypass provided the popliteal vein is healthy and draining most of the blood from the calf.[62,105]

All the published series of this operation have been done for post-thrombotic occlusions and the results have been poor (see page 424). May performed 16 of these operations;[75] in three patients immediate graft thrombosis occurred, but in 13 patients an improvement in calf pump function was seen when assessed by foot vein pressure studies. Gruss has performed 12 operations (five patients had a simultaneous Palma operation).[48] Three of the popliteal femoral bypasses thrombosed; in four patients the results of calf function tests deteriorated but in five patients they improved and the symptoms decreased. The combination of these two studies shows that some improvement occurred in 18 out of 28 patients.

When an operation is performed so rarely by experts in the field one must suspect that they doubt its value or find it difficult to decide when to do it. We are sure that both reasons are valid and consider that the difficulty in deciding about the suitability of a patient for this operation lies in the inability of our preoperative tests either to distinguish the relative importance of deep vein obstruction from calf pump inefficiency and communicating vein reflux or to indicate whether the long saphenous vein is already acting as an important collateral channel.

The deterioration of the calf pump function tests in four of the patients operated on by Gruss suggests that the popliteal vein had thrombosed. Such an event might cause a severe deterioration of symptoms and is the principal risk that has deterred us from using this procedure.

As in all cases of post-thrombotic damage, ligation of incompetent communicating veins is likely to produce the most clinical improvement, even though the deep vein damage restricts the duration of the improvement.

PALLIATIVE TREATMENT OF THE POST-THROMBOTIC CALF PUMP FAILURE SYNDROME

The pressure that affects the state and function of the wall of a hollow tube is not solely the pressure within it but the difference between the pressure inside and the pressure outside – the transmural pressure. A high transmural pressure will dilate a vein, venule, or venular capillary, open the inter-endothelial pores, and make the small vessels more permeable.

A high transmural pressure can be reduced by lowering the intraluminal pressure or increasing the extraluminal pressure. All of the reconstructive surgical techniques described above are designed to lower the intraluminal venous pressure, which *pari passu* reduces the transmural pressure. When surgical methods cannot reduce intraluminal pressure, an alternative method of reducing transmural pressure is to increase the extraluminal pressure. This can be done by bandaging, elastic hosiery or pneumatic leggings. External compression is the mainstay of the treatment of the many patients with calf pump failure that cannot be cured by surgery.

Although many of the effects of venous hypertension on the tissues will not regress when the transluminal pressure is reduced, further deterioration can be prevented.

The palliative treatment of the post-thrombotic syndrome therefore has two objectives:

- to reduce the transmural pressure
- to reverse the tissue changes, particularly the interstitial oedema.

Elastic compression

The transmural pressure in the veins of the foot when standing is 90–100 mmHg; at the knee it is 60–70 mmHg and at the groin it is 30–40 mmHg. The pressure applied by an elastic stocking should take account of this gradual reduction of pressure along the limb to avoid overcompressing the veins in the thigh and prevent the stocking acting as a tourniquet.[61,67,73] Modern elastic stockings are designed to apply a known pressure at the ankle which gradually reduces along the length of the leg; this is known as graduated compression. The pressure exerted by a stocking varies according to the tension and content of the elastic material in the stocking and the size and fitting of the stocking.

The pressure in the arteriolar capillaries – when the leg is horizontal – is 40 mmHg; when standing it is 130 mmHg at the ankle but proportionately less higher up the leg.[12] Skin blood flow, when measured with xenon clearance, is reduced by external compression greater than 40 mmHg when the leg is horizontal but is not affected when the leg is vertical until the compression reaches 80 mmHg.[70]

Studies of the skin blood flow beneath an elastic stocking with the patient supine, using laser Doppler fluximetry[1] have shown that compression pressures up to 20 mmHg produce a 33% increase of flux, a 79% median increase of blood cell velocity and 27% decrease in the concentration of moving blood cells. Greater pressures cause a decrease in all measurements. When the leg is dependent, these measurements of blood flow do not begin to decrease until the compression reaches 60 mmHg. These observations confirm the older studies.[70] The laser Doppler flux is greater in limbs with lipodermatosclerosis because of the presence of dilated elongated capillaries and venules but the effect of compression is similar to that seen in normal subjects and patients with uncomplicated varicose veins. The principal cause of the increase in laser Doppler flux is the increase in blood cell velocity. The most logical explanation of these observations is that compression reduces the diameter of the venules and so increases the velocity of flow just as it does in the larger subcutaneous veins.[95] If the rate of blood flow in the capillaries in any way causes the skin changes of the calf pump failure syndrome – perhaps through the activation of white cells – then compression is clearly beneficial.

In a normal limb the foot vein pressure falls from 90 to 30 mmHg during exercise. This is the effect that we wish stockings to mimic. A stocking pressure of 40 mmHg at the ankle reduces the transmural pressure in the lower leg, when standing, to 50 mmHg. This has little effect on the arterial inflow but helps an inefficient calf pump to reduce foot vein pressure to 20–30 mmHg during exercise instead of 60–70 mmHg. The stocking must therefore exert a pressure which has a worthwhile effect on the venous system when the patient is standing or walking without having a deleterious effect on tissue perfusion.[46,86,99] This is difficult to achieve because each patient's requirement is different. A stocking pressure at the ankle of 40 mmHg seems to be the best compromise in patients with the calf pump failure syndrome. A lower pressure may be adequate when the calf pump abnormality is confined to the superficial veins.

Of importance, equal to the reduction of venular transmural pressure, is the effect of external compression on interstitial oedema.

The interstitial spaces consist of cells – fibroblasts and fat cells, plus collagen and elastic fibres between which is free-flowing interstitial fluid and fluid in an interstitial polysaccharide phase bound to hyaluronic acid.[69] Pressures in the subcutaneous interstitial space normally range from –5 to –1 mmHg.

The resistance of the interstitial space to deformation and the resistance to movement of fluid through the space vary according to the fluid content of the space. The interstitial pressure of waterlogged compressible oedematous tissue is greater than 1 mmHg. Tissues with a negative interstitial pressure are relatively 'dry' and incompressible.[49]

Clinically detectable oedema is a feature of advanced calf pump failure but subclinical oedema is present in the skin and subcutaneous tissues of most patients with early or moderate calf pump failure and can be seen as pericapillary halos on capillaroscopy.[38] The widening of the distances between the nutritive capillaries and the cells of the dermis and epidermis must impair their nutrition, especially if that space is filled with abnormal large molecules such as polymerized fibrin. *Reducing oedema is therefore a vital part of the treatment of calf pump failure.*

Nehler *et al.*,[81] using the subcutaneous wick technique, have assessed the effect of external compression on the tissue pressures 1.5 cm below the skin of the perimalleolar area.

The resting pressures in normal subjects, patients with superficial venous incompetence, and patients with chronic venous insufficiency without oedema were all negative (–1.2 to 0.1 mmHg) whereas the

Table 17.1 The effect of external compression on supine perimalleolar subcutaneous tissue pressures

	Tissue pressure, mmHg (SEM)		
Subjects	Resting level	With 20–30 mmHg external compression	With 30–40 mmHg external compression
Normal legs (8)	–0.1 (0.67)	0.6 (0.24)	1.2 (0.54)
Superficial vein incompetence (5)	–1.2 (1.69)	5.7 (1.97)	8.0 (3.9)
Deep vein incompetence without clinically detectable oedema (8)	–0.8 (0.72)	4.2 (1.69)	4.1 (1.6)
Deep vein thrombosis with clinically detectable oedema (8)	4.7 (1.24)	12.9 (2.13)	14.7 (2.6)

Based on Nehler *et al.*[81]

pressure in patients with venous insufficiency with clinically detectable oedema was positive (4.7 mmHg).

The application of 20–30 mmHg external compression had no effect on the tissue pressure of the normal legs whereas the pressure increased in all patient groups but to a highly significant level in those with oedema (Table 17.1).

Increasing the external compression from the 20–30 mmHg range to the 30–40 mmHg range had no significant effect.

The effect of external compression on leg volume and ankle circumference is shown in Figure 17.5. These figures are similar to those of Belcaro[14] who conducted an identical study (Table 17.2).

Thus the application of 20 mmHg external compression directly reduces the capillary and venular transmural pressure by 15–20 mmHg, so reducing vessel distension and the inter-endothelial cell gaps. Both responses reduce capillary permeability and interstitial fluid production and at the same time increase interstitial pressure by 5–15 mmHg. These responses also vary according to the degree of initial oedema. This double effect of stockings, reducing filtration and increasing reabsorption has an immediate clinical effect.

The patient usually notices an immediate reduction of the ache and discomfort in the leg,[1,27] which provides a good clinical indication that the veins are the source of the symptoms. Oedema takes a few days to reduce and rarely goes completely. Varicose veins often become a little smaller but revert to their original size within 24 hours of removing the stocking. It is possible, but unlikely, that some of the valves of incompetent veins become competent while they are compressed. The effect of compression on interstitial fibrinolysis is described later.

At the first consultation graduated elastic compression stockings which give a pressure of at least 30 mmHg at the ankle should be prescribed for all patients with calf pump failure.[41] There is no evidence that stockings that stretch above the knee are of value unless there is marked thigh swelling. Stockings are known to help the calf pump, their effect on the thigh pump has not been studied.

Stockings should be put on before the patient gets out of bed and not removed until bedtime. Two pairs should be prescribed to allow for washing, and they must be replaced every 6 months as frequent washing and wearing causes a loss of elasticity.[93] Most manufacturers make a wide range of garments which will fit most sizes and shapes of leg but the best compression is obtained by made-to-measure stockings based on measurements at six levels.[45] A leg which is an unusual shape always needs a 'made-to-measure' stocking.

Table 17.2 The effect of the enhancement of fibrinolysis by defibrotide on lipodermatosclerosis (LDS)

Treatment	Area of LDS	Leg circumference	tcPO_2	Dilute blood clot lysis time	Symptom score
Elastic stockings for 3 months (16)	–42%	–5.3%	+22%	–17%	–47%
Defribotide plus elastic stockings for 3 months (16)	–18%	–3.5%	+13%	–0.5%	–18%

After Belcaro and Marelli.[14]

Stockings can be worn over dressings but a bulky mass beneath the stocking disturbs its contour and alters its compressive effect (see Chapter 20, page 593). The legs of patients who have ulcers which need frequent dressings are best supported with some form of bandage because ulcer exudate can damage the fibres of a stocking.

Elderly and fat people often have difficulty in reaching their feet and pulling on a tight stocking and may need to be helped by a friend or nurse or use a stocking applicator frame. Some people prefer elastic or impregnated bandages.

Some patients develop allergies to the elastic material, be it rubber, latex or polymer. They first notice an itching and then develop a dermatitis. They should stop using the stocking immediately. An attempt should then be made to discover the cause of the allergy so that stockings without the allergen can be prescribed.

Bandages

A multitude of ribbon-like and tubular bandages are used on patients with calf pump failure. Only those bandages capable of exerting and maintaining compression are worth using.

A heavy elastic bandage is often easier to apply than a stocking to legs of an unusual shape or a leg with an ulcer but it must be applied carefully in a way that will exert an even and, if possible, a graduated compression. Studies of the skill of nurses and doctors at bandaging reveal that this is not such a simple task as it first may seem (see Chapter 20).

Impregnated bandages are designed for use when the patient has an ulcer (Chapter 20, page 579). It is not advisable to use them when the skin is intact (even when there is severe lipodermatosclerosis) except for the occasional elderly patient who cannot put on a stocking or apply a bandage and who may be more comfortable and active when wearing an impregnated bandage renewed every 2 or 3 weeks; the skin must, however, be tolerant of the medicament in the bandage.

The regimen for the use of bandages should be the same as that for the use of stockings; they must be worn whenever the patient is out of bed.

Elevation

Standing still for prolonged periods is the worst thing that a patient with venous disease of the lower limbs can do, as it is the position in which the venous pressure in the lower part of the leg is at its highest. If patients have to stand for long periods, they must exercise their calf muscles by walking, tiptoeing or bracing the knees in order to reduce the venous pressure.

When the legs are above heart level, the venous pressure falls to zero and tissue fluid is absorbed. This relieves the aching pains and reduces the swelling. Patients should raise the foot of their bed on 12 inch (30 cm) blocks and sleep with no more than two pillows so that their legs are above the level of their heart throughout the night. This discipline can produce a marked improvement in symptoms.[55]

During the day the legs should be kept 'up' as much as possible – elevated on a stool when sitting, or on pillows when lying down. If the patient can spend 15–30 minutes in the middle of the day resting with the legs elevated at 90° (legs propped up against a wall with the patient lying on the floor), they will notice a reduction of pain and tightness in the legs during the afternoon. We have had one patient who kept his legs in excellent condition by doing 'bicycling exercises', while standing on his head, assisted by a padded head and shoulder support! Exercise with the legs above heart level is the best physiological way of reducing oedema. Unfortunately, the whole of life cannot be conducted in this position, and the amount of time spent like this depends on the patient's occupation and hobbies!

Massage and passive movements

Gentle but firm massage of the skin and subcutaneous tissues with the fingers and a little bland oil in a centripetal direction together with passive movements of the ankle joint has five effects.

1. It spreads the oedema through the tissues, moving it up the leg to areas where it is more likely to be absorbed.
2. It softens the subcutaneous tissues which makes them respond to the compression of the elastic stocking.
3. It breaks up some of the fibrin deposited in the tissue; this softens the tissues and helps to reduce the fibrous reaction.
4. The oil keeps the skin soft and reduces hyperkeratosis, but the patient must be careful not to make the skin so soft that it is more susceptible to trauma.
5. Moving the ankle reduces the chance of ankle stiffness and ensures that reduced ankle movements do not add to the inefficiency of the calf pump.

Diuretics

Diuretics do not help the oedema of chronic venous hypertension. The patient may notice a slight reduction in swelling after the first course of diuretics but the effect is short-lived.[50,54] Diuretics affect the whole body, not just the swollen limb, and may increase the chance of a deep vein thrombosis or superficial thrombophlebitis if they cause haemo-concentration.[54]

Antibiotics

In the mistaken belief that the redness, heat and tenderness of acute lipodermatosclerosis indicate infection, some practitioners prescribe antibiotics. There is no infection present and antibiotics have no value. The role of antibiotics in the treatment of venous ulceration is discussed in Chapter 20.

Sympathectomy

The skin and subcutaneous tissue changes of calf pump failure are not caused by a reduction of arterial inflow, consequently sympathectomy has no place in the treatment of its symptoms.

Venotonic/oedema reducing drugs

A number of drugs have been shown to increase venous tone and reduce capillary permeability. The drugs are mainly derived from the flavonoids. The most studied are O-(β-hydroxyethyl)-ruto-side[44,52,56,88] and diosmin.[30] These drugs are better known by their many commercial names such as Venoruton, Paroven and Daflon. They have all been shown in experimental animals to increase venous tone[8,74] and/or reduce capillary hyperpermeability[18] but their clinical effect in man is debatable. A number of placebo controlled clinical trials[33,36,82] have shown that these drugs reduce the severity of symptoms such as heaviness, tiredness, tingling, paraesthesiae, restlessness and cramps, but although those treated with the active drug had a better response than those receiving the placebo, some studies had a placebo response of 40–50%.[103]

Such a placebo response in subjective symptoms which are almost impossible to quantify make us extremely doubtful about the clinical value of these drugs. Nevertheless, objective measurements conducted in parallel with the clinical assessments have shown a reduction of oedema, an increase of $tcPo_2$ and an increase of venous tone.[36] It has also been shown that, in the sheep, Daflon increases lymph flow and the frequency of contraction of lymphatics.[79]

Thus, although most clinicians believe that similar and better results may be obtained from a simple elastic stocking,[82] the potential effect of these and similar drugs should not be ignored. Better drugs and better clinical trials are needed before their place in the treatment of calf pump failure can be clearly established. They are likely to

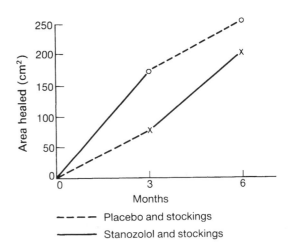

(a)

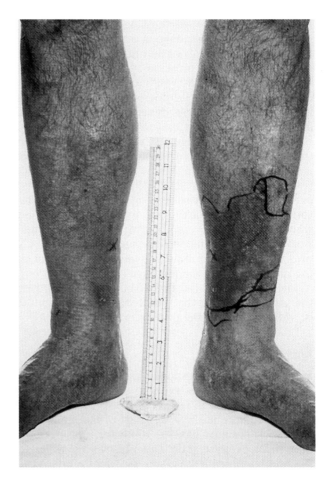

(c)

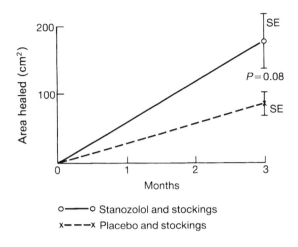

(b)

Figure 17.4 The effect of elastic compression plus placebo and compression plus stanozolol on the healing of lipodermatosclerosis.[22] (a) The areas of lipodermatosclerosis healed in the two groups of our double blind crossover study.[22] (b) The results of the two crossover groups combined. The healing rate of the patients given stanozolol was twice that of those given placebo, a difference that was significant at the 8% level. (c) Before treatment. The area of tenderness and thickening has been outlined and measured. (d) After 3 months of treatment with stanozolol (5 mg b.d.) the tenderness had gone and the area of lipodermatosclerosis had reduced in size. (e) After 6 months, the skin was not red or tender and the pigmentation was significantly less.

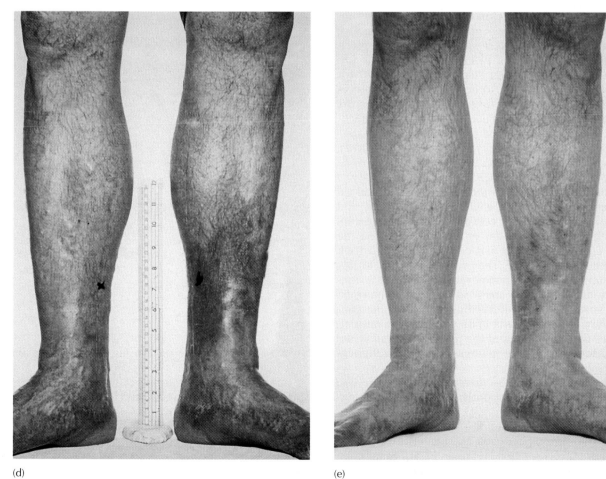

(d)

(e)

have a place in treating patients whose calf pump is beyond surgical repair.

Stimulation of fibrinolysis

If the fibrin barrier/physiological shunt hypothesis (Chapter 15) is correct, removal of the fibrin should improve tissue nutrition.[20,26] We have performed two studies to test this thesis, a pilot study[21] and a double blind crossover trial.[22] In the pilot study, 14 patients with active lipodermatosclerosis secondary to venous insufficiency who had failed to respond to elastic compression and surgical treatment of their varicose veins were given stanozolol for 3 months. Stanozolol, an anabolic steroid, now unfortunately withdrawn from the market because of its misuse by athletes, was at that time the most effective of the few drugs that lower plasma fibrinogen concentration and increase blood fibrinolytic activity.

The blood fibrinolytic activity increased and the plasma fibrinogen fell significantly during treatment. The mean area of lipodermatosclerosis, which had been unaltered for many months before treatment began, fell from 219 cm² to 58 cm². These results encouraged us to undertake a controlled clinical trial. Thirty-four legs of 23 patients with active lipodermatosclerosis were studied. Half were given elastic stockings and a placebo for 3 months followed by stockings and stanozolol 5 mg b.d. for another 3 months. The other half were treated in reverse order (i.e. the active drug was given after the placebo). Leg circumference, leg volume, skin thickness, skin biopsies stained for fibrin, foot vein pressures, routine haematology and liver function tests, plasma fibrinogen, and dilute blood clot lysis time were measured at intervals throughout the study.

The mean area of lipodermatosclerosis reduced in response to both the elastic compression and placebo and the elastic compression and stanozolol but the reduction in the group who received the active drug was twice that of the group who took placebo (Figure 17.4). The probability value of this difference being a chance event was 0.08. It is conventional to consider any *P* value greater than 0.05 as statistically insignificant but in view of the consistency of these results in all patients, the difficulties of measurement and the pilot study results, we considered that these changes were clinically significant.

The difference in the measurements of the two groups over the first 3 months of treatment was statistically significant, *P* = 0.03.

The leg volume and the ankle circumference were significantly reduced by the elastic stockings in the placebo group (Figure 17.5). Stanozolol causes mild water retention which abolished the

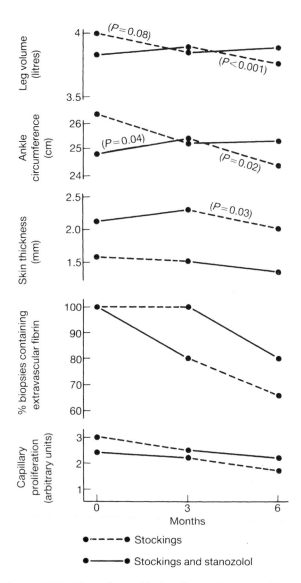

Figure 17.5   The effect of below-knee elastic stockings (with and without stanozolol) on the leg volume, ankle circumference, skin thickness, and extravascular fibrin and capillary proliferation of limbs with lipodermatosclerosis (calf pump failure syndrome). The stockings alone produced significant effects on leg volume, ankle circumference and skin thickness.[22]

effect of the stockings on the leg swelling during treatment with the active drug (Figure 17.5).

Stanozolol produced the expected 50% reduction of dilute blood clot lysis time and 25% reduction of plasma fibrinogen (Figure 17.6).[32] The amount of perivascular fibrin was less in the post-treatment biopsies (Figure 17.5). In this study stanozolol caused no serious side-effects but it may cause headaches, amenorrhoea and virilizing symptoms.

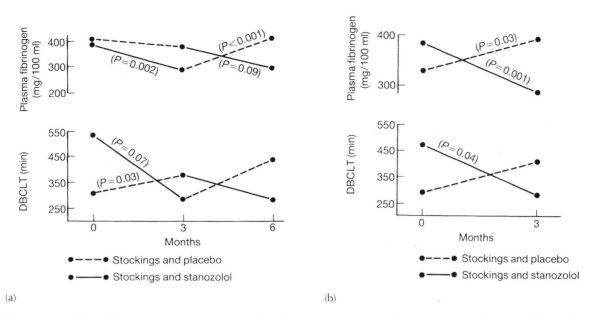

Figure 17.6 The effect of elastic compression plus placebo and compression plus stanozolol on the dilute blood clot lysis time (DBCLT) and plasma fibrinogen.[22] (a) The changes in the blood in the two groups of our double blind crossover study.[22] (b) The changes in the blood of the two crossover groups combined. The stanozolol caused a significant fall in dilute blood clot lysis time (DBCLT) and plasma fibrinogen. The levels reverted to pretreatment values within 3 months of stopping the stanozolol (a).

Groenewald[47] also found that the induration of lipodermatosclerosis improved in 17 of 22 patients given stanozolol compared with nine of 22 patients given placebo, and discoloration improved in 16 of 22 patients given the active drug compared to eight of 22 patients given a placebo.

The pain and tenderness in the affected area settles in 2–5 weeks. After 3 months the redness, heat and induration begin to go, and in many of our patients a 9-month course of treatment (including good quality stockings) caused the skin to return to normal, including a reduction of skin pigmentation.

Twenty of the patients in our 1976 trial were assessed in 1982,[25] 6 years after treatment; 13 of these patients had had frequent recurrent ulceration before entering the trial. All patients but one were still using elastic compression. Nineteen patients thought that their skin was better than it was in 1976. Two patients had had recurrent episodes of ulceration throughout the 5 years. Four of the patients who said that their skin had improved had had one short period of ulceration lasting less than 3 months

One patient had died. Thirteen patients had had no further ulceration. These long-term results suggest that the incidence of recurrent ulceration was reduced, but this needs further clinical evaluation.

Stanozolol has three effects: it is mildly androgenic, it stimulates fibrinolysis and reduces plasma fibrinogen, and is a weak steroid. It is possible that the latter property, which might be mildly anti-inflammatory, might be responsible for the reduction of pain but, as there are not that many inflammatory cells in lipodermatosclerotic tissues, this is unlikely. It is difficult to perceive how the androgenic properties would help the skin and so we are left with the conclusion that the beneficial effect of stanozolol comes from the stimulation of defective fibrinolysis. This would fit and support our hypothesis but the problem needs to be studied further; more investigations of the treatment of active lipodermatosclerosis and studies on the chronic, non-painful, 'burnt-out' variety are required.

If a patient is resistant to stanozolol, a similar effect on fibrinolysis may be obtained with ethyloestrenol and phenformin.[39,64]

Defibrotide is another drug that has profibrinolytic activity[13,104] whose value in the treatment of lipodermatosclerosis has been examined by Belcaro and Marelli.[14] They measured the effect of defibrotide with elastic compression and elastic compression alone on the area of lipodermatosclerosis, leg circumference, laser Doppler fluximetry, microangiopathy, capillary permeability and symptoms and signs in a crossover study similar to ours.[22]

Their results were remarkably similar to ours. Three months of treatment with defibrotide reduced the area of lipodermatosclerosis by 42% whereas elastic stockings only produced an 18% reduction. When the two crossover groups were combined, the overall effect of the drug was a 41% reduction; the stockings caused a 12% reduction. We did not include any patients with active ulceration in our study; Belcaro[14] showed a 96% reduction in ulcer size in patients taking defibrotide and using stockings compared with a 19% reduction in those using stockings alone. Leg circumference reduction was enhanced by the defibrotide as were the measurements of skin blood flow. Defibrotide reduced plasma fibrinogen levels by approximately 20% and decreased the dilute blood clot lysis time.

These results are summarized in Table 17.2. Together with our studies with stanozolol they strongly suggest the potential value of seeking more effective ways of stimulating natural fibrinolysis as a way of preventing the tissue damage caused by prolonged calf pump failure. It has been claimed that elastic compression helps stimulate the release of endothelial activators of fibrinolysis. We examined this hypothesis some years ago when studying the effect of external compression on deep vein thrombosis but could not confirm it (see Chapter 11).

Berridge *et al.*[16] measured the post-occlusion euglobulin lysis times of blood from the arms and the legs and, although confirming a greater fibrinolytic potential in the arm, could find no evidence of potentiation of fibrinolysis by external compression worn for up to 3 months. It seems that elastic stockings work through their effect on oedema and transmural pressure, not by stimulating endothelial cells to release plasminogen activator.

Surgical excision of damaged skin

It is sometimes worthwhile excising and replacing skin which has become scarred, hyperpigmented and hyperkeratotic with split skin grafts. This operation also divides and ligates all the communicating veins. It is rarely indicated when there has not been recurrent ulceration but sometimes non-ulcerated skin and subcutaneous tissues become so painful and tender that the patient begs for something to be done and excision may be the only answer. The surgeon's natural inclination to preserve adjacent moderately good looking skin should be resisted; if not, the patient will complain of similar problems in the skin surrounding the graft 2–3 years later.

An alternative to split skin grafting is a cross leg flap or a vascularized free skin flap with arterial and venous microanastomoses. These operations should be reserved for intractable problems in

young adults, usually the result of the combination of compound fractures of the tibia and deep vein thrombosis.

Achilles tendon lengthening

Pain in and around the ankle may cause permanent joint stiffness and a secondary shortening of the Achilles tendon, producing a fixed plantar flexion deformity.

If the joint is not completely fixed, the pain can be relieved and the condition of the skin improved by lengthening the Achilles tendon. It is not always easy to find a patch of healthy skin for the operative incision, and the operation should be preceded by a joint consultation between the vascular and the orthopaedic surgeon.

References

1. Abu-Own A, Shami SK, Chittenden SJ, Farrah J, Scurr JH, Coleridge-Smith PD. Microangiopathy of the skin and the effect of leg compression in patients with chronic venous insufficiency. *J Vasc Surg* 1994; **19:** 1074–83.
2. Ackroyd JS, Browse NL. The investigation and surgery of the post thrombotic syndrome. *J Cardiovasc Surg* 1986; **27:** 5.
3. Akesson H, Brudin L, Cwikiel W, Ohlin P, Plate G. Does the correction of insufficient superficial and perforating veins improve venous function in patients with deep venous insufficiency. *Phlebology* 1990; **5:** 113–23.
4. Allen S. The treatment of chronic venous disorders of the leg. *Practitioner* 1970; **205:** 221.
5. Arnoldi CC. The heredity of venous insufficiency. *Dan Med Bull* 1958; **5:** 169.
6. Arnoldi CC, Haeger K. Ulcus cruris venosum-crux medicorum. *Lakartidningen* 1967; **64:** 149.
7. Ballard MG, Brett GA, Watenpaugh DE, Hargen AP. Intramuscular pressures beneath elastic and inelastic leggings. *Ann Vasc Surg* 1994; **8:** 543–8.
8. Barbe R, Auriel M. Pharmacodynamic properties and therapeutic efficacy of Daflon 500 mg. *Phlebology* 1992; **Suppl 2:** 41–4.
9. Bauer G. Division of the popliteal vein in the treatment of so-called varicose ulceration. *Br Med J* 1950; **2:** 318.
10. Bauer G. Indications for popliteal vein ligation. *J Cardiovasc Surg* 1963; **4:** 18.
11. Bauer G. The aetiology of leg ulcers and their treatment by resection of the popliteal vein. *J Int Chir* 1948; **8:** 937.
12. Beaconsfield P, Ginsberg J. Effect of changes in limb posture on peripheral blood flow. *Circ Res* 1955; **3:** 478.
13. Belcaro G, Legnini M, Gianchetti E, *et al.* Clinical evaluation of defibrotide in the treatment of arter-

ial and venous vascular disease. *Panminerva Med* 1989; **31:** 34–41.

14. Belcaro G, Marelli C. Treatment of venous lipodermatosclerosis and ulceration in venous hypertension by elastic compression and fibrinolytic enhancement with defibrotide. *Phlebology* 1990; **4:** 91–106.

15. Bentley RJ. The obliteration of perforating veins of the leg. *Br J Surg* 1972; **59:** 199.

16. Berridge DC, Westby JC, Makin GS, Hopkinson BR. Do compression stockings potentiate the fibrinolytic capacity of the lower limbs. *Phlebology* 1989; **4:** 161–6.

17. Bertelsen S, Gammelgaard A. Surgical treatment of post-thrombotic leg ulcers. *J Cardiovasc Surg* 1965; **6:** 452.

18. Blumberg S, Clough G, Michel C. Effects of hydroxyethyl rutosides upon the permeability of single capillaries in the frog mesentery. *Br J Pharmacol* 1989; **96:** 913–19.

19. Browse NL. Venous ulceration. *Br Med J* 1983; **286:** 1920.

20. Browse NL, Burnand KG. The cause of venous ulceration. *Lancet* 1982; **2:** 243.

21. Browse NL, Jarrett PEM, Morland M, Burnand KG. The treatment of liposclerosis of the leg by fibrinolytic enhancement: a preliminary report. *Br Med J* 1977; **7:** 434.

22. Burnand KG, Clemenson G, Morland M, Jarrett PEM, Browse NL. Venous lipodermatosclerosis, treatment by fibrinolytic enhancement and elastic compression. *Br Med J* 1980; **280:** 7.

23. Burnand KG, Lea Thomas M, O'Donnell T, Browse NL. Relationship between postphlebitic changes in the deep veins and results of surgical treatment of venous ulcers. *Lancet* 1976; **2:** 936.

24. Burnand KG, O'Donnell TF, Lea Thomas M, Browse NL. The relative importance of incompetent communicating veins in the production of varicose veins and venous ulcers. *Surgery* 1977; **82:** 9.

25. Burnand KG, Pattison M, Browse NL. The results of a course of Stromba treatment on lipodermatosclerosis of skin of the lower leg. A five year follow up. In: Davidson JF, ed. *Progress in Fibrinolysis*, Vol VI. Edinburgh: Churchill Livingstone, 1983; 526.

26. Chilvers AS. *A Study of the Effect of Long Term Stimulation of Fibrinolysis by a Biguanide and an Anabolic Steroid on the Deposition of Fibrin in Arteries.* MCh Thesis, Cambridge University, 1971.

27. Cockett FB. Management of the postphlebitic leg. *Br J Hosp Med* 1971; **6:** 767.

28. Cockett FB, Elgan Jones DE. The ankle blow out syndrome. *Lancet* 1953; **1:** 17.

29. Cristian V. Resection of the superficial femoral vein in the treatment of post-phlebitic syndrome. Renewal of therapeutic interest. *Phlebologie* 1974; **27:** 103.

30. Daflon. *Phlebology* 1992; **Suppl 2:** 1.

31. Dale WA. Crossover vein grafts for relief of iliofemoral venous block. *Surgery* 1965; **57:** 608.

32. Davidson JF, Lockhead M, McDonald GA, McNichol GP. Fibrinolytic enhancement by stanozolol: a double blind trial. *Br J Haematol* 1972; **22:** 543.

33. Diehm C. The role of oedema protective drugs in the treatment of chronic venous insufficiency. A review. *Phlebography* 1996; **11:** 23–9.

34. Dodd H. The diagnosis and ligation of incompetent perforating veins. *Ann R Coll Surg Engl* 1964; **34:** 186.

35. Dodd H, Cockett FB, eds. *The Pathology and Surgery of the Veins of the Lower Limb.* Edinburgh: Churchill Livingstone, 1956.

36. Dormandy J. 'Venoruton'. *Phlebology* 1990; **5(Suppl):** 1–48.

37. Edwards JM. Shearing operation for incompetent perforating veins. *Br J Surg* 1976; **63:** 885.

38. Fagrell B. Microcirculatory disturbances – the final cause for venous ulcers? *Vasa* 1982; **11:** 101–3.

39. Fearnley GR, Chakrabarti R, Evans JF. Mode of action of phenformin plus ethyloestrenol on fibrinolysis. *Lancet* 1971; **1:** 723–5.

40. Fegan WG. Treatment of varicose veins by injection compression. In: Hobbs JE, ed. *Treatment of Venous Disorders.* Philadelphia, PA: JB Lippincott, 1977.

41. Fentem PH, Goddard M, Gooden BA, Yeung CK. Control of distension of varicose veins achieved by leg bandages as used after sclerotherapy. *Br Med J* 1976; **2:** 725.

42. Ferris EB, Kistner RL. Femoral vein reconstruction in the management of chronic venous insufficiency. *Arch Surg* 1982; **117:** 1571.

43. Field P, Van Boxall P. The role of the Linton flap procedure in the management of stasis dermatitis and ulceration of the lower limb. *Surgery* 1971; **70:** 920.

44. Fitzgerald D. A clinical trial of Froxerutin in venous insufficiency of the lower limb. *Practitioner* 1967; **198:** 406.

45. Gerwen D. *Pressure Gradient Tolerance in Compression Hosiery.* MD Thesis, N.V. Varitex, Haarlem. ISBN 90-9007345-0.

46. Gjöres JE, Thülesius O. Compression treatment in venous insufficiency evaluated with foot volumetry. *Vasa* 1977; **6:** 364.

47. Groenewald J. Communication to the International Vascular Symposium, London. Sept 1981.

48. Gruss JD. The sapheno-popliteal bypass for chronic venous insufficiency. In: Bergan JJ, Yao JST, eds. *Surgery of the Veins.* Orlando, FL: Grune & Stratton, 1985.

49. Guyton AC. Interstitial fluid pressure. II. Pressure–volume curves of the interstitial space. *Circ Res* 1965; **16:** 452-60.

50. Haeger K. Hypostatic oedema. *Zentralbl Phlebol* 1971; **10:** 192.

51. Haeger K. Indications for surgery in ankle perforator insufficiency. *Zentralbl Phlebol* 1969; **8:** 158.

52. Haeger K. The debatable value of flavinoids in venous insufficiency. *Zentralbl Phlebol* 1967; **6:** 526.

53. Haeger K. The treatment of the severe post-thrombotic state. *Angiology* 1968; **19:** 439.

54. Haeger K. The treatment of venous hypostatic oedema and its complications. *Zentralbl Phlebol* 1970; **9:** 23.

55. Haeger K. Treatment of the post thrombotic state in elderly patients. *Zentralbl Phlebol* 1971; **10**: 178.

56. Halborg-Sorenson A, Hansen H. Chronic venous insufficiency treated with hydroxyethylrutosides. *Angiologica* 1970; **7**: 192.

57. Halliday P. The place of subfascial ligation of perforating veins in the treatment of the postphlebitic syndrome. *Br J Surg* 1971; **58**: 104.

58. Halliday P, Harris J, May J. Femoro-femoral crossover grafts. A long term follow-up study. In: Bergan JJ, Yao JST, eds. *Surgery of the Veins.* Orlando, FL: Grune & Stratton, 1985.

59. Hansson LO. Venous ulcers of the lower limb. *Acta Chir Scand* 1964; **128**: 269.

60. Homer J, Fernandes E, Fernandes J, Nicolaides AN. Value of graduated compression stockings in deep venous insufficiency. *Br Med J* 1980; **1**: 820.

61. Homer J, Lowth LC, Nicolaides AN. A pressure profile for elastic stockings. *Br Med J* 1980; **1**: 818.

62. Husni EA. *In situ* sapheno-popliteal bypass graft for incompetence of the femoral and popliteal veins. *Surg Gynecol Obstet* 1970; **130**: 279.

63. Hyde GL, Hull DA. Long term results of subfascial vein ligation for venous stasis disease. *Surg Gynecol Obstet* 1981; **153**: 683.

64. Isacson S, Nilsson IM. Effect of treatment with combined phenformin and ethyloestrenol on the coagulation and fibrinolytic systems. *Scand J Haematol* 1970; **7**: 404–8.

65. Johnson ND, Queral LA, Flinn WR, Yao JST, Bergan JJ. Late objective assessment of venous valve surgery. *Arch Surg* 1981; **116**: 1461.

66. Johnson WC, O'Hara ET, Corey C, Widrich WC, Nabseth DC. Venous stasis ulceration. Effectiveness of subfascial ligation. *Arch Surg* 1985; **120**: 797.

67. Jones NAG, Webb PJ, Rees RI, Kakkar VV. A physiological study of elastic compression stockings in venous disorders of the leg. *Br J Surg* 1980; **67**: 569.

68. Kistner R. Deep venous reconstruction. *Int Angiol* 1985; **4**: 429.

69. Laurent TC. The ultrastructure and physical-chemical properties of interstitial connective tissue. *Pflugers Arch* 1972; **336(Suppl)**: 521–42.

70. Lawrence D, Kakkar VV. Graduated, static, external compression of the lower limb: a physiological assessment. *Br J Surg* 1980; **67**: 119.

71. Linton RR. The communicating veins of the lower limb and the operating technique for their ligation. *Ann Surg* 1938; **107**: 582.

72. Linton RR. The post thrombotic ulceration of the lower extremity: its aetiology and surgical treatment. *Ann Surg* 1953; **138**: 415.

73. Lipmann HI, Briere J-P. Physical basis of external supports in chronic venous insufficiency. *Arch Phys Med Rehabil* 1971; **52**: 555.

74. Markwardt F. Pharmacology of oedema protective drugs. *Phlebology* 1996; **11**: 10–15.

75. May R. Der Femoralis bypass bein postthrombotischen Zustandsbild. *Vasa* 1972; **1**: 267.

76. May R, Nissl R. The post thrombotic syndrome. In: May R, ed. *Surgery of the Veins of the Leg and Pelvis.* Stuttgart: Georg Thieme, 1979.

77. Mayberry JC, Moneta GL, Frang RD, Porter JM. The influence of elastic compression stockings on deep venous insufficiency. *J Vasc Surg* 1991; **13**: 91–100.

78. McEwan AJ, McArdle CS. Effect of hydroxyethylrutosides on blood oxygen levels and venous insufficiency symptoms in varicose veins. *Br Med J* 1971; **1**: 138.

79. McHale NG, Hollywood MA. Control of lymphatic pumping. Interest of Dafron 500 mg. *Phlebology* 1994; **Suppl 1**: 23–5.

80. Negus D, Friedgood A. The effective management of venous ulceration. *Br J Surg* 1983; **70**: 623.

81. Nehler MR, Moneta GL, Woodard BS, *et al.* Perimalleolar subcutaneous tissue pressure effects of elastic compression stockings. *J Vasc Surg* 1993; **18**: 783–8.

82. Neumann HAM, Brock MFB. A comparative clinical trial of graduated compression stockings and *O*-(β hydroxethyl)-rutosides in the treatment of chronic venous insufficiency. *Phlebologie* 1995; **24**: 78–81.

83. Nicolaides AN, Schull K, Fernandes JF, Niles C. Ambulatory venous pressures. New information. In: Nicolaides AN, Yao JST, eds. *Investigation of Vascular Disorders.* New York: Churchill Livingstone, 1981.

84. Nielubowicz J, Szostek M, Staszkiewicz W. Late results of Linton flap operation. *J Cardiovasc Surg* 1977; **18**: 561.

85. O'Donnell TF, Burnand KG, Clemenson G, Lea Thomas M, Browse NL. Doppler examination vs clinical and phlebographic detection of the location of incompetent perforation veins. *Arch Surg* 1977; **112**: 31.

86. O'Donnell TF Jr, Rosenthal DA, Callow AD, Ledig BL. Effect of elastic compression on venous hemodynamics in postphlebitic limbs. *JAMA* 1979; **242**: 2766.

87. Pierson S, Pierson D, Swallow R, Johnson G Jr. Efficacy of graded elastic compression in the lower leg. *JAMA* 1983; **249**: 242.

88. Prerovsky I, Roztocil K, Hlavova A, Koleilat A, Razgova L, Oliva I. The effect of hydroxyethylrutosides after acute and chronic oral administration in patients with venous diseases. *Angiologica* 1972; **9**: 408.

89. Psathakis N. Ein neues operatives verfahren sur rationallen Behandlung des Insuffiziensyndroms der tiefen Beinvenen. *Chirurg* 1964; **35**: 79.

90. Psathakis ND, Psathakis DN. Rationale of the substitute valve operation by technique II in the treatment of chronic venous insufficiency. *Int Angiol* 1985; **4**: 397.

91. Queral N, Whitehouse WM, Flinn WR, Neiman HL, Yao JST, Bergan JJ. Surgical correction of chronic deep venous insufficiency by valvular transposition. *Surgery* 1980; **87**: 688.

92. Quill RD, Fegan WG. Reversibility of femoro-saphenous reflux. *Br J Surg* 1971; **58**: 388.

93. Raj TB, Goddard M, Makin GS. How long do compression bandages maintain their pressure during

ambulatory treatment of varicose veins. *Br J Surg* 1980; **67:** 122.

94. Rose SS. A report on the use of hydroxyethylrutosides in symptoms due to venous back pressure and allied conditions of the lower limb. *Br J Clin Pract* 1970; **24:** 4.

95. Sabri S, Roberts VC, Cotton LT. Effects of externally applied pressure on the haemodynamics of the lower limb. *Br Med J* 1971; **3:** 503–8.

96. Sanberg I, Haeger K. The value of deep venous resection (Bauer's popliteal resection) for deep venous insufficiency. *Acta Chir Scand* 1966; **131:** 50.

97. Schanzer H, Peirce EC II. A rational approach to surgery of the chronic venous stasis syndrome. *Ann Surg* 1982; **195:** 25.

98. Silver D, Gleysteen JJ, Rhodes GR. Surgical treatment of the refectory post phlebitic ulcer. *Arch Surg* 1971; **103:** 554.

99. Somerville JJF, Brow GO, Byrne PJ, Quill RD, Fegan WG. The effect of elastic stockings on superficial venous pressures in patients with venous insufficiency. *Br J Surg* 1974; **61:** 979.

100. Stemmer R. Ambulatory elastocompressive treatment of the lower extremities particularly with elastic stockings. *Z Arztl Fortbild (Jena)* 1969; **63:** 1.

101. Taheri SA, Heffner R, Meenaghan MA, Budd T, Pollack LH. Vein valve transplantation. *Int Angiol* 1985; **4:** 425.

102. Taheri SA, Lasar L, Elias SM. Surgical treatment of post phlebitic syndrome. *Br J Surg* 1982; **69(Suppl):** 59.

103. Tsonderos Y. Efficacy of Daflon 500 mg in the treatment of chronic venous insufficiency. *Phlebology* 1992; **Suppl 2:** 42–5.

104. Verstraete M. Prevention of thrombosis in arteries: novel approaches. *J Cardiovasc Pharmacol* 1985; **7(Suppl 3):** S191–205.

105. Warren R, Thayer TR. Transplantation of the saphenous vein for post-phlebitic stasis. *Surgery* 1954; **35:** 867.

106. Wheeler HB, Anderson FA. The diagnosis of venous thrombosis by impedance plethysmography. In: Bernstein EF, ed. *Non-invasive Diagnostic Techniques in Vascular Disease.* St Louis, MO: CV Mosby, 1985.

107. Widmer LK. *Peripheral Venous Disorders.* Bern: Hans Huber, 1978.

108. Wismer R. The actions of tri-hydroxyethylrutoside on the permeability of the capillaries in man. *Praxis* 1963; **52:** 1412.

CHAPTER 18

Venous ulceration: pathology

Prevalence and incidence of venous ulceration	505	The pathology of a venous ulcer	521
Aetiology of venous ulceration	508	References	525

Definition

A venous ulcer of the lower limb is a solution of the continuity of the skin caused by an abnormality of the veins draining the limb. There is no single venous abnormality that is always associated with ulceration, and most of the pathological changes in the skin and ulcer base are non-specific.[62,137,153] A venous ulcer is usually situated in the 'gaiter' region of the leg (the lower third between the ankle joint and the swelling of the calf muscle) and is invariably surrounded by thickened, pigmented and fibrotic skin which we have called lipodermatosclerosis (see Chapter 16).[25,26,32]

'Varicose ulcer', 'gravitational ulcer', 'stasis ulcer' and 'hypostatic ulcer' have been used in the past as alternative names for venous ulcers. All these terms are semantically incorrect and should be abandoned.

Prevalence and incidence of venous ulceration

It is difficult to obtain accurate figures of the prevalence of venous leg ulcers because the diagnosis is so imprecise. A number of epidemiological surveys have, however, now been carried out in a variety of countries and though these all have certain deficiencies, they provide relatively uniform results.

In 1931, Dickson Wright[57] suggested that a quarter of a million patients in the United Kingdom had leg ulcers (a prevalence of 0.5%), but the means by which this figure was obtained were not given. Linton[106] took Dickson Wright's figures and extrapolated them to the USA, to produce an estimate of between 300 000 and 400 000 patients with venous ulcers in North America.

Lockhart-Mummery and Smitham[109] used Bauer's figures from Denmark[7] (which, incidentally, he derived from Roholm and it is not known how Roholm obtained his data) to estimate that there were at any one time between 100 000 and 200 000 patients with 'varicose ulcers' in England and Wales, a prevalence of 0.25–0.5%.

Boyd et al.,[21] from their experience of patients with leg ulcers referred to hospitals in the Manchester region, estimated that 5/1000 of the population were affected; surprisingly this is an identical figure to that of Dickson Wright. Hellgren[82] in Sweden found, however, that only approximately 3000 men and 15 000 women had ulceration of the leg in a population of 7.5 million (a prevalence of less than 0.1%). Bobek et al.,[18] found a much higher incidence of approximately 1%, but obtained their data from subjects with evidence of venous disease.

Widmer and his co-workers[170,171] investigated the prevalence of venous and arterial disease in 4376 workers in the Basle chemical industry. They found that 1.3% of this cohort had suffered or currently suffered from leg ulceration – 1.1% of the men and 1.4% of the women.

Ruckley's group carried out an important survey[36,37,136] on leg ulceration in the West Lothian and Forth Valley regions of Scotland, based on patients located through a postal survey of district nurses, physiotherapists, general practitioners, long-stay hospitals and hospital outpatients during a defined period. They found just under 1500 patients with ulcers in a population of approximately 1 million (a point prevalence of 0.15%). Even in this well conducted study, however, the numbers of true venous ulcers are difficult to obtain, as it was only possible to investigate and confirm the diagnosis in a cohort of subjects. Patients with ulcers not under the care of nurses or doctors went undetected. The investigations that were performed on the sample population were clinical tests and Doppler ultrasound arterial ankle pressure measurements. Even this group of well investigated subjects did not have any tests of calf pump function or studies of venous anatomy with duplex ultrasound or phlebography. The diagnosis of venous ulceration was therefore based on 'typical clinical appearances' and an absence of another cause for the ulceration.

A similar study of a defined population in northwest London by Lewis and Cornwall[46] was also based on patients obtained through general practitioners, district nurses and residential homes. They detected 357 patients with 424 leg ulcers in a population of approximately 200 000 (giving a point prevalence of 0.18%). In this survey an attempt was made to differentiate the patients with venous disease and ulcers by the use of non-invasive techniques of venous investigation on a sample of 100 patients with 117 ulcerated limbs. Venous disease was assessed by continuous wave ultrasound and by photoplethysmography (see Chapter 4). The other 257 patients were not formally examined.

Sixty-three of the 117 ulcerated limbs had evidence of venous disease alone, 36 had signs of superficial venous incompetence and 27 had superficial and deep vein incompetence. Another 132 limbs had abnormal calf pump function and Doppler evidence of venous reflux, but they also had evidence of ischaemia, defined by a reduced arterial ankle pressure index (less than 0.9). Fourteen of these 32 'ischaemic' limbs had evidence of superficial venous incompetence and 18 had signs of coexisting deep vein incompetence. Twelve of the ulcerated limbs had no evidence of any venous abnormality but had a reduced ankle pressure index indicative of arterial ischaemia, and in 10 limbs with ulcers all the tests proved normal. This study suggests that 80% of all leg ulcers have some evidence of venous disease within the affected limb but this is combined with arterial disease in nearly a third.

Since the first edition of this book we are aware of two other important epidemiological studies on the prevalence of venous ulcers. Baker, Stacey *et al.*, working in Western Australia,[6] used similar methods to the Lothian study and found very similar results.

A more ambitious project, the Swedish Ulcer Survey,[127,128] was again based on a postal questionnaire which was sent out to 12 000 randomly selected inhabitants between the ages of 59 and 89 in two regions of Sweden. The response rate was excellent at 91% although the questionnaire was only sent to 7% of the total population within the age interval. Open ulcers were reported by 306 subjects and 143 (47%) were subsequently examined.[127] Only 82 of these were found to have ulceration, giving a high false-positivity rate (43%). The point prevalence estimated from these findings was 0.63 (95% confidence interval 0.54–6.72). The overall prevalence was estimated at 2% rather than the 1% expected from previous studies. This implies that many patients with ulcers carry out self-care and has led to a considerable underestimation of the problem in previous surveys. Venous disease still caused the largest proportion of leg ulcers – 50% (including mixed venous and arterial) – while arterial disease was responsible for 21%. This survey also found that 13% of ulcers were caused by diabetes, 3% by trauma and 9% were decubitus (pressure induced). The rest were largely multifactorial or unclassifiable. Most of the false-positive results were caused by patient misdiagnosis of skin disorders such as eczema.

Comment

As no venous or arterial abnormality could be found in 10 of the ulcerated limbs investigated by Cornwall and Lewis[46] (all tests were normal), and a small proportion of the other studies, it is reasonable to maintain a sceptical attitude to all the published figures of the incidence of 'venous ulceration'.

Nevertheless, on the basis of the two British surveys[37,46] and the western Australian survey,[6] at least 1% of the population have, or have had leg ulceration, with perhaps a quarter of this figure (0.25%) having active ulceration at any one time. The Swedish data[128] suggests that this is a considerable underestimation and the figure is closer to 2%. Between 50 and 75% of all leg ulcers are associated with venous disease. The incidence increases with age[37,46] and is greater in the female population (nearly 3:1, women:men). It also increases if arterial disease or rheumatoid arthritis develops.[36] Venous ulceration appears to be common in all countries and does not appear to have any definite racial predilection.

Incidence of superficial vein incompetence, deep vein incompetence and calf communicating vein incompetence in the genesis of venous ulceration

This has been discussed in Chapter 15, but those studies which have specifically attempted to evaluate the role of these three main sites of valvular incompetence in the genesis of venous ulceration are discussed again here.

Table 18.1   Incidence of post-thrombotic ulceration

Authors	Method of diagnosis	No. of ulcerated limbs	No. of post-thrombotic limbs	% of post-thrombotic limbs
Birger[10]	History	432	173	40
Bauer[7]	Ascending phlebography	38	34	87
deTakats and Graupner[55]	History			
	Ascending phlebography	100	46	46
Anning[3]	History	1026	738	75
Cockett[42]	History			
	Clinical signs	182	38	20
Arnoldi and Haegar[4]	Ascending phlebography	1092	486	45
Burnand et al.[29]	Ascending phlebography	41	23	55
Negus and Friedgood[125]	Ascending phlebography Doppler ultrasound			
	Photoplethysmography	109	44	40
Sethia and Darke[148]	Ascending and descending phlebography	60	20	33
Cornwall and Lewis[46]	Photoplethysmography			
	Ultrasound	99	45	46
Shami et al.[149]	Duplex ultrasound	79	37	47
Nicolaides et al.[129]	Duplex ultrasound	83	42	51

Estimates of the incidence of post-thrombotic damage and superficial venous incompetence as a cause of venous ulceration vary considerably between hospitals and between countries.[9,29,107,125,149,158] These estimates also depend upon the method used to assess deep vein damage (see Chapters 4 and 16) and upon the skill of the clinician examining the superficial veins. The methods that have been used to assess incompetence of the calf communicating veins (which have already been discussed in Chapters 4 and 6) are known to be inaccurate and open to individual interpretation.

Table 18.1 shows the incidence of past deep vein thrombosis or evidence of a deep vein abnormality (valvular incompetence or post-thrombotic changes) which has been reported in patients with venous ulcers.[129,149] The methods used to make the diagnosis of post-thrombotic limb are also shown. Two recent studies using duplex scanning to assess the deep veins both showed that nearly half the venous ulcers were associated with deep venous reflux.[129,149]

A past history of thrombosis can be obtained from at least 20% of all patients with venous ulcers, and 'objective tests' of deep vein function or anatomy double this figure. Between 40 and 50% of the patients with venous ulcers therefore have objective evidence of post-thrombotic damage, though this figure varies considerably in different studies.[29,125,129,149,158]

Table 18.2 shows the incidence of incompetence of the calf communicating veins in patients with venous ulceration. These figures must be viewed

Table 18.2   Incidence of lower leg communicating vein incompetence in limbs with venous ulcers

	Techniques	Limbs	Incompetent communicating veins	
			No.	%
Dodd and Cockett[59]	Operative exploration	135	96	71
Thomas et al.[158]	Operative exploration	44	43	99
Sethia and Darke[148]	Operative exploration	60	59	99
Hoare et el.[86]	Ultrasound	80	71	88
Negus[126]	Operative exploration	109	108	99
Haeger[73]	Operative exploration	54	54	100
Arnoldi and Haeger[4]	Operative exploration	509	509	100

with some scepticism because of the inaccuracy of the methods used to assess incompetence of the calf communicating veins. They do suggest, however, that incompetence of these veins is usually present in limbs with venous ulceration.

Comment

Haegar[73] has stated that the calf communicating veins are always incompetent in limbs with venous ulceration, and saphenous vein incompetence on its own can never cause venous ulceration. We do not believe that this dogma is correct, as the words 'never' and 'always' rarely apply to biological phenomena; in general, however, venous ulceration is uncommon in limbs with pure saphenous vein incompetence.[86]

Whereas it is true that incompetence of the calf communicating veins is found in 'most' limbs with venous ulcers, it is equally true that this abnormality often coexists with superficial (saphenous) vein incompetence and with post-thrombotic damage of the deep veins, in limbs without ulcers. We need to know much more about the normal and abnormal physiology of the communicating veins.

Aetiology of venous ulceration

CALF PUMP DYSFUNCTION

The first appreciation of the association between varicose veins and venous ulceration is attributed to Hippocrates (460–377 BC). In Adam's translation of the ancient Greek book *De Ulceribus*, Hippocrates (or members of his School) stated

when the points adjoining to an ulcer are inflamed, the ulcer is not disposed to heal until the inflammation subside, nor when the surrounding parts are blackened by mortification, nor when a varix occasioned an overflow of blood in the part, is the ulcer disposed to heal, unless you bring the surrounding parts into a healthy condition.

The association between varicose veins and venous ulcers became clearly established in the sixteenth and seventeenth centuries[79,172] and a number of authors in the early nineteenth century[24,45,49,85,88,91,95] stressed the importance of varicose veins in the aetiology of leg ulceration.

In 1867, John Gay[70] gave two Lettsonian lectures entitled *On varicose discolouration, induration and ulcer*. In these lectures he recorded the findings of the dissections he had made in 24 cadavers with clinical evidence of venous disease of the leg. He stated that the relatively small number of observations make his conclusions of 'doubtful validity' and

regarded his work as a 'pioneering party' – presumably what we would now call a 'pilot study'.

In nine of the limbs he found simple external varicosities around normal skin, but in 10 limbs the varicosities were associated with discoloration of the skin and ulceration, and in one limb there were varicosities, ulceration and skin induration but no discoloration (i.e. nine legs had simple uncomplicated varicose veins and in 11 legs varicose veins were complicated by lipodermatosclerosis). He noted that the worst varicosities were often not associated with skin changes and, conversely, some of the worse skin changes were found in limbs with the least varicosities. These findings caused him to question the accepted association between varicose veins and ulceration. He went on to show that coagula (presumably new and old thrombi) were present in the short saphenous veins of three patients and in the deep veins of six of the nine patients with the cutaneous changes of lipodermatosclerosis (bronzing and induration of the skin with or without ulcers). Interestingly, some arterial disease was present in six of the limbs.

Gay states 'ulceration is not a direct consequence of varicosity but of other conditions of the venous system with which varicosity is not infrequently a complication, but without which neither of the allied skin conditions is met with'.

The presence of communicating veins between the deep and superficial compartments of the calf was probably first described by Verneuil[165] who stated that 'deep varices are more common than subcutaneous varices'. He drew the following inferences from 21 dissections:

the primitive seat of phlebectasy resides in the deep veins. These first suffer dilatation for reasons which anatomy and physiology render imperative; and from there it passes to the subcutaneous veins. The extension takes place by various anatomical channels which exist between the superficial and deep veins. I affirm that if you find in any part of the limb, a spot ever so limited in which the superficial veins are serpentine, if you trace them with care you will find that they communicate by large tracts with the deep or intramuscular branches.

Gay[70] confirmed the findings of Verneuil[165] in his cadaver dissections and drew particular attention to the communicating veins of the medial calf which he called 'perforating veins'. These are well shown in a number of illustrations which accompany the text (see Chapter 1, Figures 1.11–1.14). He also reported a series of experiments to look at the venous return in cadavers, and in a dog model after the femoral vein had been ligated. He concluded that 'obstruction of the femoral vein is followed by saphenous repletion, repletion of the intercommunicating veins, and capillary cutaneous injection'. He regarded the communicating veins as an alternative means for venous return.

A specific role for incompetence of the valves in the communicating veins of the calf (the perforating veins of Gay) in the genesis of ulceration was first suggested by John Homans in 1918[90] who, apparently ignorant of Gay's work, recognized two varieties of ulcer – the first associated with surface varices and the second associated with surface varices complicated by varicosity of the ankle communicating veins including post-thrombotic varices. He suggested that the location of ulceration in the gaiter region was the result of the location of the medial calf communicating veins in the gaiter region of the leg. He then subdivided incompetence of the communicating veins into those associated with and presumably caused by the varicose process, and those secondary to a thrombosis. He believed that the latter 'develop as an overflow or safety vent from the deep veins'.

In his conclusions based on a series of illustrated cases he states the following.

1. Varicose ulcers take origin in profound nutritional disturbances attributable to varicose veins (influenced by trauma, infection and surface stasis).
2. Varicose ulcers arising from surface varicosities are generally healed by adequate removal of varicose veins.
3. Varicose ulcers dependent upon a post-phlebitic varix are always intractable to palliative treatment, generally incurable by the removal of varicose veins alone and must be excised to be cured.

Homan's hypothesis of two causes of incompetence of the communicating veins remains valid. Phlebographic studies have confirmed that there are certainly two groups of patients with incompetence of the communicating veins – those who have no phlebographic evidence of past deep vein thrombosis and those with post-thrombotic damage (Figure 17.3).[4,7,29,52,73]

Calf pump function in limbs with incompetent calf communicating veins with phlebographically normal deep veins is often just as poor as in those limbs with unequivocal evidence of deep vein damage.[30] Furthermore, the function of the calf pump cannot be restored to normal by ligating the communicating veins even in limbs with apparently normal deep veins, which suggests, providing our tests are accurate, that there is subtle damage to the deep veins which is undetectable by phlebography. This is now being confirmed by duplex scanning.[100] It is conceivable that post-thrombotic damage may be responsible for all the valvular changes within the communicating veins but this is unlikely and a dual aetiology, from varicose veins or deep vein thrombosis remains a teleologically more attractive hypothesis.

The role of incompetence of the calf communicating veins in the genesis of ulceration has been amplified by Turner Warwick,[162] Linton[106–108] and Cockett.[41–43] These authors have all observed that saphenous vein incompetence, incompetence of the calf communicating veins and post-thrombotic damage commonly coexist, and it has proved difficult to unravel which of these mechanisms is dominant in ulcer development. The Linton and Cockett schools have argued[4,5,48,65,125,126,158] that incompetence of the calf communicating veins must be present before ulceration can occur.

The pressure flow studies of Bjordal[11–15] have cast doubt on the importance of the communicating veins in affecting calf pump function, but unfortunately have never been repeated or confirmed. Bjordal showed that reflux through the ankle communicating veins has only a minor adverse effect on calf pump function compared with the effect of saphenous vein incompetence. We also found that ligation of the medial calf communicating veins produced a relatively small improvement in the function of the calf pump, whereas the surgical abolition of saphenous reflux almost always returns the calf pump function to the normal range.[30] The fact that correcting the superficial reflux has the greatest effect on our measurement of calf pump function does not, however, mean that superficial reflux is the cause of the ulceration.[144] The reduction in the local superficial venous pressure produced by abolishing reflux through the calf communicating veins may be more important than producing an overall improvement in calf pump function, and rates of pressure change may be more important than absolute or mean levels. The effects of incompetence in the superficial and lower leg communicating veins are probably complementary.

Comment

By definition, a venous ulcer cannot exist in the presence of normal calf pump function but confusion (fuelled by inadequate methods of investigation) still exists as to which of the three main venous abnormalities is responsible for, or is the most important cause of, a venous ulcer. All three are anatomical sites of incompetence (deep vein damage, lower leg communicating vein incompetence and saphenous incompetence) and can and, in many limbs, do coexist. At the same time there are certainly some limbs with ulcers in which the calf communicating veins are not incompetent.[37,86,100]

Several papers have shown that the diagnosis of simple long saphenous vein incompetence is often inaccurate even when duplex ultrasound is used;[31,118] this makes the crude intraoperative assessment of lower leg communicating vein incompetence even more suspect. If we cannot diagnose the physiological abnormality correctly, we will never be able to assess its importance.

In view of these difficulties it is, at present, impossible to determine which site of valvular incompetence is of major or sole importance. There is some evidence that the role of communicating vein incompetence in the genesis of ulceration has been overstressed. This has partly stemmed from general dissatisfaction with the results of lower leg communicating vein ligation in preventing recurrent ulceration in the post-thrombotic limb,[29,107,108] even though there are many studies which show that this operation is very effective in limbs without post-thrombotic damage.[22,53,54,125,148,156,158] In recent years a greater emphasis has been attached to deep vein obstruction and reflux in the genesis of ulceration, and this has led to the development of surgical techniques to reconstruct, repair, or transplant valves into incompetent veins,[97,98,135,166] or techniques to bypass occluded segments,[51,116,167] but there is little evidence that this type of surgery is any more effective than ligation of the communicating veins in preventing the recurrence of post-thrombotic ulceration[131] (see Chapters 12, 13 and 17).

Most patients with uncomplicated and isolated long saphenous vein incompetence do not develop venous ulceration but there is little doubt that there exists a small group of patients without evidence of lower leg communicating vein incompetence who do get ulcers.[87] Nevertheless, the majority of patients with venous ulcers do have incompetent communicating veins.

The relative importance of each site of valvular incompetence will only be identified when random cohorts of patients with healed ulcers are treated by ligation of the communicating veins in isolation and the results compared with those of other groups treated by saphenous vein surgery alone and deep vein repair alone. These studies have still not been carried out, but the development of endoscopic perforator surgery may enable surgeons to correct this major gap in our knowledge.

A defective calf pump is essential to the development of ulceration, but it is not known if there is a critical level of increased ambulatory pressure that will always lead to ulceration, or if the development of lipodermatosclerosis is related to a certain time span of abnormal pressure, Nicolaides *et al.*[129] suggest that ulceration is rare if the venous pressure drops below 30 mmHg during exercise but common if it stays above 50 mmHg. We do not still know if an ambulatory pressure in the superficial veins that is always above 50 mmHg will inevitably lead to ulceration, if elastic compression is not worn. Large scale prospective clinical natural history studies are required to answer this type of question. Ruckley's group[22] have suggested that popliteal valvular incompetence is the major factor in venous ulcers but this has not been studied prospectively.

It may be that the genesis of lipodermatosclerosis and ulceration is a product of the level of venous pressure and the time that the tissues are exposed to this high pressure. Perhaps skin changes and ulceration develop rapidly in tissues exposed to high pressures, while lower absolute pressures only produce damage after prolonged exposure. We do not know if a constant high pressure is more harmful or less harmful than short episodes of very high pressure. We do not even know whether the absolute amount, type or persistence of the pressure matter at all! Perhaps it is the tissue reaction to the pressure that matters – sensitive tissues responding to minor changes, insensitive tissues withstanding gross changes. All these questions remain to be answered by properly planned prospective human surgical research. These questions have not yet been answered in the 10 years since the first edition of this book.

CHANGES IN THE MICROCIRCULATION AND TISSUE ANOXIA

The mechanism by which calf pump failure causes lipodermatosclerosis and ulceration is just as poorly understood as the type of venous lesion which is responsible for pump failure. Several theories have been proposed to explain how a disordered calf pump causes tissue death (Figure 18.1):

- Stasis within the cutaneous microcirculation
- The opening of arteriovenous shunts
- An interstitial barrier
- White cell blocking (trapping)
- Free radical damage
- Growth factor blockade
- Simple vasoconstriction

All these theories assume that these changes are secondary to the calf pump failure but even that assumption is debatable.

Capillary and venular stasis

Homans[90] was the first person to suggest that defective venous return from the lower limb, caused by post-thrombotic deep vein damage or varicose veins, might result in 'venous stasis'. He thought that the resulting stagnant anoxia was responsible for the tissue death seen as cutaneous ulceration. This theory has been repeated and accepted in countless publications on venous ulceration, though the concept of 'stasis' has been discredited by measurements of the

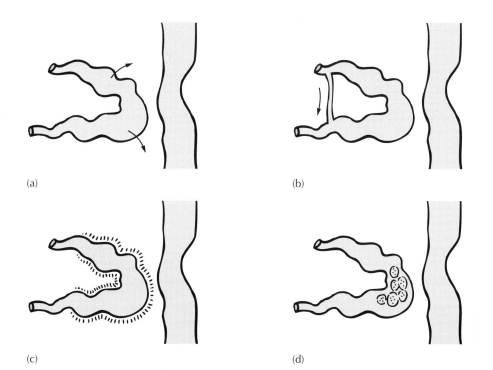

Figure 18.1 A diagrammatic representation of the four 'theories' of ulcer development. (a) Pressure and stasis. This theory postulates that the high venous pressure and slow venous blood flow of calf pump failure cause stagnant anoxia and/or pressure necrosis of the overlying skin. (b) Arteriovenous shunts. This theory postulates that arteriovenous shunts open up in the dermal capillary bed as a result of a persistently high venous pressure. These shunts, by diverting oxygenated blood away from the overlying skin, cause skin ischaemia and ulceration. (c) The fibrin diffusion block. This theory postulates that the high venous pressure present during exercise in the calf pump failure syndrome is transmitted back to the capillary bed which distends and elongates. The inter-endothelial pores enlarge, allowing large molecules, including fibrinogen, to escape into the tissues where an associated reduction in fibrinolytic capacity is thought to enable polymerization of fibrin to occur unimpeded. The pericapillary fibrin then acts as a diffusion barrier or interferes with local tissue metabolism. The eventual cause of ulceration is the reduced skin oxygenation caused by the diffusion barrier. (d) White cell trapping and activation. This theory postulates that white cells become both trapped and activated in the venular capillaries when there is capillary hypertension, so impeding the circulation, damaging the endothelium and causing an inflammatory reaction, all of which damages the surrounding tissues and leads to tissue death.

oxygen content of the venous and capillary blood and in the tissues of ulcerated limbs.

The first study which described the oxygen content of venous blood[56] reported that the venous blood oxygen content was lower in blood sampled from a varicose vein than in samples taken from the antecubital vein of the same patient. One year later, however, Blalock[16] repeated these studies and found conflicting results. He showed that the oxygen content of femoral venous blood was highest during recumbency and declined rapidly when the patient stood. He considered that differences in posture at the time of sampling could account for the conflicting results of these two studies. He also showed that the oxygen content of the femoral venous blood was higher in a limb with

varicose veins than its normal counterpart and that this difference was accentuated when ulceration was present. Blalock concluded that his findings suggested that the total blood flow through limbs with venous ulceration was increased.

A number of subsequent studies have confirmed Blalock's findings,[17,64,89,133] and only one study[117] has been contradictory. There is therefore little doubt that the venous blood leaving an ulcerated limb has a normal or high oxygen content.

The blood flow in ulcerated limbs has also been measured. Dye injected into the femoral artery appears more rapidly in the veins of the patients with ulcerated limbs than in normal 'controls'[76,77,133,166] and plethysmographic studies have also shown an increased blood flow in ulcerated limbs.[1]

The development of transcutaneous oxygen electrodes, which measure oxygen diffusion across the skin, has enabled the tissue oxygen in lipodermatosclerotic skin to be measured and compared with that in control sites. Using a probe heated to 45°C, it has been shown that the tissue oxygen concentration is reduced in areas of lipodermatosclerosis.[40,113,153]

Dodd et al.,[60] using an unheated probe over the anterior tibial compartment, found higher oxygen tensions in patients with active or past venous ulceration. The strange siting of the electrode and the small number of patients included in this study make it difficult to assess. Others, using laser Doppler and xenon clearance, have also argued that there is no demonstrable perfusion block.[39,155]

Hopkins et al.[93] used positron emission tomography to measure blood flow and oxygen utilization in the skin of a group of 11 patients with venous ulceration and five patients with lipodermatosclerosis. They found that there was an increased blood flow with a reduced tissue extraction of oxygen in areas of lipodermatosclerosis and in the abnormal skin around open ulcers. These results indicate that there is no venous stasis but a local functional shunting of blood through an abnormal microcirculation.

All these findings refute the concept of stasis as an important factor in the genesis of venous ulceration, but it is conceivable that there is local slowing of blood flow through the cutaneous capillary bed of the periulcer skin while there is rapid blood flow through other areas of the limb.[138–140] Videomicroscopy[19] has provided some support for this concept, though such a change could be an effect of the ulceration rather than its cause. The case for 'venous stasis' as a cause of venous ulceration is not entirely discredited.

Arteriovenous shunting

Holling et al.[89] stated that it was possible that 'a shunt of blood directly from the arterioles to the venules, largely avoiding the capillary bed' might explain their findings of high oxygen levels in the venous blood of ulcerated limbs. This idea was extended by Piulachs and Vidal-Barraquer,[133] who suggested that arteriovenous communications opened up in response to venous obstruction or other causes of defective venous return. Fontaine[68] provided further support for this hypothesis when he reported higher oxygen tensions in the venous blood samples from the limbs of 95 patients with varicose veins than in samples taken from healthy control subjects.

Gius[71] said that he had seen histological evidence of abnormal arteriovenous communications in the skin of the calves of patients undergoing varicose vein surgery whilst using an operating microscope. He conceded, however, that the vessels that he had seen were indistinguishable from thick-walled capillaries. His work has never been confirmed. Schalin[142] has also suggested that all varicose veins are caused by arteriovenous fistulae (see Chapter 5).

Ryan and Copeman[140] postulated that the normal temperature-regulating arteriovenous fistulae present within the dermis might open up as a result of raised venous pressure, and that these fistulae might be responsible for the arteriovenous shunting that appeared to exist in patients with ulceration.

The reduction in the time taken for radio-opaque contrast medium to traverse arteries and reach the veins in patients with ulcers,[76,77,166] together with an increase in the cutaneous temperature which has been recorded in post-thrombotic limbs[75] all lent additional support to the concept of abnormal 'shunts' opening up in limbs with severe venous dysfunction. The concept of functional arteriovenous shunting was, however, strongly challenged by the work of Partsch and his colleagues.[105,110] They used isotopically labelled macroaggregates of albumin to assess the size of any functional arteriovenous shunt that might be present in limbs with venous ulceration and compared this with similar measurements made in normal healthy limbs. No evidence of physiological shunting was found in the vicinity of an ulcer, though the authors did find some evidence of an increased blood flow in the feet of ulcerated limbs. In fact, their gamma camera scans of ulcerated limbs demonstrated an increased trapping of the aggregates in the ulcer-bearing skin – a finding which contradicts the hypothesis that there are arteriovenous shunts. These findings were confirmed by Hehne et al.,[81] who, using a similar technique, also failed to demonstrate evidence of shunting in patients with venous ulceration.

An interstitial diffusion barrier caused by increased capillary permeability and a deficiency of tissue fibrinolysis (see Chapter 15)

Our late colleague, Ian Whimster, originally observed that patients with severe chronic venous disease in their lower limbs appeared to have an increased number of capillaries in biopsies taken from the 'gaiter skin'.[168] He suggested that the capillary bed had proliferated in response to the persistently elevated venous pressure.

Other investigators,[65,104] have suggested that dermal capillary loops elongate and become tortuous rather than increase in actual number, and Ryan[138] has suggested that a rise in venous pressure

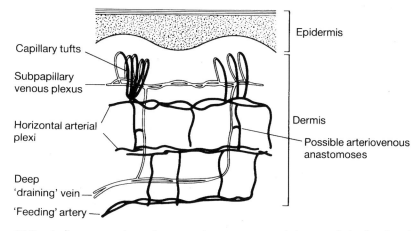

Figure 18.2 A diagram to show the normal arrangement of the vessels in the dermis. The possible sites of arteriovenous fistulae are shown. The 'elongation' or 'proliferation' that is seen in patients with chronic venous hypertension occurs in the capillary tufts that drain into the subpapillary venous plexus. The perivascular fibrin cuff is found around these capillaries.

causes dilatation of the horizontal subpapillary venous plexus (Figure 18.2), with grossly 'coiled' elongated papillary (dermal) capillaries, and a reduction in the number of capillaries supplying the

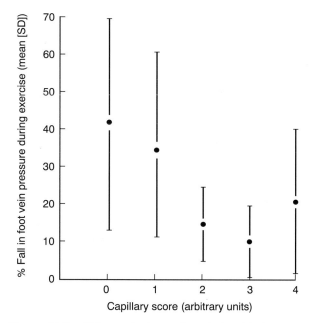

Figure 18.3 This graph shows the relationship between the capillary 'proliferation' seen in biopsies taken from the ulcer-bearing skin of legs with varying degrees of calf pump failure and the maximal fall in foot vein pressure during exercise. It can be seen that limbs with mild or absent capillary 'proliferation' (scores 0 and 1) had much more efficient calf pumps than limbs with moderate or severe capillary 'proliferation' (scores 2, 3 and 4). This difference was highly significant ($P < 0.001$).[32]

epidermis. Corrigan and Kakkar[47] observed that the endothelial cells of capillaries within the ankle skin of patients with the post-thrombotic syndrome were often swollen and contained large vacuoles. They also reported that the basement membrane of these capillaries was often irregular and thickened.

All these studies suggest that lipodermatosclerosis and ulceration might be caused by an alteration in the local capillary bed in response to calf pump failure. We confirmed this when we found a significant correlation between the number of capillaries seen on histological sections of the 'gaiter area' skin and the extent of the venous pressure fall found during exercise (Figure 18.3).[25] We then showed, in an animal model, that venous hypertension increased capillary permeability and the concentration of fibrinogen in lymph.[8,33,103] Fibrinogen, a large molecule, was found to escape significantly faster from the capillary bed of the skin and subcutaneous tissues in limbs with a high venous pressure.[33,63]

This led us to re-examine the ulcer-bearing skin of patients with severe venous disease and cutaneous complications to see if there was any evidence of fibrinogen or fibrin deposition within the tissues. Biopsies of skin were taken from patients with severe lipodermatosclerosis and were stained for fibrinogen/fibrin with phosphotungstic acid haemotoxylin (PTAH) (Figure 18.4) and also treated with rabbit raised antihuman fibrin/fibrinogen antibodies and then examined with fluorescent labelled markers (Figure 18.5). Both techniques showed the presence of pericapillary fibrin/fibrinogen.

A controlled study showed that these changes were only present in limbs with lipodermatosclerosis and were associated with a significantly larger

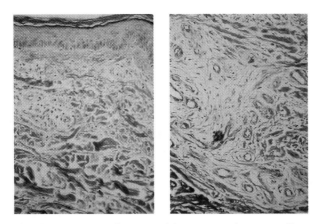

Figure 18.4 Capillary 'proliferation and pericapillary protein'. These two photomicrographs stained with phosphotungstic acid haematoxylin (PTAH) show the difference between the number of capillaries in the skin of a normal leg (left-hand panel) and the skin of a leg subjected to chronic venous hypertension (right-hand panel). There are very few capillaries in the dermis of the normal skin but many in the abnormal skin. This is mainly caused by elongation and tortuosity of existing capillaries, not by growth of new capillaries. Fibrin/fibrinogen stains blue with PTAH. The capillaries in the right-hand panel are surrounded by a 'blue' fibrillary material.

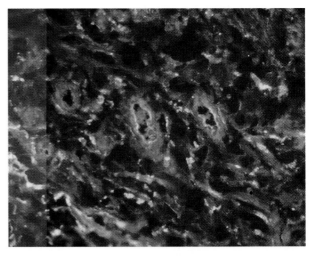

Figure 18.5 Pericapillary fibrin/fibrinogen. This section of skin, taken from an area of lipodermatosclerosis, has been stained with fluorescent antibodies to fibrin/fibrinogen. The areas of yellow–green fluorescence around the capillaries are deposits of fibrin/fibrinogen.

dermal capillary bed and a significantly reduced venous pressure fall on exercise (Figure 18.6).[32]

The deposition of fibrin within the tissues is normally prevented by the interstitial fibrinolytic system. We found, however, that patients with lipodermatosclerosis had a significant reduction in both systemic and tissue fibrinolytic activity.[27]

We felt that the pericapillary fibrin/fibrinogen deposition that we had seen in the ulcer-bearing skin might be the result of a persistently elevated venous pressure which distended the capillary bed and dilated the inter-endothelial pores (Figure 18.7).[132,151] These changes could be expected to increase the concentration of fibrinogen and other large plasma molecules in the intestital fluid where the fibrinogen/fibrin might become fixed within the tissues around the capillaries because of the defective tissue fibrinolytic activity capacity of these patients. This pericapillary 'cuff' might then act as a diffusion barrier (Figure 18.7).

The presence of pericapillary fibrils which stain with PTAH has also been reported in the abnormal skin of patients with arteriovenous fistulae formed for renal dialysis access in the upper limb.[173] This is the human equivalent of our animal model.

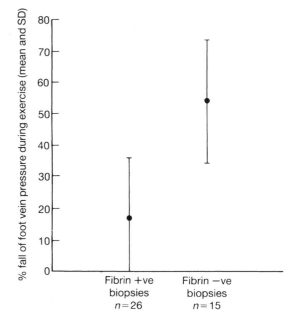

Figure 18.6 This figure shows the mean maximum fall of foot pressure during exercise in 26 limbs in which the skin biopsies had evidence of pericapillary fibrin (fibrin-positive biopsies) and in 15 limbs in which no fibrin was seen (fibrin-negative biopsies). The limbs with evidence of pericapillary fibrin in the ulcer-bearing skin had significantly worse calf pump function than those whose skin contained no pericapillary fibrin.[33]

Normal   Venous hypertension

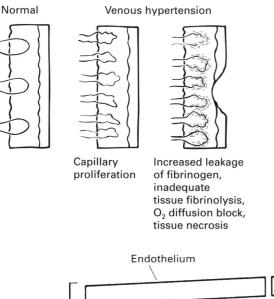

Capillary   Increased leakage
proliferation   of fibrinogen,
                   inadequate
                   tissue fibrinolysis,
                   O₂ diffusion block,
                   tissue necrosis

(a)

Figure 18.7 (a) A diagrammatic representation of the development of the pericapillary fibrin cuff. The permanently elevated venous pressure (which is not reduced by the calf pump) distends and enlarges the capillary bed (capillary 'proliferation'). The distended inter-endothelial pores allow the normally 'pore bound' fibrinogen to escape and this polymerizes and becomes fixed around the capillaries. The inadequate fibrinolytic capacity of these patients interferes with the removal of the fibrin and the subsequent reduction in the metabolism and oxygenation of the tissues nurtured by these capillaries leads to necrosis and ulceration.[26] (b) Our original illustration of the mechanisms that produce the pericapillary fibrin cuff.

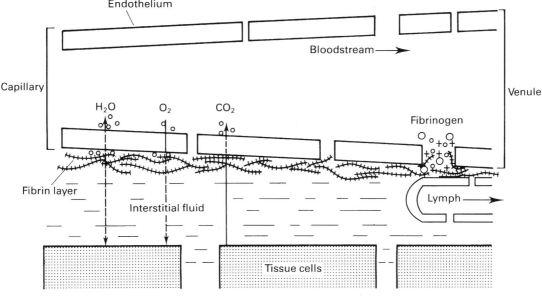

(b)

The presence of pericapillary fibrin/fibrinogen deposition in the skin of more than 90% of patients with lipodermatosclerosis has been confirmed by Marks,[114] Partsch,[130] and Eaglestein.[61] Immunofluorescent pericapillary fibrin has been found in the lipodermatosclerotic skin around venous ulcers but not in the skin adjacent to ulcers of different aetiology.[61,84,164]

Electron microscopic analysis (Figure 18.8) and monoclonal antibodies against cross-linked fibrin have shown that the pericapillary material is not necessarily pure cross-linked fibrin. The concept of a mechanical 'fibrin' block may not be correct.[161] There is no doubt that there is a pericapillary cuff of fibrin/fibrinogen but it may be behaving as a tissue metabolic block of indeterminate origin and not simply as a mechanical obstruction to diffusion.

Our own studies of the effect of chronic venous hypertension on the microcirculation of the lower limb was presaged by Arnoldi and Linderholm[5] who in 1968 concluded a study on venous pressure measurements with the following statement:

Dilatation of capillaries causes an increase in permeability of capillary walls. Proteins escape easily into the interstitial fluid[65] and after prolonged anoxaemia even blood corpuscles may penetrate the capillary wall.[174] These observations may explain the high protein content of interstitial fluid observed in patients with leg ulcers[80] and the discolouration of the skin of the ankle by haemosiderin which is an almost constant finding in these patients.

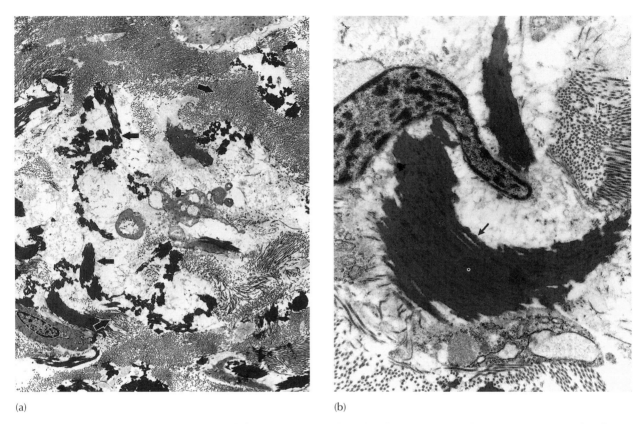

(a)   (b)

Figure 18.8 Two electron micrographs of the tissue in the edge of a chronic venous ulcer. (a) Many normal collagen fibrils are visible (white edged arrows) but there is also some electron dense material which appears to be coarsely fibrillary (black arrows). (b) A higher power magnification shows this fibrillary material more clearly. This is probably the material described by Adair, which he thought was degenerating collagen (see page 521). (These figures were kindly supplied by Gillian Bullock and Paul Sibson of Ciba Geigy.)

An important histological study from Manchester[84] confirmed that pericapillary fibrin was almost always present in the tissues surrounding venous ulcers, but was not the only protein within the cuff. Fibronectin, laminin and deposits of collagen were seen, confirming the studies of Neumann. The capillaries were again found to be thick walled. Stacey has elegantly shown that fibrin cuffs precede the development of any skin changes and their extent correlates well with the levels of local tissue hypoxia.[153] Therefore the principal challenge to the fibrin cuff theory has come from the calculations of Charles Michel,[120] who has estimated that the layer of fibrin would have to be several millimetres thick to interfere with the passage of oxygen from the capillaries to the tissues. The whole of this work is based on interstitial diffusion constants and takes little account of the protein nature of the 'cuffs' nor the generated thickening of the capillary wall and basement membrane that develops in patients with venous hypertension (see Figure 18.8). There is considerable disagreement over whether or not there is a diffusion block. Certainly the tcPo_2 is reduced but xenon diffusion does not appear to be affected.[39,121,153,155]

White cell trapping

Shortly after the publication of the first edition of this book two papers which proposed a new mechanism for the development of venous ulceration were published simultaneously in the *British Medical Journal*. The first paper from Thomas *et al.*[159] showed passive leg dependency caused greater 'loss' of white cells from the venous blood of patients with lipodermatosclerosis (30%) than from subjects with normal limbs (7%). This paper was accompanied by a second paper by Coleridge Smith *et al.*[44] proposing a 'new theory for venous ulceration', which was based on the findings of the first paper and supported by additional videomicroscopic observations which showed that the number

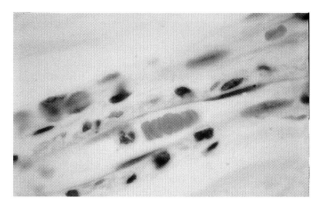

Figure 18.9 A normal venular capillary containing one leucocyte and a rouleaux of erythrocytes. The white cell trapping theory postulates that clumps of activated leucocytes adhere to the capillary endothelium, block the capillary and so cause tissue anoxia. This phenomenon has never been visualized. The variation of this hypothesis postulates that the activated leucocytes damage the capillary endothelium, disrupt permeability and initiate an inflammatory reaction. (We are grateful to H.J. Scott and P. Coleridge Smith for this illustration.)

of patent cutaneous capillary loops decreased on dependency. The authors argued that this indicated occlusion of capillaries by trapped white cells (Figure 18.9). This line of research followed the original physiological observation that white cells accumulated in the feet of subjects during periods of dependency.[122]

The original 'trapping' concept has, however, undergone modification in the light of their further studies.[147] It is no longer postulated that the white cells caught in the capillaries are causing an hypoxic (ischaemic) injury, but that they are causing damage by release of local toxic products. The authors of this hypothesis have been unable to confirm that there are white cells blocking the capillary bed (Figure 18.9) and have had difficulty reproducing the studies of Thomas.[145,146] Their modified theory concentrates on the damage done to the venous epithelium by activated white cells.[150] Neutrophil granulation has been shown to be inappropriate in patients with venous disease,[169] but the stimulus to this activation is still far from clear. Distension of the capillary bed and venous hypertension are obvious candidates but it is difficult to understand how toxic substances released from activated white cells in venular capillaries which will be washed out by the circulation into the larger venules can affect the permeability of the arteriolar nutritive capillaries.

The difficulties with all the observations to date are that they have been made in patients who already have cutaneous changes and it is difficult therefore to determine whether they are a cause or a result of the local inflammatory process. It would be interesting to know whether any measurable changes in white cell behaviour preceded skin changes in a high risk group, such as patients who have had a deep vein thrombosis. The other problem is to extrapolate short-term acute experiments (venous 'stasis' caused by dependency or application of a tourniquet) to the changes produced by years of chronic venous hypertension. The white cell trapping activation theory still has its advocates but it has already been considerably modified in the light of further work and cannot explain the site of predilection for ulcers or the healing achieved by compression.

Growth hormone trapping

In the light of Michel's theoretical objections to fibrin interfering with oxygen diffusion, Falanga *et al.*[66] suggested that the pericapillary cuffs might interfere with the diffusion of growth factors which are essential for skin and tissue repair. This might well explain why ulcerated or damaged tissues fail to heal but it is more difficult to explain why a loss of these factors might lead to the tissue inflammation and death that presents as lipodermatosclerosis and ulceration.

Reperfusion injury and free radical release

McCollum's group,[62] who have studied arterial reperfusion injury, have suggested that signs of venous hypertension (during standing) constitute a repeated reperfusion injury to the skin. This is supported by others.[141] There is again little explanation why this damage should be limited to the lower third of the leg. The toes and bottom of the feet should be more susceptible.

Overactivation of the venoarterial reflex causing venoconstriction and reduced tissue perfusion

This 'physical cause' of venous ulceration has again recently been resurrected by Holan.[88] It is difficult to believe in reduced tissue perfusion as a cause of ulceration when, as the author points out, 'compression heals venous ulcers'. The importance of venous 'hypertension' or lack of hypotension is conceded but the exact physical mechanism by which this through a vascular reflux causes lipodermatosclerosis and ulceration in the gaiter skin is far from clear.

Comment

The mechanism by which the cutaneous changes of lipodermatosclerosis and ulceration develop in response to prolonged venous hypertension remains open to speculation (see Chapter 15 and above).

There is no satisfactory animal model of the venous ulcer. Marks *et al.* have produced slowly healing 'sores' in experimental animals by injecting sodium tetradecylsulphate subcutaneously,[115] but this does not exactly mimic the human venous ulcer. Other investigators[163] have found that frogs' legs subjected to intensive external compression develop oedema, capillary dilatation, haemorrhage and, eventually, small areas of cutaneous ulceration. It is not clear how long these ulcers take to heal. Until we have a satisfactory 'ulcer model' further progress in understanding both the aetiology and pathology of venous ulceration will be delayed.

In the first edition we wrote that we awaited further studies on the cause of venous ulceration 'with interest'. There certainly has been a plethora of such studies and much interest, especially in the microcirculation, but as yet there are no definitive answers. Further work is still required. It is still our belief that the answer will lie in the balance between calf pump function and the microcirculatory response to venous hypertension, a balance which varies considerably between patients, in both the absolute level of the abnormalities and the sensitivities of the tissues.

THE CAUSE OF SKIN BREAKDOWN

Injury

It is not known if localized tissue anoxia can in itself cause the skin to ulcerate. Minor trauma, possibly as little as rubbing an itchy patch of skin, is probably necessary for ulceration to begin. It is impossible to prove or disprove the concept that local injury is always the final initiating factor in the genesis of a venous ulcer. Certainly, many of our patients describe an episode of trauma before their ulcers developed, and we advise all patients to protect their legs from injury when their ulcers have healed.

Tissue anoxia may cause the death of skin and its replacement with scar tissue without ulceration. The white scars of 'atrophie blanche' are commonly seen in areas of chronic lipodermatosclerosis. This observation suggests that something else is required to change the slow death with simultaneous repair (atrophie blanche) into the rapid skin death of ulceration.

We recently carried out a survey in our ulcer clinic of the patients' recollection of ulcer development. Three-quarters of a consecutive cohort of 120 patients remembered an injury at the time of onset. Supermarket trolleys were responsible for only 3%.

Oedema

Local tissue oedema has, for some time, been thought to play a part in the development of ulcers;[20,52,74,123,137] however, Myers *et al.* have shown that the presence of oedema does not delay ulcer healing,[124] and that its elimination does not ensure healing. Very few of our patients with lymphoedema develop ulceration of the skin, but we have shown that the combination of lymphoedema and lipodermatosclerosis is usually associated with evidence of defective fibrinolysis.[154] Many of our patients with venous ulceration have no signs of oedema although Mortimer found that 55% of his patients had some oedema.[134] There is therefore no clear evidence that oedema of the tissues is an important factor in initiating ulceration, although it may delay healing.[134]

Infection

The role of infection in the genesis of a venous ulcer is still confused. There is little doubt that venous ulcers all become secondarily infected[139,143] but it is much more difficult to know if bacteria play any part in promoting or perpetuating the ulcer. Some studies have suggested that the numbers of organisms may perpetuate ulceration; high colony counts represent significant infection and low counts represent simple commensal colonization.[139]

Anaerobic colonization of venous ulcers may have been underestimated, because we have found pathogenic anaerobic organisms in nearly half the ulcers we have examined. It is not known if these bacteria are important and it is doubtful if infection ever acts as a primary cause of venous ulceration.

Ischaemia

Ischaemia is, like trauma, a potent cause of ulceration in its own right, and it will be discussed further in Chapter 19 as a differential diagnosis of venous ulcers. It was, however, pointed out by Dodd and Cockett[59] that the skin of the anteriomedial aspect of the lower leg has an extremely poor blood supply, which increases the risk of skin breakdown if an additional noxious stimulus is present. Ischaemia and venous skin damage may therefore combine to cause necrosis and ulceration, and in some patients it may be difficult to distinguish the relative importance of calf pump failure from that of arterial ischaemia in the development of ulceration;[136] Doppler ultrasound ankle pressure measurements and arteriography may be required to define the role of ischaemia in ulcers of mixed aetiology.[46,127,128,136]

Obesity

This is reported to be an important predisposing factor in the development of ulceration[139] but it does not appear to be an initiating factor. It does, of course, make ulcer healing more difficult. Many patients with ulcers may become obese because of the reduced activity caused by their ulcer, and perhaps very obese subjects are more likely to develop varicose veins and deep vein thrombosis (see Chapters 5 and 8).

Malfunction of the calf muscles

Nerve damage, local muscle damage or joint abnormalities all cause malfunction of the calf muscle pump.[112] This is seen in patients with poliomyelitis, after severe soft tissue and bony injury and in association with osteoarthritis of the knee or ankle. Although these conditions may predispose to ulceration, we are not aware of any evidence that they cause ulceration in their own right. The fixed equinus deformity of the ankle that develops in some patients with severe long-standing ulceration around the ankle certainly impedes healing and predisposes to further ulceration by preventing normal calf pump function. Loss of ankle movement in patients with chronic venous ulcers has recently been quantified by Helliwell and Cheesbrough,[83] but it was not known if this was relevant to ulcer development or purely a result.

Erect stance and height

Ulcers do not develop in other members of the animal kingdom, and the assumption of the erect posture by man is obviously important in the development of ulceration.[69] The resting hydrostatic foot vein pressure increases with the height of the individual but, though it is a clinical impression that tall people develop ulcers, there is a low incidence of both varicose veins and ulcers in the Bantu[58] who are an exceptionally tall race. We have no knowledge on the incidence of ulceration in Pygmies!

Intersex states

There is an unexplained relationship between varicose veins, venous ulceration and Klinefelter's syndrome (XXY).[6,38,94,96] We have seen three patients with this chromosomal pattern who have resistant ulceration of the leg with normal venous physiology and anatomy (Figure 18.10). We have also seen resistant ulceration in association with other chromosomal abnormalities. It is possible that defective fibrinolysis may play a part in the development of these ulcers.

General health, cleanliness and personal hygiene

Poor general health does not cause venous ulceration, but may be the result of long-standing ulceration with its associated anaemia and protein depletion.[144] Lack of cleanliness and personal hygiene may be associated with poor compliance to treatment, but is unlikely to be an important cause of venous ulceration.

Psychological factors

Some patients appear to need a focus around which to live their lives, and an ulcer together with the medical and nursing care required for its management may provide just such a focus. The role of psychological factors in the development of venous ulceration and its persistence remain unproven but many patients tamper with their compression treatment.

In mediaeval times ulcers were thought to be necessary to allow the escape of 'evil humours', and healing was actively prevented.[3] This belief is not entirely extinct, and some patients still believe that their ulcer serves a useful purpose and that their general health will deteriorate if it heals.

THE CAUSE OF ASSOCIATED SKIN CHANGES

'Atrophie blanche' is an area of white stellate scarring (Figure 18.11) which often accompanies chronic lipodermatosclerosis and may precede venous ulceration. In an area of atrophie blanche the skin becomes shrivelled and scarred rather than thick and hard as in lipodermatosclerosis. The reason for this difference is open to speculation. Is atrophie blanche the result of cutaneous ischaemia, perhaps from capillary thrombosis, or is it just an extreme example of the effect of chronic hypoxia caused by the diffusion barrier? The two apparently dissimilar conditions – lipodermatosclerosis and atrophie blanche – may be the result of different levels of venous hypertension and tissue fibrinolysis. We do not know how the same mechanism, calf pump failure, can produce such different skin reactions.

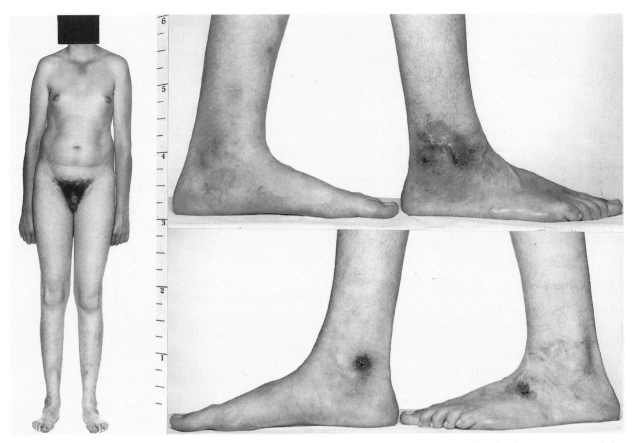

Figure 18.10 A patient with Klinefelter's syndrome (XXY) (left-hand panel) associated with ulceration around the ankles. This relationship is well recognized, but the aetiology of the ulceration remains obscure. The low level of male sex hormones in these patients may be associated with defect of fibrinolysis. This particular patient was also exceptionally tall.

THE RELEVANCE OF THE GAITER REGION TO THE AETIOLOGY OF ULCERATION

Most venous ulcers occur in the gaiter region of the leg, between the malleoli and the level of the lower muscle fibres of the gastrocnemius muscle. Venous ulcers have been described in the upper calf[3] (but we have never seen them) and they can also occasionally occur on the foot, though these are very rare. Ulcers on the foot are more often caused by different mechanisms.

Why then are venous ulcers confined to the 'gaiter skin'? The answer must lie in the relationship between this skin and the large medial calf communicating veins of the calf pump.[90] The calf pump generates pressures of up to 200 mmHg within the fascia,[112] and the high pressure developed within the soleal sinusoids and venae comitantes of the calf is transmitted directly into the surface veins

and local capillary bed if the valves within the calf communicating veins are incompetent. Waves of high pressure may reach the superficial veins during calf pump systole, especially if there is obstruction to the pump outflow tract. Although there are foot pumps and thigh pumps, these do not usually generate the same amount of pressure[112] and, consequently, skin changes seldom occur in the skin of the thigh or foot. We have seen lipodermatosclerosis of the sole of the foot in three patients who had total congenital valvular agenesis in their deep veins, and we have seen one case of true lipodermatosclerosis of the thigh in a patient with severe post-thrombotic disease.

All the evidence indicates that the site of the incompetent communicating veins determines the site of development of lipodermatosclerosis and venous ulceration. The poor arterial blood supply of the skin of the lower leg may increase skin ischaemia, but local venous hypertension is the root cause of the ulcer.

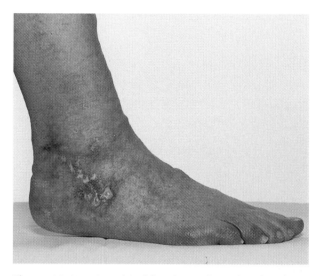

Figure 18.11 Atrophie blanche. When skin has been completely replaced with scar tissue it has a white shiny appearance. This is known as atrophie blanche. It frequently appears without passing through a stage of ulceration but a healed ulcer may present a similar appearance.

The pathology of a venous ulcer

Ulcer development

The pathological changes of lipodermatosclerosis have already been discussed (see Chapter 15). When ulceration begins there is partial skin loss in an already abnormal area of skin and subcutaneous fat. If this does not heal rapidly, the remaining layers of skin usually necrose to produce full-thickness skin loss. There is invariably some attempt at healing by the underlying tissues, and granulation tissue consisting of capillary loops and fibrous tissue starts to develop from the dermal vascular plexus, if this is still present, or from vessels in the subcutaneous fat[3,137] (Figure 18.12).

Tissue necrosis with cellular death can occasionally extend into the subcutaneous fat and even down to the deep fascia, muscles and the periosteum of the tibia or fibula. The granulation tissue is scanty and the local inflammatory reaction is variable if the ulcer is rapidly extending.

ULCER REPAIR

Once the ulcer has stopped enlarging (i.e. the skin necrosis has stopped) and the dead tissue has separated, granulation tissue begins to develop. The natural history of the ulcer is initially determined by the balance between the development of granulation tissue formation and continuing necrosis, and then by the rate of epithelial growth over the granulation tissue. Fibrin, polymorphonuclear leucocytes and phagocytes all appear around the newly formed capillaries and, providing that healing progresses, the granulation tissue extends upwards to 'fill in' the defect left by the necrosis. The fibrin exudate stimulates collagen deposition[99] and the white blood cells attack micro-organisms and digest dead tissue.

RE-EPITHELIALIZATION

The edges of the ulcer cicatrize, thus reducing the size of the skin defect, and epidermal cells are stimulated to migrate across the granulation tissue.[2] There is no evidence that epithelial cell mitosis and migration is reduced in the edges of poorly healing venous ulcers but Adair[2] has suggested that the failure of ulcers to heal may be associated with an increased loss or reduced adhe-

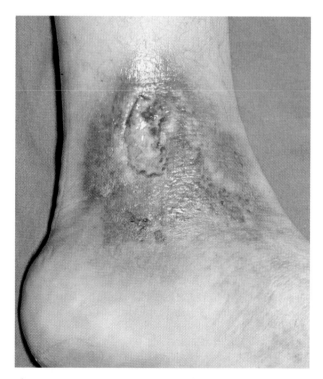

Figure 18.12 A young venous ulcer. This ulcer is only 2 weeks old. It was exuding purulent fluid and was extremely painful. The acute lipodermatosclerosis which preceded it can be seen in the surrounding skin. Some granulation tissue is just beginning to appear.

sion of epithelial cells as they attempt to migrate across the granulation tissue. Adair also found less collagen in the dermis beneath ulcers than in normal skin and an increase in the number of fibroblasts. Some new capillaries were always present, usually in large numbers. In the region of the epithelial migration in poorly healing ulcers, Adair found coarse extravascular fibrillary material (Figure 18.8) which had the high electron density usually associated with structurally normal collagen fibrils. He suggested that this material was degenerating collagen.

Adair also noted cytoplasmic vacuolation in the epidermal cells of non-healing ulcers. These vacuoles were found in the granular layers of the epidermis and were associated with a lack of collagen fibrils in the papillary dermis which were replaced by a fine fibrillary material. He did not draw any inferences from these observations but suggested that although local hypoxia does not influence epidermal division and migration,[119] it may well affect epidermal survival and be responsible for the changes that he had observed. It is possible that the fine fibrillary material which he saw within the papillary dermis was fibrin.

THE ULCER 'BASE'

In rapidly extending ulcers the necrotic epidermis and dermis may remain as a thick slough lying on top of the granulation tissue in the ulcer base. There may be a considerable volume of moist exudate comprised of oedema fluid and dead polymorphonuclear leucocytes. The bacteria contaminating the surface of the ulcer rarely invade the subcutaneous fat.

Peripheral nerve endings may be directly involved in the inflammatory process and give rise to considerable local pain, but it is surprising how seldom pain is a major symptom in some of the largest and most infected ulcers. It is impossible to equate the pathological features of the ulcer with the presence or absence of pain, though small sloughing young ulcers are often very painful. Perhaps pain is more related to the local release of kinins and other chemical stimuli than to the direct extension of the ulcer into the local nerve endings.

Once an ulcer is clean, its base becomes covered with bright red velvety granulation tissue (Figure 18.13), provided the base is not fibrous and ischaemic. Ulcers which develop in areas of chronic lipodermatosclerosis often have a white fibrous base with scanty granulation tissue; this is an indication that the ulcer will be slow to heal (Figure 18.14).

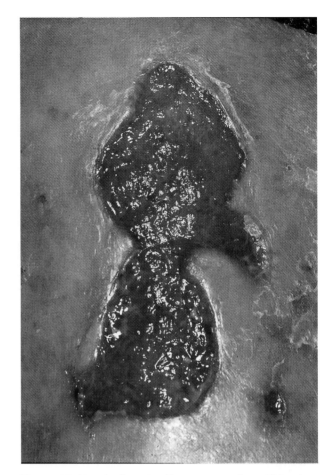

Figure 18.13 A clean healing venous ulcer. This ulcer is healing because it has a base of healthy granulation tissue and a sloping edge of new epithelium growing over the granulation tissue. The surrounding skin also looks healthy.

DEVELOPMENT AND CONTROL OF RE-EPITHELIALIZATION

Ulcers usually heal by cicatrization and epithelial migration over the granulation tissue from the skin edge. Occasionally, epithelialization develops from multiple islands of epithelium that appear over the whole surface of the granulation tissue (Figure 18.15). It is not known whether these islands of epithelium originate from deep remnants of the skin and its appendages which were not destroyed when the ulcer developed, or from cells which have migrated from the ulcer edge before becoming fixed. A third possibility is that fibroblasts and other totipotent cells may undergo squamous metaplasia but this seems unlikely. Growth factors control epithelial mitosis, migration and repair, and

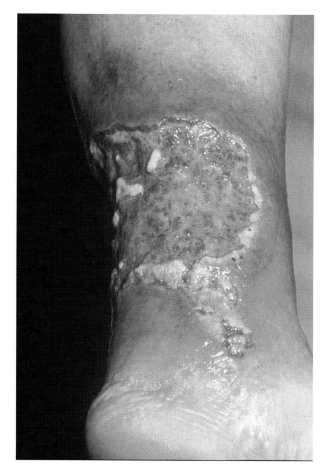

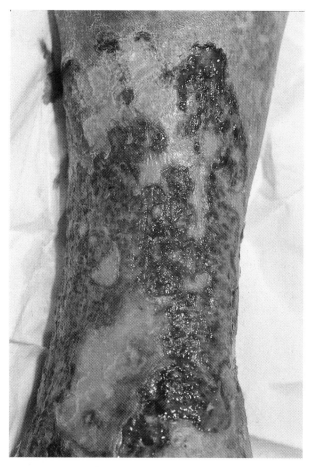

Figure 18.14 A chronic venous ulcer in long-standing lipodermatosclerosis which has already produced a circumferential constriction – the champagne bottle leg. This large ulcer had been present for 2 years. It was not painful but showed no signs of healing. The base is a mixture of fibrous tissue and small nodules of granulation tissue covered with exudate and slough. The edge is 'punched out' and the surrounding skin is pigmented and sclerotic.

Figure 18.15 An ulcer that is healing from multiple islands of epithelium that have survived the initial microcirculatory damage that caused the ulcer.

we have found that transforming growth factor β and fibroblast growth factor are probably relevant in the process of ulcer healing.[101,102] Inspection of the ulcer edge usually gives a good indication of its propensity for healing. If the edge is shallow and sloping with thin purple–pink new epithelial cells extending onto the granulation tissue, healing will proceed (Figure 18.13). When the skin is overhanging the base of the ulcer and there is no evidence that new epithelium is appearing, the ulcer will be slow to heal, especially if the granulation tissue in the base is sparse or fibrotic (Figure 18.16). This type of ulcer may need to be excised before satisfactory granulation tissue will develop and

epithelialization can follow. The factors that are responsible for transforming an acute wound into a chronic wound are still poorly understood.

MICRO-ORGANISMS IN VENOUS ULCERS

This subject is discussed in detail in Chapters 19 and 20. Most of the micro-organisms found in ulcers are commensals taking the opportunity of growing on an ideal culture medium.[139] Hopkins and Jamieson[92] have shown that antibiotics can permeate ulcer exudate and that their concentration in the exudate varies with both posture and the state of the ulcer. More studies are still needed on the relationship between ulcer exudate and microbial flora and on the influence of these factors on ulcer healing. It

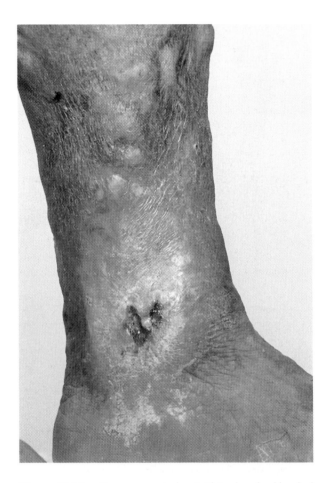

Figure 18.16 'A permanent ulcer'. This ulcer had healed and broken down many times. Its base was entirely fibrous with no granulation tissue. Epithelial growth and cicatrization are making the edge overhang the base and give a false impression of healing. The only effective treatment is excision of all the diseased skin and subcutaneous tissue and replacement with split skin grafts followed by correction of the underlying venous abnormality.

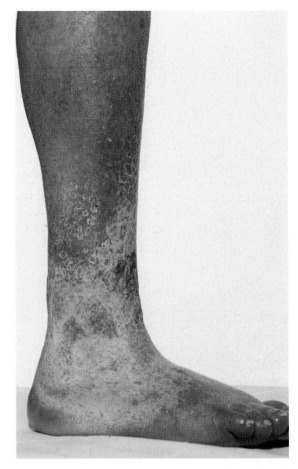

Figure 18.17 A healed venous ulcer with marked hyperkeratinization of the skin. The cause of this abnormality is obscure. It is similar to the skin changes of long-standing lymphoedema and may be caused by the damage done to the dermal lymphatic plexus by the preceding chronic ulceration.

may be important to relate events such as ulcer healing and extension to the type of micro-organism that is growing on the ulcer at the time; as far as we know this has still not been done; it would, however, help to establish the role of infection in the natural history of ulceration. It has been repeatedly observed that though venous ulcers are always covered in micro-organisms, spreading infection, cellulitis, lymphangitis or septicaemia is extremely rare. Perhaps the fibrous tissue in the ulcer base prevents the access of organisms to the lymphatics or bloodstream.

Organisms presumably reach the ulcer from the general environment and from other areas of the patient's skin that harbour bacteria. Staphylococci and streptococci may be transferred from the upper respiratory tract and nasal passages while Gram-negative bacteria and anaerobes may pass to the ulcer from the perineal area.

Cross-contamination can occur when the ulcer is dressed by medical attendants (doctors, nurses and physiotherapists). Despite this possibility, cross-infection does not appear to be of clinical importance in ulcer clinics or hospital wards provided the normal precautions of hand washing and the use of fresh sterile instruments and dressings for each patient are taken. The relevance of high concentrations of organisms and combinations of different types of organisms in the pathology of ulceration remains to be clarified.

THE SCAR (THE HEALED ULCER)

When epithelium finally covers all the granulation tissue in the ulcer base, the ulcer is healed. The new pink epithelium is fragile and unstable. Until it matures and becomes more stable, it easily breaks down or becomes detached if it is not protected from inadvertent injury. As the new skin matures it becomes paler and thicker and the granulation tissue beneath the epithelium contracts and becomes less vascular and more fibrous as the collagen matures. Sometimes the keratin in the skin over the healed surface of the ulcer increases in thickness. The mechanism of this 'hyperkeratinization' is obscure (Figure 18.17). The depth and extent of the scar tissue beneath the endothelium depends upon the inital size and depth of the ulcer.

THE GENERAL EFFECTS OF ULCERATION

These are discussed in more detail in the section on the natural history of ulceration at the beginning of Chapter 20 but they are summarized here.

- Venous ulcers are rarely life threatening, as systemic septicaemia almost never occurs.
- Ulcers may cause much morbidity from pain, discomfort and discharge.
- Ulcers never appear to cause secondary amyloid disease but can cause chronic anaemia and hypoproteinaemia.
- Very occasionally, ulcers may undergo malignant change (Marjolin's ulcer, see Chapter 19, page 541).
- Ulcers may have serious economic and psychological effects (see Chapter 20, page 572).
- Ulcers are a considerable drain on medical resources – their treatment requires considerable amounts of medical time and revenue.

References

1. Abramson DI, Fierst SM. Arterial blood flow in extremities with varicose veins. *Arch Surg* 1942; **45:** 964–8.
2. Adair HM. Repair in acute and chronic ulcers. *Ann R Coll Surg Engl* 1978; **60:** 393–8.
3. Anning ST. *Leg Ulcers: their Causes and Treatment.* London: Churchill, 1954.
4. Arnoldi CC, Haegar K. Ulcus cruris venosum – crux medicorum. *Lakartidningen* 1967; **64:** 2149–57.
5. Arnoldi CC, Linderholm H. On the pathogenesis of the venous leg ulcer. *Acta Chir Scand* 1968; **134:** 427–40.
6. Baker SR, Stacey MC, Jopp-McKay AG, Hoskin SE, Thompson PJ. Epidemiology of chronic venous ulcers. *Br J Surg* 1991; **78:** 864–7.
7. Bauer G. A roentgenologic and clinical study of the sequels of thrombosis. *Acta Chir Scand Suppl* 1942; **86:** 74.
8. Beard RC. *Factors affecting the Composition of Renal Lymph.* MCh Thesis, Cambridge University, 1982.
9. Berquist D. *Post-operative Thromboembolism.* Berlin: Springer-Verlag, 1983.
10. Birger I. Ulcus cruris. *Nord Med* 1941; **12:** 3542.
11. Bjordal RI. Blood circulation in varicose veins of the lower extremities. *Angiology* 1972; **23:** 163–73.
12. Bjordal RI. Circulation patterns in incompetent perforating veins in the calf and in the saphenous system in primary varicose veins. *Acta Chir Scand* 1972; **138:** 251–61.
13. Bjordal RI. Circulation patterns in the saphenous system and the perforating veins in the calf in patients with previous deep venous thrombosis. *Vasa Suppl* 1974; **3:** 1–41.
14. Bjordal RI. Pressure patterns in the saphenous system in patients with venous leg ulcers. *Acta Chir Scand* 1971; **137:** 495–501.
15. Bjordal RI. Simultaneous pressure and flow readings in varicose veins of the lower extremity. *Acta Chir Scand* 1970; **136:** 309–17.
16. Blalock A. Oxygen content of blood in patients with varicose veins. *Arch Surg* 1929; **19:** 898–905.
17. Blumoff RL, Johnson G. Saphenous vein pO2 in patients with varicose veins. *J Surg Res* 1977; **23:** 35–6.
18. Bobek K, Cajzl L, Cepelak V, Slaisova V, Opatzny K, Barcal R. Etude de la fréquence des maladies phlébologiques et de l'influence de quelques facteurs étiologiques. *Phlebologie* 1966; **19:** 217–30.
19. Bollinger A, Jager K, Geser A, Sgier F, Seglias J. Transcapillary and interstitial diffusion of Na fluorescein in chronic venous insufficiency with white atrophy. *Int J Microcirc Clin Exp* 1982; **1:** 5–17.
20. Bourne IHJ. Vertical leg drainage of oedema in treatment of leg ulcers. *Br Med J* 1974; **2:** 581.
21. Boyd AM, Catchpole N, Jepson RP, Rose SS. Some observations on venous pressure estimations in the lower limb. *J Bone Joint Surg* 1952; **4:** 599–607.
22. Bradbury AW, Brittenden J, Allan PL, Ruckley CV. Comparison of venous reflux in the affected and non-affected leg in patients with unilateral venous ulceration. *Br J Surg* 1996; **83:** 513–15.
23. Brakman M, Faber WR, Kerckhaert JA, Kraaijenhgen RJ, Hart HCh, Hulshof MM. Immunofluorescence studies of atrophie blanche with antibodies against fibrinogen, fibrin, plasminogen activator inhibitor, factor VIII-related antigen and collagen type IV. *Vasa* 1992; **21(2):** 143–8.
24. Brodie BC. Observations on the treatment of varicose veins of legs. *Med Chir Trans* 1816; **7:** 195–210.
25. Browse NL. Venous ulceration. *Br Med J* 1983; **286:** 1920–2.

26. Browse NL, Burnand KG. The cause of venous ulceration. *Lancet* 1982; **2:** 243–5.

27. Browse NL, Gray L, Jarrett PEM, Morland M. Blood and vein wall fibrinolytic activity in health and vascular disease. *Br Med J* 1977; **1:** 478–81.

28. Burnand KG, Clemenson G, Whimster I, Gaunt J, Browse NL. The effect of sustained venous hypertension on the skin capillaries of the canine hind limb. *Br J Surg* 1982; **69:** 41–4.

29. Burnand KG, O'Donnell TF Jr, Lea Thomas M, Browse NL. The relationship between postphlebitic changes in the deep veins and results of the surgical treatment of venous ulcers. *Lancet* 1976; **1:** 936–8.

30. Burnand KG, O'Donnell TF Jr, Lea Thomas M, Browse NL. The relative importance of incompetent communicating veins in the production of varicose veins and venous ulcers. *Surgery* 1977; **82:** 9–14.

31. Burnand KG, Pattison M, Powell S, Lea Thomas M, Browse NL. Can we diagnose long saphenous incompetence correctly? In: Negus D, Jantet G, eds. *Phlebology '85.* London: Libbey, 1986.

32. Burnand KG, Whimster I, Clemenson G, Lea Thomas M, Browse NL. The relationship between the number of capillaries in the skin of the venous ulcer-bearing area of the lower leg and the fall in foot vein pressure during exercise. *Br J Surg* 1981; **68:** 297–300.

33. Burnand KG, Whimster I, Naidoo A, Browse NL. Pericapillary fibrin in the ulcer-bearing skin of the leg: the cause of lipodermatosclerosis and venous ulceration. *Br Med J* 1982; **285:** 1071–2.

34. Callam M. Prevalence of chronic leg ulceration and severe chronic venous disease in western countries. *Phlebology (Suppl)* 1992; **1:** 6–12.

35. Callam MJ, Harper DR, Dale JJ, Ruckley CV. Arterial disease in chronic leg ulceration: an underestimated hazard? Lothian and Forth Valley leg ulcer study. *Br Med J* 1987; **294:** 929–31.

36. Callam MJ, Ruckley CV, Dale JJ, Harper DR. Chronic leg ulcer. The incidence of associated nonvenous disorders. In: Negus D, Jantet G, eds. *Phlebology '85.* London: Libbey, 1986.

37. Callam MJ, Ruckley CV, Harper DR, Dale JJ. Chronic ulceration of the leg: extent of the problem and provision of care. *Br Med J* 1985; **290:** 1855–6.

38. Campbell WA, Newton NS, Price WH. Hypostatic leg ulceration and klinefelter's syndrome. *J Ment Defic Res* 1980; **24(2):** 115.

39. Cheatle TR, McMullin GM, Farrah J, Coleridge-Smith PD, Scurr JH. Skin damage in chronic venous insufficiency: does an oxygen diffusion barrier really exist? *J R Soc Med* 1990; **83:** 493–4.

40. Clyne CAC, Ramsden WH, Chant ADB, Webster JH. Oxygen tension on the skin of the gaiter area of limbs with venous disease. *Br J Surg* 1985; **72:** 644.

41. Cockett FB. Diagnosis and surgery of high pressure venous leaks in the leg: a new overall concept of surgery of varicose veins and venous ulcers. *Br Med J* 1956; **2:** 1399–403.

42. Cockett FB. The pathology and treatment of venous ulcers of the leg. *Br J Surg* 1955; **43:** 260–78.

43. Cockett FB, Jones DE. The ankle blow-out syndrome. A new approach to the varicose ulcer problem. *Lancet* 1953; **1:** 17–23.

44. Coleridge Smith PD, Thomas P, Scurr JH, Dormandy JA. Causes of venous ulceration: a new hypothesis. *Br Med J* 1988; **296:** 1726–7.

45. Cooper AP. *Lectures on the Principles and Practice of Surgery.* London: Cox & Portwine, 1835.

46. Cornwall JV, Lewis JD. Leg ulcer revisited. *Br J Surg* 1983; **70:** 681.

47. Corrigan TP, Kakkar VV. Early changes in the postphlebitic limb: their clinical significance. *Br J Surg* 1973; **60:** 808–13.

48. Cranley JJ, Krause RJ, Strasser ES. Chronic venous insufficiency of the lower extremity. *Surgery* 1961; **49:** 48–58.

49. Critchett G. *Lectures on the Causes and Treatment of Ulcers of the Lower Extremity.* London: Churchill, 1849.

50. Dale JJ, Callam MJ, Ruckley CV, Harper DR, Berry PN. Chronic ulcers of the leg: a study of prevalence in a Scottish community. *Health Bull* 1983; **41:** 310–14.

51. Dale WA. Venous bypass surgery. *Surg Clin North Am* 1982; **62:** 391–8.

52. Dale WA, Foster JH. Leg ulcers. *Trans South Surg Assoc* 1963; **775:** 399.

53. Darke SG, Penfold C. Venous ulceration and saphenous ligation. *Eur J Vasc Surg* 1992; **6:** 4–9.

54. DePalma RG. Do primary varicose veins lead to ulceration. *Vasc Surg* 1996; **30(1):** 1–3.

55. de Takats G, Graupner GW. Division of the popliteal vein in deep venous insufficiency of the lower extremities. *Surgery* 1951; **29:** 342–57.

56. de Takats G, Quint H, Tillotsen BI, Crittenden PJ. The impairment of the circulation in the varicose extremity. *Arch Surg* 1929; **18:** 671–86.

57. Dickson Wright A. The treatment of indolent ulcer of the leg. *Lancet* 1931; **1:** 457–60.

58. Dodd HJ. The cause, prevention and arrest of varicose veins. *Lancet* 1964; **2:** 809.

59. Dodd H, Cockett FB. *The Pathology and Surgery of the Veins of the Lower Limb.* Edinburgh: Livingstone, 1956.

60. Dodd HJ, Gaylarde PM, Sakarny I. Skin oxygen tensions in venous insufficiency of the lower leg. *J R Soc Med* 1985; **78:** 373–6.

61. Eaglestein WH. Personal communication, 1985.

62. Edwards AT, Herrick SE, Suarez-Mendez VJ, McCollum CN. Oxidants, antioxidants and venous ulceration. *Br J Surg* 1992; **79(5):** 443–4.

63. Ersek RA, Jones MH, Tilak SP, Howard JM. Studies of peripheral lymphatics following femoral vein occlusion in the dog. *Surgery* 1965; **57:** 269.

64. Fagrell B. Local microcirculation in chronic venous incompetence and leg ulcers. *Vasc Surg* 1979; **13:** 217–25.

65. Fagrell B. Vital capillary microscopy. A clinical method for studying changes of the nutritional skin capillaries in legs with arteriosclerosis obliterans. *Scand J Clin Lab Invest Suppl* 1973; **133:** 2–50.

66. Falanga V, Eaglestein WH. The 'trap' hypothesis of venous ulceration. *Lancet* 1993; **341:** 1006–8.

67. Field P, Van Boxel PV. The role of the Linton flap procedure in the management of stasis dermatitis and ulceration in the lower limb. *Surgery* 1971; **70:** 920–6.

68. Fontaine R. Remarks concerning venous thrombosis and its sequelae. John Homans memorial lecture. *Surgery* 1957; **41:** 6–25.

69. Foote RR. *Varicose Veins.* London: Butterworths, 1954.

70. Gay J. *Varicose Disease of the Lower Extremities and its Allied Disorders: Skin Discoloration, Induration and Ulcer.* London: Churchill, 1868.

71. Gius JA. Arteriovenous anastomoses and varicose veins. *Arch Surg* 1960; **81:** 299–308.

72. Greenwood JE, Edwards AT, McCollum CN. The possible role of ischemia-reperfusion in the pathogenesis of chronic venous ulceration. *Wounds* 1995; **7(6):** 211–19.

73. Haeger K. Three to six year results with standardized surgical therapy of venous ulcers. *Vasc Dis* 1966; **3:** 106–8.

74. Haeger K. Diuretic treatment of postthrombotic and varicose oedema in the lower extremities. *J Cardiovasc Surg* 1961; **2:** 367–75.

75. Haeger KH, Bergman L. Skin temperature of normal and varicose legs and some reflections on the etiology of varicose veins. *Angiology* 1963; **14:** 473–9.

76. Haimovici H. Abnormal arteriovenous shunts associated with chronic venous insufficiency. *J Cardiovasc Surg* 1976; **17:** 473–82.

77. Haimovici H, Steinman C, Caplan LH. Role of arteriovenous anastomosis in vascular diseases of the lower extremity. *Ann Surg* 1966; **164:** 990–1002.

78. Halbert AR, Stacey MC, Rohr JB, Jopp-McKay A. The effect of bacterial colonization on venous ulcer healing. *Australas J Dermatol* 1992; **33:** 75–80.

79. Harvey W. *Exercitatio Anatomica de Motu Cordis et Sanguinis in Animalibus.* Frankfurt: W Fitzer, 1628.

80. Haxthausen H. Om pathogensen af ulcus cruris varicosum. *Nord Med Tidshv* 1936; **12:** 1665–70.

81. Hehne HJ, Locher JT, Waibel PP, Fridrich R. Zur Bedeutung arteriovenöser Anastomosen bei der primaren Varicosis und der chronisch-venosen Insuffizienz. *Vasa* 1974; **3:** 396–8.

82. Hellgren L. *An Epidemiological Survey of Skin Diseases, Tattooing and Rheumatic Diseases.* Uppsala: Slinquist Wiksell, 1967.

83. Helliwell PS, Cheesbrough MJ. Arthropathica ulcerosa: a study of reduced ankle movement in association with chronic leg ulceration. *J Rheumatol* 1994; **21(8):** 1512–14.

84. Herrick SE, Sloan P, McGuric M, Freak L, McCollam CN, Ferguson MW. Sequential changes in histologic patterns and extracellular matrix deposition during the healing of chronic venous ulcers. *Am J Pathol* 1992; **141:** 1085–95.

85. Hilton J. A course of lectures on pain and the therapeutic influence of mechanical and physiological rest in accidents and surgical disease. *Lancet* 1861; **2:** 245–7.

86. Hoare MC, Nicolaides AN, Miles CR, *et al.* The role of primary varicose veins in venous ulceration. *Surgery* 1982; **92:** 450.

87. Hodgson J. *A Treatise on Diseases of the Arteries and Veins.* London: Underwood, 1815.

88. Holan V. Relation between aetiology and treatment of leg ulcers. *Br J Surg* 1996; **83:** 249–50.

89. Holling HE, Beecher HK, Linton RR. Study of the tendency to oedema formation associated with incompetence of the valves of the communicating veins of the leg. Oxygen tension of the blood contained in varicose veins. *J Clin Invest* 1938; **17:** 555–61.

90. Homans J. The etiology and treatment of varicose ulcer of the leg. *Surg Gynecol Obstet* 1917; **24:** 300–11.

91. Home E. *Practical Observations on the Treatment of Ulcers of the Leg, Considered as a Branch of Military Surgery.* 2nd edition. London: Bulmer, 1801.

92. Hopkins NFG, Jamieson CW. Antibiotic concentration in the exudate of venous ulcers. A measure of local arterial insufficiency. *Br J Surg* 1982; **69:** 676.

93. Hopkins NFG, Spinks TJ, Rhodes CG, Ranicar ASO, Jamieson CW. Positron emission tomography in venous ulceration and liposclerosis: a study of regional tissue function. *Br Med J* 1983; **6:** 9–14.

94. Howell R. Hypostatic ulceration and Klinefelter's syndrome. *Br Med J* 1978; **2:** 95–6.

95. Hunt T. *A Guide to the Treatment of Diseases of the Skin: with Suggestions for Their Prevention.* 4th edition. London: Richards, 1859.

96. Jancar J. Hypostatic ulceration and male sex chromosomal abnormalities. *Br Med J* 1971; **1:** 434.

97. Johnson ND, Queral LA, Flinn WR, Yao JST, Bergan JJ. Late objective assessment of venous valve surgery. *Arch Surg* 1981; **116:** 1461–6.

98. Kistner R. Primary venous valve incompetence of the leg. *Am J Surg* 1980; **140:** 218–24.

99. Knighton DR, Hunt TK, Thakral KK, Goodson WH. The role of platelets and fibrin in the healing sequence: an *in vivo* study of angiogenesis and collagen synthesis. *Ann Surg* 1982; **196:** 379–88.

100. Labropoulos N, Giannoukas AD, Nicolaides AN, Ramaswami G, Leon M, Burke P. New insights into the pathophysiologic condition of venous ulceration with color-flow duplex imaging: implications for treatment? *J Vasc Surg* 1995; **22(1):** 45–50.

101. Lagatolla NR, Paul Clarke M, Burnand KG. Growth factors in venous ulcers. *Phlebology* 1995; **10:** 802–4.

102. Lagatolla NR, Stacey MC, Burnand KG, Gaffney PG. Growth factors, tissue and urokinase-type plasminogen activators in venous ulcers. *Ann Cardiol Angiol* 1995; **44:** 299–303.

103. Leach RD, Browse NL. Effect of venous hypertension on canine hind limb lymph. *Br J Surg* 1985; **72:** 275–8.

104. Leu HJ. The prognostic significance of cutaneous and microvascular changes in venous leg ulcers. *Vasc Dis* 1965; **2:** 77–80.

105. Lindemayr W, Loefferer O, Mostbeck A, Partsch H. Arteriovenous shunts in primary varicosis? A critical essay. *Vasc Surg* 1972; **6:** 9–14.

106. Linton RR. The communicating veins of the lower leg and the operating technics for their ligation. *Ann Surg* 1938; **107:** 582.

107. Linton RR. The post-thrombotic ulceration of the lower extremity: its etiology and surgical treatment. *Ann Surg* 1953; **138:** 415.

108. Linton RR, Hardy IB. Post-thrombotic syndrome of the lower extremity. Treatment by interruption of the superficial femoral vein and ligation and stripping of the long and short saphenous veins. *Surgery* 1948; **24:** 452–68.

109. Lockhart-Mummery HE, Smitham JH. Varicose ulcer: study of the deep veins with special reference to retrograde venography. *Br J Surg* 1951; **38:** 284–95.

110. Löfferer O, Mostbeck A, Partsch H. Arteriovenose Kurzseblüsse der Extremitaten nuclearmedizinische untersuchungen mit besonderer Berücksichtigung des postthrombotischen Unterschenkelgeschwüs. *Zentralbl Phlebol* 1969; **8:** 2–22.

111. Lookingbill DP, Miller SH, Knowles RC. Bacteriology of chronic leg ulcers. *Arch Dermatol* 1978; **114:** 1765–8.

112. Ludbrook J. *Aspects of Venous Function in the Lower Limbs.* Springfield, IL: Thomas, 1966.

113. Mani R, Gorman FW, White JE. Transcutaneous measurements of oxygen tension at the edges of leg ulcers: preliminary communication. *J R Soc Med* 1986; **79:** 650–4.

114. Marks R. Personal communication, 1981.

115. Marks R, Williams D, Pearse AD. Models to study function and disease of the skin. In: Plewig G, Marks R, eds. *Skin Models.* Berlin: Springer-Verlag, 1985.

116. May R. Der Femoralis bypass bein postthrombotischen zustandsbild. *Vasa* 1972; **1:** 267.

117. McEwan AJ, McArdle CS. Effect of hydroxyethylrutosides on blood oxygen levels and venous insufficiency symptoms in varicose veins. *Br Med J* 1971; **2:** 138–41.

118. Mclrvine AJ, Corbett CRR, Aston NO, Sherriff EA, Wiseman PA, Jamieson CW. The demonstration of sapheno-femoral incompetence: doppler ultrasound compared with standard clinical tests. *Br J Surg* 1984; **71:** 509–10.

119. Medawar PB. The behaviour of mammalian skin epithelium under strictly anaerobic conditions. *Q J Microsc Sci* 1947; **88:** 27–37.

120. Michel CC. Aetiology of venous ulceration. *Br J Surg* 1990; **77:** 1071.

121. Moosa HH, Falanga V, Steed DL, *et al.* Oxygen diffusion in chronic venous ulceration. *J Cardiovasc Surg* 1987; **28:** 464–7.

122. Moyses C, Cederholm-Williams C, Michel CC. Haemoconcentrations and the accumulation of white cells in the feet during venous stasis. *Int J Microcirc Clin Exp* 1987; **3:** 311–20.

123. Myers MB, Cherry G. Pathophysiology and treatment of stasis ulcers of the leg. *Am Surg* 1971; **37:** 167–74.

124. Myers MB, Richter M, Cherry G. Relationship between edema and the healing rate of stasis ulcers of the leg. *Am J Surg* 1972; **124:** 666–8.

125. Negus D, Friedgood A. The effective management of venous ulceration. *Br J Surg* 1983; **70:** 623–7.

126. Negus D. Prevention and treatment of venous ulceration. *Ann R Coll Surg Engl* 1985; **67:** 144–8.

127. Nelzen O, Bergqvist D, Lindhagen A. The prevalence of chronic lower limb ulceration has been underestimated: results of a validated population questionnaire. *Br J Surg* 1996; **83:** 255–8.

128. Nelzen O, Bergqvist D, Lindhagen A, Hallbrook T. Chronic leg ulcers: an underestimated problem in primary health care among elderly patients. *J Epidemiol Community Health* 1991; **45(3):** 184–7.

129. Nicolaides AN, Hussein MK, Szendro G, Christopoulos D, Vasdekis S, Clarke H. The relation of venous ulceration with ambulatory venous pressure measurements. *J Vasc Surg* 1993; **17(2):** 414–19.

130. Partsch H. Investigations on the pathogenesis of venous leg ulcers. *Acta Chir Scand* 1988; **544:** 25–9.

131. Perrin M, Bayon JM, Castells-Ferrer P, Hiltbrand B. Résultats de la chirurgie restauratrice dans les reflux veineux profonds à l'étage sous inguinal. A propos de 93 interventions. *Phlebologie* 1992; **45:** 315–30.

132. Pietra GG, Szidon JP, Leventhal MM, Fishman AP. Haemoglobin as a tracer in haemodynamic pulmonary oedema. *Science* 1969; **166:** 1643–6.

133. Piulachs P, Vidal-Barraquer F. Pathogenic study of varicose veins. *Angiology* 1953; **4:** 59.

134. Prasad A, Ali-Khan A, Mortimer P. Leg ulcers and oedema: a study exploring the prevalence, aetiology, and possible significance of oedema in venous ulcers. *Phlebology* 1990; **5:** 181–7.

135. Queral LA, Whitehouse WM, Flinn WR, Nieman HL, Yao JST, Bergan JJ. Surgical correction of chronic deep venous insufficiency by valvular transposition. *Surgery* 1980; **87:** 688–95.

136. Ruckley CV, Callam MJ, Harper DR, Dale JJ. The Lothian and Forth Valley survey. Part 4. Arterial disease. In: Negus D, Jantet G, eds. *Phlebology '85.* London: Libbey, 1986.

137. Rutter AG. Chronic ulcer of the leg in young subjects. *Surg Gynecol Obstet* 1954; **98:** 291–301.

138. Ryan TJ. The epidermis and its blood supply in venous disorders of the leg. *Trans St John's Hosp Dermatol Soc* 1969; **55(1):** 51–63.

139. Ryan TJ. *The Management of Leg Ulcers.* Oxford: Oxford Medical Publications, 1983.

140. Ryan TJ, Copeman PMW. Microvascular patterns and blood stasis in skin diseases. *Br J Dermatol* 1970; **8:** 563–73.

141. Salim A. The role of oxygen-derived free radicals in the management of venous ulceration: a new approach. *World J Surg* 1991; **15:** 264–9.

142. Schalin L. Arteriovenous communications localized by thermography and identified by operative microscopy. *Acta Chir Scand* 1981; **147:** 409–20.

143. Schraibman IG. The significance of B-haemolytic streptococci in chronic leg ulcers. *Ann R Coll Surg Engl* 1990; **72:** 123–4.

144. Schraibman IG, Stratton FJ. Nutritional status of patients with leg ulcers. *J R Soc Med* 1985; **78:** 39–42.

145. Scott HJ, Coleridge Smith PD, Scurr JH. Histological study of white blood cells and their

association with lipodermatosclerosis and venous ulceration. *Br J Surg* 1991; **78:** 210–11.

146. Scott HJ, McMullin GM, Coleridge Smith PD, Scurr JH. Venous ulceration: the role of the white blood cell. *Phlebology* 1989; **4:** 153–9.

147. Scurr JH, Coleridge Smith PD. Pathogenesis of venous ulceration. *Phlebology Suppl* 1992; **1:** 13–16.

148. Sethia KK, Darke SG. Long saphenous incompetence as a cause of venous ulceration. *Br J Surg* 1984; **71:** 754–5.

149. Shami SK, Sarin S, Cheatle TR, Scurr JH, Coleridge-Smith PD. Venous ulcers and the superficial venous system. *J Vasc Surg* 1993; **17(3):** 487–90.

150. Shields DA, Andaz S, Abeysinghe RD, Porter JB, Scurr JH, Coleridge-Smith PD. Plasma lactoferrin as a marker of white cell degranulation in venous disease. *Phlebology* 1994; **9:** 55–8.

151. Shirley HH, Wolfram CG, Wasserman K, Mayerson HS. Capillary permeability to macromolecules: stretched pore phenomenon. *Am J Physiol* 1957; **190:** 189–93.

152. Smirk FH. Observations on causes of oedema in congestive heart failure. *Clin Sci* 1936; **2:** 317–35.

153. Stacey MC, Burnand KG, Layer GT, Pattison M. Transcutaneous oxygen tensions in assessing the treatment of venous ulcers. *Br J Surg* 1990; **77:** 1050–4.

154. Stewart GJ, Pattison M, Burnand KG. Abnormal fibrinolysis: the cause of lipodermatosclerosis or 'chronic cellulitis' in patients with primary lymphoedema. *Lymphology* 1984; **17:** 23–7.

155. Stibe E, Cheatle TR, Coleridge-Smith PD, Scurr JH. Liposclerotic skin: a diffusion block or a perfusion problem? *Phlebology* 1990; **5:** 231–6.

156. Sutton R, Darke SG. Stripping the long saphenous vein peroperatively. Retrograde saphenography in patients with and without venous ulceration. *Br J Surg* 1986; **73:** 305–7.

157. Taheri SA, Lazar L, Elias S, Marchand P, Hefner R. Surgical treatment of postphlebitic syndrome with vein valve transplantation. *Am J Surg* 1982; **144:** 221–4.

158. Thomas AMC, Tomlinson PJ, Boggon RP. Incompetent perforating vein ligation in the treatment of venous ulceration. *Ann R Coll Surg Engl* 1986; **68:** 214–15.

159. Thomas PRS, Nash GB, Dormandy JA. White cell accumulation in the dependent legs of patients with venous hypertension. A possible mechanism for trophic changes in the skin. *Br Med J* 1988; **296:** 1693–5.

160. Tibbs DJ, Fletcher EWC. Direction of flow in the superficial veins as a guide to venous disorders in the lower limbs. *Surgery* 1983; **93(6):** 758–67.

161. Tronnier M, Schmeller W, Wolff HH. Morphological changes in lipodermatosclerosis and venous ulcers: light microscopy, immunohistochemistry and electron microscropy. *Phlebology* 1994; **9:** 48–54.

162. Turner Warwick W. *The Rational Treatment of Varicose Veins and Varicocele (with notes on the application of the obliterative method of treatment to other conditions).* London: Faber & Faber, 1931.

163. Van Limborgh J, Boersma W, Van der Lugt L. Experimental production of ulcus cruris venosum conditions in frogs. *Zentralbl Phlebol* 1966; **5:** 66–74.

164. Vanscheidt W, Lanff H, Wokalek H, Niedner R, Schopf E. Pericapillary fibrin cuff: a histological sign of venous leg ulceration. *J Cutan Pathol* 1990; **17:** 266–8.

165. Verneuil A. Du siège réel et primitif des varices des membres inférieurs. *Gaz Méd Paris* 1855; **10:** 524.

166. Vogler E. Angiographische Beitrage zur Enstehung von Gefasserkrankungen und Durchblutungsstrorungen unter besonderer Berücksichtigung der terminalen Strombahn. *Fortschr Roentgenstr* 1954; **81:** 479–97.

167. Warren R, Thayer TR. Transplantation of the saphenous vein for postphlebitic stasis. *Surgery* 1954; **35:** 867–76.

168. Whimster I. Cited in: Dodd H, Cockett FB. *The Pathology and Surgery of the Veins of the Lower Limb.* Edinburgh: Livingstone, 1956.

169. Whiston RJ, Hallett MB, Davies EV, Harding KG, Lane IF. Inappropriate neutrophil activation in venous disease. *Br J Surg* 1994; **81:** 695–8.

170. Widmer LK. *Peripheral Venous Disorders. Basle Study III.* Bern: Hans Huber, 1978.

171. Widmer LK, Plechl SC, Leu HJ, Boner H. Venenerkraunkungen bei 1800 Berufstatigen, Basier Studie II. *Schweiz Med Wochenschr* 1967; **97:** 107–10.

172. Wiseman R. *Eight Chirurgical Treatises.* London: Tooke & Meredith, 1705.

173. Wood ML, Reilly GD, Smith GT. Ulceration of the hand secondary to a radial arteriovenous fistula: a model for varicose ulceration. *Br Med J* 1983; **297:** 1167–8.

174. Zwiefach BW. The structural basis of permeability and other functions of blood capillaries. *Cold Spring Harbor Symp Quant Biol* 1940; **8:** 216–23.

CHAPTER 19

Venous ulceration: diagnosis

The clinical features of venous ulceration 531
Investigations 537
Differential diagnosis of leg ulcers 539
Investigation of a venous ulcer 562
References 566

The clinical features of venous ulceration

History

Leg ulcers may develop slowly or suddenly. The patient often remembers that an area of skin became thickened and discoloured and then, for no apparent reason, began to blister or weep before rapidly breaking into an open sore. Trauma is often the precipitating factor if the onset of ulceration is sudden. The supermarket trolley, an inadvertent knock or kick, or an insignificant scratch or scrape may all cause a break in the continuity of the skin which becomes an ulcer. The patient often reports that varicose veins were present before the ulcer developed, and may recollect a prior episode of deep vein thrombosis.

The association of pain and ulceration is well recognized, but this does not help to differentiate the cause of the ulcer unless there is a clear history of persistent ischaemic rest pain in the foot. Some small ulcers are very painful while some large ulcers are painless, although the reverse is also true. A complete absence of pain should suggest the possibility of a gumma or a neuropathic ulcer.

When a patient is seen with a first-time ulcer a detailed history must be taken of its onset and development. A history of trauma must be sought and enquiry must be made into any possible venous abnormality or skin changes noticed by the patient before the ulcer appeared. Direct questions should be asked about the presence of varicose veins, and any previous investigations or treatment for any venous problems, especially deep vein thrombosis. Patients must be asked specifically whether they have ever had leg swelling after an operation or pregnancy, an event which can easily slip from the patient's memory. A complicated or difficult operation, a fracture of the lower limb treated by a plaster cast, or prolonged bedrest may cause a silent deep vein thrombosis which may subsequently cause post-thrombotic skin changes (see Chapter 8). Patients must also be questioned about episodes of chest pain, haemoptysis or a known history of pulmonary embolism. Whenever possible, the objective evidence that supported the diagnosis of deep vein thrombosis or pulmonary embolism should be obtained. Treatment with anticoagulants is only indirect evidence of a thrombosis or embolism and is not completely reliable,[42,44] whereas a phlebogram or duplex ultrasound scan demonstrating thrombus or an isotope lung scan showing a ventilation–perfusion mismatch provide strong evidence.

Many patients with ulcers have a history of previous ulceration.[20] The number of episodes of ulceration, the time taken for each ulcer to heal, the period that the patient has been free from ulceration, the methods of treatment and any means used to prevent recurrence must all be recorded. Particular attention must be paid to previous operations or sclerotherapy to obliterate varicosities, and the use of elastic stockings. Very rarely, deep vein reconstruction may have been carried out in an

Table 19.1 The common causes of leg ulcer

Cause of ulcer	Incidence (%)
Venous insufficiency	70–90
Arterial insufficiency	5–20
Rheumatoid arthritis	5
Trauma	2
Neoplastic change	1
Others	0.05–2

attempt to prevent recurrence, but this may become a more common feature in the future.

A list of the common causes of leg ulcers and their approximate incidence is shown in Table 19.1. Many of the causes of leg ulcer are rare, and direct questions designed to elucidate the precise aetiology of the ulcer are usually unhelpful. Arterial, rheumatoid, diabetic and traumatic ulcers are, however, common, and specific questions should be put to confirm or refute these diagnoses. An 'atypical' ulcer may lead to further questions, for instance a history of diarrhoea may suggest pyoderma gangrenosum complicating ulcerative colitis.

A history of intermittent claudication, rest pain, transient ischaemic attacks or cerebral infarction, supports a diagnosis of underlying arterial disease as does a history of angina pectoris or myocardial infarction. A history of diabetes, treated by oral hypoglycaemic drugs or insulin injections, should raise the suspicion of infective or neuropathic ulceration. Heavy smokers and diabetics are particularly prone to develop ischaemic ulceration.

Joint pain, swelling and restricted movement suggest a diagnosis of rheumatoid ulcer. Any anti-inflammatory drugs taken by the patient for rheumatoid arthritis should be recorded. A clear history of injury in the absence of any preceding skin changes favours a diagnosis of traumatic ulceration but does not exclude other causes of ulceration.

In addition to obtaining a careful history of the ulcer and these specific enquiries, a full general inquiry must be made into all systems, including past medical conditions, drugs, allergies and the patient's social circumstances.

PHYSICAL SIGNS

The physical examination should be carried out with the patient fully undressed, except for underpants in a man, and brassière and pants in a woman. There is no place for simply examining a patient's leg by rolling up a trouser leg or lifting a skirt while the patient remains seated with all their other clothes in place, prohibiting examination of the groins, the abdomen and the rest of the body.

The examination should commence with the undressed patient lying comfortably on a couch in a warm, well-lit room. Blankets should be provided for additional warmth and modesty.

General examination

The general examination is designed to detect evidence of systemic disease. Anaemia, polycythaemia, cyanosis, jaundice, myxoedema, scleroderma, rheumatoid arthritis and Klinefelter's syndrome are some of the many conditions that may be found that might be relevant to the ulcer. Inspection of the hands can be especially valuable, revealing clubbing of the nails, koilonychia, rheumatoid changes, gouty tophi or the spindle-shaped fingers of scleroderma. A few patients with venous ulcers have Klinefelter's or XYY syndrome. Tall men with small genitalia should have their chromosomes tested (see page 519). Palpation of the pulse may reveal atrial fibrillation, and measurement of the blood pressure detects hypertension. Abdominal examination and rectal examination should be performed on all patients. Even simple inspection of the abdomen may reveal distended superficial veins indicative of an iliocaval obstruction. It is not appropriate to describe the full general examination of a patient in this book, but it is necessary to stress that *leg ulcers are so often a manifestation of distant disease that a complete medical examination is essential in all patients.*

Local examination

Both lower limbs should be examined with the patient lying and standing. It is easier to begin with the leg horizontal and then ask the patient to stand.

The ulcer

The site and the number of ulcers should be recorded. It is helpful to draw the areas of ulceration on an outline plan of the leg together with their maximum dimensions. An instant polaroid photograph of the ulcer with a centimetre rule attached to the leg allows later measurement of its surface area and comparison with future appearances.[70]

Many other techniques have been used for estimating ulcer size. The outline of the ulcer can be traced on plastic sheeting or tracing paper with an indelible pen,[47] a mould can be made to fill in the area of the ulcer and direct computerized measurements of the surface area using a light pen and a

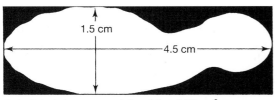

Calculated ulcer area = 1.5 × 4.5 = 6.75 cm²

Figure 19.1 A diagram to show why the product of the greatest width and the greatest length overestimates the surface area of an ulcer. Fortunately, most ulcers are oval in shape and this makes the overestimate (the black area) quite small (10–20% on average).[88]

sonic digitizer[28] or complex stereo photographs (stereo-photogrammetry) have been advocated.[14] A stereographic system is now commercially available but is very expensive. Whether the introduction of these expensive techniques into the science of ulcer measurement is of value remains to be seen. The simplest and cheapest way of assessing the area of an ulcer and its response to treatment is to calculate the product of accurate measurements of the maximum width and breadth (Figure 19.1). This has been shown to correlate well with more complex forms of measurement (Figure 19.2) even though it slightly overestimates ulcer size.[88]

Site

The site of an ulcer gives an indication of its cause. Venous ulcers typically occur in the lower third of the lower leg, the 'gaiter' region (Figure 19.3a). They can probably occur on the foot or higher up the calf in exceptional circumstances but other causes should be excluded before attributing ulceration in these areas to venous disease (Figure 19.3b). Venous ulcers tend to be situated on the medial or lateral surfaces of the leg; solitary ulcers on the front or the back of the leg, even though they are in the 'gaiter' area, may not be venous.

Size

The size of the ulcer gives little indication of its aetiology but does, of course, have considerable bearing on its treatment and must therefore be carefully recorded. We have shown that ulcer size correlates well with its time to healing[88] so size must be clearly specified in any study of ulcer healing.

Shape

Venous ulcers can appear in many different shapes. They are mostly oval or circular but may become irregular if they enlarge rapidly.

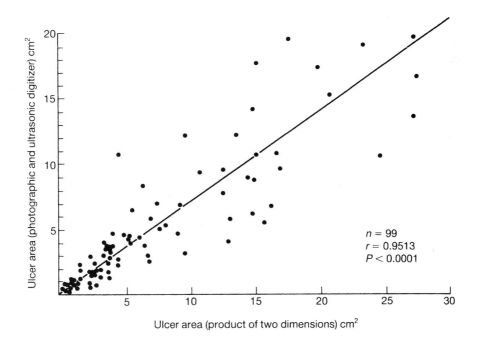

$n = 99$
$r = 0.9513$
$P < 0.0001$

Figure 19.2 This graph compares the areas of 99 ulcers, estimated by the product of the two greatest diameters, with their areas, measured with an ultrasonic digitizer from scaled polaroid photographs. The correlation is very good but the simple product method invariably overestimates the true area of the ulcer.[88]

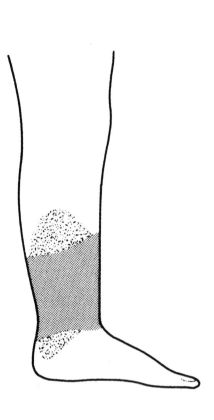

(a)

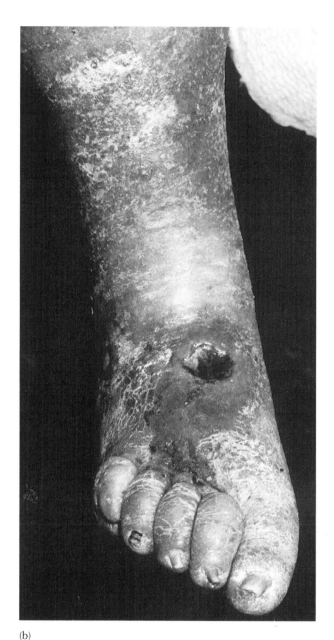

(b)

Figure 19.3 (a) The ulcer-bearing area of the lower leg is often called the 'gaiter' area. The hatched area is the 'gaiter area' but ulcers may also occur in the stippled area. (b) This ulcer on the foot looked like a venous ulcer because there was also eczema and pigmentation but the patient had normal veins and polycythaemia rubra vera. Even if an ulcer on the foot appears 'venous' other causes must be excluded.

Edge

An established venous ulcer with a granulating base which is trying to heal has a pale pink–purple sloping edge of new epithelium (Figure 19.4) but a young actively extending ulcer often has a punched-out edge and a slough covered base (Figure 19.5). *Any elevation of the ulcer edge should arouse suspicions of malignant change.*[56] Tuberculosis should be considered if the ulcer edge is undermined.

Surface (base)

The appearances of the base of a venous ulcer depend more upon the state of development of the ulcer than on its cause. An extending, infected ulcer is usually covered with slough and has a copious exudate hiding any granulation tissue from view (Figure 19.5). A chronic ulcer of many years' standing often has a pale pink or white fibrous base with little or no granulation tissue, indicating extensive fibrosis and a poor blood supply (Figure 19.6). A

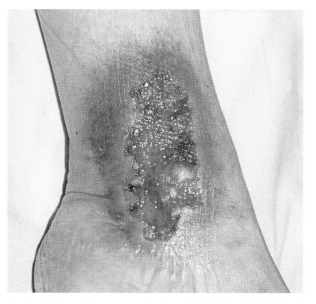

Figure 19.4 This venous ulcer is in the process of healing. The healthy looking granulation tissue in the base is being rapidly covered by a thin layer of new 'pink' epithelium.

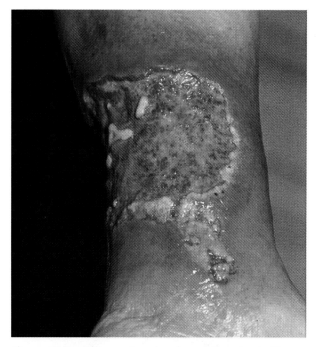

Figure 19.6 This venous ulcer has a base of pale fibrous tissue (arrowed), indicating that it has been present for some time and that it will be very slow to heal unless the fibrous tissue is excised.

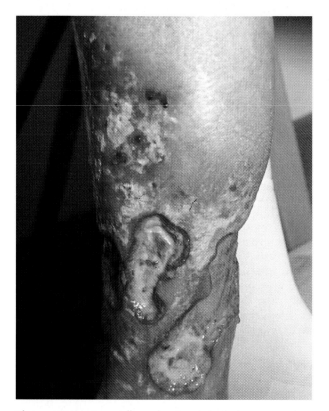

Figure 19.5 A rapidly enlarging infected venous ulcer with a punched-out edge and a base covered by thick yellow slough. No granulation tissue can be seen and there are no signs of healing.

surface of bright red, velvety granulation tissue that bleeds when touched or wiped indicates a good blood supply and good healing potential (Figure 19.7). Healing is occurring when there is a thin layer of pink epithelium growing over the granulation tissue at the edge of the ulcer (Figure 19.7). Very occasionally, the granulation tissue proliferates and rises above the level of the surrounding skin.

The tissues beneath the visible surface of the ulcer, the true base, can only be seen when the surface exudate, slough or granulations have been removed; they consist of a mixture of granulation tissue and fibrous tissue. The more chronic the ulcer, the more fibrous is its base. The fibrosis, and sometimes the ulceration itself, can extend down into the fascia, periosteum and even the underlying muscle or tendon but venous ulcers never extend into bone. If there is evidence of cortical bone involvement as opposed to periostitis, then osteomyelitis, ischaemia, neoplasia or trauma must be responsible.

Surrounding tissues

Venous ulcers usually arise within a much larger area of pigmented, thickened and indurated skin

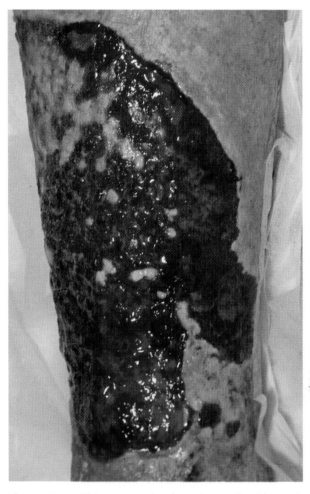

Figure 19.7 This venous ulcer has a base of healthy 'red' granulation tissue and a healthy edge. It is likely to heal rapidly from both its edge and the small islets of epithelium within it.

and subcutaneous fat. This is often also inflamed and may be incorrectly diagnosed as cellulitis (see Figures 16.3 and 16.5, pages 476 and 478). In the past these changes have been called 'post-thrombotic', even though they can occur in the absence of clear-cut evidence of deep vein damage (see Chapter 15), or 'fat necrosis', even when in the majority of cases there is no histological evidence of fat necrosis (in our view this term should be reserved for the rare situation when there is histological confirmation of dead fat cells, a complication which does undoubtedly occur in a few limbs with venous ulceration), or 'panniculitis',[71] even though there is often no inflammatory response either clinically or histologically.

For these reasons we coined the term 'lipodermatosclerosis' to described the pre-ulcer state.[12,15,16]

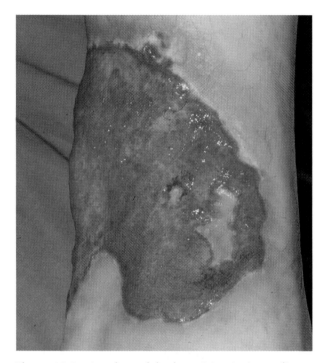

Figure 19.8 An ulcer of the leg arising in 'normal' surrounding skin. It is very difficult to decide on clinical grounds, in the absence of any pigmentation or lipodermatosclerosis in the adjacent skin, whether this ulcer is venous or not. In fact the patient had a normal venous system but was suffering from AIDS.

The word implies that the process is sclerotic and involves both the skin and the fat, and we have shown that the deposition of pericapillary fibrin which leads to fibrosis and collagen deposition is invariably found in biopsies from this abnormal tissue (see Chapters 15 and 18). The term lipodermatosclerosis can be shortened to liposclerosis or abbreviated to LDS.

The absence of the characteristic changes of lipodermatosclerosis around an ulcer should immediately raise the suspicion that the ulcer is not caused by venous disease (Figure 19.8), but does not exclude a venous aetiology.

Dilated intradermal venules at the ankle

The significance of a patch of dilated intradermal venules, usually in the skin over the ankle, below the ulcer, the 'ankle flare', was stressed by Cockett (Figure 6.10).[25] It is also called the 'corona phlebectatica' and is the clinical manifestation of a persistently elevated venous pressure which causes dilatation and elongation of the capillaries and venules (Chapters 15, 16 and 18).[18] Lipodermatosclerosis is commonly associated with an ankle flare.

The subcutaneous veins

Large subcutaneous varicosities may be seen close to an ulcer but, though their presence lends support to a diagnosis of venous ulceration, it is not diagnostic, and the absence of abnormal veins certainly does not exclude the diagnosis. The presence of 'blow-out veins', large varices overlying an incompetent communicating vein (Figure 6.11),[25] is usually significant, but superficial venous dilatation is often only seen some distance from an ulcer because the lipodermatosclerosis prevents the veins within it from dilating, with the exception of those that are very close to the skin. Ulcers on the lateral side of the leg are often associated with short saphenous vein incompetence.

Long saphenous, short saphenous and calf communicating vein incompetence must be sought and excluded in every limb with ulceration. Tourniquet tests and Perthes' walking test (see Chapter 6) should be performed to obtain an immediate rough indication of the major sites of venous incompetence in limbs with visible superficial varicosities followed by objective information from duplex scanning of both the superficial and the deep veins.

When an ulcer is associated with oedema, lipodermatosclerosis and dilated veins, the cause is likely to be venous, but venous ulcers can develop in an apparently otherwise normal limb (Figure 19.8). In these circumstances an abnormality of the veins must be confirmed with objective tests (see Chapters 4 and 6) and other causes of ulceration must be excluded.

Regional lymph glands

The lymph glands in the groin and popliteal fossa should always be palpated. The possibility of malignant change in the ulcer must be considered if they are enlarged and hard but this is a rare event; the most common cause of inguinal lymphadenopathy is infection from the ulcer.

Arterial circulation

All the pulses of the limb should be palpated, especially the dorsalis pedis and posterior tibial pulses, though the latter may be difficult to feel if the artery lies directly beneath the ulcer. A Doppler ultrasound flow detector should be used to measure the ankle-to-arm pressure index in all patients with ulcers. The normal pressure index is between 1 and 1.2 (the pressure in the leg being equal to or slightly higher than that in the arm) but the level which is indicative of arterial insufficiency is open to dispute. Some investigators have proposed that a pressure index below 0.9 is indicative of an arterial influence in the development of ulceration.[29,82] A pressure index of less than 0.7 is certainly significant and, in the absence of any venous abnormality, may indicate that arterial insufficiency is the sole cause of the ulceration.

Doppler ultrasound pressure measurements are undoubtedly helpful in assessing the role of the arterial supply of the leg but venous disease may still be the main cause of an ulcer, even when the pressures are significantly reduced.[82] It can be extremely difficult to decide which factor is playing the major role in the genesis of an ulcer, and it can be still more difficult to decide which abnormality to correct first, though a pressure index below 0.7 usually means that the arterial problem must be corrected before the contribution of the venous abnormality can be properly assessed or successfully treated.

It is important to differentiate between venous and arterial ulcers as standard compression treatment is contraindicated if there is evidence of arterial insufficiency. Stress has therefore been laid on the Doppler pressures as an important aid to clinical diagnosis and management.[82]

Comment

In the absence of severe ischaemia or another obvious cause, ulcers can be treated as 'venous' while awaiting the results of further investigations. Remember that arterial calcification, common in diabetics, causes falsely high measurements of ankle pressure.

Investigations

An erythrocyte count should be obtained to exclude anaemia or polycythaemia. Sickle cell disease or trait should be considered in all patients likely to be susceptible to this erythrocyte abnormality. Rheumatoid autoantibodies and antinuclear factor levels should be measured if there is a suspicion of rheumatoid arthritis, vasculitis or any of the other autoimmune diseases.

Serological tests for syphilis (e.g. the *Treponema pallidum* haemagglutination test) must be obtained if the ulceration is typical of syphilis (a 'punched-out' edge with a 'wash-leather' base). These tests should also be obtained if a syphilitic aetiology is suspected from the history, or if the ulcer is 'atypical'.

A biopsy of the ulcer may have to be taken under local anaesthetic, if it is felt that the ulcer is neither venous nor arterial. *When in doubt a biopsy should be performed*; it will often provide a definite diagnosis and will not cause any harm provided there is no arterial insufficiency. Eaglestein has suggested that the presence of perivascular fibrin in the skin around an ulcer may be diagnostic of a venous ulcer (see Chapters 15 and 18) but Stacey *et al.* found that these changes were not pathognomonic.[89]

TESTS OF VENOUS FUNCTION (SEE CHAPTERS 4–6)

There is no single test that diagnoses venous ulceration with total confidence but the demonstration of a functional or anatomical abnormality of calf pump function strengthens the certainty of the diagnosis and helps in planning treatment. Our present preference in order of simplicity and cost effectiveness is given below.

1. *Venous directional Doppler ultrasound.* This is a quick, easy outpatient method for confirming long saphenous vein incompetence but it is not accurate enough to assess the state of the deep or communicating veins (see Chapters 4 and 6).

2. *Duplex ultrasound scanning.* This can assess deep and superficial vein patency and valvular incompetence more effectively than the simple directional Doppler methods (see Chapters 4 and 6). The precise stimulus used to promote reflux and the significance of reflux time measurements is still disputed. The segments of vein in each limb that exhibit reflux can be documented.

3. *Foot volume measurements during exercise.* This method is inexpensive, simple to perform and non-invasive. Other clinicians prefer photoplethysmography or strain-gauge plethysmography. We think foot volume measurements are closer to foot vein pressure studies than the other methods[74] and are quantitative not just qualitative (see Chapters 4 and 6).

4. *Ascending phlebography.* This gives important information about the pathology of the deep veins, which is not always detected by duplex scanning[6] (see Chapters 4 and 6) (Figure 19.9). Descending venography has largely been

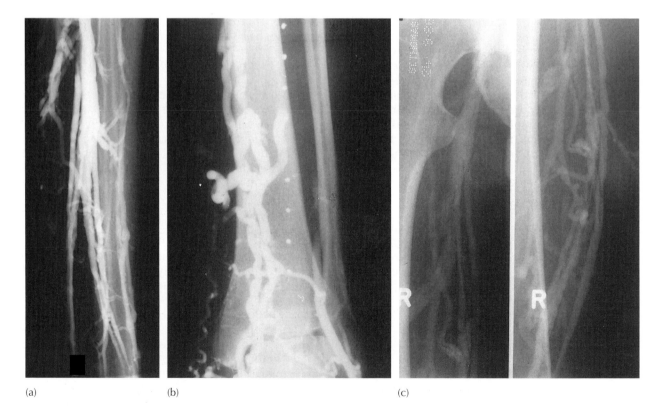

(a)   (b)   (c)

Figure 19.9 Three ascending phlebographs showing the changes that may accompany venous ulceration. (a) Normal deep veins and no incompetent communicating veins. (b) Incompetent lower leg communicating veins. (c) Severe post-thrombotic deep vein damage with synechiae and collaterals.

superseded by duplex scanning with which it agrees well[6] and is much more acceptable to patients.

5. *Varicography.* This is useful when the anatomy of the superficial veins is in doubt, or abnormal superficial-to-deep communications are suspected. It is particularly useful when planning short saphenous vein surgery and before operating on patients with recurrent varicose veins (see Chapters 4 and 6).

6. *Air plethysmography.* This has recently been rediscovered as a technique following simplification of the equipment and is now commercially available. The ejection fraction and the refilling time give some indication of deep venous obstruction and venous reflux, similar to the results of photoplethysmography and foot volumetry. Performing the test with and without tourniquets may indicate the sites of superficial reflux. This technique is still being assessed and opinions vary on its value (see Chapter 4).

7. *Photoplethysmography and light reflection rheography.* These techniques simply look at refilling times as an indicator of calf pump function (deep vein reflux). We have not found them as useful as foot volumetry.

Comment

Apart from the Doppler or duplex ultrasound assessment, the other confirmatory tests are best performed when the ulcer is healed. This means that a diagnosis of venous ulceration and its subsequent treatment must be conducted on the basis of the clinical findings and preliminary tests with final confirmation awaiting more complex investigations after the ulcer has healed. It is our opinion that an ulcer cannot be considered to be venous if the calf pump function tests of the leg with the ulcer are normal.

Differential diagnosis of leg ulcers

Although the preceding section on the diagnosis of venous ulcers has mentioned some of the other causes of leg ulceration, the following paragraphs discuss these causes in detail.

Ulcers caused by arterial insufficiency

An ischaemic ulcer on the tip of a toe which is itself blue and painful offers little difficulty in diagnosis, but the diagnosis is less obvious when the ulcer is

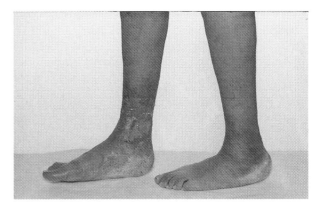

Figure 19.10 This ulcer in the 'gaiter' region of the leg was caused by arterial ischaemia. The deep and superficial veins were normal but the arterial ankle pressures, measured by Doppler ultrasound, were severely reduced. Arteriography confirmed severe arterial disease. The appearance of this ulcer and the surrounding skin made it clinically indistinguishable from a venous ulcer but objective tests excluded venous disease and confirmed the presence of severe arterial insufficiency.

in an area of lipodermatosclerosis in a leg with impalpable foot pulses (Figure 19.10). As already discussed, assessing the relative importance of combined venous and arterial disease can be extremely difficult.

A history of intermittent claudication, rest pain, or of other symptoms of vascular disease in other systems, indicates that vascular insufficiency may be the cause of the ulcer.

Pain made worse by elevation of the leg is often a feature of ischaemic ulceration, whereas the discomfort of venous disease is almost always relieved by elevation. Ischaemic ulcers are often on the feet and toes (Figure 19.11a, b), an uncommon site for venous ulcers, but they can develop anywhere on the leg and have no truly specific features except that the granulation in the ulcer base may be pale (Figure 19.12) and show little evidence of proliferation. The diagnosis is usually suspected when the pulses are found to be absent and the Doppler arterial pressure at the ankle is reduced.

Arteriography is often indicated to confirm the diagnosis and decide upon the best method of management. Femoral arteriography may give sufficient information if there is a good femoral pulse and distal disease is suspected but it is usually wise to obtain information about the aorta and iliac arteries by direct aortography with digital subtraction (Figure 19.12), even when the femoral pulse feels normal.

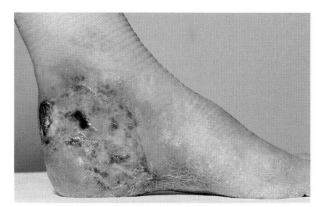

(a)

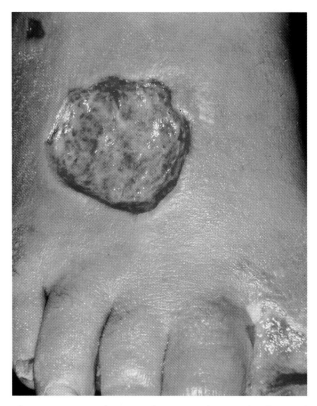

Figure 19.11 Ischaemic ulcers are often on the feet and toes. This diabetic patient had ischaemic ulceration between the toes and on the forefoot. There were also ulcers on the outer side of the heel. Ulceration such as this is almost always ischaemic in origin.

A vascular reconstruction or a lumbar sympathectomy may be required to improve the blood flow to an ischaemic ulcer to enable skin grafts to take or encourage natural healing. A prostaglandin infusion may also accelerate ulcer healing. Once the arterial circulation of the limb has been improved, it is safe to treat any venous abnormality that is causing symptoms.

Traumatic ulcers

This diagnosis is easy to make when there is a clear history of a direct injury followed immediately by obvious damage to the skin (e.g. bruising, laceration). Examination usually reveals a sharply demarcated area of ulceration in otherwise normal skin (Figure 19.13). The combination of pre-existing venous or arterial disease in association with trauma must, however, always be borne in mind, and the presence of lipodermatosclerosis, obvious surface varices or absent foot pulses demands further investigation.

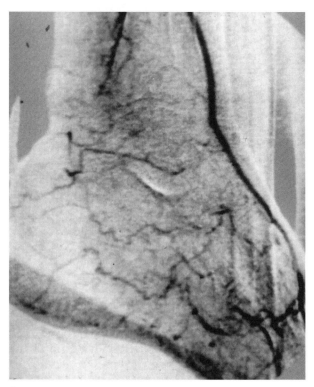

(b)

Figure 19.12 (a) An ischaemic ulcer of the heel. The patient was referred with a diagnosis of self-mutilation because the ulcer was in an unusual site and had failed to heal with elastic compression and skin grafting. (b) The digital subtraction arteriogram showed a total occlusion of the posterior tibial artery, confirming the diagnosis of an ischaemic ulcer.

Minor trauma is often the initiating factor in the development of both venous and arterial ulcers. For a confident diagnosis of traumatic ulcer to be made, the patient must give a clear history of the accident and have no other cause for the ulceration.

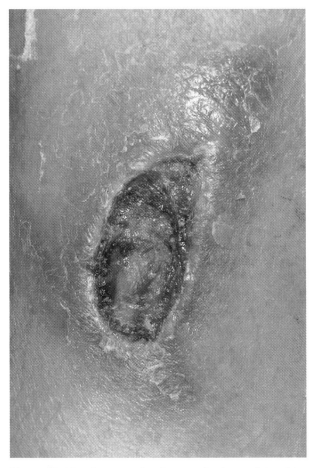

Figure 19.13 A traumatic ulcer on the front of the shin. The ulcer is surrounded by normal skin and in a site which is frequently injured. This ulcer followed a football injury and healed rapidly.

The common site for a traumatic ulcer is the front of the shin. Ulcers frequently follow a shearing injury which produces a distally based v-shaped flap which undergoes ischaemic necrosis. The skin and subcutaneous tissues of the shin are known to have a poor blood supply and heal slowly.[26] Traumatic ulcers can follow an injury to normal skin but the frail tissues of the elderly, especially those with thin skin following treatment with systemic steroids are especially susceptible to minor injury. In this latter category fall many patients with rheumatoid arthritis. The cause of the trauma varies but the supermarket trolley is now high on the list of injurious agents.

Treatment is by compression bandaging or skin grafting. Healing of the ulcer should not be followed by recurrence unless further injuries occur or other abnormalities coexist.

Basal cell carcinoma (rodent ulcers)

Basal cell carcinomata are most often found on the face, in the triangle between the eye, the ear and the mouth; a rodent ulcer that develops on a limb is therefore often misdiagnosed because it is not considered in the differential diagnosis. Every year we see at least two basal cell carcinomata on the legs in which the correct diagnosis has never been considered, an error which has resulted in a considerable delay in initiating treatment.[1]

Patients who have closely observed the skin tumour during its early stages describe the typical behaviour of a basal cell carcinoma – normally intermittent episodes of ulceration and apparent healing. As time passes, it continues to grow and becomes a persistent ulcer. Basal cell cancers on the limbs rarely have the classical 'rolled, pearly' edge seen on the face (Figure 19.14). Careful inspection may reveal some of the typical appearances with overlying telangiectasis but the centre is often slightly raised and covered with bright red granulation tissue which bleeds easily. This change can sometimes be so prominent that it leads to a misdiagnosis of pyogenic granuloma, even though the long history belies this diagnosis. The skin surrounding the ulcer is usually normal and the foot pulses are invariably palpable. Difficulties arise when a basal cell carcinoma develops is an area of lipodermatosclerosis.[56] When a basal cell carcinoma is suspected, a biopsy should be taken of the edge of the ulcer unless the diagnosis is beyond doubt when it should be treated by an excision biopsy with skin grafting if necessary. It can also be treated by incisional biopsy and radiotherapy, if this treatment is more appropriate. It is important to think of the possibility of basal cell carcinoma when examining any atypical ulcer that has failed to heal.[56] These cancers can occasionally arise in a long-standing venous ulcer[100] or in an area of irradiated skin.

Squamous cell carcinoma

This diagnosis must also be considered as a possible cause of any leg ulcer of doubtful aetiology. A squamous cell carcinoma usually presents as an ulcer with a raised everted edge arising in normal skin (Figure 19.15a) but, like basal cell carcinomata, this typical appearance is often not seen in the leg and a high level of suspicion must be maintained if the correct diagnosis is to be made.

Squamous cell carcinomata on the leg may be nodular, irregular, often have a sloping edge, grow insidiously, and do not respond to treatment (Figure 19.15b). They are not usually painful even when being dressed but they produce an excessive amount of exudate and slough. The inguinal lymph nodes are often enlarged, sometimes as a result of

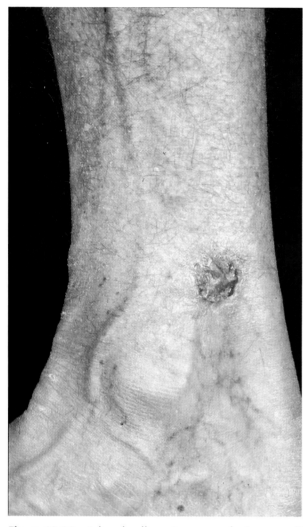

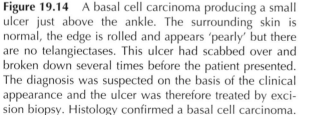

Figure 19.14 A basal cell carcinoma producing a small ulcer just above the ankle. The surrounding skin is normal, the edge is rolled and appears 'pearly' but there are no telangiectases. This ulcer had scabbed over and broken down several times before the patient presented. The diagnosis was suspected on the basis of the clinical appearance and the ulcer was therefore treated by excision biopsy. Histology confirmed a basal cell carcinoma.

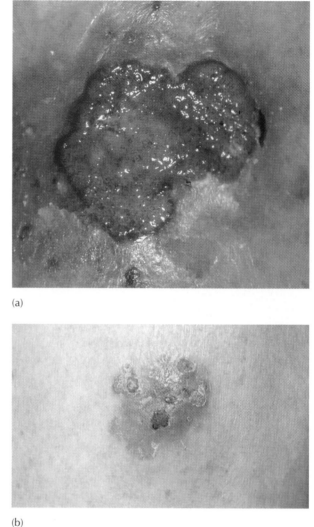

(a)

(b)

Figure 19.15 (a) A squamous cell carcinoma arising in the skin of the calf. It does not have the raised or everted edge typical of a squamous cell carcinoma. This ulcer arose in normal skin and no predisposing factor could be found. (b) A squamous cell carcinoma arising in a patch of Bowen's disease. It was misdiagnosed clinically as a basal cell carcinoma because it had a rolled, not a raised everted edge.

tumour deposits, but more commonly as a result of secondary infection.

When a squamous cell carcinoma develops in a chronic venous ulcer it is traditionally called a Marjolin's ulcer,[10,54] though Marjolin[63] originally reported squamous cell carcinomata arising in the scars of old burns. Malignant change in a venous ulcer is a rare complication. A large review reported only three cases out of 2000 ulcers,[84] and we have only seen 10 cases in 30 years.[56] A Marjolin's ulcer should be suspected if one area of a venous ulcer starts to proliferate and rise above the surface of the rest of the ulcer (Figure 19.16) or if the nature of the ulcer changes so that it starts to exude and smell.[59] A biopsy should be taken of any long-standing ulcer that displays an unusual

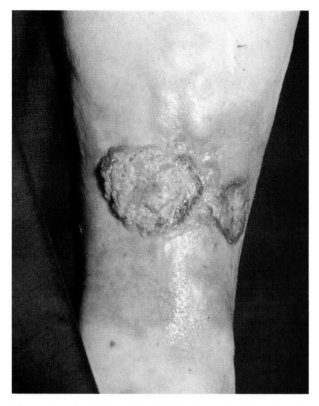

Figure 19.16 This patient had a long-standing chronic ulcer of the leg which suddenly enlarged, became offensive and developed exuberant 'granulations'. The whole change represented a squamous cell carcinoma developing in a chronic venous ulcer, the so-called Marjolin's ulcer. The chronic lipodermatosclerosis and dilated veins caused by the long-standing calf pump failure are clearly visible.

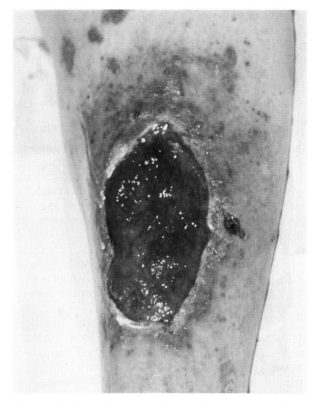

Figure 19.17 A rheumatoid ulcer. This extensive ulcer developed in a woman who had severe rheumatoid arthritis affecting all her joints, producing almost total immobility. There was no obvious venous abnormality, the phlebographs were normal, and the ankle pressures measured by Doppler ultrasound were normal. Rheumatoid ulcers are presumably caused by arteriolar arteritis and thrombosis.

appearance or enlarges despite apparently satisfactory treatment.[1,56]

Squamous cell carcinomata are treated by wide excision and skin grafting, or radiotherapy.

Rheumatoid ulcers

These ulcers are discussed separately from the other forms of vasculitis which cause ulceration because they are common and extremely difficult to manage.[4,19,72,97]

Ulcers may appear at any site on the legs of patients with rheumatoid arthritis but, interestingly, they still most commonly occur in the gaiter region and therefore must be distinguished from venous ulcers (Figure 19.17). They are not usually surrounded by lipodermatosclerosis and, if this change is present, the ulcer may be of mixed aetiology.

Rheumatoid ulcers have no special characteristics but look more like ischaemic ulcers than venous ulcers with poor quality granulation tissue in their base.

The diagnosis is made by finding the characteristic changes of rheumatoid arthritis in the hands and other joints and no evidence of venous or large artery disease in the legs. Very rarely, these ulcers occur in the absence of abnormalities of the joints and soft tissues; it is therefore our policy to request serological tests for rheumatoid disease on all new patients presenting with ulceration. We have had a number of patients with ulcers difficult to heal whose serological tests eventually turned positive and several years later the joints became swollen and deformed. The erythrocyte sedimentation rate (ESR) is commonly elevated. For similar reasons we refer those patients who have a seronegative arthritis to a rheumatologist for confirmation of the diagnosis. Histology of a rheumatoid ulcer has no specific features; it usually shows small vessel endarteritis and round cell infiltration.

The arterial blood supply of the leg must be carefully assessed as severe rheumatoid arthritis may affect the small arteries of the calf and foot and produce distal ischaemia. An attempt may be made to heal the ulcer by compression if the blood supply appears to be satisfactory, but great care must be taken to avoid making the ulcer worse. Many rheumatoid ulcers fail to respond to conservative treatment, and patients have to be admitted for long periods of bedrest, cleansing, ulcer excision and repeated skin grafting. Skin grafts often fail to take, and procedures that increase blood flow, such as an adjuvant prostacyclin infusion or a chemical sympathectomy, may help.[51] Unfortunately, bedrest makes joint stiffness worse and often causes a prolonged decrease in mobility despite intensive physiotherapy.

Elastic stockings should be worn once the ulcer is healed, as much for protection as to prevent breakdown. It is not known if anti-inflammatory drugs reduce the risk of re-ulceration, but most patients now receive this form of treatment from rheumatologists and anecdotally it seems to reduce ulcer recurrence.

Neuropathic ulcers

Neuropathic ulcers occur wherever there is pressure on the denervated skin. The areas subjected to the most pressure lie under the first metatarsophalangeal joint and the heel, over the base of the fifth metatarsal where the shoes press and rub against the toes, and over the malleoli (Figure 19.18). The gaiter region of the leg is rarely affected. These ulcers are painless, punched-out and deep and, though they often have a slough in their base, they are rarely heavily infected. A neurological examination should confirm absence of pain sensation which is often accompanied by other sensory abnormalities such as a loss of vibration or position sense.

Diabetes is one of the most common causes of neuropathy, but even when a diabetic patient presents with an ulcer which is thought to be neuropathic in site and appearance, it is important to exclude infection and arterial insufficiency as causes, both of which commonly coexist. The urine of all patients presenting with leg ulcers should be routinely tested for sugar, and we also routinely request a random blood glucose.

Treatment consists of avoiding further trauma, usually by prescribing complete bedrest, treating infection, controlling the diabetes and improving

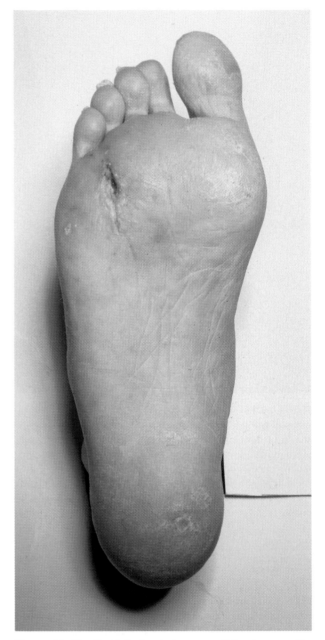

Figure 19.18 Partially healed neuropathic ulcers on the plantar surface of the foot. This patient sustained a traumatic division of the sciatic nerve in a previous accident. Neuropathic ulcers are found in skin which bears weight during standing – in this case on the anterior and posterior aspect of the sole of the foot.

the blood supply, if it is necessary or possible. The judicious use of a well-padded plaster cast is sometimes very effective.[78]

Spina bifida, spinal injury, syringomyelia, tertiary syphilis, transverse myelitis, peripheral neuropathy

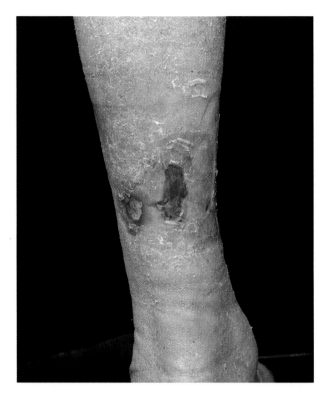

Figure 19.19 These neuropathic ulcers occurred in a patient who had to wear calipers because the limb had been partially paralysed by poliomyelitis. The calipers had rubbed against the skin and caused the ulceration.

and stroke are among the numerous other causes of neuropathic damage. In many patients with these diseases it is the pressure of calipers (Figure 19.19) or the struts of wheelchairs that cause the ulceration. The presence of a large, painless ulcer over an area which is subjected to pressure when the patient is in bed (e.g. the back of the heel, the side of knee or over the greater trochanter) should also arouse suspicion of a neuropathic ulcer.

When neurological disease has not been previously recognized, the patient should undergo a detailed clinical examination to confirm the neurological problem. Electromyography, spinal radiographs, myelography, and computerized tomography may be required to elucidate the underlying pathology.

The skin and subcutaneous tissues should be protected against further trauma; this can be extremely difficult. Neuropathic ulcers will heal if protected from further pressure but healing may be accelerated by applying split skin grafts or by bringing in new skin by the plastic surgical techniques of rotation flaps or vascularized free flap grafts.

Tuberculous ulcers

Tuberculosis of the skin is now rare in Europe and North America but it is still common in Africa, India and the Far East.

Primary tuberculosis of the skin presents as an indurated plaque which has a transparent appearance which makes it look like 'apple jelly' (Figure 19.20) but it is rarely seen in the lower leg.[35] True tuberculous ulcers of the skin (scrofula) are uncommon on the legs. These ulcers have an irregular, bluish, friable, undermined edge and a grey–pink base. The ulcers are often multiple, and the patient usually has evidence of systemic, pulmonary, abdominal or skeletal tuberculosis (Figure 19.20).

Erythema induratum scrofulosorum (Bazin's disease) occurs in the skin of the calf of middle-aged women. It starts as either a single nodule or multiple nodules which gradually turn purple and then break down to form deep undermined ulcers. The regional lymph nodes may enlarge and caseate. It tends to occur on the back of the calf, and this gives the best clue to the diagnosis. Patients with Bazin's disease show hypersensitivity to Mantoux testing. A biopsy of the ulcer edge shows tuberculous granulomata containing Langerhan's giant cells. Tubercle bacilli may be found by Ziehl–Neelsen staining of the biopsy, or may be isolated from the surface of the ulcer if great care is taken with the sample collection. Treatment is by a combination of specific antituberculosis agents.

Erythrocyanosis frigida (curum puellarum) and chilblains (lupus pernio)

Chilblains characteristically occur on the tips of the ears, the fingers and the toes but they can also occur over the Achilles tendon. They normally develop during cold weather and represent the effect of a prolonged period of cutaneous ischaemia, which is usually transitory but sometimes permanent (an infarct), caused by excessive vasospasm of the arterioles. Chilblains begin as an area of induration and oedema but then the overlying skin may ulcerate. If they develop in warm weather, the possibility of sarcoidosis should be considered. This can be confirmed by biopsy and Kveim testing.

Erythrocyanosis frigida is a condition which is found in young women with fat legs and rather thick ankles. It consists of thickened patches of erythematous skin that are mottled and cyanotic at all times (not only in cold weather), and which may very occasionally break down to form areas of superficial, painful ulceration (Figure 19.21). This ulceration is not preceded by oedema. The diagnosis is based on the clinical appearance of a cool-reddish/blue patch of indurated skin and fat over

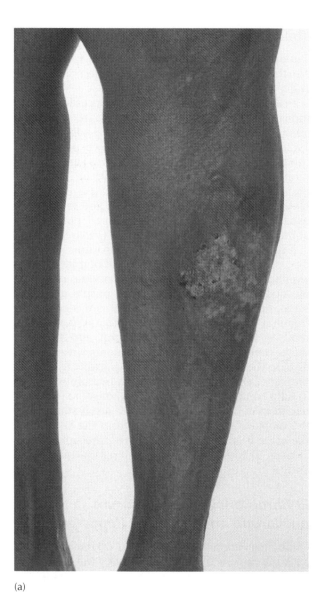

(a)

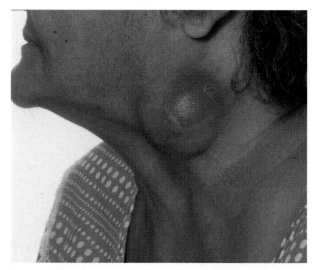

(b)

Figure 19.20 'Apple jelly' nodules in the skin of the leg (a) in a lady with a proven tuberculous node in the neck (b). The skin lesion resolved when the patient was treated with systemic antituberculosis drugs.

the lower, usually posterior, third of the leg (Figure 19.21). Although the skin discoloration is similar to that seen over a chilblain, this condition is persistent, not spasmodic and is not closely related to temperature changes. Its cause is unknown. It may be vasospastic, but it is not always relieved by sympathectomy and may therefore have a different aetiology.

The diagnosis may be more difficult to make when the skin has ulcerated but it may be suspected if the surrounding skin shows the characteristic appearances described above. The rest of the limb may have a bluish discoloration (acrocyanosis), a mixture of red and blue changes (erythrocyanosis) or may undergo the white, blue and red changes of Raynaud's phenomenon.

Similar appearances develop in limbs with neurological abnormalities particularly after poliomyelitis. These changes often occur 10 or 20 years after the attack of poliomyelitis and are particularly liable to cause ulceration over the Achilles tendon on the posterior aspect of the leg.

The object of treatment is to keep the limb warm and to encourage healing with conservative measures. Recurrent ulceration and ulcers that will not heal may be improved by vasodilator drugs or sympathectomy. Sympathectomy produces a prolonged almost permanent improvement in patients with chilblains and post-poliomyelitis vasospasm but does not always help the patient with idiopathic erythrocyanosis and may make this type of leg oedematous.

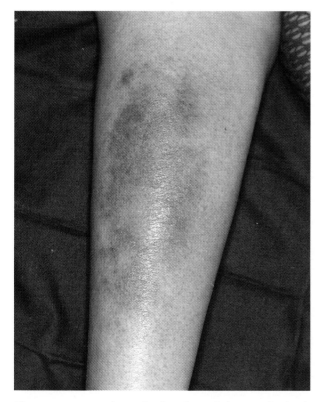

Figure 19.21 Red–purple discoloured skin on the back of calf typical of erythrocyanosis. These areas get chilblains and sometimes ulcerate. (We are grateful to Dr David McGibbon for this illustration.)

Vasculitic ulcers (scleroderma, systemic lupus erythrematosus, non-specific vasculitis)

The common vasculitic ulcer, the 'rheumatoid ulcer' is discussed on page 543; the other diseases associated with cutaneous vasculitis are far less common than rheumatoid disease but are equally resistant to treatment and it is equally important to diagnose them correctly.

The most common collagen disease causing leg ulceration is scleroderma. Ulceration rarely precedes the other manifestations of this disease but these may have passed unnoticed. Close questioning may reveal that the patient has suffered from Raynaud's phenomenon, arthritis, dysphagia or constipation, and clinical examination may detect spindle-shaped fingers, telangiectases on the face, a puckered mouth and a shiny skin tightly drawn over the facial muscles destroying facial expression.

Ulceration on the lower limb usually appears in a reddened area of skin with surrounding telangiectases (Figure 19.22a). The ulcers are small, often multiple, painful, penetrate through the full thickness of the skin and show little evidence of healing. They are usually on the toes but may extend onto the foot. Isolated ulcers on the lower limb can also occur (Figure 19.22b). Sometimes the ulcer forms over a large plaque of calcium which may prevent the ulcer from healing. The diagnosis is usually confirmed if there are high titres of antinuclear antibodies in the serum, and other autoantibodies may also be present. The erythrocyte sedimentation rate is invariably elevated, and a barium swallow may show defective peristalsis with a rigid oesophagus.

There is no definitive treatment for scleroderma. Some ulcers can be healed by regular cleansing, dressing, and compression bandaging. Other ulcers need prolonged periods of bedrest and may be helped by prostacyclin infusions, sympathectomy and skin grafting. Curettage of subcutaneous calcium may enhance healing in some instances. The role of plasmapheresis and immunosuppressive agents in treatment is not yet established. Unfortunately, sclerodermatous ulcers have a great tendency to break down, and there is little evidence that elastic support, immunosuppressive drugs or systemic steroids prevent this from happening.

Small, chronic, recurrent and multiple cutaneous ulcers also complicate systemic lupus erythematosus (SLE). These ulcers may appear anywhere on the leg in otherwise normal skin, though there may be evidence of abnormal skin vessels (telangiectases) and other stigmata of vasculitis. There may be a butterfly rash across the face and evidence of multisystem disease.

Cutaneous vasculitis often starts as a raised erythromatous nodule or collection of nodules which coalesce before developing intradermal haemorrhages. The skin over the nodules then breaks down to form single or multiple small ulcers (Figure 19.22b).

Lupus antibodies may be present in the blood of patients with SLE. Skin biopsies show an arteriolitis with a non-specific round cell infiltration through the whole thickness of the vessel wall. Treatment is as ineffective for lupus as it is for scleroderma, though the ulcers sometimes heal with prolonged bedrest and immunosuppressive therapy.

Dermatologists recognize another type of non-specific cutaneous vasculitis in which there is no systemic disorder (Figure 19.22c). Skin biopsies show the round cell infiltration of the vessel wall described above with a perivascular deposit of gammaglobulin. The aetiology of this condition remains obscure and there is no specific treatment. Areas of non-specific vasculitis can break down to form small painful ulcers on the legs and feet. The diagnosis is made from immunohistochemical stains of

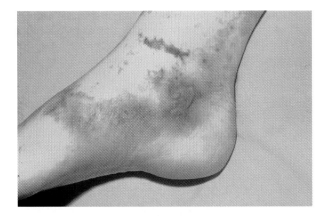

(a)

Figure 19.22 (a) The clinical features of vasculitis on the dorsal surface of the foot. The skin is red and thickened, and the skin capillaries are dilated. (b) An ulcerated and gangrenous patch of skin on the calf. This proved to be caused by a severe vasculitis which extended over the whole of the lower leg and, despite all forms of treatment, the patient rapidly deteriorated and died. (c) An abnormal area of skin on the calf; biopsy of this area revealed an allergic vasculitis. (We are grateful to Dr Martin Black for this illustration.)

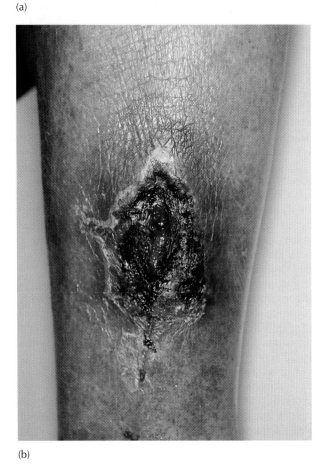

(b)

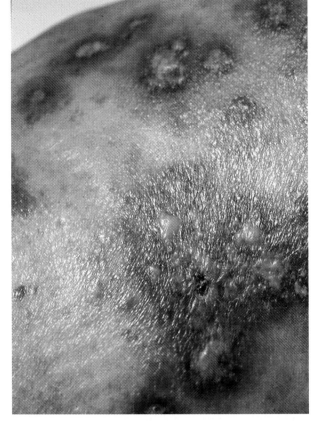

(c)

skin biopsies. Vasculitis is occasionally brought on by drugs, e.g. diltiazem has been implicated in one case of leg ulceration which resolved when the drug was stopped.[21]

Ulcers over osteomyelitis

Chronic osteomyelitis of the tibia may discharge through single or multiple sinuses which may be misdiagnosed as ulcers and referred to an ulcer clinic (Figure 19.23). The patient often gives a history of bone infection and had previous treatment with antibiotics. The skin surrounding a sinus in the lower leg is usually firmly attached to the underlying bone and, if the tract is probed, bone may be felt beneath the granulation tissue. A plain radiograph often shows evidence of bone destruction and new bone formation (Figure 19.23).

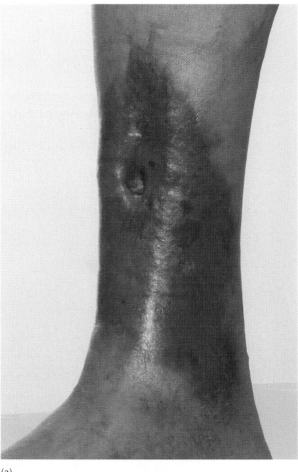
(a)

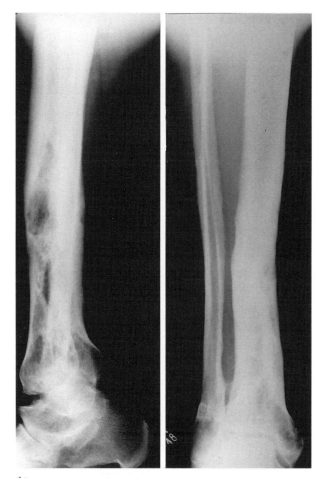
(b)

Figure 19.23 (a) This ulcer looked like a venous ulcer surrounded by severe lipodermatosclerosis, but the skin appeared to be adherent to the front of the tibia. The patient's history revealed that he had had a previous bone infection. (b) The x-ray of the tibia showed clear evidence of past osteomyelitis. The phlebographs obtained to exclude a post-thrombotic syndrome (which may be a complication of osteomyelitis) were normal.

Difficulty occasionally occurs in distinguishing the periosteal reaction that can occur beneath a long-standing chronic venous ulcer from the periostitis over osteomyelitis. An isotope bone scan may show increased uptake in the infected bones but is usually normal with simple periostitis.

Syphilitic ulcers

Syphilis is now a rare cause of leg ulceration, though it has been an important diagnosis in past centuries. Syphilitic ulcers are usually the result of the skin breaking down over a subcutaneous gumma. The rash that accompanies secondary syphilis is widespread and rarely ulcerates, it should therefore not be mistaken for a venous ulcer. Primary chancres on the leg do not occur.

Gummata begin as red, painless nodules. If the overlying skin becomes necrotic and sloughs, it leaves a circular punched-out ulcer through the whole thickness of the skin, with a 'wash-leather' slough in its base (Figure 19.24a). Despite the depth of the ulcer, it is always painless and must be distinguished from a neuropathic ulcer. The nodules and ulcers may be multiple and may coalesce to produce a serpiginous lesion. Syphilitic ulcers tend to occur on the upper outer aspect of the lower leg or high on the calf, sites not commonly frequented by venous ulcers.

We still request serological tests for syphilis on all patients with new 'atypical' ulcers (Figure

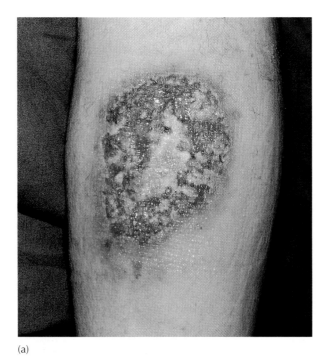

(a)

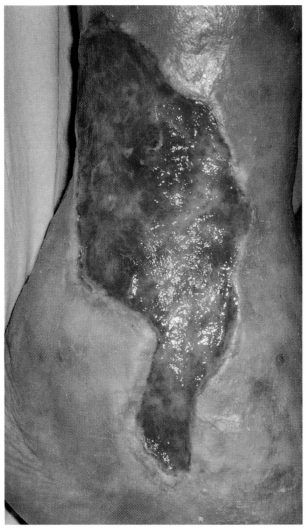

(b)

Figure 19.24 (a) A gumma on the calf which had broken down and ulcerated. The base does not really have the appearance of a 'wash-leather'. Serological tests were strongly positive, and the ulcer healed after treatment with penicillins. (b) An ulcer which looked like a venous ulcer but serological tests confirmed active syphilis and the ulcer healed after antibiotic treatment. (We are grateful to Dr Martin Black for these illustrations.)

19.24b) but this is probably unnecessary because they are invariably negative. Antibiotic treatment produces rapid healing of syphilitic ulcers, leaving the patient with the characteristic 'tissue paper' scars.

Martorell's ulcer

There is considerable doubt about the specificity and even the existence of this ulcer. Martorell[64] described a specific type of ulcer that occurred in the lower leg of patients with severe hypertension, which he believed resulted from local skin ischaemia produced by the arteriolar narrowing that accompanied and perhaps caused the hypertension.

An alternative suggestion is that the cause of this type of ulcer is similar to those of, 'trash foot' which

results from embolization of arterial debris into the skin of the lower limb at the time of peripheral vascular reconstruction, in patients with severe peripheral vascular disease.

The ulcer is said to present as a dark red area of skin at the junction of the lower and middle thirds of the calf on the back of the lower leg which becomes black (gangrenous) and then ulcerates[3] (Figure 19.25). The ulcer has a sloping edge and a red base. It is characteristically very painful, necrotic, ischaemic, superficial and dry. All the foot pulses are present and it is said to be more common in hypertensive women. There is often a symmetrical ulcer on the other leg. Histology of the base shows thickening and hyalinization of the tunica media of the arterioles of the dermis. It is probably rare today as there are few patients with untreated hypertension.

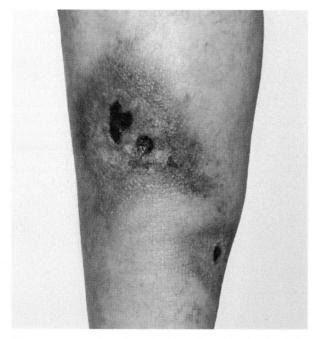

Figure 19.25 This ulcer developed on the back of the calf of an obese woman who had hypertension. Phlebograms and physiological tests of calf pump function were normal, and there was no evidence of arterial insufficiency. Some clinicians would classify this as a Martorell's ulcer, others would just consider it to be the result of a local vasculitis or embolism.

Sympathectomy is thought to be the best treatment for these ulcers. This may be combined with excision and grafting.[1,4,64,65]

Ulcers associated with blood dyscrasias

Several 'blood diseases' are associated with ulceration of the legs. In many instances the mechanism that causes the ulceration is obscure but in some cases it is probably venous thrombosis or capillary sludging. The ulcers of sickle cell disease, thalassaemia, thrombotic thrombocythaemia and polycythaemia rubra vera are all probably caused by a combination of venous thrombosis and local capillary thrombosis; it is interesting that sickle cell ulcers rarely develop during a sickle 'crisis'.

Leukaemia may also cause local capillary sludging, but the mechanisms by which congenital spherocytosis (acholuric jaundice), elliptocytosis, and pernicious anaemia cause ulceration are unknown.

Leg ulcers associated with abnormalities of the blood have no diagnostic features (Figure 19.26). They are usually on the lower third of the leg, superficial, painful and multiple. Lipodermatosclerosis is rarely present unless post-thrombotic

changes coexist. Koilonychia, a smooth tongue, peripheral neuropathy, a palpable spleen or lymphadenopathy may all be detected on general examination.

We routinely examine the blood and check for sickle cell trait when appropriate in all patients with new or obscure ulcers.

In many instances the main causative factor is a previous deep vein thrombosis; this should be investigated in the usual way while correcting the blood abnormality. Ulcers that are healed by conservative treatment or by skin grafting will break down again if the blood abnormality remains untreated. An exchange transfusion may improve the healing time of ulcers associated with capillary sludging or abnormal plasma constituents. Elastic stockings may be of benefit in preventing reulceration but we do not know why.

Self-induced (artefactual) ulceration

The psychological abnormalities that drive patients to self-mutilation are not understood. Depression or a craving for attention in a hysterical personality are two possible mechanisms. Frank schizophrenia or mental subnormality may be present[30] and patients often have a poor relationship with their parents. We see one or two patients every year with this diagnosis but there are probably others who, by tampering with their dressings, prevent their genuine ulcers from healing. Nurses and other members of the health care professions are quite commonly affected. Sleep disorders such as insomnia may be an aetiologically associated factor.

Suspicion is often first aroused by the shape and position of the ulcer, and supported by finding dressings that have been loosened or removed. The onset of the ulcers is often poorly described. A bizarre ulcer shape with normal surrounding skin (Figure 19.27), often on the anterior surface of the leg at a site which can be easily reached, is highly suggestive. A long history with multiple admissions to other hospitals for treatment of an ulcer that defies all attempts at healing should also arouse suspicion.

Oedema may be produced by applying a constricting band around the limb, and this may eventually cause pressure necrosis and ulceration beneath it.

Healing beneath a plaster of Paris cast, in hospital, under close inspection is the only way to give credence to the diagnosis which can otherwise be extremely difficult, if not impossible, to confirm.

Psychiatrists seem to agree that confronting the patient with the suspected diagnosis is not advisable but they rarely give positive advice about the correct course of action. When we are certain of the

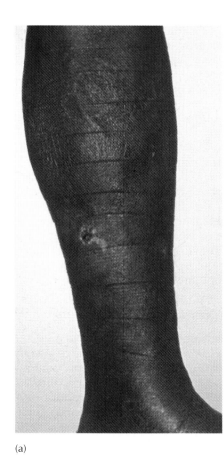

(a)

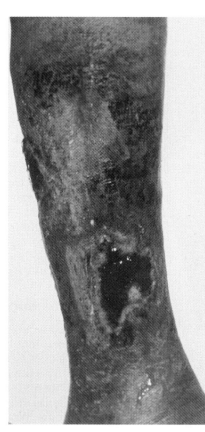

(b)

Figure 19.26 Ulcers associated with haematological disease. (a) An ulcer in a young woman with sickle cell disease. Ascending phlebography did not reveal any post-thrombotic changes or incompetent calf communicating veins. (b) This ulcer, which looks like a typical venous ulcer, was associated with haemosiderosis. The veins were normal.

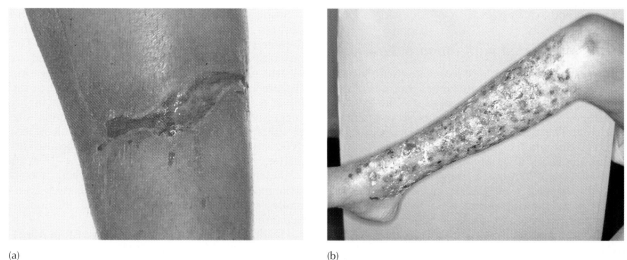

(a)

(b)

Figure 19.27 Artefactual ulcers. (a) This ulcer failed to respond to all attempts at healing in a local hospital, but it healed when the dressings were protected with plaster of Paris. The strange horizontal linear appearance is not compatible with any form of pathological ulcer. (b) This leg has the appearance usually associated with self-inflicted multiple cigarette burns, but the patient was actually producing caustic burns on the leg. The reason for this self-mutilation was obscure. (We are grateful to Dr Martin Black for this illustration.)

diagnosis, we favour some form of confrontation but only in close consultation with the family doctor and close relatives who have a detailed knowledge of the patient's home and personal circumstances. Great care must be taken not to diagnose self-mutilation in error, as nothing is more certain to upset the doctor–patient relationship and lead to litigation. It is better to delay making a diagnosis and await events than to make a wrong diagnosis of artefactual ulceration. The differential diagnosis is usually from a vasculitic ulcer (see above).

Pyoderma gangrenosum

This condition was first described by Brunsting *et al.* in 1930.[13] It begins as a sterile pustule or patch of necrotic skin which rapidly progresses to an ulcerated area with surrounding erythema. The ulcers are boggy, indurated and may become gangrenous (Figure 19.28). Sometimes a large area of skin and subcutaneous tissue around the original patch of necrotic skin becomes necrotic and secondarily infected.

Some patients with severe ulcerative colitis develop multiple pustules and areas of skin necrosis on their calves.

Pyoderma gangrenosum occasionally occurs in patients with Crohn's disease, and may also be associated with minor trauma, arthritis, leukaemia and other malignancies.

Successful treatment of the underlying condition is usually associated with an improvement in the pyoderma. Systemic steroids and gammaglobulin have produced healing in some patients and the necrotic areas can also be excised and successfully mesh grafted.

Pressure ulcers on the legs (bed sores or decubitus ulcers)

Pressure ulcers occur at sites where the weight of the body is transmitted through skin that is not adapted to weight bearing. These ulcers are most common in immobile patients in bed, hence the term 'bed sores'. They occur in the same positions on the leg as the neuropathic ulcers of bedridden

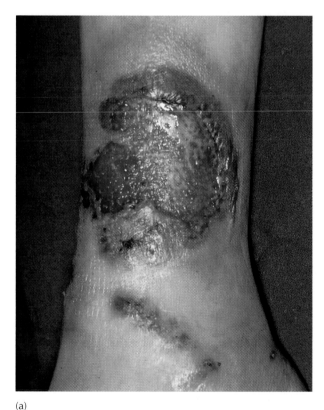

(a)

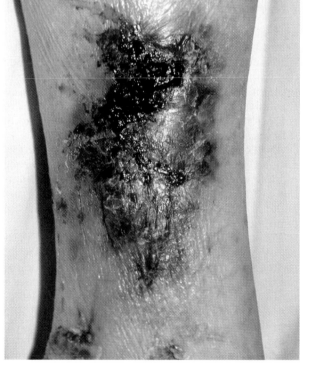

(b)

Figure 19.28   Two examples of pyoderma gangrenosum. Both patients had diarrhoea and were passing blood and mucus. A diagnosis of ulcerative colitis was confirmed by sigmoidoscopy and biopsy. The skin lesions improved when the colitis responded to treatment. (We are grateful to Dr Martin Black for these illustrations.)

patients (i.e. over the back of the heel, the head of the fifth metatarsal and the malleoli) but they are painful. Whereas the diagnosis of an ulcer over the heel is rarely in doubt, pressure ulcers in other sites have to be differentiated from venous ulcers.

The diagnosis is usually obvious if the ulcer develops after the patient has had a period of prolonged bedrest but in an elderly demented patient this history may be difficult to obtain, and a history taken from a relative or nurse may be very helpful. The diagnosis depends upon the history because, apart from its site, the appearance of the ulcer is not specific.

Pressures ulcers should not occur in patients admitted to hospital. They should be prevented by frequent position changes and careful nursing. This counsel of perfection is not always achieved in hospital and can never apply to the frail elderly person living alone.

Most pressure ulcers heal spontaneously if further damage can be prevented. Deep ulcers may have to be excised and grafted, the choice of skin replacement depending upon the site and size of the ulcer. Ulcers on the legs usually accept a split-skin graft, whereas ulcers on the buttocks can sometimes only be covered by complex rotation flaps.

Ulcers in lymphoedematous limbs

Skin ulceration in lymphoedematous limbs is rare. When ulceration does occur, it may be associated with defective fibrinolysis.[93] Inadequate clearance of lymph leads to the accumulation of plasma proteins within the interstitial spaces and, if tissue fibrinolysis is defective, lipodermatosclerosis develops. Subsequent trauma or infection may lead to skin breakdown (Figure 19.29).

An ulcer in an oedematous limb must be differentiated from a post-thrombotic ulcer. The absence of subcutaneous varicosities and dilated intradermal venules, an increased skin thickness, and oedema of the toes should suggest the diagnosis of lymphoedema.

This diagnosis can be confirmed by isotope or x-ray lymphography[92] but, though the presence of normal lymphatic function excludes lymphoedema, the finding of abnormal lymphatics does not necessarily exclude an alternative cause for the ulceration. Post-thrombotic deep vein damage and lymphoedema can occur in the same leg, and in these patients the venous anatomy and venous function must be studied with phlebography and plethysmography before a final diagnosis can be made.

Ulcers in lymphoedematous limbs can be treated by occlusion and compression in the same way that venous ulcers are treated. Once the ulcers have

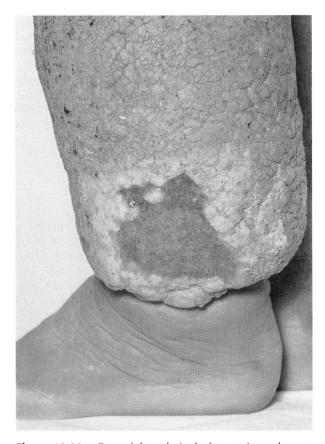

Figure 19.29   One of the relatively few patients that we have had under our care with extensive ulceration complicating gross lymphoedema. There was no evidence of venous disease.

healed, the lymphoedema can be alleviated by compression, bypass surgery, or by an excisional operation.[46,49,53]

Tropical ulcers

Texts on the differential diagnosis of venous ulceration all contain a reference to tropical ulceration. A number of organisms have been incriminated as a cause of these ulcers. Anaerobes (*Fusobacterium*) are said to be present in 35% and coliforms in 60% and these may act in synergy.[2] Actinomycosis, epidermophytosis, blastomycosis, mycetoma (Madura foot), leishmaniasis, moniliasis, syphilis and yaws can all cause ulceration and are all more common in, but not exclusive to, tropical climates.[33,42]

'Buruli boil' is a particularly virulent form of ulcer, otherwise known as 'Oriental sore' or 'Baghdad boil', which is caused by *Mycobacterium ulcerans*.[69] It begins as an indurated papule which

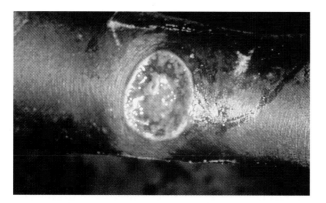

Figure 19.30 A tropical ulcer. Well-defined circular, often multiple ulcers that appear on the legs and sometimes arms of children and young adults in tropical countries (particularly West Africa and Papua New Guinea) are a distinct clinical entity justifying the descriptive term 'tropical ulcer' even though their aetiology is unknown. (We are indebted to Dr R Hay for this illustration.)

later ulcerates. The ulcer is classically very painful with undermined edges. Scrapings of the ulcer reveal the organism and confirm the diagnosis. Treatment is by excision and grafting.

Quist[80] states that 'tropical ulcers are common in barefoot young men (and women)' and are 'the result

of trauma in the presence of chronic malnutrition and anaemia'. Work from Papua New Guinea has suggested that the fusiform organism lives in salt water lagoons and in the shallow water inside coral reefs. In Africa trauma from thorn bushes may be important.[40] Figure 19.30 shows a typical circular tropical ulcer in an area of normal skin.

Ulceration following burns or insect bites

Any area of damaged skin can necrose and so become an ulcer.

Burns are usually remembered but a hot water bottle burn occurring during deep sleep may pass unnoticed and this can cause difficulties in diagnosis.

Insect bites are often not recalled by the patient, which makes a diagnosis at the stage of secondary infection and ulceration difficult. As in traumatic ulcers, the surrounding skin is normal and the ulcer is usually small with no specific features. Diagnosis relies on surmise or an appropriate history, itching often being a feature before and during the early stages of ulceration following an insect bite.

Necrobiosis lipoidica

This condition is found in diabetic patients (Figure 19.31) and represents an area of fat necrosis followed by infection and necrosis of the overlying

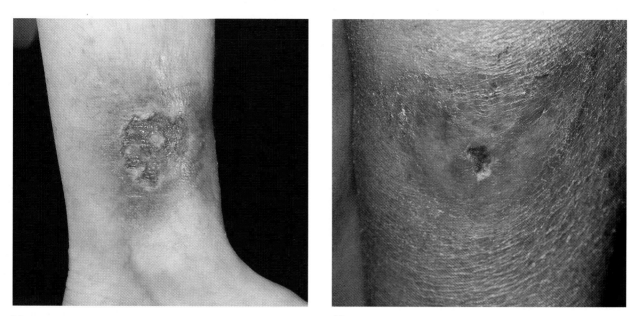

(a) (b)

Figure 19.31 These two ulcers could have been attributed to any cause but they occurred in diabetic patients without any evidence of venous disease and were thought to be caused by necrobiosis lipoidica.

skin. The underlying pathological cause of the fat necrosis is uncertain. Treatment is by antibiotics and dressings, with appropriate control of the diabetes.

Meleney's ulcer[66] (synergistic bacterial gangrene)

This is a rapidly progressive superficial gangrene produced by a synergistic infection of a micro-aerophilic non-haemolytic streptococcus combined with either a staphylococcus, a Gram-negative bacillus, a bacteroides or clostridial organism. Recently it has been suggested that this condition is caused by cutaneous amoebiasis.[32] The combination of two species of bacteria has been shown to have a synergistic effect causing a rapid extension of the infection through the skin and subcutaneous tissues.[52] The infection causes thrombosis of the small vessels in the skin which in turn causes gangrene. There is some debate as to whether there is a difference between Meleney's ulcer and necrotizing fasciitis. They are possibly the same condition.

The initial infection is often trivial but spreads rapidly along the fascial planes with the overlying erythematous skin quickly becoming insensitive and gangrenous before it necroses (Figure 19.32) and separates to leave a large area of ulceration. There are signs of toxaemia, pyrexia, malaise, poor cerebration and prostration. Treatment is urgent and consists of excising the gangrenous

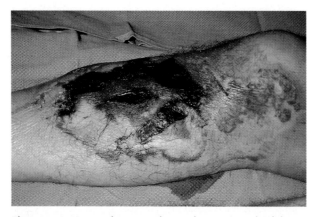

Figure 19.32 Meleney's ulcer. This patient had been holding a road-breaking drill against his calf and developed an area of erythematous skin which necrosed and then became a large area of superficial spreading gangrene. Bacteriological cultures grew a micro-aerophilic streptococcus and a bacteroides. The patient was treated by wide excision of the skin and subcutaneous tissue followed by skin grafting.

tissues and giving large doses of penicillin. Once the infection is under control, the large areas which have been denuded of skin can be covered with skin grafts.

Ulceration caused by arteriovenous fistulae

Arteriovenous fistulae may be either congenital or acquired. The lower limb is the most common site for congenital fistulae. Fistulae may be localized (single) or diffuse (multiple). A cutaneous vascular abnormality or naevus may have been present for many years before the ulcer developed.

Ulceration may occur without overt signs of a fistula. Clinical suspicion should be aroused by the youth of the patient, the presence of a capillary or cavernous naevus in the skin, and an increase in the length of the limb. Peripheral oedema, an increase in skin temperature, prominent or pulsatile surface veins, a palpable thrill, an audible machinery murmur and a positive Branham's sign may also be present.

Acquired fistulae are often caused by trauma at the groin or knee but may occasionally follow the spontaneous rupture of an atheromatous artery into its accompanying vein. Accidental iatrogenic fistulae are uncommon but they sometimes complicate percutaneous arterial catheterization or arterial surgery.

Fistulae deliberately formed to produce venous dilation suitable for venepuncture and renal dialysis, or to provide an increased venous flow after a venous reconstruction, are the most common forms of iatrogenic fistula. The histological changes of pericapillary fibrin deposition have been seen in the abnormal skin (lipodermatosclerosis) that occasionally develops after the formation of a Brescia–Cimino fistula at the wrist.[103] Other causes of skin ischaemia may be the shunting of blood away from the skin through multiple arteriovenous fistulae[77] or the high venous pressure impairing calf pump function and producing ulceration by some other, as yet unidentified, mechanism.

The ulcers that develop in a limb containing arteriovenous fistulae often look like venous ulcers (Figure 19.33) except that they often occur outside the gaiter region of the leg because their site depends upon the location of the fistula. Although the increased blood flow may make the limb hot and hypertrophic, the ulcers have poor granulation tissue, do not always bleed vigorously and are usually very painful.

The increased limb blood flow can be measured with plethysmography, and, arteriography may show the sites of abnormal arteriovenous communications and early filling of the veins (Figure 19.34).

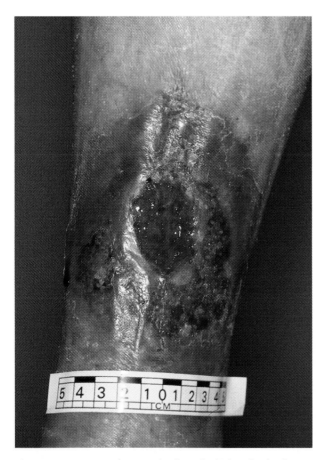

Figure 19.33 An ulcer on the leg of a lady who had varicose veins and lipodermatosclerosis but the skin on her calves was abnormally warm on palpation. The limb contained multiple arteriovenous fistulae. Part of the ulcer was also abnormal in appearance – it had an area with a raised edge. Biopsy of this area revealed a basal cell carcinoma. This may be an example of malignant change in a chronic venous ulcer or of malignant change in skin subjected to the irradiation which was part of the patient's treatment 20 years previously.

These ulcers heal when the fistula or fistulae are closed. Localized fistulae may be treated by surgical excision of the abnormal vessels or therapeutic embolization. Diffuse fistulae are difficult to treat, but operations designed to remove all the side branches (skeletonization) may be beneficial. Amputation should be reserved for diffuse fistulae which occur throughout the limb and cause congestive cardiac failure or painful incurable ulceration.

Primary skin diseases

We see many patients with contact dermatitis, psoriasis, bullous pemphigoid, impetigo and tinea who

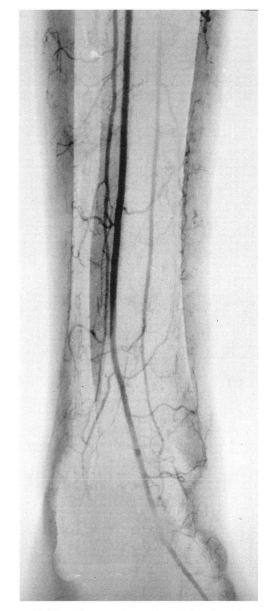

Figure 19.34 The arteriograph of the leg shown in Figure 19.33. It shows multiple small arteriovenous fistulae in the skin and subcutaneous tissues.

have been referred with a diagnosis of venous ulceration (Figure 19.35a–d). The opinion of a dermatologist should be sought whenever the nature of an ulcer is in doubt, and skin biopsies should be obtained from all atypical ulcers. Livido reticularis (Figure 19.36) and atrophie blanche (Figure 19.37) are two forms of cutaneous vasculitis which may break down to give small painful superficial ulcers[91] in areas of red–brown or white

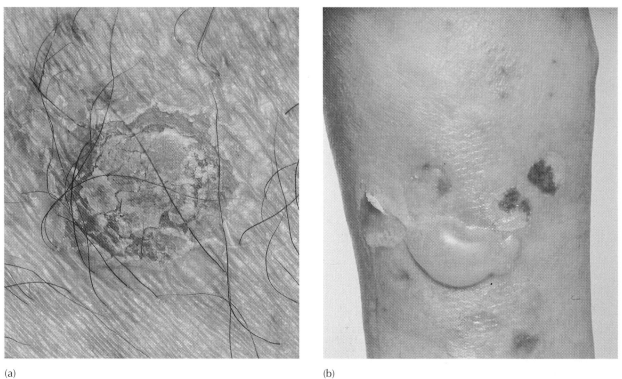

(a)   (b)

Figure 19.35 Ulcerated skin disease. (a) Ulceration in a patch of psoriasis. (b) A bullous skin eruption which had progressed to ulceration.

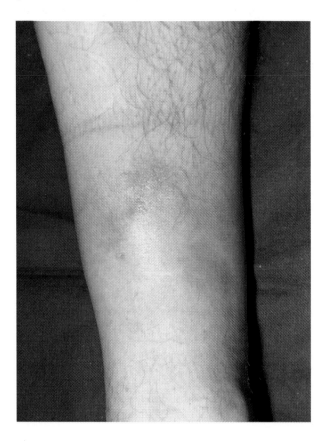

Figure 19.36 This limb has livedo vasculitis. There are patches of red–brown localized vasculitis, which may break down into shallow ulcers. (We are grateful to Dr Martin Black for this illustration.)

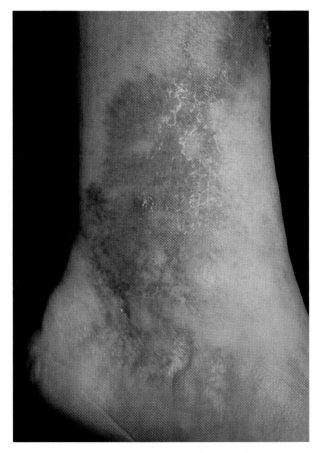

Figure 19.37 Areas of atrophie blanche throughout a wide area of cutaneous vasculitis. The white areas are scars which have slowly replaced dead skin without going through a phase of ulceration. (We are grateful to Dr Martin Black for this illustration.)

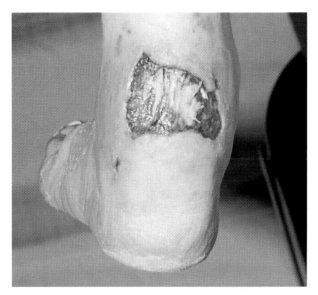

Figure 19.38 A biopsy of this unusual ulcer over the Achilles tendon showed evidence of urate crystals in the skin. The patient's serum urate level was elevated, and the cause of the ulcer was cutaneous necrosis over a gouty tophus.

skin. These conditions are common around the ankle, and the ulcers are often misdiagnosed as being venous.

The newly recorded disease of superoxide dismutase deficiency and the rare Ehlers–Danlos syndrome must be remembered as unusual causes of ulceration. These conditions, together with the cutaneous vasculitides, should be referred to a dermatologist for diagnosis and treatment.

Summer ulcers

Summer ulcers appear in the summer months on the ankle and dorsum of the feet of young women. They are sometimes associated with areas of livedo reticularis and Raynaud's phenomenon, but they heal in the cold weather. The aetiology is obscure but we have found that some of these patients have exceptionally high plasma fibrinogen levels and a reduced plasma fibrinolysis. Some of our patients' summer ulceration has been prevented by the pharmacological enhancement of fibrinolysis with stanozolol (a drug which, unfortunately, is no longer freely available).

Pyogenic granuloma

This usually presents as a raised rapidly growing patch of exuberant granulation tissue but it may be difficult to diagnose if attempts have been made to remove the proud tissue. Diagnosis and treatment consists of excision biopsy if the diagnosis is uncertain or simple curettage.

Gouty tophi and subcutaneous calcification

Persistent ulcers may develop from pressure necrosis in the skin stretched over an underlying gouty tophus (Figure 19.38). The uric acid crystals presumably delay healing by acting as a foreign body.

Subcutaneous calcification[86,96] may act in a similar manner. This may occur in long-standing lipodermatosclerosis or may be the result of metastatic calcification in systemic sclerosis (CREST syndrome) or rheumatoid arthritis.

The crystals or calcification must be excised or curetted out before healing can occur.

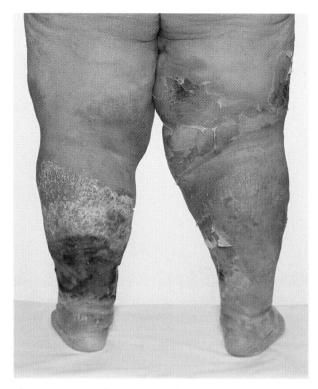

Figure 19.39 This patient developed massive ankle oedema secondary to congestive cardiac failure. The skin blistered. The blisters became secondarily infected and then broke down to expose areas of superficial ulceration. These ulcers usually heal quickly, unless there has been full-thickness skin loss.

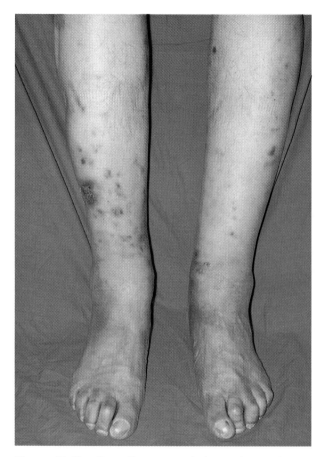

Figure 19.40 Kaposi's sarcoma is becoming an important differential diagnosis in patients with leg ulceration since the advent of AIDS. Multiple cutaneous red–purple nodules in a known homosexual are an indication for HIV antibody screening. Suspicious lesions should be biopsied to confirm the diagnosis. In this patient one lesion on the lateral side of the right leg and one on the medial side of the left leg have broken down and become ulcers. (We are grateful to Dr Martin Black for this illustration.)

Infected blisters

Patients who develop gross oedema of the lower limbs as a result of congestive cardiac failure, nephrotic syndrome, hyperalbuminaemia, or pelvic tumours, occasionally develop large intradermal blisters. When the outer layer of the blister separates, it leaves a shallow but sometimes an extensive area of ulceration which often becomes infected (Figure 19.39).

Treatment of the oedema and any secondary infection produces rapid healing, unless there has been full-thickness skin loss in which case skin grafting is required.

AIDS ulcers

We have seen a number of patients with AIDS who have developed severe multiple painful leg ulcers which were eventually healed by grafting. These ulcers were first described by Bayley.[7,8]

Ulcerating mesodermal tumours and lymphomas

Kaposi's sarcoma (Figure 19.40), histiocytic sarcoma, malignant fibroma, lymphangiosarcoma (Figure 19.41), and bone tumours can all rarely present as cutaneous ulceration.[7–9] They should not be a diagnostic problem, provided an ample biopsy is performed as part of the routine investigation of all atypical ulcers.

Lymphomas may also occasionally present as ulceration of the leg.

Injection ulcers (see Chapter 7)

The most common 'injection ulcer' on the lower leg follows extravasation of sclerosant during injection sclerotherapy for varicose veins. Sodium tetradecylsulphate (3%) is probably the most popular sclerosant used in the United Kingdom even though the newer sclerosants Variglobin and Sclerovein are said to cause fewer problems if they are injected outside the vein.

Injection ulcers do not occur if care is taken to ensure that the needle is inside the vein at the time of injection. Further injection of sclerosant must be abandoned if the needle slips out of the vein. There is no evidence that the damage caused by a sclerosant that has been injected outside the vein can be reduced by dilution with water or saline, or dispersal by hyaluronidase.

Injection ulcers are often indolent and can take many months to heal. It may be best to advise the patient to accept a local excision of the ulcer with a sutured primary closure.

Other hypertonic solutions can also cause ulceration if delivered outside the vein. These include hyperosmolar radiographic contrast media and cytotoxic drugs (Figure 19.42), though it is unusual for cytotoxic drugs to be injected into leg veins. Healing of these ulcers may also be slow, and excision with or without a skin graft may be necessary.

Nutritional ulcers

Patients with severe deficiency disease, such as beri-beri, scurvy, pellagra or kwashiorkor, may develop leg ulcers which will not heal until the nutritional deficiency has been corrected. The mechanism that causes the skin to necrose is obscure but it may be poor cellular regeneration after a minor injury.

Cryoglobulinaemia and macroglobulinaemia

These conditions cause small vessel 'sludging' accompanied by vasospasm which occasionally causes ulceration. These ulcers rarely occur on the leg and are usually found on the upper limb. The blood of any patient with Raynaud's syndrome and unusual skin ulceration should be sent for a cryoglobulin assay and protein electrophoresis to exclude these abnormalities.

Yaws, leprosy and anthrax

These are uncommon causes of ulceration of the legs. Yaws usually affects the lower limb and

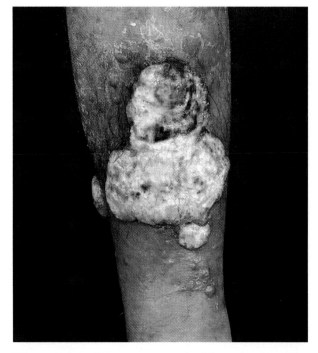

Figure 19.41 This young man had long-standing lymphoedema of the leg. He developed an area of cutaneous erythema which was initially thought to be cellulitis but this rapidly extended and ulcerated. The skin of the rest of the leg then developed multiple small haemorrhagic vascular nodules; biopsies showed these to be Stewart–Treves lymphangiosarcoma.

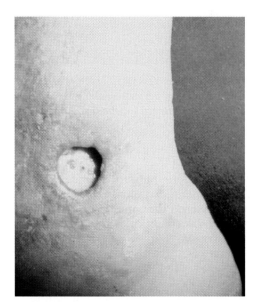

Figure 19.42 An injection ulcer on the lateral side of the ankle following the extravasation of a sclerosant material. Injection ulcers may take many weeks to heal and are sometimes best treated by excision and primary suture.

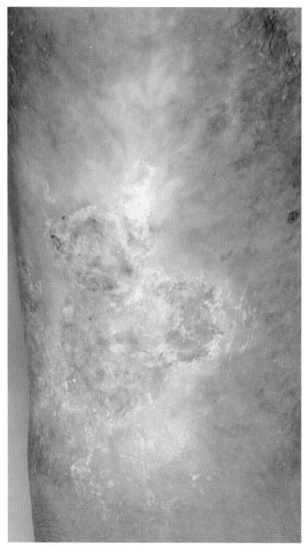

Figure 19.43   Yaws. Yaws is a spirochaetal infection which often causes skin papules which break down into superficial ulcers. (We are indebted to Dr D McGibbon for this illustration.)

often starts before puberty (Figure 19.43). The *Treponema pallidum* immobilization and VDRL (Venereal Disease Research Laboratory) tests are positive and the condition has to be differentiated from syphilis.

Lepromatous ulceration is usually neuropathic and associated with thickened nerves and the cutaneous changes of lepromatous or tuberculoid leprosy. Acid-fast bacilli are seen in skin biopsy.

Anthrax or woolsorters' disease presents as a black (malignant) pustule but rarely occurs on the lower limb. The bacillus should be seen in fluid aspirated from the vesicle.

Cutaneous necrosis secondary to warfarin or activated protein C resistance

Warfarin is a well-known cause of skin necrosis especially when associated with protein C, protein S and anti-cardiolipin antibodies.[31,62,75] The skin necrosis heals when the warfarin is withdrawn.

Tularaemia, blastomycosis and sporotrichosis

These are all theoretical rather than real causes of ulceration of the leg. They can be distinguished on bacteriological examination.

Recurrent panniculitis secondary to pancreatitis

This can produce changes that are very similar to lipodermatosclerosis and venous ulceration.[24]

Investigation of a venous ulcer

The tests designed to exclude other diagnoses have been mentioned in the previous section on differential diagnosis and are summarized in Table 19.2. Once the diagnosis of venous ulceration has been made, the investigations have two objectives:

1. Assessment of the ulcer
    *   size
    *   bacteriology
    *   nutrition
    *   histology
2. Assessment of the nature and the severity of the venous disease (Table 19.3).

TESTS DESIGNED TO ASSESS THE ULCER

Whatever the cause of the ulcer, certain tests must be carried out so that the initial state of the ulcer can be fully defined and the effect of treatment assessed.

Size

The only absolute measurement of healing is the time taken for the ulcer to heal completely. This measurement has the advantage of a reasonably clear end point. All the crust and scab must be removed to allow direct inspection and confirmation

Table 19.2 Tests that are helpful when investigating the cause of a leg ulcer

Blood investigations
    Haemoglobin*
    White cell count*
    Packed cell volume (PCV)*
    Erythrocyte sedimentation rate (ESR)*
    Rheumatoid factor*
    Rose–Waaler
    Latex
    Antinuclear factor*
    Blood sugar
    TPHA (*Treponema pallidum* haemagglutination)*
    Cryoglobulins*
    Plasma protein and strip*
    LE (lupus erythematosus) cells
Urine test (sugar)*
Bacteriological swabs*
Arm and ankle blood pressure index (Doppler
    ultrasound)*
Arteriography
Barium swallow
Isotope lymphography
Nerve conduction studies
Biopsy

*These are routine tests; the others are only performed if clinically indicated.

Table 19.3 The tests that we routinely use to assess the presence and severity of venous disease

Full clinical examination
Tourniquet tests
Doppler ultrasound flow detection of superficial vein
    reflux
Ascending phlebography
Foot volumetry
and in some cases
Varicography
Descending phlebography

of complete epithelialization before healing is accepted. Inadequate inspection will blur the end point.

The larger the area of the ulcer at the start of treatment, the longer will be the healing time (Figure 19.44).[88] An initial assessment of the ulcer area is therefore desirable for prognosis and stratification if the patient is participating in a clinical trial. The methods available for this are as follows:

1. *Tape measurement of the two largest diameters.* If the measurements of the two largest diameters (at right angles to each other) are multiplied

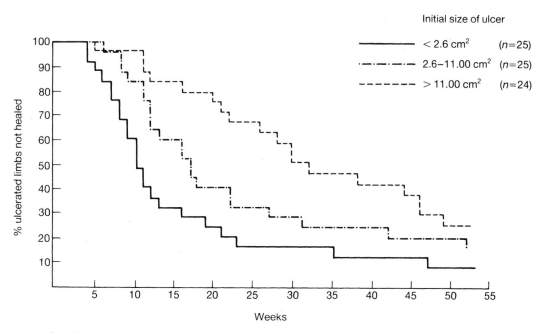

Figure 19.44 The relationship between ulcer size and ulcer healing. Ulcers have been divided into three groups based on their size at presentation. It can be seen that the largest ulcers take longer to heal but there is considerable variation in the time taken by individual ulcers to heal.[88]

together, the area of the ulcer is converted to the equivalent of a rectangle. This overestimates the area of most ulcers, as the majority are oval or irregular in shape (see Figure 19.1), but it has a surprisingly good correlation with more accurate methods of measurement described below and is probably adequate for most clinical trials.[88]

2. *Tracing out the perimeter.* The perimeter of the ulcer area can be traced on to transparent paper or polythene sheeting using an indelible pen. The marked out area on the paper can then be cut out and weighed if the paper is of standard thickness, or converted into square centimetres using a planimeter. Alternatively, an ultrasonic digitizer can be used with a light pen linked to a computer program to convert the traced ulcer area to square millimetres.[88] This is now commonly available.

3. *Photography.* Serial photographs against a scale can be used in association with one of the techniques described above to measure the exact surface area of the ulcer.[70] A normal camera does not allow for the convexity of the limb, and therefore this method of measurement will be inaccurate if the ulcer extends around more than one aspect of the leg. A complicated and expensive system of stereo-photogrammetry was developed to overcome the distortion caused by the convex limb surface and which, in the hands of its users, is claimed to give highly reproducible results.[14] It has not achieved widespread acceptance.

4. *Mould.* None of the methods described above makes any attempt to measure the depth of the ulcer. Some investigators have advocated the use of quick-setting moulds to take account of all three dimensions of the ulcer. This technique has not been adopted because it is debatable whether it provides much additional information to the measurement of surface area.

Comment

Ulcer measurements allow the doctor or nurse to assess treatment from week to week. It is important that measurements are made to avoid the standard comment 'healing well' which often appears month after month in the patient's records. Some workers have suggested that the healing rate in the first 6 weeks is an indication of successful treatment[14] but this has not been our experience (Figure 19.45). We find that the initial measurements do no more than allow us to make a crude estimate of the time to total healing. It is important, however, to have a crude initial size estimate as this allows stratification of ulcer healing studies.[88]

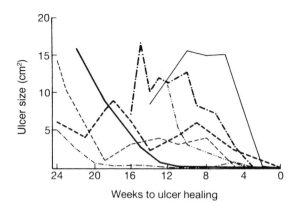

Figure 19.45 The variability of ulcer healing. This graph plots the healing of seven different ulcers and reveals how variable it can be. This variability means that assessment of treatment by measuring ulcer healing over a short period is a meaningless exercise. The only reliable method of describing healing is the time taken from the commencement of treatment to complete healing.

Other methods used to assess ulcer healing capability, based on the measurement of skin blood flow, have usually been used to assess ischaemic ulcers. These methods include injection of radioactive microspheres, skin fluorescence, and ^{99m}Tc phosphate imaging.[58] They have not yet found a place in the assessment of venous ulcer healing.

Bacteriology

Little is known about the role of bacteria in the genesis and maintenance of venous ulcers. It is assumed that high concentrations of organisms are associated with delayed healing and the rejection of skin grafts but there is little evidence that the elimination of infection or a reduction in the number of bacteria enhances healing.

Several studies[37–39,60,67,81,82,84,97] have shown that the organisms listed in Table 19.4 are commonly found on ulcers, and our own findings in 62 new ulcers are shown in Table 19.5. These organisms may simply be surface contaminants. Our own cultures of tissue biopsies taken from the ulcer base have not shown consistent evidence of infection spreading deeply into the granulation tissue. We have specifically looked for anaerobic organisms and found them in 44% of ulcer cultures; this is a much greater incidence than reported in other studies. It may be that anaerobic organisms adversely affect healing because metronidazole (Flagyl) has been reported to speed the healing of some ulcers.[5] These findings have, however, never been confirmed.

We no longer recommend routine bacteriological examination of ulcers for aerobic and anaerobic

Table 19.4 Bacteriology of venous ulcers

Organisms	Study 1 (62 ulcers),* no. of ulcers infected	Study 2 (47 ulcers),† no. of ulcers infected
Staphylococcus aureus	15	27
Staphylococcus epidermidis	12	–
Streptococcus		
Group A	–	2
Group B	1	2
Group C	–	3
Group D	4	–
Viridans	3	–
Escherichia coli	4	1
Proteus mirabilis	1	2
Enterobacter	3	1
Pseudomonas aeruginosa	5	1
Pseudomonas maltophilia	1	1
Clostridium perfringens	–	1
Corynebacterium	4	–
Acinetobacter calcoaceticus	3	–
Klebsiella pneumoniae	3	–
Citrobacter freundii	1	–
Yeast	2	–
Normal skin flora	–	4
No growth	–	2

*Study 1 – Friedman SJ, Su WPD. Management of leg ulcers with hydrocolloid occlusive dressing. *Arch Dermatol* 1984; **120:** 1329.
†Study 2 – Eriksson G. Bacterial growth in venous leg ulcers – its clinical significance in the healing process. In: *Royal Society of Medicine, International Congress and Symposium Series*, 1985; **No 88:** 45.

Table 19.5 Bacterial flora of 63 consecutive new leg ulcers

Organism	No. of ulcers with organism	Percentage
Staphylococcus aureus	32	51
Streptococcus faecalis	20	31
Staphylococcus epidermidis	12	19
Proteus mirabilis	12	19
Pseudomonas aeruginosa	12	19
β-Haemolytic streptococci	10	16
Diphtheroid	10	16
Escherichia coli	4	6
Proteus vulgaris	4	6
Non-haemolytic streptococci	3	5
Enterobacter cloacae	3	5
Klebsiella	3	5
α-Haemolytic streptococci	2	3
Acinetobacter anitratus	2	3
Morganella morganii	2	3
Streptococcus milleri	1	2
Pseudomonas putrefaciens	1	2
Haemophilus parainfluenzae	1	2

organisms and only give antibiotics in the rare case where bacterial cellulitis or lymphangitis complicate the ulcer.

Hopkins and Jamieson[47] have shown that systemically administered antibiotics can reach the surface of the ulcer but we do not know if they influence healing. Ryan[84] has argued that all organisms are not necessarily bad. For example, he has suggested that coliforms which use up oxygen may encourage the growth of anaerobes, which in turn may protect the aerobes from phagocytosis. Some organisms may remove slough while others may prevent invasion by more virulent microbes. Halbert *et al.*[43] have suggested that β-haemolytic streptococci, *Staphylococcus aureus* and coliforms do delay ulcer healing. There are still no good prospective studies which have compared healing in 'standardized' and heavily colonized ulcers, which might support the use of antimicrobial agents.

Comment

The bacteriology of venous ulcers deserves closer study. At present, no firm conclusions can be drawn from the published work about the significance of

bacteria on ulcer healing or the value of their eradication.

Nutrition

Anaemia

An association between certain anaemias and
ulceration has already been discussed but all varieties of chronic ulceration may cause anaemia.
Blood loss and chronic infection can combine to
give a mixed picture of bone marrow depression
and iron deficiency anaemia. Schraibman and
Stratton[87] found significantly lower haemoglobin
and ferritin levels in 30 patients with leg ulcers
compared with a similar number of age- and sex-
matched controls. The patients with ulcers also had
lower levels of protein and albumin but these
reductions did not reach statistical significance.

   The nutritional status of all patients with ulcers
should be assessed from anthropomorphic measurements and blood studies.

Trace elements

Much attention has been paid to the effect of zinc
deficiency and its replacement in leg ulceration.[41,44,102] Serum zinc levels have been found to be
low in some patients but it has been shown that
serum zinc does not correlate well with total body
zinc which is better assessed by measuring intracellular leucocyte zinc.[51] Confirmation that patients
with venous ulcers have a true tissue zinc depletion
is essential before attempting to show that systemically or locally administered zinc improves healing.

Tissue oxygenation

There is one small study that looked at a number
of different types of ulcer and showed that ulcers
that healed or improved had higher transcutaneous
oxygen levels than ulcers that remained static.[61]

Histology

The principal objective of ulcer biopsy is to exclude
non-venous causes of ulceration. We are not aware
of any studies that have used repeated biopsies to
access ulcer healing or healing potential.

   Clinicians are naturally averse to performing a
biopsy when an ulcer is showing signs of healing, in
case it delays or reverses the healing process. A
further biopsy when an ulcer fails to show signs of
healing might explain why this is happening.
Ultimately, the clinical behaviour of ulcers must be
related to a knowledge of the pathological changes
occurring in the skin, some of which can only be

assessed by biopsy. The role of growth factors in
ulcer healing is now being studied in greater detail.
Our own studies have shown that fibroblast growth
factor and transforming growth factor β may have
an important role in epithelial migration and adhesion. This factor may be related to urokinase which
appears to be present in abundant amounts in
healing ulcers.[89]

TESTS USED TO ASSESS CALF PUMP FUNCTION

These tests are discussed in detail in Chapter 4. The
tests that we commonly use are listed in Table 19.3.

References

1. Ackroyd JS, Young AK. Leg ulcers that do not heal. *Br Med J* 1983; **286:** 207–8.
2. Adrians B, Hay R, Drasar B, Robinson D. The infectious aetiology of tropical ulcer – a study of the role of aerobic bacteria. *Br J Dermatol* 1987; **116:** 31–7.
3. Alberdi J, Ma Z. Hypertensive ulcer: Martorell's ulcer. *Phlebology* 1988; **3:** 139–42.
4. Anning ST. *Leg Ulcers. Their Causes and Treatment.* London: J & A Churchill, 1954.
5. Baker PG, Haig G. Metronidazole in the treatment of chronic pressure sores and ulcers. A comparison with standard treatments in general practice. *Practitioner* 1981; **225:** 569–73.
6. Baker SR, Burnand KG, Sommerville KM, Lea Thomas M, Wilson NM, Browse NL. Comparison of venous reflux assessed by duplex scanning and descending phlebography in chronic venous disten-sion. *Lancet* 1993; **341:** 400–3.
7. Bayley AC. A surgical pathology of HIV lesions from Africa. *Br J Surg* 1990; **77:** 863–7.
8. Bayley AC. Kaposi's sarcoma – old and new pat-terns. *Surgery* 1988; 1404–8.
9. Berth-Jones J, Graham-Brown RAC, Fletcher A, Henderson HP, Barrie WW. Malignant fibrous his-tiocytoma: a new complication of chronic venous ulceration. *Br Med J* 1989; **298:** 230–1.
10. Black W. Neoplastic disease occurring in varicose ulcers or eczema: report of 6 cases. *Br J Cancer* 1952; **6:** 120–6.
11. Bliss MR. Acute pressure area care: Sir James Paget's legacy. *Lancet* 1992; **339:** 221–3.
12. Browse NL, Jarrett PEM, Morland M, Burnand KG. Treatment of liposclerosis of the leg by fibri-nolytic enhancement: a preliminary report. *Br Med J* 1977; **2:** 434–5.
13. Brunsting LA, Goeckerman WH, O'Leary PA. Pyoderma (echthyma) gangrenosum. *Arch Dermatol Syphilol* 1930; **22:** 655–80.
14. Bulstrode CJK, Goode AW, Scott PJ. Stereo-photogrammetry for measuring rates of cutaneous

healing: a comparison with conventional techniques. *Clin Sci* 1986; **71:** 437–43.

15. Burnand KG, Browse NL. The postphlebitic limb and venous ulceration. In: Russell RCG, ed. *Recent Advances in Surgery.* Edinburgh: Churchill Livingstone, 1982.

16. Burnand KG, Clemenson G, Morland M, Jarrett PEM, Browse NL. Venous lipodermatosclerosis: treatment by fibrinolytic enhancement and elastic compression. *Br Med J* 1980; **280;** 7–11.

17. Burnand KG, Clemenson G, Whimster I, Gaunt J, Browse NL. The effect of sustained hypertension in the skin capillaries of the canine hind limb. *Br J Surg* 1982; **69:** 41–4.

18. Burnand KG, Whimster IW, Clemenson G, Lea Thomas M, Browse NL. The relationship between the number of capillaries in the skin of the venous ulcer bearing area of the lower leg and the fall in foot vein pressure during exercise. *Br J Surg* 1981; **68:** 297–300.

19. Callum MJ, Ruckley CV, Dale JJ, Harper DR. Chronic leg ulcer. The incidence of associated non-venous disorders. In: Negus D, Jantet G, eds. *Phlebology '85.* London: Libbey, 1986.

20. Callum MJ, Ruckley CV, Harper DR, Dale JJ. Chronic ulceration of the leg: extent of the problem and provision of care. *Br Med J* 1985; **290:** 1855.

21. Carmichael AJ, Paul CJ. Vasculitic leg ulcers associated with diltiazem. (letter) *Br Med J* 1988; **297:** 562.

22. Carr AJ, Percival RC, Rogers K, Harrington CT. Pyoderma gangrenosum after cholecystectomy. *Br Med J* 1986; **292:** 729–30.

23. Chambers M, Thornes RD, McKernan M. Necrosis of skin induced by coumarin. (letter) *Br Med J* 1989; **298:** 755.

24. Cheng KS, Stansby G, Law N, Gardham R. Recurrent panniculitis as the first clinical manifestation of recurrent acute pancreatitis secondary to cholelithiasis. *J R Soc Med* 1988; **89:** 105–6.

25. Cockett FB. Diagnosis and surgery of high pressure venous leaks in the leg. A new overall concept of surgery of varicose veins and venous ulcers. *Br Med J* 1956; **2:** 1399–406.

26. Cockett FB, Elgan Jones DE. The ankle blow out syndrome. A new approach to the varicose ulcer problem. *Lancet* 1953; **1:** 17–23.

27. Coleridge-Smith PD. Investigation of patients with venous ulceration. *Phlebology Suppl* 1992; **1:** 17–21.

28. Coleridge-Smith PD, Scurr JH. A direct method for measuring venous ulcers. *Br J Surg* 1989; **76:** 689.

29. Cornwall JV, Lewis JD. Leg ulcer revisited. *Br J Surg* 1983; **70:** 681.

30. Cotterill JA. Self-stigmatization: artefact dermatitis. *Br J Hosp Med* 1992; **47(2):** 115–19.

31. Craig A, Taberner DA, Fisher AH, Foster DN, Mitra J. Type 1 protein S deficiency and skin necrosis. *Postgrad Med J* 1990; **66:** 389–91.

32. Davson J, Jones DM, Turner L. Diagnosis of Meleney's synergistic gangrene. *Br J Surg* 1988; **75:** 267–71.

33. Dodd H, Cockett FB. *The Pathology and Surgery of the Veins of the Lower Limb.* Edinburgh: Livingstone, 1965.

34. Eaglestein WH. Personal communication, 1985.

35. Ellis H. Leg, ulceration of. In: Hart FD, ed. *French's Index of Differential Diagnosis.* 12th edition. Bristol: Wright, 1985.

36. Fowkes FGR, Callam MJ. Is arterial disease a risk factor for chronic leg ulceration? *Phebology* 1994; **9:** 87–90.

37. Friedman SA, Gladstone JL. The bacterial flora of peripheral vascular ulcers. *Arch Dermatol* 1969; **100:** 29–32.

38. Friedman SJ, Su WP. Management of leg ulcers with hydrocolloid occlusive dressings. *Arch Dermatol* 1984; **120:** 1336.

39. Geronemus RG, Mertz PM, Eaglestein WG. Wound healing: the effects of topical antimicrobial agents. *Arch Dermatol* 1979; **115:** 1311–14.

40. Goodacre TEE. Tropical ulcers. (letter) *Lancet* 1987; 1152.

41. Greaves MW, Boyde TR. Plasma zinc concentrations in patients with psoriasis, other dermatoses, and venous leg ulceration. *Lancet* 1967; **2:** 1019–20.

42. Haegar K. Leg ulcers. In: Haegar K, ed. *Venous and Lymphatic Disorders of the Leg.* Lund: Scandinavian University Books, 1966.

43. Halbert AR, Stacey MC, Rohr JB, Jopp-McKay A. The effect of bacterial colonization on venous ulcer healing. *Australas J Dermatol* 1992; **33:** 75–80.

44. Halsted JA, Smith JC. Plasma zinc in health and disease. *Lancet* 1970; **1:** 322–4.

45. Hohn L. Age-related rather than ulcer-related impairment of venous function tests in patients with venous ulceration. *Dermatologica* 1990; **180:** 73–5.

46. Homans J. Treatment of elephantiasis of the legs; preliminary report. *N Engl J Med* 1936; **215:** 1099–104.

47. Hopkins NFG, Jamieson CW. Antibiotic concentration in exudate in venous ulcers; the prediction of ulcer healing rate. *Br J Surg* 1983; **70:** 532.

48. Hudson-Peacock MJ, Regnard CFB, Farr PM. Liquefying panniculitis associated with acinous carcinoma of the pancreas responding to octreotide. *J R Soc Med* 1994; **87:** 361–2.

49. Hurst PA, Kinmonth JB, Rutt DL. A gut and mesentery pedicle for bridging lymphatic obstruction. *J Cardiovasc Surg* 1978; **19:** 589–96.

50. Jones DM, Davson J, Turner L. Meleney's synergistic gangrene. (letter) *Lancet* 1988; **1:** 828–9.

51. Keeling PWN, Jones RB, Hilton PJ, Thompson RPH. Reduced leucocyte zinc in liver disease. *Gut* 1980; **21:** 561–4.

52. Kingston D, Seal DV. Current hypotheses on synergistic microbial gangrene. *Br J Surg* 1990; **77:** 260–4.

53. Kinmonth JB, Hurst PA, Edwards JM, Rutt DL. Relief of lymph obstruction by use of a bridge of mesentery and ileum. *Br J Surg* 1978; **65:** 829–33.

54. Knox LC. Epithelioma and the chronic venous ulcer. *JAMA* 1925; **85:** 1046–51.

55. Kulkarni J. Pressure sores. (correspondence) *Br Med J* 1994; **309:** 1436.

56. Lagatolla NRF, Burnand KG. Chronic venous disease may delay the diagnosis of malignant ulceration of the leg. *Phlebology* 1994; **9**: 167–9.

57. Landra AP. The tropical ulcer. *Surgery* 1988; 1402–3.

58. Lawrence PF, Syverud JB, Disbro MA, Alazraki N. Evaluation of technetium-99m phosphate imaging for predicting skin ulcer healing. *Am J Surg* 1983; **146**: 746–50.

59. Liddell K. Malignant changes in chronic varicose ulceration. *The Practitioner* 1975; **215**: 335–9.

60. Lookingbill DP, Miller SH, Knowles RC. Bacteriology of chronic leg ulcers. *Arch Dermatol* 1978; **114**: 1765–8.

61. Lucarotti M, Lancaster J, Hewitt H, Leaper D. Multiple physiological indices in the management of chronic leg ulcers. *Phlebology* 1988; **3**: 247–50.

62. McGhee WG, Klotz TA, Epstein DJ, Rapaport SI. Coumarin skin necrosis associated with hereditary protein C deficiency. *Ann Intern Med* 1984; **100**: 59–60.

63. Marjolin JN. *Ulcere diet de med (practique)*. 2nd edition. Paris, 1846.

64. Martorell F. Hypertensive ulcer of the leg. *Angiology* 1950; **1**: 133–40.

65. Martorell F. Obituary. *J Cardiovasc Surg* 1985; **26**: 319–20.

66. Meleney FL. *Clinical Aspects and Treatment of Surgical Infections*. London: Saunders, 1949.

67. Mitchell AAB, Pettigrew JB, MacGillvray D. Varicose ulcers as reservoirs of hospital strains of *Staph. aureus* and *Pseudomonas pyocyanea*. *Br J Clin Pract* 1970; **24**: 223–6.

68. Moffatt CJ, Oldroyd MI, Greenhalgh RM, Franks PJ. Palpating ankle pulses is insufficient in detecting arterial insufficiency in patients with leg ulceration. *Phlebology* 1994; **9**: 170–2.

69. Muelder K, Nourou A. Buruli ulcer in Benin. *Lancet* 1990; **336**: 1109–11.

70. Myers MB, Cherry G. Zinc and the healing of chronic leg ulcers. *Am J Surg* 1984; **120**: 77.

71. Naschitz JE, Yeshurun D, Schwartz H, Croitrou S, Shajrawi I, Misselevich I, Boss JH. Pathogenesis of lipodermatosclerosis of venous disease: the lesson learned from eosinophilic fasciitis. *Cardiovasc Surg* 1993; **5**: 524–9.

72. Negus D, Friedgood A. The effective management of venous ulceration. *Br J Surg* 1983; **70**: 623.

73. Nelzen O, Bergqvist D, Lindhagen A. Venous and non-venous leg ulcers: clinical history and appearance in a population study. *Br J Surg* 1994; **81**: 182–7.

74. Northeast ADR, Eastham D, Donald A, Paul-Clarke M, Burnand KG. A comparison between foot plethysmography and light reflection rheography in patients with healed venous ulcers. *Phlebology* 1994; **9**: 132.

75. O'Neill A, Gatenby PA, McGaw B *et al*. Widespread cutaneous necrosis associated with anticardiolipin antibodies. *J Am Acad Dermatol* 1990; **22**: 356–9.

76. Perkins W, Downie I, Keefe M, Chisholm M. Cutaneous necrosis in pregnancy secondary to activated protein C resistance in hereditary angioedema. *J R Soc Med* 1995; **88**: 229–30.

77. Piulacks P, Vidal-Barraquer F. Pathogenic study of varicose veins. *Angiology* 1953; **4**: 59–100.

78. Pollard JP, LeQuesne LP. Method of healing diabetic forefoot ulcers. *Br Med J* 1983; **286**: 436–7.

79. Prentice AG, Lowe GDO, Forbes CD. Diagnosis and treatment of venous thromboembolism by consultants in Scotland. *Br Med J* 1982; **285**: 630–2.

80. Quist G. *Surgical Diagnosis*. London: Lewis, 1977.

81. Ramsay LE. Impact of venography on the diagnosis and management of deep vein thrombosis. *Br Med J* 1983; **286**: 698–9.

82. Ruckley CV, Callum MJ, Harper DR, Dale JJ. The Lothian and Forth Valley leg ulcer survey. Part 4 Arterial disease. In: Negus D, Jantet G, eds. *Phlebology '85*. London: Libbey, 1986.

83. Ryan TJ. *The Management of Leg Ulcers*. Oxford: Oxford Medical Publications, 1983.

84. Ryan TJ, Wilkinson DS. Diseases of the veins and arteries – leg ulcers. In: Rook A, Wilkinson DS, Ebling FJG, eds. *Textbook of Dermatology*. 4th edition. Oxford: Blackwell Scientific Publications, 1985.

85. Sacks DL, Kenney RT, Kreutzer RD, *et al*. Indian kala-azar caused by *Leishmania tropica*. *Lancet* 1995; **345**: 959–61.

86. Sarkany I, Kreel L. Subcutaneous ossification of the legs in chronic venous stasis. *Br Med J* 1966; **2**: 27–8.

87. Schraibman IG, Stratton FJ. Nutritional status of patients with leg ulcers. *J R Soc Med* 1985; **78**: 39–42.

88. Stacey MC, Burnand KG, Layer GT, Pattison M, Browse NL. Measurement of the healing of venous ulcers. *Aust N Z J Surg* 1991; **61**: 844–8.

89. Stacey MC, Burnand KG, Mahmoud-Alexandroni N, Gaffney PJ, Bhogal BS. Tissue and urokinase type plasminogen activators in the environs of venous and ischaemic leg ulcers. *Br J Surg* 1993; **80**: 596–9.

90. Stacey-Clear A, Cornwall JV, Lewis JD. Intravenous prostacyclin (PEI2) and skin grafting for rheumatoid leg ulcers. In: Negus D, Jantet G, eds. *Phlebology '85*. London: Libbey, 1986.

91. Stevanovic DV. Atrophie blanche: a sign of dermal blood flow occlusion. *Arch Dermatol* 1974; **109**: 858–62.

92. Stewart GJ, Gaunt JI, Croft DN, Browse NL. Isotope lymphography: a new method of investigating the role of the lymphatics in chronic limb oedema. *Br J Surg* 1985; **72**: 906–9.

93. Stewart GJ, Pattison M, Burnand KG. Abnormal fibrinolysis: the cause of lipodermatosclerosis or 'chronic cellulitis' in patients with primary lymphoedema. *Lymphology* 1984; **17**: 23–7.

94. Thurtle OA, Cawley MID. The frequency of leg ulceration in rheumatoid arthritis; a survey. *J Rheumatol* 1983; **10**: 507–9.

95. Tibbs CJ. Hepatitis B, tropical ulcers and immunisation strategy in Kiribati. *Br Med J* 1987; **294**: 537–40.

96. Van der Molen HR. Calcifications sous-cutanees phlebopathiques. *Phlebologie* 1975; **28**: 551–8.

97. Van Duyn J. Proteus/staphylococcal synergism in punched out ulcers. *Plast Reconstr Surg* 1967; **40:** 86–8.

98. Visvanathan R. Madura foot: a surgical cure. (letter) *Br Med J* 1991; **303:** 994.

99. Vohra RK, McCollum CN. Pressure sores. *Br Med J* 1994; **309:** 853–7.

100. Walkden V, Black MM. Basal cell carcinomatous changes of the lower leg: an association with chronic venous stasis. *Br J Dermatol* 1981; **105(Suppl 9):** 9.

101. Wilson IAI, Henry M, Quill RD, Byrne PJ. The pH of varicose ulcer surfaces and its relationship to healing. *Vasa* 1979; **8:** 339–42.

102. Withers AFD, Baker H, Musa M, Dormandy TL. Plasma-zinc in psoriasis. *Lancet* 1968; **2:** 278.

103. Wood ML, Reilly GD, Smith GT. Ulceration of the hand secondary to a radial arteriovenous fistula: a model for varicose ulceration. *Br Med J (Clin Res Ed)* 1983; **287:** 1167–8.

CHAPTER 20

Venous ulceration: natural history and treatment

Natural history	571	Prevention of ulcer recurrence	591
Treatment	573	References	598

Natural history

Epidemiological studies[45,60] have shown that some patients live in symbiosis with their leg ulcers for many years without much discomfort but without achieving any period of healing, whereas other patients have ulcers that are so painful and extensive that they beg for an amputation. In the United Kingdom, approximately 100 limbs are amputated for venous disease every year,[134] 1 in every 700 000 of the population.

Many studies have described excellent early results of ulcer treatment by a number of different techniques but there are few long-term follow-up studies. We have been unable to find any studies reporting the results of ulcer treatment over periods of 10 or 20 years with adequate follow-up. The position is similar to that for breast carcinoma 20 years ago when there were many 5-year follow-up studies but none of 10 or 20 years.

The need for long-term studies is highlighted by our own experience in trials of ulcer treatment. We have conducted a number of studies on ulcers confirmed to be of venous aetiology by special investigations. Over 80% of these ulcers have been healed within 1 year of presenting to the clinic by a combination of bandages and compression. The remainder have been successfully healed with split skin grafts. Thus if patients with venous ulceration agree to treatment, it is possible to achieve healing by conservative or surgical means in almost every case. *The problem is to maintain healing.* Ten to twenty per cent of venous ulcers referred have broken down within 18 months of healing.[127]

Why do some ulcers continually break down when others remain healed? The logical answer is that venous ulcers will recur if the underlying pathophysiological abnormality is not corrected. But this explanation is probably not the whole answer as the physiological tests of calf pump function in patients whose ulcers remain healed are very similar to those of patients whose ulcers break down. We need to know much more about the factors that cause ulceration, as well as improve our methods of correcting calf pump function, before we can hope to treat all venous ulcers successfully.

The natural history studies of venous ulceration reveal the following information.

1. They represent a potentially insoluble problem from the moment they first develop until the patient dies.[31,129,130]
2. The number of patients presenting for treatment is the tip of an iceberg.[45,153]
3. In only the patients with ulceration caused by pure superficial vein incompetence is long-term cure possible.[36]
4. We need long-term follow-up studies to assess which of the treatments for post-thrombotic ulcers is the most successful in preventing recurrence.

5. Untreated venous ulcers often remain unhealed for many years.[45]
6. Without permanent prophylactic measures many venous ulcers recur.[36,38]
7. Almost all venous ulcers can be healed with good medical treatment but universal prevention of recurrence cannot yet be achieved.[31]
8. Our immediate aim must be to develop treatments that prevent ulcer recurrence. Our long-term aim must be to prevent the venous and tissue changes that precede ulceration by preventing deep vein thrombosis and developing techniques that fully correct calf pump dysfunction.

Effect on the patient

Ulcers are often painful and smelly. They require frequent dressings and visits to or by medical personnel. They therefore interfere with work and holidays and restrict the lifestyle of the patient. As a result, patients with this problem may develop personality disorders, even severe depression and paranoia.

The patient's daily life may come to revolve around the ulcer and it may provide the only reason for contact with the inhabitants of the world outside the home for a depressed, aged and immobile patient. Chronic ulcers cause shortening of the Achilles tendon with the development of an equinus deformity (Figure 20.1). This in turn may cause pain and further reduce mobility. Chronic anaemia is another reason for loss of general well-being.[184]

Bathing is a problem when the leg is wrapped with dressings, making it difficult to maintain personal hygiene. This may add to a sense of social isolation. The significance of ulceration of the leg is clouded by ignorance and hearsay. Some patients still believe that healing of an ulcer leads to certain death; this belief is presumably a relic from the theory that ulcers let out evil humours, a theory that was in vogue from the time of Hippocrates to the end of the Dark Ages.[4]

An inability to stay at work because of frequent visits to the doctor or the hospital may inflict a considerable economic burden on the patient. The cost of drugs, dressings and elastic stockings is an additional financial burden. Bosanquet[26] has estimated that we spend approximately £550 000 a year on treating ulcers for every quarter of a million of the population, giving a bill in the region of £230-400 million/year for the whole population at 1990–91 prices. All these factors make venous ulceration a miserable experience which is the reason why many patients are so grateful when their doctor shows some enthusiasm and interest in their care. When

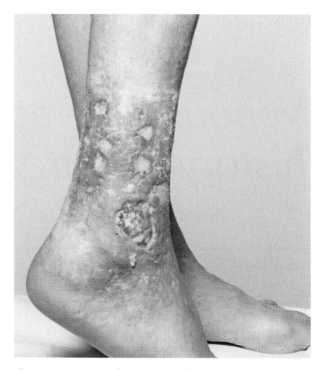

Figure 20.1 Lateral view of an ulcerated leg showing an equinus deformity causing 4 cm of apparent shortening as a result of periarticular inflammation, fibrosis, and shortening of the Achilles tendon.

ulcer care is delegated to junior doctors or community nurses whose knowledge and experience does not compare with that of their seniors, many patients are given conflicting and wrong advice; not surprisingly, the patients decide to take over the management of their ulcers themselves.

Effect on medical services

It has been estimated that every unhealed ulcer costs the community £1667 per ulcer per year in dressings and medical time.[105] In-patient admissions costing approximately £300/day are also expensive, making ulcer treatment a major drain on scarce medical resources. A study from Melbourne[98] suggests that it costs 1200 Australian dollars (approximately £6000) for every ulcer admitted to hospital. Any measure which successfully prevents recurrence is therefore bound to be cost effective.

Many hospitals have now developed ulcer clinics to concentrate expertise at a single site, and it is hoped that improvements in treatment will follow. At present most ulcer treatment is undertaken by overworked general practitioners, and community nurses.[26,45,95] There are now a number of studies showing that introduction of community-based ulcer clinics leads to improved ulcer healing, reducing costs. We do have slight concerns over the diagnostic expertise available in these community clinics where all ulcers not shown to be ischaemic are called 'venous'. A little knowledge can be a dangerous thing! One-stop hospital clinics when specialist diagnostic expertise is available may be a better solution.

Treatment

The treatment of venous ulceration has two objectives:

- To heal the ulcer
- To prevent recurrence of the ulcer.

Treatments designed to heal the ulcer are as follows.

1. Compression (normally by bandages or stockings) combined with dressings
2. Bedrest with leg elevation
3. Surgical excision of slough and ulcer base
4. Topical applications to the ulcer
   (a) antiseptics
   (b) antibiotics
   (c) cleaning agents to dissolve slough
   (d) agents to promote healing
5. Applications for the surrounding skin
6. Systemic medication
   (a) to promote healing
   (b) to sterilize the surface of the ulcer
7. Physical methods
   (a) to promote healing
   (b) to clean the ulcer
8. Application of skin substitutes to promote healing
   (a) human amnion
   (b) lyophilized pigskin
9. Skin grafting
   (a) split skin grafts
   (b) pinch grafts
   (c) full-thickness grafts
   (d) pedicle grafts
   (e) vascularized free flap grafts
10. Ulcer excision followed by skin grafting
11. Correction of calf pump malfunction
    (a) injection/compression sclerotherapy
    (b) surgical ligation of the superficial and lower leg communicating veins
    (c) surgical reconstruction of the deep veins or valves
    (d) elastic compression stockings
12. Miscellaneous treatments

COMPRESSION WITH BANDAGES OVER DRESSINGS

The value of compressing the limb with bandages has been recognized for many years. In addition to its therapeutic value, it helps to avoid hospital admissions and is therefore inexpensive. This treatment also allows the patient to continue their normal life, apart from the time devoted to changing the dressings and reapplying or adjusting the compression bandages or stocking.

Celsus[47] described the use of plasters and linen roller bandages to treat leg ulcers in AD 25; many other dressings and many different methods of bandaging have been described since that time. In 1783, Underwood[208] described the first use of modified elastic (Welsh flannel) but this was not generally accepted. In 1866, Spender[196] wrote 'the proper application of the bandage is of such great importance in the treatment of varicose ulcers of the legs that it should, when possible, be executed by the surgeon in attendance'. He felt that 'compression answers every objective to be gained by the recumbent posture'. Widespread use of 'elastic compression' followed the description of an adhesive elastic bandage by Dickson Wright[71] in 1930, and the development of the strong elastic webbing bandage described by Bisgaard[19] in 1948.

Stockings offer an alternative means of compression. In the early 1600s William Lee of Oxford developed a loom for weaving stockings.[7] Richard Wiseman[220] described a compression stocking for treating leg ulceration in 1676 (Figure 20.2). It was made of soft leather and could be laced up to differing degrees of tightness to alter the degree of compression. As it was also shaped to the contour of the leg, it probably represents the first attempt to produce a graduated compression stocking. It was not, however, until the advent of elastic fibres that could be woven into stockings that true elastic stockings became widely used as an alternative to bandages.

Since bandaging began, dressings have been placed over the ulcer to absorb the exudate and prevent soiling of the compressing bandage. The earliest dressings were leaves soaked in wine[90] but leaves were replaced by linen, wool and gauze as these materials became freely available. More recently, colloidal silver, aluminium foil[100,101] and living membranes[16,104] have all been used with varying degrees of success.

Modern methods of compression

Sigg[188] credited Van der Molen[211] with the idea of progressively reducing (graduating) the degree of compression along the leg so that the maximum

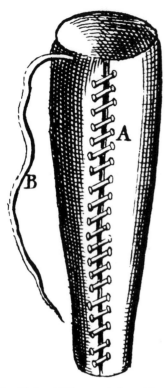

Figure 20.2   Richard Wiseman's laced leather stocking. It was shaped to be narrower at the ankle and wider over the calf. The lace allowed the stocking to be tightened to apply the correct amount of pressure; this was the forerunner of the modern elastic stocking. (From Heister L. 1768. *A General System of Surgery*. London: Whiston, 1768.)

compression is applied at the ankle and minimum compression is applied to the knee or thigh. Graduated compression stockings aim to prevent venous capillary transudation for different degrees of venous pressure fall during exercise.[200,201] Pressures of 40–50 mmHg are required at the ankle to balance the Starling equation[199] in limbs with a severe post-thrombotic syndrome and no reduction in superficial vein pressure during exercise (see Chapter 17). Graduated compression also increases the velocity of blood flow in the deep veins.[187] All methods of compression stimulate the release of fibrinolytic activity[49] and reduce discomfort by preventing oedema and venous distension. These beneficial effects of graduated compression are lost if the compression weakens or is poorly applied, or if a tourniquet effect develops anywhere along the leg.[58]

The history of compression has been fully reviewed by Marmasse and Ruckley.[137,178]

The methods of compression currently available are:

- compression bandages
- elastic stockings
- inflatable pneumatic leggings.

Compression bandages

Bandages are probably the most popular form of compression because they are relatively inexpensive and can therefore be discarded when they become soiled by ulcer exudate. The problems associated with their use include:

- failure to stay in place
- variations in the skill (and consequently the compression) with which they are applied
- loss of compression after washing.

It has been shown that bandaging techniques vary considerably from doctor to doctor and from nurse to nurse.[66] The use of a stocking tester may help the development of greater uniformity in bandaging techniques,[167] but a recent attempt to produce a standard amount of compression by printing rectangles on the surface of a bandage which become square when the bandage is pulled to its correct tension (STD, Thusane) did not appear to reduce variability when we tested the bandaging efficiency of inexperienced volunteers.[167] Despite this, the concept of a 'built-in' regulator of compression seems attractive and has been taken up by other manufacturers (Seton).

The elastic compression bandages most commonly used are:

- The red-line Bisgaard bandage (JG Marlow and Son)
- Elastoweb (Smith & Nephew)
- Bilastic (Steviseal Ltd)
- Blue-line webbing (Seton HC)
- Elset (Seton HC)
- Lastobind (Paul Hartmann)
- Rowden Foote Bandages (Hospital Management Supplies)
- Setopress (Seton HC)
- Tensopress (Smith & Nephew)
- Thusane (STD)
- SurePress (ConvaTec)

The conforming stretch bandages commonly used are:

- Creplax (Grant and Co)
- Gauzelast (Molimer)
- Gauzex (BDF)
- J Fast (Johnson & Johnson)
- Lastotel (Paul Hartmann)
- Lastocrepe (BDF)
- Mollelast (Lohman)
- Nephlex (Smith & Nephew)
- Tensofix (Smith & Nephew)
- Transelast (Lohman)

The light compression bandages commonly used are:

- Comprilan (BDF)
- Coplus (Smith & Nephew)
- Elastovic (Goent & Co)
- Rayvic (Goent & Co)
- Tensolastic (Smith & Nephew)
- Varicrepe (Sherwood)

The tubular bandages commonly used are:

- Tubigrip (Seton)
- Tensogrip (Smith & Nephew)
- Sigura (Sigma)

The adhesive bandages commonly used are:

- Coban (3M)
- Coplus (Smith & Nephew)
- Lestraflex (Seton)
- Liteflex (Johnson & Johnson)
- Veinoplast (Steriseal)
- Zoplaband (Hinders Leslies)

The Blue- or Red-line bandages, which are made of elastic webbing, give very good compression but tend to slip and are unsightly because they are very thick.

Elastocrepe is widely used but has been shown to lose its elasticity when washed[66] or reapplied.[167] It only provides an adequate amount of compression when it is combined with a paste bandage or covered by Tubigrip.

Lestraflex is an inelastic self-adhesive bandage that can cause sensitivity rashes when applied directly to the skin but its adhesive property does prevent it from slipping. It is now seldom used because of skin reactions, unless it is applied over the top of another bandage.

J Fast provides a very low degree of compression and is of doubtful value for ulcer treatment.

Coban also provides low levels of compression and is difficult to apply correctly. It is self-adhesive and can be used to prevent other underlying bandages coming undone.

Tubigrip provides poor compression on its own but is useful if used with Elastocrepe and paste bandages.

Thusane is a strong elastic bandage which provides good levels of compression but tends to slip down.

Tensopress is a relatively new elastic bandage which also provides a good level of compression.

Setopress is similarly a new bandage with good compression levels.

Elset is another type of elasticated bandage.

McCollum has suggested that criteria should be laid down to classify bandages in the same way that the British Standard applies to elastic stockings. This has not yet been accepted. One study[203] which compared six of the bandages discussed above on a stocking tester showed that only the blue-line bandage applied satisfactory sustained pressure.

Application of a compression bandage

The art of bandaging has almost disappeared as surgical wound dressings have become lighter or non-existent. The one place where bandaging skill is essential is in the ulcer clinic. In 1859, Hunt[114] wrote that the problems with bandaging arose because 'the application of a bandage is looked upon as an easy and simple operation which may be satisfactorily entrusted to a nurse or the patient'. He went on to state that 'a correctly applied bandage on an ulcer patient must be applied from the toes to the knee, with all parts of the leg being equally supported'. Hunt was the first person to suggest including pads beneath the bandage to fill out any depressions in the leg (Figure 20.3), and he also said

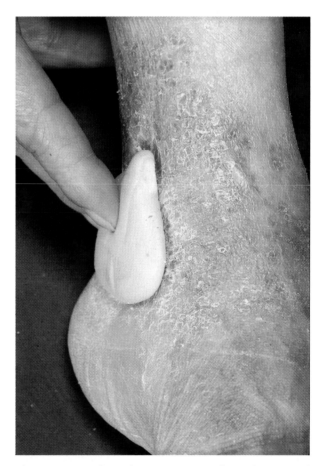

Figure 20.3 This ulcer was situated in the natural hollow just behind and below the medial malleolus. In order to compress this area of skin after the ulcer had healed the hollow was filled with a Silastic pad applied beneath the stocking.

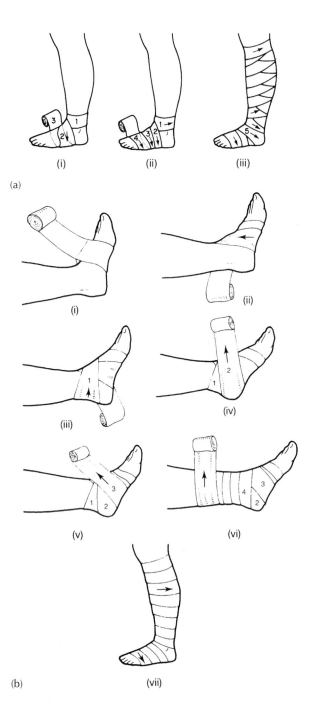

(a)

(b)

Figure 20.4 (a) Dale's technique for applying a bandage to the leg. (i) The first turn is placed around the ankle to fix the bandage. (ii) The bandage is then taken down over the ankle to compress the foot. (iii) The bandage is then taken up over the initial turn to cover the lower leg to knee level using an overlapping figure-of-eight technique. (b) The standard bandaging technique. (i) The first turn is placed around the dorsum of the foot. (ii) The bandage is then brought up over the ankle. (iii–v) The ankle is then enclosed as shown. (vi) The remainder of the leg is bandaged by simple overlapping turns. (vii) The final appearance.

that, if a bandage caused pain, it should be taken off and reapplied.

Dale has shown that bandaging is an acquired skill.[66] She recommends that the first turn should be around the ankle before working down to the foot. This starts the bandage well and prevents slipping at the ankle (Figure 20.4).

The three basic rules of bandaging are:

1. Apply the outside of the roll to the leg
2. Bandage from the medial to the lateral side
3. Bandage from below upwards.

The bandage should roll away from the hand and must be evenly spaced with, if possible, a slightly greater tension (compression) applied at the ankle. A figure-of-eight overlapping technique (Figure 20.4) prevents the bandage slipping down. A layer of stockinette (Tubigrip) applied over the bandage prevents the edges of the bandage rucking up. Alternatively, an adhesive bandage may be applied over the top. Simple crepe bandages or stockinette used on their own do not apply satisfactory compression.[203]

The elastic bandages currently available that can be recommended are the Bisgaard bandage, a combination of Elastocrepe and Tubigrip, Tensopress, Setopress, Medivip, Elset and Thusane.

Elastic stockings

We have not found it practical to use elastic stockings when there is an open ulcer because it is difficult to pull a stocking up over a dressing without disturbing the dressing. Also, the exudate soils the stocking which consequently has to be washed frequently and elasticity is lost. Some stains are not easily removed and the elastic fibres of the stocking may be weakened by the exudate. We only replace bandages with a stocking when the ulcer reaches an advanced stage of healing or becomes covered by a firmly fixed dry scab. The advantages of stockings are that the degree of compression they apply is known and constant and that they do not slip down or become loose as easily as bandages. Others have used elastic stockings and dressings with success.[164] The types of elastic hosiery available and the methods of testing stockings are discussed in detail in the section on the prevention of ulcer recurrence (see page 591).

Intermittent pneumatic compression

Intermittent positive pressure applied by inflatable leggings has been advocated for ulcer healing. These boots were originally designed to prevent the development of postoperative deep vein thrombosis[109] but it has been suggested that they might enhance ulcer healing.[14,53,169,222] Their use usually entails the admission of the patient to hospital because the equipment is expensive, and this, together with the risk of cross-infection, has prevented their routine use for the treatment of ulcers. There is one small trial[53] of this technique in ulcer healing but the control and test groups did not receive identical treatment.

Ulcer dressings

Dressings applied directly to ulcers should ideally exhibit certain properties. They should be non-adherent so that removal is painless and does not damage new fragile epithelium which is beginning to grow in across the surface of the ulcer. The dressing should be highly absorbent while maintaining the moisture of the wound and not degrading or altering its characteristics in response to changes in temperature or humidity, or when soaked with exudate. The dressing should be safe, non-toxic and non-antigenic. Dressings must be readily available, sterile, conformable and cost effective.[105,119] Morgan[144] has pointed out that a dressing fulfilling all these characteristics does not exist.

There are four main types of dressing that can be applied to an ulcer:

1. Absorbent dressings
2. Impregnated dressings
3. Occlusive dressings
4. Impregnated bandages.

Absorbent dressings

The materials that have been used to absorb ulcer exudate include linen, cotton wool, gauze (open-weave cotton), Non-adherent Dressings (N-A) (Johnson & Johnson), Tricolex (Smith & Nephew), Melolin (Smith & Nephew), and gamgee pads.

Gauze is the only dressing that is universally acceptable as it is non-allergic and does not produce a sensitivity reaction. Unfortunately, it commonly adheres to the surface of the ulcer and is painful to remove.

Melolin (Smith & Nephew) is a non-adherent dressing but has poor absorbing properties and can cause maceration, allergy, rashes and skin maceration.

N-A (non-adherent) Dressings (Johnson & Johnson) are viscose and also relatively poor at absorbing exudate and can cause skin maceration when used alone.

Perfron and Release II (Johnson & Johnson) are two new low adherent dressings which are alternatives to Melolin and gauze.

Telfa (Kendall) is a similar to Perfron and Release II.

Tricotex (Smith & Nephew) is similar to N-A dressings and also made of viscose.

Actisorb (Johnson & Johnson) is charcoal cloth enclosed in a porous envelope.

Allevyn is a foam absorbent dressing produced by Smith & Nephew.

Sofwick (Johnson & Johnson), *Multisorb* (Smith & Nephew), *Pharmocclusive* (Pharma) and *Lestra* (Molynec) are some of the newer absorbent dressings.

Impregnated dressings

The majority of impregnated dressings consist of a blanched cotton or rayon cloth impregnated with petroleum jelly (Vaseline) often with the addition of an antibacterial agent:

- Paraffin gauze, plain (Jelonet, Tulle Gras – Smith & Nephew; Paranet – Seton)
- Paraffin gauze + chlorhexidine (Bactigras – Smith & Nephew; Clorhexitulle – Roussel)
- Paraffin gauze + framycetin (Sofra-Tulle – Roussel)
- Paraffin gauze + fusidic acid (Fucidin, Intertulle – Leo)

There is little evidence to justify the addition of an antibacterial agent to the paraffin gauze. All the antibiotic and antiseptic tulles can cause local sensitivity reactions and encourage colonization by resistant bacteria. In our opinion they should never be used.

A single layer of paraffin gauze covered by ordinary gauze has good non-adherent and absorbent qualities and is painless on removal. It can be used at any stage in the management of an ulcer but is most suitable when the ulcer is clean and healing. The paraffin gauze must be applied to the ulcer, not to the surrounding skin, to avoid skin maceration. There is no evidence that the petroleum jelly delays or enhances healing. This is still one of the most popular forms of dressing but is being increasingly replaced by viscose dressings.

A number of dressings are impregnated with charcoal to help reduce the smell of the ulcer; these include Actisorb (Johnson & Johnson), Carbonet (Smith & Nephew) and Kaltrocarb (BritCair Labs).

Absorbent and occlusive dressings

There are many occlusive wound dressings which have been devised as ulcer dressings. They are all absorbent but in some the fluid in the dressing is prevented from evaporating so the dressing stays moist and does not adhere. Examples of occlusive wound dressings are given below.

Hydrogels/alginates

- Vigilon – an insoluble cross-linked polyethylene oxide copolymer (Seton)
- Geliperm – a polyacrylamide composite hydrogel, which comes in wet, dry and granulated gel forms (Geistlich)
- Sorbsan – a biodegradable, hydrophilic gel of an alginate (NI Medical)
- Kaltostat – a calcium alginate fibre (BritCair)
- Comfeel – alginate (Coloplast)
- Synthaderm – a polyurethane foam, hydrophilic on one side and hydrophobic on the other side (Armour)

Plastic sheets

- Opsite (Smith & Nephew)
- Tegaderm (3M)
- Oproflex (Lohmann)
- Dermafilm (Vygon)
- Dermocclude (BritCair)
- Ensure (Becton-Dickinson)

Polyurethane dressings

- Coraderm – a modified polyurethane which is an improvement on Synthaderm (Seton HC)
- Allevyn (Smith & Nephew)
- Omiderm (Paul Hartmann)
- Spryosorb (BritCair)

Hydrocolloids

- Granuflex – a polymeric dressing with an adhesive face and a water-proof backing which makes it impermeable (Squibb, Surgicare)
- Dermiflex – a methylcellulose base with a foam backing (Johnson & Johnson)
- Biofilm (CliniMed)
- Dermasorb (Johnson & Johnson)
- Intrasite (Smith & Nephew)
- Tegasorb (3M)

Polyurethane sheets

Opsite (Smith & Nephew), Bioclusive (Johnson & Johnson), Steridrape (3M), Transigen (Smith & Nephew), and Tegaderm (3M), are all semipermeable and non-absorbent.

Foam dressings

- Silastic foam – a silicon base with a catalyst (Calmic) – has now been withdrawn.
- Lyofoam – a polyurethane foam which can be made with added carbon (Seton HC)
- Allevyn (Smith & Nephew)
- Cavi-Care (Smith & Nephew)
- Dalzofoam (Seton HC)
- Nuprene and Silicofoam (Hindersleslies)

The majority of these dressings have been developed over the past 10 years. They have still not been tested in large-scale controlled clinical trials of ulcer healing, and their acceptance must therefore await further studies.[142] The use of these dressings is supported by the results of animal wound healing studies but such studies may not be relevant to human venous ulceration.

Impregnated bandages

These are gauze bandages impregnated with zinc, calamine, ichthyol, oxyquinoline or tar. Although they are sold on the basis of their incorporated medicament, they probably work because they set into a semi-hard cast which acts as a very effective form of inelastic external compression. The paste simply allows the bandage to mould to the shape of the limb. Whether the medicament has any intrinsic effect on ulcer healing is debatable.

Impregnated bandages are marketed as:

- Calaband (calamine) (Seton)
- Viscopaste PB7 (zinc oxide) (Smith & Nephew)
- Quinaband (oxyquinoline) (Dalmas)
- Zipzoc (Perstop-Pharma)
- Zincaband (zinc oxide) (Seton)
- Icthaband (ichthyol) (Seton)
- Steripaste (zinc) (Seton)
- Coltapaste (Smith & Nephew).

Paste bandages are amongst the most popular form of ulcer dressing in the United Kingdom and have replaced the Unna paste boot.[209] We have carried out as yet unpublished clinical trials of the use of paste bandages and in our experience a combination of Calaband or Steripaste covered with Elastrocrepe and Tubigrip heals between 70 and 80% of venous ulcers within 1 year of beginning treatment (Figure 20.5). Many other workers have reported similar results, for example only 19 out of 173 patients required hospital admission for failed treatment in Monroe-Ashman and Wells' series.[148] Nevertheless, it is desirable to undertake controlled studies to compare paste bandages with some of the newer forms of dressing described above.

Paste bandages can cause damage to the leg if they are incorrectly applied, and they can also cause sensitivity reactions (Figure 20.6). The bandage must be removed – immediately if a sensitivity reaction occurs – and replaced by a simple dressing with compression bandages.

McCollum and his colleagues[25] introduced a multilayered bandaging regimen in which a non-adhesive dressing was covered by a cotton wool layer, a crepe bandage (Elset) and finally Coban to hold it in place. They claimed 80% ulcer healing within 12 weeks, but excluded all ulcers above 10 cm^2 and had

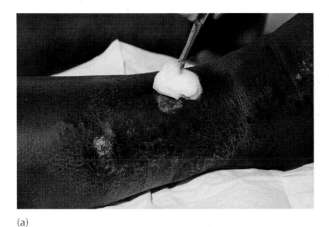

(a)

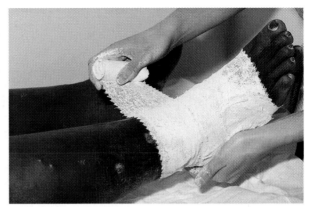

(b)

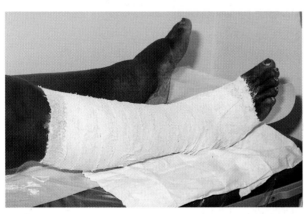

(c)

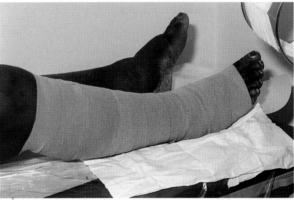

(d)

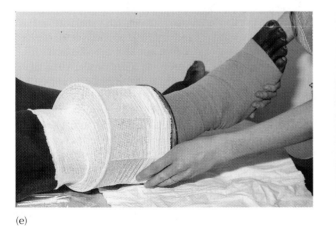

(e)

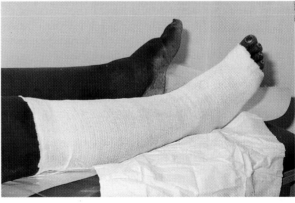

(f)

Figure 20.5 (a) Before applying a paste bandage (Calaband, Seton), the exudate must be wiped off the ulcer. If the base contains soft slough it should be removed. (b) and (c) The paste bandage is then applied directly onto the ulcer and covered by Elastocrepe, (d) and then a Tubigrip bandage, (e and f). Thusane or Tensopress bandages are alternatives.

no control group. Ruckley *et al.*[178] have found their results to be improved by a four-layer dressing when compared with a hydrocolloid dressing without external support. We have carried out a controlled trial of Elastocrepe and Tubigrip applied over Viscopaste compared with Viscopaste covered by Tensopress and Tubigrip. We were unable to show that the higher compression bandage (Tensopress)

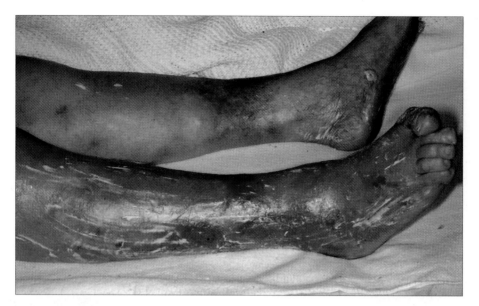

Figure 20.6   The skin of this leg has developed an allergy to a paste bandage. The skin is erythematous and eczematous. The paste bandage must not be used again. Propaderm should be applied and the paste bandage replaced with gauze dressings and a simple bandage.

increased healing. These results differ from those of Ruckley *et al.*[178] who showed a minor advantage in ulcer healing in a group treated by Tensopress and dressings compared with Elastocrepe paste and Tubigrip (non-elastic) (54% vs 28% at 12 weeks). These two trials are not quite comparable as the elastic bandages were applied over the paste bandages in our study. Partsch[163,164] has, however, shown that his so-called, 'short stretch' bandages performed better than an elasticated regimen.

There are three randomized trials of dressings – one[178] showing that Allevyn is no better than N-A, another[177] which showed no difference between Duoderm and Viscopaste and one[182] which, whilst finding no difference in healing rates between a four-layer regimen and a short stretch bandaging, suggested that the paste regimen gave poor healing.

BED REST WITH LEG ELEVATION

Hippocrates[110] stated that 'in the case of an ulcer it is not expedient to stand, more especially if the ulcer be situated in the leg', and Ambrose Paré[162] also felt that those who have 'an ulcer in the leg ought neither to stand or sit but lie on a bed'. Both Petit in 1790[168] and Hunter in 1835[115] suggested that bed rest at home or in a hospital was beneficial to healing. Sharp[186] and Brodie[30] suggested that the leg should be kept horizontal with the body. Anning[4] recognized that elevation of the leg above the level

of the heart was even more effective but Foote,[88] while agreeing with this approach, pointed out its high cost, if it meant admitting all patients with ulcers into hospital beds. Today this is especially true everywhere in the world.

Dodd and Cockett[74] regarded bed rest as an essential preliminary to successful grafting of a venous ulcer, and Fegan[85] and Bourne[27] both advocated periods of leg elevation as part of their outpatient treatment regimen. We are not aware of a comparison of bed rest alone against bed rest combined with local ulcer dressings but we accept that a period of bed rest with leg elevation is a highly successful way of healing ulcers. The main reason this treatment is now rarely used is the lack of hospital beds and its cost. Cottonot *et al.*[61] showed that the cost of healing an ulcer by hospital admission was 20 times greater than the cost of outpatient treatment. In 1849 Crichett[63] had pointed out that there were many practical objections to prolonged in-patient treatment, not only social and economic disadvantages but the risk of joint stiffness and the risk of a further deep vein thrombosis.

The policy of most clinicians supervising ulcer care is to continue outpatient treatment for as long as possible, but there is a small group of patients whose ulcers will never heal while they are walking about and who have to be admitted to hospital.[99] When this group with intractable ulceration is added to the group in whom surgical treatment (e.g. skin grafting) is indicated to speed up the healing process, we find that a significant number of patients still need to be admitted to hospital for the treatment of venous ulceration. A period of bedrest with maximal leg elevation is an integral part of our initial management of these patients.

SURGICAL EXCISION OF SLOUGH

Hippocrates[110] suggested that ulcers healed better after they were 'scarified'. Since then many other workers have suggested that the excision of all dead tissue speeds ulcer healing.[76,88,182] Excision can be done with a scalpel or a sharp pair of scissors, but this may be very painful. If excision is done with care when the slough is ready to separate, it can be done without anaesthesia, but if the slough is firmly adherent, a local or general anaesthetic is required. Local anaesthetics applied topically to the ulcer base or infiltrated by a fine needle through the base of the ulcer can be helpful but may fail to produce analgesia because of fibrosis in the ulcer base. For ulcer excision under general anaesthesia the patient should normally be admitted to hospital. This procedure should be reserved for ulcers that either fail to heal or enlarge during outpatient management.

TOPICAL APPLICATIONS

Many agents have been applied topically in an attempt to improve the healing of ulcers. These substances tend to fall into three major categories – antiseptics, antibiotics and desloughing (cleansing) agents. A fourth minor category consists of miscellaneous agents thought to stimulate ulcer healing.

Antiseptics

These include:

- hypochlorite solutions (Eusol, Milton and Chlorasol) (Schering)
- cetrimide (Savlon, Savloclens, Savlodil)
- chlorhexidine (Hibitane)
- hydrogen peroxide 3% (Hioxyl – Stuart Pharmaceuticals)
- benzoyl peroxide (Benoxyl – Stiefel; Quinoderm)
- povidone iodine (Betadine, Napp Laboratories; Disadine, Stuart Pharmaceuticals)
- cadexomer iodine (Iodosorb) (Stuart Pharmaceuticals)
- aqueous gel containing brilliant green and lactic acid (Variclene)
- mercurochrome 1–2%
- potassium permanganate (1:10 000 gentian violet)
- gentian violet in alcohol

- proflavine
- acetic acid
- ethyl alcohol
- phenoxyethanol
- silver nitrate
- Sterigel (Seton HC), a carbohydrate hydrogel

Hypochlorite, hydrogen peroxide, and even chlorhexidine have been shown in a series of animal studies[29] to damage granulation tissue and slow wound healing. They should therefore not be applied when an ulcer is healing but can be used in the early stages before healing begins. They are all, especially hypochlorite, effective agents for cleaning and removing slough. Antiseptics have never been shown to promote ulcer healing and they can cause allergic skin reactions[158] and perhaps delay ulcer healing.[76]

The reports on the efficacy of povidone iodine are purely anecdotal.[33] Iodosorb appeared to reduce healing time in two controlled trials in patients with venous ulcers,[157,192] but this conclusion has been challenged by other investigators[59,149] because the standard treatment used in the original trials may have delayed healing in the control group in which ulcers appeared to take an excessively long time to heal.

Topical antibiotics

A number of antibiotics have been applied to the surface of ulcers but there is little justification for their use because there are few controlled trials that show them to be beneficial. Bacterial resistance and skin sensitivity reactions are real risks, and topical antibiotics should be abandoned as a treatment for venous ulceration.

Some topical antibiotics that have received anecdotal support include:

- silver sulphadiazine (Flamazine) (Smith & Nephew)
- neomycin–bacitracin (Cicatrin) (Wellcome)
- mupirocin 2% (Bactroban) (Beecham)
- neomycin and gramicidin (Graneodin) (Squibb)

We are not aware of any new trials which show that topical antibiotics speed ulcer healing and they always carry the risk of inducing sensitivity.

Cleansing agents used to dissolve slough

These substances are mainly chemicals or naturally derived enzymes that are proteolytic or fibrinolytic.

- Aserbine – a mixture of malic, benzoic and salicylic acids (Bencard)
- Malatex – similar to Aserbine (Norton)
- Varidase – a mixture of streptokinase and streptodornase (Lederle)

- Sutilains (Travase) – a fibrinolytic agent with a liquifying agent (Flint)
- Dextranomer (Debrisan) – hydrophilic dextran (Pharmacia)

The active ingredient of Aserbine and Malatex is a malic acid ester. Varidase is a streptokinase–streptodornase mixture,[39] and Travase is a fibrinolytic agent mixed with a substance that liquefies pus.[56] Debrisan, a three-dimensional network of dextran polymers, showed some encouraging early results in cleansing ulcers[143,146] but failed to heal them more swiftly than standard treatments.[96,97] The cost of Debrisan makes its general acceptance into clinical practice unlikely unless it can be shown to significantly reduce the healing time.

All these preparations can be used to deslough dirty ulcers if patients will not tolerate surgical cleansing because of pain. They must be applied two or three times each day and can be extremely effective; sloughs will liquefy in 2 or 3 days. There is no firm evidence that they promote ulcer healing. A sharp scalpel or Eusol (hypochlorite) may be a more effective means of desloughing ulcers.

Agents thought to encourage ulcer healing

Many agents have been thought to promote ulcer healing by a local or general action but all the published studies contain serious flaws. Agents that have been claimed to promote healing include:

- hyaluronic acid
- *N*-acetyl hydroxyprolene
- collagen gel
- lysozyme
- napthaquinine
- anthrocyanosides
- paw-paw
- zinc
- steel foil
- aluminium foil
- amino acid solution.

Little can be said about most of these preparations when the evidence justifying their use is mostly anecdotal and unconfirmed.[67,84,91,117,136,140,160,161]

DERMATOLOGICAL PREPARATIONS FOR THE SURROUNDING SKIN

The skin around the ulcer may be treated for eczema and contact sensitivity with Lassar's paste, potassium permanganate, gentian violet or local steroids (Dermovate, Propaderm, Betnovate, hydrocortisone or clobetasol).[182] We use Propaderm or Dermovate ointment to treat excoriated eczema-

tous skin around an ulcer. These agents are highly effective in resolving eczema but great care must be taken to avoid applying the cream to the ulcer surface, because steroids may delay ulcer healing.[82] Excessive and continuous use of corticosteroids on eczematous skin may cause it to thin and atrophy and should be avoided.[213] Growth factors are known to promote keratinocytic division, migration and adhesion and may therefore have an in-patient role in ulcer healing. They may also promote granulation tissue and fibrosis. Platelet derived growth factor, fibroblast growth factor and transforming growth factor β have all been thought to have a putative role in promoting healing and are at present being evaluated.

SYSTEMIC MEDICATIONS

Medicaments thought to promote healing

The process of healing is extremely complex and needs an adequate supply of protein, vitamins, trace metals and oxygen. Medicaments that have been tried include:

- zinc
- stanozolol
- urokinase
- oxpentifylline
- aspirin
- prostaglandins
- oxyrutosides
- diuretics
- vasodilators
- growth hormone.

Zinc
Serum zinc was found to be low in some patients with chronic venous ulceration,[93,94,103,149] and systematically administered zinc was reported to improve ulcer healing in patients with low serum zinc levels.[170] Serum zinc does not, however, correlate well with cellular zinc deficiency, and therefore the relevance of serum zinc estimation is extremely doubtful.[25] Zinc can be given as effervescent tablets and does no harm but probably does little good.

Stanozolol (Stromba)
This fibrinolytic enhancing agent has been used in the treatment of pre-ulcerative lipodermatosclerosis. It has been shown to significantly enhance the resolution of the lipodermatosclerosis[34,139,154] but has not influenced the rate at which ulcers heal.[127]

Urokinase
This has been administered by infusion and produced excellent healing in one small series.[81]

Oxpentifylline (Trental)

Oxpentifylline is known to enhance fibrinolysis and increase capillary perfusion by reducing blood viscosity and increasing red cell deformability. An initial open study of venous ulcer healing revealed apparently good results,[216] though the percentage of ulcers healed was similar to the number healed in other studies using paste bandages. There have now been three controlled blind trials. In the first, 44% of the ulcers in the control group improved compared with 86% of the ulcers of the patients receiving oxpentifylline. The end points of this first trial are weak and the healing rate in the control group is extremely poor. A second study also showed a highly significant advantage for the active drug but again the healing rates were poor and all the benefit came from one of the three centres admitting patients.[54] A third much longer study from Edinburgh has shown a trend in favour of the active drug but failed to reach statistical significance. These studies taken together indicated that Trental may have a beneficial role in healing ulcers but good compression appears to mask any benefit that it may confer.

Prostaglandins

The prostaglandins are powerful vasodilators. Prostaglandin infusions are claimed to improve the healing of severe rheumatoid ulcers[198] and prostaglandin E_1 is said to be of value in both venous and arterial ulcers;[13] four out of five patients with venous ulcers responded to a prostaglandin infusion compared with one out of five who responded to a saline infusion. There is only one double blind controlled trial that we are aware of[179] which confirmed a statistically significant improvement in ulcer healing (8/20 healed with prostaglandin compared with 2/20 in the control group). Unfortunately, the drug still has to be given by intravenous infusion, although an oral preparation may soon become available.

Oxyrutosides (Paroven)

Paroven reduces capillary permeability and white blood cell migration and has been shown, in controlled trials, to reduce the symptoms of chronic venous insufficiency[174] and improve tissue oxygenation.[40,155] It has not been shown to improve ulcer healing.

Diuretics

Diuretics may be of occasional value in patients with an ulcer in a very swollen leg, usually caused by congestive cardiac failure. They do not directly promote ulcer healing but reduction of the oedema probably improves the capillary circulation and the efficacy of the calf muscle pump.[150]

Vasodilators

There is no evidence that vasodilators help the healing of venous ulcers.

Sucralfrate

There is one short report on the benefit of this compound in ulcer healing.[207]

Aspirin

One recent paper has suggested that this may be of benefit in ulcer healing.[118]

Systemic antibiotics

Virtually every antibiotic that has ever been produced has been used to treat venous ulcers but there is very little evidence that antibiotics improve ulcer healing and we do not give them unless the ulcer is contaminated by a single pathogenic organism (see page 565, Chapter 19) or there is associated cellulitis, which in our experience is extremely rare. The organisms most commonly found colonizing venous ulcers include staphylococci, streptococci, *Pseudomonas*, *Klebsiella*, *Escherichia coli* and *Proteus* (see Tables 19.4 and 19.5).

The role of anaerobic organisms in delaying ulcer healing has been neglected. Our own data suggest that these organisms are much more common than the results of standard bacteriological tests suggest, and good controlled trials of antibiotics known to be effective against anaerobic bacteria should be encouraged. Our clinical impression is that metronidazole reduces both the odour and the purulent exudate of dirty ulcers.

PHYSICAL METHODS OF TREATMENT

Physical methods of treatment include:

- massage
- short-wave diathermy
- ultraviolet light
- vibratory electromagnetic waves
- laser
- pneumatic compression.

Massage

This was first recommended by White[218] but was later championed by Bisgaard[19] as an adjunct to compression bandaging. There are no controlled trials of its use. Gentle massage around an ulcer disperses oedema and may increase blood flow but some authors have reported poor results from massage.[8,64]

Ultraviolet light

Ultraviolet light may cause vasodilation and increase tissue oxygenation as well as killing bacteria.[8,75] There are no good trials which show its benefit.

Ultrasound

This increases the local blood flow and may break down interstitial fibrin and fibrous tissue. There are controlled trials which suggest that ultrasound accelerates ulcer healing[42,79] but the rate of healing of the 'control arm' ulcers was poor in these trials. A more recent study[176] failed to show any advantage.

Electromagnetic waves

There is still only one publication[46] on the value of this treatment in leg ulcers. It is difficult to draw any conclusions from one enthusiastic report.

Laser

There are some uncontrolled studies which show that LASER light may stimulate granulation tissue and healing.

Pneumatic compression

There is one study that suggests that this is better than other forms of compression but the control patients did not have to spend an equal time on bedrest.[53]

SKIN SUBSTITUTES

Human amnion

Human amnion was first used to dress venous ulcers by Hansen[104] who claimed that it promoted healing if left in undisturbed contact with the ulcer for 6–10 weeks. It has not been widely used, perhaps because of difficulties in procurement as it has to be applied relatively fresh.[206] Amnion has the advantage of being a biological tissue whose lack of surface tissue antigens protect it from rejection,[5] and it is thought to contain substances that stimulate angiogenesis.[80]

Three studies[16,80,195] have reported that amnion successfully healed leg ulceration but all these studies were uncontrolled and therefore of doubtful validity.

No recent controlled studies on the use of amnion have been published that we are aware of.

A recent study suggests that human placental extract may be valuable in healing ulcers because it contains a lot of growth factors.[12]

Porcine dermis (lyophilized freeze-dried porcine epidermis) (Corethium – Ethicon)

The initial open studies[121,180] with porcine skin suggested that it doubled the healing rate of venous ulcers when compared with conventional treatment.

A subsequent double blind trial showed a 33% reduction in the healing time of the porcine-treated ulcers which only just reached statistical significance.[181] The sample size in this study was small, and a type II error is possible. The cost of this material can hardly justify its use if the time saved in healing is so small.[172] A Medline search failed to discover any recent studies on porcine dermis and its use appears to have declined, probably on the basis of cost against value.

SKIN GRAFTS (AUTOGRAFTS)

Skin grafting is the treatment of choice for ulcers that will not heal with conservative treatment, but few, if any, clinicians feel that skin grafting is the best method of treating all venous ulcers, and some feel that it has no place in treatment.

When a decision is taken to graft an ulcer, the choice has to be made between pinch grafts and split skin grafts. Each method has its advocates.[3,10,41,48,74,131,132,143,152,171,172]

Pinch grafts are usually taken and applied under local anaesthetic in an outpatient clinic.[48,172] Although split skin grafting can be managed in this way, it is more usual to give the patient a general anaesthetic.[132,152] General anaesthesia has the advantage of allowing the ulcer to be simultaneously excised or curetted, thus the skin graft can be applied to healthy tissue and there is a better chance of achieving satisfactory 'graft take'.

Excision of the ulcer base and application of split skin mesh grafts (Thiersch grafts)[3,74,131,132,152,172] (Figures 20.7, 20.8)

Small split skin grafts can be taken after local anaesthetic infiltration in the outpatient clinic. For large grafts the patient is usually given a general anaesthetic before being prepared with chlorhexidine and draped to expose the ulcer. The front of the thigh of the same leg, which is the normal donor site, is also prepared. The base of the ulcer is excised down to healthy tissue.

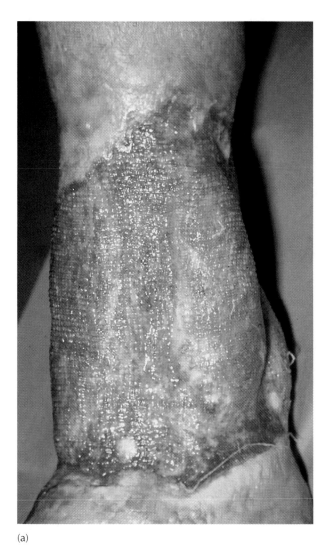

(a)

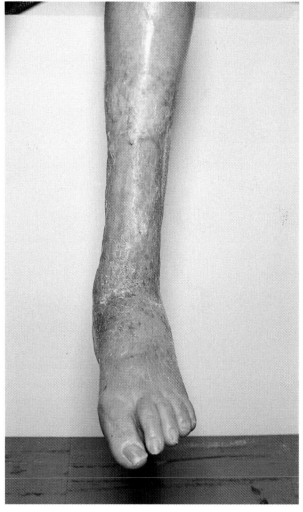

(b)

Figure 20.7 (a) A large circumferential venous ulcer that is obviously too large to treat conservatively. (b) The base of the ulcer was excised and covered with split skin grafts. This resulted in complete healing.

Skin grafts only 'take' when they have an adequate supply of blood and oxygen. The changes that precede ulceration affect the subcutaneous tissues as well as the skin (see Chapters 11 and 13). After many years of calf pump malfunction, the skin and subcutaneous tissues can be completely replaced by fibrous tissue with a minimal, almost non-existent, blood supply. Ulcers in this type of tissue have a grey-white base peppered with a few pale pink capillary loops (see Chapter 19, Figure 19.6). They never produce sufficient granulations to nurture and hold a skin graft. This is the type of ulcer that fails to heal with medical treatment and rejects split skin grafts applied to its surface.

Once the lack of blood supply is recognized, it is wise to accept that all the diseased tissue beneath and around the ulcer must be excised in order to find tissue with an adequate blood supply. Sometimes the excision has to include the deep fascia.[171] Care must be taken to preserve periostium and paratenon during excision. Excision is best performed using a Humby or Braithwaite dermatome which allows a series of slices to be removed from the ulcer base. Bleeding is controlled by firm pressure, diathermy and under-running with absorbable sutures.

Total excision of an ulcer and its base has a major advantage; any incompetent communicating veins

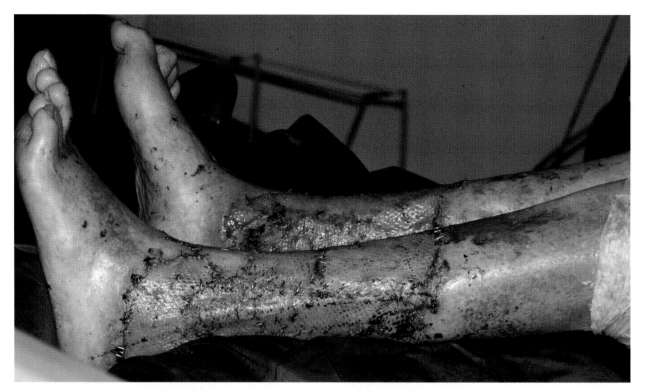

Figure 20.8 Extensive split skin grafts to bilateral venous ulcers (fixed with staples). This illustrates the fact that a 90%+ take can be expected provided the ulcer is clean and has a good base of healthy granulation tissue.

beneath the ulcer are automatically ligated and divided. The excision can also be combined with ligation of other incompetent communicating veins (see Chapter 7); this treats the immediate cause of the ulceration and improves the chance of long-term success (see Figure 20.10).

We do not know of any trials comparing direct application of split skin to the ulcer base against excision and grafting but we now never apply split skin grafts to an ulcer base without carrying out a radical excision first. We are sure that this policy has dramatically increased our success.

The skin graft is then taken with an electric dermatome or some type of Humby knife. For all except the smallest ulcers we prefer to use the dermatome because it cuts a more even graft than can be achieved by hand. We always take more skin than is required to cover the ulcer. Grafts should be approximately 0.1 mm thick as thin grafts take better than thick ones. When the graft has been cut it is spread out on a plastic sheet and measured. It is then cut to the shape of the ulcer and applied to the ulcer providing the base is clean, healthy and not bleeding excessively. It is stapled into place and held firmly applied to its base by a pressure dress-

ing of paraffin gauze, gauze, cotton wool and a crepe bandage.

If the ulcer base is bleeding excessively or is not as clean as anticipated, we wrap the graft in a moistened saline swab, place it in a sterile airtight container and keep it in a refrigerator at 4°C until the ulcer base is considered to be satisfactory. The ulcer is inspected daily, and when it is clean enough the graft is applied in the ward without anaesthesia.

Grafts may be held in place by tissue glue,[111] or a firm dressing or left completely uncovered. We have not performed a proper comparison of these methods of application but prefer to apply grafts at operation and keep them covered with dressings and bandages. The donor site is covered by an Opsite (Smith & Nephew), or Steridrape (3M), plastic dressing held in place by a crepe bandage.

Grafts are not inspected for 5–7 days unless the patient is in pain or develops a pyrexia. When the dressings are taken off, the grafted area is cleaned, any pieces of skin that have failed to adhere are removed and new pieces of split skin from the excess stored in the refrigerator are applied, unless further cleansing of the ulcer base is necessary. Skin remains viable in the refrigerator for up to 2 weeks, and we have occasionally found that skin that has been kept for 3 weeks has been accepted. Patience and perseverance are demanded to obtain complete skin cover. Refractory ulcers may require three or four applications, over a period of 3–4 weeks.

Until complete healing has been achieved, the patient must remain on strict bedrest with the foot of the bed elevated. The ulcer must be *completely* healed before the patient is allowed to stand up or walk.

Results

There are few reports which detail the success of split skin grafting in healing venous ulcers. Holm and Holmsted[111] reported 75% success (32 of 40) with tissue glue. Wood and Davies have recently reported poor results (20%). We have had much better results (effectively 100%) with persistence and repeated applications of skin. We have only failed when an element of arterial ischaemia has been present. Ulcers that are heavily colonized with *Staphylococcus aureus* or *Pseudomonas pyocyanea* are probably best treated by initial excision and subsequent grafting.[92]

Pinch grafts[10,41,48,143,172]

The skin of the thigh is prepared with chlorhexidine 0.5% in 70% spirit and draped. The ulcer is then cleaned and prepared in the same manner. The ulcer base may have to be anaesthetized with topical anaesthetic jelly before being gently freshened with a curette to remove all the slough and necrotic tissue. For a full excision of the ulcer base a general anaesthetic is invariably required and for this reason we rarely use pinch grafts.

A strip of skin along the anterior surface of the thigh is infiltrated with an intradermal local anaesthetic. A medium-sized hypodermic needle is then inserted into the anaesthetized skin to 'pick it up' before a circular slither of skin beneath the needle is cut off with a scalpel. The centre of each circle of skin is between 0.5 mm and 1.0 mm thick and the diameter of each piece is approximately 1 cm. It is important not to cut through the full thickness of the dermis at the centre of the 'circle', but at this point the graft should be almost full thickness. Multiple pinch grafts are applied to cover the whole of the ulcer, leaving less than 1 mm between each circle of skin if possible.

When the grafts are in place they are covered with paraffin gauze, cotton dressing gauze, cotton wool and a firmly applied Elastocrepe bandage. The donor site is also dressed. Patients are allowed to be mobile at home but are encouraged to rest with the leg up as much as possible before return-

ing in 7–10 days for the grafted ulcer to be inspected. At this time any grafts which have not taken may be replaced with additional pinch grafts.

Once the ulcer is covered with grafts that have 'taken', it should be covered with non-adherent cellulose dressings and bandages which should be renewed at weekly intervals until complete healing has occurred.

Results

Using this technique, Monk and Sarkany[143] and Poskitt *et al.*[172] were able to obtain early healing of between 60% and 90% of their venous ulcers. However, Monk and Sarkany[143] found that nearly 80% of ulcers treated in this way recurred within 1 year, compared with a 60% recurrence rate in those healed by conservative methods; both groups of patients were given elastic stockings after successful healing. The high recurrence rate is probably related to the fact that only a small proportion of their patients underwent surgical correction of their underlying venous abnormality.

Comment

We reserve skin grafting for ulcers that are resistant to orthodox outpatient compression bandaging techniques. We admit such patients to hospital, keep them on strict bedrest (except for toilet requirements once or twice a day) and apply antiseptic dressings of dry gauze soaked in hydrogen peroxide, Hibitane or normal saline four times a day until the ulcer is clean. These regular dressing changes are combined with mechanical cleaning by scraping and cutting off slough and necrotic debris. A course of antibiotics is given if there is a heavy growth of a single organism.

We excise the whole ulcer, including the unhealthy surrounding skin and all the subcutaneous tissue, once the base of the ulcer is looking cleaner and apply split skin grafts as described above.

We have successfully healed all the venous ulcers of patients who we have admitted to our wards over the last 10 years by diligently following this regimen, but because we have sometimes been unable to correct the underlying venous abnormality, a proportion of these, 'healed ulcers' have rapidly recurred.

Full-thickness skin grafts

We have not used full-thickness skin grafts on venous ulcers. It is of interest to note that Bergan[17] recommended removal of irreparably damaged skin and its replacement with firm and elastic skin; the illustration in this publication appears to show a full-thickness graft.

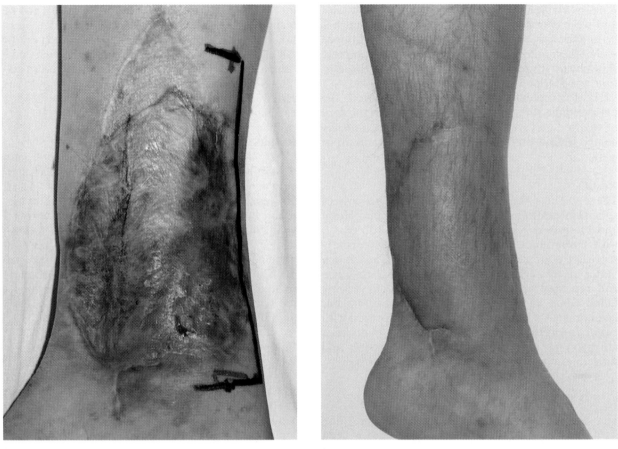

(a)   (b)

Figure 20.9 This post-thrombotic venous ulcer failed to respond to outpatient treatment. Surgery to the communicating veins and deep veins had failed, and the ulcer kept recurring even though the patient wore elastic support stockings constantly. (a) The ulcers were healed by split skin grafting after a period of bedrest and cleaning. The abnormal lipodermatosclerotic skin was then marked out and excised. (b) A cross-leg flap from the opposite calf was used to cover the skin defect. After separation of the flap the defect on the healthy limb was covered with split skin grafts. This ulcer remains healed 20 years later.

This technique has not, to our knowledge, been recommended by any other investigator.

Flaps

When a patient has had repeated ulcers which have irreparably damaged the skin and subcutaneous tissues which are scarred, and avascular, we collaborate with our plastic surgical colleagues to excise the abnormal tissues and replace them with full-thickness normal skin from another site.

Figure 20.9 shows a patient who underwent a *cross-leg flap* for persistent venous ulceration lasting for more than 15 years that had not been helped by communicating vein ligation, deep venous reconstruction or continuous use of graduated elastic stockings. After the cross-leg flap was performed, the ulcer remained healed and the transferred skin remained in good condition after 20 years.

Vascularized free flap grafts

Most patients who have chronic venous ulceration that fails to respond to the medical and surgical treatments outlined above have post-thrombotic deep vein damage. This makes the use of vascularized free flap grafts[122] questionable because it is difficult to find a healthy deep vein for the venous anastomosis and there is an increased risk of thrombosis of the pedicle vein.

Nevertheless, we have successfully treated a few patients with severe intractable post-thrombotic ulceration in this way. Patients are given anticoagulants postoperatively and one patient developed a large haematoma beneath the flap which required repeated aspiration but the flap survived. This type of operation is a major undertaking and should only be used as a last resort.

A report of six patients with excision of ulceration and replacement by fasciocutaneous free flaps suggested that good long-term results could be achieved by this therapy.[78]

CORRECTION OF CALF PUMP MALFUNCTION

The techniques used to diagnose and correct calf pump malfunction are described in Chapters 7 and Chapter 17.

Some have advocated the use of these methods to accelerate healing of the ulcer, others have only used them to prevent recurrence once the ulcer has healed. This latter policy is discussed in the section on ulcer prophylaxis (page 592). As other methods of ulcer healing are invariably combined with some definitive treatment of the venous abnormality, an assessment of the independent value of the correction of calf pump malfunction is extremely difficult.

The methods used to correct the venous abnormality include:

- sclerotherapy
- surgical ligation of the superficial and lower leg communicating veins
- surgical reconstruction of the deep veins or valves
- elastic compression stockings.

Sclerotherapy

Fegan's group[85] originally claimed that injection compression sclerotherapy (see Chapter 7 for the technique) combined with ulcer dressing successfully maintained ulcer healing for more than 4 years in 82% of a consecutive group of 82 women presenting with venous ulcers. There was no control group treated by compression and dressings without injections, and it is not clear if some ulcers healed, broke down and were then healed by a second course of treatment. Henry et al.[108] from the same Dublin clinic subsequently reported that ulcer dressings were totally ineffective unless combined with sclerotherapy. It is difficult to interpret these latter results because the results of standard treatment are so bad and because the study lacked controls. Dinn and Henry[72] appeared to have abandoned the early use of sclerotherapy in favour of elastic stockings and we know of few other centres that recommend early sclerotherapy to heal ulcers.

Surgical ligation of the superficial and lower leg communicating veins

Linton and Hardy,[130] in a review of the surgical treatment of the post-thrombotic syndrome, advocated healing all associated venous ulcers before ligating the communicating veins and treating any other sites of superficial vein incompetence (see Chapter 7, page 231 for techniques). In 1953, Linton reiterated this opinion[129] but in the same year Cockett and Elgan Jones[51] reported, in the *Lancet*, two cases in whom they had simultaneously ligated the lower leg communicating veins and grafted an associated venous ulcer with good results. In a postscript to this publication they recorded 20 additional successes.

In 1955, Cockett[50] was advocating ulcer excision combined with communicating vein ligation followed 4 or 5 days later by the application of split skin grafts to the granulating area left by the ulcer excision. However, no results of this change in policy were presented. In the same year Dodd et al.[73] reported their results of ankle communicating vein ligation for the venous ulcer syndrome. Unfortunately, it is impossible to ascertain from this paper whether the ulcers were healed or open at the time of the surgery.

Lofgren's[132] review of 129 patients with 'stasis' ulcers treated by skin grafting and surgery to the superficial veins does not clearly state whether the skin grafts and the surgery were performed simultaneously or if the vein surgery was carried out after the ulcer had healed. In a further review in 1974, Lofgren[131] commented that 'vein surgery and skin grafting can be done as a combined procedure or vein surgery alone may be sufficient if the ulcer is small or nearly healed'. A follow-up of between 3 and 12 years showed that 70% of the ulcers treated in this way had remained healed, but the majority of patients were wearing elastic stockings as an additional treatment.

Cockett's idea of operating on the veins before healing the ulcer[50] was taken up by Pickerill et al. in 1970.[171] They suggested that 1 week after 'appropriate surgery to the superficial and communicating veins the patient should be taken back to the operating theatre for a radical excision of the ulcer including the damaged surrounding skin with immediate application of split skin grafts'. No numbers or results are quoted in this paper.

In 1974, De Palma[69] again described a synchronous operation to ligate the communicating veins and apply split skin grafts to the ulcer. Yet again, neither long-term nor short-term results[152] are recorded.

In 1983, Negus and Friedgood[152] reported that of more than 100 ulcers the majority (77–80%) were healed by conservative treatment before operation. In those that did not heal (20%), split skin grafts were applied at time of vein surgery. The success rates of the sequential and simultaneous procedures were not presented separately.

The whole question of the role of ligating incompetent communicating veins to accelerate the healing of venous ulcers is being revisited with the advent of endoscopic ligation of the calf communicating veins (see Chapters 7 and 17). Many careful controlled clinical trials will be needed before the precise role of the communicating vein ligation is defined.

Pertibial fasciotomy may also encourage healing.[212]

Comment

Although this review of some of the publications that have studied the effect of the simultaneous treatment of venous ulceration and calf pump malfunction shows that surgical correction of superficial venous incompetence can be satisfactorily performed in the presence of an ulcer, there is still little evidence that this accelerates the healing of the ulcer, unless the ulcer is treated by simultaneous or subsequent split skin grafting. There is, no evidence that split skin grafts are more or less likely to adhere to an ulcer base when they are applied at the same time as venous surgery, but we have already mentioned our own satisfactory results with this method of healing ulcers that are resistant to conservative forms of treatment.

There is little evidence that ulcers that are treated by skin grafting are more liable to break down than those healed by compression bandages.

We still prefer to heal the ulcer first as it is often difficult even with duplex ultrasound to define the disorder of the calf pump in the presence of an active ulcer and it is therefore difficult to decide on the best method of treatment until the ulcer is healed. Furthermore, if the ulcer is healed, the operation can take place in a sterile field, thus avoiding the high risk of wound infection that is known to be greater after simultaneous operations performed in the presence of an open ulcer (Figure 20.10).[121,143]

It is essential that proper comparisons are made between the many combinations of sclerotherapy, surgery to the superficial veins, surgery to the communicating veins (including new endoscopic surgery), surgery to both the superficial and communicating veins, and preoperative, peroperative

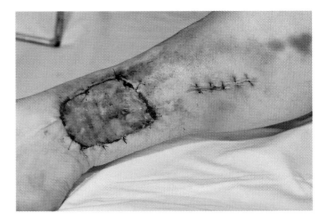

Figure 20.10   This ulcer has been excised and covered with a split skin graft. The medial calf communicating veins have been ligated at the same time. An additional incision above the ulcer (combined with the ulcer excision) has allowed all the communicating veins to be explored. A small skin bridge has been left between the two incisions.

and postoperative skin grafting. Such studies would allow the best combination of these procedures to be selected and, if only incompetent saphenous or communicating veins were treated, it would be possible to discover which of these two abnormalities has the major role in the genesis of ulceration.

Surgical reconstruction of the deep veins or valves

The operations used to reconstruct the deep veins or repair their valves (see Chapters 8 and 9 for details) include:

- femoral valve reconstruction[125]
- valve transposition operations[126]
- popliteal to femoral vein, saphenous vein bypass operations[116,214]
- sapheno-femoral bypass operations[159]
- femoro-caval bypass operations[65]
- brachial valve transplantation[202]
- the gracilis sling operation.[173]

These operations have all been used to reconstruct or bypass damaged deep veins and have all been claimed to heal ulcers or prevent the recurrence of ulcers.[18] They have almost always been combined with other operations on the superficial veins of the lower leg or with prolonged periods of bedrest. All these procedures require further evaluation but if they are to be used, it is probably preferable that any ulceration should be healed first. They may have a place in the prevention of ulcer recurrence but they do not have a role in accelerating ulcer healing.

There is little evidence that ligation of the femoral vein to prevent deep venous reflux promotes ulcer healing.[70,130]

Elastic compression stockings

In 1994, Partsch and Harkova[164] found that Sigvaris stockings healed ulcers significantly faster than a short-stretch regimen (84%, 21 of 25 compared with 82%, 13 out of 25).

MISCELLANEOUS TREATMENTS

Many ancillary treatments have been tried, for example:

- hyperbaric oxygen
- lumbar sympathectomy
- weight reduction, diuretics and vitamins
- acidification.

Hyperbaric oxygen

The low tissue oxygen found in association with venous ulceration has already been described (Chapter 18). Bass[9] reported a series of patients with venous ulcers who were treated with hyperbaric oxygen given for 2 hours every day, 5 days of the week. The only additional treatment was a gauze dressing. Seventeen of the ulcers treated in this way healed in a mean of 6 weeks but, unfortunately, the initial ulcer size was not given, and there was no control group. A similar study[86] without controls also reported good results. A properly controlled study is still required to assess the value of this treatment; until this has been carried out it cannot be recommended. It is no longer recommended as standard treatment for venous ulcers.

Lumbar sympathectomy

Opinions concerning the value of lumbar sympathectomy in the treatment of venous ulceration are conflicting. Fontaine[87] provided anecdotal evidence for its value as an adjuvant treatment in the management of chronic ulcers of the leg, but both Linton and Hardy[130] and Dodd and Cockett[74] strongly condemned its use for venous ulceration.

A more recent paper has suggested that lumbar sympathectomy may be effective in healing venous ulcers which have proved resistant to treatment by conventional means.[165] Eighty of the ulcers treated

by sympathectomy remained healed between 2 years and 11 years after treatment. A controlled trial is required before sympathectomy can be advocated for the treatment of venous ulceration.

Weight reduction, diuretics and vitamins

Haeger[102] has championed the value of diuretics and weight reduction in the healing of ulcers, but there is little hard evidence to justify the value of either form of treatment.

Acidification

One small study that used a healing equation found that acidification of the ulcer surface promoted healing.[219] We are not aware that this work has been repeated.

Psychological stress may also delay healing.[124]

COMMENT

Most ulcers felt to be venous are probably best treated initially by some form of compression bandaging regimen. This may be either a modified Unna's boot (a medicated impregnated bandage with overlying compression bandages), a multilayer system or dressings beneath elastic stockings. Very large ulcers (greater than 100 cm²) invariably take more than a year to heal and early surgical excision and grafting is probably indicated in these ulcers. Scalpel debridement is quick, effective and inexpensive. Topical antibiotics and antiseptics are of little, if any, value. A number of drugs have been thought to speed ulcer healing but of these only oxpentifylline is being actively promoted. Its benefits are marginal. The role of growth factors and early surgery is still being assessed.

Prevention of ulcer recurrence

A review of all the treatments described above shows that most studies report that between 60% and 90% of all 'new ulcers' can be healed within 3–12 months of presentation with conservative treatment. The factors which may influence this 'time to total healing' include:

- the size of the ulcer at presentation and the number of years that the ulcer has been present
- the time that the ulcer has remained unhealed and the nature of the underlying venous disease.

These prognostic factors were developed into a more sophisticated index by Skene *et al.* (1992).[191]

Smaller initial ulcer area, shorter duration of ulcer, younger age and no deep vein abnormality were all independent variables.

The ulcers that do not heal with medical treatment can be healed by skin grafting. The challenge remains to maintain healing.

METHODS OF PREVENTING ULCER RECURRENCE

The techniques used to prevent ulcer recurrence are listed.

1. Sapheno-femoral or sapheno-popliteal ligation with stripping and local avulsions
2. Ligation or interruption of the lower leg communicating veins
3. A combination of 1 and 2
4. Deep vein bypass or reconstruction
5. Injection compression sclerotherapy
6. Elastic stockings
7. Fibrinolytic enhancement
8. Permanent use of compression bandages

Superficial vein surgery

The value of occluding incompetent superficial-to-deep communications depends upon the role that each site of incompetence plays in the genesis of calf pump malfunction. Most patients have long or short saphenous vein incompetence but the value of correcting this abnormality alone is not known. Our own clinical experience suggests that saphenous ligation on its own, in the presence of lower leg communicating vein incompetence, does not prevent ulcer recurrence, but other investigators do not agree with us.[185]

None of the proponents of ligation of the lower leg communicating veins[50,51,129,130,151,152] has carried out this operation without simultaneously correcting incompetence of the saphenous veins, if this is present. We have found that ligation of the incompetent communicating veins alone fails to restore the foot vein pressure fall during exercise to normal,[37] and Bjordal[20–24] has shown that saphenous incompetence has a greater influence on calf pump function than communicating vein incompetence.

The inadequacy of the studies that have been published on this subject has been discussed already but a prospective trial of ligation of the communicating veins alone without saphenous surgery would be unlikely to obtain the approval of an ethical committee, despite its apparent importance.

The operation chosen by most surgeons is the combination of communicating vein ligation with sapheno-femoral and sapheno-popliteal ligation.[6,50,51,62,69,73,74,129,130,151,152,204]

In our experience[34] this is a good operation to perform in limbs with phlebographically 'normal' deep veins but it is relatively ineffective in limbs with clear-cut phlebographic evidence of deep vein damage. All the patients with post-thrombotic ulcers in one of our series treated by operation alone developed at least one ulcer recurrence within 5 years of operation. The patients in this study were not provided with elastic stockings. Negus's prospective, but uncontrolled, study[151,152] of identical surgery combined with permanent elastic stocking support[8] had a much lower incidence of recurrence during a mean of 3 years' review.

We have compared the results of superficial vein surgery followed by elastic stockings, after healing, with the results achieved in a randomly selected group of control patients treated with stockings and stanozolol (fibrinolytic enhancement) after ulcer healing. There was no significant difference in ulcer recurrence between the two treatments (about 90% at 5 years).

The evidence suggests that a combination of surgery followed by permanent support with elastic stockings is more certain to prevent ulcer recurrence than surgery alone. It is to be hoped that similar studies will be set up to assess endoscopic perforator surgery.

The cause of ulcer recurrence after superficial venous surgery

Finding the cause of an ulcer that has recurred after surgery is a difficult clinical problem because it is always possible that the initial surgery was inadequate or incorrect (e.g. an incompetent communicating vein or the long saphenous vein may have been missed or not properly divided), or that the surgery was adequate and a new cause of ulceration has developed.

Nielubowitcz and Szostek[156] investigated a small group of 11 patients whose ulcers recurred with phlebography to try to discover if communicating veins had been missed at the original operation. They found evidence of communicating vein incompetence in four limbs, but found it impossible to decide whether these were new communicating veins that had developed since the operation or communicating veins that had been missed at the original operation.

Incompetent communicating veins that recur should be treated surgically and we have many patients on whom we have performed this operation three or four times over 10–15 years. We also have some patients where re-exploration has failed to reveal any incompetent communicating veins and we have been unable to define the cause of their recurrent ulcer.

Deep vein bypass or reconstruction

A description of these techniques[18] is given in Chapter 13. Their place in accelerating the healing of ulcers has been briefly mentioned above. As most of these techniques have been developed within the last 5–10 years, their role in the prevention of ulcer recurrence has not yet been established.

In 1994, Masuda and Kistner[138] reviewed the long-term results of valvular reconstruction on ulcer recurrence and calf pump function. Their 10-year success was significantly better in patients with primary valvular malfunction than in those with post-thrombotic valve damage (73% vs 43%). Of the 49 limbs with class three disease preoperatively, 17 (35%) had developed ulcer recurrences. Many of these recurrences were associated with failure of the valve reconstruction.

Injection compression sclerotherapy

New evidence has been added to the uncontrolled study of Henry *et al.*[108] which suggested that sclerotherapy sustained the long-term healing of ulcers.

Elastic support stockings

Many authors[6,17,62,129,130] have recommended the continued use of permanent elastic support in limbs with severe post-thrombotic damage. This recommendation has in the past been based more on theoretical considerations than on proven efficacy but a recent controlled randomized prospective study by Stacey[197] has now shown that patients who wear stockings after ulcer healing have a significantly lower recurrence rate than those who do not.

The older type of compression stocking has now been superseded by the graduated compression stocking, but this change is also the result of theoretical arguments rather than practical experience.[189,211] Stemmer[200,201] has calculated that the ideal external compression should exactly match, and therefore overcome, the increase in venous pressure that causes the loss of capillary transudate into the tissues.[199] The higher venous pressure at the ankle therefore demands a greater external compression pressure to prevent transudation than the lower venular pressure at the knee. Sigg's argument[188,189] for graduated compression was more straightforward; he simply believed that the greatest pressure should be applied over the 'ulcer bearing skin'.

A number of measurements of calf pump function have shown that graduated compression is more effective in promoting venous return than standard uniform compression stockings.[57,75,120,163]

Indirect evidence of the value of graduation is provided by two studies. Firstly, graduated compression stockings alone or in combination with fibrinolytic enhancement have been shown to reduce areas of lipodermatosclerosis.[33,139] Secondly, surgery to the communicating veins combined with graduated compression has produced better results than those reported with surgery alone[36,151,152] Our controlled trial comparing prescription stockings (class II) with hospital prescribed (potentially better) stockings in preventing ulcer recurrence showed no difference in recurrence rates, which are still nearly 50% at 3 years – almost all in the post-thrombotic limbs.

External compression has two other effects: it increases the rate of blood flow in the deep veins[187] and it may encourage the release of fibrinolytic activator from the venous endothelium,[49] though this is probably not important.

Standardization of stockings

A number of methods are used to test the elastic tension at different sites in a stocking. The tension can then be converted to a compression pressure by Laplace's equation (pressure = tension × radius). Techniques which use testing rigs are indirect methods; direct methods measure the pressure beneath the stocking when it is on the patient's leg.

Indirect measurements of tension

The Ingstron tester measures the tension in a section of a stocking held between two movable T-pins. It is simply a standard form of tensiometer.

The Hatra tester involves placing the stocking on a 'leg former' and then stretching it by pulling out a movable bar to a predetermined site. A measuring head is then applied to the stretched stocking to obtain the fabric tension at the desired position.

The Hohenstein tester is a computerized device which measures the tension between numerous points marked on a stocking stretched over an expandable leg former.

Direct measurements of tension

The original Sigg balloon tester[189] has been superseded by the testing system devised by Borgnis and Bollinger.[210] The Borgnis system overcomes the defect of the original balloon tester which gave false results because the inflated balloon between the leg and the stocking increased the curve of the leg, and so reduced the radius, thus artificially increasing the measured tension.

The Borgnis medical stocking tester (the MST) consists of a long thin plastic envelope containing four pairs of carbon electrodes on its two inside opposing surfaces which make contact when the envelope is empty (Figure 20.11). When the probe

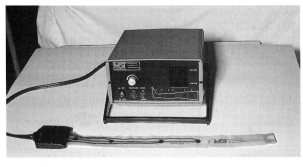

(a)

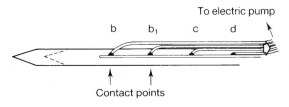

(b)

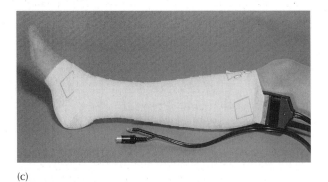

(c)

Figure 20.11 The Borgnis tester. (a) The envelope (probe) containing the four circular carbon contacts is in the foreground; the pump with the pressure dial is behind. When the pump is turned on, air is blown into the envelope. The pressure at which the contacts separate is equal to the compression pressure of the stocking at the point of measurement. This is recorded on the digital display. (b) This diagram shows the circuits inside the envelope. (c) The Borgnis tester beneath a Thusane bandage.

is placed on the limb beneath the stocking the carbon contacts meet and complete four independent circuits which light four indicator lights on the pump. Air is then slowly pumped into the plastic envelope by an electric pump. When the pressure in the envelope exceeds the pressure applied by the stocking, the contacts separate, the circuit is broken and the indicator light is extinguished. The pressure in the envelope at the moment that each

of the contacts break is recorded on a digital dial which provides a series of pressure measurements from four points beneath the stocking. The amount of air required to separate the contacts within the envelope is so small that the curvature of the overlying stocking is not changed and the true tension which the stocking is imparting to the limb can be recorded.

Other substocking pressure monitors have been described, but we have found them to be just as 'temperamental' and no real advance on the MST.

Which tester? Which stocking? It is important to state the type of test used when publishing data on stocking tensions because the indirect methods give different values to those of the direct methods.[217] The British Standards Committee have chosen the Hatra system as their reference test.[35]

The advantage of the Borgnis tester is that it measures the actual pressure developed by the stocking on an individual limb. This often differs from the manufacturer's specification (almost always lower);[39] this is hardly surprising as artificial formers are very different from real legs. The MST probe is, however, very temperamental. It can be markedly affected by minor adjustments to the overlying stocking and, unfortunately, has a short life; the carbon wears off the contacts after approximately 100 tests. The MST probe is, however, a valuable tool for testing the accuracy of stocking fitting and for carrying out studies on the durability of stockings.[39]

We have found that stockings tested by this method rarely achieve the pressures claimed by the manufacturers using their laboratory methods of testing and that stockings which are subjected to normal wear and tear and regular washing lose their elasticity after 6–12 months. We now give each patient four pairs of stockings every year so that each pair is actually used for no more than 3 months.

There is no substitute for a good quality, inevitably expensive, elastic stocking. Each clinician must decide which stockings provide the best compression, using the Borgnis tester, and which are the most cosmetically acceptable. In the United Kingdom we prescribe either Sigvaris 503 or 504 (Ganzoni), or Venosan 2000 (Credenhill) because we have tried and tested these two makes of stocking against others and found them to be superior in quality and acceptability. There are, however, many other makes such as MEDI and Scholl which are probably equally efficacous.

We prescribe only below the knee stockings for patients with the calf pump failure syndrome (Figure 20.12) because we are unaware of any studies that have shown full length stockings to be more effective, though some patients with oedema of the whole leg caused by iliac vein obstruction

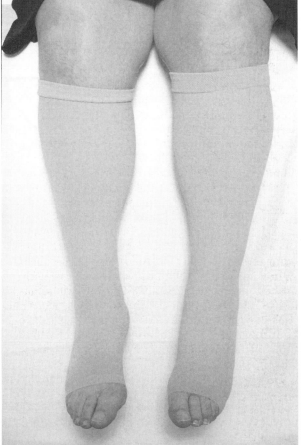

Figure 20.12   A patient fitted with a pair of below-knee medium compression (503) Sigvaris stockings. These provide good quality graduated compression and, with normal care and usage, last approximately 6 months.

prefer full length stockings. Stockings must be put on before getting out of bed every morning and worn every day, all day, until the patient goes to bed. This must be impressed upon each patient. Pulling on a stocking is quite difficult, especially for the patient who is elderly, obese, or who has arthritis of the hands. If possible, we arrange for these patients to be helped with application, removal, washing and reapplication of their stockings by their spouse, other relatives, a neighbour or through regular visits by a community nurse.

A frame has been developed over which the stocking can be stretched open to allow the patient to push his/her leg into the stocking, as if putting on a boot, without bending down. Some patients definitely find this a great help.

Although continuous use of stockings may be dangerous in ischaemic limbs, the inability to put on stockings may well allow the development of another ulcer. Under these circumstances it may be better for the patient to wear the stockings constantly, day and night or wear bandages continually, having them reapplied by the community nurses every few weeks.

Stocking care
Elastic stockings must be looked after properly, otherwise they do not retain their elasticity. They must be washed in soap, not in detergent, and each patient needs to have at least two pairs to allow for regular washing after wear. Patients are provided with a silk sock to help the stocking slide over the foot, and they should wear rubber gloves when pulling the stocking up the leg to avoid damaging the fabric of the stocking with the finger nails.

When a stocking is easy to apply, it needs to be replaced. If a stocking tester is not available, feeling the tension by picking up the stocking off the leg and inspecting its external appearance is often enough to indicate the need for replacement. It is better to err towards unnecessary replacement than to have a patient with a recurrent ulcer.

Comment
The wearing of elastic stockings has now been shown to reduce the incidence of recurrent venous ulceration. There is, however, no prospective controlled evidence that wearing a graduated compression stocking after a deep vein thrombosis prevents the development of lipodermatosclerosis and ulceration although most clinicians believe that it does. Much more information is required on the role of elastic stockings in ulcer prevention.

If rubber sensitivity develops, stockings made of 'lycra' should be prescribed for the patient.

Some patients who have severe post-thrombotic syndrome get an unbearable amount of pain and discomfort when wearing a high compression stocking. These patients are very difficult to treat.

Fibrinolytic enhancement

The value of the anabolic steroid stanozolol, which enhances blood and tissue fibrinolytic activity, in the treatment of lipodermatosclerosis is discussed in Chapter 17 (page 498). A review of a group of patients with lipodermatosclerosis treated with a course of fibrinolytic enhancement has shown that they developed statistically fewer ulcers in the 5 years following treatment than in the 5 years preceding the treatment.[38] All these patients, however, wore elastic stockings for the second 5 years, and it is possible that the stockings rather than the fibrinolytic enhancement may have prevented the ulcers recurring. Nevertheless, these observations indicate that we need to find out whether the resolution or prevention of lipodermatosclerosis does reduce the risk of subsequent ulceration or re-ulceration.

Although stanozolol is no longer licensed for this treatment because it can cause virilization and liver damage, there are other safer drugs with similar actions (see Chapter 17). Further study of the fibrinolytic properties of the microcirculation and interstitial space would be worthwhile.

Permanent use of compression bandages

We have some patients who are incapable of wearing elastic stockings who we treat with 'permanent' compression (usually a Steripaste bandage, covered by Elastocrepe and Tubigrip bandages or a four-layer bandage), changed at weekly or monthly intervals by the community nurse. This regimen has been extremely effective in keeping the skin healthy and the oedema under control.

Commentary on ulcer healing and prevention

In 1953 Cockett and Elgan Jones[51] argued that ligation of the communicating veins, when post-thrombotic skin changes were just appearing, would reduce the incidence of ulceration. This approach seems to be logical but there have not been any prospective studies which have properly tested whether elastic stockings or early surgical correction of superficial venous incompetence prevents ulceration in limbs with post-thrombotic deep vein damage. We recommend that all patients who have had an extensive deep vein thrombosis, involving more than just one or two calf veins, should wear below-knee, graduated, compression stockings for the rest of their lives.

We prescribe a course of a fibrinolytic enhancing drug, e.g. defibrotide, for 6–9 months if lipodermatosclerosis develops while the patient continues to wear stockings, until the maximum resolution has been achieved.

When a patient presents with a typical venous ulcer, we try to heal it conservatively, with Calaband, Elastocrepe and Tubigrip or with dry dressings and compression, and then investigate the limb to ascertain whether the superficial, communicating, or deep veins are at fault. Trials now in progress may indicate whether early surgery enhances ulcer healing.

We operate to eradicate long and short saphenous vein incompetence if the deep veins are normal, and routinely ligate all medial lower leg communicating veins through a subfascial approach though we are investigating the role of duplex ultrasound guided endoscopic surgery in these patients as an alternative.

If there is evidence of severe post-thrombotic deep vein damage, we assess the role of the superficial veins by using tourniquet tests, duplex ultrasound assessment and foot volumetry and tailor our surgery according to the findings of these tests in combination with the anatomical information provided by a phlebogram. If the post-thrombotic damage is mainly in the calf veins and there is ultrasound-confirmed superficial or communicating vein incompetence and tourniquets improve the expelled foot volume, we ligate the sites of deep-to-superficial reflux and prescribe permanent stockings. If there is severe post-thrombotic damage confined to the thigh or pelvis, causing a significant degree of outflow obstruction with no improvement in the expelled foot volume with tourniquets and poor collateral vessels, we would consider the feasibility of a 'Palma' bypass[159] or a femoro-caval reconstruction,[65] together with ligation of the incompetent communicating veins (see Chapter 13).

If there is extensive post-thrombotic damage at all levels throughout the limb, we try to avoid surgery and rely on elastic stockings plus fibrinolytic enhancement if there is severe lipodermatosclerosis.

We consider that this is a logical approach to ulcer prophylaxis but other clinicians would simply ligate all the incompetent communicating veins of all patients with ulcers and provide elastic stockings. These clinicians must, however, expect a 10–15% incidence of recurrence every year. Careful identification of those situations likely to cause a recurrence should lead to better treatment of these patients and possibly a lower incidence of recurrence.

TREATMENT OF THE COMPLICATIONS OF VENOUS ULCERATION AND ITS ASSOCIATED CONDITIONS

Eczema

Venous ulcers are commonly associated with eczema in the skin near the ulcer or at distant sites around the body (e.g. the opposite leg, the upper limb, and even the face and the trunk). The aetiology of the eczema is obscure. It may be the result of local skin sensitivity to lesser degrees of the damage which causes lipodermatosclerosis and ulceration.

The eczema may be treated with local or systemic steroids, and it usually disappears when the ulcer heals or the venous abnormality is repaired.

There is nothing specific about venous eczema and the diagnosis is simply suspected when varicose veins and eczema coexist. The diagnosis is confirmed when the eczema clears after the veins have been treated.

Contact dermatitis

Although this dermatitis is similar to venous eczema it is worth thinking of contact dermatitis as a separate entity because it is often caused by the treatment of the ulcer[78] rather than by an underlying skin abnormality. Eighty per cent of patients who have had an ulcer for more than 5 years are sensitive to at least one agent that has been applied to their skin during this period.[182] The presence of contact dermatitis appears to delay the healing of the ulcer.

Causes of contact dermatitis include:[182] bandages containing dyes or rubber, adhesive plasters, antibiotics, antiseptics, coal-tars, local anaesthetics, antihistamines, soaps, spirits, ointment preservatives and stabilizers (e.g. lanolin), wood alcohols, diachylon, parabens, mercuric chloride and chlorocresol.

Patients who have contact dermatitis that does not subside when the allergen is withdrawn should be referred for a dermatological opinion and possible patch testing.

Treatment of contact dermatitis is by withdrawal of the sensitizer and application of local steroid creams (Propaderm or Dermovate). Systemic steroids may occasionally be required.

Cellulitis, lymphangitis and septicaemia

Ulcers can serve as the portal of entry for bacteria that cause cellulitis, but this is surprisingly rare. Acute lipodermatosclerosis is often misdiagnosed as cellulitis.

Treatment with systemic antibiotics is indicated if a patient develops a hot, red, tender area of skin or swollen subcutaneous tissue, sometimes associated with lymphangitis, lymphadenitis and pyrexia. The exudate from the ulcer and the blood should be cultured but antibiotics should be started before the results of the cultures and bacteriological sensitivities are available. A combination of amoxycillin and flucloxacillin, Augmentin, or a cephalosporin are alternatives.

Haemorrhage

A brisk spontaneous haemorrhage may arise from a venous ulcer. The ulcer is often small and relatively uncontaminated. Treatment is by applying pressure on the bleeding point and elevating the limb until the bleeding stops. The patient should lie down with the leg elevated on a bed or chair, and a pad should be applied to the ulcer with a firm bandage. If patients are alone they should lie down, raise the leg and press on the bleeding point. Occasionally, the haemorrhage is profuse and the patient has to be admitted to hospital for a blood transfusion. The definitive treatment is to heal the ulcer. If the bleeding recurs during treatment, the ulcer is best treated by excision and skin grafting. Local veins can be sclerosed or excised.

'Champagne bottle' legs, ankylosis and equinus deformity of the ankle

The contraction of the fibrous tissue that follows the healing of severe lipodermatosclerosis or ulceration often constricts the tissues around the ankle to give the leg the appearance of an inverted 'champagne' bottle. This affects the function of the calf muscle pump by interfering with ankle movements and causes oedema of the foot.

Dodd and Cockett[74] described a 'gusset' operation for this condition, in which a vertical incision is made through the thickened tissue to allow it to retract and the resulting gap is closed by a split skin graft. This operation gives the limb a better shape but there is no evidence that it leads to better calf pump function.

The combination of persistent pain, recurrent ulceration and fibrosis often causes plantar flexion at the ankle (equinus) and eventually a fibrous ankylosis in plantar flexion (see Figure 20.1). Movement of the ankle joint is painful and the patient therefore walks on the ball of the foot, with the ankle and knee flexed and without contracting the calf muscles at all. The development of the equinus deformity is accelerated if the Achilles tendon is involved in the base of the ulcer.

If the deformity is mild, it may be simply treated by raising the heel of the shoe. If the deformity is severe, the function of the ankle joint may only be regained by lengthening the Achilles tendon; it is preferable to heal the ulcer before undertaking such an operation. Skin breakdown at the site of the incision is common. If the tendon can be successfully lengthened and joint mobility regained, the function of the calf muscle pump improves.

Anaemia

This topic has been discussed in Chapter 19. Anaemia may be the result of iron deficiency or marrow depression. It responds to oral administration of iron and healing of the ulcer.[41] Blood transfusions are rarely required.

Malignant change

This problem is discussed in detail in Chapter 19. Marjolin's ulcer is extremely rare but overgrowth of any part of a long-standing venous ulcer with the development of a foul-smelling odour should arouse suspicion. If a biopsy shows a squamous cell or even a basal cell carcinoma, the ulcer should be widely excised and the defect in the skin covered with a skin graft. Radiotherapy to skin damaged by chronic venous insufficiency may cause skin necrosis.

Amputation

More than 50 limbs are amputated, each year, for chronic painful venous ulcers in the United Kingdom.[134] If all medical and surgical measures fail in a leg severely damaged by deep vein thrombosis and which is the cause of constant pain, amputation may have to be considered. Artificial legs are never as satisfactory as natural limbs, and most natural limbs even with a large chronic ulcer are preferable to a prosthesis. We try to avoid amputation, but have had to resort to this treatment on two occasions in the past 25 years.

Conclusion

The care of venous ulcers is often delegated to junior surgeons who are commonly ill-equipped to cope with their care. Ulcers require careful assessment, and their management must also be closely monitored. When an ulcer is healed, the venous abnormality must be defined and corrected. There is still truth in both of the following statements.

The clinical evaluation of the patient's leg is more satisfactory than any artificial means. The patient's history is written on the skin of his leg. It is there to be read by those who wish to read it.[17]

Correct anatomical and pathophysiological diagnosis of leg ulcers leads to better treatment. The patient may have the problem for life.[31]

Our aim must be to achieve palliation, to look for a cure and hope that better methods of preventing and treating deep venous thrombosis will eventually lead to the eradication of venous ulceration.

References

1. Ackroyd JS, Browse NL. The investigation and surgery of the post-thrombotic syndrome. *J Cardiovasc Surg* 1986; **27:** 5.
2. Allen S. Varicose ulcers: preliminary report on a new material to assist regranulation. *Curr Med Res Opin* 1973; **1(10):** 603.
3. Anderson MN, Donald KE. Results of surgical therapy of severe stasis ulceration of the legs. *Ann Surg* 1963; **157:** 281.
4. Anning ST. *Leg Ulcers. Their Causes and Treatment.* London: Churchill, 1954.
5. Arkle CA, Adinolfi M, Welsh KI, Leibowitz S, McColl I. Immunogenicity of human amniotic epithelial cells after transplantation into volunteers. *Lancet* 1981; **2:** 1003.
6. Arnoldi CC, Haeger K. Ulcus cruris venosum – crux medico rum? *Lakartidningen* 1967; **64:** 2149.
7. Aubrey J. William Lee. *The Worlds of John Aubrey.* London: The Folio Society, 1988; Chapter 7.
8. Bartholomew A. Short account of the treatment by physiotherapy of gravitational ulcers. *Br J Phys Med* 1952; **15:** 289.
9. Bass BH. The treatment of varicose leg ulcers by hyperbaric oxygen. *Postgrad Med J* 1970; **46:** 407.
10. Battle R. *Plastic Surgery.* London: Butterworths, 1964.
11. Bauer G. The etiology of leg ulcers and their treatment by resection of the popliteal veins. *J Int Chir* 1948; **8:** 937.
12. Beaconsfield T, Genbacev O, Taylor RS. The treatment of long-standing venous ulcers with an extract of early placenta – a pilot study. *Phlebology* 1991; **6:** 153–8.
13. Beitner H, Hammar H, Olsson AG, Thyresson N. Prostaglandin E1 treatment of leg ulcers caused by venous or arterial incompetence. *Acta Dermatol Venereol (Stockh)* 1980; **60:** 425.
14. Belcaro GV, Coen F. Pneumatic intermittent compression treatment of venous ulcerations caused by venous hypertension. In: Negus D, Jantet G, eds. *Phlebology '85.* London: Libbey, 1986.
15. Belcaro G, Marelli C. Treatment of venous lipodermatosclerosis and ulceration in venous hypertension by elastic compression and fibrinolytic enhancement with defibrotide. *Phlebology* 1989; **4:** 91–106.
16. Bennett JP, Mathews R, Page-Faulk W. Treatment of chronic ulceration of the legs with human amnion. *Lancet* 1980; **1:** 1153.
17. Bergan JJ. Ulcers of the leg. *Ind Med Surg* 1967; **36:** 253.
18. Bergan JJ, Yao JST, Flinn WR, McCarthy WJ. Surgical treatment of venous obstruction and insufficiency. *J Vasc Surg* 1986; **3:** 174.
19. Bisgaard H. *Ulcers and Eczema of the Leg Sequels of Phlebitis.* Copenhagen: Munksgaard, 1948.
20. Bjordal RI. Simultaneous pressure and flow recordings in varicose veins of the lower extremity. *Acta Chir Scand* 1970; **136:** 309.
21. Bjordal RI. Pressure patterns in the saphenous system in patients with venous leg ulcers. *Acta Chir Scand* 1971; **137:** 495.
22. Bjordal RI. Blood circulation in varicose veins of the lower extremities. *Angiology* 1972; **23:** 163.
23. Bjordal RI. Circulation patterns in incompetent perforating veins in the calf and in the saphenous system in primary varicose veins. *Acta Chir Scand* 1972; **138:** 251.
24. Bjordal RI. Circulation patterns in the saphenous system and the perforating veins of the calf in

patients with previous deep venous thrombosis. *Vasa Suppl* 1974; **3**: 1–41.

25. Blair SD, Wright DDI, Backhouse CM, Riddle E, McCollum C. Sustained compression and healing of chronic venous ulcers. *Br Med J* 1988; **297**: 1159–61.

26. Bosanquet N. Costs of venous ulcers. From maintenance therapy to investment programmes. *Phlebology Suppl* 1992; **1**: 44–6.

27. Bourne IHJ. Vertical leg drainage of oedema in treatment of leg ulcers. *Br Med J* 1974; **2**: 581.

28. Brearley S. Extensible bandages. Should be dispensed with more information on performance. *Br Med J* 1992; **304**: 520–1.

29. Brennan SS, Leaper DJ. Antiseptics and wound healing. *Br J Surg* 1985; **72**: 780.

30. Brodie BC. *Lectures Illustrative of Various Subjects in Pathology and Surgery.* London: Longmans, 1846.

31. Browse NL. Venous ulceration. *Br Med J* 1983; **286**: 1920.

32. Browse NL, Jarrett PEM, Morland M, Burnand K. Treatment of liposclerosis of the leg by fibrinolytic enhancement: a preliminary report. *Br Med J* 1977; **2**: 434–5.

33. Burke HB, Kuglar W, Oriti J, Seidenspinner C, Lockwood B, Buskey A. The use of gelfoam powder and betadine-saturated gauze in treatment of chronic ulcerations. *J Foot Surg* 1981; **20**: 76.

34. Burnand KG, Clemenson G, Morland M, Jarrett PEM, Browse NL. Venous lipodermatosclerosis: treatment by fibrinolytic enhancement and elastic compression. *Br Med J* 1980; **280**: 7–11.

35. Burnand KG, Layer G. Graduated elastic stockings. *Br Med J* 1986; **293**: 224.

36. Burnand KG, O'Donnell TF, Lea Thomas M, Browse NL. Relation between post-phlebitic changes in the deep veins and results of surgical treatment of venous ulcers. *Lancet* 1976; **1**: 936.

37. Burnand KG, O'Donnell TF, Lea Thomas M, Browse NL. The relative importance of incompetent communicating veins in the production of varicose veins and venous ulcers. *Surgery* 1977; **82**: 9.

38. Burnand KG, Pattison M, Browse NL. The results of a course of Stromba treatment on lipodermatosclerosis: a five year follow-up. In: Davidson JF, Bachmann F, Bouvier CA, Kruithof EKO, eds. *Progress in Fibrinolysis.* Vol 6. Edinburgh: Churchill Livingstone, 1983; 526.

39. Burnand KG, Pattison M, Layer GT. How effective and long lasting are elastic stockings? In: Negus D, Jantet G, eds. *Phlebology '85.* London: Libbey, 1986.

40. Burnand KG, Powell S, Bishop CCR, Stacey M, Pulvertaft T. The effect of paroven on skin oxygenation in patients with varicose veins. *Phlebology* 1989; **4**: 15–22.

41. Burns DA, Sarkany I. Management of stasis ulcers by pinch graft. *Br J Dermatol* 1976; **95(Suppl 14)**: 82.

42. Callam MJ, Dale JJ, Ruckley CV, Harper DR. Trial of ultrasound in the treatment of chronic leg ulceration. In: Negus D, Jantet G, eds. *Phlebology '85.* London: Libbey, 1986.

43. Callam MJ, Harper DR, Dale JJ, *et al.* Lothian and Forth Valley Leg Ulcer Healing Trial, Part 1: Elastic versus non-elastic bandaging in the treatment of chronic leg ulceration. *Phlebology* 1992; **7**: 136–41.

44. Callam MJ, Harper DR, Dale JJ, *et al.* Lothian and Forth Valley Leg Ulcer Healing Trial, Part 2: Knitted viscose dressing versus a hydocellular dressing in the treatment of chronic leg ulceration. *Phlebology* 1992; **7**: 142–5.

45. Callam MJ, Ruckley CV, Harper DR, Dale JJ. Chronic ulceration of the leg: extent of the problem and provision of care. *Br Med J* 1985; **290**: 1855.

46. Carion J, Debelle M, Goldschmidt JP. New therapeutic measures for the treatment of ulcers. *Phlebologie* 1978; **31(4)**: 339.

47. Celsus AC. *Of Medicine in Eight Books.* Grieve J, trans. London: Wilson, 1756.

48. Chilvers AS, Freeman GK. Outpatient skin grafting of venous ulcers. *Lancet* 1969; **2**: 1087.

49. Clarke RL, Orandi A, Cliffton EE. Tourniquet induction of fibrinolysis. *Angiology* 1960; **11**: 367.

50. Cockett FB. The pathology and treatment of venous ulcers of the leg. *Br J Surg* 1955; **43**: 260.

51. Cockett FB, Elgan Jones D. The ankle blow-out syndrome; a new approach to the varicose ulcer problem. *Lancet* 1953; **1**: 17.

52. Coleridge-Smith PD, ed. Consensus paper on venous leg ulcers. The Alexander House Group. *Phlebology* 1992; **7**: 48–58.

53. Coleridge Smith P, Sarin S, Hasty J, Scurr JH. Sequential gradient pneumatic compression enhances venous ulcer healing, a randomized trial. *Surgery* 1990; **108**: 871–5.

54. Colgan MP, Dormandy JA, Jones PW, Schraibman IG, Shanik DG, Young RAL. Oxpentifylline treatment of venous ulcers of the leg. *Br Med J* 1990; **300**: 972–5.

55. Conrad P. Treatment of varicose veins and venous ulcers. *Med J Aust* 1977; **1**: 144.

56. Coopwood TB. Evaluation of a topical enzymatic debridement agent. Sutilains ointment: a preliminary report. *South Med J* 1976; **69**: 834.

57. Cornwall JV, Doré C, Lewis JD. To graduate or not? The effect of compression garments on venous refilling time. In: Negus D, Jantet G, eds. *Phlebology '85.* London: Libbey, 1986.

58. Cornwall JV, Doré CJ, Lewis JD. Graduated compression and its relation to venous filling time. *Br Med J* 1987; **295**: 1087–90.

59. Cornwall JV, Gilliland EL. Controlled trial of Iodosorb in chronic venous ulcer (Letter). *Br Med J* 1985; **291**: 902.

60. Cornwall JV, Lewis JD. Leg ulcers re-visited. *Br J Surg* 1983; **70**: 681.

61. Cottonot F, Carton FX, Tessler L, *et al.* Incidences économiques du mode de traitement des ulcères de jambe. *Phlebologie* 1979; **32**: 333.

62. Cranley JJ, Krause RJ, Strasser ES. Chronic venous insufficiency of the lower extremity. *Surgery* 1961; **49**: 48.

63. Crichett G. *Lectures on the Cause and Treatment Of Ulcers of the Lower Extremity.* London: Churchill, 1849.

64. Curwen IHM, Scott BO. The ambulant treatment of the complications resulting from varicose veins and allied conditions. *Arch Phys Med Rehabil* 1953; **1:** 17.

65. Dale WA. Peripheral venous reconstruction. In: Dale WA, ed. *Surgical Problems.* New York: McGraw-Hill, 1985; 493.

66. Dale J, Callam M, Ruckley CV. How efficient is a compressive bandage? *Nurs Times* 1983; **79(46):** 49–51.

67. Daniel F, Foix C, Zaegel R. Le collagène approche physiologique de la cicatrization cutanée. Son application dans la traitement pratique des ulcères de jambe. *Sem Hop Paris* 1978; **54:** 833.

68. DeFriend DJ, Edwards AT, McCollum C. Treatment of venous ulceration – when is surgical management indicated? *Phlebology Suppl* 1992; **1:** 33–7.

69. De Palma RG. Surgical therapy for venous stasis. *Surgery* 1974; **76:** 910.

70. de Takats G, Graupner GW. Division of the popliteal vein in deep venous insufficiency of the lower extremities. *Surgery* 1951; **29:** 342.

71. Dickson Wright A. Treatment of varicose ulcers. *Br Med J* 1930; **2:** 996.

72. Dinn E, Henry M. Treatment of venous ulceration by injection sclerotherapy and compression hosiery: A 5-year study. *Phlebology* 1992; **7:** 23–6.

73. Dodd H, Calo AR, Mistry M, Rushford A. Ligation of the ankle communicating veins in the treatment of the venous ulcer syndrome of the leg. *Lancet* 1957; **2:** 1249.

74. Dodd H, Cockett FB. *The Pathology and Surgery of the Veins of the Lower Limb.* London: Churchill Livingstone, 1976.

75. Dodd HJ, Tatnall FM, Gaylarde PM, Sarkany I. The effect of ultraviolet irradiation on skin oxygen tension and its potential role in the management of venous leg ulcers. In: Negus D, Jantet G, eds. *Phlebology '85.* London: Libbey, 1986.

76. *Drug and Therapeutics Bulletin.* Local applications to wounds – I Cleansers, antibacterials, debriders. *Drug Ther Bull* 1991; **29(24):** 93–5.

77. Duby T, Hoffman D, Cameron J, *et al.* A randomized trial in the treatment of venous leg ulcers comparing short stretch bandages, four layer bandage system, and a long stretch–paste bandage system. In: *Wounds – A Compendium of Clinical Research and Practice* 1993; **5(6):** 276–9.

78. Dunn RM, Fudem GM, Walton RL, Anderson FA, Malhotra R. Free flap valvular transplantation for refactory venous ulceration. *J Vasc Surg* 1994; **19:** 525–31.

79. Dyson M, Franks C, Suckling J. Stimulation of healing of varicose ulcers by ultrasound. *Ultrasonics* 1976; **14:** 232.

80. Egan TJ, O'Driscoll J, Thakar DR. Human amnion in the management of chronic ulceration of the lower limb: a clinico-pathological study. *Angiology* 1983; **34:** 197.

81. Ehrly AM, Schenk J, Bromberger U. Venous leg ulcers: Microcirculatory improvement with low-dose, long-term urokinase therapy. *Proceedings of the Vth European American Symposium on Venous Disease.* Vienna: 1990. (Unpublished abst).

82. Evans CD, Harman RRM, Warin RP. Varicose ulcers and the use of topical corticosteroids. *Br Med J* 1967; **2:** 482.

83. Falanga V, Kirsner RS, Eaglestein WH, Katz MH, Kerdel FA. Stanozolol in treatment of leg ulcers due to cryofibrinogenaemia. *Lancet* 1991; **338:** 347–8.

84. Famulari C, Monaco M, Versaci A, Perri S, Terranova ML, Cuzzocrea D. L'azione della N-acetil-idrossiprolina nella guarigione della lesion ulcerative cutanee. *Ann Ital Chir* 1979; **51:** 527.

85. Fegan WG. *Varicose Veins and Compression Sclerotherapy.* London: Heinemann, 1971.

86. Fischer BH. Treatment of ulcers of the legs with hyperbaric oxygen. *J Dermatol Surg* 1975; **1:** 55.

87. Fontaine R. Remarks concerning venous thrombosis and its sequelae. *Surgery* 1957; **41:** 6.

88. Foote RR. *Varicose Veins.* London: Butterworths, 1954.

89. Franks PJ, Moffatt CJ, Connolly M, *et al.* Community leg ulcer clinics: effect on quality of life. *Phlebology* 1994; **9:** 83–6.

90. Galen C. *Ad Scripti Libri.* Venice: Vincentium Valgrisium, 1562.

91. Gallaso U, Fiumano F, Cloro L, Strati V. L'uso dell acido ialuronico nella terapia delle ulcere varicose degli arti inferior. *Minerva Chir* 1978; **33:** 1581.

92. Gilliland EL, Nathwani N, Doré CJ, Lewis JD. Bacterial colonisation of leg ulcers and its effect on the success rate of skin grafting. *Ann R Coll Surg Engl* 1988; **70:** 105–8.

93. Greaves MW, Ive FA. Double blind trial of zinc sulphate in the treatment of chronic venous leg ulceration. *Br J Dermatol* 1972; **87:** 632.

94. Greaves MW, Ive FA, Skillen AW. Effects of long continued ingestion of zinc sulphate in patients with venous leg ulceration. *Lancet* 1970; **2:** 889.

95. Greenhalgh R, McCollum C. Community leg ulcer clinics: cost-effectiveness. *Health Trends* 1993; **25(4):** 146–8.

96. Groenewald JH. An evaluation of dextranomer as a cleansing agent in the treatment of postphlebitic stasis ulcer. *S Afr Med J* 1980; **57:** 809.

97. Groenewald JH. The treatment of varicose stasis ulcer. A controlled trial. *Praxis* 1981; **70:** 1273.

98. Gruen RL, Chang S, Maclellan DG. Optimising the hospital management of ulcers. *Aust N Z J Surg* 1996; **66:** 171–4.

99. Gupta PD, Saunders WA. Chronic leg ulcers in the elderly treated with absolute bedrest. *Practitioner* 1982; **226:** 1611.

100. Haeger K. Preoperative treatment of leg ulcers with silver spray and aluminium foil. *Acta Chir Scand* 1963; **125:** 32.

101. Haeger K. Topical treatment of varicose ulcers. *Br J Med* 1930; **2:** 996.

102. Haeger K. *Venous and Lymphatic Disorders of the Leg.* Copenhagen: Scandinavian University Books, 1966.

103. Hallbook T, Lanner E. Serum-zinc and healing of venous leg ulcers. *Lancet* 1972; **2:** 780.

104. Hansen ET. Amniotic grafts in chronic skin ulceration. *Lancet* 1950; **1:** 850.

105. Harkiss KJ. Cost analysis of dressing materials used in venous leg ulcers. *Pharm J* 1985; **31:** 268.

106. Harms W. Lokale therapie insbensondere der Ulzera. *Hautarzt* 1979; **30:** 210.

107. Hellgren L. Cleansing properties of stabilized trypsin and streptokinase–streptodornase in necrotic leg ulcers. *Eur J Clin Pharmacol* 1983; **24:** 623.

108. Henry MEF, Fegan WG, Pegum JM. Five year survey of the treatment of varicose ulcers. *Br Med J* 1971; **2:** 493.

109. Hills NH, Pflug JJ, Jeyasingh K, Boardman L, Calnan JS. Prevention of deep vein thrombosis by intermittent compression of calf. *Br Med J* 1972; **1:** 131.

110. Hippocrates 460 BC. *'De Ulceribus' – The Genuine Works of Hippocrates.* Adams F, trans and ed. London: Sydenham Society, 1849.

111. Holm J, Holmstedt B. Skin transplantation of venous ulcers using a fibrinogen glue. In: Negus D, Jantet G, eds. *Phlebology '85.* London: Libbey, 1986.

112. Horner J, Fernandes J, Fernandes E, Nicolaides AN. Value of graduated compression stockings in deep venous insufficiency. *Br Med J* 1980; **280:** 820–1.

113. Humzah MD, Marshall J, Breach NM. Eusol: the plastic surgeon's choice? *J R Coll Surg Edinb* 1996; **41:** 269–70.

114. Hunt T. *A Guide to the Treatment of Diseases of the Skin: with Suggestions for their Prevention.* 4th edition. London: Richards, 1859.

115. Hunter J. *The Works of John Hunter FRS.* Palmer JF, ed. London: Longman, 1835.

116. Husni EA. Venous reconstruction in postphlebitic disease. *Circulation* 1971; **43(Suppl):** 147.

117. Hutinel B, Raider P. Le gel de collagène: un nouveau traitement dans la cicatrisation des ulcères de jambe. *Phlebologie* 1977; **30:** 317.

118. Ibbotson SH, Layton AM, Davies JA, Foodfield MJ. The effect of asprin on haemostatic activity in the treatment of leg ulcers. *Br J Dermatol* 1995; **132:** 422–6.

119. Johnson A. The economics of modern wound management. *Br J Pharm Pract* 1985; **7:** 294.

120. Jones NAG, Webb PJ, Rees RI, Kakkar VV. A physiological study of elastic compression stockings in venous disorders of the leg. *Br J Surg* 1980; **67:** 569.

121. Kaisary AV. A temporary biological dressing in the treatment of varicose ulcers and skin defects. *Postgrad Med J* 1977; **53:** 672.

122. Kartik I, Gulyas G. A lab boerhianyainak potolasa arteria dorsalis pedis szigetlebennyl. *Magy Traumatol Orthop* 1979; **22:** 146.

123. Keeling PWN, Jones RB, Hilton PJ, Thompson RPH. Reduced leucocyte zinc in liver disease. *Gut* 1980; **21:** 561.

124. Kiecolt-Glaser JK, Marucha PT, Malarkey WB, Mercado AM, Glaser R. Slowing of wound healing by psychological stress. *Lancet* 1995; **346:** 1194–6.

125. Kistner RL. Surgical repair of the incompetent femoral vein valve. *Arch Surg* 1975; **110:** 1336.

126. Kistner RL, Sparkuhl MD. Surgery in acute and chronic venous disease. *Surgery* 1979; **85:** 31.

127. Layer GT, Stacey MC, Burnand KG. Stanozolol and the treatment of venous ulceration – an interim report. *Phlebology* 1986; **1:** 197–203.

128. Leaper DJ. Eusol: still awaiting proper clinical trials. *Br Med J* 1992; **304:** 930–1.

129. Linton RR. The post-thrombotic ulceration of the lower extremity: its etiology and surgical treatment. *Ann Surg* 1953; **138:** 415.

130. Linton RR, Hardy IB. Post-thrombotic syndrome of the lower extremity. Treatment by interruption of the superficial femoral vein and ligation and stripping of the long and short saphenous veins. *Surgery* 1948; **24:** 452.

131. Lofgren KA. Stasis ulcer: diagnosis and treatment. *Minn Med* 1974; **57:** 135.

132. Lofgren KA, Lauvstad WA, Bonnemaison MFE. Surgical treatment of large stasis ulcer: review of 129 cases. *Mayo Clin Proc* 1965; **40:** 560.

133. Lucarotti ME, Morgan AP, Leaper DJ. The effect of antiseptics and the moist wound environment on ulcer healing: an experimental and biochemical study. *Phlebology* 1990; **5:** 173–9.

134. Luff R. Personal communication, 1986.

135. Mann RJ. A double blind trial of oral O,β-hydroxyethyl rutosides for stasis leg ulcers. *Br J Clin Pract* 1981; **35:** 79–81.

136. Margraf HW, Covey TH. A trial of silver-zinc-allantoinate in the treatment of leg ulcers. *Arch Surg* 1977; **112:** 699.

137. Marmasse J. La méthode compressive à travers les ages. *Phlebologie* 1979; **32:** 119.

138. Masuda EM, Kistner RL. Long term results of venous valve reconstruction: a four to twenty one year follow-up. *J Vasc Surg* 1994; **19:** 391–403.

139. McMullin GM, Watkin GT, Coleridge-Smith PD, Scurr JH. Efficacy of fibrinolytic enhancement with stanozolol in the treatment of venous insufficiency. *Aust N Z J Surg* 1991; **61(4):** 306–9.

140. Mian E, Currie SB, Lietti A, Bombardelli E. Antocianosidi e parete dei microvasi nuovi aspetti sul modo d'azione dell effetto protettivo nelle sindromi da abnorme fragilita a capillare. *Minerva Med* 1977; **68:** 3565.

141. Moffatt CJ, Franks PJ, Oldroyd MI, Greenhalgh RM. Randomized trial of an occlusive dressing in the treatment of chronic non-healing leg ulcers. *Phlebology* 1992; **7:** 105–7.

142. Moffatt CJ, Oldroyd MI, Franks PJ. Personal communication, 1992.

143. Monk BE, Sarkany I. Outcome of venous stasis ulcers. *Clin Exp Dermatol* 1982; **7:** 397.

144. Morgan DA. *The Care and Management of Leg Ulcers.* UKCPA Boot's Award, 1984.

145. Morris WT, Lamb AM. The Auckland hospital varicose veins and venous ulcer clinic: a report on six years' work. *N Z Med J* 1981; **93:** 350.

146. Morrison JD. Debrisan. An effective new wound cleanser. *Scott Med J* 1979; **23:** 277.

147. Moss C, Taylor A, Shuster S. Controlled trial of Iodosorb in chronic venous ulcers. *Br Med J* 1985; **291:** 902.

148. Munro-Ashman EJ, Wells RS. The treatment time for varicose ulcers. *Br J Clin Pract* 1968; **22:** 129.

149. Myers MB, Cherry G. Zinc and leg ulcers. *Am J Surg* 1970; **120:** 77.

150. Myers MB, Richter M, Cherry G. Relationship between edema and the healing rate of stasis ulcers of the leg. *Am J Surg* 1972; **124:** 666.

151. Negus D. Prevention and treatment of venous ulceration. *Ann R Coll Surg Engl* 1985; **67:** 144.

152. Negus D, Friedgood A. The effective management of venous ulceration. *Br J Surg* 1983; **70:** 623.

153. Nelzen O, Bergqvist D, Lindhagen A, Hallbrook T. Chronic leg ulcers an understimated problem in primary health care among elderly patients. *J Epidemiol Community Health* 1991; **45:** 184–7.

154. Neumann HAM, van den Broek MJTB. Stanozolol and the treatment of severe chronic venous insufficiency. *Phlebology* 1988; **3:** 237–46.

155. Neumann HAM, van den Broek MJTB. Evaluation of *O*-(β-hydroxyethyl)-rutosides in chronic venous insufficiency by means of non-invasive techniques. *Phlebology* 1990; **5(Suppl):** 13–20.

156. Nielubowitcz J, Szostek M. Recurrences after the Linton flap operation. *J Cardiovasc Surg* 1979; **20:** 49.

157. Ormiston MC, Seymour MTJ, Venn GE, Cohen RI, Fox JA. Controlled trial of Iodosorb in chronic venous ulcers. *Br Med J* 1985; **291:** 308.

158. Osmundsen PK. Contact dermatitis to chlorhexidine. *Contact Dermatitis* 1982; **8(2):** 81.

159. Palma EC, Esperon R. Sapheno-femoral bypass. Vein transplants and grafts in the surgical treatment of the post-phlebitic syndrome. *J Cardiovasc Surg* 1960; **1:** 94.

160. Palmieri B, Boraldi F. Trattamento topico di alcune lesioni distrofiche a flogistiche della cute e dei tissuti molli. *Arch Sci Med (Torino)* 1977; **134:** 481.

161. Papageorgiou VP. Wound healing properties of naphthaquinone pigments from Alkanna tinctoria. *Experientia* 1978; **34:** 1499.

162. Paré A. *The Works of the Famous Chirurgian Ambrose Paré.* Johnson T, trans and ed. London: Cotes et Du Gard, 1649.

163. Partsch H. Do we need firm compression stockings exerting high pressure? *Vasa* 1984; **13:** 52.

164. Partsch H, Horakova MA. Compression stockings in the treatment of lower leg venous ulcer.*Wien Med Wochenschr* 1994; **144:** 242–9.

165. Patman RD. Sympathectomy in the treatment of chronic venous leg ulcers. *Arch Surg* 1982; **117:** 1561.

166. Patton MA. Eusol: the continuing controversy. (letter) *Br Med J* 1992; **304:** 1636.

167. Pattison M, Stacey MC, Layer GT, Burnand KG. Which elastic bandage gives the best compression? Personal observations, 1987.

168. Petit JL. *Traites des Maladies Chirurgicales.* Vol II. Paris: Mequignon, 1790.

169. Pflug JJ. Intermittent compression of the swollen leg in general practice. *Practitioner* 1975; **215:** 69.

170. Phillips A, Davidson M, Greaves MW. Venous leg ulceration: evaluation of zinc treatment, serum zinc and rate of healing. *Clin Exp Dermatol* 1978; **2:** 395.

171. Pickrell K, Thompson L, Nichol T, Kasdan M. The surgical treatment of varicose ulcers. *Am Surg* 1970; **36:** 55.

172. Poskitt KR, James AH, Lloyd-Davies ER, Walton J, McCollum C. Pinch grafting of porcine dermis in venous ulcers: a randomised trial. *Br Med J (Clin Res Ed)* 1987; **294:** 674–6.

173. Psathakis N. Has the 'substitute valve' at the popliteal vein solved the problem of venous insuffiency of the lower extremity? *J Cardiovasc Surg* 1968; **9:** 64.

174. Pulvertaft T. Paroven in the treatment of chronic venous insufficiency. *Practitioner* 1979; **223:** 838.

175. Rasmussen LH, Avnstorp C, Karlsmark T, Peters K, Horslev-Petersen K. Dose-response study of human growth hormone in venous ulcers: influence on healing and synthesis of collagen types I and III. *Phlebology* 1994; **9:** 92–8.

176. ter Riet G, Kessels AG, Knipschild P. Randomised clinical trial of ultrasound treatment for pressure ulcers. *Br Med J* 1995; **310:** 1040–1.

177. Robinson BJ. Randomized comparative trial of DuoDERM vs Viscopaste PB7 bandage in the management of venous leg ulceration and cost to the community. In: Ryan TJ, ed. *Beyond Occlusion: Wound Care Proceedings.* Royal Society of Medicine Services International Congress and Symposium series No 136. London: RSM Services Ltd, 1988.

178. Ruckley CV. Treatment of venous ulceration. *Phlebology Suppl* 1992; **1:** 22–6.

179. Rudofsky G. Intravenous prostaglandin E1 in the treatment of venous ulcers – a double-blind, placebo-controlled trial. *Vasa* 1989; **28(Suppl):** 39–43.

180. Rundle JSH, Cameron SH, Ruckley CV. New porcine dermis dressing for varicose and traumatic leg ulcers. *Br Med J* 1976; **2:** 216.

181. Rundle JSH, Elton RA, Cameron SH, Watson N, Gunn AA, Ruckley CV. Porcine dermis in varicose ulcers: a clinical trial. *Vasa* 1981; **10:** 246.

182. Ryan T. *The Management of Leg Ulcers.* Oxford: Oxford Medical Publishers, 1983.

183. Sawyer PN, Dowbak G, Sophie Z, Feller J, Cohen L. A preliminary report of the efficacy of Debrisan (dextranomer) in the debridement of cutaneous ulcers. *Surgery* 1979; **85:** 201.

184. Schraibman I, Stratton FJ. Nutritional status of patients with leg ulcers. *J R Soc Med* 1985; **78:** 39.

185. Sethia KK, Darke SG. Long saphenous incompetence as a cause of venous ulceration. *Br J Surg* 1984; **71:** 754.

186. Sharp S. *A Treatise on the Operations of Surgery.* 7th edition. London: Tonson, 1758.

187. Sigel B, Edelstein AL, Savitch L, Hasty JH, Felix WR. Types of compression for reducing venous stasis. *Arch Surg* 1975; **110:** 171.

188. Sigg K. Compression with pressure bandages and elastic stockings for prophylaxis and therapy of

venous disorders of the leg. *Fortschr Med* 1963; **15:** 601.

189. Sigg K. *Varizen, Ulcus Cruris and Thrombose*. 3rd edition. Berlin: Springer, 1968.

190. Simon DA. Community leg ulcer clinics: a comparative study in two health authorities. *Br Med J* 1996; **312:** 1648–51.

191. Skene AI, Smith JM, Dore CJ, Charlett A, Lewis JD. Venous leg ulcers: a prognostic index to predict time to healing. *Br Med J* 1992; **305:** 1119–21.

192. Skog E, Arnesjo B, Troeng T, *et al*. A randomized trial comparing cadexomer iodine and standard treatment in the out-patient management of chronic venous ulcers. *Br J Dermatol* 1983; **109:** 77.

193. Slavin J, Nash JR, Kingsnorth AN. Effect of transforming growth factor beta and basic fibroblast growth factor on steroid-impaired healing intestinal wounds. *Br J Surg* 1992; **79:** 69–72.

194. Slavin J, Nash JR, Kingsnorth AN. The effect of platelet derived growth factor (PDGF) on steroid impaired intestinal wounds. *Surg Res Commun* 1991; **11:** 233–8.

195. Somerville PG. The possible use of amniotic membrane in chronic leg ulcers. *Phlebologie* 1982; **35:** 223.

196. Spender JK. *A Manual of the Pathology and Treatment of Ulcers and Cutaneous Diseases of the Lower Limbs*. London: Churchill, 1866.

197. Stacey MC, Vandongren N, Trengove S, Hoskins S, Thompson P, Pearce C. The effectiveness of compression in healing venous ulcers. *Phlebology Suppl* 1995; **1:** 929–31.

198. Stacey-Clear A, Cornwall JV, Lewis JD. Intravenous prostacyclins (PGI$_2$) and skin grafting for rheumatoid leg ulcers. In: Negus D, Jantet G, eds. *Phlebology '85*. London: Libbey, 1986.

199. Starling EH. On the absorbtion of fluid from the connective tissue spaces. *J Physiol (Lond)* 1896; **19:** 312.

200. Stemmer R. Ambulatory elasto-compressive treatment of the lower extremities particularly with elastic stockings. *Der Kassenarzt* 1969; **9:** 1.

201. Stemmer R, Marescaux J, Furderer C. [Compression therapy of the lower extremities particularly with compression stockings.] *Hautarzt* 1980; **31:** 355–65.

202. Taheri SA, Lazar L, Elias SM, Marchand P. Vein valve transplant. *Surgery* 1982; **91:** 28.

203. Tennant WG, Park KGM, Ruckley CV. Testing compression bandages. *Phlebology* 1988; **3:** 55–61.

204. Thomas AMC, Tomlinson PJ, Boggon RP. Incompetent perforating vein ligation in the treatment of venous ulceration. *Ann R Coll Surg Engl* 1986; **68:** 214.

205. Travers JB, Makin GS. Reduction of varicose vein recurrence by use of postoperative compression stockings. *Phlebology* 1994; **9:** 104–7.

206. Trelford JD, Trelford-Sauder M. The amnion in surgery, past and present. *Am J Obstet Gynecol* 1977; **134:** 835.

207. Tsakayannis D, Li WW, Razvi S, Spirito N. Sucralfate and chronic venous stasis ulcers. *Lancet* 1994; **343:** 424–5.

208. Underwood M. *A Treatise upon Ulcers of the Legs*. London: Mathews, 1783.

209. Unna PG. *Die Histopathologie der Hautkrankheiten*. Berlin: Verlag Hirschwald, 1894.

210. Van den Berg E, Borgnis FE, Bollinger AA, Wupperman T, Alexander K. A new method for measuring the effective compression of medical stockings. *Vasa* 1982; **11:** 117.

211. Van der Molen HR. The choice of compressive methods in phlebology. *Phlebologie* 1982; **35:** 73.

212. Vanscheidt W, Peschen M, Kreitinger J, Schopf E. Paratibial fasciotomy: a new approach for treatment of therapy-resistant venous ulcers. *Phlebologie* 1994; **23:** 45–8.

213. Vin F. Corticothérapie locale ablusive en phlébologie. A propos d'une observation. *Phlebologie* 1982; **35:** 819.

214. Warren R, Thayer TR. Transplantation of the saphenous vein for post-phlebitic stasis. *Surgery* 1954; **35:** 867.

215. Weitgasser H. The use of pentoxifylline (Trental 400) in the treatment of leg ulcers: results of a double-blind trail. *Pharmatherapeutica* 1983; **3:** 143–51.

216. Weitgasser H, Schmidt-Modrow G. Trental forte in der Ulcus Cruris – Therapie. Ergebnnis einer Feldstudie. *Z Hautkr* 1982; **57:** 1574–80.

217. Westlake BC, Hasty JH. An analysis of factors to be addressed in the measurement of elastic compression. In: Negus D, Jantet G, eds. *Phlebology '85*. London: Libbey, 1986.

218. White RP. Ulcers of the legs, miscalled varicose: a clinical review. *Br J Dermatol* 1918; **30:** 138.

219. Wilson JAI, Henry M, Quill RD, Byrne PJ. The pH of varicose ulcer surfaces and its relationship to healing. *Vasa* 1979; **8:** 339.

220. Wiseman R. *Eight Chirurgical Treatises*. London: Tooke & Meredith, 1676.

221. Wright DDI, Franks PJ, Blair SD, Backhouse CM, Moffatt C, McCollum CN. Oxerutins in the prevention of recurrence in chronic venous ulceration: randomized controlled trial. *Br J Surg* 1991; **78:** 1269–70.

222. Zelikowski A, Argranat A, Sternberg A, Haddad M, Urca I. The conservative treatment of stasis ulcer. *Angiology* 1978; **29:** 832.

CHAPTER 21

Pulmonary embolism

Pulmonary thromboembolic disease	605	Prophylaxis of pulmonary embolism	622
Investigations	610	Some other special situations in pulmonary	
Diagnosis	616	embolic disease	623
Differential diagnosis	616	Other forms of pulmonary embolism which	
Natural history and prognosis	616	may mimic thromboembolism	624
Treatment	617	References	625

Pulmonary thromboembolic disease

Definition

Pulmonary thromboembolic disease is any condition in which the pulmonary arteries become obstructed by thrombus. Nearly always this thrombus has formed in the venous system or right heart and then embolized into the pulmonary arteries. If there have been no previous episodes and the right ventricle was normal prior to the embolism, the pulmonary artery pressure only rises to a limited degree because the normally thin-walled right ventricle cannot generate a high pressure in the face of obstruction.[107] The effects of the embolic episode may be worsened by thrombosis *in situ*.

Evidence of deep venous thrombosis (DVT) is found in at least 70–80% of patients who have had a pulmonary embolus (PE),[18,65] whereas studies of the natural history of DVT have established that PE occurs in up to 50% of patients with proximal vein thrombosis, and is less likely when the thrombus is confined to the calf veins.[30,62,63,109,112] The factors

predisposing to PE and DVT are the same, except in very special situations, and broadly fit Virchow's famous triad of venous stasis, injury to the vein wall and enhanced coagulability of the blood; often a definite predisposing factor can be identified, although occasionally DVT and PE occur for no apparent reason. Immobility is important and seems to be much more powerful when it is combined with trauma, surgery, or some other serious illness that enhances thrombosis. Other factors include neoplasia,[122] cardiac failure, oestrogen-containing oral contraceptives (the new low-oestrogen preparations have reduced this risk substantially) and pregnancy, which combines hormonal changes with venous stasis (PE remains one of the most frequent causes of maternal mortality during both pregnancy and the puerperium;[7] Table 21.1). Obesity is also an important risk factor,[45] which may operate alone but often seems particularly potent in combination with another factor such as the contraceptive pill or surgery. Occasionally, thromboembolic disease is due to abnormalities which increase clotting such as thrombocythaemia, cystinuria, antiphospholipid antibodies,[39,133] and the rare familial conditions of antithrombin, protein C and protein S deficiency[59,116] and factor V Leiden[21,141] (which is relatively common in the population compared with the other abnormalities mentioned), as well as defective fibrinolysis.[50] Paradoxically the thrombocytopenia associated with heparin therapy

*This chapter has been written by Roger Hall, BA, MD, FRCP, FESC, Professor of Clinical Cardiology, RPMS and Hammersmith Hospital.

Table 21.1 Risk factors for thromboembolic disease

Immobility
Trauma (and surgery)
Neoplasia
Prior history of thromboembolism
Reduced cardiac output
Clotting abnormalities, e.g. antithrombin deficiency,
    protein C or S deficiency, thrombocythaemia,
    elevated plasminogen-activator inhibitor
Obesity
Pregnancy and oestrogen-containing contraceptive pill
Indwelling catheters and electrodes in great veins and
    right heart

(HITS – the 'heparin induced thombocytopenia syndrome'[36]) also leads to increased coagulation. A risk factor that has emerged in recent years is thrombosis in association with indwelling catheters in the superior vena cava or right heart used for parenteral nutrition, chemotherapy, fluid infusion, pressure monitoring or occasionally pacing.[108] These techniques are often used in debilitated or immobilized patients who already have an increased risk of thrombosis. Risk factors are summarized in Table 21.1.

EPIDEMIOLOGY

The true incidence and mortality of PE in the population is unknown because the clinical diagnosis of both PE and DVT is extremely unreliable, many events are asymptomatic, the autopsy rates are low and death certification is inaccurate. Despite these problems, some authors have attempted to estimate the incidence using many tenuous assumptions.[23] The practising physician or surgeon is, however, in no doubt about the importance of this condition and its potentially disastrous effects. With increased awareness the mortality seems to be falling.[28,130] For instance, death from PE in surgical patients actually decreased from 8.8% of the total deaths in 1966 to 2.3% in 1980. The overall case fatality rate has also declined to about 13%,[3,14,42] being less than 5% in treated patients who are haemodynamically stable at presentation but approximately 20% in those who have persistent hypotension.

The prevalence of PE in hospitalized patients increases with age and is more common among men than women.[3,93] It may occur in as many as 25–50% of high-risk patients, i.e. after trauma, pelvic or orthopaedic surgery and even following myocardial infarction.[15,72]

Evidence of recent or old PE is detected in 25–30% of routine autopsies; with special techniques, this figure may exceed 60%.

PATHOLOGY

In the majority of patients the thrombi form in the veins of the leg, frequently beginning in the sinuses of the venous valves.[55] Whilst the majority of ilio-femoral thrombi develop as an extension of calf vein thrombi, those that develop as isolated proximal DVT are most often associated with hip surgery. In cases of massive fatal PE, the emboli mostly originate from the femoral and iliac veins.[130] They may also originate in the pelvis, particularly after gynaecological procedures. Thrombosis of the superior vena cava is becoming more common as a result of indwelling central venous catheters. The right atrial appendage has been incriminated as a source of emboli in chronic silent thromboembolism.[73] Fresh thrombi are susceptible to fragmentation in transit through the contracting right ventricle and often produce multiple smaller emboli.

In massive PE, the lumen of the pulmonary trunk and main pulmonary arteries is occluded or partially obstructed by thrombi, which may even fill the right ventricular cavity. The presence of organized thrombus in the pulmonary artery indicates that the patient has survived previous thromboembolic episodes. Recanalization of organized thrombus occurring over a long time produces fibrous bands and webs. In chronic thromboembolic pulmonary hypertension, the walls of the pulmonary trunk and main pulmonary arteries are hypertrophied and may contain atherosclerotic plaques.

PATHOPHYSIOLOGY AND CLINICAL FEATURES

The pathophysiology and clinical features of PE are so closely related that they are considered together. The effects of a PE depend mainly on the extent to which the embolus obstructs the pulmonary circulation, the duration over which that obstruction accumulates, and the pre-existing state of the patient. Although humoral factors and neural reflexes play a role in determining the severity of haemodynamic responses to PE in experimental animals, their role in man is uncertain. Some mediators (e.g. serotonin or thromboxane released from activated platelets) are probably capable of producing both bronchoconstriction and vascular spasm in non-embolized segments of the lung. As a result, a degree of pulmonary hypertension may

Table 21.2 Classification of pulmonary embolism

Pulmonary embolism	History	Degree of pulmonary artery obstruction (%)
Acute minor	Short	<50
Acute massive	Short	>50
Subacute massive	Several weeks	>50
Chronic thromboembolic hypertension	Months or years	Usually >50

develop that is disproportionately great for the amount of vasculature which is mechanically occluded. In general, a patient who has pre-existing cardiopulmonary disease, or who is old, frail or debilitated, will be more sensitive to the effects of an embolus than a patient who was well until the embolic event occurred. Most emboli are multiple. Small emboli are often asymptomatic.[109,157] As both the extent and chronicity of obstruction vary so widely, PE can produce widely differing clinical pictures. It is convenient to consider PE under four main headings (Table 21.2), but these are arbitrary divisions and some patients do not fit precisely into this classification.

Acute minor pulmonary embolism

If an embolus obstructs less than 50% of the pulmonary circulation, it is regarded as minor and often produces no symptoms. If symptoms do occur these are mainly some degree of dyspnoea due disturbed ventilation of the embolized area and possibly symptoms of pulmonary infarction with pleuritic chest pain, haemoptysis and fever. Pulmonary infarction occurs in only about 10% of patients without pre-existing cardiopulmonary disease because in 90% of patients the bronchial blood supply is sufficient to maintain the viability of the lung. If, however, the embolized segment is already compromised, because either the bronchial arterial supply or the airways are abnormal as a result of pre-existing cardiopulmonary disease, then the incidence of infarction rises to 30%.[130]

If there are any physical signs, they are those of pulmonary infarction. The patient is often distressed, with rapid shallow breathing because of the pleuritic pain, but is not cyanosed because the disturbance of gas transfer is only slight. Fever is common due to infarcted lung, and is sometimes such a prominent feature that it is difficult to differentiate a PE from an infective cause of pleurisy. The fever and pain often produce a sinus tachycardia. Pulmonary artery mean pressure rarely exceeds 20–25 mmHg. Since minor PE does not compromise the right ventricle, cardiac output is well main-

tained, hypotension does not occur and the venous pressure and heart sounds are usually normal. The P2 is not loud despite a commonly held belief to the contrary and although atrial fibrillation can occur the rhythm is usually sinus. Signs of pulmonary infarction may be found in the lungs – a mixture of consolidation and effusion, possibly with a pleural rub. In about 20% of patients, there will also be signs of a DVT which sometimes reveal themselves after the PE has occurred.

Acute massive pulmonary embolism

When >50% of the pulmonary circulation is suddenly obstructed, the pathophysiology and clinical signs become dominated by the acute and severe derangement of cardiac and pulmonary function and this situation is termed acute massive PE. This form of PE is much less common than minor PE. The right ventricle is a thin-walled structure designed to work against the normally low pulmonary vascular resistance; consequently, it performs poorly against a sudden obstruction. As a result, it dilates and fails so that there is only a moderate rise in the right ventricular and pulmonary artery systolic pressure which rarely exceeds 50–60 mmHg.[107] Cardiac output falls and the patient suddenly becomes hypotensive. This may occur so rapidly that syncope is either the presenting feature[46] or easily induced by a relatively minor cardiovascular stress, such as sitting up or the vasodilatation consequent on getting into a warm bath. If the degree of obstruction is sufficient, death occurs almost immediately. The right ventricular end-diastolic pressure and right atrial pressure rise as the ventricle fails, and they are often of the order of 15–20 mmHg. Acute right ventricular dilatation leads to tricuspid regurgitation. In the final stages, the fall in aortic pressure and the rise in right ventricular diastolic pressure cause ischaemia of the right ventricle through a critical reduction of right coronary perfusion.[153]

Severe hypoxaemia develops which correlates roughly with the extent of embolism.[101,123,126] Although massive PE without hypoxaemia has

Table 21.3 Symptoms and signs of acute massive pulmonary embolism

	Symptoms	Signs
Previous minor pulmonary embolism	Pleuritic chest pain, haemoptysis	Pleural rub, signs of pleural fluid and pulmonary consolidation
Severe V/Q disturbance	Dyspnoea, anginal chest pain	Central cyanosis
Obstruction to right ventricular outflow	Postural hypotension, syncope, angina	Hypotension, tachycardia (sinus), peripheral circulatory shutdown and cyanosis; jugular venous pressure increased, S3 (left sternal border), wide splitting of S2

Table 21.4 Frequency of presenting symptoms and physical signs of acute massive pulmonary embolism

Symptoms/signs	Frequency (%)
Symptoms	
Acute onset dyspnoea	87
Syncope/'collapse'	70
Central chest pain	22
Physical signs	
Sinus tachycardia, small sharp pulse, low blood pressure, low urine flow, peripheral vasoconstriction = 'Shock'	90
Gallop rhythm LSE	87
Raised central venous pressure	79
Central cyanosis	62
Single second heart sound (S2)	60
Widely split S2	40

LSE, left sternal border (edge).

been reported,[74] it must be regarded as being so rare that if the arterial oxygen tension is normal an alternative diagnosis should be seriously considered. The combination of respiratory and circulatory failure results in a critical situation.

The mechanisms leading to the severe hypoxaemia of acute massive pulmonary embolism are incompletely understood, mainly because this is a very difficult situation in which to carry out studies to clarify the situation. The main factors[25,61,98,126] seem to be ventilation–perfusion mismatch, intrapulmonary shunting and shunting via a patent foramen ovale[76] if one is present (20–30% of the population have one), a very low mixed venous oxygen saturation caused by the severely reduced cardiac output so that there is not enough transit time in the lung for complete oxygenation to occur, and miscellaneous other factors among

which is bronchospasm which can sometimes be severe.[159]

The clinical features of acute massive PE can be explained in terms of these pathophysiological changes (Table 21.3). The frequency of the symptoms and the physical signs are shown in Table 21.4. Usually the patient becomes acutely distressed, severely short of breath, and may be syncopal as a result of the combination of hypoxaemia and low cardiac output. Anginal-type chest pain may be caused by the combination of hypotension, hypoxaemia and increased cardiac work, although it is usually a much less prominent symptom than the dyspnoea. The physical signs are those of reduced cardiac output, i.e. marked sinus tachycardia, hypotension and a cool periphery, sometimes with confusion and oliguria. In addition, the patient is nearly always obviously dyspnoeic (but not orthopnoeic), cyanosed both centrally and peripherally and has signs of acute right heart strain, consisting of a raised venous pressure, which is often difficult to appreciate because of the respiratory distress, a gallop rhythm at the right sternal border and a widely split second heart sound caused by the delayed right ventricular ejection, which is often difficult to detect because of the accompanying tachycardia. The pulmonary component of the second heart sound is usually normal and not loud because the pulmonary artery pressure is only moderately raised. In addition to these features, there may be symptoms and signs of a preceding minor embolus that produced pulmonary infarction.

Subacute massive pulmonary embolism

Subacute massive PE is even less common than acute massive pulmonary embolism but is an important condition caused by multiple emboli of moderate or small size that accumulate (usually over several weeks) to obstruct the pulmonary circulation. Because this obstruction occurs slowly, there is time for the right ventricle to adapt and for some hypertrophy to develop; consequently, the right ventricular and pulmonary artery pressures are higher than those in the acute forms of PE.[53] The main symptoms are insidiously increasing dyspnoea and falling exercise tolerance. There is often an associated cough. Normally, the most prominent physical sign is shortness of breath which is out of proportion to all other findings, and there may be central cyanosis. The blood pressure and pulse rate are usually normal because the cardiac output is well maintained. Commonly, the venous pressure is raised and a third heart sound is audible at the right sternal border which may be accentuated by inspiration. The pulmonary component of the second heart sound is sometimes loud.[53] In some cases, all these right heart signs are absent. There may also be intermittent symptoms and signs of the pulmonary infarction that occurred during the build-up of the obstruction. In advanced cases, right heart failure develops and eventually the cardiac output falls. A further pulmonary embolus may change the clinical picture to one that resembles acute massive PE. An obvious predisposing factor may be detected (see Table 21.1) but less often than in the acute forms of PE.[53]

Chronic thromboembolic pulmonary hypertension

Chronic thromboembolic pulmonary hypertension[111] is the least common form of thromboembolic disease and is only mentioned here for the sake of completeness. Large and medium-sized pulmonary vessels become obstructed with organized, fibrotic masses in a haphazard fashion. It has been assumed that this form of obstruction is the result of single or recurrent unresolved emboli, initially overlooked and untreated, occurring over months to years, resulting in symptoms of pulmonary hypertension rather than symptoms of repeated symptomatic PE. However, in many cases, the evidence for this mechanism is weak because often there are no identifiable thromboembolic episodes in the history.[129,140] No strong evidence has as yet been provided to indicate that patients who fail to resolve emboli have a recognized disorder of coagulation. It is possible that in some cases thrombosis *in situ* may be an important mechanism, causing retrograde propagation of the initial emboli. Chronic thromboembolic pulmonary hypertension is pathologically, but not necessarily clinically, quite distinct from primary pulmonary hypertension, in which the obstructing lesions (often non-thrombotic) appear in the small, distal pulmonary arteries.

The main pathophysiological features are those of impaired gas exchange and obstruction to the output of the right heart, which produce exertional dyspnoea and reduced exercise tolerance with the physical signs of severe pulmonary hypertension combined with cyanosis. As bronchial arterial collateral blood flow increases substantially with persistence of pulmonary arterial obstruction, the flow to the capillary bed and thus surfactant production and alveolar stability is retained, and the patients do not suffer permanent parenchymal injury to the lung. As with other causes of severe pulmonary hypertension, there may be classical angina of effort. A chronic non-productive cough and recurrent haemoptysis may occur. Tachypnoea, persisting during sleep, is an prominent feature. The pulse rate and blood pressure are normal until a very late stage of the disease. The systolic murmur of tricuspid regurgitation is common. As identifiable episodes of pulmonary infarction are unusual, abnormal physical signs in the lungs are not a feature of this condition. Sometimes, however, the murmur (or murmurs) caused by the partial obstruction of the pulmonary arteries is heard over the lung fields.[110] Obvious predisposing factors are often absent, but some patients have long-standing and severe venous thrombosis of the lower limb(s).[129] The illness usually develops insidiously over several years and consequently its onset is difficult to identify. The average time from onset of the non-specific symptoms to diagnosis exceeds 3 years.[5] Ultimately, the condition leads inexorably to right heart failure and death.[129,140] These patients require long-term anticoagulation and if, as they often are, they are very disabled the possibility of thromboarterectomy of the obstructed pulmonary arteries should be considered. This operation, in experienced hands, has a hospital mortality in the region of 13%, which is less than the mortality of heart–lung transplantation which is the only other possibility. The late results have been good with a sustained fall in the pulmonary artery pressure and reduction in symptoms[22,110,111]

Investigations

ELECTROCARDIOGRAM

ECG changes, although common in PE, are usually non-specific.[139] In acute minor PE, there is no real haemodynamic stress and therefore the only finding is sinus tachycardia. In acute massive PE, evidence of right heart strain may be seen, but the classic and indeed specific S1Q3T3 pattern (Figure 21.1) occurs in only a limited number of cases; similar changes are seen in subacute massive PE but they are less common and sometimes the ECG is normal. The main value of ECG is in excluding other potential diagnoses, such as myocardial infarction. In chronic thromboembolic pulmonary hypertension, there is nearly always evidence of right ventricular hypertrophy by the time the condition is a clinical problem.

CHEST RADIOGRAPH

The chest radiograph findings are also non-specific but they may be helpful. A normal film is compatible with all but chronic thromboembolic pulmonary hypertension and in fact, a normal film in a patient with severe acute dyspnoea and hypoxaemia without clinical signs of bronchospasm is very suspicious of PE.[137] In all types except chronic thromboembolic pulmonary hypertension, the heart shadow is normal and the lung fields may show evidence of pulmonary infarction, either single or multiple; peripheral opacities, sometimes but not always wedge-shaped; linear shadows, which may radiate out from the hila; pleural effusions, and elevation of the diaphragm(s) are the most common signs. In minor PE, the main branches of the pulmonary artery are normal. In acute massive PE, a plump pulmonary artery shadow may be seen, particularly in the right hilum, but the main pulmonary artery is normal, whereas in subacute massive PE it is occasionally enlarged when the pulmonary artery pressure is elevated. It may be possible to detect areas of oligaemia in the parts of the lung affected by emboli[78] (particularly in acute massive PE), but this is difficult, not particularly accurate and almost impossible on the type of portable film that is usually available in the acute situation. Very occasionally, patchy pulmonary oedema is seen on the chest radiograph.

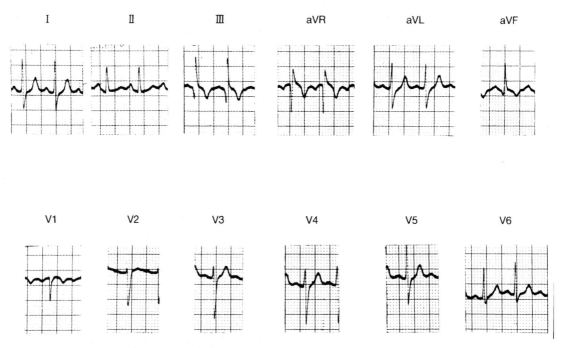

Figure 21.1   Acute massive pulmonary embolism. Electrocardiogram showing typical 'S1, Q3, T3' pattern. In this patient there is T wave inversion in lead V1; more typically T wave inversion extends to leads V3 or V4.

The chest radiograph is especially valuable in excluding other conditions mimicking acute PE (pneumothorax, pneumonia, left heart failure, rib fracture, massive pleural effusion, mediastinal emphysema) and is also necessary for the proper interpretation of the lung scan.

In chronic thromboembolic pulmonary hypertension, the main pulmonary artery and the large arteries in the hila are very prominent due to the severe and long-standing pulmonary hypertension and cardiomegaly is common.

ECHOCARDIOGRAPHY

Transthoracic echocardiography rarely enables direct visualization of the pulmonary embolus but may reveal thrombus floating in the right atrium or ventricle.[70,81,94] In acute massive PE the right ventricle is obviously dilated.[12] With transoesophageal echocardiography, it is possible to visualize massive emboli in the main pulmonary artery, proximal left pulmonary artery, and somewhat further down the proximal right pulmonary artery.[99,120,160] The Doppler technique may allow the pulmonary artery systolic pressure to be measured.[125,148] Although echocardiography is of limited use in the diagnosis of PE, it may be helpful in excluding or suggesting alternative causes for cardiovascular collapse (aortic dissection, pericardial tamponade, etc.).

BLOOD GASES

The characteristic changes are a reduced PaO_2, and a $PaCO_2$ that is normal, or is reduced because of hyperventilation.[61,123] There is a rough correlation between the extent of hypoxaemia and embolism if there is no prior cardiopulmonary disease.[20,101] The PaO_2 is almost never normal when a patient with massive PE (acute, subacute or chronic) is breathing room air but can be occasionally normal in minor PE, if the patient is hyperventilating.

LUNG FUNCTION TESTS

These have little place in the acute situation but may be very useful for distinguishing patients with chronic and subacute embolic pulmonary hypertension from those in whom airways obstruction or lung restriction is the true diagnosis.[13,25,61,128,132]

BIOCHEMISTRY

There is no blood test that will diagnose thromboembolic disease. Although intravascular thrombosis is indicated by the sensitive thrombin-antithrombin III (T-AT) complex assay[84], and fibrinolysis by the assay of cross-linked fibrin degradation products (D-dimer),[92,134] these tests have a low specificity and are positive not only when there is PE or DVT but also in the presence of disseminated intravascular coagulation, malignant neoplasms and after surgery. However, it has been suggested that negative tests may be strong enough evidence that clotting has not occurred and that anticoagulants can be withheld.[27,155]

LUNG SCANS

Perfusion lung scan with Tc-99m albumin macroaggreggates or microspheres is very sensitive in detecting PE and modern diagnosis and management is heavily based on their results. A normal perfusion lung scan essentially excludes the diagnosis because all types of occlusive PE produce a defect of perfusion (Figure 21.2).[67] However, many conditions other than PE, such as tumours, consolidation, vasculitis, bullous lesions and chronic obstructive airways disease, may also produce perfusion defects. The addition of a ventilation scan, obtained by the inhalation of a radioactive tracer (Xe-133, Xe-127, Kr-81m or an Tc-99m aerosol), greatly increases the specificity of this technique. PE produces a defect of perfusion but not of ventilation (Figure 21.2) whereas most of the other conditions mentioned above produce a ventilation defect in the same area as the perfusion defect. The extent and severity of the pulmonary embolism is reflected in the degree of abnormality of the lung scan (Figure 21.3). PE can also produce 'matched defects' when infarction has occurred, but in this situation the chest radiograph is nearly always abnormal, showing shadowing in the area of lung scan defect. In both acute massive PE and subacute massive PE the perfusion defects are always extensive.

The lung scan is an indirect method of diagnosis since it does not detect the embolus itself but only its main consequence, the perfusion abnormality. The probability that perfusion defects have been caused by PE can be assessed as high, intermediate or low, depending on the type of scan abnormality.[9,102,143,154] If the scan is of a high probability type (basically multiple large perfusion defects with a normal ventilation scan) there is an 85% chance that the patient has PE. However, 60% of patients with PE do not have high probability scans and instead have scans that suggest either low or medium probability.[66,143] Taking the clinical circumstances into account improves diagnostic accuracy slightly (Table 21.5). Although the

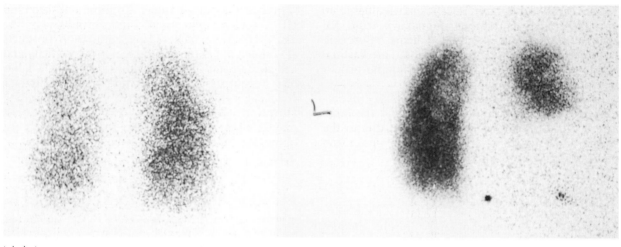

Inhalation   Posterior

Figure 21.2   The ventilation–perfusion (V/Q) scans of a patient with a large single pulmonary embolus. Ventilation (V) on left; perfusion (Q) on right. These posterior views show a large defect of perfusion at the base of the right lung, caused by a pulmonary embolus, while ventilation in that area remains normal.

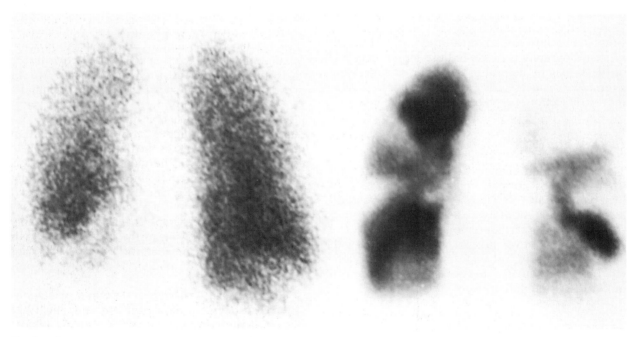

First breath   Posterior

Figure 21.3   The ventilation–perfusion (V/Q) scans of a patient with multiple pulmonary emboli (ventilation on left; perfusion on right). These posterior views show multiple perfusion defects in both lungs while ventilation in these areas remains normal. This appearance is typical of multiple pulmonary emboli.

lung scan is often an imprecise guide, it is extremely useful in clinical decision making. A normal scan means that treatment for suspected PE can be withheld and a high probability scan means that treatment is mandatory. Clinical judge-ment combined with objective tests for DVT and pulmonary angiography must be used to decide on the therapy for those patients who are between these extremes and in whom the probability is assessed as low or medium.

Table 21.5 Occurrence of angiographically proven pulmonary emboli (in %) according to scan category and clinical probability[72]

V/Q scan probability	Clinical probability			
probabilities	Low	Medium	High	All
Normal	2	6	0	4
Low	4	16	40	14
Intermediate	16	28	66	30
High	56	88	96	87
Any abnormal scan	9	30	68	33

Follow-up scans may be helpful retrospectively. The majority of abnormalities caused by PE will show some change in the perfusion pattern within 1 week,[123] although failure to change does not exclude the diagnosis.[1] The lung scan also serves as a guide to suspicious areas if pulmonary angiography is required. A follow-up scan at the time of discharge is helpful in establishing a new baseline for subsequent episodes of suspected PE.

In chronic thromboembolic pulmonary hypertension, one or more segmental mismatched defects are always present, but unlike the relatively close correlation between the findings on perfusion scans and angiograms in acute PE, the scan in chronic thromboembolic pulmonary hypertension consistently and often dramatically underestimates the extent of major vessel obstruction revealed by angiography.

RIGHT HEART CATHETERIZATION AND PULMONARY ANGIOGRAPHY

The pulmonary angiogram is the only technique that can diagnose PE with certainty (Figures 21.4 and 21.5) and as such its main role is when there is important diagnostic doubt particularly when the empirical use of anticoagulation would have very significant disadvantages. As a technique it has disadvantages, the most important of which are its limited availability and a small but definite mortality (<0.5%).[8,138] This risk gets higher the more seriously ill the patient is, and is particularly great when there is significant pulmonary hypertension due to chronic thromboembolic pulmonary hypertension. Pulmonary angiography should not be carried out in the radiology department of a hospital that does not perform cardiac angiography routinely because it is essential to apply the skill that arises from the everyday use of invasive cardiology to the acutely ill patient.

Miller *et al.*[107] developed a convenient angiographic scoring system to assess the severity of PE using a combination of the number of vessels involved by embolus and the degree to which perfusion is reduced. In patients with no underlying cardiopulmonary disease this score correlates directly with the severity of pulmonary hypertension and hypoxaemia.

The changes in the right heart pressures that occur in PE are summarized in Table 21.6. It is very helpful to obtain right heart pressures and oxygen saturations before angiography so that the haemodynamic situation, including cardiac output and any intracardiac shunting, can be identified. Occasionally, if the precatheter diagnosis is wrong, the haemodynamic data may suggest the correct diagnosis and lead to appropriate therapy.[8]

After angiography, attempts can be made to fragment and dislodge the acute embolus more peripherally using the angiographic catheter with a guide wire.[11,60] An alternative approach is to aspirate embolic material with a specially designed catheter.[147] This technique is technically difficult, partly because the catheter is very large, making the whole procedure so technically demanding that very few people attempt it.

OTHER IMAGING TECHNIQUES

Digital subtraction angiography (DSA) may be adequate for showing proximal arterial occlusions,

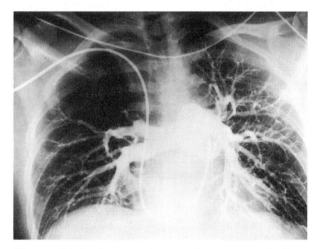

Figure 21.4 Acute minor pulmonary embolism. Pulmonary arteriograph showing occlusion of the right upper lobe pulmonary artery. There was no haemodynamic disturbance.

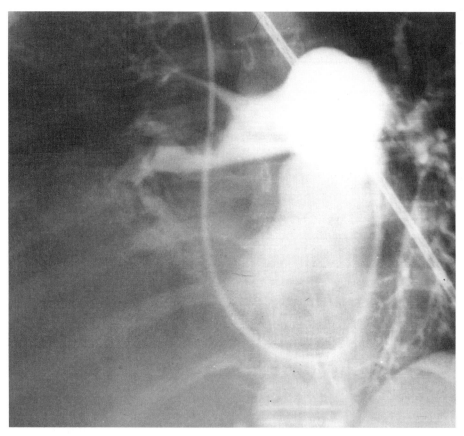

Figure 21.5 Acute massive pulmonary embolism. Pulmonary arteriograph. There is a 'saddle embolus' astride the bifurcation of the right pulmonary artery causing a convex filling defect typical of acute (recent) embolism.

Table 21.6 Typical right heart pressures in thromboembolic disease

	Pressures (mmHg)			
	RA	RV	PA	Comment
Minor pulmonary embolism	5	30/0–5	30/15	Normal pressures
Acute massive pulmonary embolism	12	45/0–12	45/20	Severe pulmonary hypertension does not occur. Systolic PAP rarely >50 mmHg. RAP and RVEDP usually raised
Subacute massive pulmonary embolism	6	70/0–6	70/35	RAP and RVEDP may be raised. RV and PA systolic range 50–90 mmHg
Chronic thromboembolic pulmonary hypertension	6	90/0–6	90/50	RAP and RVEDP higher when patient develops congestive cardiac failure

PA, pulmonary artery; PAP, pulmonary artery pressure; RA, right atrium; RAP, right atrial pressure; RV, right ventricle; RVEDP, right ventricular end-diastolic pressure.

but is generally rather disappointing and PE cannot be excluded on the basis of a normal DSA.[113] The new technique of spiral CT looks promising but its place has yet to be defined.[150]

SEARCH FOR DEEP VENOUS THROMBOSIS

Phlebograms will show thrombus in the deep venous system in at least 70% of patients who have sustained PE, but thrombus will often be present in patients who have not.[18,65] Consequently, phlebograms and other methods for detecting thrombus in the deep veins, such as serial impedance plethysmography,[2,41,62,68] or duplex ultrasound[37] have limited value in making the definitive diagnosis of PE. Furthermore, phlebography is costly and difficult to carry out in the acutely ill patient. However, the detection of DVT gives further information on which to base the decision to treat or not,[68] particularly when the lung scan suggests an intermediate or even low probability of PE; for example, the chance of a serious PE is very low with a low-risk lung scan and normal veins and anticoagulation can be omitted, whereas if there is definite DVT this demands therapy in its own right regardless of the lung scan result.[41,66] This approach needs caution if the patient is likely to remain immobile or if there could be an embolic source elsewhere (e.g. right atrium or vena cava).

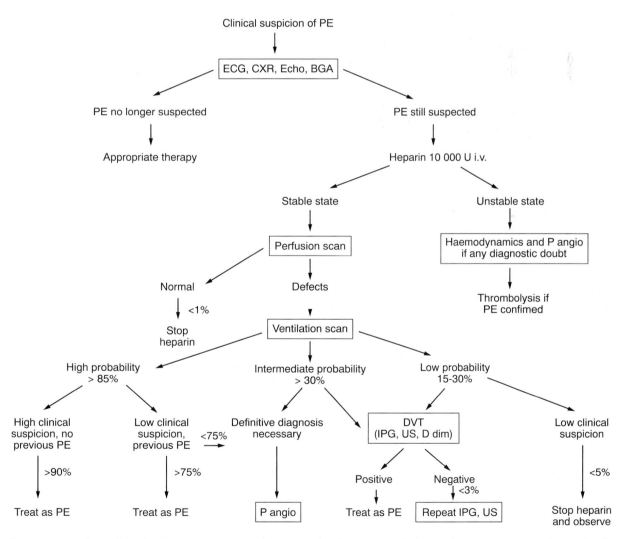

Figure 21.6 Flow chart for the management of suspected pulmonary embolism. The percentages indicate the frequency of proven pulmonary embolism in each group. BGA, blood gas analysis; CXR, chest x-ray; D-dim, D-dimer; DVT, deep vein thrombosis; ECG, echocardiogram; IPG, impedance plethysmography; P angio, pulmonary angiogram; PE, pulmonary embolism; US, duplex ultrasound.

Diagnosis (Figure 21.6)

An accurate diagnosis of PE is important to prevent excessive morbidity and mortality from either failure to treat when necessary or inappropriate anticoagulation. It is important to remember that the consequences of missing the diagnosis can be fatal in an otherwise fit patient, the overall risk of therapy has a mortality of less than 0.1%, and that in some studies up to 75% of the patients who have the diagnosis suspected do not have the condition. The clinical diagnosis of PE is often difficult,[33] particularly when there is coexisting heart or lung disease[32,94,131] and it is notoriously inaccurate when based on clinical signs alone.[30,56,126,130,149] The diagnostic difficulties arise because most of the symptoms and signs are non-specific. The diagnosis requires a high level of clinical suspicion and the judicious use of investigations to confirm or refute this suspicion. Normal blood gases make the diagnosis unlikely (but not impossible). As ECG and chest radiograph abnormalities in PE are non-specific, absent, transient, or delayed, they cannot be used to confirm the diagnosis although they may add to suspicion.[139] Echocardiography may occasionally show the embolus but more often gives indirect information by giving information about the pulmonary artery pressure and the state of the right ventricle. Thus none of these investigations is reliably diagnostic but may give some useful information and, together with clinical history and examination, provide reasonably good predictions. If there are no contraindications to anticoagulation it is prudent to begin heparin while undertaking the necessary tests.[77,126]

The lung scan plays a central role in diagnosis; in about one-third of cases it either rules out the diagnosis by being normal[67] or suggests a high enough likelihood of PE (Table 21.5) that therapy can be undertaken on the basis of its results and no further studies are necessary unless the findings do not fit the clinical situation. However, an uncritical assumption that an intermediate or a low-probability scan excludes PE is unwarranted and potentially dangerous. If significant doubt remains after the lung scan, there are three possible approaches:

1. to carry out pulmonary angiography
2. to start treatment while accepting some degree of uncertainty
3. to obtain some additional evidence of thromboembolism.

Some authorities advocate strongly the more widespread use of pulmonary angiography,[8,103] but the value of such an expensive approach is dubious and may have little or no advantage over accepting

moderate degrees of doubt and only using angiography in particularly difficult cases.

The value of looking for other confirmatory evidence of thrombosis in the difficult case has been discussed already. Such confirmation is usually in the form of evidence of DVT but may be based on biochemical evidence of thrombosis which is becoming far more sophisticated.

If there is no apparent predisposing cause for thrombosis, the patient should be screened for occult cancer and coagulation defects[21,39,59,116,122,133] (see Chapter 8).

Differential diagnosis

The differential diagnosis is wide.[69] For acute minor PE it consists of all forms of acute respiratory illness that can lead to any combination of pleuritic pain, fever, haemoptysis and dyspnoea (e.g. acute bronchitis, pneumonia); that of acute massive PE includes all conditions that can lead to acute circulatory collapse particularly if they are likely also to cause acute dyspnoea (e.g. cardiac tamponade, myocardial infarction, tension pneumothorax, severe asthma, dissecting aneurysm of the aorta). The conditions that have to be differentiated from subacute massive PE are those that lead to exertional dyspnoea that develops over a few weeks or months. The most important are cardiac failure and respiratory conditions, such as chronic obstructive airways disease, asthma and fibrosing alveolitis.

The differential diagnosis of chronic thromboembolic pulmonary hypertension includes all causes of severe pulmonary hypertension. The most important distinctions are from primary pulmonary hypertension and hypoxic cor pulmonale. The perfusion lung scan is usually near normal or mottled in primary pulmonary hypertension and shows gross widespread perfusion defects with normal ventilation in chronic thromboembolic pulmonary hypertension. Chronic thromboembolic pulmonary hypertension is usually easily distinguished from hypoxic cor pulmonale by lung function tests.

Natural history and prognosis

The early mortality of treated minor PE is very low. Although a small number of patients succumb to a recurrent large embolus or to haemorrhage due to anticoagulant therapy;[52,158] mortality is usually under 5%. The original study of Barritt and Jordan[6] showed a recurrence rate in the untreated control group of 35%. This risk is reduced substantially by adequate anticoagulant therapy.[28,40] Multiple small recurrent emboli occurring for several weeks after the initial episode may cause subacute massive PE, but this is rare.

The long-term prognosis in minor PE is excellent. Once the patient has recovered from the initial event, the normal outcome is complete recovery without any late sequelae.[129] Recurrent emboli months or years after the initial episode are uncommon[28,140] (the risk is about 0.5% per annum), particularly if the risk factor leading to the initial episode was identifiable and resolved. The absence of a well-defined risk factor suggests an adverse prognosis because both recurrent PE and occult malignancy are more frequent in such patients.[59] If late recurrence does occur, there is often an identifiable risk factor.

In the short term, there are several possible outcomes in acute massive PE. Most of the deaths result from the initial haemodynamic insult and occur either immediately or within a few hours. A few patients survive the initial insult but have profound hypotension which persists and leads to death as long as 24 or 48 hours later unless effective treatment is instituted. The patients who survive the initial insult run an extremely high risk of a recurrent embolus, which often proves fatal, unless they are promptly heparinized.[6] In this group of patients, the main aim of therapy is to prevent further emboli.[40]

In the majority of patients who survive the initial illness, the long-term prognosis is good[54,117] and is influenced mainly by any underlying chronic disease, of which cancer, congestive heart failure, and chronic lung disease are the most important.[28] As with minor PE, there is a small risk of recurrence, particularly if there is a chronic predisposing factor or the patient enters another high-risk situation, for example, further surgery. Chronic thromboembolic pulmonary hypertension is only a long-term sequel in a very small number of patients. These patients can be recognized at an early stage (2–3 months after the initial event) because their pulmonary artery pressure remains elevated (mean >30 mmHg), rather than returning to normal, or near normal, as is usual in the vast majority of patients.[129] A few patients with a particularly strong predisposing factor, usually malignant disease, have frequent recurrent emboli despite therapy.

There are few data on the natural history of subacute massive PE, even with therapy. It has a high (>20%) early mortality,[53] but little is known about the long-term prognosis. The results of the only studies that have been performed suggest that if the patient survives the initial episode the outcome is usually good but that chronic thromboembolic pulmonary hypertension, although uncommon, may occur.[129] As in other forms of the disease, this risk can be predicted with some accuracy by measuring the pulmonary artery pressure 2–3 months after the onset of the illness. If the mean pulmonary artery pressure is still >30 mmHg, the risk of chronic thromboembolic pulmonary hypertension developing is high.[129]

Treatment

Schemes for the management and treatment of PE are given in Figures 21.6 and 21.7, and problems related to therapy have been critically reviewed elsewhere.[36,52,71]

GENERAL MEASURES

Patients who are in pain should receive analgesia but they should be used with extreme care in the hypotensive patient. If there is hypoxaemia, oxygen should be given by face mask. When the cardiac output is reduced, the dilated right ventricle is hypoxic and already near-maximally stimulated by the high level of endogenous catecholamines, it is unlikely to respond to inotropic agents, which may do no more than precipitate arrhythmias. When absolutely necessary, the judicious use of noradrenaline titrated against a moderate increase in blood pressure might be beneficial in improving right ventricular function and systemic haemodynamics.[57] The right atrial pressure should be allowed to remain at a high level (normally 15–20 mmHg) which is necessary if the failing right ventricle is to maintain its output; if the right atrial pressure falls for any reason (e.g. dehydration or bleeding), administration of fluid while monitoring venous pressure may be helpful. Diuretics and vasodilators should be avoided at all times.

If angiography shows massive emboli in the main pulmonary arteries, it may be possible to break these up thus dispersing them more peripherally, using a pigtail catheter and a guide wire.[11,60] The rationale is that the cross-sectional area and thus obstructive capacity of an embolus is large in relation to the proximal pulmonary arteries but when fragmented is much smaller in relation to the more distal vascular bed which has a larger total cross-sectional area. Thus the same thrombus fragmented and displaced distally obstructs a smaller percentage of the vascular bed. Cardiac massage probably achieves the same beneficial effect in a small number of patients.

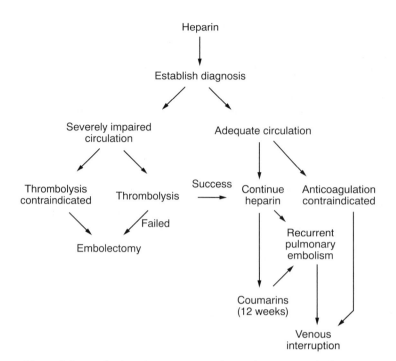

Figure 21.7   Scheme for treating acute massive pulmonary embolism.

HEPARIN

Unfractionated heparin is the mainstay of treatment for all patients who do not have severe circulatory embarrassment. The action of heparin both in reducing the risk of a further embolus and reducing mediator-induced pulmonary vascular constriction and bronchoconstriction from thrombin activation and platelet aggregation is immediate.[25] When there is a definite suspicion of PE and no strong contraindication to anticoagulation, it is wise to start therapy before the diagnosis is confirmed. If subsequent tests rule out the diagnosis then therapy can be stopped.

There is strong evidence that heparin substantially reduces mortality almost entirely by preventing recurrent PE,[6,28,40] thereby allowing the patient's native thrombolytic mechanisms to destroy the thrombus in the pulmonary arteries. The dose of heparin is often arbitrary, although sometimes adjusted in accordance with the results of the clotting tests. The findings of most studies suggest that it should be between 480 and 600 U/kg/day and that therapy should be initiated with a bolus of 10 000 units. Although the value of careful control of the level of anticoagulation for the prevention of complications and for the improvement of therapeutic efficacy is unproven, control is often attempted.[52,89] Various clotting tests are available; the most commonly used is the

activated partial thromboplastin time (aPTT). This should be maintained at 1.5–2.5 times the mean control value, which is equivalent to a plasma heparin level judged from animal experiments to be effective in preventing clot extension. Measurements of heparin levels by anti-Xa activity appears to be more sensitive than the aPTT, and will soon become widely available. A wide diurnal variation in heparin activity has been reported[26] and therefore the tests should be performed at the same time of day if possible.

The correct duration of therapy is not known, but for a major thromboembolic episode it should be at least 1 week, because this is the minimum amount of time that it takes for thrombus already present to become adherent to vein walls; therapy should be continued until the patient is ambulant. Oral anticoagulants are started 24 hours after heparin therapy is commenced and should be administered jointly with heparin for at least 4 days.

Recurrent PE may occur during the first few days of heparin therapy before the peripheral thrombus becomes adherent to the endothelium and does not constitute a therapeutic failure. About 40% of patients who suffer recurrence while receiving heparin will be found to be inadequately anticoagulated as reflected by an aPTT below the therapeutic range.[10] Increasing the dose of heparin should be the initial alteration in therapy in these patients.

Low-dose heparin has no place in the management of acute PE because it works by preventing the activation of the coagulation cascade, an event that has already occurred in such patients. It may sometimes be an alternative to the use of oral anticoagulants for preventing recurrent PE after the initial episode has been successfully treated,[64] although there is evidence that it is less effective than the use of coumarin derivatives. Its main use is in the prevention of DVT and PE.

Haemorrhagic complications occur in up to 20% of patients on full-dose heparin, but they are serious in only 4–7% and the mortality directly attributable to therapy is in the region of 0.1%.[89,158] These problems are most likely if the patient has a potential source of bleeding such as an active peptic ulcer or any of a wide variety of risk factors, the most important of which are a pre-existing bleeding tendency, uraemia, advanced age, obesity, recent surgery, severe hypertension and previous gastrointestinal haemorrhage.[52,89,158] Blood transfusion will correct massive blood loss, but protamine is the specific antidote. Heparin therapy is absolutely contraindicated if the patient has had a recent haemorrhagic stroke. Occasionally, prolonged administration of heparin will lead to osteoporosis.

Heparin causes transient mild thrombocytopenia in about 20% of patients and severe thrombocytopenia in few.[16,36] The milder variety occurs within the first 4 days of heparin administration and is the result of the direct aggregation effect of heparin on platelets. The platelet count is generally $100–150 \times 10^9/l$. The patient is usually asymptomatic and thrombocytopenia resolves spontaneously in spite of continuation of heparin therapy. The severe heparin-induced thrombocytopenia produces what has come to be known as the HITS syndrome (heparin-induced thrombocytopenia syndrome) which occurs 6–14 days after starting heparin therapy, probably as a heparin-dependent immune-mediated phenomenon, in which antibodies induce platelet aggregation leading to arterial or venous thrombus formation. It differs from other types of drug-induced thrombocytopenia as it gives rise to both arterial or venous thrombosis as well as haemorrhagic complications. The platelet count is below $100 \times 10^9/l$. In established cases, heparin should be stopped and oral anticoagulants given together with agents that inhibit platelet aggregation. In severe cases, thrombolytic therapy or surgical intervention may be necessary.[115] The complications and morbidity related to delayed heparin-induced thrombocytopenia can be prevented if the thrombocytopenia is recognized and heparin stopped immediately. It is therefore essential to monitor the platelet count in all patients receiving heparin.

Recently, low molecular weight heparin twice daily subcutaneously has been shown as effective and safe as standard full-dose unfractionated heparin in the treatment of acute minor PE.[145] The bioavailability of low molecular weight heparin after subcutaneous injection is very high and the half-life longer than that of unfractionated heparin. The anticoagulant response of a given dose correlates with body weight, so it is possible that it may be effective when given in standard doses (anti-Xa units per kg) without laboratory monitoring.[71] The treatment is convenient since it allows early mobilization and requires less nursing and laboratory supervision. Low molecular weight heparin interacts with platelets less readily and, although less likely to do so, can cause HITS. It has a great advantage as it offers the possibility of treating DVT at home.[135]

THROMBOLYTIC THERAPY

The rationale of the thrombolytic therapy of PE, followed by anticoagulation, is that it actively dissolves the thrombus, thereby returning the cardiopulmonary function towards normal as quickly as possible (Figure 21.8). By relieving pulmonary artery obstruction, thrombolysis can quickly reduce the load on the right ventricle and reverse right ventricular failure, and consequently has the potential to prevent death in the haemodynamically compromised patient who would otherwise not survive the many hours or days required for spontaneous fibrinolysis. A further potential but unproven advantage of thrombolytic therapy over heparin is that it may reduce the chance of recurrent embolism by lysing peripheral thrombus before it embolizes, and by doing so may also reduce the chances of chronic thromboembolic pulmonary hypertension developing at a later date. Thrombolysis is also the therapy of choice in those rare cases with a profound deficiency of antithrombin III, protein C, or protein S, where the effectiveness of heparin as an anticoagulant may be severely impaired.

Thrombolytic therapy is reserved mainly for use in those patients in whom there is evidence of a severely compromised circulation, for example, hypotension, impaired peripheral circulation, oliguria or severe hypoxaemia. Scientific evidence that thrombolytic therapy as opposed to heparin reduces mortality in these very ill patients is lacking and it is unlikely to be forthcoming because of the logistic problems involved in mounting such a study.[52] However, there is strong indirect evidence[4,106,146] and clinical experience combined with the rationale for their use means that they should not be denied to the very ill patient.

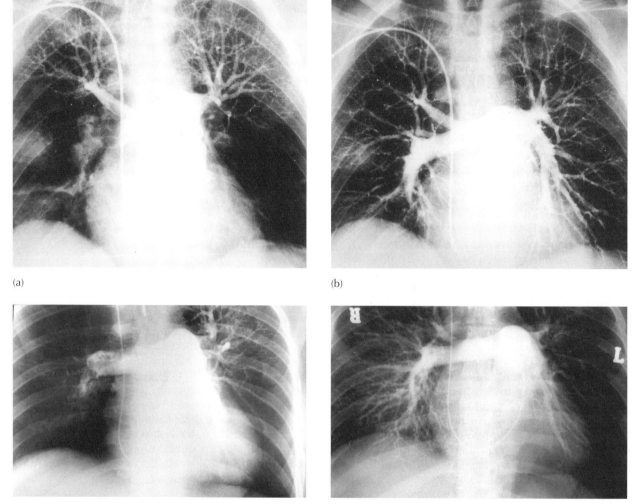

(a)

(b)

(c)

(d)

Figure 21.8   (a and b) Acute massive pulmonary embolism. Pulmonary arteriographs performed (a) at the time of admission to hospital and (b) again 72 hours later following treatment with streptokinase. There is almost complete resolution. (c & d) Pulmonary angiographs (c) before and (d) after successful lysis with rt-PA of large embolus in the right pulmonary artery.

The thrombolytic agents currently in use are streptokinase (SK), urokinase (UK), recombinant tissue plasminogen activator (rt-PA, alteplase), and anisoylated plasminogen streptokinase activator complex (APSAC, anistreplase). Accelerated early resolution of PE as compared with heparin has been proved in all these agents.[24,43,90,96,104,107,146,149,151] They are equally effective given intravenously or via a catheter in the pulmonary artery.[152]

Prior to the initiation of the thrombolytic therapy, the prothrombin time, aPTT, fibrinogen level and platelet count should be measured to make sure that there is no pre-existing coagulation disorder which would contraindicate thrombolysis. Other contraindications include intracranial or intraspinal disease, active internal bleeding, recent major surgery or trauma, and uncontrolled severe hypertension. Generally accepted fixed-dosage regimens are shown in Table 21.7. There is no need to obtain clotting tests during therapy. Experience has shown that these tests are of no value in predicting complications or adjusting dosage.

The correct duration of therapy is not established. In practice, the best approach is to treat for between 12 and 72 hours depending on the clinical response. After the conclusion of the thrombolytic

Table 21.7 Thrombolytic regimens for massive pulmonary embolism

Streptokinase	500 000 U as a loading dose over 30 min followed by 100 000 U/h for 24–48 h
Urokinase	4400 U/kg as a loading dose over 10 min followed by 4400 U/kg/h for 12–24 h
rt-PA	100 mg as a continuous infusion over 2 h

infusion, measurements of aPTT and fibrinogen are mandatory in order to determine when heparin (without a bolus) should be instituted. If the post-thrombolysis aPTT exceeds twice the upper limit of normal or fibrinogen level is under 1 g/l, these tests should be repeated every 4 hours until they reach these levels at which heparin can be started safely. After the patient has been adequately heparinized, oral anticoagulation is initiated and even if the pro-thrombin time quickly reaches the target range, it should overlap with heparin for 4 days.

Recently, the effectiveness of rt-PA (and UK) in inducing rapid lysis has been shown to be increased and bleeding to be reduced by using very high doses over a short interval.[44,46,90,118]

Conventional thrombolytic therapy is effective only when the thrombus to be lysed is fairly fresh. Once about 2 weeks have passed, the thrombus contains little or no plasminogen and will not lyse, which explains the disappointing results obtained in patients with subacute massive PE although special techniques may help in this group.[31]

EMBOLECTOMY

Pulmonary embolectomy is rarely undertaken for the treatment of acute massive PE, although it did enjoy a vogue during the 1970s. The main reason for its decline is the excellent results obtained in severely ill patients with thrombolytic agents. Emergency embolectomy can be carried out with success only by experienced cardiac surgeons in centres where cardiopulmonary bypass is immediately available (Figure 21.9). Under these circumstances, the operative mortality is low (<10%)[106] unless the patient is completely moribund and receiving cardiac massage at the time the chest is opened; even then, survivors have been reported.[105,106] Occasional patients in extremis are encountered in whom embolectomy is the correct treatment: either those with severe acute massive PE and a strong contraindication to thrombolytic therapy or those who continue to deteriorate despite thrombolytic agents.[48,105] The modified

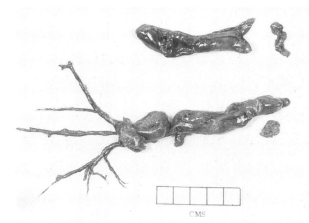

Figure 21.9 Material removed at emergency pulmonary embolectomy. Note that beyond the embolus 'thrombosis *in situ*' has formed a cast of the branching pulmonary artery.

Trendelenburg operation of embolectomy without bypass is rarely successful.

Embolectomy employing special large steerable catheters, with a suction cup to remove central emboli, usually inserted via cutdown in the femoral vein, has been used successfully in the past[147] but is rarely undertaken now. Fragmentation of the thrombus with a guide wire and catheter has already been mentioned above.[11,60]

ORAL ANTICOAGULANTS

Oral anticoagulants (coumarins) have no role in the early treatment of PE, although their effectiveness in preventing recurrence is well established. If PE occurs postoperatively, anticoagulation for 4 weeks is likely to be sufficient. For other patients, provided there is no persisting risk factor, treatment for 3 months is indicated.[40,64,83,124] Certain groups require prolonged or even indefinite treatment, including patients with subacute massive PE, particularly when there is no obvious predisposing factor, patients with tumours, with antithrombin, protein C or S deficiency[21,141] (see Chapter 8), those with proven recurrence of either PE or DVT and patients who have chronic thromboembolic pulmonary hypertension (Figure 21.10).

Coumarins do not act immediately and therefore it is essential to overlap heparin and coumarin therapy for about 4 days, even if the prothrombin time reaches the target range sooner. The dose must be controlled so that the international normalized ratio (INR) is between 2.0 and 3.0.[58,71] The risk of haemorrhage is always present and with

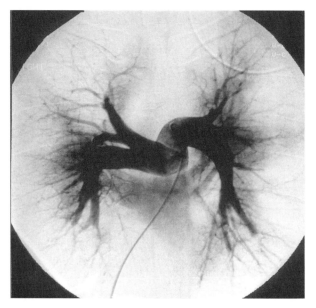

Figure 21.10   The pulmonary angiograph of a patient with chronic thromboembolic pulmonary hypertension. Note sudden cut-off of many of the third and fourth divisions of the pulmonary artery and the sparcity of vessels in the periphery of the lung.

long-term therapy the cumulative risk is not inconsiderable (6–22 per 1000 patient-months).[89,124]

VENOUS INTERRRUPTION

Venous interruption procedures are designed to prevent further emboli from reaching the lungs. Their use has a marked geographical variation: they are widely applied in some centres in the USA whereas they are seldom used in Europe. In the past the main methods were ligation, plication or the surgical application of clips to the outside of the inferior vena cava. These procedures carried an appreciable mortality (7–15% depending on the intervention) and morbidity, of which lower limb swelling after inferior vena cava ligation was the worst.[10] Nowadays the method of choice is the pervenous placement of a filter in the inferior vena cava.[29,47,49,144] There is no evidence that they have any advantages for routine prophylaxis following an acute PE because the incidence of recurrence with anticoagulation alone is so low.[40] Their place is in the rare case in which anticoagulation alone fails or adequate anticoagulation cannot be achieved because of a strong contraindication, in the presence of a large free-floating peripheral thrombus, and as a concurrent performance in pulmonary embolectomy.

Prophylaxis of pulmonary embolism

As PE is difficult to diagnose, expensive to treat, and occasionally lethal despite therapy, prophylaxis has received an enormous amount of attention. The fact that 90% of PE arise from thrombi in the proximal deep veins of the legs has important implications:

1. Prevention of DVT is the most effective approach to prevention of PE.
2. Prompt treatment of DVT may limit the frequency of PE.
3. Techniques which allow the diagnosis of DVT will allow identification of the vast majority of patients at high risk of PE.

The rationale of prophylaxis of venous thromboembolism is based on the clinically silent nature of the disease. To wait until a clinical diagnosis can be established may expose susceptible patients to unacceptable risks. The first manifestation of the disease may be fatal PE.

All prophylactic measures require supervision, extra work, organization, vigilance and money. The efficacy of many measures in preventing DVT have been assessed in clinical trials but only a few of these have assessed the incidence of fatal PE because mortality due to this complication is low. This is a very important question, since the majority of thromboses detected in trials will undergo spontaneous lysis without sequelae once mobility is re-established. One measure agreed to be simple and effective is early ambulation although it is not well proved scientifically. Once this measure alone has been taken, the incidence of fatal PE is small.

In urological, elective orthopaedic, and general surgical patients over 40 years of age who undergo anaesthesia for more than 30 minutes, prophylactic low-dose heparin (5000 U subcutaneously 2 hours before operation and every 8–12 hours afterwards), alone or combined with graded compression stockings, has been shown to prevent about two-thirds of DVTs and about a half of the fatal PEs,[7,15,17,72,156] but many hundreds of patients have to be treated to prevent one fatality. Low molecular weight heparin appears promising and its simple once-daily administration will encourage its widespread adoption as the probable method of choice; it inhibits factor Xa with only a minimal inhibition of thrombin, which is needed for local haemostasis at the site of operation. It is also less likely to cause thrombocytopenia. However, the hope that it will be free of any bleeding complications has not been fully realized.[15,80,82,85,88,91,114,142]

Prophylaxis is continued postoperatively until the patient is fully ambulant. In high-risk patients, among whom those undergoing emergency orthopaedic surgery for fractures of the femur probably constitute those with the highest risk because of the combination of trauma quickly followed by surgery, the effectiveness of these measures in preventing PE has not been established despite extensive investigation. This is probably because the clotting cascade has been activated long before the patient reaches medical attention. In these patients, oral anticoagulants with a target INR of 1.5–2.5 are effective,[119,121] but the concomitant risk of bleeding makes them unacceptable to many surgeons. Intravenous dextran is also effective,[51] but potential adverse effects include pulmonary oedema, bleeding, and, rarely, anaphylactic reactions and renal failure.

The value of other measures in preventing fatal PE, such as antiembolism stockings alone, intermittent pneumatic compression and other devices for maintaining the calf blood flow during surgery, is unproven, although it is probably an effective alternative in situations such as neurosurgery where it may be preferable to avoid heparin prophylaxis. Firm compressive stockings are cost effective in conjunction with low-dose heparin, and give symptomatic relief and reduce swelling in patients with severe DVT. Very occasionally interruption of the inferior vena cava can be considered as a preoperative measure under exceptional circumstances, e.g. in patients at a very high risk of PE who have contraindications to both pharmacological and mechanical prophylaxis.[15]

Low-dose heparin or low molecular weight heparin together with graduated compression stockings are often used in medical patients judged to be at high risk, for example, those with cardiac failure, myocardial infarction, thrombotic stroke or neoplastic disease who are likely to be immobilized for some time, but although they reduce the incidence of venous thromboembolism generally, there is little definitive evidence that they reduce the incidence of fatal PE.[15]

In all patients at risk, any suggestion of thromboembolism should be treated early and energetically with heparin in full doses while the diagnosis is established and followed by oral anticoagulants.[62,83]

Some other special situations in pulmonary embolic disease

PARADOXICAL THROMBOEMBOLISM

If an embolus originating in the venous system manages to bypass the lungs, usually via a pre-existing congenital right-to-left shunt (including pulmonary arteriovenous fistula), the patient presents with symptoms and signs of systemic embolization.[86,95] Passage to the left side of the circulation can also occur through communications between the atria[35,87] which, under normal circumstances, allow either a left-to-right shunt (atrial septal defect) or no shunt at all (patent foramen ovale, present in 20–30% of the population).[76] In order for an embolus to pass through a patent foramen ovale, the normal pressure gradient between the left and right atrium must be reversed. This occurs if there is acute or chronic pulmonary hypertension or right heart failure but may occur transiently in normal subjects during coughing or the Valsalva manoeuvre.

PULMONARY THROMBOEMBOLISM IN PREGNANCY

PE remains the second most common cause of maternal mortality during pregnancy.[7] Pregnancy causes a hypercoagulable state with increased concentrations of clotting factors, platelet turnover, and viscosity, while diminishing fibrinolysis. The venous return from the legs is decreased as the pregnant uterus obstructs the vena cava. The risk of thromboembolic disease is increased sixfold compared with the non-pregnant state, and is further increased by previous thromboembolism, obesity, and operative delivery.[100] PE during pregnancy represents a difficult diagnostic and therapeutic problem. Dyspnoea, chest pain, palpitations, fatiguability and syncope are symptoms of PE, but all are common in normal pregnant women. Chest radiographs and lung scanning involve radiation exposure and should be avoided. Consequently, diagnosis often remains uncertain, based mainly on the results of echocardiography, and impedance plethysmography and duplex ultrasound of the lower extremities. However, although fetal wellbeing should always be considered, the highest priority should be given to maternal health, and if radiological studies are required to confirm the diagnosis that is needed to preserve the mother's life, then these should be undertaken with as much radiation protection as possible. The possible consequences of failure to treat, or unnecessary use of anticoagulants, outweigh risks to the fetus of the appropriate use of radiological investigations.

Therapy is problematic since coumarins cross the placenta and reach the fetal circulation. Fetal developmental abnormalities, spontaneous abortions and stillbirth can all occur. Pregnant women with DVT or PE are best treated initially with continuous intravenous heparin[38] and then taught to self-administer full-dose subcutaneous low molecular weight heparin (in doses larger than for non-pregnant patients) once daily for the remainder of pregnancy and the puerperium. The therapy should be monitored at least once a week, with the aPTT before the next injection being at least several seconds elevated above the upper limit of normal. Measurements of therapeutic efficacy by anti-Xa (desired levels 0.5–1.0 anti-Xa U/ml) appears to be more sensitive than aPTT. Another acceptable approach is to give coumarin between the 12th and 38th weeks of gestation, and switch to intravenous heparin in hospital during the last 2 weeks of pregnancy. If the mother is admitted in premature labour while still on coumarins, she should be given fresh frozen plasma before caesarean section. Coumarin treatment can be resumed immediately after delivery. The effect of coumarin on the baby persists for 7–14 days after it is stopped and therefore the baby should be given vitamin K at delivery. Breast feeding is not contraindicated.[38]

Other forms of pulmonary embolism which may mimic thromboembolism

FAT EMBOLISM

Major trauma, usually to the large bones of the leg, the pelvis and soft tissues, may force fat droplets, mainly from the marrow, and some marrow tissue into the blood. Some of this fat may aggregate with red cells, platelets and fibrin to form larger particles and some passes through the lungs so that there is obstruction of both systemic and pulmonary circulations. The clinical effects are very variable.[34] More than 50% of patients experiencing major trauma have some evidence of fat embolism in the form of a mildly reduced Pa_{O_2}. More severe problems occur in 1–5% of trauma patients and include immediate unconsciousness, cerebral irritation, profound hypoxaemia and acute right heart failure. More often, the onset is delayed for 1–4 days and the main features are fever, dyspnoea, tachycardia, coagulation abnormalities combined with evidence of pulmonary and systemic embolization. In the pulmonary circulation, this causes acute right heart failure and reduced cardiac output; pulmonary oedema can also occur as a result of the irritant effects of the fat droplets and causes severe hypoxaemia. In fact, it is frequently difficult to distinguish between the fat embolism syndrome and the adult respiratory distress syndrome (ARDS). Therapy is supportive and includes artificial ventilation with positive end-expiratory pressure and a high Po_2,

corticosteroids, and diuretics. Early treatments included intravenous alcohol, thought to dissolve neutral fat, and heparin. Neither therapy has proved effective, and heparin might cause severe problems for patients with multiple injuries.[34]

AMNIOTIC FLUID EMBOLISM

This complication should be suspected if sudden cardiorespiratory collapse occurs during labour or soon after.[136] Amniotic fluid as well as fragments of trophoblast and decidual tissue are forced into the circulation by the vigorously contracting uterus and lodge in the lungs, causing a syndrome that closely resembles acute massive PE. The fluid is strongly thrombogenic and induces clotting in the pulmonary vasculature and elsewhere. Treatment is to evacuate the uterus immediately and support the circulation and ventilation as well as possible; there is no specific therapy and the mortality is very high (>80%). Patients who survive the initial event nearly always develop disseminated intravascular coagulation and may develop the ARDS.

AIR EMBOLISM

Air may be introduced into the venous system following trauma to the great veins usually in the neck, as a complication of central venous catheterization[75] and of a wide variety of surgical procedures, of which neurosurgery performed with the patient in the sitting position perhaps carries the highest risk. Air can enter both the venous and arterial sides of the circulation as the result of penetrating lung trauma.[79] It may also complicate any diagnostic technique that involves the insufflation of gas or air (pneumoperitoneum) and attempts to speed the rate of intravenous infusion with pressure devices.

When air enters the venous system, its most damaging effect is to obstruct the right ventricle ('air lock') and pulmonary circulation, which leads to acute cardiovascular collapse combined with severe dyspnoea and hypoxaemia. On examination, the patient is collapsed and dyspnoeic and a loud sucking sound, in time with the cardiac cycle, may be heard without the aid of a stethoscope while auscultation over the precordium reveals a churning sound said to resemble the sound of a mill wheel, produced by the air and blood in the right ventricle. When air gains access via the venous side of the circulation, the features of pulmonary obstruction are often coupled with those of cerebral disturbance because some air gets inevitably through to the systemic side of the circulation. Air in the cerebral circulation causes confusion, convulsion and loss of consciousness.

Diagnosis of air embolism depends on an awareness of the possibility, particularly in patients with chest and neck trauma who are collapsed out of proportion to their injuries. Although a chest radiograph taken in the left lateral position may show an air-fluid level within the right ventricle and echocardiography can demonstrate the presence of air in the right ventricle, obtaining these investigations is likely to lead to delay which may prove to be fatal. Treatment must be immediate. Placing the patient head down on the left side may displace the bubble of air obstructing the right ventricular outflow tract and will also discourage air from entering the cerebral circulation. Attempts should then be made to remove air from the right side of the heart either with a central venous line, Swan–Ganz catheter, direct percutaneous needle puncture of the right ventricle or cardiopulmonary bypass if necessary. Even with prompt treatment, this condition has a mortality as high as 50%, and survivors often have neurological defects.

References

1. Alderson PO, Dzebolo NN, Biello DR, *et al.* Serial lung scintigraphy: utility in diagnosis of pulmonary embolism. *Radiology* 1983; **149:** 797–802.
2. Anderson DR, Lensing AWA, Wells PS, *et al.* Limitations of impedance plethysmography in the diagnosis of clinically suspected deep-vein thrombosis. *Ann Intern Med* 1993; **118:** 25–30.
3. Anderson FA, Wheeler B, Goldberg RJ, *et al.* A population-based perspective of the hospital incidence and case-fatality rates of deep vein thrombosis and pulmonary embolism. *Arch Intern Med* 1991; **151:** 933–8.
4. Arnesen H, Hoiseth A, Ly BV. Streptokinase or heparin in the treatment of deep venous thrombosis. *Acta Med Scand* 1982; **211:** 65–8.
5. Auger WR, Fedullo PF, Moser KM, *et al.* Chronic major-vessel thromboembolic pulmonary artery obstruction: appearance at angiography. *Radiology* 1992; **182:** 393–8.
6. Barritt PW, Jordan SC. Anticoagulant drugs in the treatment of pulmonary embolism – a controlled trial. *Lancet* 1960; **1:** 1309–12.
7. Benatar SR, Immelman EJ, Jeffery P. Pulmonary embolism. *Br J Dis Chest* 1986; **80:** 313–34.
8. Benotti JR. Pulmonary angiography in the diagnosis of pulmonary embolism. *Herz* 1989; **14:** 115–25.
9. Biello DR. Radiological (scintigraphic) evaluation of patients with suspected pulmonary thromboembolism. *JAMA* 1987; **257:** 3257–9.
10. Bomalski JS, Martin GJ, Hughes RI, *et al.* Inferior vena cava interruption in the management of pulmonary embolism. *Chest* 1982; **82:** 767–74.
11. Brady AJ, Crake T, Oakley CM. Percutaneous catheter fragmentation and distal dispersion of proximal pulmonary embolus. *Lancet* 1991; **338:** 1186–9.
12. Bullock RE, Hall RJC. Left ventricular function and mitral valve opening in massive pulmonary embolism. *Br Heart J* 1982; **48:** 413–15.
13. Burki NK. The dead space to tidal volume ratio in the diagnosis of pulmonary embolism. *Am Rev Respir Dis* 1986; **133:** 679–85.
14. Carson JL, Kelley MA, Duff A, *et al.* The clinical course of pulmonary embolism. *N Engl J Med* 1992; **326:** 1240–5.
15. Clagett GP, Salzman EW, Wheeler HB, *et al.* Prevention of venous thromboembolism. *Chest* 1992; **102:** 391S–407S.
16. Cola C, Ansell J. Heparin-induced thrombocytopenia and arterial thrombosis: alternative therapies. *Am Heart J* 1990; **119:** 368–74.
17. Collins R, Scrimgeour A, Yusuf S, *et al.* Reduction in fatal pulmonary embolism and venous thrombosis by perioperative administration of subcutaneous heparin. Overview of results of randomized trials in general, orthopedic, and urologic surgery. *N Engl J Med* 1988; **318:** 1162–73.
18. Corrigan TP, Fossard DP, Spindler J, *et al.* Phlebography in the management of pulmonary embolism. *Br J Surg* 1974; **61:** 484–8.
19. Crowell RH, Adams GS, Koilpillai CJ, *et al.* In vivo right heart thrombus. Precursor of life-threatening pulmonary embolism. *Chest* 1988; **94:** 1236–9.
20. Cvitanic O, Marino PL. Improved use of arterial blood gas analysis in suspected pulmonary embolism. *Chest* 1989; **95:** 48–51.
21. Dahlback B. Inherited resistance to activated protein c, a major cause of venous thrombosis, is due to mutation in the factor V gene. *Haemostasis* 1994; **24(2):** 139–51.
22. Daily PO, Dembitsky WP, Iversen S, *et al.* Risk factors for pulmonary thromboendarterectomy. *J Thorac Cardiovasc Surg* 1990; **99:** 670–8.
23. Dalen J, Alpert J. Natural history of pulmonary embolism. *Progr Cardiovasc Dis* 1975; **17:** 259–70.
24. Dalla-Volta S, Palla A, Santolicandro A, *et al.* PAIMS 2: Alteplase combined with heparin versus heparin in the treatment of acute pulmonary embolism. Plasminogen activator Italian multicenter study. *J Am Coll Cardiol* 1992; **20:** 520–6.
25. D'Alonzo GE, Bower JS, DeHart P, *et al.* The mechanisms of abnormal gas exchange in acute massive pulmonary embolism. *Am Rev Respir Dis* 1983; **128:** 170–2.
26. Decousus HA, Croze M, Levi FA, *et al.* Circadian changes in anticoagulant effect of heparin infused at a constant rate. *Br Med J (Clin Res Ed)* 1985; **290:** 341–4.
27. Demers C, Ginsberg JS, Johnston M, *et al.* D-dimer and thrombin-antithrombin III complexes in patients with clinically suspected pulmonary embolism. *Thromb Haemost* 1992; **67:** 408–12.
28. Dismuke SE, Wagner EH. Pulmonary embolism as a cause of death. The changing mortality in hospitalized patients. *JAMA* 1986; **255:** 2039–42.

29. Dorfman GS. Percutaneous inferior vena caval filters. *Radiology* 1990; **174:** 987–92.
30. Dorfman GS, Cronan JJ, Tupper TB, *et al.* Occult pulmonary embolism: a common occurrence in deep venous thrombosis. *Am J Roentgenol* 1987; **148:** 263–6.
31. Ellis DA, Neville E, Hall RJ. Subacute massive pulmonary embolism treated with plasminogen and streptokinase. *Thorax* 1983; **38:** 903–7.
32. Fanta CH, Wright TC, McFadden ERJ. Differentiation of recurrent pulmonary emboli from chronic obstructive lung disease as a cause of cor pulmonale. *Chest* 1981; **79:** 92–5.
33. Fennerty T. The diagnosis of pulmonary embolism. *Br Med J* 1997; **314:** 125–9.
34. Fulde GW, Harrison P. Fat embolism – a review. *Arch Emerg Med* 1991; **8:** 233–9.
35. Gin KG, Thompson CR, Jue J, *et al.* Embolic occlusion of a patent foramen ovale: a cause of false negative contrast echocardiogram. *J Am Soc Echocardiogr* 1992; **5:** 444–6.
36. Ginsberg JS. Management of venous thromboembolism. *N Engl J Med* 1996; **335:** 1816–27.
37. Ginsberg JS, Caco CC, Brill-Edward PA, *et al.* Venous thrombosis in patients who have undergone major hip or knee surgery: detection with compression US and impedance plethysmography. *Radiology* 1991; **181:** 651–4.
38. Ginsberg JS, Hirsh J. Use of antithrombotic agents during pregnancy. *Chest* 1992; **102:** 385S–90S.
39. Ginsburg KS, Liang MH, Newcomer L, *et al.* Anticardiolipin antibodies and the risk for ischemic stroke and venous thrombosis. *Ann Intern Med* 1992; **117:** 997–1002.
40. Girard P, Mathieu M, Simonneau G, *et al.* Recurrence of pulmonary embolism during anticoagulant treatment: a prospective study. *Thorax* 1987; **42:** 481–6.
41. Glew D, Cooper T, Mitchelmore AE, *et al.* Impedance plethysmography and thrombo-embolic disease. *Br J Radiol* 1992; **65:** 306–8.
42. Goldhaber SZ, Hennekens CH. Time trends in hospital mortality and diagnosis of pulmonary embolism. *Am Heart J* 1982; **104:** 305–6.
43. Goldhaber SZ, Kessler CM, Heit J, *et al.* Randomised controlled trial of recombinant tissue plasminogen activator versus urokinase in the treatment of acute pulmonary embolism. *Lancet* 1988; **2:** 293–8.
44. Goldhaber SZ, Kessler CM, Heit JA, *et al.* Recombinant tissue-type plasminogen activator versus a novel dosing regimen of urokinase in acute pulmonary embolism: a randomized controlled multicenter trial. *J Am Coll Cardiol* 1992; **20:** 24–30.
45. Goldhaber SZ, Savage DD, Garrison RJ, *et al.* Risk factors for pulmonary embolism. The Framingham Study. *Am J Med* 1983; **74:** 1023–8.
46. González-Juanatey JR, Valdés L, Amaro A, *et al.* Treatment of massive pulmonary thromboembolism with low intrapulmonary dosages of urokinase. *Chest* 1992; **102:** 341–6.
47. Grassi CJ, Goldhaber SZ. Interruption of the inferior vena cava for prevention of pulmonary embolism: transvenous filter devices. *Herz* 1989; **14:** 182–91.
48. Gray HH, Morgan JM, Paneth M, *et al.* Pulmonary embolectomy for acute massive pulmonary embolism: an analysis of 71 cases. *Br Heart J* 1988; **60:** 196–200.
49. Greenfield LJ. Evolution of venous interruption for pulmonary thromboembolism. *Arch Surg* 1992; **127:** 622–6.
50. Grimaudo V, Bachmann F, Hauert J, *et al.* Hypofibrinolysis in patients with a history of idiopathic deep vein thrombosis and/or pulmonary embolism. *Thromb Haemost* 1992; **67:** 397–401.
51. Gruber UF. Prevention of fatal pulmonary embolism in patients with fractures of the neck of the femur. *Surg Gynecol Obstet* 1985; **161:** 37–42.
52. Hall R. Difficulties in the treatment of acute pulmonary embolism. *Thorax* 1985; **40:** 729–33.
53. Hall RJC, McHaffie D, Pusey C, *et al.* Subacute massive pulmonary embolism. *Br Heart J* 1981; **45:** 681–8.
54. Hall RJC, Sutton GC, Kerr IH. Long-term prognosis of treated acute massive pulmonary embolism. *Br Heart J* 1977; **39:** 1128–34.
55. Havig O. Pulmonary thromboembolism. *Acta Chir Scand Suppl* 1977; **478:** 24–37, 48–76.
56. Hildner FJ, Ormond RS. Accuracy of the clinical diagnosis of pulmonary embolism. *JAMA* 1967; **202:** 115–18.
57. Hirsh LJ, Rooney MW, Wat SS, *et al.* Norepinephrine and phenylephrine effects on right ventricular function in experimental canine pulmonary embolism. *Chest* 1991; **100:** 796–801.
58. Hirsh J, Dalen JE, Deykin D, *et al.* Oral anticoagulants; mechanism of action, clinical effectiveness, and optimal therapeutic range. *Chest* 1992; **102:** 312S-26S.
59. Hirsh J, Piovella F, Pini M. Congenital antithrombin III deficiency. *Am J Med* 1989; **87:** 34S–8S.
60. Horstkotte D, Heintzen MP, Strauer BE. Kombinierte mechanische und thrombolytische Wiedereröffnung der Lungenstrombahn bei massiver Lungenarterienembolie mit kardiogenem Schock. *Intensivmedizin* 1990; **27:** 124-32.
61. Huet Y, Lemaire F, Brun BC, *et al.* Hypoxemia in acute pulmonary embolism. *Chest* 1985; **88:** 829–36.
62. Huisman MV, Buller HR, ten Cate JW, Vreeken J. Serial impedance plethysmography for suspected deep venous thrombosis in outpatients. The Amsterdam General Practitioner Study. *N Engl J Med* 1986; **314:** 823–8.
63. Huisman MV, Buller HR, ten Cate JW, *et al.* Unexpected high prevalence of silent pulmonary embolism in patients with deep venous thrombosis. *Chest* 1989; **95:** 498–502.
64. Hull R, Delmore T, Genton E, *et al.* Warfarin sodium versus low-dose heparin in the treatment of venous thrombosis. *N Engl J Med* 1979; **301:** 855–8.
65. Hull RD, Hirsh J, Carter CJ, *et al.* Pulmonary angiography, ventilation lung scanning, and venography for clinically suspected pulmonary embolism with abnormal perfusion lung scan. *Ann Intern Med* 1983; **98:** 891–9.

66. Hull RD, Hirsh J, Carter CJ, *et al.* Diagnostic value of ventilation-perfusion lung scanning in patients with suspected pulmonary embolism. *Chest* 1985; **88:** 819–28.

67. Hull RD, Raskob GE, Coates G, *et al.* Clinical validity of a normal perfusion lung scan in patients with suspected pulmonary embolism. *Chest* 1990; **97:** 23–6.

68. Hull RD, Raskob GE, Coates G, *et al.* A new non-invasive management strategy for patients with suspected pulmonary embolism. *Arch Intern Med* 1989; **149:** 2549–55.

69. Hull RD, Raskob GE, Hirsh J. The diagnosis of clinically suspected pulmonary embolism. Practical approaches. *Chest* 1986; **89(Suppl 41):** 7S–25S.

70. Hunter JJ, Johnson KR, Karagianes TG, *et al.* Detection of massive pulmonary embolus-in-transit by transesophageal echocardiography. *Chest* 1991; **100:** 1210–14.

71. Hyers TN, Hull R, Weg JG. Antithrombotic therapy for venous thromboembolic disease. *Chest* 1992; **102:** 408S–25S.

72. International Multicentre Trial Prevention of fatal postoperative pulmonary embolism by low dose heparin. *Lancet* 1975; **2:** 45–51.

73. James TN. Thrombi in antrum atrii dextri of human heart as clinically important source for chronic microembolisation to lungs. *Br Heart J* 1983; **49:** 122–32.

74. Jardin F, Bardet FJ, Sanchez A, *et al.* Massive pulmonary embolism without arterial hypoxemia. *Intens Care Med* 1977; **3:** 77–80.

75. Kashuk JL. Air embolism after central venous catheterization. *Surg Gynecol Obstet* 1984; **159:** 249–52.

76. Kasper W, Geibel A, Tiede N, *et al.* Patent foramen ovale in patients with haemodynamically significant pulmonary embolism. *Lancet* 1992; **340:** 561–4.

77. Kelley MA, Carson JL, Palevsky HI, *et al.* Diagnosing pulmonary embolism: new facts and strategies. *Ann Intern Med* 1991; **114:** 300–6.

78. Kerr IH, Simon G, Sutton GC. The value of the plain radiograph in acute massive pulmonary embolism. *Br J Radiol* 1971; **44:** 751–7.

79. King MW, Aitchison JM, Nel JP. Fatal air embolism following penetrating lung trauma. *J Trauma* 1984; **24:** 753–5.

80. Koppenhagen K, Adolf J, Matthes M, *et al.* Low molecular weight heparin and prevention of postoperative thrombosis in abdominal surgery. *Thromb Haemost* 1992; **67:** 627–30.

81. Kronik G. The European Cooperative Study on the clinical significance of right heart thrombi. *Eur Heart J* 1989; **10:** 1046–59.

82. Kuster B, Gruber UF. Wert von Heparin-Dihydergot zur Prophylaxe thromboembolischer Komplikationen. *Schweiz Med Wochenschr* 1984; **114:** 322–32.

83. Lagerstedt CI, Olsson CG, Fagher BO, Oqvist BW, Albrechtsson U. Need for long-term anticoagulant therapy in symptomatic calf-vein thrombosis. *Lancet* 1985; **2:** 515–18.

84. Leitha T, Speiser W, Dudczak, R. Pulmonary embolism. Efficacy of D-dimer and thrombin-antithrombin III complex determinations as screening tests before lung scanning. *Chest* 1991; **100:** 1536–41.

85. Leizorovicz A, Haugh MC, Chapius F-R, *et al.* Low molecular weight heparin in the prevention of perioperative thrombosis. *Br Med J* 1992; **305:** 913–20.

86. Leonard RCF, Neville E, Hall RJC. Paradoxical embolism. A review of cases dignosed during life. *Eur Heart J* 1981; **3:** 362–70.

87. Leonard RCF, Neville E, Hall RJC. Paradoxical embolism associated with patent foramen ovale. *Postgrad Med J* 1981; **57:** 717–18.

88. Levine MN, Hirsh J, Gent M, *et al.* Prevention of deep vein thrombosis after elective hip surgery. A randomized trial comparing low molecular weight heparin with standard unfractionated heparin. *Ann Intern Med* 1991; **114:** 545–51.

89. Levine MN, Hirsh J, Landefeld S, *et al.* Hemorrhagic complications of anticoagulant therapy. *Chest* 1992; **102:** 352S–63S.

90. Levine M, Hirsh J, Weitz J, *et al.* A randomized trial of a single bolus dosage regimen of recombinant tissue plasminogen activator in patients with acute pulmonary embolism. *Chest* 1990; **98:** 1473–9.

91. Leyvraz PF, Bachmann F, Hoek J, *et al.* Prevention of deep vein thrombosis after hip replacement: randomised comparison between unfractionated heparin and low molecular weight heparin. *Br Med J* 1991; **303:** 543–8.

92. Lichey J, Reschofski I, Dissmann T, *et al.* Fibrin degradation product D-dimer in the diagnosis of pulmonary embolism. *Klin Wochenschr* 1991; **69:** 522–6.

93. Lilienfeld DE, Godbold JH, Burke GL, *et al.* Hospitalization and case fatality for pulmonary embolism in the twin cities: 1979–1984. *Am Heart J* 1990; **120:** 392–5.

94. Lippman M, Fein A. Pulmonary embolism in the patient with chronic obstructive pulmonary disease. *Chest* 1981; **79:** 39–42.

95. Loscalzo J. Paradoxical embolism: clinical presentation, diagnostic strategies, and therapeutic options. *Am Heart J* 1986; **112:** 141–5.

96. Ly B, Arnesen H, Eie H, *et al.* A controlled clinical trial of streptokinase and heparin in the treatment of major pulmonary embolism. *Acta Med Scand* 1978; **109:** 465–70.

97. MacIntyre D, Banham SW, Moran F. Pulmonary embolism – a long-term follow-up. *Postgrad Med J* 1982; **58:** 222–5.

98. Manier G, Castaing Y. Influence of cardiac output on oxygen exchange in acute pulmonary embolism. *Am Rev Respir Dis* 1992; **145:** 130–6.

99. Marber MS, deBelder BM, Pumphrey CW, *et al.* Transoesophageal echocardiography in the diagnosis of paradoxical embolism. *Int J Cardiol* 1992; **34:** 283–8.

100. McHale SP, Tilak MD, Robinson PN. Fatal pulmonary embolism following spinal anaesthesia for caesarean section. *Anaesthesia* 1992; **47:** 128–30.

101. McIntyre KM, Sasahara AA. The hemodynamic response to pulmonary embolism in patients without prior cardiopulmonary disease. *Am J Cardiol* 1971; **28**: 288–94.

102. McNeil BJ. Ventilation perfusion studies and the diagnosis of pulmonary embolism: concise communication. *J Nucl Med* 1980; **21**: 319–23.

103. Menzoian JO, Williams LF. Is pulmonary angiography essential for the diagnosis of acute pulmonary embolism? *Am J Surg* 1979; **137**: 543–8.

104. Meyer G, Sors H, Charbonnier B, *et al.* Effects of intravenous urokinase versus alteplase on total pulmonary resistance in acute massive pulmonary embolism: a European multicenter double-blind trial. The European Cooperative Study Group for Pulmonary Embolism. *J Am Coll Cardiol* 1992; **19**: 239–45.

105. Meyer G, Tamisier D, Sors H, *et al.* Pulmonary embolectomy: a 20-year experience at one center. *Ann Thorac Surg* 1991; **51**: 232–6.

106. Miller GAH, Hall JRC, Paneth M. Pulmonary embolectomy, heparin and streptokinase – their place in the treatment of acute massive pulmonary embolism. *Am Heart J* 1977; **93**: 568–74.

107. Miller GAH, Sutton GC, Kerr IH, *et al.* Comparison of streptokinase and heparin in treatment of isolated acute massive pulmonary embolism. *Br Med J* 1971; **2**: 681–5.

108. Monreal M, Lafoz E, Ruiz J, *et al.* Upper-extremity deep venous thrombosis and pulmonary embolism. A prospective study. *Chest* 1991; **99**: 280–3.

109. Monreal M, Ruiz J, Olazabal A, *et al.* Deep venous thrombosis and the risk of pulmonary embolism. *Chest* 1992; **102**: 677–81.

110. Moser KM, Auger WR, Fedullo PF. Chronic major-vessel thromboembolic pulmonary hypertension. *Circulation* 1990; **81**: 1735–43.

111. Moser KM, Auger WR, Fedullo PF, *et al.* Chronic thromboembolic pulmonary hypertension: clinical picture and surgical treatment. *Eur Respir J* 1992; **5**: 334–42.

112. Moser KM, LeMoine JR. Is embolic risk conditioned by location of deep vein thrombosis? *Ann Intern Med* 1981; **94**: 439–44.

113. Musset D, Rosso J, Petitpretz P, *et al.* Acute pulmonary embolism: diagnostic value of digital subtraction angiography. *Radiology* 1988; **166**: 455–9.

114. Nurmohamed MT, Rosendaal FR, Büller HR, *et al.* Low-molecular-weight heparin versus standard heparin in general and orthopaedic surgery: a meta-analysis. *Lancet* 1992; **340**: 152–6.

115. Obadia JF, Lancon JP, Becker F, *et al.* Thrombopénies induites par l'héparine. *Ann Chir* 1991; **45**: 729–34.

116. Pabinger I, Brücker S, Kyrle PA, *et al.* Hereditary deficiency of antithrombin III, protein C and protein S: prevalence in patients with a history of venous thrombosis and criteria for rational patient screening. *Blood Coagul Fibrinolysis* 1992; **3**: 547–53.

117. Paraskos JA, Adelstein SJ, Smith RE, *et al.* Late prognosis of acute pulmonary embolism. *N Engl J Med* 1973; **289**: 55–8.

118. Petitpretz P, Simmoneau G, Cerrina J, *et al.* Effects of a single bolus of urokinase in patients with life-threatening pulmonary emboli: a descriptive trial. *Circulation* 1984; **70**: 861–6.

119. Poller L, McKernan A, Thomson JM, *et al.* Fixed minidose warfarin: a new approach to prophylaxis against venous thrombosis after major surgery. *Br Med J* 1987; **295**: 1309–12.

120. Popovic AD, Milovanovic B, Neskovic AN, *et al.* Detection of massive pulmonary embolism by transoesophageal echocardiography. *Cardiology* 1992; **80**: 94–9.

121. Powers PJ, Gent M, Jay RM, *et al.* A randomized trial of less intense postoperative warfarin or aspirin therapy in the prevention of venous thromboembolism after surgery for fractured hip. *Arch Intern Med* 1989; **149**: 771–4.

122. Prandoni P, Lensing AWA, Büller HR, *et al.* Deep-vein thrombosis and the incidence of subsequent symptomatic cancer. *N Engl J Med* 1992; **327**: 1128–33.

123. Prediletto R, Paoletti P, Fornai E, *et al.* Natural course of treated pulmonary embolism. Evaluation by perfusion lung scintigraphy, gas exchange, and chest roentgenogram. *Chest* 1990; **97**: 554–61.

124. Research Committee of the British Thoracic Society. Optimum duration of anticoagulation for deep-vein thrombosis and pulmonary embolism. *Lancet* 1992; **340**: 873–6.

125. Riedel M, Dennig K, Henneke K-H, *et al.* Comparison of various echocardiographic methods for the estimation of pulmonary artery pressure. *Eur Heart J* 1988; **9**: 355.

126. Riedel M, Rudolph W. Hämodynamik und Gasaustausch bei akuter Lungenembolie. *Herz* 1989; **14**: 109–14.

127. Riedel M, Rudolph W. Diagnostik der Lungenembolie. *Herz* 1989; **14**: 71–81.

128. Riedel M, Stanek V, Widimsky J. Spirometry and gas exchange in chronic pulmonary thromboembolism. *Bull Eur Physiopathol Resp* 1981; **17**: 209–21.

129. Riedel M, Stanek V, Widimsky J, *et al.* Longterm follow-up of patients with pulmonary thromboembolism. Late prognosis and evolution of hemodynamic and respiratory data. *Chest* 1982; **81**: 151–8.

130. Riedel M, Urbanova D, Ruzbarsky V, *et al.* Clinicopathologic correlations in pulmonary thromboembolism. *Cor Vasa* 1980; **22**: 176–84.

131. Riedel M, Urbanova D, Ruzbarsky V, *et al.* Clinical diagnosis of pulmonary embolism in cardiac patients. *Progr Respir Res* 1980; **13**: 96–103.

132. Riedel M, Widimsky J, Stanek V. Steady-state pulmonary transfer factor in chronic thromboembolic disease. *Bull Eur Physiopathol Resp* 1980; **16**: 469–77.

133. Rosove MH, Brewer PMC. Antiphospholipid thrombosis: clinical course after the first thrombotic event in 70 patients. *Ann Intern Med* 1992; **117**: 303–8.

134. Rowbotham BJ, Egerton VJ, Whitaker AN, *et al.* Plasma cross linked fibrin degradation products in pulmonary embolism. *Thorax* 1990; **45**: 684–7.

135. Shafer AI. Low molecular weight heparin – an opportunity for home treatment of venous thrombosis. *N Engl J Med* 1996; **334:** 724–5.

136. Sperry K. Amniotic fluid embolism. *JAMA* 1986; **255:** 2183–6.

137. Stein PD, Alavi A, Gottschalk A, *et al.* Usefulness of noninvasive diagnostic tools for diagnosis of acute pulmonary embolism in patients with a normal chest radiograph. *Am J Cardiol* 1991; **67:** 1117–20.

138. Stein PD, Athanasoulis C, Alavi A, *et al.* Complications and validity of pulmonary angiography in acute pulmonary embolism. *Circulation* 1992; **85:** 462–8.

139. Stein PD, Terrin ML, Hales CA, *et al.* Clinical, laboratory, roentgenographic, and electrocardiographic findings in patients with acute pulmonary embolism and no pre-existing cardiac or pulmonary disease. *Chest* 1991; **100:** 598–603.

140. Sutton GS, Hall RJC, Kerr IH. Clinical course and late prognosis of treated subacute massive, acute minor, and chronic pulmonary thromboembolism. *Br Heart J* 1977; **39:** 1135–42.

141. Svensson PJ, Dahlback B. Resistance to activated protein C as a basis for venous thrombosis. *N Engl J Med* 1994; **330(8):** 517–22.

142. The GHAT Group. Prevention of deep vein thrombosis with low molecular-weight heparin in patients undergoing total hip replacement. A randomized trial. The German Hip Arthroplasty Trial (GHAT) Group. *Arch Orthop Trauma Surg* 1992; **111:** 110–20.

143. The PIOPED Investigators. Value of the ventilation/perfusion scan in acute pulmonary embolism. Results of the prospective investigation of pulmonary embolism diagnosis (PIOPED). *JAMA* 1990; **263:** 2753–9.

144. Théry C, Asseman P, Amrouni N, *et al.* Use of a new removable vena cava filter in order to prevent pulmonary embolism in patients submitted to thrombolysis. *Eur Heart J* 1990; **11:** 334–41.

145. Théry C, Simmonneau G, Meyer G, *et al.* Randomized trial of subcutaneous low-molecular-weight heparin CY 216 (fraxiparine) compared with intravenous unfractionated heparin in the curative treatment of submassive pulmonary embolism. A dose-ranging study. *Circulation* 1992; **85:** 1380–9.

146. Tibbut DA, Davies JA, Anderson JA, *et al.* Comparison by controlled clinical trial of streptokinase and heparin in treatment of life-threatening pulmonary embolism. *Br Med J* 1974; **1:** 343–7.

147. Timsit JF, Reynaud P, Meyer G, *et al.* Pulmonary embolectomy by catheter device in massive pulmonary embolism. *Chest* 1991; **100:** 655–8.

148. Torbicki A, Tramarin R, Morpurgo M. Role of Echo/Doppler in the diagnosis of pulmonary embolism. *Clin Cardiol* 1992; **15:** 805–10.

149. Urokinase Pulmonary Embolism Trial. A national cooperative study. *Circulation* 1973; **47 & 48:** 1–108.

150. Van Rossum AB, Treurniet FE, Kieft GJ, Smith SJ, Schepers-Bok R. Role of spiral volumetric computed tomographic scanning in the assessment of patients with clinical suspicion of pulmonary embolism and an abnormal ventilation/perfusion lung scan. *Thorax* 1996; **51:** 23–8.

151. Vander Sande J, Bossaert L, Brochier M, *et al.* Thrombolytic treatment of pulmonary embolism with APSAC. *Eur Respir J* 1988; **1:** 721–5.

152. Verstraete M, Miller GA, Bounameaux H, *et al.* Intravenous and intrapulmonary recombinant tissue-type plasminogen activator in the treatment of acute massive pulmonary embolism. *Circulation* 1988; **77:** 353–60.

153. Vlahakes GJ, Turley K, Hoffman JIE. The pathophysiology of failure in acute right ventricular hypertension: hemodynamic and biochemical correlations. *Circulation* 1981; **63:** 87–95.

154. Webber MM, Gomes AS, Roe D, *et al.* Comparison of Biello, McNeil, and PIOPED criteria for the diagnosis of pulmonary emboli on lung scans. *Am J Roentgenol* 1990; **154:** 975–81.

155. Wells PS, Brill-Edwards P, Stevens P, *et al.* A novel and rapid whole blood assay for D-dimer in patients with clinically supected deep vein thrombosis. *Circulation* 1995; **91:** 2184–7.

156. Wille-Jorgensen P, Thorus J, Fischer A, *et al.* Heparin with and without graded compression stockings in the prevention of thrombo-embolic complications of major abdominal surgery. *Br J Surg* 1985; **72:** 579–81.

157. Williams JW, Eikman EA, Greenberg S. Asymptomatic pulmonary embolism. A common event in high risk patients. *Ann Surg* 1982; **195:** 323–7.

158. Wilson JE, Bynum LJ, Parkey RW. Heparin therapy in venous thromboembolism. *Am J Med* 1981; **70:** 808–16.

159. Windebank WJ, Boyd G, Moran F. Pulmonary thromboembolism presenting as asthma. *Br Med J* 1973; **1:** 90.

160. Wittlich N, Erbel R, Eichler A, *et al.* Detection of central pulmonary artery thromboemboli by trans-oesophageal echocardiography in patients with severe pulmonary embolism. *J Am Soc Echocardiogr* 1992; **5:** 515–24.

CHAPTER 22

Prevention of pulmonary embolism

Primary prevention (through the prevention of
  deep vein thrombosis)   632

Secondary prevention (prevention of embolism
  from established thrombosis)   636

References   651

The prevention of pulmonary embolism falls into two distinct categories:

- primary prevention – preventing the thrombosis that is the source of the embolus
- secondary prevention – preventing embolism from established thrombosis.

The first approach can only be applied when the time and place of the event that might cause a thrombosis is known (e.g. a surgical operation, parturition, or the beginning of a serious illness).

The second approach is applicable to all patients with a deep vein thrombosis and in particular to those who have already had an embolism. It consists of the therapeutic removal of the peripheral thrombus or the confinement of the thrombus to the limbs by some form of venous blockade.

In the late 1960s the development of the fibrinogen uptake test provided a method for testing the efficacy of a number of pharmacological and mechanical methods of prophylaxis against deep vein thrombosis. Although one of the aims of prophylaxis is the prevention of the symptoms of a thrombosis and its post-thrombotic sequelae, the main object is to reduce the incidence of fatal pulmonary embolism. It has been assumed that any method that reduces the incidence of thrombosis will reduce the incidence of embolism, but it cannot be assumed that a technique that fails to reduce the incidence of thrombosis will *a priori* fail to reduce

the incidence of embolism; nor can it be assumed that changes in the incidence of the two events (thrombosis and embolism) will move in parallel. For example, it could be that a particular form of prophylaxis may fail to prevent the type of thrombi that are the main source of emboli, whereas those thrombi that it does prevent are the thrombi which rarely become emboli.

These arguments mean that it is essential to test the effectiveness of a prophylactic regimen in a clinical trial that is large enough to show a significant effect on a relatively uncommon event – fatal pulmonary embolism. Very few trials of this type have been performed. Unfortunately (from a scientific point of view), the results of the early trials were sufficiently suggestive of a positive effect to persuade the organizers of subsequent studies that it was unethical to include an untreated control group. This defect has led to endless discussion and disagreement over the significance of these later trials.

The results of the studies presented in this chapter are discussed in a highly critical manner. This is not meant to be a reflection on the workers who undertook the daunting task of conducting these trials but it is intended to demonstrate the difficulties that these studies present in both their conduct and their interpretation – difficulties which profoundly affect the conduct of our daily clinical practice.

Primary prevention (through the prevention of deep vein thrombosis)

ORAL ANTICOAGULANTS

The seminal study of Sevitt and Gallagher in 1959[175] showed that the administration of oral anticoagulants to patients who had suffered a hip fracture reduced the incidence of fatal pulmonary embolism from 10% to 1.3%. Although there were only 150 patients in each group, the reduction in overall mortality rate was also significant. In 1966, Eskeland[60] found similar results; fatal embolism was reduced from 7% to 1%.

As so few orthopaedic surgeons used anticoagulants, Morris and Mitchell decided to repeat this study using warfarin.[147] Their study was of similar size to that of Sevitt and Gallagher (75 patients in each group) and the effect of warfarin on fatal embolism was the same, 8% in the control group, 0% in the treated group. The difference in total mortality did not reach statistical significance, probably because the total number of patients studied was smaller.

There has, therefore, been a known, proven, effective method of reducing total mortality from fatal pulmonary embolism and deep vein thrombosis after hip fractures since 1959, yet the method has not been adopted by surgeons because of the necessity for laboratory control of the anticoagulation and the high incidence of bleeding complications. Nevertheless, these studies must be the 'gold standard' against which studies of other prophylactic agents should be compared.

HEPARIN

The International Multicentre Trial published in 1975,[8] organized by Kakkar, studied 4121 patients. Of these patients 2076 were controls, and 2045 were given 5000 units heparin subcutaneously every 8 hours. One hundred of the control patients and 80 of the test patients died. In the control group 16 deaths were caused by fatal embolism compared with two deaths in the test group. The difference in overall mortality was not statistically significant. The difference in fatal embolism was statistically significant ($P < 0.005$) (Table 22.1).

Unfortunately, only 72% of the patients who died in the control group and 66% of the patients who died in the test group had an autopsy. Furthermore, the diagnosis of death was made by many different pathologists in different parts of the world. This presents two difficulties: the obvious problem of lack of uniformity between centres but, more importantly, the fact that death from pulmonary embolism is a physiological event, difficult to diagnose at post mortem. For every patient who is dead in the autopsy room with a large embolus there is a living patient in the ward with an equally large embolus. The embolus is not the only factor that causes the patient's death; many other properties of the heart and pulmonary circulation are also involved (see Chapter 21). The pathologist cannot take these other factors into account and never sees the patients who survive large emboli.

After the publication of this study serious criticism was made about the randomization[176] and the variability of results from different centres,[92,94] yet this study remains the principal source of evidence justifying the use of low doses of heparin for the prevention of postoperative fatal pulmonary embolism.

A smaller study of the effect of low-dose heparin was published by Kiil *et al.* in 1978;[110] it involved 653 controls and 643 treated patients. They found no difference in the incidence of fatal pulmonary embolism, no difference in autopsy-detectable emboli and no difference (in a small subgroup) in the incidence of leg vein thrombosis.[111] Another subgroup was studied with ventilation–perfusion scanning and showed no benefit from the heparin.[112] The absence of an effect of heparin on

Table 22.1 The effect of low-dose subcutaneous heparin (5000 units, 8-hourly) in an International Multicentre Trial conducted between 1970 and 1975 on the incidence of postoperative pulmonary embolism[8]

	Controls (2076 patients)	Heparin (2045 patients)
Fatal pulmonary embolism	16	2
Embolism contributing to death	6	3
Other deaths	84	78
Total deaths	100	80

non-fatal lung scan-detectable pulmonary emboli has also been observed in a study from Cape Town.[92]

In a compilation of 28 studies of the effect of low-dose subcutaneous heparin on pulmonary embolism by Bergqvist,[22] the overall mortality rates for controls and treated patients were 4.4% and 3.5%, respectively, and the fatal embolism rates were 0.8% and 0.3%, respectively. In 20 of these studies, however, no patient had a fatal embolism, and in two studies the incidence was not reduced. The overall apparent reduction of fatal embolism was derived solely from two studies, the Multicentre Study already discussed[8] and a smaller study by Sagar[173] which had a 16% mortality rate in the control group.

The continuing arguments concerning the effectiveness of low doses of heparin in preventing pulmonary embolism stimulated the Clinical Trials Unit in Oxford to perform a meta-analysis of all those studies published before 1986 which were randomized and gave details concerning overall mortality, mortality from embolism and bleeding complications.[45]

They studied 74 publications. The duration of heparin administration varied from 2 to 14 days; 48 trials gave the heparin twice each day, 29 three times a day. Only five studies had more than 250 patients in each arm, thus there were many significant differences between the trials. The meta-analysis shows an incidence of fatal embolism of 0.3% (19 in 6366) in the treated group and 0.9% (55 in 6426) in the controls but once again these results are dominated by the results of the International Multicentre Trial (no fatal emboli in the treated group, 15 in the control group) and the study by Sagar (no fatal emboli in the treated group, eight in the control group), the latter having as mentioned above, an extraordinary overall postoperative mortality rate of 13.0% – 10% in the treated group and 16% in the controls. If the results of these two trials are removed from the Oxford meta-analysis the incidence of fatal pulmonary embolism in the remaining 68 trials is 0.5% (19 in 3991) in the treated group and 0.8% (32 in 4053) in the controls, i.e. not a two-thirds reduction, but a one-third reduction which statistically is only just on the borderline of significance.

In our opinion and in the opinion of others[140] these figures do not support the widely held view[171] that subcutaneous heparin is a statistically and scientifically proven method for effectively preventing pulmonary embolism in general surgical patients. Nevertheless, it is our opinion that the data are sufficiently suggestive to affect our clinical practice; this is a view shared by most surgeons.[23]

The studies so far discussed all used unfractionated heparin. It is now clearly established that low molecular weight heparin, given subcutaneously once each day, is just as effective in preventing deep vein thrombosis and probably has fewer haemorrhagic side-effects (see Chapter 11).

The introduction of low molecular weight heparin was preceded by a large number of clinical trials in which it was compared with unfractionated heparin. Although all these studies carefully measured the incidence of deep vein thrombosis with the fibrinogen uptake test or phlebography, none was designed to study the incidence of pulmonary embolism. Consequently, they describe small numbers and often make no mention of embolic events.

In a review of the 27 studies performed between 1986 and 1992 which compared low molecular weight with unfractionated heparin in general surgical patients, Bergqvist[24] found one death from pulmonary embolism amongst 5359 patients receiving low molecular weight heparin (0.02%) and seven deaths amongst 4826 patients receiving unfractionated heparin (0.15%). The overall mortality in the two groups – 1.2 and 1.4%, respectively – was not statistically significant. These figures suggest that low molecular weight heparin might be more effective than unfractionated heparin in preventing embolism but in the absence of a modern untreated control group such a deduction cannot be substantiated. It should be remembered that the incidence of fatal pulmonary embolism has been falling over the past 20 years so comparison with the data of the 1950s and 1960s is not acceptable. It is also important to note that neither form of heparin completely abolishes fatal pulmonary embolism.

Many studies have shown that subcutaneous heparin is less effective at preventing deep vein thrombosis after orthopaedic operations than after general surgical operations (see Chapter 11). One reason for this may be the higher incidence of major axial vein thrombosis, partly caused by local trauma. The German Hip Arthroplasty Trial,[73] which compared unfractionated with low molecular weight heparin in 341 patients, detected incidences of proximal vein thrombosis of 19% and 10%, respectively, in the two groups and pulmonary embolism in 3.6% and 1.2%, respectively. Once again the absence of an untreated control group makes deductions on the effect of either form of heparin on the rate of fatal embolism impossible. Many orthopaedic surgeons claim similar or lower embolism rates with no form of prophylaxis.[99] Two other reasonably sized studies[124,125] observed slightly lower incidences of embolism with both forms of heparin – 0.6% with low molecular weight heparin and 1.5% with unfractionated heparin. If these results are considered alongside the very large study by Bergqvist[24] of general surgical patients (ignoring the fact that it compared two different doses of low molecular weight heparin) and a study by Oertli[153] of the effect of low molecular weight heparin given after hip fractures which observed fatal embolism rates of 0.1% and 1.7%, respectively, it is reasonable to conclude that the fatal pulmonary embolism rate in surgical and orthopaedic patients, undergoing emergency or elective surgery, is approximately 1.0% in orthopaedic patients and 0.1% in general surgical patients if given 5000 anti-Xa units of low molecular weight heparin subcutaneously each day.

Whether this is of value depends entirely upon the incidence of fatal pulmonary embolism in unprotected patients. Between 1970 and 1975 when the International Multicentre Trial was conducted, the overall incidence of fatal embolism in 2137 unprotected general surgical patients was only 0.7%. This means that five or six lives might be saved for every 1000 patients given heparin – a significant number of whom are likely to have advanced malignant disease. Amongst orthopaedic patients one or two may be saved per 100, i.e. 10 or 20 per thousand, an effect of significantly greater value.

The vast majority of surgeons have decided that protection with low molecular weight heparin in medium- and high-risk cases is worthwhile – especially if the theoretical but as yet unproven possibility of the reduction of the post-thrombotic syndrome is added into the equation. Clinical decisions often have to made on inadequate evidence. It is unlikely that we will get better evidence on the value of subcutaneous heparin but it is always important to remember the quality of the evidence – whatever clinical course we choose – and seek new ways of testing it.

DEXTRAN

Dextran was used for the prevention of pulmonary embolism before subcutaneous heparin but has not been studied in any very large randomly allocated controlled clinical trials.

Kline *et al.*[115] studied a group of 435 control patients and 396 patients who were given dextran 70. They found 14 fatal pulmonary emboli in the control group and four in the test group, but there are some diagnostic and logistic defects in this study. Other studies of the effect of dextran on fatal embolism have been based on comparisons with historical controls.[14,114,127] These studies have shown a lower incidence of embolism during the periods of dextran administration but such analyses cannot

be considered to be hard scientific evidence because of the lack of randomly selected comparable control studies. In fact, no large study of dextran (against no treatment) has been carried out which is comparable to the quality of the heparin Multicentre International Study. We performed a study[32] in which dextran and pneumatic compression was compared with controls in which the incidence of non-fatal pulmonary embolism was assessed with ventilation–perfusion scanning. The test group had a significantly lower incidence of emboli but whether this was caused by the dextran or by the pneumatic compression is open to speculation. Bergqvist did not find that dextran reduced lung scan-detected pulmonary emboli in elective hip surgery.[26]

In a compilation of 23 studies of controls against dextran 70, Bergqvist[22] found an incidence of fatal embolism of 1.5% and 0.4%, respectively, but the statistical validity of such an exercise is open to question. When he repeated the exercise in 1994,[25] reviewing 29 studies, he found similar results. Dextran appeared to have reduced the incidence of fatal pulmonary embolism from 1.5% to 0.3%. Using the more formal methods of meta-analysis, Clagett and Reisch[42] came to the same conclusions, dextran appeared to have reduced the incidence of fatal pulmonary embolism from 1.5% to 0.27% (95% confidence interval 0.05–0.68).

The data for the effectiveness of dextran, like the data for heparin, do not prove to our scientific satisfaction that dextran is effective against embolism, but the few small controlled studies plus the sequential retrospective and meta-analyses all suggest that dextran has an effect which many consider is sufficient to affect their clinical practice. However, very few surgeons use dextran because a daily subcutaneous injection of low molecular weight heparin is far simpler and convenient to administer than 500 ml dextran intravenously, during, after and on the day following operation. Furthermore, heparin does not carry the risks of cardiac overload and anaphylactoid reactions that occasionally accompany the administration of dextran. Nevertheless, its protective effect should not be forgotten; there are times – when, for example, it is necessary to expand the blood volume – that giving dextran may be more convenient than giving heparin.

In the 1960s, the workers involved in large multicentre trials felt that the evidence that heparin and dextran reduced the incidence of fatal pulmonary embolism was so good that future studies did not need untreated control groups because they were both unnecessary and ethically unacceptable. Consequently, they embarked upon comparisons of heparin with dextran, leaving the vital question of the real effect of both drugs on fatal embolism and total mortality unanswered.

Heparin versus dextran 70

In 1980 Gruber presented a multicentre comparison of the effect of heparin and dextran in general surgical patients.[94] The dose of heparin was 5000 units, 8-hourly for 6 days; the dose of dextran was 500 ml during operation, 500 ml during the next 24 hours and 500 ml during the subsequent 24 hours. In this study, 1991 patients were given heparin and 1993 were given dextran. In the heparin group 37 patients died; 38 patients given dextran died. Eighty per cent of the patients had autopsies. In the heparin group, three patients were thought to have died of pulmonary embolism compared with five patients in the dextran group. Gruber concludes that both regimens have the same effect but this study does not show that either treatment is better than nothing at all. The main difference between Gruber's groups was the increased incidence of haemorrhage in those patients treated with heparin.

It is not valid to compare these results with the control group of a study performed 5 years previously. In the 1975 Multicentre Trial,[8] the mortality rate of the control group, excluding the fatal emboli, was 4.0%. In the heparin group, excluding the fatal emboli, the mortality rate was 3.8%. In Gruber's 1980 study,[94] the mortality rate in the heparin group, excluding the fatal emboli, was 1.8%. The patients studied in the first trial must therefore have been considerably different as their mortality rate was twice that reported in the second study. It is quite unacceptable to equate the heparin arm of a 1975 trial with the heparin arm of a 1980 trial. This means that there is no way of deciding whether Gruber's 1980 heparin and dextran comparison trial had any effect on the incidence of pulmonary embolism whatsoever.

ANTIPLATELET DRUGS: ASPIRIN

The way in which thrombus develops in a vein is undoubtedly different from the way in which it develops in an artery. Arterial thrombi begin with the deposition of platelets on a thrombogenic site and at first grow through the successive deposition of platelets and thrombus. Red cells rarely become enmeshed in this type of thrombus until it begins to obstruct and slow blood flow. Arterial thrombi are often called white thrombi because of the absence of red cells and predominance of platelets within them.

Venous thrombi, developing in a slower flowing system and often as a result of a coagulation rather than vein wall change, are mainly made up of fibrin and red cells with comparatively few platelets. They are often called red thrombi in contrast to the white thrombi formed in arteries.

Because of this difference in aetiology and composition it has been argued that antiplatelet drugs such as aspirin would be unlikely to affect the incidence of deep vein thrombosis or pulmonary embolism and the early small trials appeared to support this opinion. However, in 1994, the Antiplatelet Trialists Collaboration[9] published a meta-analysis of 53 randomized trials (8400 patients) which studied the effect of antiplatelet drugs on the incidence of deep vein thrombosis detected by phlebography or the fibrinogen uptake test. These trials also recorded the incidence of fatal and non-fatal pulmonary embolism but these diagnoses were made on clinical grounds and only sometimes confirmed by ventilation–perfusion scans or autopsy. They also studied a variety of antiplatelet agents and many different doses. Doses of aspirin varied from 600 to 1500 mg each day, mostly for 1–3 weeks after operation, and other drugs studied or used in combination included dipyridamole, sulphinpyrazone and hydroxychloroquine. The authors of the meta-analysis also sought unpublished information on events that occurred in patients withdrawn from the trials. Thus the meta-analysis was of an extremely varied group of trials and its conclusions must be treated with caution.

Nevertheless, they found that antiplatelet drugs appeared to reduce the incidence of deep vein thrombosis from 34% to 25%, non-fatal postoperative pulmonary embolism from 1.8% to 0.7% and fatal postoperative embolism from 0.9% to 0.2%. As with the meta-analyses of the effect of heparin on pulmonary embolism, we view this form of meta-analysis with considerable suspicion. Most of the trials studied had only one, two or no emboli in each arm but one study of 565 had two non-fatal emboli in the treated group and 16 in the controls, another study of 1381 had two and 10. Similarly, two studies had two and seven and one and eight fatal emboli in the treated and control groups, respectively. If these studies are omitted from the analysis, the number of non-fatal emboli changes from 42 vs 82 to 38 vs 56 and fatal emboli from 14 vs 40 to 11 vs 25.

In spite of the deficiencies of their analysis, the authors believe that aspirin – dose unclear – is of value and does little harm. As aspirin takes 48 hours to affect platelet function significantly, it would seem logical to begin its administration before the operation and we would argue that it should not replace but supplement whatever form of prophylaxis is being currently used. Aspirin does have the advantage of being easy to take and so treatment for 2 or 3 weeks after an operation may help prevent the emboli that are known to recur 2 or 3 weeks after discharge from hospital.

MECHANICAL METHODS

There are no studies of the effect of mechanical methods of prophylaxis on either fatal or non-fatal pulmonary embolism, except an early clinical study of Wilkins *et al.* in 1950 which was unsupported by autopsy, but which showed a reduction of the incidence of fatal embolism in patients who wore elastic stockings.[192,193]

CLINICAL COMMENT

The preceding paragraphs have discussed the evidence provided in the published clinical studies of the prevention of pulmonary embolism from a critical scientific point of view. Clinical medicine is rarely guided by hard scientific facts. Clinicians must make up their minds on the basis of evidence which they know will never be perfect because of the biological nature of disease and the patients it affects.

Although we have expressed grave doubts about the scientific validity of much of the evidence concerning the current methods used for preventing pulmonary embolism, this does not mean that we ignore it; rather it makes us wish to stimulate others to perform better studies, including untreated controls, and it affects our clinical practice as given below. It may never be unequivocally shown that these methods of prophylaxis truly cause a reduction in the incidence of thromboembolism because of the logistic problems of performing large clinical trials and because the incidence of the disease appears to be declining.[56,117,172] Our clinical policy is as follows.

Our primary prevention regimen

We believe that the circumstantial evidence is sufficient to justify the use of systemic and mechanical prophylactic agents against pulmonary embolism.

Patients less than 40 years old, who have no history of deep vein thrombosis, are given antithromboembolism stockings. If pneumatic compression is available, it can be used during and after operation. This attitude is based on the sound evidence that these methods reduce the incidence of deep vein thrombosis (see Chapter 11) and the knowledge that fatal pulmonary embolism is a rare complication in patients under 40 years of age.[27]

Patients over the age of 40 years who are having major operations are given antithromboembolism stockings on admission and either subcutaneous low molecular weight heparin (5000 units daily for 5 days) or, very rarely, dextran 70 (500 ml three times in 48 hours). Dextran is only used if there is a major contraindication to using heparin.

We advise orthopaedic surgeons performing hip surgery to use low molecular weight heparin or dextran. The addition of dihydroergotamine (DHE) to heparin does not confer a significant benefit and carries the disadvantage of occasionally precipitating peripheral arterial ischaemia.

For patients undergoing operations where a minor haemorrhage might jeopardize the result (ophthalmic, plastic, and neurological surgery) we prefer to use mechanical methods of preventing pulmonary embolism.

We protect patients at high risk (e.g. those with a known previous episode of pulmonary embolism) by administering oral anticoagulants or intravenous heparin starting before surgery.

Secondary prevention (prevention of embolism from established thrombosis)

Thirty per cent of patients who survive a pulmonary embolism and are given no treatment are known to have a second embolus, and 20% of these second emboli will be fatal.[18]

There will always be patients who have sporadic deep vein thrombosis because the initiating incident (e.g. an illness or an accident) begins before prophylaxis can be started. It is therefore important to ensure that a patient who has a deep vein thrombosis does not have a pulmonary embolus. It is even more important to ensure that a patient who has already had one pulmonary embolism does not have a second one which may be fatal.

There are three ways in which peripheral thrombi can be prevented from becoming emboli:

- The thrombus can be removed – surgically or pharmacologically.
- The thrombus can be 'locked in' in the limbs – either surgically or by an intravascular filter.
- The growth of new fresh thrombus can be prevented with anticoagulants with the hope that this will prevent further emboli.

The last approach is difficult to justify.

The incidence of recurrent fatal emboli during and after treatment with heparin and/or oral anticoagulants can be as high as 10% and non-fatal embolism can occur in 10–15%. A compilation of 14 studies on 2196 patients (Table 22.2) reveals an

Table 22.2 The incidence of recurrent pulmonary embolism during and after treatment with heparin. A compilation of 14 studies* on 2196 patients, performed between 1947 and 1966

	Incidence (%)	Range
Recurrent fatal embolism	2.5	0–18.6
Recurrent non-fatal embolism	8.5	1.0–19.1
Total recurrence rate	11	2–20

* References 6,17,19,37,46–48,67,68,104,108,126,149,154.

average incidence of recurrent fatal embolism of 2.5% and non-fatal embolism of 8.5% – a total recurrence rate of 11%. Although these studies were performed in the 1950s and 1960s, many recent studies have confirmed that the treatment of deep vein thrombosis with anticoagulants does not abolish recurrent pulmonary embolism.[35]

Similarly, it is commonly assumed that the prophylactic administration of low-dose subcutaneous heparin pre- and postoperatively abolishes pulmonary embolism. It may be reduced but Table 22.1 shows that 0.25% of patients so treated may still suffer a serious embolus.

A rational approach to any problem requires its definition. In order to assess whether a thrombus will fragment and embolize, it is necessary to know its size, state, and age. These features are best determined by phlebography, or less well but more easily, by duplex ultrasound. In our opinion phlebography is still the best investigation to guide the management of deep vein thrombosis but we accept that duplex ultrasound is a close second best. One or other of these tests is a mandatory investigation for all patients who have suffered a pulmonary embolus,[34] or both when loose thrombus is suspected in the iliac vein as this may be missed by duplex ultrasound.

Their object is to determine the nature of the thrombus and to assess the likelihood of further embolism. Treatment can then be conducted on a rational basis.[35] All the main veins in both legs from the ankle to the vena cava should be studied. Unilateral examination, dictated by the side of the symptoms, is not acceptable because the asymptomatic leg often contains a large non-adherent thrombus. Phlebography or duplex ultrasound which fails to delineate the iliac veins and lower vena cava is also inadequate. Sometimes these veins can only be clearly displayed by phlebography using femoral vein injection or, very rarely, pertrochanteric intraosseus injection.

A logical form of treatment cannot be planned without displaying the whole venous tree and the bottom and top of the thrombus.

The source of emboli

In 1974, in a radiological study of the leg veins of 201 patients who had suffered a pulmonary embolism,[33] we found residual thrombus in the calf of 26%, in the thigh of 23% and in the pelvis of 13%. No thrombus was seen in 28%, and 9% were excluded from the calculations because they had asymmetrical bilateral thrombi. Forty-one per cent of the legs containing thrombus had no physical signs. These findings agree with the post-mortem studies of Gibbs[74] and show that, though the calf is the most common site for thrombosis, patients with pulmonary emboli frequently have thrombi in larger veins.

In another analysis of the phlebographs of a group of 50 patients who had had one clinical episode of pulmonary embolism,[35] we found residual thrombus present in 39 patients. In 17 patients it was below the level of the knee joint, in 15 patients it was in the superficial femoral vein, in six patients it was in the common femoral and iliac veins and one patient had residual thrombus in the vena cava. This distribution of thrombi is similar to that found in the larger series mentioned above. In this study, however, particular attention was paid to the nature of the thrombus. The thrombus was fresh, non-adherent and considered to be a potential embolus in 19 of the 39 patients (38%) with residual thrombus (Figure 22.1). In one patient the embolus was thought to have come from the calf. Fourteen (of 15) of the patients had residual non-adherent femoral vein thrombi, and four (of seven) patients had residual iliac/vena caval non-adherent thrombi. Thus phlebography not only detected the presence of thrombus but indicated the likelihood of further embolism and the need for active treatment to prevent further embolism in 19 of 50 patients. Sometimes the square cut upper end of the thrombus indicated that an embolus had already occurred (Figure 22.2).

Others have obtained similar findings using duplex ultrasound. In a series of 5238 scans[15] which detected 732 cases of deep vein thrombosis, 73 patients (10%) had free-floating (non-adherent) thrombi, 13% of whom had lung scan evidence of pulmonary embolism. In the next 30 days only one-half of these thrombi became adherent. In another similar study,[28] 18% of 399 patients had free-floating thrombus. Where this loose thrombus was unilateral, 25% had evidence of pulmonary embolism but this incidence rose to 50% in those patients who had bilateral free-floating thrombus.

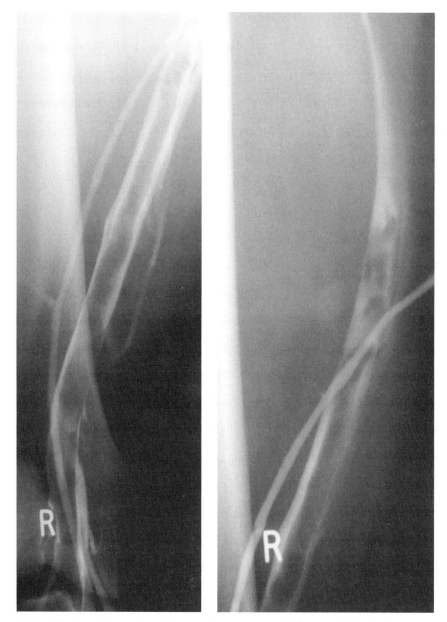

Figure 22.1 The loose thrombus that may become an embolus in spite of adequate anticoagulation. (a) An extensive fresh non-adherent thrombus in the superficial femoral vein with an irregular upper end. This size of thrombus would probably cause death if it were to break free so it should either be locked in or removed pharmacologically or surgically. (b) A fresh non-adherent femoral vein thrombus with a thin coiled loose upper end.

Overall, therefore, careful investigation of the lower limb veins in patients with deep vein thrombosis is likely to reveal at least 25% with thrombus that could easily become an embolus – indeed, one-quarter of these will have already have had an embolus.

In patients who have already had an embolus, the incidence of free-floating thrombus – and conse-quently the possibility of further embolism – may be as high as 40–50%.

THROMBECTOMY OR THROMBOLYSIS

Removing a thrombus stops it becoming an embolus. It may also relieve any venous obstruction

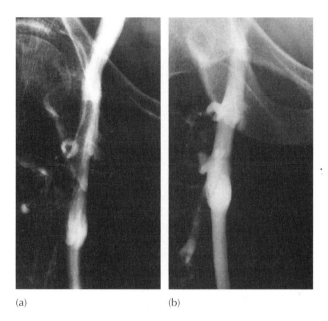

(a)   (b)

Figure 22.2 (a) The phlebograph of a patient who presented with a small pulmonary embolus. The top of the residual thrombus is 'square cut', indicating that it has recently fractured at this site. (b) The phlebograph of the same patient after 4 days of full anticoagulation with heparin, 1 day after a new episode of pleuritic chest pain. The thrombus has moved to the lungs. Heparin does not stop residual non-adherent thrombus from fragmenting and becoming a pulmonary embolus.

and possibly save the valves. These two methods of treating deep vein thrombosis are discussed in detail in Chapter 10.

Surgical removal can only be complete if the thrombus has clearly defined limits which are accessible to a balloon catheter. A thrombus confined to the femoral vein can be completely removed. A thrombus in the femoral vein that extends into many small venous tributaries in the calf cannot be completely removed, even with repeated manual compression and calf bandaging during thrombectomy. In these circumstances thrombectomy may have to be combined with a surgical 'locking-in' procedure to prevent recurrent embolism, followed by anticoagulants to prevent new thrombosis.

Pharmacological thrombolysis with streptokinase or urokinase can lyse thrombi beyond the reach of the balloon catheter, but by causing thrombi to fragment these drugs occasionally cause emboli; this is rarely a serious complication. Thrombolysis successfully prevents embolism only if it dissolves all the thrombus, which is only possible if the thrombus is very fresh.

VENOUS INTERRUPTION

Pulmonary embolism cannot occur if the veins between the thrombus and the heart are occluded.

There are two ways of deciding where to occlude the veins. The first is to ignore the site of the thrombus and occlude the outflow tract of both the limbs and the pelvis, namely the vena cava just below the renal veins. The second is to select the site of venous occlusion or partial interruption according to the site of the thrombus revealed by the venous imaging.

If a patient is having multiple small almost microscopic emboli, the vena cava must be ligated.[148,174]

Caval ligation[179]

Ligation of the vena cava in a patient with a raised pulmonary artery pressure and right heart failure can be a dangerous procedure because the sudden reduction of venous return may precipitate a cardiac arrest. We ligate the vena cava below the renal veins through a right flank extraperitoneal approach, while monitoring the cardiac output. A trial clamping of the vena cava before the ligation will confirm that it is safe to proceed.

The only indications for vena caval ligation are multiple very small emboli producing pulmonary hypertension, small septic emboli and the failure of other filter techniques to prevent embolism. The procedure should be avoided whenever possible because it is bound to produce significant lower limb oedema and post-thrombotic sequelae in at least 30% of patients.

PARTIAL OCCLUSION OF THE VENA CAVA

All except very small emboli can be prevented from reaching the lungs by partially occluding the vena cava. Some of the surgical ways of achieving this occlusion are shown in Figure 22.3. Surgical plication with multiple stitches, a grid of stitches and pericaval clips have been largely replaced by the development of filters that can be inserted transluminally, but surgeons should know about the earlier methods just in case they find themselves without a filter or an expert interventional radiologist.

Vena cava filters

Vena cava filters have been developed in an attempt to reduce morbidity and mortality in patients with pulmonary emboli and have virtually replaced surgical plication and ligation as a means of caval interruption. Since the 1960s there has

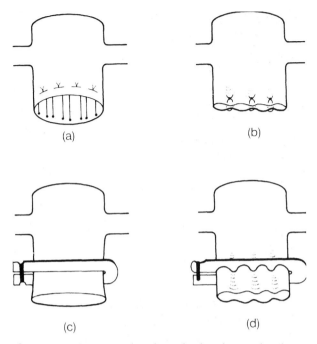

Figure 22.3 Four surgical methods of partial inferior vena cava interruption. (a) The DeWeese filter.[55] (b) The Spencer plication.[181] (c) The Moretz clip.[146] (d) The Miles clip.[139]

been continued research to develop vena cava filters that demonstrate long-term safety and are consistently effective in preventing pulmonary emboli.

The first device introduced into clinical practice was the Mobin-Uddin umbrella in 1967.[142] It was effective in preventing pulmonary emboli but had a significant caval thrombosis rate and was withdrawn in 1986. The most widely used filter is the Greenfield filter, introduced in 1972 and originally made of stainless steel. A titanium version of the same filter was introduced in 1990, of similar design, but with a smaller percutaneous delivery system. A newer stainless steel version is now available. The other caval filters currently in clinical use include the bird's nest filter, nitinol filter, Vena Tech filter, Gunther tulip filter and the Antheor filter (temporarily withdrawn in the UK due to filter migration).

A recent development is the introduction of temporary filters. These have either a wire and catheter assembly attached to the filter which is passed percutaneously, leaving the catheter end outside the patient, or have a wire assembly attached to the filter which is implanted subcutaneously next to the access vein, which can be retrieved, along with the attached filter at a later date.[150,160]

The ideal filter

Four criteria must be addressed when balancing the risk and benefit equation for vena cava filters, notably:

- effective filtration of emboli
- continued caval patency after capture of an embolus
- lack of filter thrombogenicity
- a low-risk insertion procedure.

The ideal filter would have a small introducer system, be technically easy to insert mechanically and biologically stable. It should have a low rate of short- and long-term complications, while effectively protecting against major embolic disease. While such an ideal filter has yet to be designed, the current caval filters, specifically designed for transvenous use, do represent a significant step forward in terms of ease of placement, low complications and effective filtration.

Some devices allow the passage of small emboli of up to 3 mm,[53] whereas the bird's nest filter will trap very small emboli.[66,166]

The major features of the filters in current use are summarized below.

The Greenfield filter (Figure 22.4)

This filter has six wire legs arranged in a conical shape, extending from a central hub. The base of each strut has a fine hook which hooks into the wall of the cava. The stainless steel model, introduced in 1972, requires a larger delivery system for percutaneous delivery than the titanium filter (26F sheath as opposed to 14F), consequently the titanium filter, introduced in 1990, is now used more often than the stainless steel variety although recently in 1996, a smaller 12F stainless steel Greenfield has been introduced.

The two types of filter can be employed in a vena cava measuring up to 28 mm in diameter. An alternative device must be used in a larger or megacava to avoid filter instability and migration.

The bird's nest filter (Figure 22.5)

Introduced in 1989, this filter consists of four stainless steel wires, 25 cm long, attached to two V-shaped struts. The wires are converted into a mesh in the vena cava by a series of manoeuvres by the operator. Two design modifications have taken place since its introduction to reduce filter migration after placement. A 12F delivery system is used and with its wide diameter of 60 mm it is particularly suited for megacava (above 28 mm diameter) insertion.

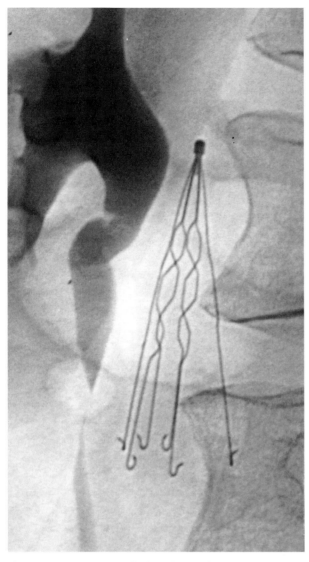

Figure 22.4 A magnified radiograph of a Greenfield filter.

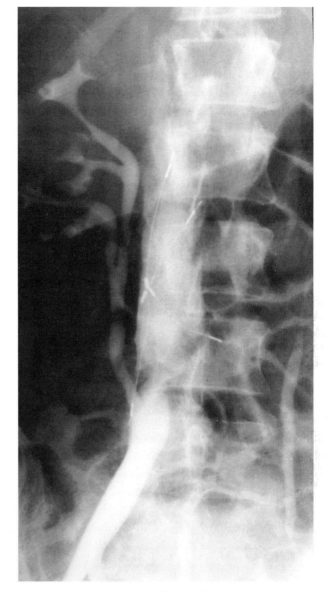

Figure 22.5 A bird's nest filter in the inferior vena cava.

The Simon nitinol filter

This filter incorporates a conical design with a petal-shaped dome of nitinol wire, which has a thermally activated shape memory property. Introduced into clinical practice in 1990, it is designed for filtering both small and large pulmonary emboli, and is deployed through a 9F delivery system. It is not big enough for mega cavae.

The Vena Tech filter

Introduced into clinical practice in 1991, this filter has a six-legged conical design with six stabilizer

bars attached to the filter legs to improve centring and stability in the vena cava. The small fixing hooks are in the stabilizer bars. It is introduced via 12F delivery system. It is not big enough for mega cavae.

The Gunther tulip filter (Figure 22.6a, b)

This filter replaced the original Gunther filter which was withdrawn from clinical use in 1990. The original filter was made of stainless steel and consisted of a wire mesh bracket and 12 anchoring

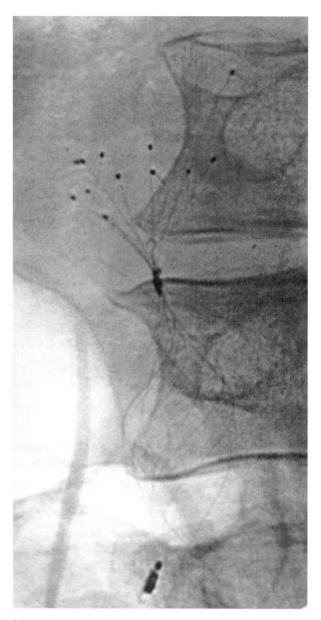

(a)

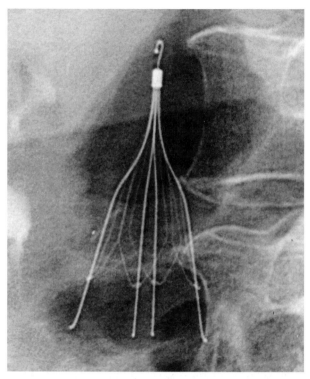

(b)

Figure 22.6 Radiographs of (a) an early Gunther filter and (b) a Gunther tulip filter with retrieval hook.

limbs. The Gunther tulip filter, introduced into clinical practice in 1993, consists of four stainless steel struts with small attached hooks. There is a stainless steel half-bracket filter above the struts and at the apex of the filter there is a small hook. This unique feature allows the filter to be retrieved percutaneously, if clinically indicated.[97] It is introduced via a 8.5F delivery system. It is not big enough for mega cavae.

The Antheor filter (Figure 22.7)

Introduced into clinical practice in 1990, this helical-shaped filter is made from a phynox alloy. Small hooks are located at the side of the filter to aid caval wall fixation.

It is introduced via an 8F delivery system. It is available in two sizes, to suit caval diameters from 10 to 28 mm and 24 to 34 mm.

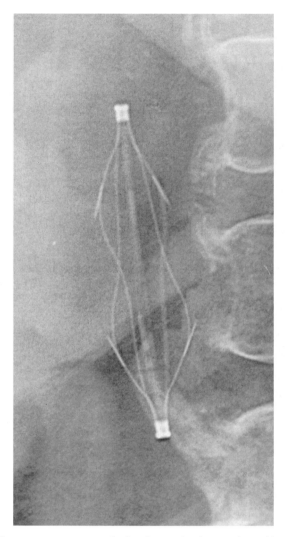

Figure 22.7 A magnified radiograph of an Antheor filter.

Both permanent and temporary designs are available. The temporary filter lacks the hooks of the permanent filter and is attached to a wire catheter assembly, the distal end of which has to be left lying on the skin close to the access vein. The Antheor filter has been temporarily withdrawn from use because of problems with filter migration following placement.

Temporary vena cava filters

The appeal of a temporary filter is that for many patients the risk from pulmonary emboli may last only a few days or weeks, especially since they are properly anticoagulated. There are obvious advantages in using a temporary filter, placed during the high-risk period, which can be removed when the risk of pulmonary embolus has passed. The patient thus obtains the protection provided by the filter but avoids the long-term complications it could cause.

The majority of temporary devices are removed by a wire permanently attached to the filter, which is either buried subcutaneously adjacent to the access vein or lies under a dressing on the skin.

The Gunther tulip filter is, as discussed, a self-contained device which can be used as a temporary or permanent filter.

The successful use of a temporary filter requires an ability to predict the moment when the risk of pulmonary embolism has passed. Failure to define this time accurately, followed by premature removal, may have fatal consequences. The problem of thrombus trapped within the filter prior to its removal must also be addressed, either by thrombolysis before filter removal or by placing a permanent filter above the temporary filter prior to its removal. Waiting for spontaneous thrombolysis to occur may exceed the time limit allowed after placement, following which removal may cause significant damage to the caval wall.

In view of these problems the role of temporary filters is likely to be limited.

Indications for filter placement

There are four absolute indications for filter placement:

- The presence of a contraindication to anticoagulation, such as overt gastrointestinal haemorrhage or risk from bleeding that would cause severe morbidity before detection, for example in vascular brain metastases.
- The development of a complication related to anticoagulation, such as gastrointestinal haemorrhage or heparin-induced thrombocytopenia.
- A failure of *adequate* anticoagulation to prevent recurrent pulmonary embolism or progressive deep vein thrombosis.
- Patients with thromboembolic disease and reduced cardiopulmonary reserve, untreated chronic pulmonary emboli, free-floating caval or iliac thrombus where other forms of treatment are contraindicated or have failed.

Other less certain indications include prophylactic filter placement, i.e. insertion of a filter in a patient[15,28] who is at increased risk of pulmonary embolism, for example, patients with major lower limb and pelvic trauma, previous pulmonary embolism, anticipated major or prolonged immobilization in the presence of severe pulmonary hypertension;[20] patients with cancer and paraplegics.[38,43,103,144] Prophylactic placement is always

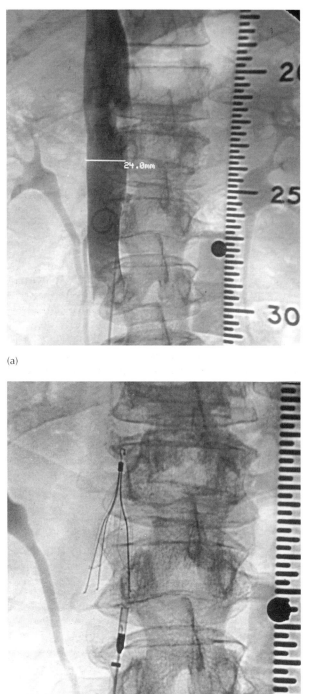

(a)

(b)

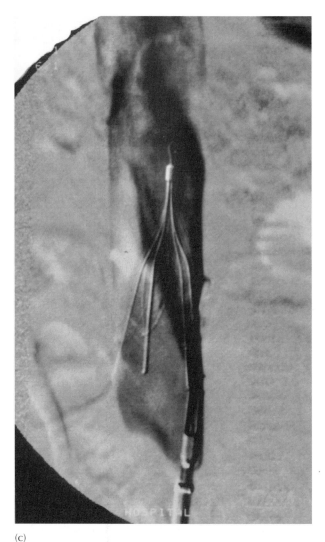

(c)

Figure 22.8 The insertion and deployment of a Gunther tulip filter. (a) An intravenous digital inferior cavagraph with electronic calipers for measuring the diameter of the vena cava. (b) The deployment of the filter from its carrying device. (c) A post-deployment cavagraph confirming the alignment and position of the filter.

difficult to justify, as it entails placing a permanent device in a patient to treat a condition that has not and might not occur. Temporary filters may have a role in these circumstances, especially if risk assessment improves.

Contraindications to filter placement

The only absolute contraindications to filter placement are complete thrombosis of the vena cava and the absence of a route for access.

Filters have no role in the treatment of patients with uncomplicated thromboembolic disease who can be safely treated with anticoagulation.[20]

Technique of filter placement (Figure 22.8)

Percutaneous access to the vena cava is usually via the internal jugular or femoral vein. Because of its familiarity, the femoral route is usually preferred by radiologists but pre-existing thrombus in the iliac vein above the site of femoral vein puncture is a contraindication to the femoral route. Filters like the Greenfield titanium filter can only be placed via the right femoral or right jugular vein, but smaller and more flexible filters, such as the Antheor filter, can be placed via either the femoral and jugular veins, as well as the left subclavian vein.

Whichever route is used, an inferior vena cava cavagram is performed via a catheter placed in the vena cava using a power injector for contrast media delivery.

These investigations are necessary for several reasons.

1. It is necessary to establish whether there is thrombus in the vena cava or renal veins because the filter needs to be placed above it.
2. The local anatomy needs to be assessed, to reveal any congenital abnormalities such as a duplicated inferior vena cava which may require two filters, one for each vena cava or accessory renal veins which could act as a conduit for emboli to bypass the filter.
3. The level at which the renal vein enters the inferior vena cava needs to be determined because infra-renal placement of the filter is preferable to supra-renal placement, unless there is extensive thrombus in the infra-renal cava which precludes caval filter placement there. Some radiologists recommend selective catheterization and visualization of the renal veins to improve detection of any renal vein anomalies that may affect filter placement.[187]
4. The diameter of the cava must be measured to ensure the placement of an appropriately sized filter or when there is a mega cava and no suitable filter size is available the insertion of two, one in each iliac vein.

Although supra-renal caval filter placement should be avoided whenever possible its use is well documented. In young women of child-bearing age, supra-renal placement may be advantageous as the filter will not be compressed by an enlarging uterus.[80,85,132,159] Furthermore, because the right ovarian vein joins the vena cava too far cephalad for an infra-renal filter to trap any thrombus within

it, and the left ovarian vein normally drains into the left renal vein, an infra-renal filter will not prevent emboli from either ovarian vein reaching the pulmonary circulation.

The pelvic veins are a well recognized site of thrombosis and source of pulmonary emboli in young women.[75] Many of the pelvic veins drain into the ovarian veins; consequently, an infra-renal filter may not be effective in this group of patients.[85]

Although a 16-year follow up[85] of 71 patients with supra-renal filters showed no serious complications, infra-renal placement is preferred because if vena cava thrombosis occurs as a late complication the renal veins will be unaffected.

The filter should always be deployed under fluoroscopic control.

A post-procedure cavagram is performed to confirm the position of the filter with regard to the position of the renal veins and any malpositioning, such as tilting, leg asymmetry and leg locking, which might reduce its filtration ability and stability.

Following removal of the filter delivery assembly, pressure is applied over the venepuncture site until any bleeding has ceased. Following this the puncture site should be kept under observation in case rebleeding causes an haematoma, particularly if the patient is anticoagulated.

The whole procedure takes approximately 45 minutes.

Although unusual, superior vena cava filter placement is technically possible. It can be performed safely and effectively prevents pulmonary embolism from upper extremity venous thrombosis. The indications for its use are the same as those given for inferior vena cava filters.[12]

Complications of vena cava filters

The improved design of filter devices, coupled with the development of percutaneous radiological deployment, has been associated with a rapid expansion in the number of caval filter devices placed. By 1992, more than 125 000 Greenfield devices had been deployed. In the USA, 13 000 caval filters are inserted annually.

While concern over the use of prophylactic filters has been expressed,[123] the major reasons for the increasing number of caval filters placed are:

- The lowering of the clinical threshold for filter placement
- The relative ease of placement of current filter designs.

The complications of vena cava filter insertion are well documented. Historically, transabdominal

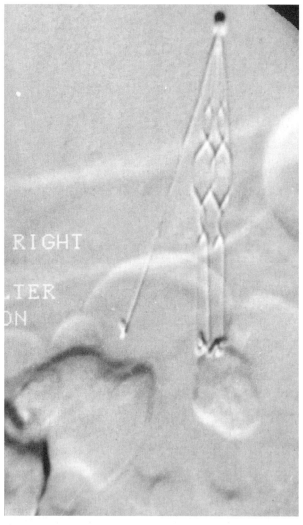

(a)

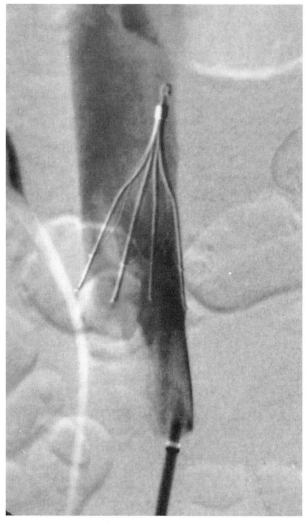

(b)

Figure 22.9 (a) A sign of poor filter deployment. The legs of this Greenfield filter are clearly asymmetrical, indicating that it is not properly anchored and has large spaces either side of the malplaced leg which could allow the passage of emboli. (b) Malalignment of a Gunther tulip filter. This inferior cavagraph shows that the filter is tilted to one side, not parallel to the direction of blood flow. The right-hand hook may have penetrated through the wall of the cava.

interruption of the inferior vena cava by ligation, plication and clipping was associated with significant morbidity. The early filters often caused vena cava thrombosis and provided only moderate protection against embolism.[132] The caval occlusion often caused chronic venous insufficiency in the lower limb. The early filters were also more prone to migrate.[44,54,101,132,134,195] The stainless steel Greenfield filter proved to be a significant advance in that it prevented embolism in 95% of patients, maintained vena cava patency in 95%,[41,80,88,90] and

had a low risk of migration. The large delivery system, however, was associated with a femoral vein thrombosis rate of up to 30%.[63,138,157] The introduction of the titanium version of the Greenfield filter has reduced the femoral vein thrombosis rate to under 10%[84] while maintaining a 97% effectiveness in preventing embolism, with a zero rate of vena cava occlusion.[83] The bird's nest filter and Vena Tech filter have a reported embolism prevention rate of over 95% and a similar caval patency rate.[49,164,165,167]

Early complications

The incidence of early minor and major complications has been reported to be between 5 and 10%.[39,88,116,168] The early mortality rate varies from 0 to 14%, but is usually due to the underlying disease.[78,82,168] Unfavourable anatomy occasionally precludes filter placement and may result in filter misplacement.[72,88,155] Tilting of a filter reduces its filtration ability, but may be corrected by subsequent manipulation[58] (Figure 22.9a, b).

More serious are complications such as caval perforation (Figure 22.10), filter migration to a position higher in the cava, to the right atrium and the pulmonary artery[136,163,187] (Figures 22.10). Other complications include bleeding, air embolism, caval and insertion site thrombosis and obstructive uropathy.[2,3,11,13,50,52,58,64,95–97,137,151,187,188]

Dislodgement of caval filters during central venous line insertion has also been reported.[128,136]

Some of these complications can be treated. Successful lysis of caval thrombus following caval thrombosis has been reported[96] as well as percutaneous removal of a malpositioned filter.[51,178,187]

Failure to prevent embolism because of filter misplacement (Figures 22.11, 22.12a, b) or incorrect deployment can often be resolved by placing a second filter above the first filter, even in the suprarenal vena cava if necessary.[2,116,157]

Operator errors during percutaneous insertion of caval filters are defined as complications specific to filter placement that are not attributable to the filter design itself. The frequency of operator errors is unknown. They can be divided into imaging errors, errors in filter selection, and errors of filter deployment[72,76,121,133,188,189] such as placement in the renal veins, iliac veins or even the aorta. Technical problems related to filter design are reported to occur in 5–20% of filter insertions.[188]

Late complications

The numerous reports of late complications of filter placement include filter migration;[16,66,177] mechanical failure of the filter;[3,113,159,161] caval wall penetration;[113,170] aortic and vena cava penetration;[3,52,75,113,119,177] bowel perforation, obstruction and bleeding;[16,36,177] caval and ilio-femoral thrombosis[39,59,65,66,77,166,168] progressing to venous stasis and gangrene;[11,16,39,89] and propagation of thrombus through the filter, resulting in recurrent embolism.[71,130]

With up to 40 000 filters being placed annually world wide,[132] meticulous long-term studies are needed to identify the frequency of each complication.[39,99] Most published studies claim a low complication rate,[88,96,120,168] but the number of patients studied this way is small.[1,10,82,89,91,129,132,143,184,191] The true late complication rate may be higher than we think. The ease of placement and this low reported

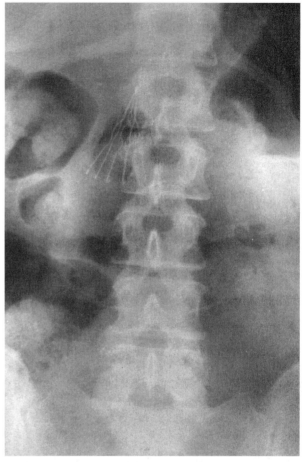

(a)

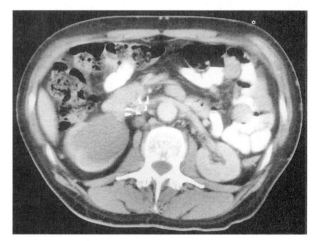

(b)

Figure 22.10 Maldeployment of a Greenfield filter. (a) A plain radiograph showing an apparent good position of a Greenfield filter. (b) The CT scan of the same patient shows that four of the legs have penetrated through the wall of the vena cava.

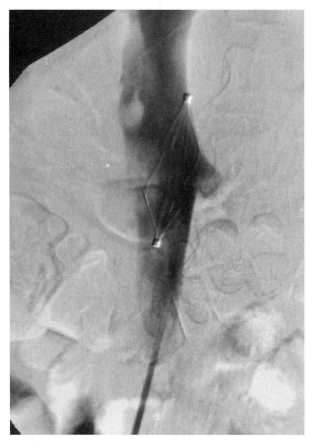

(a)

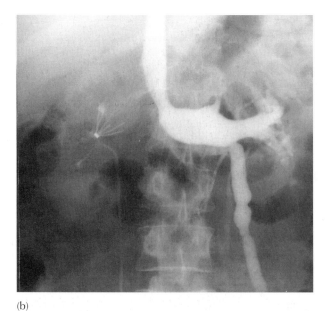

(b)

Figure 22.11 (a) Filter misplacement. This Antheor filter has been deployed too far up the vena cava because it is covering the entrance of the left renal vein. This was not apparent on the plain radiograph but is obvious on the check post-placement cavagraph. (b) A Mobin-Uddin filter inadvertently deployed in the right renal vein in a patient with a thrombus of the inferior vena cava up to the level of the renal veins. Note the very large left ovarian vein providing a collateral pathway around the occluded vena cava.

rate of complications have unfortunately encouraged clinicians to insert filters for prophylaxis.[50,109,123,157]

Up to 39% of filters are found to contain trapped emboli.[66,82,102] This observation suggests that wherever possible systemic anticoagulation should be continued, or begun, after filter placement if and when it is safe to do so because we do not yet know how much of this trapped thrombus is caused by the patient's underlying thrombotic disorder or the thrombotic properties of the filter itself.[83,116]

As Greenfield has indicated, percutaneous vena cava filters are an appropriate, effective and valuable evolutionary step in the secondary prevention of pulmonary embolism, but the indiscriminate use of filters must be discouraged.

Phlebographically based venous interruption

The results of phlebography in patients with both deep vein thrombosis and pulmonary emboli have been described earlier in this chapter. In a series of 50 patients, 19 legs contained non-adherent thrombus,[35] in 11 patients the thrombus was below the

inguinal ligament (in the superficial femoral or calf veins) and in another three patients the thrombus was below the inguinal ligament but extended into the common femoral vein. As reliable vena cava filters were not available at that time the thrombi in these 14 patients were all 'locked in' by ligating the superficial femoral vein below the groin. This is a simple procedure that can be performed under local anaesthesia. Only four patients had thrombi in their iliac veins or vena cava with a propagating non-adherent tail that could not be removed through a common femoral venotomy because it was adherent; they all had a partial surgical vena cava interruption. None of the 19 patients had emboli after their 'locking-in' procedure.

It is our experience that most of the loose residual thrombus in patients who have had a 'herald' embolus is below the groin and if it cannot be removed it can be 'locked in' by ligating the superficial femoral vein just below its junction with the deep femoral vein.

This approach was suggested many years ago by Homans[100] and was practised extensively by his surgical service and others,[5,44] but fell into disrepute

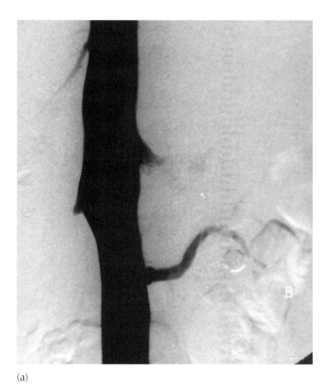

(a)

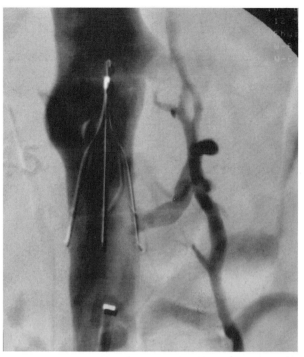

(b)

Figure 22.12 Misplacement of a Gunther tulip filter. (a) The pre-placement cavagraph shows an unusually large lumbar vein entering the vena cava a few centimetres below the left renal vein. (b) The filter has been deployed below this vein, so leaving a potential route for emboli from the azygos veins to the lungs. This potential route would become particularly significant if the filter were to become occluded with emboli, or thrombose, and the lumbar and azygos veins dilate to form large collateral channels.

because some patients had further emboli. We believe that further emboli occurred because the ligation was not preceded by a phlebogram but was carried out blindly. In some cases the ligature was probably tied around a thrombus in the femoral vein, not above the thrombus, thus making further embolism highly likely.

The ligation of the superficial femoral vein, in the presence of a pre-existing thrombosis, does not cause any additional symptoms in the legs. In a comparison[196] between patients with thrombus of a similar extent, but adherent at its upper end, treated with anticoagulants, and patients with non-adherent thrombus treated with femoral vein ligation, ligation did not increase the incidence of post-thrombotic symptoms. The symptoms score of patients with femoral vein thrombosis treated medically or surgically was the same. The percentage of patients in both groups developing the post-thrombotic syndrome 3 years later was quite high (50%), and 10% had venous ulceration. This incidence of complications is almost identical to that observed following the insertion of a Greenfield filter, which suggests that the complications are

caused by the initial thrombosis, not by the filter or the ligation.

Figure 22.13 illustrates a plan of treatment which can be used for such patients if a cava filter is contraindicated or unavailable. It is a combination of removal, locking in or anticoagulation based upon the phlebographic findings. Our early studies convinced us that this policy reduced the incidence of pulmonary embolism without increasing the incidence of post-thrombotic symptoms in the legs.

ANTICOAGULANTS

Table 22.2 shows clearly that anticoagulants will not prevent all recurrent embolism; the explanation for this is shown in Figure 22.2. Loose non-adherent thrombus will still fragment and embolize in spite of heparin. Provided anticoagulants are used as the main form of treatment only when there is adherent thrombus, recurrent embolism will not occur. In a comparison between a group of 50 patients treated with anticoagulants and a group of 31 patients who had phlebograms and anticoagulants

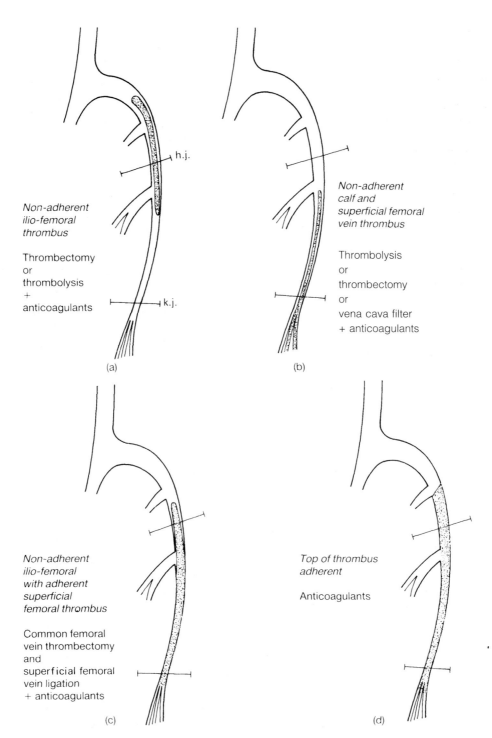

Figure 22.13   Our scheme of treatment for the prevention of pulmonary embolism, if caval blockade is contraindicated or not available, based upon the phlebographic feature of the thrombus (h.j., hip joint; k.j., knee joint). All patients are given heparin for 7–10 days followed by warfarin for 6 months.

alone only when there was no non-adherent thrombus in the veins above the calf, we found 20 recurrent emboli (seven fatal and 13 not fatal) in the first group and four small non-fatal emboli in the control group whose treatment was based on the phlebographic findings.[35] Only one of the emboli in the second group occurred within 1 month of treatment.

Our view of the significance of non-adherent thrombus, the incidence of which is discussed earlier in this chapter, has been confirmed in a study by Norris *et al.*[152] of 78 patients with deep vein thrombosis. Three of the five patients with non-adherent thrombus (60%) had pulmonary emboli compared to four of the 73 patients with adherent thrombus (5.5%).

Treatment based on phlebography therefore allows the rational use of anticoagulants alone in 60% of patients and avoids the risk of recurrent embolism. Anticoagulants should be given to all patients who have a venous thrombosis or pulmonary embolism but will only prevent recurrent embolism in those patients with adherent or calf vein thrombosis. The effect of anticoagulants in these circumstances lies in their ability to prevent the formation of new fresh non-adherent thrombus forming.

COMMENTARY

The studies discussed in the preceding section reinforce our view that no treatment of deep vein thrombosis should be undertaken without having a detailed knowledge of the state of the thrombus. Immediate anticoagulation is always indicated to prevent new thrombosis but in up to 20% of patients additional mechanical measures may be required to prevent a recurrent and possibly fatal embolism.

It has been suggested that to perform venous imaging on all patients who have had an embolus, however small, to pick up the 20% that need more than anticoagulants is not cost effective, but amongst the patients with non-adherent thrombus will be that group (4% of the total) who will have a fatal recurrent embolism. A mandatory study of both lower limbs on 100 patients, followed by adequate surgical or radiological action (if indicated) on 20 patients to save four lives seems to us to be worthwhile – until the day when deep vein thrombosis is completely abolished. Furthermore, the confirmation of the diagnosis and the subsequent avoidance of bleeding complications and death from unnecessary anticoagulation is undoubtedly worthwhile.

References

1. Aburahma AF, Robinson PA, Boland JP, *et al.* Therapeutic and prophylactic vena caval interruption for pulmonary embolism: caval and venous insertion site patency. *Ann Vasc Surg* 1993; **7:** 561–8.
2. Adye BA, Raabe RD, Zobell RL. Errant percutaneous Greenfield filter placement into the retroperitoneum. *J Vasc Surg* 1990; **12:** 60–1.
3. Alexander JJ, Gerwertz BL, Zarins CK. Intraoperative disruption of a Greenfield vena cava filter. *J Cardiovasc Surg (Torino)* 1989; **30(1):** 130–3.
4. Alexander JJ, Yuhas JP, Piotrowski JJ. Is the increasing use of prophylactic percutaneous IVC filters justified? *Am J Surg* 1994; **168:** 102.
5. Allen AW. Interruption of the deep veins of the lower extremities in the prevention and treatment of thrombosis and embolism. *Surg Gynecol Obstet* 1947; **84:** 529.
6. Allen EV, Hines EA, Kvate WF, Barker NW. The use of dicoumarol as an anticoagulant, experience in 2307 cases. *Ann Intern Med* 1947; **27:** 371.
7. Amador E, Li TK, Crane A. Ligation of inferior vena cave for thromboembolism. Clinical and autopsy correlations in 119 cases. *JAMA* 1968; **206:** 1758.
8. An International Multicentre Trial. Prevention of fatal postoperative pulmonary embolism by low doses of heparin. *Lancet* 1975; **2:** 45.
9. Antiplatelet Trialists Collaboration. Collaborative overview of randomized trials of antiplatelet therapy–III. Reduction in venous thrombosis and pulmonary embolism by antiplatelet prophylaxis in surgical and medical patients. *Br Med J* 1994; **308:** 235–46.
10. Arnold TE, Karanbinis VD, Mehta V, Dupont EL, Matsumoto T, Kerstein MD. Potential of overuse of the inferior vena cava filter. *Surg Gynecol Obstet* 1993; **177:** 463–7.
11. Aruny JE, Kandarpa K. Phlegmasia cerulea dolens; a complication after placement of a bird's nest vena cava filter. *Am J Roentgenol* 1990; **154:** 1105–6.
12. Ascer E, Gennaro M, Lorensen E, Pollina RM. Superior vena caval Greenfield filters: Indications, techniques and results. *J Vasc Surg* 1996; **23:** 498–503.
13. Athanasoulis CA. Complications of vena cava filters. *Radiology* 1993; **188:** 614–15.
14. Atik M, Broghamer W. The impact of prophylactic measures in fatal pulmonary embolism. *Arch Surg* 1979; **114:** 366.
15. Baldridge ED, Martin MA, Welling RE, *et al.* Clinical significance of free-floating venous thrombi. *J Vasc Surg* 1990; **11:** 62–9.
16. Balshi JD, Cantelmo NL, Menzoian JO. Complications of caval interruption by Greenfield filter in quadriplegics. *J Vasc Surg* 1989; **96:** 558–62.
17. Barker NW. Anticoagulant therapy in thrombosis and embolism. *Postgrad Med J* 1947; **1:** 265.
18. Barker NW, Priestley JT. Postoperative thrombophlebitis and embolism. *Surgery* 1942; **12:** 411.
19. Barritt DW, Jordan SC. Anticoagulant drugs in treatment of pulmonary embolism, controlled trial. *Lancet* 1960; **1:** 1309.
20. Becker DM, Philbrick JT, Selby JB. Inferior vena cava filters: indications, safety, effectiveness. *Arch Intern Med* 1992; **152:** 1985–94.
21. Benavides J, Noon R. Experimental evaluation of inferior vena cave procedures to prevent pulmonary embolism. *Ann Surg* 1967, **166:** 195.

22. Bergqvist D. *Postoperative Thromboembolism.* Berlin: Springer-Verlag, 1983; 102, 138.

23. Bergqvist D. The prevention of postoperative embolism in Sweden. *Thromb Haemost* 1985; **53:** 239.

24. Bergqvist D. Low molecular weight heparins for prevention of venous thromboembolism following general surgery. In: Bounameaux H. *Low Molecular Weight Heparin in Prophylaxis and Therapy of Thromboembolic Disease.* Basel: Marcel Dekker Inc., 169–85.

25. Bergqvist D. Dextran. In: Bergqvist D, Comerota A, Nicolaides A, Scurr J, eds. *Prevention of Venous Thromboembolism.* London: Med Orion, 1994; 181–98.

26. Bergqvist D, Efsing HO, Hallbook T, Hedlund T. Thromboembolism after elective and post traumatic hip surgery – a controlled prophylactic trial with dextran and low dose heparin. *Acta Chir Scand* 1979; **145:** 213.

27. Bergqvist D, Lindblad B. A 30 year survey of pulmonary embolism verified at autopsy, an analysis of 1274 surgical patients. *Br J Surg* 1985; **72:** 105.

28. Berry RE, George JE, Shaver WA. Free-floating deep venous thrombosis. *Ann Surg* 1990; **211:** 719–23.

29. Blumenberg RM, Gelfland ML. Long term follow up of vena caval clips and umbrellas. *Am J Surg* 1977; **134:** 205.

30. Brenner DW, Brenner CJ, Scott J, Wehberg K, Granger JP, Scheilhammer PF. Suprarenal Greenfield filter placement to prevent pulmonary embolus in patients with vena caval tumor thrombi. *J Urol* 1992; **147:** 19–23.

31. Browse NL, Burnand KG, Lea Thomas M. Prevention of pulmonary embolism. *Diseases of the Veins: Pathology, Diagnosis and Treatment.* London: Edward Arnold, 1989: 581–93.

32. Browse NL, Clemenson G, Bateman NT, Gaunt JI, Croft DN. Effect of intravenous Dextran 70 and pneumatic leg compression on the incidence of postoperative pulmonary embolism. *Br Med J* 1976, **2:** 1281.

33. Browse NL, Lea Thomas M. Source of non-lethal pulmonary emboli. *Lancet* 1974; **1:** 258.

34. Browse NL, Lea Thomas M, Solan MJ. The management of the source of pulmonary emboli. The value of phlebography. *Br Med J* 1967; **4:** 596.

35. Browse NL, Lea Thomas M, Solan MJ, Young AE. Prevention of recurrent pulmonary embolism. *Br Med J* 1969; **3:** 382–6.

36. Burandt TM, Jarski RW. Small bowel obstruction by adhesion secondary to caval perforation by Greenfield vena cava filter. *J Am Osteopath Assoc* 1988; **88:** 1239–41.

37. Byrne JJ. Phlebitis. A study of 979 cases at the Boston City Hospital. *JAMA* 1960; **174:** 113.

38. Cantelmo NL, Menzolan JO, Logerfo FW, *et al.* Clinical experience with vena caval filters in high-risk cancer patients. *Cancer* 1982; **50:** 341–4.

39. Carabesi RA, Moritz MJ, Jarell BE. Complications encountered with the use of the Greenfield filter. *Am J Surg* 1987; **154:** 163–8.

40. Carmichael D, Edwards S. Prophylactic inferior vena caval plication. *Surg Gynecol Obstet* 1967; **124:** 785.

41. Cimochowski GE, Evans RH, Zarins CK, Lu CT, De Meester TR. Greenfield filter versus Mobin-Uddin umbrella: the continuing quest for the ideal method of vena caval interruption. *J Cardiovasc Surg* 1980; **79:** 358–65.

42. Clagett GP, Reisch JS. Prevention of venous thromboembolism in general surgical patients. *Ann Surg* 1988; **208:** 227–40.

43. Cohen JR, Grella L, Citron M. Greenfield filter instead of heparin as primary treatment for deep venous thrombosis or pulmonary embolism in patients with cancer. *Cancer* 1992; **70:** 1993–6.

44. Colby F. The prevention of fatal pulmonary emboli after prostatectomy. *J Urol* 1948; **59:** 920.

45. Collins R, Scringeour A, Yusef S, Peto R. Reduction in fatal pulmonary embolism and venous thrombosis by perioperative administration of subcutaneous heparin. *N Engl J Med* 1988; **318:** 1162–73.

46. Coon WW, Mackenzie JW, Hodgson PK. A critical evaluation of anticoagulant therapy in peripheral venous thrombosis and pulmonary embolism. *Surg Gynecol Obstet* 1958; **106:** 129.

47. Cosgriff SW, Cross RJ, Habif DV. Management of venous thrombosis and pulmonary embolism. *Surg Clin North Am* 1948; **28:** 324.

48. Crane C. Deep venous thrombosis and pulmonary embolism. *N Engl J Med* 1957; **257:** 147.

49. Cull DL, Wheeler JR, Gregory RT, Synder SO Jr, Gayle RG, Parent FN III. The vena tech filter: evaluation of a new inferior vena cava interruption device. *J Cardiovasc Surg* 1991; **32:** 691–6.

50. Crystal KS, Kase DJ, Scher LA, Shapiro MA, Naidich JB. Utilization patterns with inferior vena cava filters: surgical versus percutaneous placement. *J Vasc Intervent Radiol* 1995; **6(3):** 443–8.

51. Cynamon J, Bakal CW, Epstein SB, Gabelman G. Percutaneous removal of a titanium Greenfield filter. *Am J Roentgenol* 1992; **159(4):** 777–8.

52. Dabbagh A, Chakfe N, Kretz JG, *et al.* Late complication of a Greenfield filter associating caudal migration and perforation of the abdominal aorta by a ruptured strut. *J Vasc Surg* 1995; **22:** 182–7.

53. Dalman R, Kohler TR. Cerebrovascular accident after Greenfield filter placement for paradoxical embolism. *J Vasc Surg* 1989; **9:** 452–4.

54. De Laria GA, Hunter JA, Serry C, *et al.* Thromboembolism and cancer: treatment with the Hunter balloon. *J Vasc Surg* 1984; **1:** 670–4.

55. De Weese MS, Hunter DC. A vena cave filter for the prevention of pulmonary emboli. *Bull Soc Int Chir* 1958; **17:** 17.

56. Dismuke SE. Declining mortality from pulmonary embolism in surgical patients. *Thromb Haemost* 1981; **46:** 17.

57. Donaldson M, Wirthlin L, Donaldson G. Thirty year experience with surgical interruption of the inferior vena cava prevention of pulmonary embolism. *Ann Surg* 1980; **191:** 367.

58. Dorfman GS. Risks and benefits of manipulation of the titanium Greenfield inferior vena cava filter

after deployment: filter facts and filter fantasies (editorial: comment). *J Vasc Intervent Radiol* 1993; **4(5):** 617–20.

59. Epstein DH, Darcy MD, Hunter DW, *et al.* Experience with the Amplatz retrievable vena cava filter. *Radiology* 1989; **172:** 105–10.

60. Eskeland G, Solheim K, Skjorten F. Anticoagulant prophylaxis, thromboembolism and mortality in elderly patients with hip fractures. A controlled clinical trial. *Acta Chir Scand* 1966; **131:** 16.

61. Feinman LJ, Meltzer AJ. Phlegmasia cerulea dolens as a complication of percutaneous insertion of a vena cava filter. *J Am Osteopath Assoc* 1989; **89:** 63–8.

62. Ferris EJ, McCowan TC, Carver DK, McFarland DR. Percutaneous inferior vena caval filters: follow-up of seven designs in 320 patients. *Radiology* 1993; **188:** 851–6.

63. Fink JA, Jones BT. The Greenfield filter as the primary means of therapy in venous thromboembolic disease. *Surg Gynecol Obstet* 1991; **172:** 253–6.

64. Flanagan D, Creasy T, Chataway F, Kerr D. Caval umbrella causing obstructive uropathy. *Postgrad Med J* 1996; **72:** 235–7.

65. Flinn WR, Yao JST, Bergan JJ. Direct vena cava interruption. In: Bergan JJ, Yao JST, eds. *Surgery of the Veins.* New York: Grune & Stratton, 1985; 497–506.

66. Fobbe F, Dietzel M, Korth R, *et al.* Gunther vena cava filter: results of a long term follow up. *Am J Roentgenol* 1988; **151:** 1031–4.

67. Fontaine R, Kiény R, Tuchmann L, Suhler A, Babin S. Quelques réflexions sur les embolies pulmonaries d'après une statistique personnelle de 409 thromboses veineuses récentes. *Ann Chir Thorac Cardiovasc* 1965; **4:** 1296.

68. Fuller CH, Robertson CW, Smithwick RH. Management of thromboembolic disease. *N Engl J Med* 1960; **263:** 983.

69. Fuller CH, Willbanks OL. Incidental prophylactic inferior vena cave clipping. *Arch Surg* 1971; **102:** 440–1.

70. Gazzaniga AG, Cahill JL, Replogle RL, Tilney NL. Changes in blood volume and renal function following ligation of the inferior vena cave. *Surgery* 1967; **62:** 417.

71. Geisinger MA, Zelch MG, Risius B. Recurrent pulmonary embolism after Greenfield filter placement. *Radiology* 1987; **165:** 383–4.

72. Gelbfish GA, Ascer E. Intracardiac and intrapulmonary Greenfield filters: a long term follow up. *J Vasc Surg* 1991; **14:** 614–17.

73. German Hip Arthroplasty Trial. Prevention of deep vein thrombosis with low molecular weight heparin in patients undergoing total hip replacement. *Arch Orthop Trauma Surg* 1992; **111(2):** 110–20.

74. Gibbs NM. Venous thrombosis of the lower limbs with particular reference to bed rest. *Br J Surg* 1957; **45:** 209.

75. Godleski JJ. Pathology of deep venous thrombosis and pulmonary embolism. In: Goldhaber SZ, ed. *Pulmonary Embolism and Deep Venous Thrombosis.* Boston, MA: Saunders, 1985; 11–25.

76. Goertzen TC, McGowan TC, Garvin KL, *et al.* An unopened titanium Greenfield IVC filter: intravascular ultrasound to reveal associated thrombus and aid in filter opening. *Cardiovasc Intervent Radiol* 1993; **16:** 251–3.

77. Goluecke PJ, Garrett WV, Thompson JE, Smith BL, Talkington CM. Interruption of the vena cava by means of the Greenfield filter. Expanding the indications. *Surgery* 1988; **103:** 111–17.

78. Gomez GA, Cutler BS, Wheeler HB. Transvenous interruption of the inferior vena cava. *Surgery* 1983; **93:** 612–19.

79. Greenfield LJ. Antiembolic filters; the state of the art. *Hosp Pract* 1992; **15:** 16.

80. Greenfield LJ. Current indications for and results of Greenfield filter placement. *J Vasc Surg* 1984; **1:** 502–4.

81. Greenfield LJ. Use and abuse of intracaval devices. *Surgery* 1986; **99:** 383.

82. Greenfield LJ. Results of catheter embolectomy and Greenfield filter insertion. In: Bergan JJ, Yao JS, eds. *Surgery of the Veins.* Orlando, FL: Grune & Stratton, 1985; 479.

83. Greenfield LJ, Cho KJ, Proctor M, *et al.* Results of a multicenter study of the modified hook-titanium Greenfield filter. *J Vasc Surg* 1991; **14:** 253–7.

84. Greenfield LJ, Delucia A, III. Endovascular therapy of venous thromboembolic disease. *Surg Clin North Am* 1992; **72(4):** 969–89.

85. Greenfield LJ, Kyung JC, Proctor MC, Sobel M, Shah S, Wingo J. Late results of suprarenal Greenfield vena cava filter placement. *Arch Surg* 1992; **127:** 969–73.

86. Greenfield LJ, Langham MR. Surgical approaches to thromboembolism. *Br J Surg* 1984; **71:** 468.

87. Greenfield LJ, McCurdy JR, Brown PHP, Elkins RC. A new intracaval filter permitting continued flow and resolution of emboli. *Surgery* 1973; **73:** 599.

88. Greenfield LJ, Michna BA. Twelve-year clinical experience with the Greenfield vena cava filter. *Surgery* 1988; **104:** 706–12.

89. Greenfield LJ, Peyton R, Crute S, Barnes R. Greenfield vena caval filter experience: Late results in 156 patients. *Arch Surg* 1981; **116:** 1451.

90. Greenfield LJ, Proctor MC. Twenty year clinical experience with the Greenfield filter. *Cardiovasc Surg* 1995; **2:** 199–205.

91. Greenfield LJ, Proctor MC, Cho KJ, *et al.* Extended valuation of the titanium Greenfield vena caval filter. *J Vasc Surg* 1994; **20(3):** 458–64.

92. Groote Schuur Hospital Thromboembolus Study Group. Failure of low dose heparin to prevent significant thromboembolic complications in high risk surgical patients. *Br Med J* 1979; **1:** 1447.

93. Gruber UF, Duckert F, Fridrich R, Tornhurst J, Rem J. Prevention of postoperative thromboembolism by Dextran 40, low doses of heparin, or xantinol nicotinate. *Lancet* 1977; **1:** 207–10.

94. Gruber UF, Saldeen T, Brokop T, *et al.* Incidences of fatal postoperative pulmonary embolism with dextran 70 and low dose heparin. An International Medicine Multicentre Trial. *Br Med J* 1980; **280:** 69.

95. Hainaut P, Luyeye B, Vincent B, Goffette P. Inferior vena cava thrombosis following percutaneous filter insertion: an unsual cause of haemodynamic compromise. *Acta Clin Belg* 1995; **50(4):** 231–7.

96. Hansen ME, Miller GL, Starks KC. Pulse spray thrombolysis of inferior vena cava thrombosis complicating filter placement. *Cardiovasc Intervent Radiol* 1994; **17(1):** 38–40.

97. Heenan SD, Grubnic S, Buckenham TM. Transjugular retrieval of a Gunther Tulip caval filter. *J Intervent Radiol* 1995; **10:** 111–14.

98. Hicks ME, Malden ES, Vesely TM, Picus D, Darcy MD. Prospective anatomic study of the inferior vena cava and renal veins: comparison of selective renal venography with cavography and relevance in filter placement. *J Vasc Intervent Radiol* 1995; **6(5):** 721–9.

99. Hirsh J, Levine M. Prevention of venous thrombosis in patients undergoing major orthopaedic surgical procedures. *Acta Chir Scand Suppl* 1990; **556:** 30–5.

100. Homans J. Thrombosis of the deep veins of the lower leg causing pulmonary embolism. *N Engl J Med* 1934; **211:** 993.

101. Hunter JA, De Laria GA. Hunter vena cava balloon: rationale and results. *J Vasc Surg* 1984; **1:** 491–7.

102. Iabloklow EG, Zubarev AR, Muradia RA. Assessment of the results of implantation of an anti-embolic cava-filter using the method of ultrasound scanning. *Klin Khir* 1989; **7:** 28–31.

103. Jarrell BE, Posuniak E, Roberts J, *et al.* A new method of management using the Kim-Ray Greenfield filter for deep venous thrombosis and pulmonary embolism in spinal cord injury. *Surg Gynecol Obstet* 1983; **157:** 316–18.

104. Jorpes JE. On the dosage of the anticoagulants, heparin and dicumarol, in the treatment of thrombosis. *Acta Chir Scand Suppl* 1950; **149**.

105. Kantor A, Glanz S, Gordon DH, Sclafani SJ. Percutaneous insertion of the Komray-Greenfield filter: incidence of femoral vein thrombosis. *Am J Roentgenol* 1987; **149:** 1065–6.

106. Kaufman JA, Geller SC. Correspondence. *Am J Roentgenol* 1995; **164:** 257.

107. Kaufman JA, Geller SC, Rivitz SM, Waltman AC. Operator errors during percutaneous placement of vena cava filters. *Am J Roentgenol* 1995; **165:** 1281–7.

108. Kernohan RJ, Todd C. Heparin therapy in thromboembolic disease. *Lancet* 1966; **1:** 621.

109. Khansarinia S, Dennis JW, Veldenz HC, Butcher JL, Hartland L. Prophylactic Greenfield filter placement in selected high-risk trauma patients. *J Vasc Surg* 1995; **22(3):** 231–5.

110. Kiil J, Kiil J, Axelsen F, Andersen D. Prophylaxis against postoperative pulmonary embolism and deep-vein thrombosis by low-dose heparin. *Lancet* 1978; **1:** 1115.

111. Kiil J, Moller JC. Postoperative deep vein thrombosis of the lower limb and prophylactic value of heparin evaluated by phlebography. *Acta Radiol Diagn (Stockh)* 1979; **20:** 507.

112. Kiil J, Taagehoj-Jensen F. Pulmonary embolism associated with elective surgery, detected by ventilation–perfusion scintigraphy. *Acta Chir Scand* 1978; **144:** 427.

113. Kim D, Porter DH, Siegel JB, Simon M. Perforation of the inferior vena cava with aortic and vertebral penetration by a suprarenal Greenfield filter. *Radiology* 1989; **172:** 721–3.

114. King R, Daly A. The prevention of postoperative pulmonary emboli with low-molecular-weight dextran. *Am J Obstet Gynecol* 1975; **123:** 46.

115. Kline A, Hughes LE, Campbell H, Williams A, Zlosnick J, Leach KG. Dextran 70 in prophylaxis of thromboembolic disease after surgery: a clinically oriented randomized double-blind trial. *Br Med J* 1975; **2:** 109.

116. Kneimeyer HW, Sandmann W, Bach D, Torsello G, Jungblut RM, Grabensee B. Complications following caval interruption. *Eur J Vasc Surg* 1994; **8:** 617–21.

117. Knight B, Zaini MR. Pulmonary embolism and venous thrombosis. A pattern of incidence and predisposing factors over 70 years. *Am J Forensic Med Pathol* 1980; **1:** 227.

118. Korwin SM, Callow AD, Rosenthal D, Ledig B, Deterling RA, O'Donnell TF. Prophylactic interruption of the inferior vena cave. *Arch Surg* 1979; **114:** 1037.

119. Kurgan A, Nunelee JD, Auer AI. Penetration of the wall of an abdominal aortic aneurysm by a Greenfield filter prong: a late complication. *J Vasc Surg* 1993; **18:** 303–6.

120. Lagatolla NRF, Burnand KG, Irvine A, Ferrar D. Twelve years experience of vena cava filtration. *Ann R Coll Surg Engl* 1994; **76:** 336–9.

121. Lahey SJ, Meyer LP, Karchmer AW, *et al.* Misplaced caval filter and subsequent pericardial tamponade. *Ann Thorac Surg* 1991; **51:** 299–301.

122. Lang W, Schweiger H, Hofmann-Preiss K. Results of long-term venacavography study after placement of a Greenfield vena caval filter. *J Cardiovasc Surg (Torino)* 1992; **3(5):** 573–8.

123. Lang W, Weingartner M, Sturm M, Schweiger H. Prophylactic use of cavafilters: is this indication justified? *Zentralbl Chir* 1994; **119:** 625–30.

124. Leyvraz P, Bachmann F, Bohnet J, *et al.* Thromboembolic prophylaxis in total hip replacement: a comparison between the low molecular weight heparinoid lomoparah and heparin-dihydroergotamine. *Br J Surg* 1992; **79(9):** 911–14.

125. Leyvraz PF, Bachmann F, Hoek J, *et al.* Prevention of deep vein thrombosis after hip replacement: randomised comparison between infractionated heparin and low molecular weight heparin. *Br Med J* 1991; **303:** 543–8.

126. Little JM, Loewenthal J, Mills FH. Venous thrombo-embolic disease. *Br J Surg* 1966; **53:** 657.

127. Ljungstrom KG. Dextran 70 as prophylaxis against lethal postoperative pulmonary embolism. *Lakartidningen* 1975; **72:** 2284.

128. Loesberg A, Taylor FC, Awh MH. Dislodgment of inferior vena caval filters during 'blind insertion of

central venous catheters. *Am J Roentgenol* 1993; **161:** 637–8.

129. Lord RSA, Benn I. Early and late results of Bird's nest filter placement in the inferior vena cava: clinical and duplex ultrasound follow up. *Aust N Z J Surg* 1994; **64:** 106–14.

130. McAuley CE, Webster MW, Jarrett F, Hirsch SA, Steed DL. The Greenfield intracaval filter as a source of recurrent pulmonary thromboembolism. *Surgery* 1984; **96:** 574–7.

131. Maas D, Demierre D, Wallsten H, Senning A. A new vena caval filter for the prevention of pulmonary embolism. *J Cardiovasc Surg* 1985; **26:** 116.

132. Magnant JG, Walsh DB, Jurzvsky LI, Cronenwett JL. Current use of inferior vena cava filter. *J Vasc Surg* 1992; **16:** 701–6.

133. Malden ES, Hicks ME, Picus D, Darcy MD, Vesely TM, Hovespian DM. Inferior vena cava cavography with and without selective renal venography in diagnosing renal vein variant anatomy and its relationship to caval filter placement (abstract). *J Vasc Intervent Radiol* 1994; **5:** 23.

134. Mansour M, Chang AE, Sindelar WF. Interruption of the inferior vena cava for the prevention of recurrent pulmonary embolism. *Am Surg* 1985; **51:** 375–80.

135. Maraan B, Taber R. The effects of inferior vena caval ligation on cardiac output, an experimental study. *Surgery* 1968; **63:** 996.

136. Marelich GP, Tharratt RS. Greenfield inferior vena cava filter dislodged during central venous catheter placement. *Chest* 1994; **106:** 957–9.

137. Mastrobattista JM, Caputo TA, Bush HS. Perforation of the inferior vena cava by a recently inserted Greenfield filter. *Gynecol Oncol* 1995; **56:** 399–401.

138. Mewissen MW, Erikson SJ, Foley WD, *et al.* Thrombosis at venous insertion sites after inferior vena cava filter placement. *Radiology* 1989; **173:** 155–7.

139. Miles RM, Chappell F, Renner O. A partially occluding vena cave clip for the prevention of pulmonary embolism. *Am Surg* 1964; **30:** 40.

140. Mitchell JRA. Can we really prevent postoperative pulmonary emboli. *Br Med J* 1979; **1:** 1523.

141. Mobin-Uddin K, McLean R, Bolooki H. Caval interruption for prevention of pulmonary embolism. *Arch Surg* 1969; **99:** 711.

142. Mobin-Uddin K, Smith PE, Martinez LD, Lombardo CR, Jude JR. A venacaval filter for the prevention of pulmonary embolism. *Surg Forum* 1967; **18:** 209.

143. Mohan CR, Hoballah JJ, Sharp WJ, Kresowik TF, Lu CT, Corson JD. Comparative efficacy and complications of vena caval filters. *J Vasc Surg* 1995; **21(2):** 235–45.

144. Moore FD Jr, Osteen RT, Karp DD, *et al.* Anticoagulants, venous thromboembolism and the cancer patient. *Arch Surg* 1981; **116:** 405–7.

145. Moretz W, Naisbitt P, Stevenson G. Experimental studies of temporary occlusion of the inferior vena cave. *Surgery* 1954; **36:** 384.

146. Moretz WH, Rhode CM, Shepherd MH. Prevention of pulmonary emboli by partial occlusion of the inferior vena cava. *Am Surg* 1959; **25:** 617.

147. Morris GK, Mitchell JRA. Warfarin sodium in prevention of deep venous thrombosis and pulmonary embolism in patients with fractured neck of femur. *Lancet* 1976; **2:** 869.

148. Mozes M, Bogokowsky H, Antebi E, Tzur N, Penchas S. IVC ligation for pulmonary embolism. Review of 118 cases. *Surgery* 1966; **60:** 790.

149. Murray G. Anticoagulants in venous thrombosis and the prevention of pulmonary embolism. *Surg Gynecol Obstet* 1947; **84:** 665.

150. Neuerburg J, Gunther RW, Rassmussen E, *et al.* New retrievable percutaneous vena cava filter: experimental in vitro and in vivo evaluation. *Cardiovasc Intervent Radiol* 1993; **16:** 224–9.

151. Newman A. Phlegmasia cerulea dolens: a complication of use of the filter in the vena cava. A case report (letter). *J Bone Joint Surg (Am)* 1995; **77(11):** 1783.

152. Norris CS, Greenfield LJ, Herrmann JB. Free floating iliofemoral thrombus. *Arch Surg* 1985; **120:** 806.

153. Oertli D, Hess P, Durig M, *et al.* Prevention of deep vein thrombosis in patients with hip fractures: low molecular weight heparin versus dextran. *World J Surg* 1992; **16(5):** 980–4.

154. Oschner A, DeBakey ME, De Camp PT, Da Rocha E. Thrombo-embolism. An analysis of cases at the Charity Hospital in New Orleans over a 12 year period. *Ann Surg* 1951; **134:** 405.

155. Otchy DP, Elliott BM. The malpositioned Greenfield filter: lesson learned. *Am Surg* 1987; **53:** 580–3.

156. Pais SO, De Orchis DF, Mirvis SE. Superior vena caval placement of Kimray-Greenfield filters. *Radiology* 1987; **65:** 385–6.

157. Pais SO, Tobin KD, Austin CB, Queral L. Percutaneous insertion of the Greenfield inferior vena cava filter; experience with ninety-six patients. *J Vasc Surg* 1988; **8:** 460–4.

158. Parrish EH, Adams JT, Pories WJ, Burget DE, De Weese JA. Pulmonary emboli following vena cava ligation. *Arch Surg* 1968; **97:** 899.

159. Perry JN, Wells IP. A long term follow-up of Gunther vena caval filters. *Clin Radiol* 1993; **48:** 35–7.

160. Pieri A, Santoro G, Duranti A, Mori F, Vannuzzi A, Benelli L. Temporary caval filters. Our experience. Preliminary analysis of 24 cases. *Phlebologie* 1993; **46(3):** 457–66.

161. Plaus WJ, Hermann G. Structural failure of a Greenfield filter. *Surgery* 1988; **103:** 662–4.

162. Ramadan F, Johnson Jr G, Burnham S. Pulmonary embolism in autopsy review. In: Veith FJ, ed. *Current Critical Problems in Vascular Surgery.* Vol. 2. St Louis, MO: Quality Medical Publishing, 1990; 125–6.

163. Ritchie AJ, Mitchell L, Forty J. Migration of a vena caval filter to the pulmonary artery. *Br J Surg* 1995; **82:** 207.

164. Roehm JOF Jr. The Bird's Nest inferior vena cava filter: progress report. *Radiology* 1988; **168:** 745–9.

165. Roehm JOF Jr. The Bird's Nest filter: a new percutaneous transcatheter inferior vena cava filter. *J Vasc Surg* 1984; **1:** 498–501.

166. Roehm JOF Jr, Gianturco C, Barth MH. Percutaneous interruption of the inferior vena cava: The bird's nest filter. In: Bergan JJ, Yao JST, eds. *Surgery of the Veins.* New York: Grune & Stratton, 1985; 487–95.

167. Roehm JOF Jr, Johnsrude IS, Barth M, Wright KC. Percutaneous transcatheter filter for the inferior vena cava. *Radiology* 1984; **150:** 255–7.

168. Rohrer MJ, Scheidler MG, Wheeler HB, Cutler BS. Extended indications for placement of inferior vena cava. *J Vasc Surg* 1989; **10:** 44–50.

169. Rosenthal D, Cossman D, Matsumoto G, Callow A. Prophylactic interruption of the inferior vena cave. A retrospective evaluation. *Am J Surg* 1979; **137:** 389.

170. Rozin L, Perper JA. Spontaneous fatal perforation of aorta and vena cava by Mobin-Uddin umbrella. *Am J Forensic Med Pathol* 1989; **10:** 149–51.

171. Ruckley CV. Protection against thromboembolism. *Br J Surg* 1985; **72:** 421.

172. Ruckley CV. Pulmonary embolism in the Edinburgh surgical audit. *Thromb Haemost* 1981; **46:** 18.

173. Sagar S, Massey J, Sanderson JM. Low-dose heparin prophylaxis against fatal pulmonary embolism. *Br Med J* 1975; **4:** 257.

174. Schauble JF, Stickel DL, Anlyan WG. Vena caval ligation for thromboembolic disease. *Arch Surg* 1962; **84:** 17.

175. Sevitt S, Gallagher NG. Prevention of venous thrombosis and pulmonary embolism in injured patients. *Lancet* 1959; **2:** 981.

176. Sherry S. Low dose heparin prophylaxis for postoperative venous thromboembolism. *N Engl J Med* 1975; **253:** 300–2.

177. Sidawy AN, Menzoian JO. Distal migration and deformation of the Greenfield vena cava filter. *Surgery* 1986; **99:** 369–72.

178. Siegel EL, Robertson EF. Percutaneous transfemoral retrieval of a free-floating titanium Greenfield filter with an Amplatz goose neck snare. *J Vasc Intervent Radiol* 1993; **4(4):** 565–8.

179. Silver D, Sabiston DC. The role of vena caval interruption in the mangement of pulmonary embolism. *Surgery* 1975; **77:** 1.

180. Simon M, Athanasoulis CA, Kim D, *et al.* Simon nitinol inferior vena cava filter: initial clinical experience. Work in progress. *Radiology* 1989; **172:** 99–103.

181. Spencer FC. Experimental evaluation of partitioning of the inferior vena cava to prevent pulmonary embolism. *Surg Forum* 1960; **10:** 680.

182. Starok MS, Common AA. Follow-up after insertion of bird's nest inferior vena caval filters. *Can Assoc Radiol J* 1996; **47(3):** 189–94.

183. Stewart JR, Peyton JWR, Crute SL, Greenfield LJ. Clinical results of suprarenal placement of the Greenfield vena cava filter. *Surgery* 1982; **92:** 1–4.

184. Stoneham GW, Burbridge BE, Milward SF. Temporary inferior vena cava filters: in vitro comparison with permanent IVC filters. *J Vasc Intervent Radiol* 1995; **6(5):** 731–6.

185. Sue LP, Davis JW, Parks SN. Iliofemoral venous injuries: an indication for prophylactic caval filter placement. *J Trauma* 1995; **39:** 693–5.

186. Tardy B, Mismetti P, Page Y, *et al.* Symptomatic inferior vena cava filter thrombosis: clinical study of 30 consecutive cases. *Eur Respir J* 1996; **9(10):** 2012–16.

187. Van Allan RJ, Hanks SE, Harrell DS, Katz MD. Percutaneous retrieval of a misplaced titanium Greenfield filter. *Cardiovasc Intervent Radiol* 1994; **17(2):** 110–12.

188. Vesely TM. Technical problems and complications associated with inferior vena cava filters. *Semin Intervent Radiol* 1994; **11:** 121–33.

189. Vesely T, Darcy M, Picus D, Hicks M. Technical problems associated with placement of the bird's nest inferior vena cava filter. *Am J Roentgenol* 1992; **158:** 875–80.

190. Wheeler CG, Thompson JE, Austin DJ, Patman DR, Stockton RL. Interruption of the inferior vena cava for thromboembolism. *Ann Surg* 1966; **163:** 199.

191. Whitehill TA. Caval interruption methods: comparison of options. *Semin Vasc Surg* 1996; **9(1):** 59–69.

192. Wilkins RW, Mixter G, Stanton JR, Litter J. Elastic stockings in the prevention of pulmonary embolism. *N Engl J Med* 1952; **246:** 360.

193. Wilkins RW, Stanton JR. Elastic stockings in the prevention of pulmonary embolism. II. A progress report. *N Engl J Med* 1953; **248:** 1087.

194. Williams BT, Roding B, Schenk WG. Experimental evaluation of haemodynamic effects of inferior vena cave ligation. *J Cardiovasc Surg* 1970; **11:** 454.

195. Wingerd M, Bernhard VM, Maddison F, Towne JB. Comparison of caval filters in the management of venous thromboembolism. *Arch Surg* 1978; **113:** 1264–71.

196. Young AK, Lea Thomas M, Browse NL. Comparison between sequelae of surgical and medical treatment of thromboembolism. *Br Med J* 1974; **4:** 127.

CHAPTER 23

Superficial thrombophlebitis

Pathology	657	Treatment	660
Diagnosis	659	References	662

Many words have been used over the past 100 years to describe venous thrombosis. 'Thrombophlebitis' and 'phlebothrombosis' were the terms in common use until 30 years ago; the former was used to describe a thrombus which was adherent to an inflamed vein wall, the latter was used to describe fresh thrombus free from or just loosely adherent to a normal non-inflamed vein wall. Both words were used for thrombosis in any vein.

As our understanding of postoperative deep vein thrombosis grew, it became apparent that neither of these terms should be used, as neither of them described the precise pathology and, even if they did, we were unable to determine the pathology *in vivo* and apply the correct word.

The generally accepted solution is to use a simple term, that does not imply a pathological mechanism, for all forms of thrombosis in the deep veins, deep vein thrombosis, and reserve the term 'thrombophlebitis' for superficial thrombosis, in most cases secondary to, but always associated with inflammatory changes in the vein wall.

Pathology

Superficial thrombophlebitis is the combination of thrombosis and phlebitis in a superficial vein in any part of the body. In most cases the thrombosis is secondary to the phlebitis but in some circumstances changes in the blood cause spontaneous thrombosis with a secondary phlebitis.

AETIOLOGY

The common causes of an inflammatory response in the vein wall are as follows.

External trauma

A blow or prolonged pressure from the edge of a tight bandage can injure a superficial vein, particularly its endothelium. The resulting oedema, leucocyte infiltration and exposure of subintimal collagen following the shedding of damaged endothelial cells stimulates thrombosis.[16,47]

Thrombophlebitis is a common complication of varicose veins possibly because their prominence makes them more vulnerable to local trauma.[11,20]

Superficial thrombophlebitis in pregnancy probably occurs because pregnancy causes varicose veins.[1] Whether venous stasis in varicose veins can cause a thrombophlebitis in the absence of a coagulation defect is extremely doubtful.[48] Thrombosis in varicose veins may be less likely to extend into the deep veins than a thrombosis in a non-varicose superficial vein.

Internal trauma

A direct injury to the endothelium causing loss of endothelial cells initiates a progression of events which is the same as that initiated by external trauma.

Physicians are by far the commonest instigators of intravenous injuries.[4,17,44] Simple venepuncture and indwelling catheters often cause phlebitis. The chemical composition of the infusion set and cannula also affect the incidence of phlebitis. The longer the catheter is in place, the higher the incidence of thrombophlebitis. Any injected substance which is not iso-osmolar and/or cytotoxic will destroy endothelium.[13,46] Many intravenous infusion fluids are both hypertonic and extremely noxious. Many drugs damage the endothelium. Common substances (e.g. pentobarbitone and diazepam) often cause a painful chemical thrombophlebitis, and the older contrast media used for phlebography sometimes caused superficial and deep phlebitis.

The slower the venous blood flow, the higher the incidence of thrombosis. Thus an injection into a vein on the dorsum of the hand is more likely to cause a thrombophlebitis than an injection into a vein in the cubital fossa. Many hypertonic phlebitis-promoting substances must be given directly into a large central vein where the blood flow is high, the catheter is in the centre of the bloodstream away from the vein wall, and the injectate is quickly diluted.

The thrombus which forms around an intravenous catheter may become infected if bacteria enter the vein through the skin puncture wound. This can give rise to a local abscess and septicaemia.[8,28,36,43]

Post-infusion and injection phlebitis is a common cause of annoying and sometimes painful symptoms in all hospital patients and can cause pulmonary embolism.

Primary vein wall inflammation

Inflammatory changes may arise spontaneously in the vein wall and cause thrombosis. The best example of this is the superficial thrombophlebitis which often precedes or accompanies thromboangiitis obliterans (Buerger's disease).[7] Although this condition is primarily an arteritis of unknown cause (but inextricably linked with smoking), many authorities will not diagnose it without clinical evidence of

venous as well as arterial thromboses. The cause of the histological changes seen in the vein wall of patients with Buerger's disease has not been elucidated. In a neurovascular bundle the inflammatory process may simply spread directly from the artery to the vein, but in the superficial veins this cannot be the case.

Inflammatory changes adjacent to a vein, whether they be caused by trauma, infection, chemical or physical processes, can spread into the vein wall and cause thrombophlebitis. Infection may also spread into a vein and cause a septic thrombophlebitis.

Vein wall infiltration

Nearby disease, particularly malignant disease, may spread into a vein, replace the endothelium and cause a thrombophlebitis. Some tumours, notably carcinoma of the kidney and primary vascular tumours, actually spread along the lumen of their draining veins and cause it to thrombose. Carcinoma of the breast can cause superficial thrombophlebitis in the breast (Mondor's sign) and in the arm.

Vein wall fibrinolytic activator deficiency (idiopathic superficial thrombophlebitis)

A small group of patients present with recurrent episodes of superficial thrombophlebitis, but no evidence of occult malignant disease, collagen disease or vascular problems such as Buerger's disease. Some of these patients also have recurrent deep vein thrombosis.

The search to find a coagulation defect in these patients is usually unsuccessful,[9] except for rare coagulation abnormalities such as antithrombin and protein S deficiencies, but abnormalities of fibrinolysis have been found (Table 23.1). These patients may have a reduced resting level of blood fibrinolytic activity, a raised plasma fibrinogen, a reduced increase in blood fibrinolytic activity following venous congestion and a reduced vein wall

Table 23.1 Mean blood and tissue fibrinolytic activity and plasma fibrinogen concentration in 16 patients with vein wall fibrinolytic activator deficiency (idiopathic superficial thrombophlebitis) and 48 normal subjects[23]

Test	Normal subjects (Mean)	Patients with superficial thrombophlebitis (Mean)	Significance of difference (*t*-test)
Dilute blood clot lysis time (min)	256	608	$P < 0.0001$
Fibrin plate lysis area (mm²)	453	240	$P < 0.0001$
Plasma fibrinogen (g/l)	2.75	4.13	$P < 0.0001$
Vein wall activator activity (units)	24	11.6	$P < 0.009$

activator production in both leg and arm veins.[5,21,33,35]

It is reasonable to assume that 'idiopathic' superficial thrombophlebitis in the presence of normal coagulation factors is a primary abnormality of vein wall fibrinolytic activator production, the cause of which remains unknown.

Primary blood changes

Thrombosis following injury is clearly caused by the vein wall damage. The superficial thrombophlebitis associated with changes in the blood may also be a primary vein wall abnormality if the blood changes are the result of a failure of the venous endothelium to produce coagulation factors or fibrinolytic activators because the production of these substances by the vein wall is not only of importance to the coagulability of the blood as a whole but is also an important local protective mechanism.

A number of diseases which alter blood coagulability are associated with superficial thrombophlebitis.

The attacks of superficial thrombophlebitis caused by occult malignant disease are usually transient and migratory. The fault appears to be primarily in the blood.[10,39,40] Coagulation changes include an increase of factor VIII.

The vein wall fibrinolytic activity of patients with advanced carcinoma has not been studied extensively but the normal decrease of blood fibrinolytic activity that follows surgical operations is greater in patients with malignant disease.[6]

Primary blood diseases such as polycythaemia,[27] thrombocythaemia and sickle cell disease[26] can cause superficial thrombophlebitis.

What initiates an episode of thrombophlebitis migrans is not clear. It may be minor unnoticed local trauma, or a blood change plus a local change such as stasis, or a local loss of the vein wall antithrombosis protective mechanism. Whatever the order of events, there is ultimately a thrombosis and a phlebitis which lasts for a few days and then resolves, sometimes with venous recanalization.

Diagnosis

CLINICAL PRESENTATION

Local

The patient presents with a tender 'worm-like' mass which is deep to the skin. The surrounding tissues may be oedematous and the overlying skin may be red and hot. The mass corresponds to the line of a vein which may be visible and slightly distended upstream from the thrombosis.

There may be evidence of previous attacks of thrombophlebitis, for example pigmented areas of skin over thickened cord-like veins, and evidence of primary venous disease (e.g. varicose veins).

The pain and tenderness develops in a few hours and can be severe. The symptoms may extend along the whole length of a vein. Long saphenous vein thrombophlebitis may spread from the ankle to the sapheno-femoral junction and cause iliac vein thrombosis.

There is often a history of local trauma – a blow or prolonged pressure. The patient may have had an intravenous injection for the induction of anaesthesia or the administration of drug therapy.

General

It is important to ask all the normal systematic questions, as these may reveal loss of appetite, loss of weight, backache, intermittent claudication or other symptoms of an underlying problem (e.g. an occult carcinoma or thromboangiitis obliterans).

Care must be taken to examine the calf muscles and the local lymph glands because the differential diagnoses include deep vein thrombosis, erysipelas, lymphangitis and acute lipodermatosclerosis.

INVESTIGATIONS

The initial investigations are directed towards finding a cause for the thrombosis (if it is not an obvious superficial thrombophlebitis in a large varicose vein) and excluding deep vein thrombosis.

Deep vein thrombosis is said to be less common when the superficial thrombophlebitis is in a varicose vein but a number of recent studies which have examined the deep veins of patients presenting with varicose veins and the signs of superficial thrombophlebitis with duplex ultrasound have shown incidences of 23%,[25] 31%,[29] and 12%.[38] Bergqvist and Jaroszewski[3] found an incidence of 40% in patients with superficial thrombophlebitis in nonvaricose veins. The absence of varicose veins on clinical examination is therefore an absolute indication for a duplex ultrasound study but, in view of the above studies it is probably wise to perform such a study in all cases to help decide upon treatment. Sometimes a study reveals a free-floating thrombus in the femoral or popliteal veins propagating from or associated with thrombus in the long or short saphenous veins – a potential embolus. Jorgensen *et al.*[25] discovered this situation in four of the 44 (9%) patients they examined. Propagation

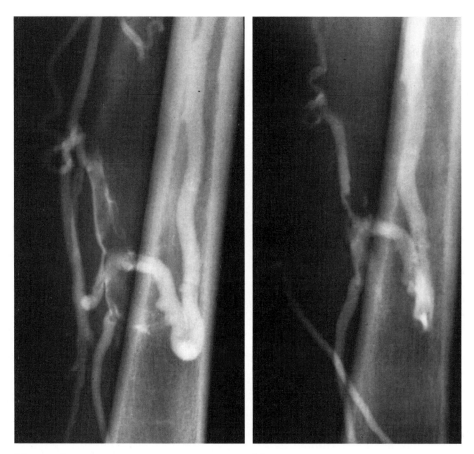

(a)   (b)

Figure 23.1 (a) Non-adherent mural thrombus in a superficial vein. (b) Adherent mural thrombus in a superficial vein.

into the calf veins via a communicating vein is more common (Figure 23.1) but of equal clinical importance because it is highly likely to cause serious long-term damage to the function of the calf pump.

Full blood investigations should always be performed if there are no varicose veins, especially coagulation factors, platelet count and platelet function studies, plasma fibrinogen and euglobulin lysis time. Blood studies may reveal a lymphoma or there may be polycythaemia, thrombocythaemia or sickle cell disease.

It may be necessary to perform x-ray contrast studies of the stomach, colon and kidney, gastrointestinal endoscopy, chest radiograph and liver and pancreas computerized tomography (CT) scans to discover clinically occult malignant disease.

Arteriography may be required to exclude thromboangiitis obliterans.

If all these investigations are negative, a histochemical study of vein wall fibrinolysis is indicated.

Treatment

The vigour of treatment depends upon the severity of the symptoms, the underlying cause and the presence and extent of any associated deep vein thrombosis.

Thrombophlebitis in varicose veins

If the thrombosis is localized and showing no signs of extending then it is best treated with a firm compression bandage and by urging the patient to walk. Sitting still or lying in bed encourages the thrombus to spread. Firm support and mild analgesia (e.g. aspirin) usually relieves the pain sufficiently to allow walking. Many physicians give stronger anti-inflammatory drugs (e.g. indomethacin) but these drugs can have serious adverse effects and should not be used for a benign self-limiting, though painful, condition. An old-fashioned treatment is to apply a bandage impregnated with glycerine and ichthyol. This makes the skin of the leg hot and acts as a counter-irritant. It also sets into a firm good quality compression bandage. Apart from the fishy smell and grey colour this treatment has much to commend it.

Very occasionally, the pain is so severe that the patient has to rest in bed for a few days. If this happens, it is wise to give the patient intravenous or subcutaneous heparin until the pain has subsided and walking can begin to prevent extension of the thrombus into the deep veins through the communicating veins.

If a patient has had a series of episodes of thrombophlebitis and/or if duplex ultrasound scanning shows the presence of thrombus in the deep veins, they should be given a 3–6 months' course of oral anticoagulation.

Occasionally, a large varix thromboses and causes a large tender mass that does not subside within a few days. The pain and swelling can be relieved immediately by expressing the thrombus from the vein through a small venotomy made under local anaesthesia. An incision 0.5 cm long into the vein allows the surgeon to express the soft red–black thrombus which reduces the tension and instantly relieves the pain. One stitch and a pressure dressing controls any tendency to bleed.

Ascending long saphenous vein thrombophlebitis

This is usually a complication of varicose veins but can accompany phlebitis of other origins. Once the thrombus passes the midpoint of the thigh, there is a risk that it will extend into the femoral and iliac veins and surgical treatment is urgently required[15,30] (Figure 23.2). The saphenous vein should be ligated at its termination and separated from the femoral vein. Before the vein is tied, it is felt carefully and opened to make sure that there is no intraluminal free-floating thrombus which a ligature might divide and turn into an embolus.

Infusion phlebitis

Most intravenous injection or infusion phlebitides resolve quickly if the injection or infusion is stopped. Although the vein is painful, it should be compressed with a firm bandage and the pain relieved with mild analgesia. The arm should not be kept in a sling.

Infusion phlebitis should not be seen in the leg because intravenous infusions should never be given into leg veins, except in extreme emergencies.

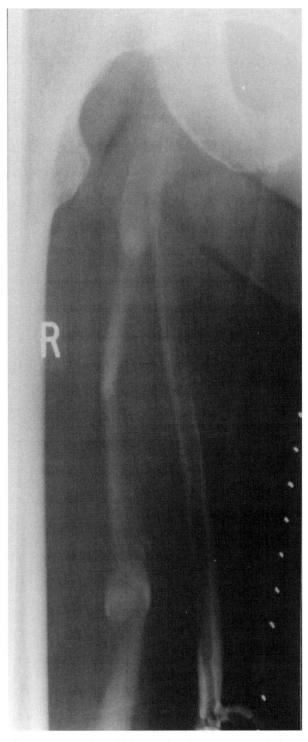

Figure 23.2 The phlebograph of a patient with long saphenous vein thrombophlebitis showing non-adherent thrombus extending up to the sapheno-femoral junction. Propagation of this thrombus into the femoral or iliac vein could produce a life-threatening embolus. This patient should be treated by ligating the saphenous vein flush with the femoral vein and full anticoagulation.

Table 23.2   The effect of stanozolol (5 mg b.d.) on the mean blood fibrinolytic activity and plasma fibrinogen of 12 patients with vein wall fibrinolytic activator deficiency (idiopathic superficial thrombophlebitis)[23]

Test	Before treatment	After treatment	Significance of difference (*t*-test)
Dilute blood clot lysis time (min)	578	172	$P < 0.003$
Fibrin plate lysis area (mm²)	247	409	$P < 0.01$
Plasma fibrinogen (g/l)	3.4	2.9	$P < 0.03$

The addition of heparin to the infusion fluid does not reduce the incidence of phlebitis[39] but the application of a heparinoid cream over the inflamed vein may produce symptomatic relief.[30]

Infusion phlebitis can be avoided by using non-irritant cannulae, iso-osmolar infusion fluids, changing the site of infusion after 24–48 hours, using large central veins for the infusion of phlebotoxic substances and taking careful antiseptic precautions.[12]

Infected superficial thrombophlebitis

If a thrombus becomes infected, the vein may have to be opened through a long longitudinal venotomy and the infected clot removed.[41] It is sometimes easier to remove the whole vein. Septicaemia caused by fragments of infected thrombus breaking free into the circulation is stopped by ligating the vein above the area of septic phlebitis and, if the thrombus in the vein is purulent, excising the vein.

Secondary thrombophlebitis migrans

Management of secondary thrombophlebitis involves treatment of the underlying cause plus palliation for the local symptoms – compression, mild support and exercise.

When thrombophlebitis migrans is associated with malignant disease this is usually advanced and inoperable; the underlying cause must, however, be sought and treated if possible.

If thrombophlebitis is caused by blood abnormalities (e.g. thrombocythaemia and polycythaemia), correction of the blood abnormality will stop the attacks of thrombophlebitis.

If a phlebogram reveals the presence of a deep vein thrombosis, the patient should be fully anticoagulated.

Vein wall fibrinolytic activator deficiency

If all investigations, except the tests of blood fibrinolysis and vein wall activator activity, are negative

then it is reasonable to assume that vein wall fibrinolytic activator deficiency is the cause of the recurrent thrombophlebitis, and the patient should be treated by enhancing blood fibrinolysis.

Many drugs stimulate natural fibrinolysis in the short term but only two substances produce a sustained long-term effect. The drug we have used is stanozolol;[9] Nilsson has used ethyloestrenol.[14,22,34] Both drugs are mild anabolic sex hormones. They both take between 3 weeks and 3 months to work but will return the tests of blood fibrinolytic activity to normal (Table 23.2). Both drugs cause mild water retention, and stanozolol, which has now been withdrawn because of abuse, has mild androgenic effects (oligomenorrhoea, acne and, very rarely, hirsutism).

In a group of 16 patients who had pure superficial thrombophlebitis, we found that stanozolol stopped the attacks in 13 patients and reduced their frequency in the other three patients.[23] The Malmo group treated 49 patients, who had a mixture of recurrent superficial and deep vein thrombosis, with ethyloestrenol. They saw no recurrent attacks over a 16-month period in the 45 patients whose blood fibrinolytic activity returned to normal levels.[18] In both these studies the close correlation between the cessation of attacks and the return of blood fibrinolytic activity to normal adds weight to the belief that the cause of the thrombophlebitis was a deficiency of fibrinolysis.

References

1. Aaro LA, Johnson TR, Juergens JL. Acute superficial venous thrombophlebitis associated with pregnancy. *Am J Obstet Gynecol* 1967; **97**: 514.
2. Albrechtsson V, Olsson CB. Thrombotic side effects of lower limb phlebography. *Lancet* 1976; **1**: 723.
3. Bergqvist D, Jaroszewski H. Deep vein thrombosis in patients with superficial thrombophlebitis of the leg. *Br Med J* 1986; **292**: 658.
4. Brown GA. Infusion thrombophlebitis. *Br J Clin Pract* 1970; **24**: 197.

5. Browse NL, Gray L, Jarrett PEM, Morland M. Blood and vein wall fibrinolytic activity in health and disease. *Br Med J* 1977; **1:** 478.

6. Browse NL, Gray L, Morland M. Changes in the blood fibrinolytic activity after surgery. The effect of deep vein thrombosis and malignant disease. *Br J Surg* 1977; **64:** 23.

7. Buerger L. The association of migrating thrombophlebitis with thromboangitis obliterans. *Int Clin* 1909; **3:** 84.

8. Collin J, Collin C, Costable FL, Johnston IDA. Infusion thrombophlebitis and infection with various cannulas. *Lancet* 1975; **2:** 150.

9. Davidson JF, Lockhead M, McDonald GA, McNichol GP. Fibrinolytic enhancement by stanozolol. A double blind trial. *Br J Haematol* 1972; **22:** 543.

10. Edwards EA. Migrating thrombophlebitis associated with carcinoma. *N Engl J Med* 1949; **240:** 1031.

11. Edwards EA. Thrombophlebitis in varicose veins. *Surg Gynecol Obstet* 1938; **66:** 236.

12. Elfring G, Hastbacka J, Tammisto T. Infusion thrombophlebitis and its prevention. *Am Heart J* 1967; **73:** 717.

13. Elfring G, Saikkn K. Effect of pH on the incidence of infusion thrombophlebitis. *Lancet* 1966; **1:** 953.

14. Fearnley GR, Chakrabarti R, Evans JF. Mode of action of phenformin plus ethyloestrenol on fibrinolysis. *Lancet* 1971; **1:** 723–5.

15. Galloway JMD, Karmody AM, Mavor GE. Thrombophlebitis of the long saphenous vein complicated by pulmonary embolism. *Br J Surg* 1969; **56:** 360.

16. Ghildyal SK, Pande RC, Mistra TR. Histopathology and bacteriology of postinfusion phlebitis. *Int Surg* 1975; **60:** 341.

17. Hastabacka J, Tammisto T, Elfving G, Tiitinen P. Infusion thrombophlebitis. *Acta Anaesthesiol Scand* 1965; **10:** 9.

18. Hedner V, Nilsson IM, Isacson S. Effect of ethyloestrenol on fibrinolysis in the vessel wall. *Br Med J* 1976; **2:** 729.

19. Hume M. Blood coagulation in deep and superficial thrombophlebitis. *Arch Surg* 1966; **92:** 934.

20. Husni EA, Williams WA. Superficial thrombophlebitis of lower limbs. *Surgery* 1982; **91:** 70.

21. Isacson S, Nilsson IM. Defective fibrinolysis in blood and vein walls in recurrent 'idiopathic' venous thrombosis. *Acta Chir Scand* 1972; **138:** 313.

22. Isacson S, Nilsson IM. Effect of treatment with combined phenformin and ethyloestrenol on the coagulation and fibrinolytic systems. *Scand J Haematol* 1970; **7:** 404–8.

23. Jarrett PEM, Morland M, Browse NL. Idiopathic recurrent superficial thrombophlebitis, treatment with fibrinolytic enhancement. *Br Med J* 1977; **1:** 933.

24. Jones MV, Craig DB. Venous reaction to plastic intravenous cannulae, influence of cannula composition. *Can Anaesth Soc J* 1972; **19:** 491.

25. Jorgensen JO, Hanel KC, Morgan AM, Hun JM. The incidence of deep venous thrombosis in patients with superficial thrombophlebitis of the lower limbs. *J Vasc Surg* 1993; **18:** 70–3.

26. Kwaan HC. Inhibitors of fibrinolysis. *Thromb Res* 1972; **2:** 31.

27. Kwaan HC, Suwanwela N. Inhibitors of fibrinolysis in platelets in polycythaemia vera and thrombocytosis. *Br J Haematol* 1971; **21:** 313.

28. Leading Article. Septic thrombophlebitis and venous cannulas. *Lancet* 1970; **2:** 406.

29. Luther KS, Rerr TM, Roedersheimer R, Lohr JM, Sampson MG, Cranley JJ. Superficial thrombophlebitis diagnosed by duplex scanning. *Surgery* 1991; **100:** 42–6.

30. Martin P, Lynn RC, Dibble JM, Aird I. *Peripheral Vascular Disorders.* Edinburgh: Livingstone, 1954.

31. Medical Research Council Trial. Thrombophlebitis following intravenous infusion. A trial of plastic and red rubber giving sets. *Lancet* 1957; **1:** 595.

32. Mehta PP, Sagar S, Kakkar VV. Treatment of superficial thrombophlebitis. A randomized double-blind trial of heparinoid cream. *Br Med J* 1975; **3:** 614.

33. Nilsson IM. Phenformin and ethylestrenol in recurrent venous thrombosis. In: Davidson JF, Samama MM, Desnoyes PC, eds. *Progress in Chemical Fibrinolysis and Thrombosis.* New York: Raven Press, 1975.

34. Nilsson IM, Hedner V, Isacson S. Phenformin and ethyloestrenol in recurrent venous thrombosis. *Acta Med Scand* 1975; **198:** 107–13.

35. Pandolfi M, Isacson S, Nilsson IM. Low fibrinolytic activity in the walls of veins in patients with thrombosis. *Acta Med Scand* 1969; **186:** 1.

36. Pruitt BA Jr, Stein JM, Foley FD, Moncrief JA, O'Neill JA. Intravenous therapy in burn patients. Suppurative thrombophlebitis and other life-threatening complications. *Arch Surg* 1970; **100:** 399.

37. Ritchie WMG, Lynch PR, Stewart GJ. Effects of contrast media on normal and inflamed canine veins. *Invest Radiol* 1974; **9:** 444.

38. Skillman J, Kent KC, Porter DH, Kim D. Simultaneous occurrence of superficial and deep thrombophlebitis in the lower extremity. *J Vasc Surg* 1990; **11:** 818–22.

39. Soong BCF, Miller SP. Coagulation disorders in cancer. III Fibrinolysis and inhibitors. *Cancer* 1970; **25:** 867.

40. Stein JM, Pruitt BA. Suppurative thrombophlebitis, a lethal iatrogenic disease. *N Engl J Med* 1970; **282:** 1452.

41. Stradling JR. Heparin and infusion phlebitis. *Br Med J* 1978; **4:** 1195.

42. Thomas ET, Evers W, Racz GB. Post infusion phlebitis. *Anesth Analg (Cleve)* 1970; **49:** 150.

43. Thomas ML, Briggs GM, Kuan BB. Contrast agent induced thrombophlebitis following leg phlebography: meglumine ioxaglate versus meglumine othalamate. *Radiology* 1983; **147:** 399.

44. Vere D, Sykes C, Armitage P. Venous thrombosis during dextrose infusion. *Lancet* 1960; **2:** 627.

45. Welch GW, McKeel DW, Silverstein P, Walker HL. The role of catheter composition in the development of thrombophlebitis. *Surg Gynecol Obstet* 1974; **138:** 421.

46. Wessler S. Thrombosis in the presence of vascular stasis. *Am J Med* 1962; **33:** 648.

47. Woodhouse CRJ. Infusion thrombophlebitis, the histological and clinical features. *Ann R Coll Surg Engl* 1980; **62:** 364.

48. Zollinger RW, Williams RD, Briggs DO. Problems in the diagnosis and treatment of thrombophlebitis. *Arch Surg* 1962; **85:** 18.

CHAPTER 24

Congenital venous abnormalities

Pathology	665	Popliteal vein entrapment	686
Congenital vena caval obstruction	670	References	686
Klippel–Trenaunay syndrome	671		

The blood vessels develop into their mature organized and remarkably constant pattern from a sponge-like collection of capillaries.[70] It is an extraordinary achievement of organization and growth, controlled by factors of which we have no knowledge or understanding. The end result is billions of humans with a remarkably similar venous anatomy. It is hardly surprising that this development occasionally falters, leaving isolated individuals with abnormal veins. These congenital abnormalities are rare but must be recognized if only because they are often best treated conservatively. The unsightliness of these abnormalities combined with ignorance of their natural history tempts surgeons to treat them surgically but as they have been present since birth, any physiological abnormality that they might cause is usually well compensated, and direct surgical treatment may make it worse.

Pathology

There are four main forms of congenital abnormality of the veins: aplasia, hypoplasia, reduplication and the persistence of vestigial vessels. Each may be associated with other abnormalities of the cardiovascular and musculoskeletal systems. The valves may, independently, be absent or abnormal. One group of abnormalities is sufficiently common to justify an eponym, the Klippel–Trenaunay syndrome.

Aplasia

Aplasia is a total absence of a vein. Failure of a segment of a vein to develop tends to occur when that vein has a complicated embryological derivation involving the union of a number of more primitive veins. For example, the vena cava has a complex derivation (see Chapter 2) and is the most common site of venous aplasia.[16,54] Inferior vena caval aplasia usually affects the hepatic portion so that its renal segment has to connect with the right atrium via collaterals.

Aplasia of the iliac vein (Figure 24.1)[31,39] and the deep veins of the leg is uncommon, except in association with the other abnormalities that form the Klippel–Trenaunay syndrome (see later). One-third of the patients with this syndrome have aplasia of the iliac, common superficial and deep femoral or popliteal veins.

The prevalence of venous aplasia has not been well documented.

Membranous occlusion

Membranes are sometimes left across a vein at the site where two primitive vessels should have connected.

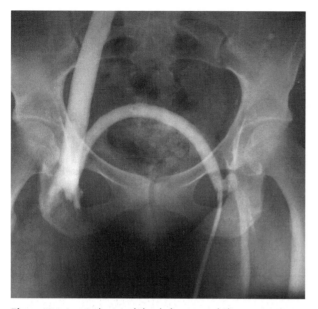

Figure 24.1 Aplasia of the left external iliac vein. X-ray contrast medium injected into the foot has ascended in the superficial femoral and saphenous veins as far as the common femoral vein. Thereafter it flowed across to the right common femoral vein. No iliac vein is visible. The patient had had a large vein across the abdomen since childhood and had never had a clinical event suggestive of deep vein thrombosis.

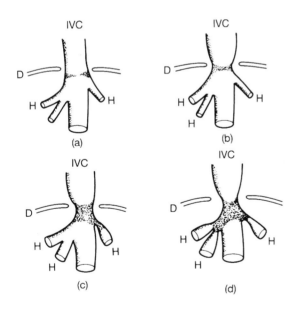

Figure 24.2 The sites of membranous occlusion of the inferior vena cava. Congenital stenosis or occlusion of the suprarenal inferior vena cava may take the form of (a) a partial membrane, (b) a complete membrane or (c and d) a membrane and thrombosis which may involve one or all of the hepatic veins. IVC, inferior vena cava; D, diaphragm; H, hepatic vein.

Membranes are commonly found just below the diaphragm at the embryological junction of the sub-cardinal and the intersubcardinal anastomoses close to the point where the ductus venosus joins the left hepatic vein (Figure 24.2).[26,55] These may be found in association with the Budd–Chiari syndrome.

It is not known whether the membrane is a failure of fetal development or an extension of the obliteration of the ductus venosus. As the membrane is sometimes small, the stenosis extensive and the histological appearance variable, it has been suggested that it might be an acquired lesion superimposed upon congenital predisposition.[7] The membrane may be complete or perforated and consists of collagen, endothelium and elastic tissue but no muscle. The majority of reports about this abnormality have come from the eastern hemisphere. The prevalence of this condition is not known.

Hypoplasia

Patients presenting with the symptoms of aplasia of the inferior vena cava or iliac veins may be shown, with phlebography, to have a very narrow channel in the correct anatomical site, suggesting that the vessel is hypoplastic, not aplastic. Without direct examination of the vessel by surgical exposure and histological analysis, it is not possible to know whether such a phlebographic appearance is truly hypoplasia or an acquired abnormality secondary to an event such as thrombosis. Nevertheless, if veins can be aplastic, they must occasionally be hypoplastic. Figure 24.3 shows a patient who appears to have a hypoplasia of the inferior vena cava.

Hypoplastic veins are often associated with other abnormalities, for example the Klippel–Trenaunay syndrome (Figure 24.4a, b).

The prevalence of venous hypoplasia is not known.

Reduplication

Reduplication of veins is common (see Chapter 2). Double inferior vena cavae, double renal veins passing in front, or behind the aorta, double superficial femoral and double saphenous veins are all well recognized (Figures 24.5, 24.6 and Figure 4.27c).

Reduplication of the vena cava results from persistence of both lumbar supracardinal veins in their entirety. The two cavae may be of equal size, or the right vena cava may be larger. The mechanism that causes reduplication of lower limb veins is unknown but it is presumably a minor failure of fetal organization, as the structure of the second vein is always identical to that of its partner.

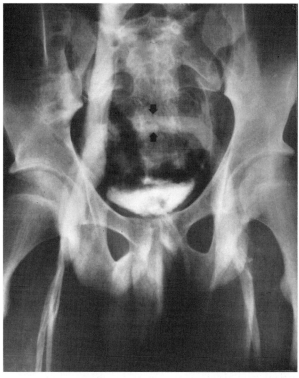

(a)

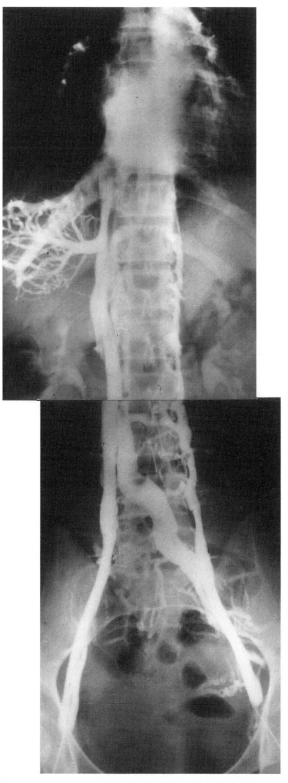

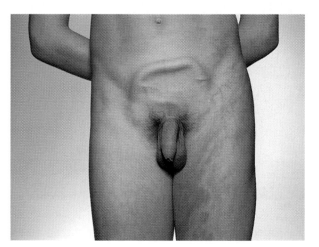

(b)

Figure 24.3 Congenital hypoplasia of the inferior vena cava. The right common iliac vein continues as a narrow hypoplastic vena cava. The left common iliac vein drains into the right and left lumbar azygos veins.

Figure 24.4 Iliac vein hypoplasia in a patient with the Klippel–Trenaunay syndrome. (a) This phlebograph shows a large collateral vessel crossing from the left to the right common femoral vein below a hypoplastic left external and common iliac vein. (b) The large collateral vein shown in the phlebograph (a) was clearly visible in the subcutaneous tissues. The patient asked for the vein to be removed. He was told that it should never be removed or ligated because it was the main venous outflow tract of his left leg.

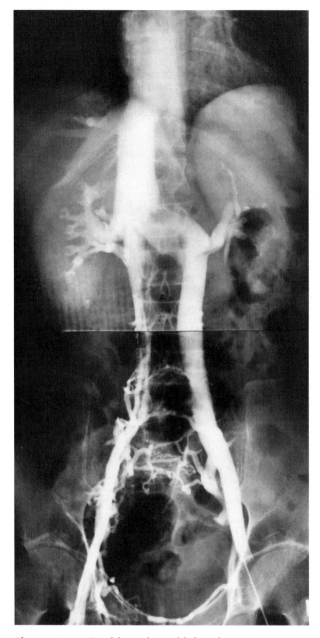

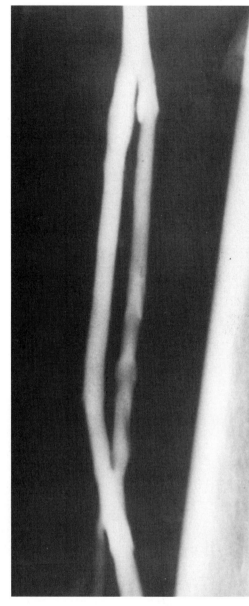

Figure 24.6   A double superficial femoral vein. This is a common anatomical variant.

Figure 24.5   Double (right and left) inferior vena cavae. The patient presented with swelling of the right leg caused by thrombosis of the right-sided vena cava following plication of this vessel to prevent recurrent pulmonary emboli. A phlebogram had not been performed before the plication. This phlebograph was obtained when the patient had further emboli via the left-sided vena cava.

Persistent fetal veins

This has already been identified as a cause of reduplication but sometimes veins that are present in the fetus in areas distant from the normal main veins may persist into adult life. The best example of this is the persistent lateral limb bud vein seen on the outer side of the leg of many patients with the Klippel–Trenaunay syndrome (see Figure 24.12a). Some venous haemangioma should be included in this category. Many of these vascular malformations are not true tumours but are hamartomas or simply areas of disorganized persistent fetal veins (see Chapter 27). These veins have the same histological structure as normal veins but are often dilated and without valves.

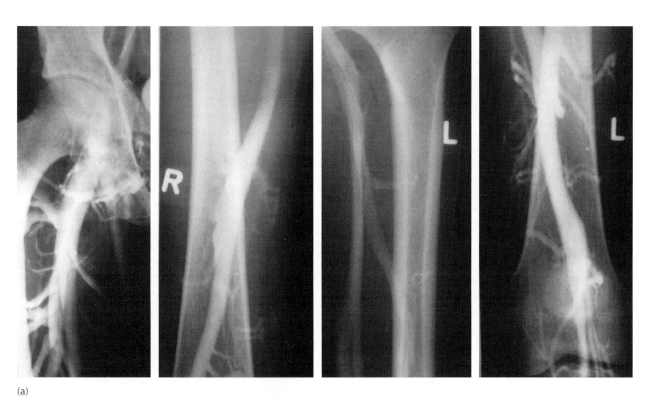

(a)

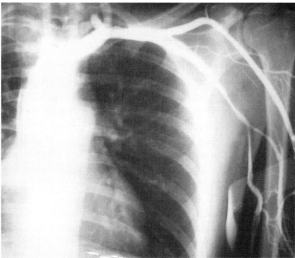

(b)

Figure 24.7 Congenital absence of the valves. (a) The descending phlebographs of a patient who had had swollen legs and recurrent ulceration since adolescence. The valve aplasia allows the contrast medium to reflux into all the tributaries. The absence of valves and valve sinuses gives the phlebograph an 'arteriogram-like' appearance. (b) There were no valves in the arm veins.

Valve abnormalities

Congenital absence of the valves is extremely rare.[6,36,48] It can affect the lower limb veins alone or the whole body. We have seen three patients with congenital absence of valves in 30 years' experience, and less than 50 cases have been reported in the literature (Figure 24.7).

Kistner has described a group of patients with *floppy valves.*[29] This abnormality is an enlarged valve cusp with a long, free edge that allows the cusp to prolapse when subjected to retrograde flow. Whether this is a congenital or an acquired abnormality is not known.

Vein wall deficiencies

The walls of varicose veins and of veins taken from relatives of patients with varicose veins but without varicose veins themselves have been found to contain more of the tissue lysosomal enzymes that control mucopolysaccharide metabolism.[50] This may be the congenital abnormality that is responsible for the abnormal collagen and polysaccharide content of varicose veins and for their tendency to be a family trait.

Varicose veins are discussed in detail in Chapters 5, 6 and 7 but are mentioned here to emphasize the fact that the primary (non-thrombotic) variety may be a congenital abnormality.

Major venous abnormalities are rarely found in association with other conditions which affect the collagen composition of the blood vessels to cause aneurysms and spontaneous rupture of arteries (e.g. Marfan's syndrome and Ehlers–Danlos syndrome), though varicose veins are said to be more common in patients with type I Ehlers–Danlos syndrome. The veins are probably affected in the same way as the arteries but the intraluminal pressure may not be sufficient to cause fatigue and distension.

Congenital vena caval obstruction

CLINICAL PRESENTATION

Aplasia

The majority of patients with aplasias or hypoplasias have few symptoms and the clinical signs are of a well compensated venous obstruction, because the abnormality has been present since birth and collateral vessels have had time to develop.

The most common complaint is of visible varicose veins in the subcutaneous tissues of the abdominal wall (Figure 14.1, page 431). These are collateral veins which run across the abdomen and chest wall to connect the veins of the lower limbs with the veins of the axilla and neck.

Iliac vein aplasia may present with large suprapubic collateral vessels (Figure 24.4b). Provided these collaterals are large enough to carry the increased blood flow that occurs during muscle exercise, the patient may have no other symptoms. If the collaterals are inadequate, the secondary changes in the upstream veins may cause aching pain, venous claudication, varicose veins, oedema, lipodermatosclerosis and ulceration.[13] The symptoms of venous outflow obstruction are discussed in detail in Chapters 12, 13, 15 and 16.

Subdiaphragmatic vena caval occlusion

The symptoms and signs of subdiaphragmatic vena caval occlusion are a mixture of the effects on the systemic venous return and hepatic blood flow.

The obstruction to blood flow from the limbs may cause oedema and venous distension. Collateral veins may be visible on the abdomen and chest wall.

If the condition is long-standing, skin changes develop in the lower leg (pigmentation, eczema, lipodermatosclerosis and even ulceration). The ulceration is often widespread and in sites other than the medial side of the lower leg.

The effect on hepatic venous drainage is similar to that of the Budd–Chiari syndrome, namely ascites, hepatosplenomegaly and portal hypertension with oesophageal varices.[51] The patient may complain of abdominal distension and/or haematemesis.

Although the obstruction is above the level of the renal veins, uraemia and renal failure are uncommon.

As this is a congenital abnormality, the collateral venous circulation for the limbs and liver is often adequate for many years and patients do not develop symptoms until they are 20–30 years old.

INVESTIGATIONS

The most important investigation is a careful phlebographic anatomical delineation of the problem. Injections are needed from below (bilateral femoral phlebography) and sometimes from above (retrograde percutaneous catheterization via an arm vein) so that the extent of the occlusion and its relation to the hepatic and renal veins are displayed. Computerized tomography (CT) with contrast enhancement[19] and, more recently, spiral CT[25] may both be used to assess IVC anomalies.

It is also essential to assess liver function (biochemically and by biopsy) and renal function. Liver function is usually normal, but there may be hypoproteinaemia if ascites and portal hypertension have been present for a long time. The liver biopsy will show centrilobular venous congestion, and possibly centrilobular cellular damage and fibrosis.

Blood coagulation should be studied if an operation involving a vascular prosthesis is contemplated.

Patients with complete aplasia of the hepatic portion of the inferior vena cava develop a large azygos vein. This usually provides an adequate outflow tract and the patient is therefore symptomless but the enlarged azygos vein may be visible on a routine chest radiograph (see Figure 14.7, page 436).

TREATMENT

Aplasia of the vena cava rarely requires treatment. Symptoms in the lower limbs can usually be controlled with elastic stockings. If the patient has severe symptoms (e.g. venous claudication), the occlusion can be treated by a bypass operation between the highest part of the iliac system that is patent and the right atrium.[43,66]

The bypass (made of externally supported PTFE, 12–18 mm in diameter) is attached to the lower vena cava using an oblique retroperitoneal approach and is passed up behind the liver, through the diaphragm, before being attached to the right atrium which is exposed through a right anterolateral thoracotomy. Alternatively, the intrathoracic end of the graft may be anastomosed to the patent azygos or hemiazygos system.[13] The blood flow is normally sufficient to maintain patency, and an arteriovenous fistula is not required. It is wise to maintain the patient on anticoagulants for 3–6 months while the pseudointima of the graft becomes established and stable.

The same operation can be used for subdiaphragmatic membranous occlusions, provided the hepatic veins are patent and can drain retrogradely down the vena cava into the bypass.

If the hepatic veins are aplastic or obstructed by the aplasia or the membrane, the subdiaphragmatic vena cava must be exposed, the membrane excised and, if necessary, the vena cava widened with a patch graft of vein or PTFE.[68]

Sometimes the membrane can be split by direct pressure from a finger inserted into the vena cava via the right atrium[27] but this gives less satisfactory results than membrane excision. Successful endovascular balloon dilatation of caval membranes has been reported[37] but experience is very limited.

A note of caution

The large azygos vein carrying blood around an aplastic or occluded inferior vena cava may be discovered during a pulmonary or cardiac operation. We, and others,[15] have seen patients, in whom this vein was ligated during the performance of the thoracic part of an oesophagectomy, die as a result of hepatic and renal failure. Thus although vena caval atresia seldom requires surgical correction, the natural collaterals can confuse interpretion of the chest radiograph and cause technical problems during the surgical exposure of other intrathoracic structures. All surgical trainees should be told that if they meet a large collateral vein within the thorax, they should never ligate it.

Klippel–Trenaunay syndrome

Definition

This syndrome was first described in 1900 by Klippel and Trenaunay in the *Archives of General Medicine of Paris*[30] when they recorded the combination of a cutaneous naevus, varicose veins and bone and soft tissue hypertrophy affecting one or more limbs. Trelat and Monad[62] had previously noted an association between tissue hypertrophy and varicose veins.

In 1907, Parkes Weber[45] described a group of patients with limb hypertrophy associated with large arteries, an increased blood flow, and varicose veins.

For a number of years many investigators considered that these two publications described two variations of the same abnormality, and many classifications have grouped them together. The main cause of confusion was the mistaken belief that tissue overgrowth was always caused by arteriovenous fistulae but when Lindenauer[35] showed that venous obstruction without a change in blood flow may cause tissue overgrowth these two syndromes became disentangled.

Klippel–Trenaunay syndrome (KTS)

This is an abnormality of the veins, skin capillaries, soft tissues and bones of the limb, without any pathological arteriovenous fistulae.

Parkes Weber syndrome

This is the congenital persistence of multiple diffuse microscopic arteriovenous fistula. All the other features of the syndrome (e.g. limb overgrowth and varicose veins) are secondary effects of the fistulae.

The KTS is therefore a diffuse mesodermal abnormality, often associated with lymphatic dysfunction and other congenital abnormalities, whereas the Parkes Weber syndrome is a pure abnormality of the arteriolar microcirculation. The prevalence of these two congenital vascular abnormalities is not known. Recently, a genetic basis for KTS has been suggested with reports of families containing several members affected by KTS or naevi and hemihypertrophy.[1,12] We have only seen three pairs of closely related patients with KTS. A single gene defect has been suggested[69] but further studies are required to confirm this.

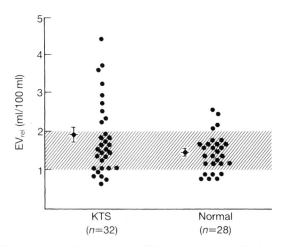

Figure 24.8 The volume of blood (EV$_{rel}$) expelled from the foot veins during knee bending exercise in 28 normal limbs and 32 limbs with the Klippel–Trenaunay syndrome (KTS). The shaded area is the normal range. The difference between the mean values is not statistically significant. (Modified from Baskerville *et al.*, 1985.[4])

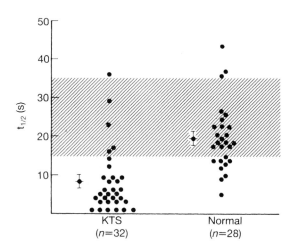

Figure 24.9 The rate of refilling (t$_{1/2}$) of the leg veins, after exercise, in 28 normal limbs and in 32 limbs with Klippel–Trenaunay syndrome (KTS); the shaded area is the normal range. The difference between the means is statistically significant. *P* <0.0005 (Mann–Whitney *U*-test). (Modified from Baskerville *et al.*, 1985.[4])

PATHOPHYSIOLOGY

The symptoms of KTS are related to disordered calf pump function and tissue hypertrophy.

Calf pump efficiency

Most patients with KTS have good calf muscles which can pump the venous blood out of the affected limb but the abnormal veins usually have incompetent valves which decrease refilling time.[4] Figure 24.8 shows the relative expelled foot volume of 32 patients with KTS compared to that of 28 normal limbs. The variation of results amongst the patients is larger than in the normal limbs, but the number of patients who have expelled volumes below the 'normal' limit is no greater than in the normal group. The very large quantities of blood expelled from the foot in some patients is a reflection of the gross distension of the veins and the strong calf muscles of young adults.

Figure 24.9 shows the 50% refilling time of the same group of 32 patients. The mean refilling time for the normal limbs was 21 seconds, and that for the KTS limbs was 8.7 seconds. The refilling time was improved but not corrected by a mid-thigh tourniquet which occluded the superficial veins. There is no doubt that the abnormal subcutaneous and deep veins in limbs with KTS are grossly

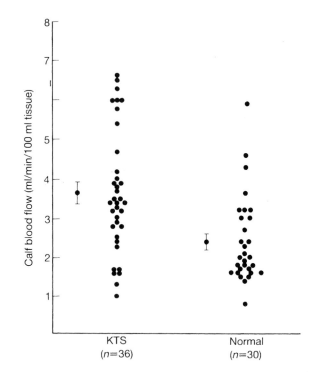

Figure 24.10 The resting calf blood flow in 30 normal limbs and 36 limbs with the Klippel–Trenaunay syndrome (KTS). All the values for the two groups lie within the normal range but the difference between the mean values is statistically significant. *P* <0.001 (Mann–Whitney *U*-test). (Modified from Baskerville *et al.*, 1985.[4])

incompetent, yet the calf pumps of this group of patients (who had a mean age of 28 years) were able to deal with the reflux.

Calf blood flow

The mean resting calf blood flow of KTS limbs, measured by venous occlusion strain-gauge plethysmography, is approximately 50% greater than that of normal limbs (Figure 24.10). The range of blood flow is wide but even the highest rates of flow are still within the normal range.[3] There is therefore no haemodynamic evidence of arteriovenous fistulae. Multiple arteriovenous fistulae would cause blood flows 10–20 times greater than normal. Nevertheless, the increased blood flow does suggest a reduced peripheral resistance. It may be that this reduced resistance resides within the naevus because the mean blood flow of the KTS limbs with small or no naevi was 2.2 ml/min/100 ml, whereas the flow in the limbs with large naevi was 3.8 ml/min/100 ml; this is a statistically significant difference. The blood flow is not related to the degree of hypertrophy.

These studies suggest that the subcutaneous venous abnormality and the naevus are congenital defects; the naevus allows an increased but not an abnormal resting blood flow. The tissue hypertrophy does not appear to be caused by either the increased blood flow (because it occurs in limbs without naevi and with normal blood flow) or the venous abnormality (because the calf pump function is usually normal). We believe it is a primary congenital abnormality of the mesoderm.

Bones and soft tissues

The bones and the soft tissues may overgrow, in some cases to a size justifying the term 'gigantism'.[63,67] Histological examination of these hypertrophic tissues reveals no abnormality. All the constituents of normal tissues are present in normal amounts.

Many believe that the bony overgrowth is related to the changes in capillary and venous blood flow but the precise causal mechanism is not known.[24,58]

Veins

The walls of the abnormal veins are thickened and contain more muscle fibres which suggests an hypertrophic and hyperplastic response to the increased venous pressure.[3,34] The production of fibrinolytic activator by the walls of these veins, assessed by incubation on a fibrin plate, is reduced but the clinical significance of this observation is uncertain.

Blood

A careful study of the clotting factors in the blood of patients with KTS has revealed an increase of thrombin activation.[5] It is not known whether this is a primary or secondary abnormality.

CLINICAL PRESENTATION

Patients usually present soon after birth with one or a combination of the three main features: the naevus, tissue hypertrophy or varicose veins.[4,21,38,49,56,64,65,71] The naevus is usually the first abnormality to be noticed by the child's parents. Hypertrophy may not become obvious for years, and varicose veins are often not noticed until the child begins to walk or sometimes many years later.

The degree and extent of each abnormality varies from patient to patient. Some patients have extensive naevi, a moderate number of varicose veins and little tissue hypertrophy. Other patients have gigantism, a few varicose veins and little or no visible naevi. In the 49 patients we have studied in detail,[4] 47 had naevi, 49 had varicose veins and 36 had noticeable hypertrophy.

The majority of patients have KTS abnormalities in one leg, either leg being equally affected. In approximately 15% of patients both legs are affected and in 5% both legs and one arm are affected. In a few patients (5%) the abnormality is confined to the arm.[10] KTS in all four limbs is very rare.

The naevus

The presence of a naevus is very common. Gloviczki *et al.*[18] found 95% of KTS patients affected. It may be a few patches on one limb, or it may involve the whole limb or the whole body (Figure 24.11a–c). Approximately 25% of patients have naevi which extend beyond the affected limb. In 50% of patients the naevus tends to fade as the years pass, and in some patients it is almost invisible by adulthood. Sometimes the surface of the naevus is rough and verrucose. Prominent nodules are susceptible to injury and may bleed freely (Figure 24.11).

Varicose veins

The varicose veins are cosmetically disfiguring and cause discomfort and swelling in 90% of patients. The pain is an aching sensation that is exacerbated by standing and gets worse as the day passes. The pain is relieved by elevating the leg and a night's rest.

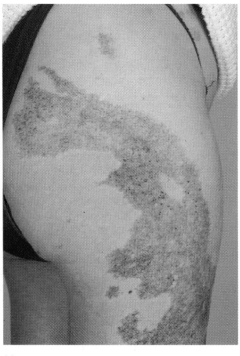

(a)

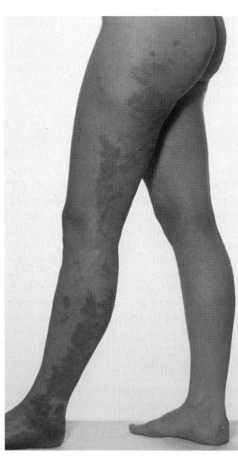

(b)

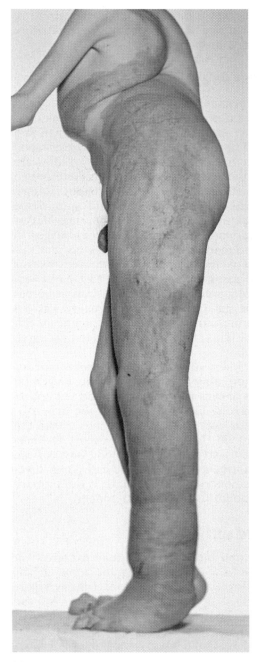

(c)

Figure 24.11 The naevus of the Klippel–Trenaunay syndrome. (a) A lateral view showing a 'metameric' appearance of the naevus. The subcutaneous veins are not prominent. (b) An extensive 'patchy' naevus. (c) A naevus extending onto the buttock and trunk.

The veins are often large and extensive and their appearance is a common reason for referral to a surgeon. Men often ignore the disfigurement as it develops slowly over many years but the combination of the prominent veins, naevus and hypertrophy leads most young women to seek treatment at an earlier stage.

The unusual distribution of the veins should alert the clinician to the possibility that they are not simple varicose veins, even if the patient presents in adult life. Although the common 'normal' variety of varicose vein can appear anywhere over the leg, the larger dilated subcutaneous veins tend to run towards the line of the saphenous veins. The veins of patients with KTS are often in unusual positions, the most common being a large vein running down the *lateral side of the limb* (Figure 24.12a, b). This is probably the fetal lateral limb bud vein which has failed to regress (the long saphenous vein is derived from the fetal medial limb bud vein). It may begin at the ankle, have many dilated tributaries and run up the whole length of the limb to the upper thigh where it either penetrates the deep fascia to connect with the deep femoral vein or disappears beneath the gluteus maximus muscle to join a tributary of the internal iliac vein. There are always many communicating veins between such a vein and the deep calf veins (see Figure 24.18 and 24.20).

Sometimes the long saphenous vein is dilated (Figure 24.12c) but it is more often small and competent. Occasionally, both the lateral and medial subcutaneous veins are abnormal.

Varicosities may be present in the pelvis and be the cause of rectal and submucosal venous congestion and haemorrhage. In our own series of patients, *20% had rectal bleeding and 10% had haematuria*; 33% had phlebographic evidence of abnormal intrapelvic veins.

Attacks of *superficial thrombophlebitis* are uncommon in adults (6%), but appear much commoner in children with 53% of patients affected in Samuel and Spitz's series. A history of chest pain, haemoptysis and collapse should be sought, as 20% of our patients had clinical evidence of *pulmonary embolism*.

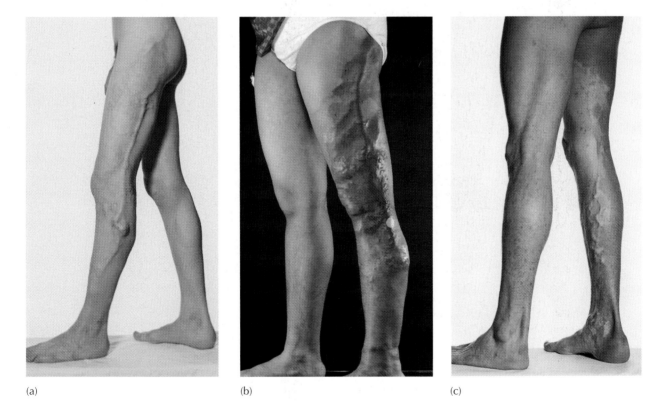

(a) (b) (c)

Figure 24.12 The varicose veins of the Klippel–Trenaunay syndrome. (a) The typical lateral vein. This vein passed beneath the gluteus maximus muscle to drain into the internal iliac vein. The 'blow-out' in the mid-calf lay over a large incompetent communicating vein. (b) A lateral vein with many varicose veins beneath the naevus some of which ran across the back of the thigh to drain into the postero-medial tributary of the saphenous vein. (c) A dilated abnormal long saphenous vein. This patient also had abnormal veins on the lateral side of the leg.

Other venous abnormalities include venous aneurysms[45] and deep vein atresia.[18]

Swelling

Most legs with KTS are slightly oedematous but it is not always easy to distinguish a mild oedema from soft tissue hypertrophy until the patient has been in bed for 24 hours and the oedema has reabsorbed.

Gross oedema is rare except when there is extensive aplasia or hypoplasia of the deep veins or associated lymphatic obliteration (Figure 24.13). Oedema caused by these abnormalities will be made worse if the superficial veins are removed.

Skin changes

Pigmentation, eczema, lipodermatosclerosis and ulceration are uncommon (10%) while the calf pump remains efficient; as the years pass the incidence of these complications increases (Figure 24.14). It is, however, unusual to find an elderly patient who has KTS with a venous ulcer.

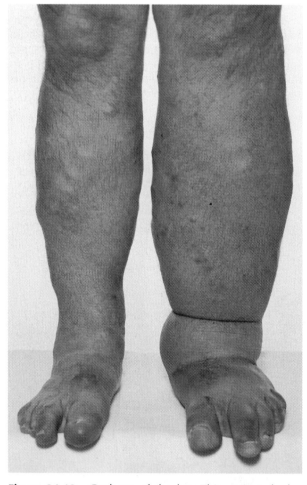

Figure 24.13 Oedema of the leg. This patient, had a swollen elongated, hypertrophic limb, with bilateral limb bud veins. The bony hypertrophy was greater on the left than the right. A lymphangiogram showed peripheral lymphatic obliteration. Some parts of the naevus were covered with lymphatic vesicles. Thus the enlargement of the limb was caused by a mixture of bone hypertrophy, extensive subcutaneous varicose veins and lymphoedema caused by lymphatic obliteration.

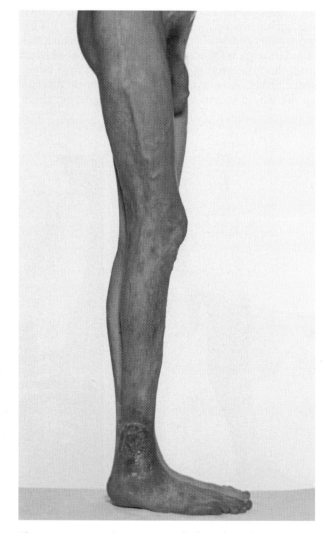

Figure 24.14 Ulceration and the Klippel–Trenaunay syndrome. Ulcers are relatively uncommon and often appear in unusual sites. This patient had an ulcer just above the lateral malleolus at the bottom of a long incompetent lateral vein. There is little pigmentation or oedema.

Bone hypertrophy

Any or all of the bones in the limb may overgrow. A discrepancy between the length of the limbs is often present at birth. This may increase during the first few years but then tends to remain static; we have not seen the leg length disparity increase after the age of 10 years. This is an important difference from the Parkes Weber syndrome in which the overgrowth gets progressively worse throughout childhood until the epiphyses fuse.

There is no pattern to the bony hypertrophy. Sometimes all the bones of a limb are involved; less commonly, hypertrophy may affect the phalanges of one toe, or the bones of the lower leg but not those of the upper leg (Figure 24.15a, b).

The difference in leg lengths may cause a lumbar scoliosis and flexion deformities of the joints of the hypertrophic limb (see Figure 24.25).

Soft tissue hypertrophy

The majority of patients with KTS have some soft tissue hypertrophy, but the skin over the hypertrophied subcutaneous tissues and bone usually looks quite normal. In two-thirds of our patients with

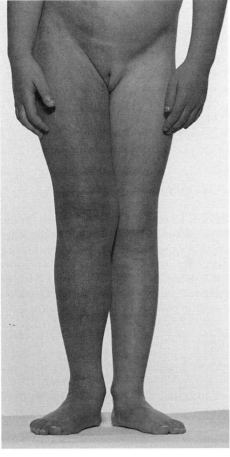
(a)

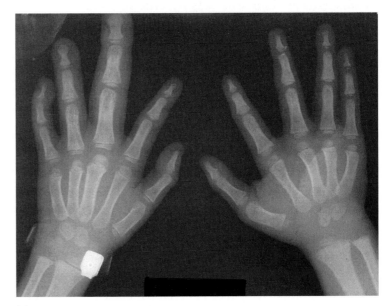

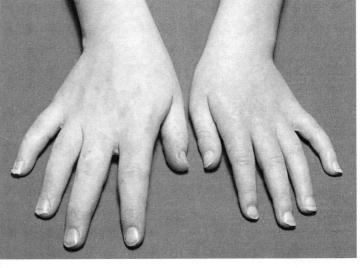
(b)

(c)

Figure 24.15 Bony hypertrophy. (a) This patient has the typical overgrowth of the whole leg. (b) Overgrowth of the whole hand. (c) A radiograph showing overgrowth of one, middle finger.

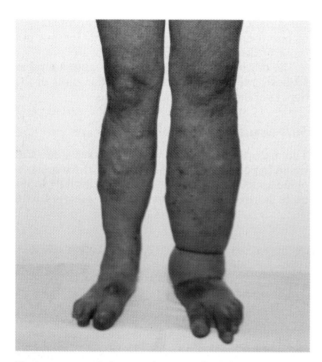

Figure 24.16 Soft tissue hypertrophy. This 30-year-old man with Klippel–Trenaunay syndrome had enlargement of both legs and the right arm. Much of the enlargement was caused by soft tissue hypertrophy. Sometimes there is plexiform neurofibromatosis. The naevus was extensive. All limbs functioned normally.

unilateral KTS the volume of the affected foot was 5–50% greater than that of the normal foot. Some of this swelling was oedema, some was caused by the dilated veins and some was hypertrophy. It is often difficult to separate these three different causes of swelling clinically, except when the soft tissue overgrowth is localized to a digit, or part of the foot (Figure 24.16).

Other abnormalities

Lymphatics

The KTS is often associated with lymphatic abnormalities.[42,71] Twenty per cent of patients have cutaneous vesicles which leak lymph. The groups of vesicles have the same clinical appearance as the vesicles of lymphangioma circumscriptum but the underlying abnormality – multiple subcutaneous lymph cysts not connected to the main lymphatics – is much more diffuse than the lesion of lymphangioma circumscriptum.

Lymphangiography revealed peripheral lymphatic obliteration in eight of 14 of our patients; the other patients were normal.[4] The lymphatic defect

is probably part of the general mesodermal abnormality but it may be an acquired abnormality secondary to the prolonged venous hypertension and high lymph flow.

Bony abnormalities

Bony abnormalities such as spina bifida, pelvic nonfusion, syndactyly and coxa vara, have each been observed in our own series of patients. Others investigators have reported digital agenesis, atresia of the ear canal, and clinodactyly.

Other congenital malformations do not seem to occur. This is surprising as cardiac abnormalities are reported in association with some forms of congenital lymphoedema.[28]

Coagulopathy

The presence of thrombocytopenia and a consumptive coagulopathy (Kasabach–Merritt syndrome) has been described in patients with KTS[41] and seems to occur more commonly in patients with extensive naevi. In Samuel and Spitz's[53] series of 47 children with KTS, 45% had Kasabach–Merritt syndrome.

INVESTIGATIONS

The diagnosis of KTS is made at the bedside on the basis of the three diagnostic abnormalities together with a history that began at birth and the absence of any evidence of arteriovenous fistulae. Any doubt about the presence of arteriovenous fistulae should be excluded by measuring the limb blood flow and, on rare occasions, by arteriography.

Foot volumetry

This investigation is useful when deciding whether the reflux is embarrassing the calf pump. Most patients can reduce their foot volume to the normal range during exercise,[4] but have an increased rate of refilling (see Figures 24.8 and 24.9).

Venous outflow

Plethysmography may define the degree of outflow obstruction in patients with deep vein atresia but the results are usually normal.

Phlebography

This is difficult but essential.[32,57,59,61]

Standard ascending phlebography should be the first investigation, because it is essential that the

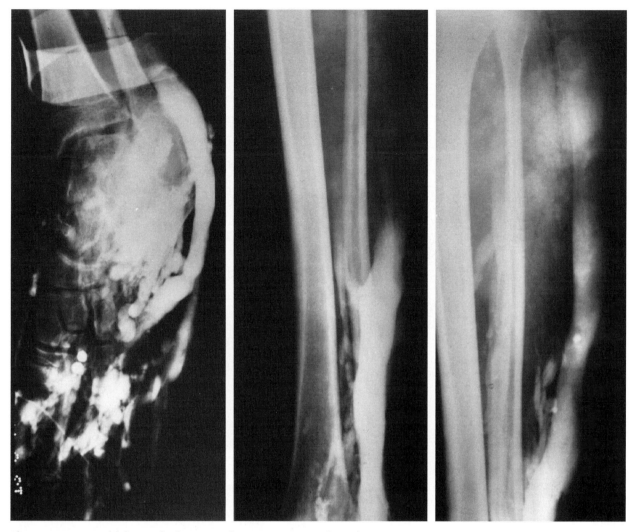

Figure 24.17   A phlebograph showing a large incompetent lateral vein.

state of the deep veins is known. The course and destination of the large subcutaneous veins is often best displayed by direct injection into an abnormal vein (Figure 24.17).

If the radio-opaque contrast medium is injected into the large veins at various points along the limb, the many sites of superficial-to-deep connections can be demonstrated (Figure 24.18).

The delineation of pelvic vein abnormalities may require direct percutaneous common femoral vein phlebography. In the rare patient whose femoral vein is absent, abnormal veins around the bladder and rectum can be demonstrated with percutaneous intraosseus trochanteric phlebography.

In our series,[3] all of the 49 KTS limbs had an abnormal lateral limb bud vein (see Figure 24.12a). This vein was connected to the deep calf veins by

large communicating veins in over 50% of limbs. The lateral vein drained into the deep thigh veins in 50% of the limbs (Figure 24.19a, b), into the gluteal veins in 33% (Figure 24.20a, b) and into the long saphenous vein in 15%.

Most limbs (80%) had normal, slightly dilated or reduplicated deep veins. Twenty per cent of limbs had deep vein atresia or hypoplasia affecting the superficial femoral vein (see Figure 24.19b), which in a few limbs also affected the common femoral and iliac veins (see Figure 24.4a).

Deep vein aplasia (Figure 24.21) is not a common finding,[18,60] and clearly cannot be the cause of either the superficial venous abnormality or the soft tissue and bony hypertrophy.

Similar phlebographic abnormalities may be found in the upper limb (Figure 24.22).

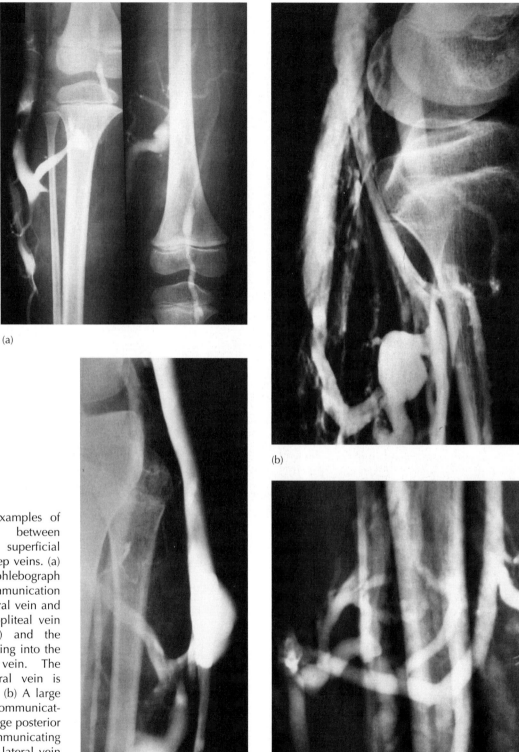

(a)

(b)

(c)

(d)

Figure 24.18 Examples of communications between the abnormal superficial veins and the deep veins. (a) An ascending phlebograph showing a communication between the lateral vein and a hypoplastic popliteal vein (left-hand panel) and the lateral vein draining into the deep femoral vein. The superficial femoral vein is also hypoplastic. (b) A large lateral mid-calf communicating vein. (c) A large posterior mid calf communicating vein. (d) A large lateral vein crossing the back of the calf to communicate with the deep veins on both sides of the calf.

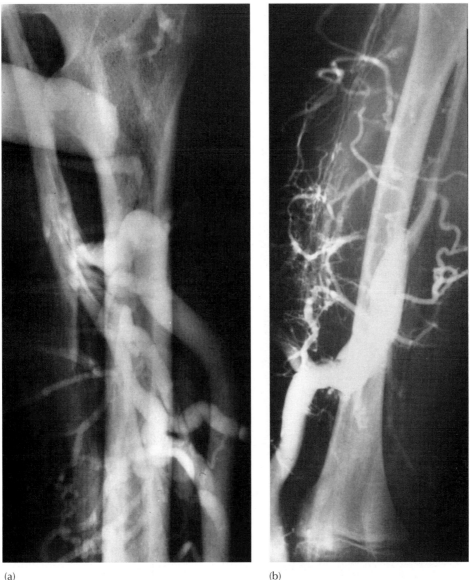

(a)   (b)

Figure 24.19 (a) A phlebograph showing a large lateral vein draining into the deep femoral vein. (b) A large lateral vein draining into the superficial femoral vein, which is hypoplastic.

Colour Doppler ultrasound scanning has been used increasingly to demonstrate the abnormal lateral venous channels, deep veins and connections between the two.[22] Arteriovenous communications can be demonstrated or excluded. Although useful, ultrasound has not supplanted good quality phlebography for the demonstration of anatomical detail because of the infinite variety and unpredictable abnormal venous patterns.

Arteriography

Arteriography and measurements of blood flow may be necessary to exclude the presence of arteriovenous fistulae.[9,44]

Scannograms

These are x-rays of the bones of the limbs taken at a fixed distance against a background graticule. A

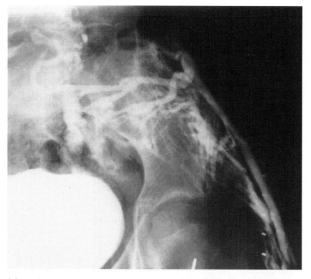

(a)

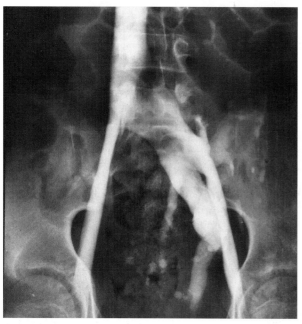

(b)

Figure 24.20   (a) A phlebograph showing a large lateral vein draining into the internal iliac vein. (b) The internal iliac vein of the same patient. Its stem and its superior gluteal tributaries are dilated and abnormal. There are phleboliths in the pelvis.

scannogram allows the exact measurement of bone length (Figure 24.23).[2] Simple bedside measurements are difficult and inaccurate when there is soft tissue hypertrophy. If these measurements are repeated over the years, the change in limb length

discrepancy can be noted and orthopaedic correction can be advised if necessary.

Chest and abdominal radiographs

A chest radiograph is an important initial investigation to exclude other congenital abnormalities and detect cardiomegaly caused by arteriovenous fistulation. An abdominal radiograph may reveal pelvic phleboliths if the veins of the pelvis are abnormal (Figure 24.24).

CT and NMR

Scans with and without radio-opaque contrast injections can outline the exact anatomical distribution of the clusters of abnormal veins in the limbs and, more particularly, in the pelvis.

Endoscopy

Symptoms such as haematuria or rectal bleeding must be fully investigated by cystoscopy, proctoscopy and sigmoidoscopy and by the usual radiographic studies. Other causes of bleeding must be excluded before attributing it to the venous malformation.

Blood investigations

In view of the increased incidence of thromboembolic complications, it is wise to perform a full study of circulating coagulation and fibrinolytic factors.

Differential diagnosis

The investigations outlined above will reveal the nature of other abnormalities often confused with the KTS (e.g. venous angiomata, gigantism, multiple arteriovenous fistulae, the post-thrombotic syndrome and lymphoedema).

TREATMENT

Many patients need no treatment for the KTS but even when the condition is symptomless we advise patients to wear elastic stockings.

Elastic stockings

The principal complaints of aching, mild swelling and visible veins are best treated by elastic compression. This treatment has brought considerable relief to all our patients. Patients must be told that they will have to wear the stockings at all times, for the rest of their lives. A full-length stocking is preferable as it compresses the vessels in the upper

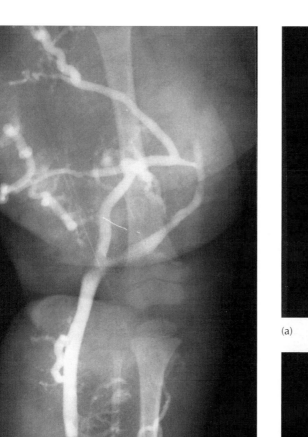

Figure 24.21 Deep vein aplasia. The ascending phlebograph of a 6-month-old child with an enlarged leg and a naevus showing a large lateral vein and no deep veins. The arteriogram and calf blood flow were normal.

thigh and prevents reflux from the gluteal or deep thigh veins. A below-knee stocking is, however, easier to put on and is adequate if the major abnormalities are below the knee.

Superficial vein surgery

Superficial veins should not be removed when there is aplasia of the deep veins.

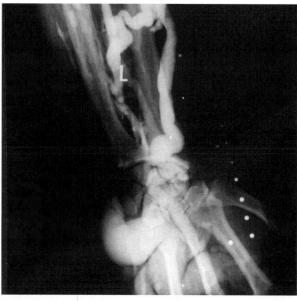

(a)

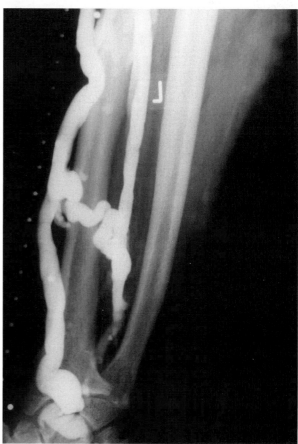

(b)

Figure 24.22 Phlebographs of the abnormal veins of a patient with the Klippel–Trenaunay syndrome affecting the left arm.

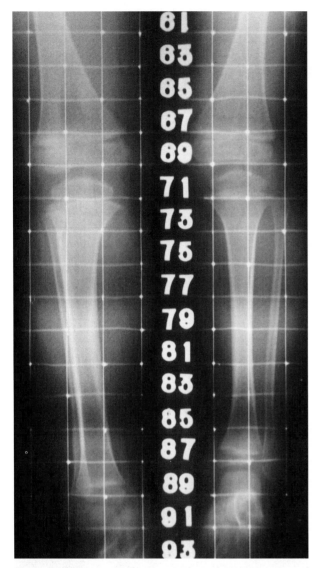

Figure 24.23 A scannogram. Clinical measurement of leg length is sufficient for the adjustment of the heel of the shoe but precise measurements of bone length are required when choosing the optimum time for epiphysiodesis. The graticules are 2 cm wide. The tibia of the right leg is 1.75 cm longer than the left tibia.

Surgery to the superficial veins should only be advised when skin changes (e.g. pigmentation, eczema or ulceration) are present.

Patients who insist on surgical removal of the large visible veins for cosmetic reasons should be told that recurrences are inevitable because of the diffuse nature of the abnormality, unless extensive excisions are performed.

If the deep veins are normal, the large subcutaneous trunks can be removed by stripping, and at the same time the incompetent communicating

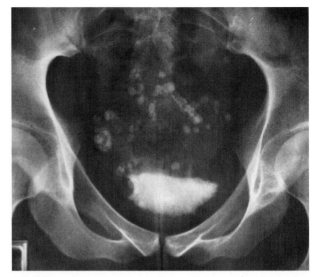

Figure 24.24 Phleboliths in the pelvis. This patient had many abnormal veins in the pelvis and had had recurrent episodes of haematuria.

veins between the abnormal surface veins and the deep veins can be ligated and divided. This is a major rather than a minor procedure but it usually alleviates the aching pains and gives a temporary cosmetic improvement. All patients must continue to wear elastic stockings after the operation. Localized subcutaneous angiomatous collections of veins, particularly those involving the skin, can be excised without complications.

Deep vein surgery

The deep vein aplasia rarely needs to be treated because the large superficial veins provide an adequate outflow tract. A total common femoral and iliac aplasia may be helped by a vein bypass once the patient is fully grown, if the aplasia is causing severe swelling and venous claudication. We have not seen a patient with these symptoms because all our patients have had adequate collateral vessels.

The naevus

Many patients ask for treatment of the naevus. It is best to reassure them that it is likely to fade and to avoid any surgical treatment.

Cosmetic creams and paints often provide good camouflage. Laser coagulation may be used for particularly dark areas but is not a practical treatment for a naevus that covers the whole limb and it may leave unsightly white scars.

Verrucose patches, caused by protruding dilated intradermal venules sometimes bleed and may become infected. These patches are best treated by local excision. Suture lines in the naevus heal normally but dilated venules often develop in the scar. Excision and skin grafting may be required for large areas of abnormal skin.

Reducing operations

Patients who have concomitant lymphatic obliteration or diffuse lymphangiomatosis sometimes develop severe swelling of the leg. If the skin vesicles become chronically infected, they may be replaced with hypertrophic bleeding granulation tissue. These patients may benefit from either a Homans' or a Charles' type of reducing operation.

The venous abnormality makes the operation difficult and bloody. Wound healing is often slow but once healing has occurred the combination of the subcutaneous excision and the ligation of the abnormal veins can reduce the limb to an acceptable size.

Amputations

Gigantism of the toes or forefoot is often best treated by local amputation because it enables the patient to wear a shoe of a normal size and to walk properly. Normal walking is important because it means that the calf muscles contract properly and venous calf pump function improves.

Control of limb growth

Careful measurements of limb length will indicate whether any length discrepancy is stable or is increasing. Mild stable differences in leg length can be treated by raising the heel of the shoe of the normal leg. Failure to correct overgrowth leads to deformities of the joints (Figure 24.25).

An increasing discrepancy should be treated by retarding growth by epiphyseal stapling or epiphysiodesis (Figure 24.26).[8,20,47] The time at which this procedure is performed must be carefully calculated from age-growth charts in consultation with an orthopaedic surgeon. The operation itself is not difficult as the venous abnormality does not extend into the bones.

Prevention of bleeding

Haematuria and rectal bleeding from submucosal vesicles and rectal veins are difficult to control. Local sclerosing injections may be helpful. We have not had to excise bowel or bladder to stop bleeding and would hesitate to do so because of the problem of defining the source of bleeding from a pelvic abnormality which is so diffuse.

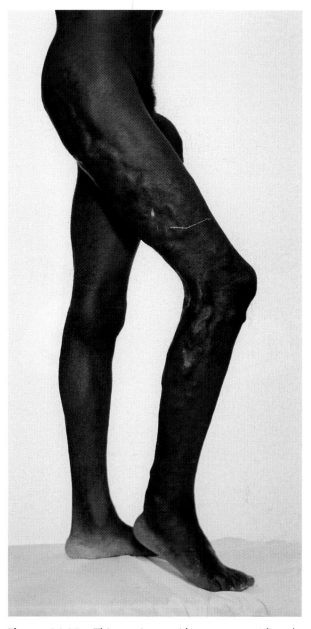

Figure 24.25 This patient with a severe Klippel–Trenaunay syndrome developed fixed flexion of the hip, knee and ankle joints because his leg length was not corrected.

Ancillary procedures

Table 24.1 lists the operations that we have performed on our patients. Many of the operations on our patients are simply 'tidying up' procedures. Although 50% of our patients have had some form of operation on the veins, the mainstay of treatment has been good elastic support.

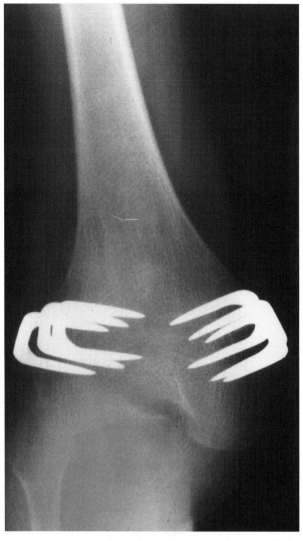

Figure 24.26   Epiphyseal staples, inserted to retard the growth of the leg.

Table 24.1   The 88 procedures performed on 38 patients with Klippel–Trenaunay syndrome[3]

Procedure	Number	%
Vein ligation and stripping	49	56
Excision of angioma	11	13
Excision of ulcer and skin graft	8	9
Excision of lymphatic vesicles	4	4.5
Amputation of digits	4	4.5
Epiphyseal stapling	4	4.5
Reducing operations	2	
Excision of fibroma	2	
Evacuation of spontaneous haematoma	2	
Injection of subcutaneous varices	1	
Injection of rectal varices	1	
Total	88	

the popliteal vein in a similar fashion to the better known popliteal artery entrapment syndrome.[11,14,52] The patient complains of intermittent swelling and discomfort brought on by exercise or presents with symptoms and signs of chronic venous insufficiency or acute deep vein thrombosis.[17] The diagnosis depends upon seeing a localized compression of the popliteal vein on phlebography or the abnormal muscle on CT scanning.[71] If the vein is not thrombosed, the symptoms can be relieved by dividing the abnormal strand of muscle. Leon *et al.*[33] demonstrated some degree of anatomical popliteal vein entrapment and functional outflow obstruction in 27% of healthy volunteers, suggesting that the abnormality is common and that only a small proportion of those affected present with symptoms.

Thrombosis prophylaxis

As patients with KTS are at increased risk of thromboembolism, they should be given prophylactic subcutaneous heparin whenever they are admitted to hospital. Once these patients have had a thrombosis, serious consideration should be given to the administration of oral anticoagulants for the rest of their lives.

Popliteal vein entrapment

Abnormalities of the insertion of the gastrocnemius muscle into the femur may cause compression of

References

1. Aelvoet GE, Jorens PG, Roelen LM. Genetic aspects of the Klippel–Trenaunay syndrome. *Br J Dermatol* 1992; **126:** 603–7.
2. Anderson M, Green WT, Messner MB. Growth and predictions of growth in the lower extremities. *J Bone Joint Surg* 1963; **45:** 1.
3. Baskerville PA, Ackroyd JS, Browse NL. The aetiology of the Klippel–Trenaunay syndrome. *Ann Surg* 1985; **202:** 624.
4. Baskerville PA, Ackroyd JS, Thomas ML, Browse NL. The Klippel–Trenaunay syndrome: clinical and haemodynamic features and management. *Br J Surg* 1985; **72:** 232.
5. Baskerville PA, Browse NL, personal observations.
6. Basmajian JW. The distribution of valves in the femoral, external iliac and common iliac vein and their relationship to varicose veins. *Surg Gynecol Obstet* 1952; **95:** 537.

7. Benbow EW. Idiopathic obstruction of the inferior vena cava, a review. *J R Soc Med* 1986; **79:** 105.

8. Blount WP, Clarke GR. Control of bone growth by epiphyseal stapling: a preliminary report. *J Bone Joint Surg (Am)* 1949; **31:** 464.

9. Bourde C. Classification des syndrome de Klippel–Trenaunay, et de Parkes Weber d'après des données angiographiques. *Ann Radiol (Paris)* 1974; **17:** 153.

10. Coget JM, Merlen JF, Arnolstan M. Klippel–Trenaunay syndrome of the upper extremity. *Phlebologie* 1983; **36:** 271.

11. Connell J. Popliteal vein entrapment. *Br J Surg* 1978; **65:** 351.

12. Craven N, Wright AL. Familial Klippel–Trenaunay syndrome: a case report. *Clin Exp Dermatol* 1995; **20:** 76–9.

13. Dougherty MJ, Calligaro KD, De Laurentis DA. Congenitally absent vena cava presenting in adulthood with venous stasis and ulceration: a surgically treated case. *J Vasc Surg* 1996; **23:** 141–6.

14. Edmonson HT, Crowe JA. Popliteal artery and venous entrapment. *Am J Surg* 1972; **38:** 657.

15. Effler DB, Greer AK, Sifers EC. Anomaly of the vena cava inferior, report of a fatality after ligation. *JAMA* 1951; **146:** 1321.

16. Elke M, Ludin H. Drainage der unteren Korperhalfte bei Agenesie und erworbenem verschluss der vena cava candalis. *Fortschr Roentgenstr* 1965; **103:** 665.

17. Gerkin TM, Beebe HG, Williams DM, Bloom JR, Wakefield TW. Popliteal vein entrapment presenting as deep venous thrombosis and chronic venous insufficiency. *J Vasc Surg* 1993; **18:** 760–6.

18. Gloviczki P, Stanson AW, Stickler AW, *et al.* Klippel–Trenaunay syndrome: the risks and benefits of vascular interventions. *Surgery* 1991; **110:** 469–79.

19. Gomes MN, Choyke PL. Assessment of major venous anomalies by computerised tomography. *J Cardiovasc Surg* 1990; **31:** 621–8.

20. Green WT. Equalization of leg length. *Surg Gynecol Obstet* 1950; **90:** 119.

21. Hollier LH. Surgical treatment of congenital venous malformations. In: Bergan JJ, Yao JST, eds. *Surgery of the Vein.* New York: Grune & Stratton, 1985; 275.

22. Howlet DC, Roebuck DJ, Frazer CK, Ayers B. The use of ultrasound in the venous assessment of lower limb Klippel–Trenaunay syndrome. *Eur J Radiol* 1994; **18:** 224–6.

23. Hunter GC, Malone JM, Moore WS, Misiorowski RL, Chvapil M. Vascular manifestations in patients with Ehlers–Danlos syndrome. *Arch Surg* 1982; **117:** 495.

24. Hutchinson WJ, Burdeaux BD. The influence of stasis on bone growth. *Surg Gynecol Obstet* 1954; **99:** 413.

25. Kim HJ, Ahn IO, Park ED. Hemiazygos continuation of a left inferior vena cava draining into the right atrium via persistent left superior vena cava: demonstration by helical computed tomography. *Cardiovasc Intervent Radiol* 1995; **18:** 65–7.

26. Kimwa C, Shirotani H, Hirooka M, Terada M, Iwahashi K, Maetani S. Membranous obliteration of the inferior vena cava in the hepatic portion. *Cardiovasc Surg* 1963; **4:** 87.

27. Kimwa C, Shirotani H, Kuma T, *et al.* Transcardiac membranotomy for obliteration of the vena cava in the hepatic portion. *J Cardiovasc Surg* 1962; **3:** 393.

28. Kinmonth JB. *The Lymphatics.* 2nd edition. London: Edward Arnold, 1982.

29. Kistner RL. Surgical repair of the incompetent femoral vein valve. *Arch Surg* 1975; **110:** 1336.

30. Klippel M, Trenaunay P. Du noevus variqueux osteo-hypertrophique. *Arch Gen Med (Paris)* 1900; **185:** 641.

31. Lea Thomas M. Agenesis of the iliac veins. *J Cardiovasc Surg* 1984; **25:** 64.

32. Lea Thomas M, Andress MR. Angiography in venous dysplasias of the limbs. *Am J Roentgenol* 1971; **113:** 722.

33. Leon M, Volteas N, Labropoulos N, *et al.* Popliteal vein entrapment in the normal population. *Eur J Vasc Surg* 1992; **6:** 623–7.

34. Leu HJ, Wenner A, Spycher MA, Brunner V. Ultrastrukturelle Veranderungen bei venoser Angiodysplasie von Typ Klippel Trenaunay. *Vasa* 1980; **9:** 147.

35. Lindenauer SM. The Klippel–Trenaunay syndrome: varicosity, hypertrophy and haemangioma with no arteriovenous fistula. *Ann Surg* 1965; **162:** 303.

36. Lodin A, Lindvall N, Gentele H. Congenital absence of venous valves as a cause of leg ulcers. *Acta Chir Scand* 1958; **116:** 256.

37. Loya YS, Sharma S, Amrapurka DN, Desai HG. Complete membranous obstruction of the inferior vena cava: case treated by balloon dilatation. *Cathet Cardiovasc Diagn* 1989; **17:** 164–7.

38. Malan E, Puglionisi A. Congenital angiodysplasias of the extremities. I: Generalities and classification, venous dysplasias. *J Cardiovasc Surg* 1964; **5:** 87.

39. Martorell F. Aplasia of the iliac vein. *Angiologia* 1971; **23:** 117.

40. Muller N, Morris DC, Nichols DM. Popliteal artery entrapment demonstrated by CT. *Radiology* 1984; **151:** 157.

41. Neubert AG, Golden MA, Rose NC. Kasabach–Merritt coagulaopathy complicating Klippel–Trenaunay syndrome in pregnancy. *Obstet Gynecol* 1995; **85:** 831–3.

42. O'Donnell TF. Congenital mixed vascular deformities of the lower limbs. *Ann Surg* 1977; **185:** 162.

43. Ohara I, Ouchi H, Takahashi K. A bypass operation for occlusion of the hepatic inferior vena cava. *Surg Gynecol Obstet* 1963; **117:** 151.

44. Paes EH, Vollmar JF. Aneurysmal transformation in congenital venous angiodysplasias in lower extremities. *Int Angiol* 1990; **9:** 90–6.

45. Parkes Weber F. Angioma formation in connection with hypertrophy of limbs and hemihypertrophy. *Br J Dermatol* 1907; **19:** 231.

46. Partsch H, Lofferer O, Mostbeck A. Zur Diagnostik von arteriovenosen Fisteln bei Angiodysplasien der Extremitaten. *Vasa* 1975; **4:** 288.

47. Phemister DB. Operative arrestment of longitudinal growth of bones in the treatment of deformities. *J Bone Joint Surg* 1933; **15**: 1.
48. Plate G, Brudin L, Eklof B, Jensen R, Ohlin P. Physiologic and therapeutic aspects in congenital vein valve aplasia of the lower limb. *Ann Surg* 1983; **198**: 229.
49. Poulet J, Ruff F. Les dysplasies veineuses congénitales des membres. *Presse Med* 1969; **77**: 163.
50. Prerovsky I, Linholt J, Dejdar R, Svejcar J, Kruw J, Vavrejn B. Research on primary varicose veins and chronic venous insufficiency. *Rev Czech Med* 1962; **8**: 171.
51. Rao KS, Gupta BK, Banerjee A, Srivastava KK. Chronic Budd–Chiari syndrome due to congenital membranous obstruction of the inferior vena cava: clinical experience. *Aust N Z J Surg* 1989; **59**: 335–8.
52. Rich NM, Hughes CW. Popliteal artery and vein entrapment. *Am J Surg* 1967; **113**: 696.
53. Samuel M, Spitz L. Klippel–Trenaunay syndrome: clinical features, complications and management in children. *Br J Surg* 1995; **82**: 757–61.
54. Sarma KP. Anomalous inferior vena cava. Anatomical and clinical features. *Br J Surg* 1966; **53**: 600.
55. Sen PK, Kinare SG, Kelkar MD, Paralkar GB, Mehta JM. Congenital membranous obliteration of the inferior vena cava. *J Cardiovasc Surg* 1967; **8**: 344.
56. Servelle M. Klippel and Trenaunay's syndrome. *Ann Surg* 1985; **201**: 365–73.
57. Servelle M. La phlebographie va-t-elle nous permettre de demembrer le syndrome de Klippel et Trenaunay et l'hémangiectasie hypertrophique de Parkes-Weber. *Presse Med* 1945; **53**: 353.
58. Servelle M. Stase veineuse et croissance osseuse. *Bull Acad Nat Med* 1948; **132**: 472.
59. Servelle M, Babillot J. Les malformations des veines profondes dans le syndrome de Klippel et Trenaunay. *Phlebologie* 1980; **33**: 31.
60. Servelle M, Zolotas E, Soulie J, Andrieux J, Cornu C. Syndrome de Klippel et Trenaunay: malformations iliaques et poplitée. *Arch Mal Coeur* 1965; **68**: 1187.
61. Thomas ML, MacFie GB. Phlebography in the Klippel–Trenaunay syndrome. *Acta Radiol Diagn (Stockh)* 1974; **15**: 43–56.
62. Trelat U, Monad A. De l'hypertrophie unilaterale partielle ou totale du corps. *Arch Gen Med* 1869; **2**: 536.
63. Van der Molen HR. Maladie de Klippel–Trenaunay et grosses jambes. *Soc Fr Phlebol* 1968; **2**: 187.
64. Van der Molen HR. Quelques remarques cliniques au sujet des dysplasies vasculaires. *Phlebologie* 1980; **33**: 43.
65. Van der Stricht J. Syndrome de Klippel et Trenaunay et phacomatoses. *Phlebologie* 1980; **33**: 21.
66. Vollmar J. Malformations of the leg and pelvic veins. In: May R, ed. *Surgery of the Veins of the Leg and Pelvis.* Stuttgart: Georg Thieme, 1974; 200.
67. Vollmar J, Vogt K. Angiodysplasie und Skeletsystem. *Chirurg* 1976; **47**: 205.
68. Watkins E, Fortin CL. Surgical correction of a congenital coarctation of the inferior vena cava. *Ann Surg* 1964; **159**: 536.
69. Whelan AJ, Watson MS, Porter FD, Steiner RD. Klippel-Trenaunay–Weber syndrome associated with a 5:11 balanced translocation. *Am J Med Gen* 1995; **59**: 492–4.
70. Woollard HH. The development of the principal arterial stems in the forelimb of the pig. *Contrib Embryol (Carnegie Inst)* 1922; **22**: 139.
71. Young AK. Congenital mixed vascular deformities of the limbs and their associated lesions. *Birth Defects* 1978; **14**: 289.

CHAPTER 25

Occlusion of the veins of the upper arm and neck

Axillary/subclavian vein thrombosis	689	References	707
Superior vena caval occlusion and thrombosis	702		

The two major problems that affect the veins of the upper arm and neck are axillary and subclavian vein thrombosis and obstruction of the superior vena cava. Primary varicose veins are never found in the upper limb except as part of a Klippel–Trenaunay syndrome, but congenital and acquired arteriovenous fistulae can cause secondary varicose veins which can be treated by eradicating the underlying cause.

The valves may be congenitally absent from the upper limb veins but this does not cause any clinical problems. In the upper limb, thrombotic complications and their sequelae are less common and less severe than in the leg. Probable reasons for this include the arm's lack of an equivalent to the soleal plexus, the insignificant hydrostatic venous pressure and the more extensive collateral circulation. In addition, the production of the activators of fibrinolysis is greater in the upper limb.[44,50] Injuries to the great veins in the upper limb, supraclavicular region and thorax do occur, and these are discussed in Chapter 26. Superficial thrombophlebitis is discussed in Chapter 23 and venous angiomata, which may also affect the upper limb, are discussed in Chapter 27.

Axillary/subclavian vein thrombosis

Thrombosis of the axillary/subclavian vein was originally described by Sir James Paget in 1875[42] and by von Schroetter in 1884;[66] it is therefore frequently called Paget–Schroetter's syndrome. It is a rare condition, accounting for 1–4% of all cases of deep venous thrombosis.[1,10,11,20,26,28,47,51]

A recent apparent rise in incidence may be attributable to the increasing use of subclavian vein catheterization and greater diagnostic awareness and availability of venography and duplex ultrasound.

AETIOLOGY

Thrombosis of the axillary vein may be a primary or secondary event, though increasingly, investigators doubt a primary aetiology and try to find a cause for all cases.

It often follows excessive or unusual physical exercise and has consequently been called 'effort thrombosis'.[34] The greater incidence of axillary vein thrombosis in men compared with that in women, and the greater incidence in the right arm,[5,34,40,65] are indicative of the relevance of physical exertion to its development.

Many workers consider that external compression of the axillary vein as it enters the thoracic inlet is a major aetiological factor[1,15,39] and some investigators have implied that thoracic inlet/outlet compression is the cause of all axillary vein thromboses.[14,17,59] There is, however, considerable disagreement over the anatomical structure that causes the obstruction. A cervical rib (Figure 25.1), a congenital web

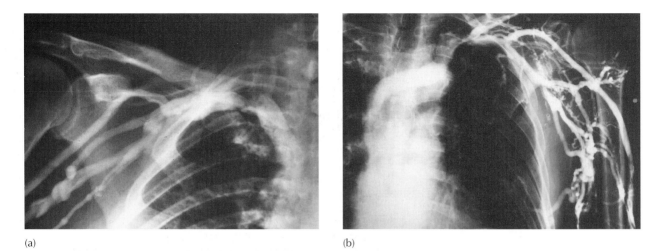

(a)   (b)

Figure 25.1   (a, b) Two examples of narrowing of the axillary/subclavian vein associated with a cervical rib.

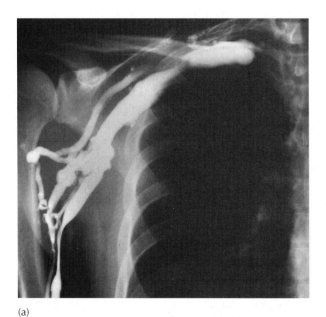

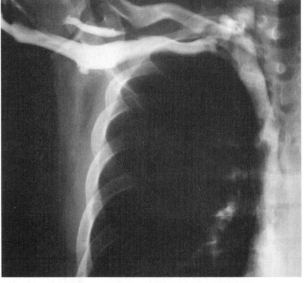

(a)   (b)

Figure 25.2   (a) An intraluminal congenital septum producing almost complete obstruction of the subclavian
vein, with the arm by the side. (b) The obstruction was
less when the arm was elevated. (c) A stenosis of the junction of the right subclavian and jugular veins in a young
man – presumably of congenital origin. A digital subtracted image.

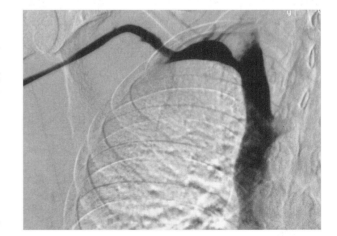

(c)

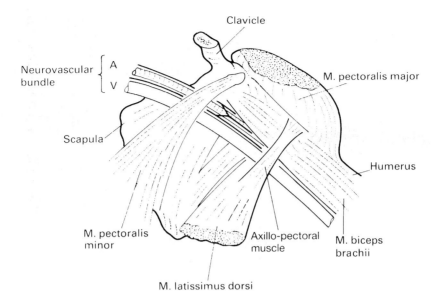

Figure 25.3 The anatomical position of a persistent axillopectoral muscle, a rare cause of axillary vein occlusion.[7,12]

(Figure 25.2), the first rib, the subclavius and scalenus anterior muscles, an anteriorly placed phrenic or accessory phrenic nerve, the pectoralis minor muscle, the clavicle or a malunited fracture of the clavicle, and a persistent axillo-pectoral muscle (Figure 25.3) have all been incriminated.[1,7,12,13,30,52,65,69] Other well recognized conditions causing secondary thrombosis are upper limb/chest wall radiotherapy (usually for breast cancer) and the use of indwelling catheters in the great veins.

A number of large reviews of axillary vein thrombosis have suggested that it is more likely that several factors, acting in combination, are responsible for its development. Hughes[29] reported one of the first and largest series in 1949 with 320 cases of symptomatic axillary/subclavian vein thrombosis. Effort thrombosis comprised 49% of cases and 34% were spontaneous (83% primary thrombosis). The incidence of secondary thrombosis was 17%, but less than 1% were attributed to anatomical factors and in this era before central venous lines, there were no catheter-related thromboses. In 1966, Coon and Willis[11] reported an incidence of secondary axillary/subclavian vein thrombosis related to intravenous catheters and irritant solutions of 10%. Tilney *et al.* in 1970[65] reported similar findings in 18% of their 48 cases.

In 1977, Campbell *et al.*[10] described eight patients with 'effort thrombosis', ten with internal injury (e.g. an intravenous catheter or infusion), six with extrinsic compression and one with a hypercoagulable state.

Sundqvist *et al.*[61] examined the blood for evidence of an abnormality of systemic fibrinolysis in 60 patients with axillary vein thrombosis and found it to be present in nearly 50% of these patients, though it is possible that this was an effect rather than a cause of the condition. Within this group of patients they also found a multitude of aetiological factors:

- evidence of coincidental leg vein thrombosis in six patients
- a family history of leg vein thrombosis in eight patients
- a history of trauma to the shoulder in two patients (one had a fracture of the clavicle)
- excessive 'effort' in five patients (including long-distance swimming and chopping down trees)
- cervical ribs in two patients
- contraceptive pill ingestion in ten patients
- pregnancy in two patients
- cancer of the breast in one patient (Figure 25.5)
- cancer of the prostate in one patient
- two patients who were severely ill in the intensive care unit
- two patients who had recently suffered a myocardial infarct (one developed pneumonia)
- two patients who were alcoholic.

Martin *et al.*[38] reported that half of their 20 patients with an axillary vein thrombosis had a demonstrable cause for the condition. The causes which they reported included breast carcinoma (Figure 25.5), a central venous pressure catheter, heroin addiction, and cervical ribs (see Figure 25.1).

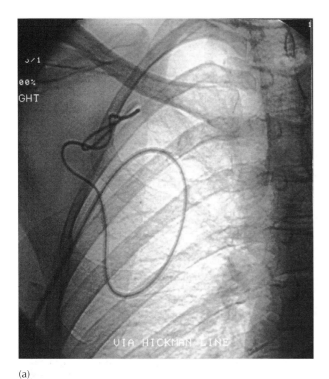

(a)

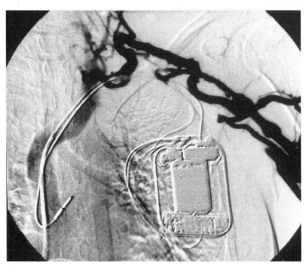

(b)

Figure 25.4   Two common causes of axillary and subclavian vein thrombosis: (a) a Hickman line; (b) a dual chamber pacing wire.

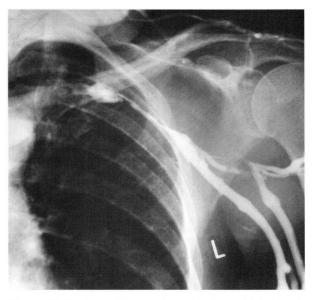

Figure 25.5   An axillary vein occlusion which developed after a mastectomy followed by radiotherapy given to treat a stage II carcinoma of the breast. The axillary vein is narrow and irregular.

In three patients presenting with venous gangrene of the hand, the initiating factors were reduced tissue perfusion, hypercoagulability and venous injury.[57]

In 1988, Horattas *et al.*[28] reviewed 33 cases of upper limb deep vein thrombosis and found that subclavian venous catheterization was the major cause, accounting for 39% of cases. They indicated that 28% of subclavian vein catheterization procedures resulted in thrombosis, often subclinical. They cite the following important factors in the development of catheter-related thrombosis:

- catheter diameter
- catheter material
- multiple venepuncture
- duration of catheter placement
- pH and osmolality of infusate
- aseptic technique
- anticoagulants.

Hill and Berry[26] studied 40 patients with subclavian vein thrombosis and found that 45% were idiopathic, effort-related or associated with anatomical anomalies. There was a 2:1 right-sided bias in this group and the average age was 39 years. Catheter-related thrombosis occurred in 32% and the average age of this group was 52 years (Figure 25.4). Radiotherapy- or cancer-related thrombosis occurred in 23% and some of these were bilateral thromboses. The average age of this group was 51 years. Pulmonary embolism affected only one patient (2.5%).

Burihan and associates,[9] reporting 52 cases of upper limb deep vein thrombosis in 1993, found that 67% of patients were male and that the mean age was 45 years. The right arm was affected in 44%. Thoracic outlet syndrome or effort thrombosis was identified in 24%, central venous catheterization in 29% and extrinsic compression (most caused by cancer) in 29%. Pulmonary embolism and phlegmasia cerulea dolens affected one patient each.

The association of axillary vein thrombosis with both malignancy and intravenous infusions, particularly long central catheters, is common to most of these studies. The operation of axillary clearance of lymph glands and radiotherapy to the axilla are both known to carry a risk of axillary vein thrombosis. This is an important cause of swelling of the arm in patients who have had treatment for carcinoma of the breast (see Figure 25.5).

Comment

As for deep vein thrombosis of the leg, the aetiology of axillary vein thrombosis is almost certainly multifactorial. Thoracic outlet compression is rarely the sole cause of 'primary' or idiopathic thrombosis. Thoracic outlet compression does, however, appear to be an important factor and should always be considered in patients presenting with this condition.

Stevenson and Parry[59] have suggested that a compression abnormality can always be detected in the opposite normal limb of patients presenting with 'idiopathic' axillary vein thrombosis, if axillary phlebographs are obtained during differing degrees of shoulder abduction (Figure 25.5). This study was inevitably open to observer bias and requires confirmation by other investigators before it can be fully accepted. In our experience, bilateral axillary vein thrombosis is extremely rare, except in patients with terminal malignant disease. This observation suggests that bilateral anatomical abnormalities are rare or their presence is insignificant.

CLINICAL FEATURES

Most series[5,9,10,40] show a male-to-female preponderance of approximately 3:2. The majority of patients are between the ages of 35 years and 45 years, and the thrombosis involves the dominant right arm in two-thirds of cases.

Swelling (98%), discoloration and collateral vein dilatation (71%) and aching (63%) are the commonest clinical features.[9] Patients complain of discomfort and weakness developing within 24 hours of excessive or unusual exercise.[5] The discomfort varies between a dull ache with a feeling of tightness to a severe pain. The hand and forearm become cold and hand and finger movements are diminished. The arm then gradually becomes swollen and blue from the fingertips to the shoulder. Enlargement of the female breast has been reported to occur on the side of the occlusion[11] if the pectoral and scapular regions become oedematous.

On examination there is usually evidence of pitting oedema of the fingers, hand and forearm, and a variable amount of oedema of the upper arm.[65] The oedema is most obvious over the dorsum of the hand. The skin has a diffuse blue tinge and is cool to the touch; there is often a clear line of demarcation between these changes and normal skin over the upper arm or shoulder. The main subcutaneous veins, the basilic and cephalic, are the first to distend but later there is a generalized distension of all the veins and venules.[3] The distended veins feel tense and do not collapse when the arm is elevated above the level of the right atrium. Collateral veins develop over the chest wall and shoulder in the weeks following a thrombosis as anastomoses open up between the tributaries of the axillary and cephalic veins and the mediastinal and intercostal veins (Figure 25.6). These may be sufficient to relieve all symptoms.

In approximately 50% of patients, the axillary vein may be palpable as a thickened tender cord high up on the lateral side of the axilla.[5] If there is extension of the thrombosis into the subclavian vein (a common event), there may be supraclavicular tenderness. The supraclavicular hollow and the subclavian dimple may also be filled in, and the face and neck may become swollen if the thrombus extends into the jugular vein or superior vena cava.[65]

The clinical diagnosis of subclavian or axillary vein thrombosis can be difficult to make and there is evidence that many catheter-related thromboses are asymptomatic.[4,8,35]

Late sequelae and complications in the arm

Many patients develop adequate collateral circulation or recanalize the thrombosed segment (Figure 25.6) and approximately 40% are free of symptoms 6 months after the thrombosis.[9] It has been recognized recently that long-term swelling and pain are commoner than had been appreciated, one study reporting late objective signs of venous insufficiency in 42% of patients.[21] Patients may complain of recurrent swelling and pain during arm exercise[5] or severe fatigue and discomfort after exercise.[10] At worst, they may develop disabling venous claudication of the arm, especially when using the arm above the shoulder level (Figure 25.7).

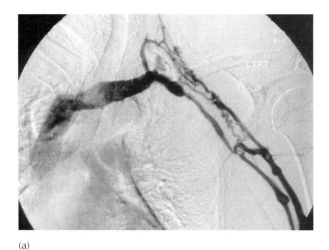

(a)

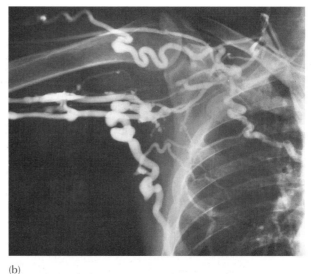

(b)

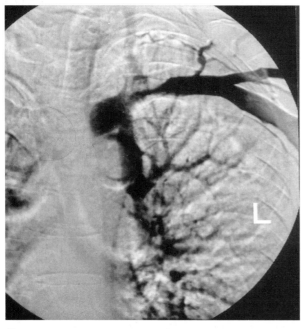

(c)

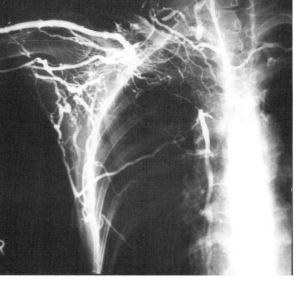

(d)

Figure 25.6 (a) Collateral formation and possibly recanalization following an axillary vein thrombosis, sufficient to relieve all the symptoms. (b) Extensive collateral vessels crossing the subcutaneous tissues of the chest wall. (c) An unusual collateral pathway via the left hemiazygos vein into the left pulmonary artery. (d) Collateral pathways through the intercostal veins into the azygos vein.

The late sequelae described above appear to be dependent as much upon the aetiology of the thrombosis[10] as the success of the treatment.[5]

Venous gangrene of the hand is a rare complication. Although only a few cases have been reported,[1,43,57] we have seen three patients with this complication, all in the terminal stages of advanced disseminated malignant disease, so it may therefore not be quite so uncommon as many texts suggest.

Differential diagnosis

In the early stages, symptoms of weakness, coldness and skin discoloration may suggest arterial ischaemia but the presence of normal pulses and the development of oedema, cyanosis and distended veins usually make the correct diagnosis apparent. External compression of the veins by malignant lymph nodes, Pancoast's tumour or soft

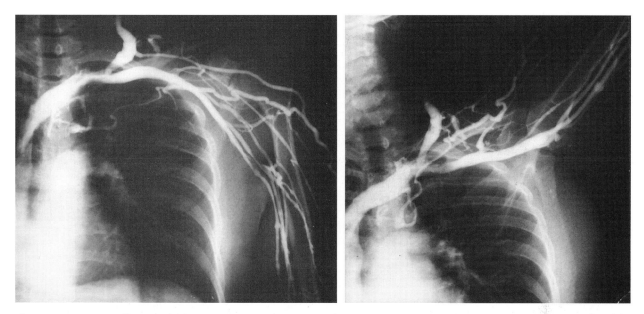

Figure 25.7 An axillary vein obstruction at the thoracic inlet (left-hand panel) which was more apparent when the arm was elevated (right-hand panel) and only caused symptoms when the arm was used above shoulder level.

tissue sarcomata (Figure 25.8) must always be excluded, and computerized tomography (CT), magnetic resonance imaging (MRI) and lymphography may be required if external compression is suspected. Lymphoedema and cellulitis are other rare causes of a painful and swollen arm.

Pulmonary embolism

Although some studies have suggested that pulmonary embolism is uncommon in association with

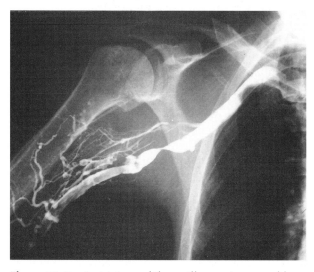

Figure 25.8 A stricture of the axillary vein caused by a myosarcoma with fresh thrombus in the brachial veins.

axillary vein thrombosis,[23,65] other workers have shown that this complication occurs in 5–12% of patients.[28,30,67] A small group of patients have repeated pulmonary emboli and develop pulmonary hypertension, but massive or fatal pulmonary embolism from an axillary vein thrombosis is extremely rare.

DIAGNOSIS AND INVESTIGATIONS

A careful history and general examination are essential to detect or exclude any of the many causes of axillary vein thrombosis outlined in the section on aetiology. Particular attention should be paid to a history of unusual exercise and recent intravenous injections or catheterizations. Careful questioning may reveal evidence of a known hypercoagulable state or a family history of thrombosis. Pregnancy or exposure to the contraceptive pill may also be relevant.

During the examination, it is important to look for evidence of malignant disease, particularly of the breast, prostate and lung and also lymphoma. There may be clinical evidence of cervical ribs or thoracic outlet syndrome, for example disappearance of the radial pulse when the arm is elevated to 180° (Adson's test).[2]

A full red and white cell count should be performed to exclude polycythaemia and leukaemia, and a platelet count should be carried out to exclude thrombocytosis (thrombocythaemia).

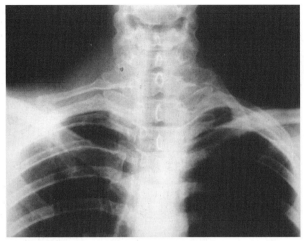

Figure 25.9 Cervical ribs are usually easy to see on a plain radiograph of the thoracic inlet.

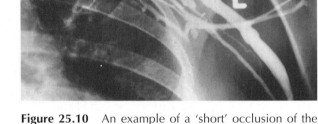

Figure 25.10 An example of a 'short' occlusion of the subclavian vein. The occlusion begins at the edge of the first rib.

A chest radiograph may reveal a carcinoma of bronchus or secondary deposits from a distant malignancy. Cervical ribs may also be seen on a chest radiograph but thoracic inlet and cervical spine films should always be requested (Figure 25.9).

Screening for hypercoagulation should include measurement of the common coagulation factors, antithrombin III, protein C, protein S and lupus anticoagulant levels, together with tests of fibrinolysis.[61] These tests take time to organize and obtain; they do not affect the initial management but may affect later care.

Non-invasive assessment with arterial and venous Doppler probes should demonstrate normal arterial wrist pressures but diminished or absent antegrade deep venous flow and loss of the Valsalva response in the peripheral arm veins. Doppler venous examination is, however, rather insensitive due to the extensive collateral circulation that may develop.[35,46] Colour duplex ultrasound is more accurate, localizing the site of the occlusion with visualization of the thrombus.

Impedence plethysmography has been reported to have good sensitivity and specificity (over 90%) when compared with phlebography in the diagnosis of axillary vein thrombosis.[43,45] Air plethysmography appears to be accurate in the diagnosis of upper limb deep vein thrombosis.[22] Strain-gauge plethysmography[70] and light reflection rheography[41] have been assessed with encouraging initial results in patients with occluded veins, but their accuracy in milder, non-occlusive thrombosis remains in doubt. Initial studies with isotope scintigraphy[24,27] and spiral CT[64] have also been encouraging.

Despite technical advances in duplex ultrasound, ascending brachial venography remains the preferred method of diagnosis as collateral veins are more easily identified and treatment with thrombolysis can be initiated where appropriate. Contrast should be introduced via the basilic vein to ensure full visualization of the subclavian/axillary vein thrombosis rather than bypassing of the thrombosis through collaterals which may occur when the cephalic vein is used.[10] Venograms should be performed with the arm in partial abduction to avoid false-positive appearances of venous occlusion. There is poor correlation between the venographic findings and the severity of symptoms.[21] Two main phlebographic patterns have been described.[5] The first pattern is a short, localized obstruction at the junction of the subclavian vein with the axillary vein (between the first rib and the clavicle) (Figure 25.10). The second pattern is a long obstruction extending distally down the axillary vein into the brachial vein (Figure 25.11). Martin *et al.*[38] reported that in over 70% of their cases the thrombosis extended into the subclavian vein, but the innominate vein was rarely involved. It is often quite difficult to determine the proximal extent of the thrombosis.

Ventilation–perfusion lung scans and pulmonary angiography may be indicated if there is a suspicion of pulmonary embolism.

Digital subtraction arteriography of the subclavian and axillary arteries in different degrees of shoulder abduction may help to confirm the presence of a thoracic outlet obstruction.

TREATMENT

Many patients present days or weeks after the onset of symptoms. By this time, conservative treatment,

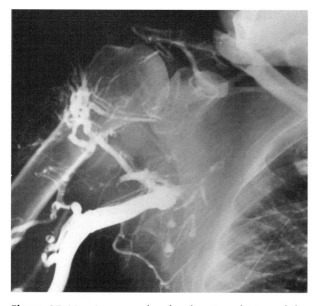

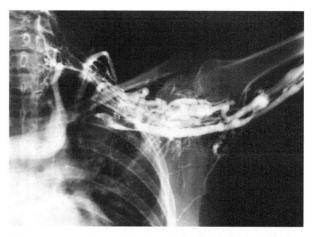

Figure 25.12 An example of the thrombus retraction and extensive collateral vessel formation that followed a subclavian vein thrombosis caused by a Hickman line. The patient had no symptoms.

Figure 25.11 An example of a 'long' occlusion of the axillary and subclavian vein. The occlusion begins at the level of the axillary skin fold.

plus careful follow-up, is the only practical method of management[69] with a view to some form of delayed venous reconstruction if severe post-thrombotic symptoms develop later.[32] Conservative treatment consists of bedrest, arm elevation, administration of anticoagulants and, very rarely, a stellate ganglion block when this is indicated.[5]

In one study, 21 out of 24 patients treated conservatively, half with anticoagulants, developed symptoms of chronic venous insufficiency,[62] and persistent symptoms were present in eight of the 31 patients reported by Tilney *et al.*,[65] who were available for long-term follow-up. Tilney concluded that new forms of treatment should be considered but our own clinical experience has not been so depressing. Two-thirds of our patients have recovered to such a degree that they have had very minor symptoms which are not incapacitating and Steed *et*

al.[58] reported spontaneous improvement in 80% of their patients without treatment.

The active measures that have been tried include thrombolysis[5] and thrombectomy,[37] alone or in combination with surgical decompression of the axillary vein or thoracic inlet,[14] patch angioplasty, segmental bypass, and balloon angioplasty with and without stent placement. Delayed venous reconstruction or bypass can be tried in patients treated conservatively who continue to have disabling symptoms.

Venous thrombectomy

Venous thrombectomy alone has been only moderately successful (Table 25.1),[14,37] and the addition of first rib resection has not appreciably improved results. In patients with catheter-induced thrombosis, conservative treatment with catheter removal, elevation and anticoagulation frequently leads to full regression of thrombus and symptoms[16] (Figure 25.12). On the other hand, a significant proportion (40–70%) of patients with

Table 25.1 Results of treatment of acute axillary thrombosis[17]

Treatment	Number of arms treated	Recanalization			Persisting symptoms	
		Complete	Partial	Nil	None	Present
Anticoagulants	42	2	8	32	13	29
Thrombectomy	9	2	4	3	3	6
Thrombectomy plus 1st rib resection	6	2	2	2	2	4
Thrombolysis	12	8	2	2	6	6
Thrombolysis plus 1st rib resection	12	10	2	0	10	2

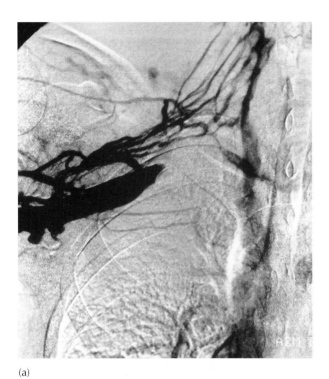

(a)

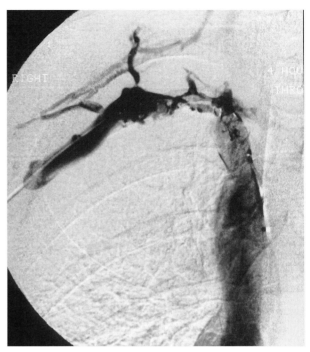

(b)

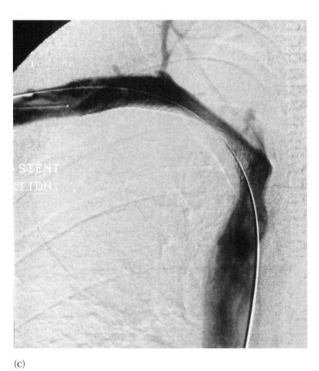

(c)

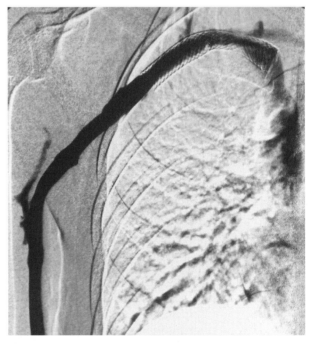

(d)

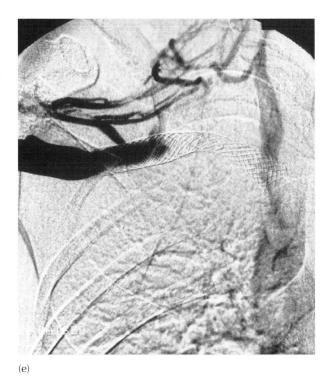

(e)

Figure 25.13 Inadequate treatment of a subclavian vein thrombosis caused by external compression. (a) The presenting acute subclavian vein thrombosis. (b) The thrombus was lysed by a 4-hour intrathrombus infusion of rt-PA. (c) A Wall stent was deployed. The symptoms were relieved. (d) A follow-up phlebograph, 2 months later, shows the stent to be patent when the arm is beside the trunk but partially compressed and kinked at the inner edge of the first rib. (e) When the arm was abducted the stent occluded. The patient still had symptoms when using the arm above shoulder level and there is a high risk that such activity may precipitate stent thrombosis. This illustrates the need to treat external compression surgically even after successful thrombolysis and stenting. Stents cannot resist the high pressures of external bony/muscular compression, especially during abduction of the arm.

effort thrombosis or thoracic outlet compression treated conservatively suffer persistent long-term symptoms.

Thrombolysis

Thrombolysis followed immediately by correction of any anatomical factors appears to improve the long-term outcome, although there are no controlled trials to confirm this widely held view. Thrombolysis may be effective up to 1–2 weeks after the initial event. Low-dose streptokinase, urokinase or tissue plasminogen activator is administered locally via the venography catheter which is advanced into the thrombus. Heparin is also given to prevent pericatheter thrombosis. Following successful lysis, the patient should be anticoagulated and there is increasing evidence that any subclavian/axillary vein stricture should be corrected by direct venous surgery or dilatation followed by the insertion of a stent and any external compressing agent removed surgically (Figures 25.13, 25.14). The optimum timing of this remains unclear but Molina claims that urgent surgery immediately after completion of lysis gives the best chance of avoiding recurrent venous strictures and long-term symptoms.[40]

First or cervical rib resection

First or cervical rib resection, excision of anomalous fibromuscular bands, division of subclavius and/or scalenus anterior and medial claviculectomy have been described for decompression of the subclavian vein (Figure 25.15). These procedures have often been combined with thrombectomy, thrombolysis and patch venoplasty and their relative merits are difficult to assess. Where thrombolysis reveals an underlying venous stricture secondary to the endothelial damage induced by the thoracic outlet compression, balloon venoplasty is effective in restoring patency.[36]

Bypass surgery and venoplasty

The overall place of venous stenting is still being examined.[51] Concern has been expressed that a stent placed in a vessel such as the subclavian/axillary vein which is subjected to frequent bending and twisting may kink and thrombose or fracture and embolize. It is argued that thrombosis can be prevented by permanent anticoagulation and incorporation of the stent into the vein wall makes embolism unlikely – nevertheless, these procedures should only be used in units that keep their patients under careful long-term surveillance and report their results. We will not know the value of these aggressive methods of treating benign axillo-subclavian vein thrombosis for at least 5 years. In patients who present too late for thrombolysis and in those with chronic symptoms of upper limb venous outflow obstruction, endoluminal or surgical reconstruction may be of benefit. Reconstructive techniques such as internal jugular vein transposition and prosthetic axillojugular bypass with temporary arteriovenous fistula[53]

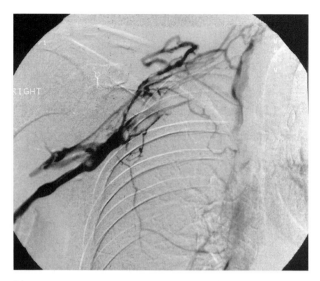

(a)

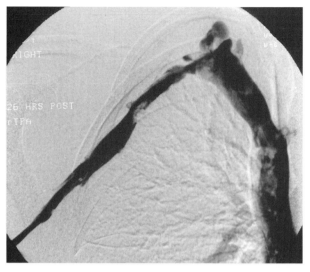

(b)

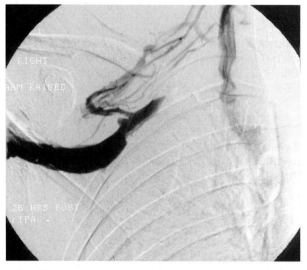

(c)

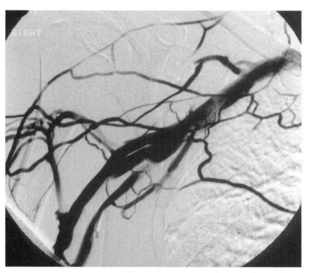

(d)

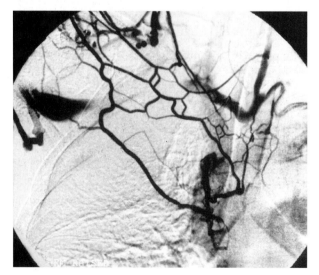

(e)

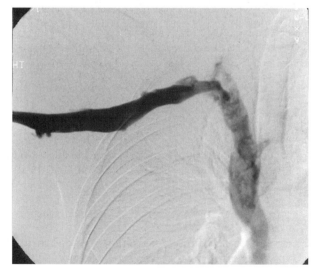

(f)

Figure 25.14 The treatment of axillary vein thrombosis by thrombolysis and surgery combined. (a) An acute axillary vein thrombosis. (b) After 26-hour infusion of rt-PA the vein was patent but still contained some residual mural thrombus. (Note the flow artefacts in the superior vena cava.) (c) Even after complete thrombolysis abduction of the arms was observed to cause complete occlusion of the junction of the axillary and subclavian veins. (d) A follow-up phlebogram, 3 months later, fortunately without further thrombosis, showed the vein to be patent when the arm was beside the trunk, but (e) the vein became totally occluded when the arm was abducted. (f) After surgical removal of a large bony protuberance on the first rib (not visible on these subtracted phlebographs) the vein remained patent during abduction of the arm.

and axillary vein–right atrial bypass[18] are being developed with encouraging early patency and resolution of symptoms. In one study reported from the Ochsner clinic, long-term symptomatic relief was greater in a surgically bypassed group than a group undergoing single venoplasty, although results in patients undergoing repeated venoplasty approached those of the surgical group.[68]

We recommend that such procedures should only be performed when the patient is severely disabled and by those skilled in the techniques of direct major vein reconstruction and that the operation should preferably be part of a properly controlled clinical study.

PROGNOSIS

Aggressive early treatment appears to give better results than conservative management although it must be acknowledged that most studies of thrombolysis, thoracic outlet decompression and venous reconstruction are small and uncontrolled with poorly defined end points. If the degree of residual disability after axillary vein thrombosis has been underestimated, late venous reconstruction by bypass may offer hope for the chronic sufferer. It is, however, surprising that there are so few complications when the brachial vein is resected for a valve transfer operation.[63] This makes us think that it is the local abnormality, the extent of the initial thrombosis and the effectiveness of the collaterals

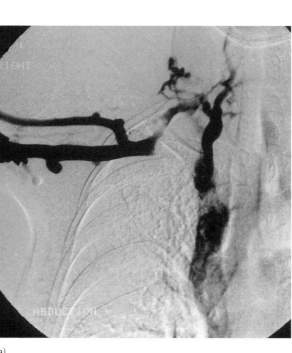

(a)

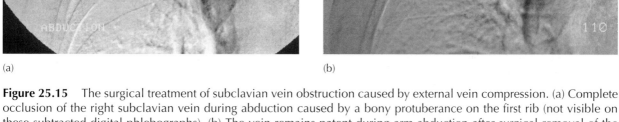

(b)

Figure 25.15 The surgical treatment of subclavian vein obstruction caused by external vein compression. (a) Complete occlusion of the right subclavian vein during abduction caused by a bony protuberance on the first rib (not visible on these subtracted digital phlebographs). (b) The vein remains patent during arm abduction after surgical removal of the bony protuberance and the patient was cured.

(Figure 25.12) that determine the late sequelae rather than the treatment. We need to know much more about these factors so that we can decide which patients need early aggressive treatment and which patients can be treated conservatively before we become too attracted to the surgical appeal of venous reconstruction.

Superior vena caval occlusion and thrombosis

Thrombosis of the superior vena cava is commonly an acute event, usually caused by a rapidly growing intrathoracic neoplasm (80–95%). This neoplasm is most often a carcinoma of the bronchus (75%) but lymphomas (25%), thymomas and carcinoma of the thyroid may also lead to occlusion (Figure 25.16). Retrosternal goitres (see Figure 25.17), rarer mediastinal tumours such as caval leiomyosarcoma and secondary deposits can also produce obstruction. In the past, syphilitic thoracic aneurysms were an important cause of thrombosis; this was the cause of the superior vena cava obstruction in the first description of this syndrome, published by William Hunter in 1747.[31] Constrictive pericarditis and mediastinal fibrosis (Figure 25.18), a condition similar to retroperitoneal fibrosis, are also recognized as rare but important conditions which may lead to thrombosis.

Spontaneous thrombosis of the superior vena cava can occur but it is rare. The increasing use of

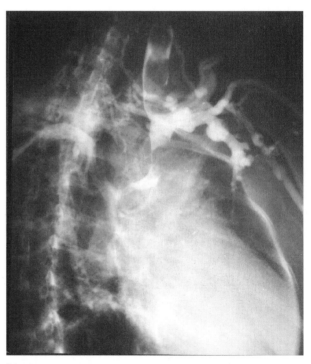

(b)

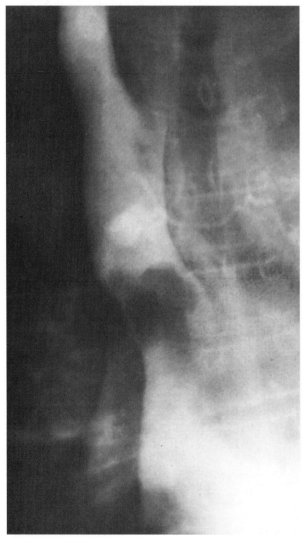

(a)

Figure 25.16   Two examples of malignant superior vena cava obstruction. (a) A carcinoma of the bronchus protruding into the vena cava. (b) Compression by lymph nodes enlarged by Hodgkin's lymphoma. Note the fresh thrombus in the brachiocephalic and jugular veins.

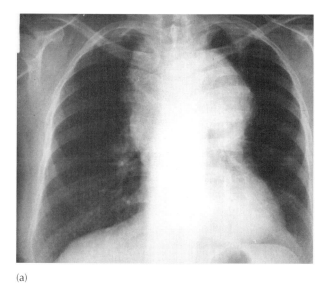

(a)

Figure 25.17 An enlarged retrosternal thyroid gland obstructing the superior vena cava. (a) The mediastinal mass. (b) A digital subtraction phlebograph showing compression and displacement of the right innominate vein and the vena cava with obstruction of the left pulmonary artery.

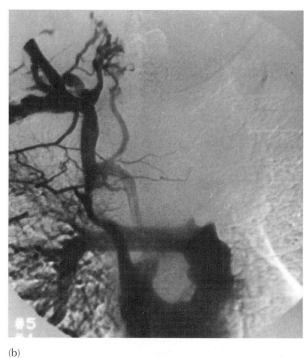

(b)

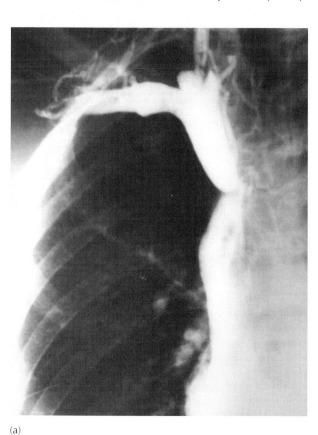

(a)

(b)

Figure 25.18 Two examples of mediastinal fibrosis causing superior vena cava obstruction: (a) a partial obstruction; (b) total occlusion.

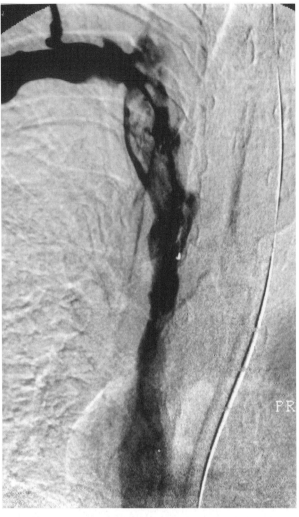

(a)

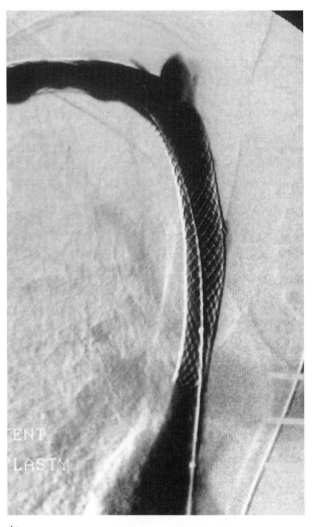

(b)

Figure 25.19   Stenting for partial malignant obstruction of the vena cava. (a) A phlebograph showing extensive infiltration and obstruction of the superior vena cava by a carcinoma of the bronchus. There is also some intraluminal mural thrombus. (b) The insertion of a Wall stent produced considerable amelioration of the symptoms.

intravenous cannulation and the injection of hyperosmolar fluids into the neck veins may cause thrombosis. The use of very low dose warfarin (1 mg/day) in patients undergoing chronic central venous cannulation reduces the likelihood of great vein thrombosis.[6] Thrombosis may also follow local injuries and iatrogenic injuries occurring during surgery to the heart and pericardium.

Normally when the superior vena cava becomes obstructed the azygos, the hemiazygos, the internal mammary, the lateral thoracic and vertebral veins act as collateral channels (see Figures 25.18 and 25.19).

CLINICAL FEATURES

Patients with superior vena caval obstruction usually present with swelling of the face and neck, and shortness of breath, which is often acute in onset. Very occasionally, patients may complain of tinnitus and deafness, epistaxis, a dry cough and dysphagia. The skin of the face is hyperaemic and cyanotic, and the jugular veins which are visibly distended do not alter in size with respiration or when the patient sits upright. If there is no hepatomegaly or ankle oedema heart failure is unlikely; but exophthalmos may occasionally be present. In the

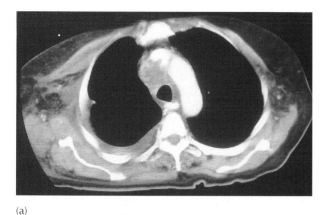

(a)

Figure 25.20 Stenting for a localized malignant stenosis of the vena cava. (a) A CT scan showing a mediastinal mass infiltrating and occluding the vena cava. (b) The superior vena cava graph showing a tight localized stenosis but still with a lumen capable of passage by a guide wire. (c) Restoration of patency by the deployment of a Wall stent.

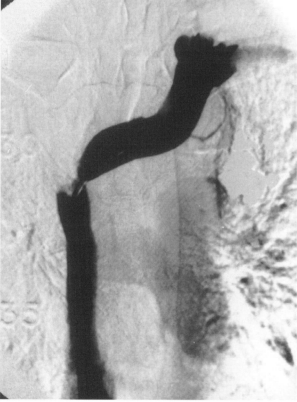

(b)

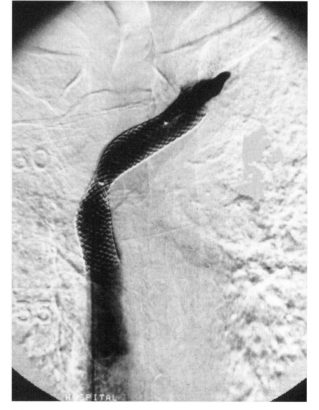

(c)

late stages patients may complain of a feeling of congestion of the head, marked confusion, restlessness, dizziness, syncope and somnolence.

INVESTIGATIONS

A chest radiograph commonly reveals the cause of the problem, if this is not clinically apparent. Mediastinal widening may also be apparent.

Computerized tomography (CT) may provide better evidence of the presence and extent of mediastinal tumours and transoesophageal echocardiography has been used to diagnose superior vena caval thrombosis and monitor response to fibrinolytic therapy.[25] A tissue diagnosis should be obtained before any treatment is begun. Non-invasive tests (e.g. ultrasonography and plethysmography) may be used in screening but phlebography is required to confirm the diagnosis of a spontaneous

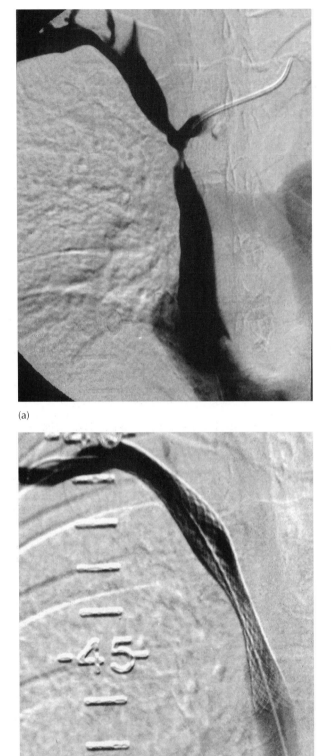

(a)

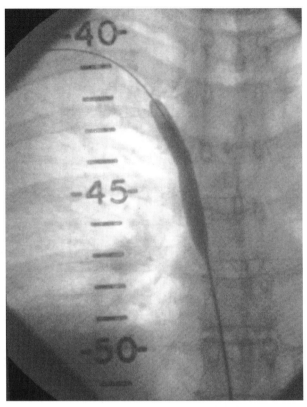

(b)

(c)

Figure 25.21 Balloon dilatation of a benign stricture of the superior vena cava. (a) This phlebograph in a young patient who complained of pain and swelling when exercising his right arm revealed this stenosis at the junction of the brachiocephalic vein and superior vena cava. Probably a congenital abnormality. (b) Balloon dilatation. (c) Wall stent deployment through the stricture. Although there is some residual wasting at the site of the stricture, the patient's symptoms were much improved.

or primary superior vena caval thrombosis. This can usually be obtained by bilateral brachial vein injections of contrast medium. The technique is described in greater detail in Chapter 4.

TREATMENT

An extensive carcinoma of the bronchus occluding the superior vena cava is best treated by irradiation. If there has been no thrombosis, irradiation often alleviates the caval obstruction and produces marked symptomatic improvement but dilatation and stenting often alleviate symptoms more rapidly and to a greater degree. As this treatment is short-term palliation, the concern expressed about the possible long-term complications of stenting are irrelevant. For patients in a terminal state with extremely unpleasant symptoms the interventional radiologist can provide valuable relief (see Figures 25.19–25.21).

Caval thrombosis is also being treated more often by fibrinolysis and expandable stent placement[19,48] but there are no large series reported and for those cases not associated with terminal malignant disease the caveats expressed about the long-term results still apply.

Individual cases have been reported where the occluded vena cava has been successfully bypassed but this operation is rarely indicated when the condition is secondary to advanced malignant disease. A venous reconstruction can be performed with a graft fashioned from panels of long saphenous vein[48] or an externally supported synthetic polytetrafluoroethylene (PTFE) prosthesis.[54,55] The bypass usually has to reach from a patent neck vein to the right atrium, superior vena cava or azygos vein. The small number of patients who have been treated by these procedures provide an insufficient basis on which to base an opinion on their long-term effectiveness.[56]

References

1. Adams JT, McEvoy RK, DeWeese JA. Primary deep venous thrombosis of the upper extremity. *Arch Surg* 1965; **91:** 29.
2. Adson AW, Coffey JR. Cervical rib. *Ann Surg* 1927; **85:** 839.
3. Aird I. The veins. In: Burnand KG, Young AE, eds. *A Companion in Surgical Studies.* London: Churchill Livingstone, 1957; Chapter 18, p. 412.
4. Balestreri L, De Cicco M, Matovic M, Coran F, Morassut S. Central venous catheter-related thrombosis in clinically asymptomatic oncologic patients: a phlebographic study. *Eur J Radiol* 1995; **20:** 108–11.
5. Becker GJ, Holden RW, Rabe FE, *et al.* Local thrombolytic therapy for subclavian and axillary vein thrombosis. *Radiology* 1983; **149:** 419.
6. Bern MM, Lokich JJ, Wallach SR, *et al.* Very low doses of warfarin can prevent thrombosis in central venous catheters. A randomized prospective trial. *Ann Intern Med* 1990; **112:** 423–8.
7. Boontje AH. Axillary vein entrapment. *Br J Surg* 1979; **66:** 331.
8. Bozzeti F, Scarpa D, Terno G, *et al.* Subclavian venous thrombosis due to indwelling catheters: a prospective study on fifty two patients. *JPEN* 1983; **7:** 560–2.
9. Burihan E, Poli de Figueiredo LF, Francisco J, Miranda F. Upper extremity deep venous thrombosis: analysis of 52 cases. *Cardiovasc Surg* 1993; **1:** 19–22.
10. Campbell CB, Chandler JG, Tegtmeyer CJ, Berstein EF. Axillary, subclavian and brachiocephalic vein obstruction. *Surgery* 1977; **82:** 816.
11. Coon WW, Willis PW. Thrombosis of the axillary and subclavian veins. *Arch Surg* 1967; **94:** 657.
12. Corning HK. *Lehrbuch der topographischen Anatomie.* 24th edition. Munich: Bergmann, 1949; 635.
13. Daskalakis E, Bouhoutsos J. Subclavian and axillary vein compression of musculo-skeletal origin. *Br J Surg* 1980; **67:** 573.
14. Denck H, Fischer M, Kasprzak P. Thrombolysis in acute axillary vein thrombosis. *Int Angiol* 1984; **3:** 161.
15. De Weese JA, Adams JT, Gaiser DL. Subclavian venous thrombectomy. *Circulation* 1970; **42:** 158.
16. Donayre CE, White GH, Mehringer SM, Wilson SE. Pathogenesis determines late morbidity of axillosubclavian vein thrombosis. *Am J Surg* 1986; **152:** 179–84.
17. Dunant JH. Subclavian vein obstruction in thoracic outlet syndrome. *Int Angiol* 1984; **3:** 157.
18. Duncan JM, Baldwin RT, Caralis JP, Cooley DA. Subclavian vein-to-right atrial bypass for symptomatic venous hypertension. *Ann Thorac Surg* 1991; **52:** 1342–3.
19. Edwards RD, Cassidy J, Taylor A. Case report: superior vena cava obstruction complicated by central venous thrombosis – treatment with thrombolysis and Gianturco-Z stents. *Clin Radiol* 1992; **45:** 278–80.
20. French GE. Spontaneous thrombosis of the axillary vein. *Br Med J* 1944; **2:** 277.
21. Galea MH, Berridge DC, Gregson RHS, Hopkinson BR, Makin GS. Axillary/subclavian vein thrombosis: a clinical and radiological evaluation of conservative management. *Phlebology* 1990; **5:** 193–9.
22. Gardner GP, Cordts PR, Gillespie DL, LaMorte W, Woodson J, Menzoian JO. Can air plethysmography accurately identify upper extremity deep venous thrombosis? *J Vasc Surg* 1993; **18:** 808–13.
23. Gillmer DJ, Mitha AS. Primary (stress) thrombosis of the upper arm associated with multiple pulmonary embolism. *S Afr Med J* 1980; **57:** 251.

24. Giordano A, Muzi M, Massaro M, Rulli F. Scintigraphic assessment of 'effort' axillary–subclavian vein thrombosis. *Clin Nucl Med* 1992; **17:** 933–5.

25. Guindo J, Montagud M, Carreras F, *et al.* Fibrinolytic therapy for superior vena cava and right atrial thrombosis: diagnosis and follow-up with biplane transoesophageal echocardiography. *Am Heart J* 1992; **124:** 510–13.

26. Hill SL, Berry RE. Subclavian vein thrombosis: a continuing challenge. *Surgery* 1990; **108:** 1–9.

27. Hirano T, Tomiyoshi K, Watanabe N, Oriuchi N, Kumakura H, Ichikawa S. Bilateral subclavian vein thromboses presenting as a superior vena cava syndrome demonstrated by radionuclide blood flow and In-111 WBC imaging. *Clin Nucl Med* 1995; **20:** 630–2.

28. Horattas MC, Wright DJ, Fenton AH, *et al.* Changing concepts of deep venous thrombosis of the upper extremity: report of series and review of the literature. *Surgery* 1988; **104:** 561–7.

29. Hughes ES. Venous obstruction in the upper extremity (Paget–Schroetter's syndrome). *Int Abstr Surg* 1949; **88:** 89–127.

30. Hughes ESR. Venous obstruction of the upper extremity. *Br J Surg* 1948; **36:** 155.

31. Hunter W. History of aneurysms of aorta with some remarks on aneurysms in general. *Med Observ Inquiries* 1747; **1:** 323.

32. Jacobson JH, Haimov M. Venous revascularization of the arm. Report of three cases. *Surgery* 1977; **81:** 599.

33. Johnson V, Eiseman B. Evaluation of arteriovenous shunt to maintain patency of venous autograft. *Am J Surg* 1969; **118:** 915.

34. Kleinsasser LJ. 'Effort' thrombosis of the axillary and subclavian veins. *Arch Surg* 1949; **59:** 258.

35. Lockich JJ, Becker B. Subclavian vein thrombosis in patients treated with infusion chemotherapy for advanced malignancy. *Cancer* 1983; **52:** 1586–9.

36. Machleder HI. Evaluation of a new treatment strategy for Paget–Schroetter syndrome: spontaneous thrombosis of the axillary–subclavian vein. *J Vasc Surg* 1993; **17:** 305–15.

37. Mahorner H, Castleberry JW, Coleman WO. Attempts to restore function in major veins which are the site of massive thrombosis. *Ann Surg* 1957; **146:** 510.

38. Martin EC, Koser N, Gordon DH. Venography in axillary–subclavian vein thrombosis. *Cardiovasc Radiol* 1979; **2:** 261.

39. McLeer RS, Kesterson JE, Kirtley JA, Love RB. Subclavian and anterior scalene muscle compression as a cause of intermittent obstruction of the subclavian vein. *Ann Surg* 1951; **133:** 588.

40. Molina JE. Need for emergency treatment in subclavian vein effort thrombosis. *J Am Coll Surg* 1995; **181:** 414–20.

41. Mukherjee D, Anderson CA, Sado AS, Bertoglio MC. Use of light reflection rheography for diagnosis of axillary or subclavian venous thrombosis. *Am J Surg* 1991; **161:** 651–6.

42. Paget J. *Clinical Lectures and Essays.* London: Longman's Green, 1875.

43. Paletta FX. Venous gangrene of the hand. *Plast Reconstr Surg* 1981; **67:** 67.

44. Pandolfi M, Robertson B, Isacson S, Nilsson IM. Fibrinolytic activity of human veins in arms and legs. *Thromb Diath Haemorrh* 1968; **20:** 247–56.

45. Patwardhan NA, Anderson FA Jr, Cutler BS, Wheeler HB. Non-invasive detection of axillary and subclavian venous thrombosis by impedence plethysmography. *J Cardiovasc Surg* 1983; **24:** 250.

46. Pollak EW, Walsh J. Subclavian–axillary venous thrombosis: role of noninvasive diagnostic methods. *South Med J* 1980; **73:** 1503–6.

47. Prescott SM, Tikoff G. Deep venous thrombosis of the upper extremity, a reappraisal. *Circulation* 1979; **59:** 350.

48. Putnam JS, Uchida BT, Antonovic R, Rosch J. Superior vena cava syndrome associated with massive thrombosis: treatment with expandable wire stents. *Radiology* 1988; **167:** 727–8.

49. Rheinlander HF. Superior vena cava replacement; report of a successful autogenous composite graft. *J Thorac Cardiovasc Surg* 1969; **57:** 774.

50. Robertson BR, Pandolfi M, Nilsson IM. Response of local fibrinolytic activity to venous occlusion of arms and legs in healthy volunteers. *Acta Chir Scand* 1972; **138:** 437–40.

51. Rochester JR, Beard JD. Acute management of subclavian vein thrombosis. *Br J Surg* 1995; **82:** 433–4.

52. Sachatello CR. The axillopectoral muscle (Langer's axillary arch): a cause of axillary vein obstruction. *Surgery* 1977; **81:** 610.

53. Sanders RJ, Cooper MA. Surgical management of subclavian vein obstruction, including 6 cases of subclavian vein bypass. *Surgery* 1995; **118:** 1342–3.

54. Sauvage LR, Gross RE. Evaluation of venous autografts and aortic homografts in canine intrathoracic venae cavae for periods of up to eight years. *J Thorac Cardiovasc Surg* 1967; **53:** 549.

55. Sauvage LR, Gross RE. Observations on experimental grafts in intrathoracic vena cavae. *Surg Gynecol Obstet* 1960; **110:** 569.

56. Skinner DB, Saltzman EW, Scannell JG. The challenge of superior vena caval obstruction. *J Thorac Cardiovasc Surg* 1965; **49:** 824.

57. Smith BM, Shield GW, Riddell DH, Snell JD. Venous gangrene of the upper extremity. *Ann Surg* 1985; **201:** 511.

58. Steed DL, Teodori MF, Peitzman AB, McAuley CE, Kapoor WN, Webster MW. Streptokinase in the treatment of subclavian vein thrombosis. *J Vasc Surg* 1986; **4:** 28–32.

59. Stevenson IM, Parry EW. Radiological study of the aetiological factor in venous obstruction of the upper limb. *J Cardiovasc Surg* 1975; **16:** 580.

60. Sullivan ED, Reece CI, Cranley JJ. Phleborheography of the upper extremity. *Arch Surg* 1983; **119:** 1134.

61. Sundqvist SB, Hedner U, Kullenberg HKE, Bergentz SE. Deep venous thrombosis of the arm: a study in coagulation and fibrinolysis. *Br Med J* 1981; **283:** 265.

62. Swinton NW, Edgett JW, Hall RJ. Primary subclavian-axillary vein thrombosis. *Circulation* 1968; **38:** 737.

63. Taheri SA, Lazar L, Elias S, Marchand P. Vein valve transplant. *Surgery* 1982; **91:** 28.

64. Tello R, Scholz E, Finn JP, Costello P. Subclavian vein thrombosis detected with spiral CT and three-dimensional reconstruction. *Am J Roentgenol* 1993; **160:** 33–4.

65. Tilney NL, Griffith HJG, Edwards EA. Natural history of major venous thrombosis of the upper extremity. *Arch Surg* 1970; **101:** 792.

66. Von Schroetter L. Erkrankungen der Gefasse. In: Nothnagel CNH, ed. *Handbuch der Pathologie und Therapie.* Vienna: Holder, 1884.

67. Weinberg G, Pasternack BM. Upper extremity suppurative thrombophlebitis and septic pulmonary emboli. *JAMA* 1978; **240:** 1519.

68. Wisselink W, Money SR, Becker MO, *et al.* Comparison of operative reconstruction and percutaneous balloon dilatation for central venous obstruction. *Am J Surg* 1993; **166:** 200–4.

69. Zimmerman R, Morl H, Harenberg J, Gerhardt P, Kuhn HM, Wahl P. Urokinase therapy of subclavian–axillary vein thrombosis. *Klin Wochenschr* 1981; **59:** 851.

70. Zufferey P, Pararas C, Monti M, Depairon M. Assessment of acute and old deep venous thrombosis in upper extremity by venous strain gauge plethysmography. *Vasa* 1992; **21:** 263–7.

CHAPTER 26

Venous injury

Incidence	711	Investigation	717
Classification	714	Treatment: general considerations	717
Clinical presentation	717	References	726

The veins are frequently injured when there is blunt or penetrating trauma and during many surgical operations. The small and medium-sized veins which are most commonly damaged can usually be ignored or ligated without causing any ill effects. Problems arise when large deep limb veins are damaged, as ligation of these vessels (which was commonly practised before the Second World War) can cause oedema, venous insufficiency, limb loss and death. It is now recognized that restoration of the continuity of the large veins of the limbs, abdomen and thorax can reduce late morbidity and preserve limbs. Unfortunately, many venous injuries pass unnoticed at the time of trauma and are only suspected later when the post-thrombotic syndrome develops. This is particularly common after fracture of the tibia (Figure 26.1), which often causes a deep vein thrombosis days or weeks after the injury and the post-thrombotic syndrome many years later.[39,56]

Incidence

For the reasons outlined above, it is very difficult to obtain an accurate assessment of the incidence of venous injuries. Many injuries pass undetected and others are recognized but not recorded. Few patients with lower limb fractures have a phlebogram on admission to hospital because the care of the fracture takes precedence, and it is only many years later when post-thrombotic symptoms

develop that a phlebogram reveals that a concomitant venous injury passed unrecognized. Veins are also frequently damaged when their accompanying artery is injured.

Many large series of vascular injuries during both peace and war have shown that the incidence of major venous injury appears to be increasing.[27,43,44,66,73,76,85,86,91,95,105] In the First World War, surgeons advocated ligation of injured arteries and veins to save life,[7] and some even suggested that ligation of undamaged limb veins might even be beneficial if the artery had to be tied off.[60] Other surgeons had observed that the chances of limb survival were reduced if the major artery and vein of the limb had both been divided.[52,61] The incidence of venous injuries was not recorded in the First World War.

In a review of vascular injuries in the Second World War, DeBakey and Simeone[23] concluded that concomitant vein ligation did not increase the chance of limb survival. No mention was made of the harmful effects of venous ligation, and the number of servicemen with venous injuries was not recorded.

In the Korean War, Hughes[47,48] reported that there were nearly as many injuries to major veins as injuries to the major arteries (Table 26.1), but in the Vietnam War the number of venous injuries was only a third of the number of arterial injuries (Table 26.2).[79,80,85] Overall, only 38% of the 936 arterial injuries which made up the Vietnam vascular registry[80] had an associated major venous injury (Table 26.3). More than 50% of the popliteal artery

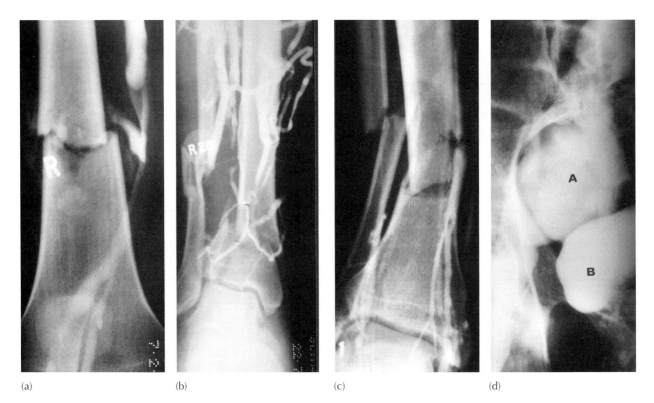

(a) (b) (c) (d)

Figure 26.1 Four examples of the damage to veins that accompanies major fractures. (a) A femoral vein torn by a fractured femur. (b) Deep veins of the lower limb disrupted by a fractured tibia. (c) A saphenous vein torn by a fractured tibia. (d) A large false aneurysm (A) arising from the external iliac vein following a fracture of the pelvis. The patient's bladder (B) is also opacified by excreted contrast medium.

Table 26.1 Incidence of venous and arterial injuries in the Korean War[46]

	Number	Percentage
Major arterial injury	79	44
Major venous injury	71	40
Minor arterial injury	30	16

Table 26.2 Incidence of venous and arterial injuries in 500 combat casualties of the Vietnam War[86]

Total number of vascular injuries	718
Total number of venous injuries	194
Number of isolated venous injuries	28
Number of combined venous and arterial injuries	166

Table 26.3 Incidence of combined venous injuries in the Vietnam War[80]

Artery injured	Number of arterial injuries	Number of concomitant venous injuries (%)
Axillary	59	20 (33.9)
Brachial	283	54 (19.1)
Iliac	26	11 (42.3)
Common femoral	46	17 (36.9)
Superficial femoral	305	139 (45.6)
Popliteal	217	116 (53.5)
Total	936	357 (38.1)

injuries were associated with a concomitant venous injury. By contrast, 80% of the venous injuries were associated with arterial injuries. In the Yom Kippur War of 1973 there were only 15 severe venous injuries out of 82 vascular injuries.[91]

The vessels most frequently injured in the early years of the 'troubles' in Northern Ireland were the popliteal artery and vein; this was a result of the practice called 'knee-capping', a particularly unpleasant and disabling form of penalty in which the popliteal fossa is deliberately shot through by a bullet.[73]

Table 26.4 Site of venous injuries

	Vollmar[108]	Gaspar and Treiman[32]	Rich et al.[86]
Traumatic (3 series)			
Inferior vena cava	2	8	–
Superior vena cava	0	1	–
Common iliac vein	2	1	11
Brachiocephalic vein	1	1	–
Brachial vein	10	7	54
Axillary vein	1	1	20
Femoral vein	5	9	156
Popliteal vein	2	4	116
Internal jugular	0	8	–
Portal	0	1	–
Iatrogenic[108]			
Inferior vena cava (nephrectomy)	2		
Inferior vena cava (aorto-iliac)	1		
External iliac vein (ureterostomy)	1		
External iliac vein (hernia)	1		
Common femoral vein (varicose veins)	1		

Sfeir *et al.*[92] reviewed 484 patients who suffered lower limb vascular injuries during the Lebanese War. At operation, there was a concomitant venous injury in 58% of femoral and 54% of popliteal arterial injuries. The great majority of these were caused by penetrating wounds with only 2% resulting from blunt trauma.

In a prospective study of vascular injuries sustained during the Afghanistan War,[95] a major venous disruption accompanied 41% of arterial injuries, the majority occurring in the lower limb as a result of land mine explosion. In the Bosnian conflict,[57] venous injuries accompanied 61% of arterial injuries. All these injuries were caused by penetrating wounds of which 87% were caused by high velocity missiles.

The incidence of venous injuries occurring in the civilian population has been steadily rising. In 1960, Gaspar and Trieman[32] reported that of 228 civilian patients with arterial injuries only 20% had concomitant venous injuries. In 1966,[105] the same group of workers reported 92 venous injuries but the proportion of venous to arterial injuries had not increased significantly. Four years later, Drapanas *et al.*[27] found a 41% incidence of concomitant venous injury in their series of civilian arterial injuries.

By 1979, Vollmar[107] reported that 66% of arterial injuries were associated with an injury to the accompanying veins, though not all the venous injuries required reconstruction. Vollmar observed that arterial injury occurred in 0.3–0.5% of patients

with major trauma, and he suggested that major venous injury was probably more common because the veins were more vulnerable. Conversely, Vollmar found that 75% of the patients presenting with venous injuries had associated arterial injuries. During a period of 8 years he reconstructed 30 venous injuries; seven of these injuries were iatrogenic. The distribution and site of the injuries is shown in Table 26.4; the series reported by Gaspar and Trieman,[32] Wiencek and Wilson[109] and Rich *et al.*[86] are shown for comparison.

Military and civilian series indicate that major venous injuries accompany arterial injuries in approximately 35–65% of cases,[15,76,95] but the pattern and frequency of the vascular damage depends on the nature of the injuring agent. In the series of 204 civilian vascular injuries reported by Pasch *et al.*,[76] the injuring agent was a single gunshot (64%), stabbing (24%) and shotgun injuries (12%), major venous injuries occurring in only 45% of patients. This contrasts with a series of 49 vascular injuries caused by close-range shotgun blasts, in which, Meyer *et al.*[64] found major deep venous damage in 82%.

Vena cava, limb and cervical venous injuries are usually caused by penetrating injuries,[14,50,74,112] whereas Hollands and Little[44] found that 95% of hepatic vein injuries were caused by blunt trauma. The growth of therapeutic laparoscopy since 1990 has not resulted in the detection of more major vascular injuries, Nordestgaard *et al.*[69] could trace only 20 reported cases in their 1995 review.

Since 1980, many series of civilian venous injuries have been reported from the USA[6,36,43,66,71,76] where the rising incidence of civilian violence has been mirrored by an increase in the number of serious venous injuries.

Classification

A vein may be injured in one of five ways (Table 26.5).

Incision or laceration

This injury is usually caused by an external force (e.g. a cut or stab from a knife, bullet, shell or bomb fragment). Iatrogenic penetrating venous injuries are also becoming more common, as vascular surgery and invasive radiology increase. The resulting laceration can be subdivided into three main types (Figure 26.2):

1. a clean cut into the lumen of the vein, often on two surfaces if the knife or bullet traverses the vein (Figure 26.2a)
2. an irregular laceration caused by a rough penetrating agent (e.g. a spicule of bone) or by the avulsion of a tributary (Figure 26.2c)
3. complete venous transection. This is really a form of incision or laceration but is classified separately in Table 26.5 because it presents special technical problems (Figure 26.2e).

Contusion

This type of injury results from a blow or crushing injury which does not disrupt the wall of the vein. The main damage is usually on the internal surface, with bruising extending through the media towards the adventitia.

The endothelial cells of the intima may be damaged or shed with no obvious external signs of injury but this can initiate mural thrombosis (Figure 26.3). The medial muscle cells may also be

damaged without external signs of injury and, in the most severe injury, cells in all layers of the vessel wall can be severely crushed and killed. If the vein wall is heavily contused and the intima is

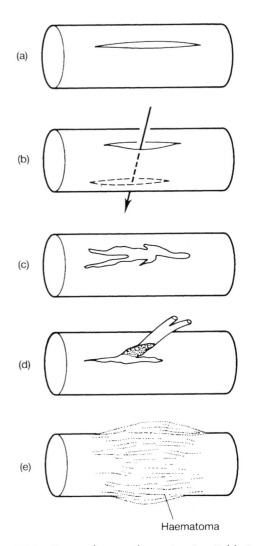

Figure 26.2 Types of venous laceration (see Table 26.5). (a) Incision. (b) Transfixion. (c) Irregular laceration. (d) Avulsion of a tributary. (e) Complete transection.

Table 26.5 Type and cause of vein injuries

Injury	Cause
Incision	Direct external and internal forces
Laceration (tear)	Direct external and internal forces or avulsion of tributaries
Contusion	Direct blunt injury
Intramural tear	Stretching (indirect force)
Complete division	Direct or indirect external or internal force

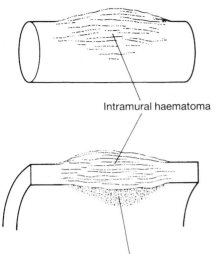

Figure 26.3 Venous contusion. All layers of the vein wall may be involved with thrombus forming on damaged intima or exposed collagen.

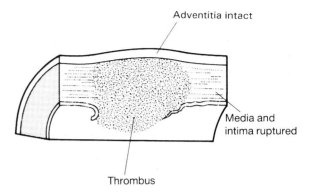

Figure 26.4 The effect of a venous stretching injury. The adventitia remains intact, but the media and intima may disrupt. Intramural haematoma distorts the lumen, damages the endothelium and causes intraluminal thrombosis.

damaged, secondary thrombosis usually follows. A vein may become bruised simply by being involved in a large fracture haematoma.

Stretching

When a vein lies close to a bone or joint which has fractured or dislocated it may be damaged by being overstretched. Dislocations of the hip, knee, and shoulder are the most common causes of this type of injury. A severe stretch may completely disrupt one or more layers of the vein wall, usually the intima and media, leaving the vessel held together by the adventitia (Figure 26.4). A less severe stretch may only damage the intima.

The exposed collagen makes thrombosis likely and, occasionally, 'false aneurysms' develop.

A severe deceleration injury can tear the inferior vena cava as it passes through the diaphragm. This injury is similar to the tear of the aortic arch that occurs in aeroplane and motor car crashes. If the vena cava is completely divided, the patient usually dies rapidly of exsanguination.

Iatrogenic injuries

These have become an important group of venous injuries with the growth and extension of vascular surgery and the increase in interventional radiology (see Table 26.4). There is a high risk of venous injury whenever a structure is being dissected off a major vein. Operative venous injuries are particularly common in the pelvis where tumours of the

bowel or aortic aneurysms may be closely applied to the iliac veins or to the inferior vena cava. Dissection of the common iliac artery from the underlying vein can be extremely difficult, and if a small tear is made in the vein because the vein wall is adherent to the artery, further traction on the artery simply enlarges the tear. Forceps should never be pushed behind the iliac artery without first dissecting a clear passage between the artery and the vein. Other common sites of surgical venous damage are in the femoral triangle and the popliteal fossa where the femoral and popliteal veins are often adherent to the adjacent artery and joined by many small tributaries.

Inadvertent ligature of a major vein is another important and, unfortunately, not uncommon iatrogenic venous injury. The femoral and popliteal veins have often been tied during varicose vein operations by inexperienced surgeons (Figure 26.5), usually because they have not fully displayed the anatomy of the sapheno-femoral or sapheno-popliteal junctions (see Chapter 7).

Major veins should not be ligated after inadvertent injury unless the haemorrhage is of such life-threatening proportions that vein ligation is the only hope for the patient's survival.

Another increasingly common form of venous injury is that which results from catheters inserted into veins by radiologists or physicians. Tears occur if the catheter happens to enter the vein in the angle between it and a tributary. Even small injuries carry an increased risk of intraluminal thrombosis with embolization of the thrombus, and if veins such as the vena cava are ruptured, severe haemorrhage may result.

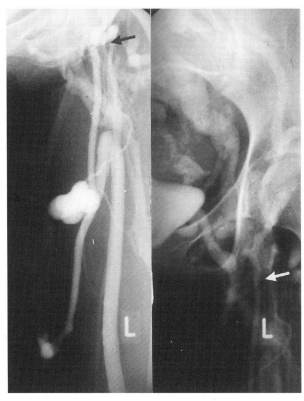

(a)

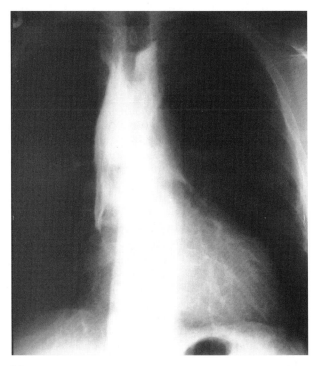

(b)

(c)

Figure 26.5 Iatrogenic venous injuries. (a) This phlebograph shows the result of inadvertently ligating the femoral vein during a varicose vein operation. The occlusion has extended below the site of the ligature (arrowed) to the entry of a large tributary and proximally to the beginning of the common iliac vein. (b and c) A CT scan and chest radiograph showing extensive mediastinal extravasation of contrast medium when a central venous catheter which had inadvertently pierced the superior vena cava was used for a pressure injection (intravenous digital subtraction angiogram, IVDSA). Catheters are a common cause of vein perforation, laceration and thrombosis.

Arteriovenous fistulae may develop if a penetrating injury traverses both a vein and an artery.[27] Arteriovenous fistulae may also complicate lumbar disc surgery if adjacent walls of the iliac artery and vein are inadvertently damaged.[37,58,63]

Badly placed sutures during an inguinal or femoral hernia repair may occlude or damage the external iliac or femoral vein as it passes beneath the inguinal ligament.

Toxic substances injected into a vein may damage the endothelium and cause thrombosis. This type of venous injury is discussed in Chapter 23, page 657.

Clinical presentation

Most venous injuries are associated with other injuries to soft tissues, arteries and bones, the symptoms of which often overshadow those of the venous injury. Massive haemorrhage can, however, occur from a penetrating wound in a vein, especially if it is associated with an open wound, during an operation. Haemorrhage from a venous injury may be more frightening and difficult to control than arterial haemorrhage because there is very little spontaneous reduction in bleeding from venous spasm. Blood escapes rapidly and continually until thrombus occludes the wound or the blood pressure falls.

Even if the connective tissues around a venous injury remain intact, a massive haematoma can occur around the lacerated vessel. The patient rapidly develops hypovolaemic shock with faintness, pallor, tachycardia and hypotension progressing to cardiac arrest, if no remedial action is taken.

Blunt trauma or stretching causing intramural bruising and oedema and intraluminal thrombosis may result in venous obstruction. The veins in the limb then become congested, the skin becomes cyanotic and the soft tissues swell. Surface veins become engorged and fail to collapse when the limb is elevated above heart level. If there is an associated injury to the artery (this occurs in 80% of patients), there may also be signs of distal ischaemia, and these signs may predominate.

Investigation

Phlebography and, more recently, duplex ultrasound scanning have been used in the investigation of venous injuries. Phlebography will demonstrate venous occlusion, compression and contrast extravasation (see Figure 26.5), whereas duplex will demonstrate surrounding haematoma, flow abnormalities and the presence of a traumatic arteriovenous fistula. If the patient is unstable and injury severe, exploration by a suitably experienced surgeon should not be delayed by time-consuming investigations.

Treatment: general considerations

Venous injuries present two main clinical problems, blood loss and vein repair.

MAJOR BLOOD LOSS

Venous bleeding from an open wound should be suspected if the blood is dark and rapidly rises from the base of the wound without evidence of pulsation. The first aid treatment is to apply local pressure to the wound and, if possible, elevate the affected part. Pressure and elevation should be maintained while the patient is being transferred rapidly to hospital. Blood is cross-matched and intravenous catheters are inserted for resuscitation.

The catheters should be put into the normal arm if there is an upper limb injury, and they should be placed in the internal jugular vein or an arm vein if the injury is in the lower limb or abdomen. In patients with major vein injuries in the superior mediastinum, a central venous catheter may have to be inserted via a femoral vein. A central venous catheter allows blood to be rapidly infused and may also be used to measure central venous pressure; it is therefore an invaluable adjunct to the management of all major venous injuries.

The patient should be anaesthetized in the operating room and the wound gently inspected. If this inspection is accompanied by further profuse haemorrhage, pressure should be reapplied to control the bleeding until an appropriate level of resuscitation has been achieved and adequate quantities of cross-matched blood are available for surgery to be commenced. Bleeding from a wound in the limb can be controlled with a pneumatic tourniquet and surgical exploration can be carried out in a bloodless field but tourniquets should not be applied indiscriminately before the patient enters hospital. A loose, badly applied tourniquet may cause venous engorgement and increase, rather than reduce, blood loss.

Wounds should be extended to allow easy access to the injured vein. Bleeding can usually be controlled by gentle direct finger pressure (Figure 26.6) on, or on either side of, the bleeding point until the vein has been dissected out and can be clamped above and below the injury (Figure 26.6). If this cannot be done, bleeding can be controlled by inserting two Fogarty balloon catheters into the vessel through the tear (Figure 26.7).

Once the damaged vein has been dissected free from its surrounding tissues, the venous injury and any associated injuries to nearby arteries and nerves should be assessed. A decision can then be made about the best method of repair. It is preferable to repair the venous injury first, even if there are other vascular injuries, though it is, of course, important to gain control of any arterial bleeding before beginning the venous repair.

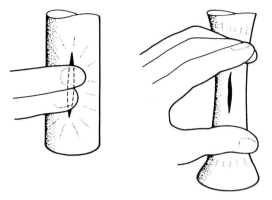

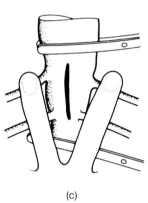

(a)   (b)

(c)

Figure 26.6 Digital methods of controlling venous haemorrhage. (a) Direct finger pressure. (b) Proximal and distal finger pressure. (c) Proximal and distal venous occlusion by clamps with finger control of the tributaries.

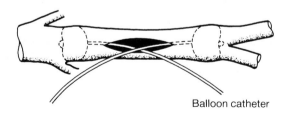

Balloon catheter

Figure 26.7 Control of venous haemorrhage by intraluminal balloon tamponade. Fogarty balloon catheters are inserted proximally and distally through the venotomy and are inflated until they stop the blood flow.

ANTICOAGULATION

Systemic heparin has not been shown to improve the long-term patency of venous repair[4,40,113] but we give heparin, 5000 units intravenously, as soon as we are ready to apply vascular clamps to the vein, except when there is extensive soft tissue contusion

and uncontrolled bleeding. Heparin should always be given if there is an associated arterial injury requiring arterial occlusion and reconstruction. Some workers have advocated the use of dextran in addition to heparin[28,40] but we find that this combination increases capillary oozing which makes the surgery more difficult and increases the risk of postoperative haematomata.

HISTORY OF VEIN REPAIR

Travers and Cooper[104] reputedly performed the first venous repair in 1816. In 1877, Eck[30] performed the first veno-venous anastomosis when he anastomosed the portal vein to the inferior vena cava, and Schede (1882)[89] was credited by Murphy[67] with the first successful venous repair by lateral suture. Kümmel in 1899[55] performed the first end-to-end venous anastomosis, and Clermont (1901)[20] successfully joined a divided inferior vena cava.

In 1903, Exner (in Rich[84]) first attempted vein grafting by transplanting segments of autogenous jugular vein in the dog. The following year, Payr (in Rich[84]) attempted to unite the divided femoral vein using his magnesium cylinder invagination technique. In 1906, Guthrie in his Nobel Prize winning work with Carrel[16,17] described many of the basic principles of vascular surgery and transplanted valve-bearing vein segments. It was not until 1947 that Johns[53] revived interest in venous surgery with a series of experiments concerning suture and non-suture methods of venous anastomosis.

Rich *et al.*[80,81,85] popularized venous repair in battle injuries and showed that this reduced limb loss and subsequent morbidity from chronic venous obstruction.

TECHNIQUES OF VEIN REPAIR

Lateral suture

A simple side-hole in a vein can be sutured with a carefully placed single or continuous vascular suture (Prolene, 5/0 or 6/0 is ideal), while the vein is occluded either side of the tear by gentle finger pressure or by a Satinsky clamp (Figure 26.8). Although this procedure may cause a little narrowing of the vein (Figure 26.8), the narrowing is unlikely to be significant if a segment of vein wall has not been lost.[32,48,96]

Vein patch

If a segment of vein wall has been lost, or if the vessel is small (e.g. the popliteal vein), it is probably better to close the defect with a vein patch to

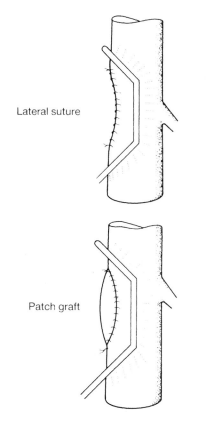

Figure 26.8 The lateral suture and patch repair of venous injuries. These repairs can often be performed with the lumen partially occluded with a Satinsky clamp.

prevent narrowing (see Figure 26.8).[17,81,106] The patch should be fashioned from a nearby tributary or a subcutaneous vein from the opposite limb. It should not be taken from a major subcutaneous vein of the injured limb (e.g. the saphenous vein) because this may later serve as an important collateral vessel if the damaged vein becomes occluded.

End-to-end anastomosis

When the vein wall is extensively damaged, transected, or a complete segment is destroyed, it usually has to be replaced by a graft. Veins can rarely be mobilized and stretched so that they can be sutured end to end, except when there is a clear incised wound.[78] In these circumstances ligation of the tributaries may be needed in order to mobilize the vein, and the anastomosis is best performed using the Carrel triangulation technique (Figure 26.9).[16]

Vein replacement

Autogenous vein is the material of choice for vein replacement.[35,73,81,86] The veins commonly used as

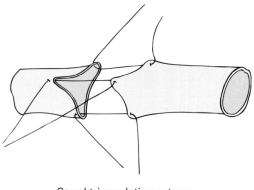

Carrel triangulation sutures

Figure 26.9 The Carrel triangulation technique of venous anastomosis. Stretching each segment of vein with the stay sutures stops the intervening continuous suture causing a stenosis.

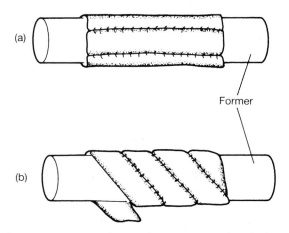

Figure 26.10 Two forms of composite grafts which can be used to bridge complete deficiencies in large veins: (a) a panel graft; (b) a spiral graft.

grafts include the long and short saphenous veins, the cephalic vein and the internal jugular vein. The internal jugular vein was first used for mesocaval bypass grafts[42] but has also been used to bypass axillary vein obstruction.[51,102] and to replace the injured femoral vein.[111] It has the advantage of being of similar size to the iliac and femoral veins. The subcutaneous veins are usually too small for a simple end-to-end anastomosis, and if the saphenous or cephalic veins are used, a composite graft must be made in order to produce a tube whose diameter is equal to that of the damaged vein (Figure 26.10). This is achieved by splitting two or three segments of vein longitudinally and sewing them together along their lateral margins.[5,29,73] The resulting wide-bore tube can then be anastomosed, end to end, to the damaged vein after excising the damaged segment.

An alternative method of producing a wide-bore tube is to split the vein and sew it as a spiral (see Figure 26.10); this has proved satisfactory in some circumstances.[26,43] End-to-end anastomoses are preferred to end-to-side anastomoses for the reconstruction. These techniques are time consuming and are not appropriate for venous reconstruction in the unstable injured patient.

Flow-enhancing arteriovenous fistulae

There is good experimental evidence that venous anastomoses have better patency rates when there is a high rate of blood flow passing through the anastomosis.[2,56,90,94,97]

The increased rate of blood flow can be achieved by forming a temporary arteriovenous fistula upstream to the anastomosis (Figure 26.11). Most authorities[68,70,81] suggest that a temporary arteriovenous fistula should be kept open for 3 months after reconstructive venous surgery. Fashioning a fistula adds time to the procedure; this is a factor that must be considered if there are other severe injuries needing treatment. Intermittent pneumatic compression applied to the distal part of the limb is an alternative method of enhancing venous flow and reducing the incidence of postoperative thrombosis.[2,110]

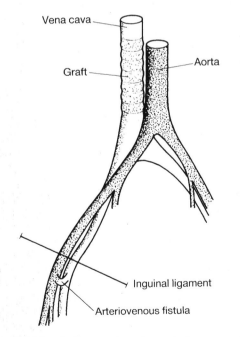

Figure 26.11 A flow enhancing arteriovenous fistula which should be used to increase venous blood flow after a venous repair (see Figure 10.9, page 333).

Manoeuvres to remove propagated thrombosis

Before the vascular clamps are removed and venous blood flow is released, the vein should be washed out with heparinized saline and, if there is any suspicion of poor blood flow from either side of the anastomosis, a Fogarty balloon catheter should be passed as far as possible in both directions.[78] If distal thrombus is suspected and the balloon will not pass beyond the nearest competent valve, an Esmarch bandage applied from the foot to the wound may be used to express thrombus. These precautions should always be taken if there has been a long interval between the injury and the operation.

Repair of concomitant injuries

When the veins have been reconstructed, the arterial injuries can be repaired, followed by internal or external fixation of fractures, suturing of torn tendons and repair of nerves. When manipulating and fixing fractures great care must be taken not to disrupt the vascular anastomoses.[73,83] All ischaemic tissue should be widely excised.

Repair of one large vein probably guarantees a sufficient outflow tract, even if there are, for example, two large popliteal veins that have been damaged. Care should be taken at all times to preserve the superficial veins in the injured limb.[78,87] If all the subcutaneous veins draining a digit, hand or foot are severed, some must be repaired as the deep veins at the wrist and ankle are often small and an insufficient outflow tract. Small veins (e.g. digital veins) may be repaired with end-to-end anastomoses or interposition vein grafts using an operating microscope.

Drainage and antibiotics

Suture lines in veins bleed more than suture lines in arteries; all wounds should therefore be closed over suction drainage. Broad-spectrum antibiotics which are effective against staphylococci and anaerobic organisms (especially clostridia) should be given for 5 days if the wound is contaminated or the tissues are extensively damaged.

Fasciotomy

The fascia enclosing the anterior and the posterior compartments of the lower limb should be divided if there has been a prolonged period of arterial ischaemia or severe venous congestion.[73,81] Fasciotomy does, however, carry its own inherent morbidity, prolongs hospital stay and is frequently performed unnecessarily. Field *et al.*[31] have thus proposed a selective approach to fasciotomy based on well-defined criteria. Where there is uncertainty, it is better to perform unnecessary fasciotomy than to risk the loss of a limb.

SPECIAL PROBLEMS

Inferior vena caval injuries

Inferior vena caval trauma comprises the majority (40–55%) of abdominal venous injuries,[50,109] most being caused by penetrating wounds.[13,50,62,75,77,98,110] Mortality rates of 30–55%[13,24,34,54,65,100,109] have been reported. The main factors influencing mortality are the presence of shock, the number of associated vascular injuries and the site of the injury[13,24,54,65,100] with trauma in the juxtahepatic position carrying the highest mortality.[44,62,72,77,98,110]

The injured segment of cava must be fully exposed, either by reflecting the root of the mesentery and fourth part of the duodenum to the patient's right (as when exposing the aorta) or by reflecting the caecum and ascending colon to the patient's left.[62] This later, almost retroperitoneal, approach gives better access to the vena cava above the right renal vein (Figure 26.12). If an abdominal incision is extended above the right costal margin and through the diaphragm to open the thorax, the liver can be turned to the patient's left and the

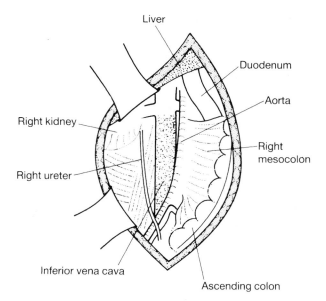

Figure 26.12 Exposure of the inferior vena cava. The duodenum and ascending colon are freed along their lateral border and are reflected to the left to expose the subhepatic inferior vena cava.

whole of the upper abdominal and the thoracic inferior vena cava exposed.[62]

The lumbar veins drain into the postero-lateral aspect of the inferior vena cava. Access to this surface of the vein is difficult because it lies directly on the vertebral column. This makes control of haemorrhage through a caval tear difficult and finger control (see Figure 26.6) or pressure with pledgets[77,98] around the tear may be all that is initially possible. With better exposure it may be possible to apply a Satinsky type of partially occluding clamp (see Figure 26.8).[110]

A simple tear is the commonest injury and this can usually be repaired with lateral venorrhaphy using continuous 5/0 Prolene. If both the anterior and posterior surfaces of the vein have been injured, the anterior tear may have to be extended after the bleeding has been fully controlled and the posterior tear may have to be closed from within, before the anterior defect is closed. If the vessel wall has been severely damaged or disrupted, the injured segment should be replaced with an end-to-end interposition graft. An externally supported PTFE graft is the material of choice for replacement of the vena cava,[22] and a high blood flow in the postoperative period is ensured by the formation of a distal arteriovenous fistula between the iliac or femoral vein and a small branch of the corresponding artery or by anastomosing a small tributary of the vein to the artery (see Figure 10.9, page 333).

Where repair or reconstruction cannot be safely undertaken, caval ligation may be necessary. Infrarenal ligation is usually accompanied by leg swelling which gradually subsides; however, suprarenal ligation markedly reduces venous return to the right heart and impairs renal function, resulting in high mortality.

Juxtahepatic caval injuries or injury to the hepatic veins are very difficult to isolate and control, resulting in a high mortality whichever method of repair is employed. Unlike caval injuries, damage to the hepatic veins is usually sustained during blunt trauma and should be suspected at laparotomy if Pringle's manoeuvre (occlusion of the vessels in the lesser omentum/porta hepatis) fails to control the bleeding. The site of avulsion is usually the right hepatic vein or its upper branch.[44]

Blood loss from the retrohepatic portion of the vena cava or the hepatic veins can be controlled by isolating the liver from its blood supply. An intraluminal atriocaval shunt may be inserted through the femoral vein, iliac vein or lower part of the cava and held in place by tapes placed above and below the liver and tightened to occlude venous flow other than through the shunt (Figure 26.13). Double balloon catheters have been produced to allow

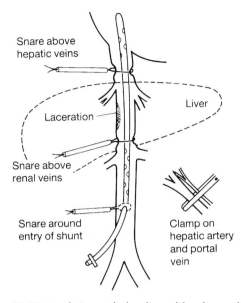

Figure 26.13 Isolation of the liver blood supply. A plastic 'shunt' containing side-holes at either end is positioned across the liver and held in place by 'snares' around the supra- and subhepatic segments of the vena cava to prevent venous blood flowing up beside the shunt. If the portal vein and hepatic artery are also occluded, all blood flow to the liver is stopped.

rapid liver and caval isolation through a femoral venous cut-down before the cava is exposed.

The use of the atriocaval shunt remains controversial and is associated with a high mortality by virtue of the injuries involved.[13,19,74,109] Many other techniques for vascular isolation of the liver have been described. Pachter *et al.*[74] advocate finger fracture dissection to the injury using portal triad compression and hepatocyte protection with hypothermia and steroids. Buechter *et al.*[12] advocate transection of the suprahepatic cava following caval and portal triad clamping to gain a posterior approach to the retrohepatic veins and cava.

Iliac vein injuries

When there is extensive damage to the iliac veins consideration must be given to direct replacement or bypass. A bypass may be placed end to side across the damaged vein, or the opposite long saphenous vein may be used as a bypass from the femoral vein below the ligated vein to the normal femoral vein (the Palma operation, see Chapter 13, page 420).[75] Both these procedures should be combined with a distal arteriovenous fistula. It is much easier to perform a Palma operation than to carry out an orthotopic replacement or bypass.

Internal iliac vein injuries

A damaged internal iliac vein should be ligated. There is no need to repair it as there are many veins that cross the floor of the pelvis that can act as collaterals. These injuries can be difficult to identify.

Left renal vein injuries

If the left renal vein is damaged between the inferior vena cava and its suprarenal tributaries, it may be tied without affecting renal blood flow or renal function. Damage to the veins in the hilum of the kidney should be repaired if possible but injuries in this area are often associated with significant arterial and pelvi-ureteric damage which may necessitate nephrectomy.

Subclavian and axillary vein injuries

The axillary and subclavian veins may be injured by penetrating wounds above and below the clavicle and by fractures of the clavicle and first rib.

Subclavian vein injuries are rare. Their significance lies in the inaccessibility of the vein, the potential for heavy blood loss and their tendency to cause air embolism. Demetriades *et al.*[25] report a 61% mortality amongst 228 South African civilians with penetrating subclavian vessel injuries, 44% of which affected the vein alone. Those with vein injury alone had an overall mortality of 81% and an operative mortality of 21%.

Exposure of the subclavian vein may be difficult, especially if there is heavy bleeding.[9,10,38,49,99] Bleeding can be reduced by inflating a tourniquet high on the arm to above systolic pressure to prevent arterial inflow to the arm and so reduce venous outflow. If the vein is not totally divided but cannot be seen, the bleeding can be controlled by passing balloon catheters proximally through an upper arm vein so that a balloon can be inflated on either side of the tear. In a desperate life-saving situation, which usually means that there is massive bleeding from the central end of a totally divided subclavian vein, the clavicle should be divided or the mediastinum opened through a sternal splitting incision to gain control of the jugular and innominate veins or superior vena cava (Figure 26.14).[110]

The subclavian and axillary veins can be ligated without risk to the viability of the limb. Tears can be sutured but it is probably not wise to attempt a resection and interposition or bypass graft in the emergency situation. Reconstructions can be considered later if the ligation causes disabling symptoms – an unusual event (see Chapter 25).

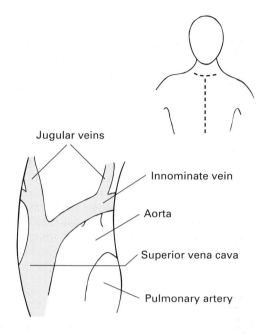

Figure 26.14 The exposure of the large veins in the root of the neck.

Iatrogenic injuries

Minor tears in veins that occur during an operation can usually be controlled by one or two carefully places sutures across the tear while the bleeding is controlled with pressure and suction. Sometimes the tear may be difficult to see, for example when an iliac vein is torn during the dissection of the iliac artery. To avoid this complication many surgeons advocate mobilizing an artery on either side and applying clamps without putting a snare around the artery. In difficult circumstances access may be improved by transecting the artery to reveal the anterior surface of the vein behind it.

Venous occlusion by accidental ligation or secondary thrombosis

This is another form of venous injury most often caused by an inexperienced surgeon mistakenly ligating a deep vein or accidentally including a deep vein in a mass ligature. The presence of a major vein obstruction is indicated by swelling of the limb, distension of the veins and generalized tightness and pain in the muscles. If this complication is suspected, its presence may be confirmed by duplex ultrasonography but if this investigation is inadequate the precise site of the occlusion should be demonstrated by ascending phlebography before surgical exploration is undertaken (see Figure 26.5).[33]

The occluded vein is explored through an appropriately sited incision which is usually the incision of the previous operation. The vein is inspected and palpated to determine the level of the occlusion and the presence of distal thrombosis.

Heparin is administered systemically, tapes are placed around the vessel above and below the damaged area and vascular clamps are applied. Any obstructing ligatures are removed and a venotomy is made in the contused or thrombosed vein. Thrombus can be gently removed with a Fogarty catheter, and the presence of intact intima can be confirmed before the venotomy is closed. If there is intimal damage with loss of endothelium, the segment should be replaced by one of the techniques described above. Consideration should also be given to forming a distal arteriovenous fistula to help maintain patency. Flow may also be encouraged by applying intermittent pneumatic compression to the legs. Systemic anticoagulants (heparin followed by warfarin) should be given for 4–6 weeks.

POSTOPERATIVE MONITORING

In the early postoperative stages flow through the vein should be assessed with a Doppler ultrasound flow detector. Duplex ultrasound scanning or phlebography should be performed if there is any indication that the vein has reoccluded, a complication which may be treated by venous thrombectomy if a thrombosis is confirmed. Duplex ultrasound scanning or phlebography should be performed in the early postoperative period to confirm patency, and it should be repeated a few months later to document long-term success. The venous phase of a digital subtraction arteriogram may provide useful information about the patency of any associated large vein repairs.

RESULTS

The simultaneous repair of a venous injury associated with an arterial injury has been shown to improve limb survival.[18,46,79,85,87,96,101] Ligation of venous injuries, particularly in the popliteal vein, can result in limb swelling, impairment of calf pump function and chronic venous insufficiency.[1,47,83,87] Venous reconstruction is the ideal in the haemodynamically stable patient, although some authors have reported minimal morbidity with ligation rather than reconstruction.[103,112] Success following reconstruction is dependent on the site of the injury and the nature of the repair with simple lateral suture achieving higher patency rates than complex reconstructions.[1,7] Early post-reconstruction patency rates of 45–65% have been reported.[7,71,93] The substantial rate of thrombosis following reconstruction probably accounts for the relatively small benefit of reconstruction versus ligation noted by some authors.

These injuries are becoming commoner with increasing military and civilian conflict, but large series are still scarce and long-term follow-up is inevitably poor.

COMPLICATIONS OF VENOUS INJURIES AND THEIR REPAIR

The common complications of venous injuries are: air embolism, arteriovenous fistula, pulmonary embolism, post-thrombotic limb, secondary infection and bleeding.

Air embolism

This is usually a complication of injuries of the veins of the head, neck and upper limb. It may also be seen in association with a tension pneumothorax combined with an intrathoracic venous injury. The most common cause is careless manipulation of the vein during exploration of a venous injury. Air must always be prevented from entering the vein by downstream compression, lowering the level of the damaged vein beneath that of the right atrium, and asking the anaesthetist to apply strong positive pressure ventilation. Since the introduction of positive pressure ventilation, air embolism is a rare occurrence.[107]

Arteriovenous fistula

This is usually caused by a penetrating injury that passes through an adjacent artery and vein. A fistula develops immediately through the incisions or through a haematoma between the two vessels.

Traumatic arteriovenous fistulae have been reported after lumbar disc surgery if the rongeur passes through the anterior longitudinal ligament into the iliac vessels.[37,58,63] Fistulae may also follow penetrating injuries in the groin (e.g. knife wounds or cardiac catheterization) (Figure 26.15) if both the femoral artery and femoral vein are inadvertently punctured.[82] Ligation of the renal artery and vein or of both the splenic vessels in a mass ligature is a reported cause of traumatic arteriovenous fistulae.[45]

The diagnosis of an arteriovenous fistula is made by finding distended pulsating veins, a palpable thrill and loud bruit and a positive Branham's sign.[8] There may be signs of right-sided congestive heart failure or high output left heart failure with engorged neck veins, crepitations in the lungs and ankle oedema.[68]

The site of the fistula should be localized by arteriography (see Figure 26.15) or duplex ultrasound and then closed by surgical suture. The artery should be controlled above the fistula before the vein and the artery are dissected. The vessels can then be separated and the communication closed. It may be necessary to open the artery and close the hole into the vein from the luminal side of the artery or even replace the involved segment of artery.[45] The techniques of the interventional radiologists, balloons, springs and emboli may be used when it is not essential to maintain the patency of the artery and vein involved.

Pulmonary embolism

Cook and Haller[21] suggested that pulmonary embolism was likely to be a common complication of vein repair, because if the repair was unsuccessful, it would thrombose and the thrombus might propagate proximally from the site of the repair before breaking off and embolizing to the lungs. This has not been borne out by clinical experience,[16,56] and the incidence of thromboembolism is said to be higher after popliteal vein ligation than after vein repair.[83] Nevertheless, pulmonary emboli will inevitably occasionally follow any form of direct deep vein surgery.

Post-thrombotic syndrome

Despite the early enthusiastic reports of improved limb salvage by combining venous and arterial repair, the success of venous repair may be as low as 30%,[42] though this figure may have increased with improvements in technique.[43]

The long-term results of venous repair are not known. Many of the 'successful repairs' probably thrombose in the postoperative period. A proportion will then recanalize, giving the patient a better outlook than if the vein had been ligated[88] but it is not unreasonable to expect that almost half of patients who have had a venous reconstruction will develop a post-thrombotic syndrome. No reliable figures are available to confirm or refute this prediction.

Secondary infection

The use of autogenous tissues for grafts, careful excision of devitalized tissue, antibiotic prophylaxis, and the use of delayed primary suture should reduce secondary infection to a minimum.[59] Delayed primary suture is a vital part of the management of gunshot wounds but major arteries and

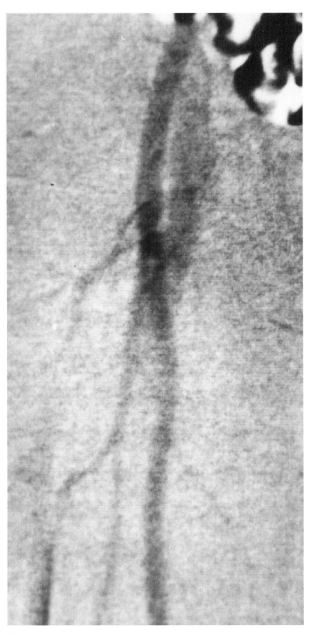

(a)

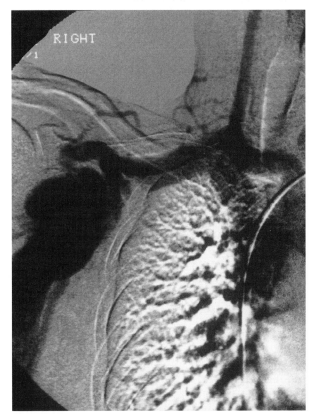

(b)

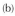

(c)

Figure 26.15 Traumatic arteriovenous fistulae. (a) This is a digital subtraction arteriogram showing contrast medium passing down the femoral artery and entering the femoral vein rather than passing distally down the limb. It followed a femoral artery puncture for cardiac catheterization. (b) A plain radiograph showing a calcified venous aneurysm in the right axilla. (c) An intravenous digital angiograph showing the innominate, carotid and subclavian arteries and almost simultaneous blood flow into the aneurysmal right axillary vein and aneurysm (shown in b) with early opacification of the subclavian vein and superior vena cava. This A-V fistula and subsequent aneurysm was caused by a previous penetrating injury.

veins must not be left uncovered in the base of a wound.[23] The skin should not be closed but some tissue, preferably muscle, should be mobilized to cover the vessels, especially if they contain suture lines closed with non-absorbable materials.

Limb loss

Gangrene only follows a major vein injury when there is an associated arterial occlusion or when all the veins of the limb have been transected or occluded. The latter situation occurs with traumatic amputations, usually at the level of the knee where the popliteal vein is the only effective outflow when even multiple venous anastomoses can be insufficient to allow an adequate circulation. If arterial insufficiency can be corrected, a limb should survive even if its main axial vein is occluded. The limb may become swollen and discoloured,[48] and oedema of muscles enclosed within tight compartments may make them and their adjacent nerves ischaemic.[27,73,80] The importance of careful clinical observation of the anterior and posterior deep compartments of the leg and the flexor compartments of the forearm cannot be overemphasized. Any swelling, tenderness, induration, pain or loss of function should be treated by immediate and extensive fasciotomy.[27,73] An adequate vein repair should reduce the incidence of compartment compression syndromes when there is extensive soft tissue and major vein damage, and should also reduce the incidence of distal gangrene.

COMMENT

Venous damage to small vessels is common and unimportant. Major vein damage from trauma occurs mainly in armed conflicts but has become common in civilian practice where terrorism and violence are prevalent. Careful venous repair or reconstruction is important, especially following injury to the popliteal vein. It is important to try to keep the blood flow through a repaired vein as high as possible, but collateral veins, however small, must not be sacrificed. The incidence of long-term sequelae after venous injuries and reconstruction is not known but basic principles[78] insist that it is preferable to repair rather than to ligate a major vein.[36,43,66]

The surgeons of North America, Israel, South Africa and Northern Ireland[48,73,78] have shown the value of successful venous repair in avoiding amputation and severe venous congestion (Table 26.6). Although many of the initial reports were mainly on missile injuries, more recent studies have shown that military principles can be translated to civilian

Table 26.6 Success of venous repair[73]

	Number	Success	Amputation
Lateral suture	12	9	2
Panel grafts	6	6	0
Vein graft (delayed)	5	2	1
Vein patch (delayed)	7	6	0
End-to-end anastomosis	3	1	1
Ligation	3	0	1

practice.[36,43,66] The technique of lateral suture should be used whenever possible, but when there is extensive vein wall damage, the panel-graft or spiral graft techniques are valuable, using the contralateral long saphenous vein to make the composite grafts. Although generally being preferable to venous ligation, lengthy reconstructive techniques should not be used in unstable patients with multiple injuries who are bleeding heavily.

Venous injuries rarely occur in isolation, and it is difficult to assess the results of treatment without taking into consideration the scale and extent of the other injuries, both their management and an appraisal of their results.

References

1. Aitken RJ, Matley PJ, Immelman EJ. Lower limb vein trauma: a long-term clinical and physiological assessment. *Br J Surg* 1989; **76**: 585–8.
2. Andrews BT, Sommerville KM, Austin S, Wilson NM, Browse NL. Effect of foot pump compression on the velocity and volume of blood flow in the deep veins. *Br J Surg* 1993; **80**: 189–200.
3. Aschberg S, Hindmarsh T. Distal arteriovenous shunts in autotransplantation of canine venous valves. *Acta Chir Scand* 1971; **137**: 503–10.
4. Baird RJ, Lipton IH, Miyagishima RT, Labrosse CJ. Replacement of the deep veins of the leg. *Arch Surg* 1964; **89**: 797.
5. Benvenuto R, Rodman FSB, Gilmour J, Phillips AF, Callagham JC. Composite venous graft for replacement of the superior vena cava. *Arch Surg* 1962; **89**: 100.
6. Blumoff RL, Powell T, Johnson G. Femoral venous trauma in a university referral center. *J Trauma* 1982; **22**: 703.
7. Borman KR, Jones GH, Snyder WH. A decade of lower extremity venous trauma: patency and outcome. *Am J Surg* 1987; **154**: 608–12.
8. Branham HH. Das arteriellvenose Aneurysma. *Arch Klin Chir* 1896; **33**: 1.
9. Brawley RK, Murray GF, Crisler C, Cameron JL. Management of wounds of the innominate, subclavian

and axillary blood vessels. *Surg Gynecol Obstet* 1970; **131:** 1130.

10. Bricker DL, Noon GP, Beall AC, DeBakey ME. Vascular injuries of the thoracic outlet. *J Trauma* 1970; **10:** 1.

11. Brooke B. Surgical applications of therapeutic venous obstruction. *Arch Surg* 1929; **9:** 1.

12. Buechter KJ, Gomez GA, Zeppa R. A new technique for exposure of injuries in the confluence of the retrohepatic veins and the retrohepatic vena cava. *J Trauma* 1990; **30:** 328–31.

13. Burch JM, Feliciano DV, Mattox KL. The atriocaval shunt. Facts and fiction. *Ann Surg* 1988; **207:** 555–68.

14. Burch JM, Feliciano DV, Mattox KL, Edelman M. Injuries of the inferior vena cava. *Am J Surg* 1988; **156:** 548–52.

15. Cargile JS, Hunt JL, Purdue GF. Acute trauma of the femoral artery and vein. *J Trauma* 1992; **32:** 364–70.

16. Carrel A. La technique opératoire des anastomoses vasculaires et la transplantation des viscères. *Lyon Méd* 1902; **98:** 859.

17. Carrel A, Guthrie CC. Uniterminal and biterminal venous transplantation. *Surg Gynecol Obstet* 1906; **2:** 266–86.

18. Chandler JG, Knapp RW. Early definitive treatment of vascular injuries in the Vietnam conflict. *JAMA* 1967; **202:** 960.

19. Ciresi KF, Lim RC. Hepatic vein and retrohepatic venacaval injury. *World J Surg* 1990; **14:** 472–7.

20. Clermont G. Suture latérale et circulaire des veins. *Presse Med* 1901; **1:** 229.

21. Cook FW, Haller JA. Penetrating injuries of the subclavian vessels with associated venous complications. *Ann Surg* 1962; **155:** 370.

22. Dale WA. Peripheral venous reconstruction. In: Dale WA, ed. *Management of Vascular Surgical Problems.* New York: McGraw-Hill, 1985.

23. DeBakey ME, Simeone FA. Battle injuries of the arteries in World War II: an analysis of 2471 cases. *Ann Surg* 1946; **123:** 534.

24. Degiannis E, Velhamos GC, Levy RD, Souter I, Benn CA, Saadia R. Penetrating injuries of the abdominal inferior vena cava. *Ann R Coll Surg Engl* 1996; **78:** 485–9.

25. Demetriades D, Rabinowitz B, Pezikis A, Franklin J, Palexas G. Subclavian vascular injuries. *Br J Surg* 1987; **74:** 1001–3.

26. Doty DB, Baker WH. Bypass of the superior vena cava with a spiral vein graft. *Ann Thorac Surg* 1976; **22:** 490.

27. Drapanas T, Hewitt RL, Weichert RF, Smith AD. Civilian vascular injuries: a critical appraisal of three decades of management. *Ann Surg* 1970; **172:** 351.

28. Eadie DGA, de Takats G. The early fate of autogenous vein grafts in the canine femoral vein. *J Cardiovasc Surg* 1966; **7:** 148.

29. Earle AS, Horsley JS, Villavicencio JL, Warren R. Replacement of venous defects by venous autografts. *Arch Surg* 1960; **80:** 119.

30. Eck NVK. Voprosu o perevyazkie vorotnoi veni. Predvaritelnoye soobshtshjenye. *Voen Med J* 1877; **130:** 1.

31. Field CK, Senkowsky J, Hollier LH, *et al.* Fasciotomy in vascular trauma: is it too much, too often? *Am Surg* 1994; **60:** 409–11.

32. Gaspar MR, Treiman RL. The management of injuries to major veins. *Am J Surg* 1960; **100:** 171.

33. Gerlock AJ, Muhletaler CA. Venography of peripheral venous injuries. *Radiology* 1979; **133:** 77.

34. Graham JM, Mattox KL, Beall AC, DeBakey ME. Traumatic injuries of the inferior vena cava. *Arch Surg* 1979; **113:** 413–18.

35. Haimovici H, Hoffert PW, Zinicola N, Steinman C. An experimental and clinical evaluation of grafts in the venous system. *Surg Gynecol Obstet* 1970; **131:** 1173.

36. Hardin WD, Adinolfi MF, O'Connell RL, Kerstein MD. Management of traumatic peripheral vein injuries. *Am J Surg* 1982; **144:** 235.

37. Hernando FJS, Paredero VM, Solis JV, *et al.* Iliac arteriovenous fistula as a complication of lumbar disc surgery. *J Cardiovasc Surg* 1986; **27:** 180.

38. Hewitt RL, Smith AD, Becker ML, Lindsey ES, Dowling JB, Drapanas T. Penetrating vascular injuries of the thoracic inlet. *Surgery* 1974; **76:** 715.

39. Hjelmstedt AU, Bergvall S. Phlebographic study of the incidence of thrombosis in the injured and uninjured limb in 55 cases of tibial fracture. *Acta Chir Scand* 1968; **134:** 229.

40. Hobson RW, Croom RD, Rich NM. Influence of heparin and low molecular weight dextran on the patency of vein grafts in the venous system. *Ann Surg* 1973; **178:** 773.

41. Hobson RW, Lee BC, Lynch TG, *et al.* Use of intermittent pneumatic calf compression in femoral venous reconstruction. *Surg Gynecol Obstet* 1984; **159:** 284.

42. Hobson RW, Wright CB, Swann KG, Rich NM. Current status of venous injury and reconstruction in the lower extremity. In: Bergan JJ, Yao JST, eds. *Venous Problems.* Chicago, IL: Year Book Medical Publishers, 1978.

43. Hobson RW, Yeager RA, Lynch TG, *et al.* Femoral venous trauma: techniques for surgical management and early results. *Am J Surg* 1983; **146:** 220.

44. Hollands MJ, Little JM. Hepatic venous injury after blunt abdominal trauma. *Surgery* 1990; **107:** 149–52.

45. Hollman E. *Abnormal Arteriovenous Communications.* 2nd edition. Springfield, IL: Thomas, 1937.

46. Hughes CW. Acute vascular trauma in Korean casualties. *Surg Gynecol Obstet* 1954; **99:** 91.

47. Hughes CW. Arterial repair during the Korean war. *Ann Surg* 1958; **157:** 155.

48. Hughes CW. Vascular surgery in the armed forces. *Milit Med* 1959; **124:** 30.

49. Hunt TK, Blaisdell FW, Okimoto J. Vascular injuries of the base of the neck. *Arch Surg* 1969; **98:** 586.

50. Jackson MR, Olson DW, Bekett WC, Olsen SB, Robertson FM. Abdominal vascular trauma: a review of 106 injuries. *Am Surg* 1992; **58:** 622–6.

51. Jacobson JH, Haimov M. Venous revascularization of the arm. Report of three cases. *Surgery* 1977; **81:** 599.

52. Jacobson WHA. In: Rowlands RP, Turner P, eds. *The Operations of Surgery*. 6th edition. London: J & A Churchill, 1915; 843.

53. Johns TPN. A comparison of suture and nonsuture methods for the anastomosis of veins. *Surg Gynecol Obstet* 1947; **84:** 939–42.

54. Kudsk LA, Bongard F, Lim RC. Determinants of survival after vena caval injury. *Arch Surg* 1984; **119:** 1009–12.

55. Kümmel H. Abkürzung des Heilungsverlaufs Laparatomierter durch frühzeitiges Aufstehen. *Verh Dtsch Ges Chir* 1908; **37:** 1.

56. Kunlin J, Kunlin A, Richard S, Tregovet T. Le rétablissment de la circulation veineuse par greffe en cas d'oblitération traumatique ou thrombophlébitique. *Mem Acad Clin* 1953; **79:** 109.

57. Leutic V, Sosa T, Tonkovic I, *et al*. Military vascular injuries in Croatia. *Cardiovasc Surg* 1993; **1:** 3–6.

58. Linton RR, White PD. Arteriovenous fistula between the right common iliac artery and inferior vena cava: a report of its occurrence following operation for ruptured intervertebral disc with cure by operation. *Arch Surg* 1945; **50:** 6.

59. Livingstone RH, Wilson R. Gunshot wounds of the limbs. *Br Med J* 1975; **1:** 667.

60. Makins GH. *On Gunshot Injuries to the Blood Vessels*. Bristol: John Wright, 1919.

61. Matas R. Surgery of the vascular system. In: Keen WW, ed. *Surgery, its Principles and Practice by Various Authors*. Philadelphia, PA: WB Saunders, 1921.

62. Mattox KL. Abdominal venous injuries. *Surgery* 1982; **91:** 497.

63. May ARL, Brewster DC, Darling RC, Browse NL. Arteriovenous fistula following lumbar disc surgery. *Br J Surg* 1981; **68:** 41.

64. Meyer JP, Lim LT, Schuler JJ, *et al*. Peripheral vascular trauma from close-range shotgun injuries. *Arch Surg* 1985; **120:** 1126–31.

65. Milikan JS, Moore EE, Cogbill TH, Kashuk JL. Inferior vena cava injuries – continuing challenge. *J Trauma* 1983; **23:** 207–12.

66. Mullins RJ, Lucas CE, Ledgerwood AM. The natural history following venous ligation for civilian injuries. *J Trauma* 1980; **20:** 737.

67. Murphy JB. Resection of arteries and veins injured in continuity: end to end suture. Experimental and clinical research. *Med Rec* 1897; **51:** 73.

68. Nicalodoni C. Phlebarteriectasie der rechten oberen extremitat. *Arch Klin Chir* 1875; **18:** 252.

69. Nordestgaard AG, Bodily KC, Osborne RW, Buttorff JD. Major vascular injuries during laparoscopic procedures. *Am J Surg* 1995; **169:** 543–5.

70. Nylander GH, Semb C. Veins of the lower part of the leg after tibial fractures. *Surg Gynecol Obstet* 1972; **134:** 974.

71. Nypaver TJ, Schuler JJ, McDonnell P, *et al*. Long term results of venous reconstruction after vascular trauma in civilian practice. *J Vasc Surg* 1992; **16:** 762–8.

72. Ochsner JL, Crawford ES, DeBakey ME. Injuries of the vena cava caused by external trauma. *Surgery* 1961; **49:** 397.

73. O'Reilly NJG, Hood JM, Livingston RH, Irwin JWS. Penetrating injuries of the popliteal vein: a report on 34 cases. *Br J Surg* 1980; **67:** 337.

74. Pachter HL, Spencer FC, Hofstetter SR, Liang HC, Coppa GF. The management of juxtahepatic venous injuries without an atriocaval shunt: preliminary clinical observations. *Surgery* 1986; **99:** 569–75.

75. Palma EC, Esperon R. Vein transplants and grafts in the surgical treatment of the post-phlebitic syndrome. *J Cardiovasc Surg* 1950; **1:** 94.

76. Pasch AR, Bishara RA, Lim LT, Meyer JP, Schuler JJ, Flanigan DP. Optimal limb salvage in penetrating civilian trauma. *J Vasc Surg* 1986; **3:** 189–95.

77. Quast DC, Shirkey AL, Fitzgerald JB, Beall AC, DeBakey ME. Surgical correction of injuries of the vena cava: an analysis of 61 cases. *J Trauma* 1965; **5:** 3.

78. Rich NM. Principles and indications for primary venous repair. *Surgery* 1982; **91:** 492.

79. Rich NM. Vascular trauma in Vietnam. *J Cardiovasc Surg* 1970; **11:** 368.

80. Rich NM, Baugh JH, Hughes CW. Acute arterial injuries in Vietnam: 1000 cases. *J Trauma* 1970; **10:** 359.

81. Rich NM, Collins GV, Anderson CA, McDonald PT. Autogenous venous interposition grafts in repair of major venous injuries. *J Trauma* 1977; **17:** 512.

82. Rich NM, Hobson RW, Collins GJ. Traumatic arteriovenous fistulas and false aneurysm: a review of 558 lesions. *Surgery* 1975; **78:** 817.

83. Rich NM, Hobson RW, Collins GJ, Anderson CA. The effect of acute popliteal venous interruption. *Ann Surg* 1976; **183:** 365.

84. Rich NM, Hobson RW, Wright CB. Historical aspects of direct venous reconstruction. In: Bergan JJ, Yao JST, eds. *Venous Problems*. Chicago, IL: Year Book Medical Publishers, 1978.

85. Rich NM, Hughes CW. Vietnam vascular registry: a preliminary report. *Surgery* 1969; **65:** 218.

86. Rich NM, Hughes CW, Baugh JH. Management of venous injuries. *Ann Surg* 1970; **171:** 724.

87. Rich NM, Jarstfer BS, Greer TM. Popliteal artery repair: causes and possible prevention. *J Cardiovasc Surg* 1974; **15:** 340.

88. Rich NM, Sullivan WG. Clinical recanalization of an autogenous vein graft in the popliteal vein. *J Trauma* 1972; **12:** 919.

89. Schede M. Einige Bemerkungen Über die Naht von Venenwunden, nebst Mittheilung eines Falles von geheilter Naht der Vena cava inferior. *Arch Klin Chir* 1892; **43:** 338.

90. Scheinin TM, Jude JR. Experimental replacement of the superior vena cava: effect of a temporary increase in blood flow. *J Cardiovasc Surg* 1964; **48:** 781.

91. Schramek A, Hashmonai M. Vascular injuries in the extremities in battle casualties. *Br J Surg* 1977; **64:** 644.

92. Sfeir RE, Khoury GS, Kenaan MK. Vascular trauma to the lower extremity: the Lebanese war experience. *Cardiovasc Surg* 1995; **3:** 653–7.

93. Sharma PV, Shah PM, Vinzons AT, Pallan TM, Clauss RH, Stahl WM. Meticulously restored lumina of injured veins remain patent. *Surgery* 1992; **112:** 928–32.

94. Shenk WG, Martin JW, Leslie MB, Portin BA. The regional haemodynamics of chronic experimental arteriovenous fistulas. *Surg Gynecol Obstet* 1960; **110:** 44–50.

95. Sherif AA. Vascular injuries: experience during the Afghanistan war. *Int Surg* 1992; **77:** 114–17.

96. Spencer FC, Grewe RV. The management of acute arterial injuries in battle casualties. *Ann Surg* 1955; **141:** 304.

97. Stansel HC Jr. Synthetic inferior vena cava grafts. Influence of increased flow. *Arch Surg* 1964; **89:** 1096.

98. Starzl TE, Kaupp HA, Beheler EM, Freeark RJ. The treatment of penetrating wounds of the inferior vena cava. *Surgery* 1962; **51:** 195.

99. Steenberg RW, Ravitch MM. Cervico-thoracic approach for subclavian vessel injury from compound fracture of the clavicle: considerations of sub-clavian-axillary exposures. *Ann Surg* 1963; **157:** 839.

100. Stewart MK, Stone HH. Injuries of the inferior vena cava. *Am Surg* 1986; **51:** 9–13.

101. Sullivan WG, Thornton FH, Baker LH, La Plante ES, Cohen A. Early influence of popliteal vein repair in the treatment of popliteal vessel injuries. *Am J Surg* 1971; **122:** 528.

102. Thompson BW, Read RC, Casali RE. Interposition grafting for portal hypertension. *Am J Surg* 1975; **130:** 733.

103. Timberlake GA, Kerstein MD. Venous injury: to repair or ligate, the dilemma revisited. *Am Surg* 1995; **61:** 139–45.

104. Travers B, Cooper A. *On Wounds and Ligature of Veins. Surgical Essays.* London: 1818; **1:** 243.

105. Treiman RL, Doty D, Caspar MR. Acute vascular trauma. A fifteen year study. *Am J Surg* 1966; **111:** 469.

106. Vollmar J. Plastiche eingriffe an den tiefen Venen. In: Kappert A, May R, eds. *Das postthrombotische Zustandsbild der extremitd ten.* Bern: Hueber, 1968.

107. Vollmar J. Venous trauma. In: May R, ed. *Surgery of the Veins of the Leg and Pelvis.* Stuttgart: Georg Thieme, 1979.

108. Vollmar J. Venous trauma. *Maj Prob Clin Surg* 1977; **134:** 25.

109. Wiencek RG, Wilson RF. Abdominal venous injuries. *J Trauma* 1986; **26:** 771–8.

110. Wood M. Penetrating wounds of the vena cava, recommendations for treatment. *Surgery* 1966; **60:** 311.

111. Woodson J, Rodriguez AA, Menzonian JO. The use of internal jugular vein as interposition graft for femoral vein reconstruction following traumatic venous injury: a useful approach in selected cases. *Ann Vasc Surg* 1990; **4:** 494–7.

112. Yelon JA, Scalea TM. Venous injuries of the lower extremities and pelvis: repair versus ligation. *J Trauma* 1992; **33:** 532–6.

113. Zincola N, Hoffert PW, Haimovici H. Autogenous vein bypass grafts in the venous system; an experimental evaluation. *Bull Soc Int Chir* 1962; **21:** 265.

CHAPTER 27

Venous tumours

Cystic degeneration of the vein wall	731	Leiomyoma and leiomyosarcoma of the vein wall	742
Venous (cavernous) haemangioma	732	References	745

In this chapter the word 'tumour' is interpreted literally as a *mass* so that three rare conditions of the veins can be discussed – cystic mucoid degeneration of the vein wall, cavernous haemangioma and leiomyoma/leiomyosarcoma. All these conditions may present as a palpable mass or with the sequelae of major vein obstruction. Only the leiomyoma/leiomyosarcoma is a true neoplasm.

Cystic degeneration of the vein wall

Cystic degeneration in the wall of an artery was first reported in 1947[6] in the external iliac artery and has since been observed in the popliteal, radial, ulnar and other small arteries. It was first described in a vein in 1963.[39]

PATHOLOGY

All reports describe this lesion as a cystic swelling in the wall of a vein containing a transparent gelatinous material which is similar to that found in a subcutaneous ganglion.

The cyst lies between the media and adventitia and has a collagenous wall. Collections of acid mucin-like material are also found between the fibromuscular tissues as well as in the cavity of the cyst. The wall on the luminal side of the cyst retains an endothelial covering (Figure 27.1).

No analyses of vein cyst contents have been reported but the analysis of the contents of popliteal artery adventitial cysts shows the material to be a mucoprotein with little or no hydroxyproline; this finding suggests that it is not derived from collagen.[31] The true origin and nature of these cysts is yet to be determined. The veins reported to have been affected are the iliac veins,[18] the common femoral vein,[4,20,23] and the subcutaneous veins at the ankle and wrist.[3,13] All these sites are close to joints; this is a feature of subcutaneous ganglions, and it has been suggested that the common subcutaneous ganglion may begin in a very small blood vessel.[21]

CLINICAL PRESENTATION

The patient presents with a lump or with the symptoms of venous obstruction. The lump itself is not usually painful or tender. It is often impalpable and is usually too deep for fluctuation to be felt. Cysts on subcutaneous veins may be single or multiple and cause few problems other than mild aching pain and disfigurement. Cysts on the femoral vein tend to present with venous obstruction (swelling, superficial venous distension and venous claudication) before the patient notices a lump.

INVESTIGATION

The diagnosis of venous compression or obstruction is first made by duplex ultrasound scanning and/or phlebography. The vein may be stenosed or

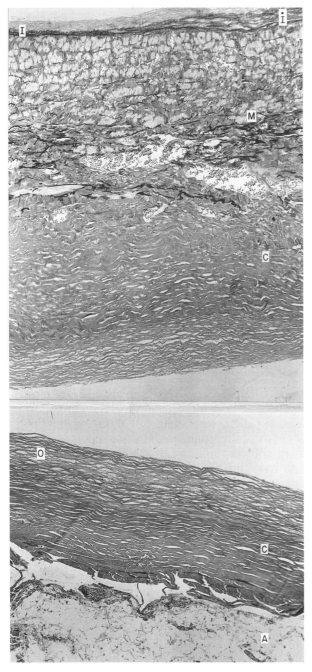

Figure 27.1 Photomicrographs of the inner (I) and outer (O) walls of a femoral vein wall cyst. The inner wall consists of intima (i) and medial smooth muscle (M); the outer wall consists of adventitia (A) and laminae of collagen (C), suggesting that the cyst developed between the adventitial and medial layers.

totally occluded. Occlusion or compression indicates the site of the problem and the ultrasound image may reveal a fluid-filled mass. A stenosis, especially if it is asymmetrical, suggests an external

lesion and should raise the suspicion of a vein wall cyst, even though extrinsic lesions (e.g. lymphadenopathy) are far more likely causes of venous compression.

Although the presence of a cystic mass can often be seen on an ultrasound scan, it is best displayed with computerized tomography (CT) scanning. The combination of a CT scan and a phlebogram should pinpoint the size and position and likely nature of the lesion. Together these two investigations provide the best anatomical information on which to plan a surgical excision.

Lymphangiography may be required to exclude venous compression by enlarged lymph nodes. Cystic degeneration must be differentiated from leiomyosarcomata and extrinsic compression because its treatment is so different.

TREATMENT

The lesion should be explored and fully exposed. Two methods of treatment are possible, total excision of the whole vein and vein replacement or evacuation and partial excision of the cyst. At operation these cysts feel cystic and look bluish in colour. If the CT scan shows a mass with a radiolucent fluid-like content, it is safe to confirm the diagnosis at operation by aspiration or frozen section. If jelly-like material is obtained, the lumen can be restored by removing either the outer wall of the cyst, without opening the vein, or the inner wall of the cyst, through a venotomy. The latter approach is advisable if there is any suggestion of intraluminal thrombus at the site of the venous constriction. Removing the outer wall without opening the vein reduces the risk of postoperative thrombosis. The patient should be given a course of heparin after the operation.

There is a small chance of recurrence if only one wall of the cyst, inner or outer, is removed because the mucoid degeneration has usually spread into the tissues around the cyst (see Figure 27.1).

If there is any doubt about the pathology of the lesion, it should be treated as if it was a neoplasm and completely excised together with the adjacent segment of vein. The vein may then have to be reconstructed with a vein graft or prosthesis.

Venous (cavernous) haemangioma

Venous haemangiomata are formed from venular capillaries, venules and large veins. Those derived from venules form skin lesions (e.g. the port wine

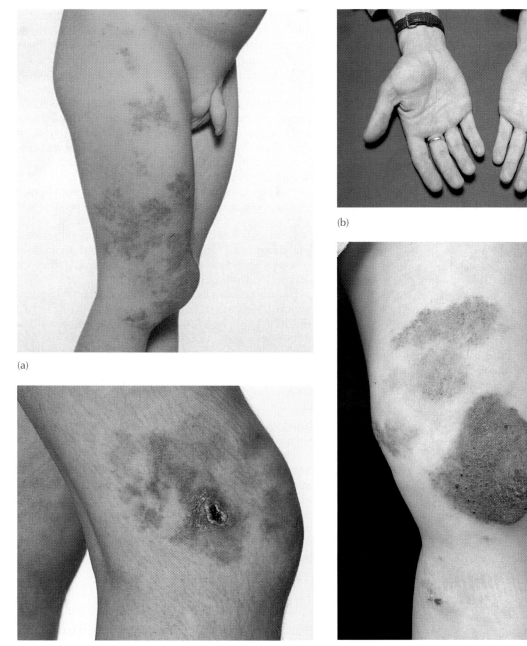

(a)

(b)

(c)

(d)

Figure 27.2 Four examples of venous angiomata. (a) Multiple, soft, subcutaneous venous angiomata on the thigh. (b) A venous angioma involving the skin, subcutaneous tissues and muscles of the thenar eminence and the thumb. (c) A venous angioma involving the skin and subcutaneous tissues over the right knee but not extending into the knee joint or quadriceps femoris muscle, but with some superficial ulceration. (d) A venous angioma involving the skin and subcutaneous tissues over the lateral medial aspect of the knee joint. The lesion extended into the knee joint, causing pain and recurrent haemarthoses.

stain). Malformations of large veins often occur in association with other congenital abnormalities, for example the Klippel–Trenaunay syndrome, but in such cases they are commonly connected to other abnormal veins in the limb and not usually an independent abnormality (see Chapter 24).

Venous haemangiomata which occur in an otherwise normal limb present a distinct clinical problem.

PATHOLOGY

The blood vessels in early fetal life form a network of undifferentiated tubes. Between the fifth and tenth weeks of intrauterine life the vessels begin to organize into the system which we recognize in adult life.[48] It is believed that most vascular abnormalities begin as a failure of organization in this period. A venous haemangioma is a collection of large dilated disorganized veins which drain into a normal venous system. They are not true neoplasms and would be better described as hamartomata than as angiomata. They do not undergo malignant change. We are not aware of any reports of malignant venous haemangiosarcomas. They commonly occur in the subcutaneous tissues and between the muscles of the limbs but often extend into adjacent skin, muscle, and, occasionally, into bone. The upper and lower limbs are equally affected. They fluctuate in size but tend to progressively distend and enlarge. Thrombophlebitis and calcification of the thrombus to produce 'phleboliths' are common complications. It is unusual for these tumours to seriously affect the function of adjacent or even extensively involved muscles but muscular exercise may damage the veins and precipitate thrombosis or haemorrhage. Joint movements may be affected. Flexion deformities may develop if the veins protrude into the joint cavity and cause recurrent haemarthroses or if repeated episodes of thrombosis cause muscle fibrosis and contractures. The overall size of the limb is not affected, as it is in the Klippel–Trenaunay syndrome.

The arteries of the limb are normal. Some venous angiomata of the skin are associated with lymphatic dilatation and lymph reflux.

CLINICAL PRESENTATION

Most patients present in their early years when they or their parents notice a variable swelling in the limb with dilated veins in or under the skin or a bluish discoloration of the overlying skin (Figure 27.2).[5]

When a venous haemangioma is deep within the limb, there may be no visible mass and the only complaint is of pain.

The nature of the pain varies. It is usually a dull ache which may be present at all times, but worse when the limb is dependent and relieved by elevation. This type of pain is probably caused by the tension of venous distension.

Sharp tingling sensations or areas of cutaneous sensory loss may occur if a haemangioma involves a nerve.

Episodes of haemorrhage or thrombophlebitis, which are usually related to local trauma, can cause severe pain. Haematomata and bruising may appear, and tender masses of venous thrombosis may be palpable. These painful episodes usually subside within 5–10 days.

The pain may be exacerbated by exercise if the haemangioma is infiltrating a muscle or bulging into a joint. An extensive haemangioma in the quadriceps femoris muscle can cause so much pain on walking that a child may develop a fixed flexion deformity of the knee.

Sudden swelling and stiffness of a joint, commonly the knee joint, may be caused by an acute serous effusion or bleeding into the joint.

Repeated knee or hip joint irritation may cause muscle spasm, deformity, limping, and secondary scoliosis and back pain; all these complications are severely disabling (Figure 27.3).

Examination reveals a soft compressible mass which collapses when raised above the level of the heart but becomes tight and distended when dependent or if its downstream veins are occluded with a tourniquet. There may be a venular naevus in the overlying skin (Figure 27.2). If the lesion is in the subcutaneous tissues, it will give the skin a dark blue tinge. Although the mass is compressible, there may be hard nodules within it – the remnants of episodes of thrombosis.

The muscles and arteries of the limb are usually normal but nearby joints may contain an effusion and joint movements may be limited. Venous angiomata may involve nerves and cause motor and sensory neurological defects. Multiple venous haemangiomata are uncommon, in contrast to multiple capillary haemangiomata (strawberry naevi) which are common.

INVESTIGATION

The most useful information is obtained from plain and contrast radiography. A plain film may show the mass and many phleboliths (Figure 27.4). Nearby bone may show translucent areas if there are dilated veins within it (Figure 27.5).

A Doppler ultrasound flow detector is useful when delineating the extent of the lesion and excluding arteriovenous fistulae, Duplex ultrasound cannot usually display the fine anatomical details of a lesion.

Ascending phlebography usually shows normal axial veins but may fail to fill the haemangioma. It is, however, important to know that the deep axial veins are normal before considering surgical excision (Figure 27.6a, b).

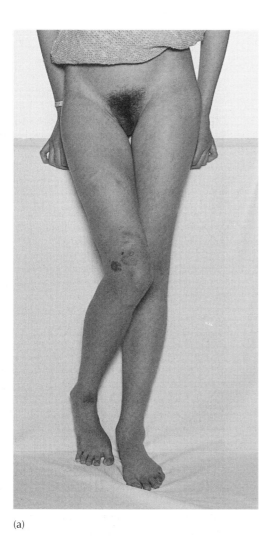
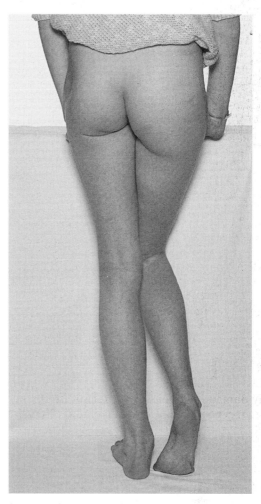

(a)   (b)

Figure 27.3   This patient has an extensive venous angioma involving the knee joint and quadriceps femoris muscle. Recurrent episodes of pain and haemarthroses have caused a fixed flexion deformity of the knee and ankle joints. The knee joint had to be arthrodesed and the Achilles tendon had to be lengthened to restore walking to normal.

The extent and the size of the haemangioma are best displayed by a direct injection into one of its veins (Figure 27.7a, b). This is easy to carry out when the lesion is subcutaneous and visible, but not as easy to perform when it lies deep beneath the muscles; in these circumstances the venous phase of an arteriogram may reveal the full extent of the lesion more clearly. An arterial phlebogram using digital subtraction angiography is sometimes helpful (Figure 27.8).

A CT scan after the intravenous injection of a radio-opaque contrast medium will show the relationships between the lesion and nearby muscles, arteries, nerves and joints (Figure 27.9). Neurovascular bundles are often closely related to deep intermuscular venous haemangiomata.

Magnetic resonance phlebography provides valuable information and may well replace CT scanning (Figure 27.10).

Arthrography and arthroscopy are important investigations if there are joint symptoms. The filling defects caused by veins bulging into the joint can be enhanced by a tourniquet placed around the limb to produce venous congestion. Joint involvement may also be seen on the venous phase of an arteriogram (Figure 27.11). At arthroscopy (through an unaffected part of the synovium) the veins can be seen to bulge into the joint making the synovium bosselated and blue.

Arteriography and lymphography are not indicated, unless there is some clinical indication of an arterial or lymphatic abnormality.

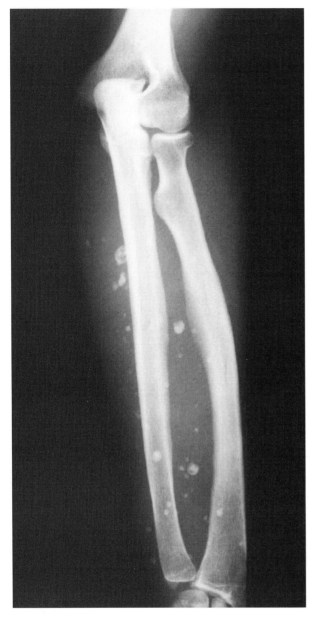

Figure 27.4 A plain radiograph of a forearm with an extensive deep venous angioma containing many phleboliths.

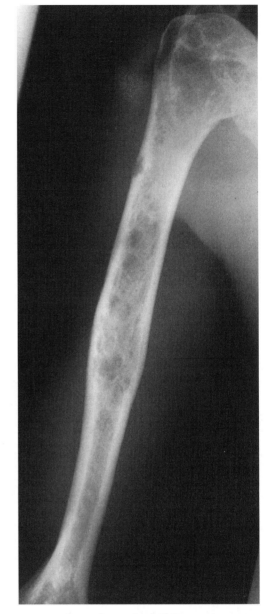

Figure 27.5 The radiograph of a humerus in an arm with a deep intramuscular and intraosseus venous angioma. The large veins in the bone are visible as multiple x-ray-lucent areas.

Any weakness of the limb should be investigated with a careful neurological examination and, if indicated, electromyography. Clinical examination and phlebography usually exclude the main differential diagnoses (e.g. arteriovenous fistulae, other vascular tumours, lymphangioma circumscriptum and simple varicose veins). When in doubt, all the investigations mentioned above may be necessary, followed, on rare occasions, by an incisional biopsy even though this is an haemorrhagic and difficult procedure.

TREATMENT

Venous haemangiomata are difficult to excise but complete excision is the best form of treatment. Sclerotherapy with irritant chemicals or boiling water is risky and fails because of the capaciousness of the veins. Venous haemangiomata do not have a large arterial blood supply and therefore embolization is of no help.

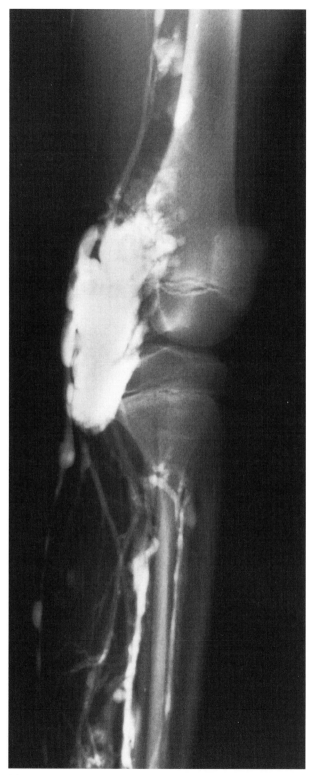

(a)

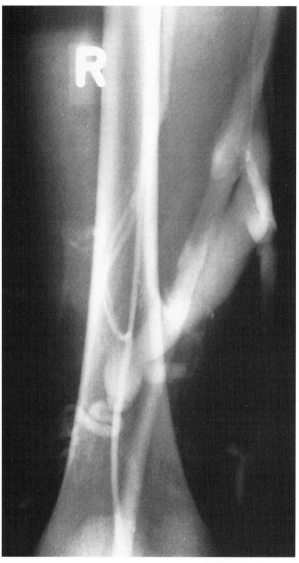

(b)

Figure 27.6   (a) An ascending phlebograph filling a large venous angioma behind the knee and some abnormal veins in the mid calf. (b) An ascending phlebograph filling the large draining vessel of a venous angioma in the lower thigh but failing to fill the many veins draining into it.

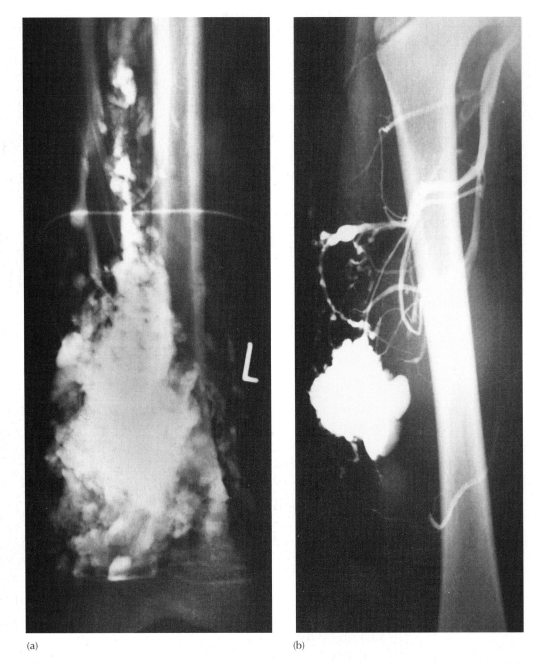

(a) (b)

Figure 27.7 (a) A direct injection into a venous angioma on the medial side of the lower thigh showing that the lesion extends to the lateral side of the femur and far higher up the thigh than the visible mass had suggested. (b) A direct injection into a venous angioma on the lateral aspect of the thigh showing that it drains into tributaries of the deep femoral vein.

Before excision is contemplated, the major axial veins should be shown to be normal and the extent and anatomical relationships of the lesion should be defined as accurately as possible. The patient must be fully appraised of the size of the operation and any likely sequelae (e.g. nerve or joint damage).

Superficial lesions

Superficial lesions are best excised through a longitudinal incision over the mass and through a bloodless field provided by a tourniquet.[33,46] It is important to mark the extent of the lesion before

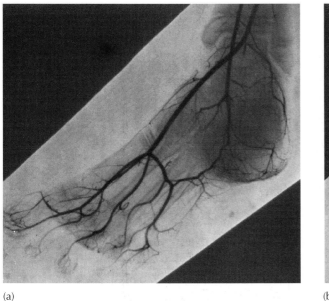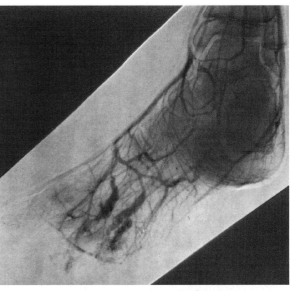

(a)   (b)

Figure 27.8 (a) The arterial and (b) venous phases of an intra-arterial digital subtraction angiogram. The venous phase reveals the large draining veins of a venous angioma lying deep in the foot between the metatarsal bones.

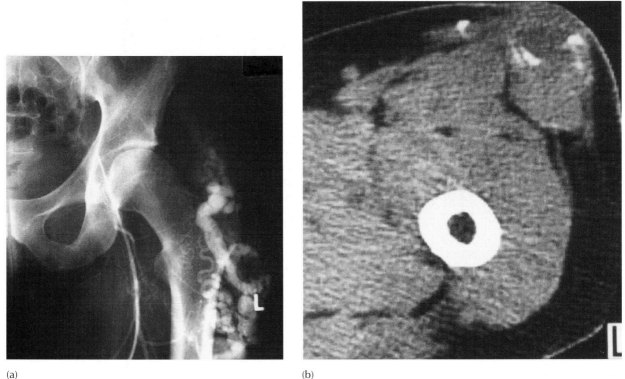

(a)   (b)

Figure 27.9 (a) The venous phase of a femoral arteriogram showing an extensive venous angioma in the upper thigh. (b) The CT scan with vascular enhancement of the same patient showing that the lesion is entirely subcutaneous. Some of the large veins can be seen filled with contrast medium.

Pain in the wound is an indication for early wound inspection. If a large haematoma is found, it should be evacuated as soon as possible. Skin necrosis is an important and undesirable complication. It is usually caused by tension in the skin, secondary to a haematoma or a misguided attempt to achieve a primary closure when too much skin has been excised. Necrotic skin must be excised and the defect covered with a split skin graft after the tendency of the tissues to bleed has stopped and some healthy granulation tissue has formed. Grafting onto any tissue that contains residual haemangioma that might bleed or ooze serum carries a high risk of a further haematoma developing beneath the graft. If a large area of skin has to be excised, the defect can be covered with a rotation or pedicle skin flap or with a vascularized free skin flap.

Deep lesions

Deep venous haemangiomata should also be explored through a bloodless field. A long incision should be made, extending beyond the limits of the lesion, so that the deep compartment of the limb can be opened to identify, isolate and protect any major blood vessels or nerves that may be passing through or near to the angioma.

The superficial and lateral surfaces of the angioma are then exposed, until it is possible to see if the angioma can be separated from the surrounding structures, whether any major arteries or nerves pass through it and whether any muscle is extensively involved.

Intermuscular angiomata can usually be removed; the last phase is the careful dissection of the mass from any adjacent artery and veins. In the upper limb, deep veins such as the brachial vein can be removed because the superficial veins provide an adequate outflow tract. In the lower limb the main axial veins above the knee should be preserved if possible; below the knee one or two pairs of the crural veins can be excised without affecting calf pump function.

Intramuscular angiomata are difficult to remove without excising the muscle, and the symptoms rarely justify excising a whole muscle (e.g. the biceps humeris or quadriceps femoris). When a large mass of veins occupies a major part of an important muscle we prefer to obliterate the whole mass with large continuous encircling stitches of a non-absorbable material, for example silk or braided polyethylene. The mass must be dissected clear on three sides, and the deep aspects must not contain a major nerve or artery. A large continuous stitch is then placed around the whole mass. The encircling turns should be approximately 1 cm apart

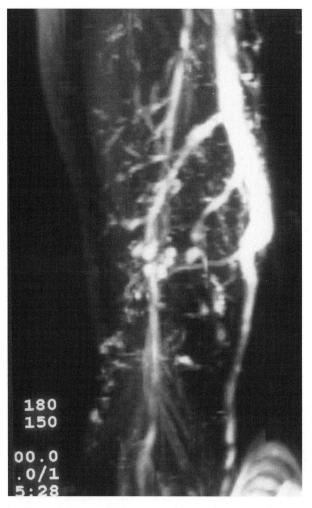

Figure 27.10 An MR coronal two-dimensional TOF phlebograph showing a venous angioma in the left thigh and its draining vessels.

applying the tourniquet, as it may not be visible once the limb is exsanguinated. Involved skin and all the subcutaneous tissue containing the large veins can be excised within the limits imposed by the blood supply of the skin flaps. If it is not possible to remove the whole haemangioma, it can be transected, its cut edge oversewn to prevent bleeding, and the residual abnormality removed through another incision at a second-stage operation, 3–6 months later. Subcutaneous nerves are difficult to identify in the middle of a mass of veins and may have to be excised, leaving small patches of anaesthetic skin on the limb. This is not a serious complication, provided the nerves at the wrist and ankle, which supply the hand and foot, are not damaged. The skin must be closed over suction drainage and compressed firmly to reduce the considerable chance of haematoma formation.

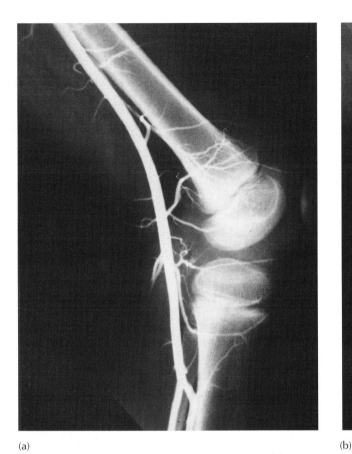

(a)

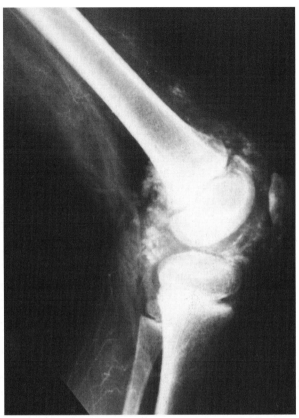

(b)

Figure 27.11 (a) The arteriograph of a patient with a large venous angioma around the knee. The arteries are normal; this confirms that no arteriovenous fistulae are present. (b) The venous phase of the same arteriograph showing an extensive angioma closely related to the synovium of the joint and extending into the quadriceps femoris muscles.

and run the whole length of the mass. The object is to compress the lesion and make it thrombose, yet retain some muscle function and the contours of the limb. When the procedure is completed, the mass looks like a tied up roll of meat. We have found this method to be an effective way of obliterating the mass and stopping the pain, yet preserving function. The same approach can be used on the remnant of a haemangioma if only part of it can be excised.

When the angioma involves a nerve, individual bundles of nerve fibres may be separated by the veins and may be difficult to see. The surgeon must then decide whether to excise the nerve or leave haemangiomatous tissue inside the nerve. The symptoms rarely justify excising a major nerve.

A venous haemangioma which is bulging into a joint should be excised if it is causing recurrent effusions or haemarthroses. It is unusual to be able to excise all the angioma and leave the synovium intact but, fortunately, most of the synovium can be removed from a joint without seriously affecting joint mobility, provided the patient has vigorous postoperative physiotherapy to restore full movement.

In our experience, the joint most often involved is the knee joint, in association with a venous haemangioma in the quadriceps muscles of the thigh. In this situation the abnormal veins in the fat, deep to the rectus femoris muscle, the synovium of the suprapatella pouch, and the synovium on either side of the patella down to the level of the knee joint can be excised with the overlying subcutaneous veins without damaging knee movements. Extensive involvement of the vastus medialis or lateralis is treated by the encircling suture technique. After releasing the tourniquet, it is essential to obtain perfect haemostasis to prevent blood collecting in the joint. Suction drainage and compression are mandatory. Quadriceps exercises must start the day after the operation, but joint movements should not begin for 4–5 days. We have not seen a venous angioma involving the ankle, hip or shoulder joint but we have seen two venous angiomata in the back of the arm which impinged upon the elbow joint.

Some young patients who have extensive haemangiomata in and around the knee joint experience severe pain and muscle spasms and develop secondary flexion deformities of the knee joint which cannot be overcome with physiotherapy (see Figure 27.3). In four patients with this problem we have had to arthrodese the knee joint because the limb shortening resulting from the fixed flexion of the knee was causing a progressing flexion deformity of the hip and ankle and a lumbar scoliosis.

Leiomyoma and leiomyosarcoma of the vein wall

Tumours of smooth muscle are rare; this is surprising in view of the ubiquity of smooth muscle, especially in the vascular system. Leiomyosarcomata arising from veins are reported to be more common than those arising from arteries.

The distinction between a benign and low-grade malignant smooth muscle tumour is a histological nicety which accounts for the fact that between 1871 and 1984, 93 leiomyosarcomata were reported[29] whereas only one leiomyoma was described.[34] For practical purposes, it is wise to assume that all smooth muscle tumours arising in veins are sarcomas with differing degrees of malignancy.

PATHOLOGY

The incidence of leiomyosarcomata of the inferior vena cava found incidentally at post mortem is probably less than 1 in 25 000;[1,26] the clinical incidence is far less. Most vascular surgeons see only one or two of these tumours in a lifetime. Tumours in the inferior vena cava seem to be more common than tumours in other veins.[27] Tumours in the superior vena cava are very rare.[5] Vena caval tumours are said to occur more often in females than in males but tumours in other veins occur equally in the two sexes.[8,27]

Leiomyosarcomata have a lobulated, grey–pink appearance with a thin fibrous capsule. Histologically, they look like uterine fibroids because they consist of whirls of smooth muscle cells. They contain a variable but small number of large, densely staining nuclei at various stages of mitosis which betrays their malignant potential (Figure

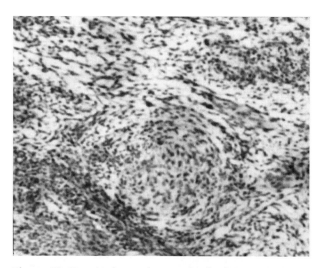

Figure 27.12 A photomicrograph of a leiomyosarcoma that arose from the wall of the deep femoral vein. It shows the typical whorls of cells with nuclei in different stages of mitosis.

27.12). They tend to grow away from their origin in the wall of a vein, displacing nearby structures rather than infiltrating them, but they can grow along the vein wall and spread within its lumen in a downstream direction. This form of spread blocks the mouths of the tributary veins but the tumour rarely spreads down the lumen of a tributary against the blood flow. Although these tumours are slow growing, they are malignant and ultimately metastasize; only 14 of the 35 patients reviewed by Kieffer were alive 2 years after operation.[27] These tumours must therefore be considered highly malignant, whatever their histological appearance.

Leiomyosarcomata arising in the wall of the uterus or a uterine myoma occasionally spread into the lumen of the vena cava and may be mistakenly diagnosed as primary vena cava leiomyosarcomata.[7,11] There is a difference of opinion between the pathologists as to whether tumours of this type which spread along the lumen of major veins – often described as intravenous leiomyomatosis – are derived from the smooth muscle of veins[28] or the uterus.[43] Whatever the source, leiomyoma with this form of spread are very slow growing and at the very benign end of the spectrum of malignancy.[14,38,42]

CLINICAL PRESENTATION

The symptoms and signs depend upon the site of the tumour and its effect on its vein of origin.

Leiomyosarcomata of the inferior vena cava

These tumours grow slowly and may not cause symptoms for many years. Abdominal pain is a common feature and is often misinterpreted as indigestion. The pain may radiate to the groin or loin. The patient may complain of swelling of the legs, dilated veins on the abdominal wall and abdominal distension caused by compression or, rarely, by thrombosis of the vena cava.[22]

Examination reveals leg oedema, collateral veins, sometimes an upper abdominal mass slightly to the right-hand side, hepatomegaly and ascites.

When the tumour is below the renal veins the symptoms are mainly of pain and vena caval obstruction. The most common site of origin of inferior vena caval tumours is the segment between the renal and hepatic veins. This causes pain and sometimes the symptoms and signs of vena caval obstruction, but it rarely causes uraemia or renal failure, as the slow occlusion of the renal veins allows time for collaterals to develop.

A high tumour at or above the hepatic veins can cause the Budd–Chiari syndrome – ascites, hepatomegaly and jaundice.[10,32,36] Leiomyosarcomata occasionally present with a pyrexia.[17]

Leiomyosarcomata of the iliac and femoral veins

These present with pain, a mass, or signs of venous obstruction – oedema and distended veins.[30,45] When a mass is palpable it is usually painful and tender. The patient illustrated in Figure 27.13 had pain in the upper part of the thigh for 10 years, and three surgical explorations of the groin were carried out in different hospitals before a mass appeared and a fourth exploration revealed a leiomyosarcoma arising from a deep tributary of the deep femoral vein. The pain which the patient had experienced for 10 years had been caused by a stretched obturator nerve.

The venous obstruction may cause oedema, but it is often asymptomatic, as it develops slowly and the collaterals are usually good. Venous claudication is rarely seen as a presenting symptom.

It is unusual for patients with leiomyosarcomata to present with debility and weight loss, but these tumours can spread to the lungs and ultimately death is caused by disseminated secondary disease.

INVESTIGATIONS

Phlebography, CT and MRI scanning are the most useful investigations (Figure 27.13a, b). Phlebography defines the venous anatomy, the site of origin of the tumour and the extent of the collateral circulation. CT and MRI define the size of the tumour and its relationship to the surrounding structures.

Gastrointestinal investigations which are ordered because of an incorrect diagnosis of indigestion may reveal a retroperitoneal mass displacing the duodenum, stomach or kidney. Ultrasound can detect a retroperitoneal mass but does not provide the anatomical detail provided by a CT scan.[41,48]

Retrograde catheterization of the vena cava via an arm vein may be needed to obtain a phlebograph that shows the veins above a caval occlusion.

Careful renal and liver function studies must be carried out in patients with vena caval tumours. It may be necessary to measure portal vein pressure and to obtain a liver biopsy.

These tumours are not very vascular and arteriography is therefore not helpful.[15,40] The other causes of similar symptoms (e.g. gastroenterological problems, retroperitoneal tumours and vena caval thrombosis) should be detected by the above investigations.

In spite of the possibility of making a preoperative diagnosis on the basis of all these investigations, the symptoms and signs of vena caval tumours can be so vague that the diagnosis is first made at a laparotomy. When this occurs it is wise to obtain a biopsy and stop the operation so that detailed investigations can be performed and a planned approach to treatment can be formulated.

TREATMENT

Leiomyosarcomata arising from peripheral limb veins should be treated by wide excision as for any other low-grade sarcoma, if possible by compartmentectomy.[30,45] This is often difficult, as these tumours arise from blood vessels that are commonly between, not within, the fascial compartments of the limb. Fortunately, most leiomyosarcomata have a capsule and rarely infiltrate adjacent muscle and bone; they can therefore be dissected free of the surrounding tissues, even though the vessel from which they arise must be excised. This may mean excising the femoral or iliac vein. If the vein is already totally occluded and the symptoms of the venous occlusion are not severe, the excised vein does not need to be replaced provided the collateral veins are not disturbed. If swelling or bursting pain becomes a problem after the operation and all of the tumour has been excised, the excised segment of vein may be replaced with a segment of autogenous vein (e.g. saphenous vein) or a prosthesis (e.g. supported PTFE).

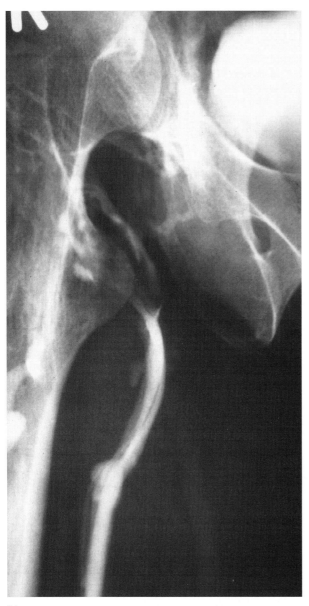

(a)

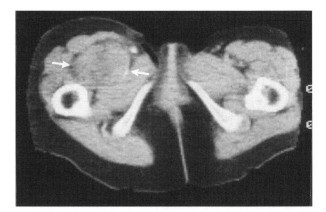

(b)

Figure 27.13 (a) The phlebograph of a patient with a large leiomyosarcoma in the thigh. The deep femoral vein is stretched around the mass, and the upper part of the common femoral vein contains projecting tumour thrombus. (b) The CT scan of the same patient showing a large homogeneous mass in the upper thigh.

Residual tumour should be irradiated, though these tumours are not very radiosensitive. Leiomyosarcomata are not sensitive to chemotherapy.

Leiomyosarcomata of the inferior vena cava

These tumours have become susceptible to surgical treatment since the advent of venous bypass grafting.

Tumours below the renal veins can be excised with removal of as much of the vena cava as necessary. If a pedunculated tumour is excised with a small piece of vein wall, the vena cava can be sutured or repaired with a patch. The whole infrarenal vena cava can be ligated and excised if necessary.[37] After this operation the patient is likely to develop bilateral leg oedema but this is a relatively small price to pay for complete excision of the tumour. It is better not to replace the vena cava with a prosthesis at the time of the excision to avert the risk of postoperative graft thrombosis and pulmonary embolism. Replacement of the vena cava should be carried out at a later date with a PTFE prosthesis if the patient has symptoms and when it is clear that the patient has no recurrent disease.[27]

By the time they are discovered, tumours between the renal and hepatic veins are usually large and have to be treated by a complete resection of the vena cava from its origin to just below the hepatic veins. The right kidney may have to be removed if its pedicle is involved in the tumour. If the pedicle is not involved, both it and the left renal vein can be tied without causing renal failure because genital, adrenal, and lumbar veins dilate to act as collateral vessels, provided the vein is ligated on the caval side of these vessels.[3,9,13,25,35] Sometimes the left renal vein can be anastomosed to the upper or lower stump of the vena cava. A healthy right kidney that has to have part of its vein excised can be transplanted into the iliac fossa. Reconstruction of the vena cava with a prosthesis and implantation of the renal veins into the prosthesis is rarely indicated.[2]

Tumours at or above the hepatic veins are usually impossible to remove because the tumour has usually spread into the hepatic veins or the liver. Hepatic lobectomy and upper vena caval replacement has been performed when one of the hepatic veins was free of tumour. The success of liver transplantation now presents the possibility of performing a liver and upper vena caval transplant after complete excision of the tumour mass.

When the tumour cannot be excised and the patient has the Budd–Chiari syndrome, some form of portal–systemic shunt should be considered (e.g. a portal or mesenteric–atrial shunt).[12]

Intravenous leiomyomatosis

The form of treatment described in the preceding paragraphs refer to tumours that are arising from the wall of the inferior vena cava and often, by the time of presentation, spreading into surrounding tissues. They can only be treated by extensive excision.

Pelvic – probably uterine – tumours which spread along the lumen of the iliac veins and vena cava do not invade the vein wall and can often be removed through a venotomy with forceps or a balloon catheter. Tumours extending from the pelvis to the right side of the heart have been removed in this way.[24] It may be necessary to perform a hysterectomy and to clear out the vena cava in stages. Although some tumour must be left behind after this type of operation, recurrence is uncommon and may not appear for many years,[14] presumably because this type of tumour spread is associated with a very low grade of malignancy.

References

1. Abell MR. Leiomyosarcoma of the inferior vena cava. *Am J Clin Pathol* 1957; **28:** 272.
2. Adebonojo SA, Atil PC, Christiansen KH, Stainback WC, Williams KR. Acute ligation of inferior vena cava above renal veins. A clinical and experimental appraisal of graft replacement of inferior vena cava above renal veins. *J Cardiovasc Surg* 1973; **14:** 508.
3. Annetts DL, Graham AB. Cystic degeneration of the femoral vein. *Br J Surg* 1980; **67:** 287.
4. Arland R. Venous angiomas. *Phlebologie* 1980; **33:** 547.
5. Atkins HB, Key JA. A case of myxomatous tumour arising in the adventitia of the left external iliac artery. *Br J Surg* 1947; **34:** 426.
6. Baggish MS. Mesenchymal tumours of the uterus. *Clin Obstet Gynaecol* 1947; **17:** 51.
7. Bailey RV, Stribling J, Weitzner S, Hardy JD. Leiomyosarcoma of the inferior vena cava. *Ann Surg* 1976; **184:** 169.
8. Beck AD. Resection of the suprarenal inferior vena cava for retroperitoneal malignant disease. *J Urol* 1979; **121:** 112.
9. Brewster DC, Athanasoulis CA, Darling RC. Leiomyosarcoma of the inferior vena cava. *Arch Surg* 1976; **111:** 1081.
10. Cameron AEP, Graham JC, Cotton LT. Intracaval leiomyomatosis. *Br J Obstet Gynaecol* 1983; **90:** 272.
11. Cameron JL, Herlong HF, Sanfoy H, *et al.* The Budd–Chiari syndrome: treatment by mesenteric–systemic venous shunts. *Ann Surg* 1983; **198:** 335–46.
12. Caplan BB, Halasz NA, Bloomer WE. Resection and ligation of the suprarenal inferior vena cava. *J Urol* 1964; **92:** 25.
13. Chauhan MA, Smith PL, Ferris EJ, Murphy K, Westbrook K, Slayden JE. Leiomyosarcoma of the inferior vena cava: angiographic and computed tomography findings. *Cardiovasc Intervent Radiol* 1981; **4:** 209.
14. Clement BP. Intravascular leiomyomatosis of the uterus. *Pathol Annu* 1988; **23(Pt2):** 153–83.
15. Couinaud C. Tumeurs de la veine cava inférieure. *J Chir (Paris)* 1973; **105:** 411.
16. Flores Torre M, Merino Angulo J, Villanueva Marcos R, Aguirre Errasti C. Leiomyosarcome de la veine cava inférieure revelé par un syndrome fébrile. *Nouv Presse Med* 1981; **10:** 3493.
17. Frileux CI, Le Baleur A, Uzan E. Obstruction of the iliac vein by mucoid cyst. *J Cardiovasc Surg* 1979; **20:** 517.
18. Fujiwara Y, Cohn LH, Adams D, Collins JJ. Use of Gore-Tex grafts for replacement of the superior and inferior venae cavae. *J Thorac Cardiovasc Surg* 1974; **67:** 774.
19. Fyfe NCM, Silcocks PB, Browse NL. Cystic mucoid degeneration in the wall of the femoral vein. *J Cardiovasc Surg* 1980; **21:** 703.

20. Ghadially FN, Mehta PN. Multifunctional mesenchymal cells resembling smooth muscle cells in ganglia of the wrist. *Ann Rheum Dis* 1971; **30:** 31.

21. Goerttler U, Noldge G, Baumeister I, Bohn N. Cava Verschluss-Syndrome durch ein Leiomyosarkom der Vena Cava inferior. *Radiologie* 1977; **17:** 350.

22. Gomez-Ferrer F. Cystic degeneration of the wall of the femoral vein. *J Cardiovasc Surg* 1966; **7:** 162.

23. Greenfield LJ, Peyton JWR, Crute S. Hemodynamics and renal function following experimental suprarenal vena caval occlusion. *Surg Gynecol Obstet* 1982; **155:** 37.

24. Grella L, Arnold TE, Kvilekval KHU, Giron F. Intravenous leiomyomatosis. *J Vasc Surg* 1994; **20:** 987–94.

25. Hallock CJ, Watson CJ, Berman L. Primary tumour of the vena cava with clinical features suggestive of Chiari's disease. *Arch Intern Med* 1940; **66:** 50.

26. Kevorkian J, Cento DP. Leiomyosarcoma of large arteries and veins. *Surgery* 1973; **73:** 390.

27. Kieffer E, Berrod JL, Chometter G. Primary tumours of the inferior vena cava. In: Bergan JJ, Yao JS, eds. *Surgery of the Veins.* Orlando, FL: Grune & Stratton, 1985; 423.

28. Knauer E. Beitrag zur anatomie der uterusmyome. *Beitr Geburtshilfe Gynakol* 1903; **1:** 695–735.

29. Larmi TKI, Niinimaki T. Leiomyosarcoma of the femoral vein. *J Cardiovasc Surg* 1974; **15:** 602.

30. Lewis GJT, Douglas DM, Reid W, Kennedy Watt J. Cystic adventitial disease of the popliteal artery. *Br Med J* 1967; **2:** 411.

31. Lintner F, Faust U, Nowotny C. Ein maligner entartetes primares Leiomyom der Vena Cava inferior (Leiomyosarkom) unter dem klinishen Bild des Chiari–Buddschen Syndromes. *Wien Klin Wochenschr* 1978; **90:** 485.

32. Lofgren EP, Lofgren KA. Surgical treatment of cavernous haemangiomas. *Surgery* 1985; **97:** 474.

33. Mandelbaum I, Pauletto FJ, Nasser WK. Resection of a leiomyoma of the inferior vena cava that produced tricuspid valvular obstruction. *J Thorac Cardiovasc Surg* 1974; **67:** 561.

34. McCombs PR, Delaurentis DA. Division of the left renal vein: guidelines and consequences. *Am J Surg* 1979; **138:** 257.

35. McDermott WV, Stone MD, Bothe A Jr, Trey C. Budd–Chiari syndrome. Historical and clinical review with an analysis of surgical corrective procedures. *Am J Surg* 1984; **147:** 463–7.

36. Melchior E. Sarkom der Vena Cava inferior. *Dtsch Z Chir* 1928; **213:** 135.

37. Mentha C. La degenerescence mucoide des veines. *Presse Med* 1963; **71:** 2205.

38. Norris HJ, Parmley T. Mesenchymal tumours of the uterus. V. Intravenous leiomyomatosis. A clinical and pathologic study of 14 cases. *Cancer* 1975; **36:** 2164–78.

39. Nyman U, Hellekant C, Jonsson K. Angiography in leiomyosarcoma of the inferior vena cava. *Br J Radiol* 1979; **52:** 273.

40. Picard JD, Denis P, Chambeyron Y, *et al.* Leiomyosarcomes de la veine cava inférieure. *Chirurgie* 1983; **109:** 306.

41. Rutner R. Pathologie Radiologie und Chirugie de zystischen adventitia degeneration peripher blutgefasse. *Vasa* 1977; **6:** 94.

42. Shida T, Yoshimura M, Chihara H, Nakamura K. Intravenous leiomyomatosis of the pelvis with re-extension into the heart. *Ann Thorac Surg* 1986; **42:** 104–6.

43. Sitzenfry A. Ueber venenmyome des uterus mit intravaskularem wachstum. *Z Geburtshilfe Gynakol* 1911; **68:** 1–25.

44. Taheri SA, Conner GW. Leiomyosarcoma of the iliac veins. *Surgery* 1983; **94:** 516.

45. Trout HH, McAllister HA, Giordano JM, Rich NM. Vascular malformations. *Surgery* 1985; **97:** 36.

46. Van Der Molen HR. Use of Doppler ultrasound in the examination of the extent of venous angiomas. *Phlebologie* 1976; **29:** 9.

47. Woollard HH. The development of the principal arterial stems in the forelimb of the pig. In: *Contributions to Embryology.* Washington, DC: Carnegie Institute of Washington, 1921; **14(70):** 141.

48. Young R, Friedman AC, Hartman DS. Computed tomography of leiomyosarcoma of the inferior vena cava. *Radiology* 1982; **145:** 99.

Index

Abdominal radiographs in Klippel–Trenaunay
    syndrome 681
Abdominal tumours
    deep veins obstruction by, thrombosis distinguished
        from 297
    inferior vena cava obstruction by 430
Absorbent dressings 577
    occlusive and 577–8
Aches, varicose veins 164–5
Achilles tendon lengthening 500
Achilles tendonitis 299
Acidification of ulcer surface 591
Actisorb 577
Activated partial thromboplastin time, heparin dose
    and 341
Activated protein C resistance, *see* Protein C
Adenosine diphosphatase 260
Adhesion molecules, leucocyte (in thrombosis
    aetiology) 258–9
Adhesive bandages 575
Admission for varicose vein surgery, duration 231
Adrenergic innervation 52–3
Adventitial coat (tunica adventitia) 27
Aetius of Amida 3
Afghanistan War 712
Age
    calf muscle pump failure syndrome and 467
    thrombosis and 270
    valve changes with 387
    varicose veins and 153
AIDS ulcers 560
Air embolism 624
    phlebography risk 101
    with venous injuries 724
Air plethysmography 118–20
    ulcers 539
Alberti, Saloman 5
Albumin microaggregates, Tc-99m-labelled 307
Alginates 578
Allergic reactions
    elastic materials 495
    sclerosants 235
    thrombolytics 322
    see also Sensitivity reactions

Allevyn 577, 580
Allografts, valve, experimental 403–4
Alopecia with heparin 344
Ambulation in thrombophylaxis 368
American Vascular Society, classification of clinical
    severity of signs/symptoms of chronic venous
    insufficiency 70
American Venous Forum, classification of clinical
    severity of signs/symptoms of chronic venous
    insufficiency 70–1
Amnion, human 584
Amniotic fluid embolism 624
Amputation
    with chronic venous ulcers 598
    in Klippel–Trenaunay syndrome 685
    thrombosis risk following 254
    traumatic 726
Amynos, Doctor 1, 2
Anabolic steroids
    in lipodermatosclerosis 497, 498–500, 582, 595–6
    in superficial thrombophlebitis 662
    with ulcers 582
        in preventing recurrence 595–6
Anaemia and ulceration 566, 597
Anaesthesia
    sapheno-femoral junction ligation 196
    thrombectomy 330
Analgesia after varicose vein surgery 231
Anaphylactic reactions to sclerosant 235
Anastomosis
    arteriovenous fistula improving patency rates
        719–20
    end-to-end 719
    history 718
Anatomy 30–47
    in CEAP classification (of clinical severity of
        signs/symptoms of chronic venous insufficiency)
        70
    Leonardo da Vinci's drawings 4
    radiographic 30–47
    Vesalius' description 5
    see also specific structures
Aneurysms, aortic, inferior vena cava obstruction with
    430

Angiography, *see* Arteriography; Digital subtraction
     angiography; Magnetic resonance imaging;
     Phlebography; Pulmonary angiography
Angioma/haemangioma, venous (cavernous
     haemangioma) 668, 732–42
  clinical presentation 734
  investigation
     CT 108, 735
     MRI phlebography 105, 106, 107, 735
  pathology 734
  treatment 736–42
Angioplasty, *see* Dilatation (surgical)
Ankle
  'blow-out veins' 19–20
  dilated intradermal venules 536–7
  joint stiffness in calf pump failure syndrome 478
  oedema 166, 167–8
     thrombosis distinguished from 299
     thrombosis-related 292
  plantar flexion, *see* Plantar flexion
  saphenous vein pressure measurement at 19
Ankle flare (corona phlebectatica) 171, 172, 536–7
  in calf pump failure syndrome 459
  varicose vein diagnostic pathways regarding 186–7
Ankylosis 597
Antero-lateral approach to calf (duplex ultrasound) 83
Antero-lateral superficial veins of thigh 39
  ligation at sapheno-femoral junction regarding 201
Antheor filter 642–3
  misplacement 648
Anthrax 562
Antibiotics
  calf pump failure 496
  venous ulcers
     systemic 565, 583
     topical 581–2
  venous wounds 720
Antibodies, *see* Autoantibodies; Monoclonal antibodies
Anticardiolipin antibody 268
Anticoagulants (drugs)
  pulmonary embolism prevention, *see subentries below*
  pulmonary embolism therapy 618–19, 621–2
     oral, *see* Oral anticoagulants
     parenteral, *see* Heparin
  thrombosis prophylaxis (=primary prevention of
        pulmonary embolism) 360–7, 632–4, 635
     oral, *see* Oral anticoagulants
     parenteral, *see* Heparin
  thrombosis therapy (=secondary prevention of
        pulmonary embolism) 320, 340–51, 649–51
     oral, *see* Oral anticoagulants
     parenteral, *see* Heparin
     thrombolytics compared with 328
  venous injury 718
Anticoagulants (endogenous) in thrombosis aetiology
     260–1
  lupus 268
Antiphospholipid antibodies 267–9
Antiplatelet activity, thrombosis aetiology and
     reduction in 259–60
Antiplatelet drugs in thrombosis prevention 367–8,
     635–6
  postoperative 269, 368, 635–6

Antiseptics, ulcers 581
Antithrombin deficiency 265
Aortic aneurysms, inferior vena cava obstruction with
     430
Aplasia (absence)
  valves 148, 387, 669
  veins 665
     deep 679, 681
     inferior vena cava 24, 26, 670
     pelvic 413
Arm phlebography 87–8
  for valve transplant 393
  see also Upper limb veins
Artefactual ulceration 551–2
Arteriography
  arterial ulcers 539
  haemangioma 735
  in Klippel–Trenaunay syndrome 681
  pulmonary, *see* Pulmonary angiography
Arteriovenous fistula 556–7
  accidentally manufactured 716
  adjuvant/deliberately manufactured
     in iliac vein bypass 420
     in thrombectomy 333, 338
     venous anastomosis patency improved by 719–20
  calf pump failure distinguished from 480
  phlebography risk 101
  thrombosis distinguished from 299
  traumatic 716, 724, 725
  ulceration caused by 556–7
  varicose veins and 152
Arteriovenous shunts
  in calf pump failure syndrome 465
  ulceration and 511, 512
Arteritis, differentiation from calf pump failure 480
Artery/arteries
  iliac veins compressed by 409, 411–12, 417
  injury/damage
     in varicose vein surgery 204, 210
     venous injury associated with 711–12, 713
  insufficiency 537, 539–60
     stripping of long saphenous vein contraindicated in
        210
     ulcers caused by 537, 539–60
  ischaemia (acute), thrombosis differentiated from 297
  peripheral
     disease, differentiation from calf pump failure
        479–80
     pulse, loss 293–4
  puncture wounds (recent), thrombolytics
     contraindicated with 322
  sclerosant injected accidentally into 236
  veins and, recognition of differences 3
  see also specific arteries
Artery forceps, fine, for vein avulsion 224, 225
Arthritis
  calf pump failure syndrome distinguished from 481
  knee, distinguished from thrombosis 299
  rheumatoid, *see* Rheumatoid arthritis
Arthrography, haemangioma 735
Arthroplasties (joint replacement), thrombophylaxis
  mechanical 370
  pharmacological 360, 362, 365–6, 633

Arthroscopy, haemangioma 735
Ascites, inferior vena cava obstruction with 430
Aserbine 581, 582
Aspirin
  thrombophylactic 367–8, 635–6
  with venous ulcers 583
Atrial pressure with pulmonary embolism, right 617
Atriocaval shunt in inferior vena caval injury 721–2
Atrophie blanche 557, 559
  causes 477, 518
    calf pump failure syndrome 461, 465, 477
    varicose veins 173, 174
    other 481
Attenuation of sound waves in Duplex ultrasound
    79
Auscultation 70
  varicose veins 176
Autoantibodies to phospholipids 267–9
Autografts
  skin
    in calf pump failure 500
    ulcers 584–9
  valve, experimental 402–3
  veins, for injury repair 719
Autopsy evidence of thrombosis/pulmonary embolism
    epidemiology 251–2
Avicenna 3
Avulsion of varicose veins 222–6
Axial vein thrombosis
  thrombectomy, postoperative phlebography 336
  thrombolytics 329
    vs. anticoagulants 328
Axillary vein
  anatomy 44, 45
  thrombosis 689–702
    aetiology 689–93
    clinical features 693–4
    diagnosis/investigations 695–6
    differential diagnosis 694–5
    prognosis 701–2
    treatment 696–701
  ultrasound 81
Azygos vein 46–7
  anatomy 46–7
  development 24
  dilated/enlarged 436, 670

Bacillus anthracis (anthrax) 562
Bacteria in venous ulcers 523–4, 564–6, 583
Bacterial gangrene, synergistic 556
Baghdad boil 554–5
Baker's cyst, ruptured 296
Ballie M 9
Balloon catheter in thrombectomy 331
Balloon dilatation, *see* Dilatation
Bandages 573–7, 578–80
  in calf pump failure 495
  elastic, *see* Elastic compression bandages
  for ulcers 573–7, 578–80
    compression, *see* Compression bandages
    paste, *see* Paste bandages
  see also Dressings
Basal cell carcinomas 541, 598

Basilic vein
  anatomy 44
  ultrasound 81
Basle definition of varicose veins 145
Baynton T 10
Bazin's disease 545
Bed rest
  thrombosis and 20
  ulcers healed by 580–1
    historical accounts 12, 20, 580
Bed sores 553–4
Behçet's syndrome, thrombosis risk 271
β₂-glycoprotein I 268
Biochemistry, pulmonary embolism 611
Biopsy (and subsequent histology)
  in lipodermatosclerosis 483
  liver/kidney, thrombolytics contraindicated with 322
  lymph node 435
  ulcer 538, 542–3, 566
Birch sprigs/twigs, *see* Intradermal venules, dilated
Bird's nest filter 640–1
Bisgaard regimen 19
Blancardus 9
Blastomycosis 562
Bleeding, *see* Haemorrhage; Haemorrhagic/bleeding
    disorders
Blister(s), infected 560
Blistering/bullous disorders 557, 558
Blood, Harvey's observations on circulation 6, 7
Blood dyscrasias/diseases
  superficial thrombophlebitis with 659
  ulcers associated with 551
Blood flow, calf, in Klippel–Trenaunay syndrome 673
Blood flow, venous 52
  assessment 262
    ultrasound, *see* Ultrasound
  obstruction, *see* Obstruction
  respiration and 59, 122
  see also Outflow
Blood gases, pulmonary embolism 611
Blood pool scintigraphy 102–3
Blood pressure, raised, *see* Hypertension
Blood tests
  calf pump failure syndrome 483
  inferior vena cava obstruction 435
  Klippel–Trenaunay syndrome 681
  thrombosis 308, 435
  ulcers 563
Blood volume, venous 51
  in calf, isotope plethysmography measuring 129
'Blow-out/blow-down veins' 19–20, 458, 474
  ulcers and 537
Blue leg 293
Blue-line bandages 575
Boil, Buruli/Baghdad 554–5
Bone
  fracture, *see* Fracture
  in Klippel–Trenaunay syndrome 673
    malformation 678
    overgrowth/hypertrophy 673, 677
  puncture/injection for phlebography, *see* Intraosseous
    phlebography
Borgnis system 593–4, 594

Bowel habit and varicose veins 154
Boyd's (communicating) vein 43
  ligation 221
Brachial vein
  anatomy 44
  phlebography in axillary/subclavian vein thrombosis
    696
  ultrasound 81
Brachiocephalic vein
  anatomy 44, 45
  development 23
    anomalies/variations 26, 28, 45
  ultrasound 81
Breast cancer treatment, axillary vein thrombosis
    associated with 693
Briquet, Paul 10
Brodie B 10
Brodie–Trendelenburg test, *see* Tourniquet test
Bronchial carcinoma, superior vena cava obstruction
    with 702, 704, 707
Budd–Chiari syndrome
  bypass operation 439
  leiomyosarcoma causing 743, 745
Buerger's disease, thrombosis risk 271
Bullae, *see* Blister; Blistering disorders
Burns
  carcinoma arising in old (Marjolin's ulcer) 542, 598
  thrombosis risk 254
  ulceration following 555
Buruli boil 554–5
Bypass operation
  axillary/subclavian vein 699–701
  deep vein
    grafts for, *see* Grafts
    historical accounts 20
    iliac vein, *see* Iliac vein
    inferior vena cava 439–40, 671
    superficial femoral vein 20, 422–5, 492
    in ulcer recurrence prevention 593
  superior vena cava 707

Calcification
  subcutaneous 559
  in varicose veins 156, 157
  see also Phleboliths
Calf (lower leg)
  blood flow in Klippel–Trenaunay syndrome 673
  blood volume, isotope plethysmography measuring 129
  compression/squeezing, thrombus and risk of
    detachment with 122
  tenderness
    palpation for 292
    thrombosis-related 292
Calf muscle
  electrostimulation in thrombophylaxis 370
  thrombosis-related induration 292
  varicose vein-related changes in 158
  venous ulceration and malfunction of 519
Calf muscle pump 55–61
  chamber, *see* Deep compartment
  first description 6
  function (physiology) 57–9
    anatomy related to 55–7

  in Klippel–Trenaunay syndrome 672
  thrombosis affecting 454–8
  functional assessment 481–2
    foot vein pressure in 58, 112–14
    plethysmography in 115–21, 131
    ulcers and 566
    value of various tests 131
  outflow tract, *see* Outflow tract
Calf muscle pump failure syndrome (inclusive of post-
    thrombotic syndrome) 443–503, 508–10
  causes 59–61, 443
  clinical presentation 473–9
  diagnosis 474–9
    differential 479–81
  first description 18
  investigations 479–83
  natural history 485–6
  pathology 443–71
  prevalence 466–7
  prevention (of post-thrombotic sequelae)
    heparin 328, 348
    oral anticoagulants 351
    thrombectomy 337
    thrombolytics 328
  severity of disease in, assessment 481–3
  treatment 486–92, 589–91
    palliative 492–500
  ulceration associated with 479, 508–10, 589–91
  venous reconstruction and risk of 724
Calf veins
  communicating 43
    incompetence, comparison of various location
      methods 175
    incompetence, ulceration and 506–8
    medial, ligation 215–21
  deep, anatomy 31–3
  incompetence 456, 458
    calf pump function and effects of 456, 458
    combined with outflow tract
      obstruction/incompetence 458
    communicating, *see subheading above*
  obstruction
    combined with outflow tract
      obstruction/incompetence 458
    thrombotic, *see subheading below*
  superficial 37–40 *passim*
  thrombosis 83, 449–50
    phlebography 97
    plethysmography's inability to detect minor
      thrombosis 128
    reopening after 447
    sequelae 449–50, 456
    thrombolytics 326, 329
    treatment plan 353
    ultrasound 83
  ultrasound 83
  varices, diagnostic pathways with 187
Calipers, neuropathic ulcers with 545
Callender GW 14–15
Camera
  gamma, in lung scintigraphy 108
  light photography 73
Canadian Sickness Survey, varicose veins 146

Canano, Gian Battista 5
Cancer, *see* Malignant tumours
Capillaries (venular)
    in calf pump failure 459–61, 465, 510–12
    permeability, *see* Permeability
    pressure measurement, historical account 17
    stasis, ulceration and 510–12
Carcinomas
    breast, axillary vein thrombosis associated with
        treatment for 693
    bronchial, superior vena cava obstruction with 702,
        704, 707
    cutaneous, ulcerating 541–3, 598
    renal, inferior vena cava obstruction with 429, 436
Cardinal veins
    anterior, development 23
    posterior, development 23
        anomalies 25
Cardiolipin, autoantibodies 268
Cardiovascular reflexes 54
Carrel triangulation technique 719
Catheter(s)
    balloon, in thrombectomy 331
    venous injuries caused by 715
Catheterization
    right heart 613
    subclavian vein, causing thrombosis 692
Caudad compression 124
Caval veins, *see* Vena cava
Cavernous haemangioma, *see* Angioma
CEAP classification 70–1
Cellulitis
    lipodermatosclerosis distinguished from 481
    lymphoedema with, differentiation from thrombosis
        296
    misdiagnosis 477, 478, 536
    with ulcers 597
Celsus AC 3
Cephalad compression 124
Cephalic vein
    anatomy 44
        variations 45
    ultrasound 81
Cervical rib 689, 690
    resection 699
'Champagne bottle' legs 597
Chapman HT 12
Chest infection, varicose vein surgery 230
Chest radiography
    axillary/subclavian vein thrombosis 696
    in Klippel–Trenaunay syndrome 681
    pulmonary embolism 610–11
Chilblains 545–6
Children, thrombosis prevention 367
Chinese (ancient) 2
Cinephlebography, thrombosis 304
Circulation of blood, Harvey's observations 6, 7
Claudication, venous
    in chronic deep venous incompetence 389
    pain of 474
Cleanliness, venous ulcers and 520
Cleansing agents to dissolve slough (with venous ulcers)
    581–2

Climate and thrombosis 270
Clinical examination, *see* Examination
Clip, caval, inferior vena cava compression by 435
Clothing and varicose veins 155
Clotting, *see* Coagulation system
Coagulation system
    deficiencies, *see* Haemorrhagic/bleeding disorders
    endothelium and 54
    failure
        death causing, historical account 9
        fright causing, historical account 9
    fibrinolytic and, balance between 19
    in Klippel–Trenaunay syndrome 673
    in thrombosis aetiology, changes
        in axillary/subclavian vein thrombosis 696
        in deep venous thrombosis 264
    see also Hypercoagulability
Coagulopathy in Klippel–Trenaunay syndrome
    678
Coban 575
Cockett's operation 219
Cockett's veins 43
Collagen
    thrombosis aetiology and 256
    in varicose veins 156, 157
        content 151–2
Collateral circulation
    in obstruction 415–16, 448
        caused by thrombosis 448
        of common iliac vein 415
        of external iliac vein 34, 35
        of inferior vena cava 36–7, 38, 415–16
    phlebography (following thrombosis) 97
Colour Doppler ultrasound 80
    deep vein reflux 127
    in Klippel–Trenaunay syndrome 679–81
    thigh veins 82
    thrombosis 305–6
Colour photography 73
Communicating vein(s)
    ligation (lower limb) 215–22, 488–90
        in calf pump failure syndrome treatment 488–90,
            589–90
        complications 221
        historical account 18
        medial calf communicating vein 215–21
        other vein(s) 221
        in ulcer recurrence prevention 592
    lower limb 42–3, 56–7
        anatomy 45–6
        calf, *see* Calf vein(s)
        foot, *see* Foot
        incompetence, *see* Communicating vein
            incompetence
        ligation, *see subheading above*
    shearing 490
    thrombosis 455
    upper limb, anatomy 45–6
    valves 29–30, 52, 56
    varicosities over 171, 172
Communicating vein incompetence/reflux 61, 175–6,
    191–2, 482, 488–91
    definition 192

Communicating vein incompetence/reflux (*contd*)
  investigation/tests
    fluorescein test 129–30
    palpation 175–6
    phlebography 92, 181, 482
    thermography 76
    ultrasound 124–6, 179–82, 482
  post-thrombotic 474
  in pump outflow tract obstruction 448
  recurrence 229
  skin changes related to 191–2
  surgical correction 488–91, 589–90
  ulceration and 506–8, 589, 592
Compression (pathological), deep vein 409–12
  differentiation from thrombosis 297
  imaging 416–17
  inferior vena cava thrombosis secondary to 430
Compression (technique) 573–80
  pneumatic, *see* Pneumatic compression
  squeezing (venous), in ultrasound measurement 122
    downstream 124
    upstream 124
  ulcers 573–80
    in preventing recurrence 593–5, 596
Compression bandages
  elastic, *see* Elastic compression bandages
  postoperative varicose vein surgery 231
    after stripping of long saphenous vein 210
  sclerotherapy with, *see* Sclerotherapy
  for ulcers 574–6
    application 575
    elastic, *see* Elastic compression bandages
    historical accounts 4, 4–5, 11, 15, 573
    medicated 11
    in preventing recurrence 596
Compression stockings
  care 595
  deep venous incompetence 394
  deep venous obstruction 419
  elastic, *see* Elastic compression stockings
  historical account 7
  inferior vena cava occlusion 439
  Klippel–Trenaunay syndrome 682–3
  standardization 593–5
  ulcers 574, 576, 591
    in preventing recurrence 593–5
  varicose veins 237
Computed tomography
  pulmonary arteries 111–12
  spiral, *see* Spiral CT
  veins (CT venography) 103–4
    angioma 108, 735
    cystic mass 732
    inferior vena cava obstruction 433
    in Klippel–Trenaunay syndrome 681
    superior vena cava obstruction 705
Conforming stretch bandages 574
Congenital bony abnormalities in Klippel–Trenaunay
  syndrome 678
Congenital venous abnormalities 665–81
  anatomical anomalies/variations 23–7, 34, 40, 40–1,
    665–70
    in Klippel–Trenaunay syndrome, *see*
      Klippel–Trenaunay syndrome

  valves 148, 387, 669
  see also specific veins
  pathology 665–70
  thrombosis risk 271
Congenital web 689, 690
Consent, informed, contrast media use 99
Consumptive coagulopathy in Klippel–Trenaunay
  syndrome 678
Contact dermatitis and ulcers 597
Continuous wave ultrasonic Doppler equipment 79
Contrast media
  phlebography 87
    adverse reactions 87, 99–100
    calf compression during injection 89
    historical 20
  pulmonary angiography 110, 111
Contusions, venous 714–15
Cooper, Astley 10
Coraderm 578
Coralline thrombus 273
Corethium 584
Corona phlebectatica, *see* Ankle flare
Cosmetic aspects of varicose veins 163–4
  treatment aimed at 193
Cost, economic, venous ulcers 572
Cough impulse test 70, 174
Coumarins, *see* Oral anticoagulants
Cross-leg flap 588
Cross-linked fibrin degradation products, assay 611
Crural veins, ultrasound 83
Cryoglobulinaemia 562
Curum puellarum, *see* Erythrocyanosis frigida
Cusps of valves 51
  floppy, *see* Floppy valve cusps
  mechanical properties 52
  surgery 395–6
  thrombosis destroying 389
Cyst, Baker's, ruptured 296
Cystic degeneration of venous wall 731–2
Cytokines and thrombosis aetiology 259

D-dimer assay 611
da Vinci, Leonardo 4
Dale's technique for applying compression bandage 576
Davies DD 10
De Carnibus 1–2
de Mondeville, Maitre Henri 4
De Motu Cordis 6, 7
De Ulceribus 2
Death certificate, thrombosis/pulmonary embolism
  epidemiological information from 251
Debrisan 582
Decompression, iliac veins 422
Decubitus ulcers 553–4
Deep compartment of calf pump (pump chamber) 55,
  56–7
  communications with superficial compartment 56–7,
    57
  contraction 59
Deep fascia, short saphenous vein piercing 212
Deep veins (in general)
  accidental ligation 723
  aplasia in Klippel–Trenaunay syndrome 679, 683

bypass operation, *see* Bypass operation
in calf pump failure
    role of 482–3
    surgical reconstruction 590–1
    surgical reconstruction of valves of 590–1
compression (pathological), *see* Compression
connections between superficial and
    eradication of all 194–5
    in Klippel–Trenaunay syndrome, abnormal 679,
      680
    surgical exploration (with recurrent varicosities)
      229–30
haemangioma 736, 740–2
incompetence (and reflux – in general/post-
    thrombotic) 389, 404–5
    connection with superficial vein incompetence 11
    correction 394–404, 404, 405
    post-thrombosis 448–9
    ultrasound 127
    value of various tests of 131
    venous ulceration and 506–8
incompetence, chronic 385–408
    clinical presentation 389–90
    diagnosis 389–93
    investigations 390–3
    pathology, *see* Valves
    pathophysiology 389
    treatment 394–404, 404, 405
insufficiency, first operation for 15
in Klippel–Trenaunay syndrome
    abnormal connections between superficial and 679,
      680
    surgery 684
lower limb, anatomy
    calf 31–3
    sole 31
    thigh, *see* Thigh
obstruction (non-thrombotic/in general) 409–28
    aetiology/pathology 409–14
    chronic 409-28
    clinical presentation 415–16
    investigation/tests 15, 131, 416–19
    treatment 419–26
obstruction (thrombotic), *see* Thrombosis
reflux, *see* Reflux
thrombosis, *see* Thrombosis; Thrombus
upper limb
    anatomy 44, 45
    ultrasound 81
valves
    defects 148
    surgical reconstruction 590–1
varicose, special investigations 178–82
with venous ulceration
    reconstructive surgery 590–1, 593
    role of incompetence in genesis 506–8
see also specific veins
Defibrinogenation 351
Defibrotide in lipodermatosclerosis 499–500
Denmark, Sickness Survey of, varicose veins 146
Dermatan sulphate 367
Dermatitis (eczema)
    in calf pump failure syndrome 459, 474–7

contact 597
    ulcers and, association 596–7
    with varicose veins 169, 173
    other causes 480–1
Dermatological preparations for surrounding skin of
    ulcer 582
Dermiflex 578
Dermis, porcine 584
Dermovate 582
Development 23–7
    anomalies/variations, *see* Congenital venous
      abnormalities *and specific veins*
Dextran 367, 634–5
Dextranomer 582
Diabetes, ulcers associated with 544, 555–6
Diastole, calf pump in 58–9
    see also End-diastolic volume
Diathermy sclerosis 237
Diet/nutrition
    ulcers and 561, 566
    varicose veins and 154
Digital subtraction angiography 88, 99
    haemangioma 735, 739
    pulmonary embolism 613–15
    thrombosis 304
      axillary vein 696
      subclavian vein 100, 696
Dihydroergotamine and heparin prophylaxis 363
Dilat(at)ion (pathological)
    azygos vein 436, 670
    examination for 69
    intradermal venules, *see* Intradermal venules, dilated
    saphenous vein, *see* Saphenous vein; Saphenous vein,
      long
    valve ring 388
    in varicose veins 149–50
      as definition of varicose veins 145
      inspection for 173
      location/site (and its determination) 149, 178
    see also Distension
Dilat(at)ion (surgical), endovascular (angioplasty)
    deep veins 422
    superior vena cava 706, 707
Diosmin 496
Discharge from hospital, *see* Hospital
Discomfort, varicose veins 164–5
Disfigurement, varicose veins, *see* Cosmetic aspects
Distension
    collateral veins 415–16
    superficial veins, thrombosis-related 293
    see also Dilatation
Diuretics
    calf pump failure 495–6
    ulcers 583, 591
Doctor Amynos 1, 2
Dodd's/Hunterian (communicating) veins 43
    ligation 221
Doppler ultrasound, *see* Duplex ultrasound; Ultrasound
Dorsiflexion test 293
Double (reduplicated) veins 666
    inferior vena cava 24, 25, 666, 668
Downstream compression 124
Drainage, venous wounds 720

Drapes/towelling
  sapheno-femoral junction ligation 196–7
  sapheno-popliteal junction ligation 211–12
Dressings for ulcers 573, 577–80
  historical accounts 4–5, 573
  see also Bandages
Drugs
  calf pump failure palliation 495–6, 498–500
  injected, phlebitis caused by 716
  interacting with oral anticoagulants 349
  varicose vein palliation 237
  see also specific (types of) drugs
Duplex ultrasound 78–87, 126–7
  colour, *see* Colour Doppler ultrasound
  compared with other imaging techniques 86–7
  equipment/instrumentation 79, 79–80
  incompetence, venous
    communicating 179–82, 482
    deep 390–1
  lower limb (generally) 82–3
  normal veins on 80–7
  obstruction
    deep veins 417
    inferior vena cava 433
  physics 78–9
  sclerotherapy guidance by 235
  superficial thrombophlebitis 659
  thrombosis 81, 305
    accuracy 310
    in pulmonary embolism patients 637
    in thrombolysis monitoring 323
  ulcers 538
  upper limb (generally) 81–2
  varicose veins
    deep 183
    superficial 179
Dysfibrinogenaemia, hereditary 266

Ebers papyrus 1
ECG, pulmonary embolism 610
Echocardiography, pulmonary embolism 611
Economic cost, venous ulcers 572
Eczema, *see* Dermatitis
Egyptians (ancient) 1
Ehlers–Danlos syndrome 557
  varicose veins and 670
Ejection volume (of one calf contraction), assessment 119
Elastic compression bandages
  in calf pump failure syndrome 495
    plus stanozolol 497, 498, 499
    transmural pressure reduction with 195
  for ulcers 574, 575
    historical account 15
Elastic compression stockings
  calf pump failure syndrome 493–5
  care 595
  deep venous obstruction 419
  inferior vena cava occlusion 439
  Klippel–Trenaunay syndrome 682–3
  standardization 593–5
  in thrombophylaxis 368–9
  ulcers 576, 591, 593–5
    in preventing recurrence 593–5

varicose veins 237
Elastin content of varicose veins 151–2
Elastocrepe 575, 579–80
Electrical stimulation of calf muscle in thrombophylaxis 370
Electrocardiogram, pulmonary embolism 610
Electromagnetic wave treatment, ulcers 584
Elevation of limb/leg 70
  calf pump failure syndrome 495
  in thrombophylaxis 368
  ulcers healed by 580–1
    historical accounts 12, 580
Elset 575
Embolectomy 621
Embolism
  air, *see* Air embolism
  amniotic fluid 624
  fat 624
  pulmonary, *see* Pulmonary embolism
Embolus, paradoxical 291, 623
Embryology 23–7
Employment, *see* Occupation
End-diastolic volume
  increased 59
  reduced 59
End-to-end anastomosis 719
Endoscopic ligation of medial communicating veins, subfascial 217, 218, 219
Endoscopy in Klippel–Trenaunay syndrome 681
Endothelin in thrombosis aetiology 260
Endothelium/endothelial cell 54, 255–62, 462–3
  activation in calf pump failure syndrome 462
  activation (in thrombosis aetiology) 257–63
    changes 258–9
    intracellular mechanisms underlying 262
  functions 257
  injury/damage to
    in calf pump failure syndrome 462–3
    in thrombosis aetiology 255–7
Endovascular dilatation and stenting, *see* Dilatation (surgical); Stenting
Enzymatic changes in varicose vein walls (and of patients' relatives) 157–8, 669–70
Epidermis, porcine 584
Epigastric vein, superficial inferior, ligation at sapheno-femoral junction regarding 201
Epiphyseal stapling in Klippel–Trenaunay syndrome 685
Epithelium in venous ulceration 521–2, 522–3
Equinus deformity, *see* Plantar flexion
Erasistratos 3
Erect stance and venous ulcers, 519–20
  see also Posture
Erythema induratum scrofulosum 545
Erythrocyanosis frigida (curum puellarum) 545–6
  lipodystrophy with 296–7
Erythrocytes, Tc-99m-labelled 306
Ethnicity, *see* Race
Ethyloestrenol in superficial thrombophlebitis 662
Examination, clinical/physical 69–72
  axillary/subclavian vein thrombosis 695
  calf pump failure syndrome 481
  ulcers, *see* Ulcers
  varicose vein patient 169–77

Excisional operations
  tumours
    cystic degeneration of vein wall 732
    haemangioma 736–42
    inferior vena cava-obstructing 440
  varicose veins
    of all visible varices, symptom relief via 194
    of tributaries 222–5
  venous ulcers
    slough 581
    of ulcer base 584–7
Exercise
  foot vein pressure changes during, *see* Foot veins
  foot volumetry in, *see* Foot volumetry
  venous emptying during, assessment of pump
    function via 481–2
  venous refilling after, strain-gauge plethysmography
    in assessment of 118
Exercise phlebography 89
Extrafascial ligation of medial communicating veins 219
Extravasation of contrast media into skin 99, 101

Fabricius, H 5–6
Factor VIII
  elevated 267
  endothelium and 54
Factor XII deficiency 267
Fallopius (Fallopio) 5, 6
Family history of varicose veins 155, 169, 670
Fascia
  deep, short saphenous vein piercing 212
  palpation for defects 175–6
  see also Extrafascial ligation; Subfascial ligation;
    Subfascial shearing
Fasciitis, necrotizing 556
Fasciotomy 720–1
Fat embolism 624
Fat necrosis 536
Feet, *see* Foot
Femoral arteriography with ulcers 539
Femoral artery damage in varicose vein surgery 204
Femoral veins (generally/unspecified)
  blood flow, respiration affecting 122
  compression (Gullmo's phenomenon) 412–13
    phlebography 417
  ligation, *see* Ligation
  ligation of long saphenous vein and its tributaries
    flush with, *see* Saphenous vein, long
  percutaneous access to vena cava via 645
  phlebography 93
  pressure measurement 114–15, 419
  thrombosis, imaging 85, 97
    see also Ilio-femoral thrombosis
  valves
    absence 148
    cusps, mechanical properties 52
  wall
    cyst 732
    leiomyosarcoma 743
  see also under Sapheno-femoral
Femoral veins, common
  anatomy 34
  damage in varicose vein surgery 204

  stenting 424
  thrombosis, reopening after 447
Femoral veins, deep (profunda)
  anatomy 33–4
  anomalies 34
  transposition (for valve replacement) 398, 399
  ultrasound
    duplex 83
    in incompetence 390
  valves 29
Femoral veins, superficial
  anatomy 33
  anomalies 34
    in Klippel–Trenaunay syndrome 679, 681
  incompetence 457–8
    combined with iliac vein obstruction/incompetence
     457–8
    surgery 398, 399
    ultrasound 390
  ligation, thrombosis 'locked in' by 648–9
  obstruction 457–8, 492
    bypass operation, *see* Bypass operation
    combined with iliac vein obstruction/incompetence
     457–8
    by thrombosis, *see subheading below*
  thrombosis
    management 338
    reopening after 447
  ultrasound
    duplex 82
    in incompetence 390
  valves 29
Femoro-femoral bypass operation 420–2
  historical account 20
Fetal toxicity, oral anticoagulants 350
Fetal veins, persistent 668
  in Klippel–Trenaunay syndrome 675, 679
Fever with thrombosis 294
'Fibrin barrier hypothesis'
  in calf pump failure syndrome 465
  ulceration and 511, 512–16
Fibrin degradation products, cross-linked, assay 611
Fibrinogen
  in lymph, venous hypertension and 460
  Tc-99m-labelled 307
  see also Dysfibrinogenaemia
Fibrinogen uptake test 76–8, 306
  accuracy 77–8
  application 77
  development 21
  method 76–7
Fibrinolytic activator, vein wall 658–9
  deficiency 658–9, 662
    management 662
  production 20, 54
Fibrinolytic activity/fibrinolysis (endogenous)
  in calf pump failure syndrome 498–500
    drugs enhancing 494, 498–500
    reduced 463
  coagulation and, balance between 19
  excessive, postoperative 17
  historical mentions 11, 17, 19
    of physiological fibrinolysis 18–19

Fibrinolytic activity/fibrinolysis (endogenous) (*contd*)
  in lipodermatosclerosis treatment, drugs stimulating
    368
  in superficial thrombophlebitis
    drugs enhancing 662
    reduced 658–9
  in thrombotic disease aetiology 261–2, 264
    in axillary vein thrombosis 691
    reduced 54, 261–2, 454
  in thrombotic disease prevention, drugs stimulating
    368
  in thrombotic disease sequelae 454
  with ulcers
    drugs enhancing 582, 595–6
    reduced 512–16
  in varicose veins 454
Fibrinolytic drugs, *see* Thrombolysis
Fibrosis, retroperitoneal, *see* Retroperitoneal fibrosis
Filters, vena cava 622, 639–48
  complications 645–8
  contraindications 644–5
  indications 643–4
  placement technique 645
  temporary 643
  types 640–3
Finger, sliding, over incompetent communicating veins
  176
First rib resection 699
First World War, venous injuries 711
Fistula
  arteriovenous, *see* Arteriovenous fistula
  lymph 228–9
Flaps, skin
  in calf pump failure 500
  for ulcers 588–9
Floppy valve cusps 388, 669
  correction 395–6
Fluid, tissue, principle underlying production, historical
  explanations 15
Fluorescein test 129–30
Foam dressings 578
Foot
  'trash' 550
  weight-bearing in calf pump failure syndrome 478
Foot veins
  anatomy 30–1
  communicating veins 31, 42
    valves 30
  pressure measurements during exercise 58, 112–14
    post-valve repair 396
Foot volumetry 120–1
  calf pump assessment via 482
  deep venous incompetence and 391–3
  in Klippel–Trenaunay syndrome 678
  saphenous vein reflux and 482
  ulcers and 538
Forceps, fine artery, for vein avulsion 224, 225
Fractures
  pathological, thrombosis distinguished from 298
  thrombosis after 253
    prophylaxis 360, 362
  see also Injury
Franklin KJ 16

Free radicals in ulcer aetiology 517
Function (physiology) of veins 49–65
  first description 1
  investigations/tests 112–30, 131
    historical 19
    in venous obstruction 417–19
    in venous ulceration 538–9
  thrombosis affecting 444–54

Gaiter region/skin, ulcers in 533, 534
  aetiology of 520–1
Galen of Pergamum 3
Gamma camera in lung scintigraphy 108
Gangrene
  synergistic bacterial 556
  venous
    deep venous thrombosis-related 293
    historical descriptions 6, 17
    of upper extremity 694
  venous injury complicated by 726
Gas(es), blood, pulmonary embolism 611
Gastrocnemius muscle
  torn 296
  veins 28, 29
    communicating vein, ligation 221
    thrombosis, ultrasound 83
Gastrointestinal ulcers, thrombolytics contraindicated
  with 323
Gauze 577
Gay, John 12–13, 508
Geliperm 578
Gender
  thrombosis and 270
  varicose veins and 153
General anaesthesia
  sapheno-femoral junction ligation 196
  thrombectomy 330
Genetics, *see* Inherited disorders; Inherited factors
β_2-Glycoprotein I 268
Goitre, retrosternal 702, 703
Gouty tophi 559
Graduated compression in prevention of ulcer
  recurrence 593
Grafts
  for bypass operations
    experimental 425–6
    for iliac vein bypass 420–2
    for superficial femoral vein bypass 422–5, 492
  skin
    in calf pump failure 500
    ulcers 584–9
  veins, for injury repair 719
Granuflex 578
Granulation tissue, healing ulcer 534, 535, 536
Granuloma, pyogenic 559
'Gravitational'/'varicose' ulcers, historical accounts 7,
  13, 16, 505, 509
Gravity 9
Greece (ancient) 1–2
Greenfield filter 640
  maldeployment 646, 647
Groin, recurrent varices 226
  re-exploration for 228–9

Growth, lower limb, control in Klippel–Trenaunay syndrome 685
Growth hormone trapping 517
Gullmo's phenomenon, *see* Femoral veins
Gummata 549
Gunther tulip filter 642, 643
  malaligned/misplaced 646, 649
Gynaecological surgery, thrombosis after 253
  mechanical prophylaxis 369, 370
  pharmacological prophylaxis 360, 362, 365
    new drugs 367

Haemangioma, *see* Angioma
Haematological disorders, *see* Blood dyscrasias
Haematuria in Klippel–Trenaunay syndrome 675, 685
Haemodilution, thrombosis risk 271
Haemodynamics and varicose veins 152
Haemophilia, thrombolysis contraindicated in 323
Haemorrhage/bleeding 717
  heparin-induced 342, 343–4, 362–3, 619
  from injured veins 717
  rectal, in Klippel–Trenaunay syndrome 675, 685
  in thrombectomy 334
  with thrombolytics 321–2
  thrombosis and, differentiation 297
  from varicose vein 168
  with varicose vein surgery
    in long saphenous vein ligation/division 202–4
    in long saphenous vein stripping 208–9
    in medial communicating vein ligation 221
  with venous ulcers 597
Haemorrhagic/bleeding disorders (diatheses) as contraindication
  to stripping of long saphenous vein 210
  to thrombolysis 323
Haemosiderin deposits in calf pump failure syndrome 475
Haemostatic abnormalities 263–4
Hair loss with heparin 344
Hale, Stephen 9
Haller A 9
Hand gangrene, axillary/subclavian vein thrombosis 694
Harvey, William 6, 7
Hatra tester 593, 594
Health (general)
  of varicose vein patient 169
  venous ulcers and 520
Health services and effects of venous ulcers 572–3
Heart
  catheterization of right 613
  peripheral, calf muscle as 57
  thrombus in 323
Height
  varicose veins and 154
  venous ulcers and 519–20
Hemi-azygos vein, anatomy 46, 47
Heparan sulphate and thrombosis aetiology 260
Heparin (general aspects), complications 342, 343–4, 619
  thrombocytopenia 344, 363, 605–6, 619
Heparin (pulmonary embolism treatment) 618–19
  low-molecular weight subcutaneous 618
  unfractionated 618–19

Heparin (thrombosis prevention = primary prevention of pulmonary embolism) 361–7, 623, 632–4, 635
  dextran 70 compared with 635
  with dihydroergotamine 363
  first account of use 17
  in Klippel–Trenaunay syndrome 686
  low-molecular weight subcutaneous 363–7, 633–4
    characteristics/properties 364
  postoperative 361–2, 364–6, 633, 636
    historical accounts 18, 19
  unfractionated 361–3, 632–3
    intravenous 363
    low-dose subcutaneous 361–3, 632, 633
Heparin (thrombosis treatment = secondary prevention of pulmonary embolism) 340–8
  administration 342
    intravenous 342
    subcutaneous 342
  dose 341–2
  duration 343
  historical accounts 18
  indications (in treatment of thrombosis) 348
  inferior vena cava thrombus 438
  low molecular weight 344–5
  monitoring 342–4
  preoperative 330
  results 344–8, 350
    post-thrombotic syndrome prevention 328, 348
  thrombolytics followed by 324
Heparin cofactor II deficiency 267
Hepatic vein
  drainage in subdiaphragmatic vena caval occlusion 670
  leiomyosarcoma at/above 743, 745
  leiomyosarcoma between renal and 745
Heredity, *see* Inherited disorders; Inherited factors
Herophilos 3
Hexosamine content of varicose veins 151–2
Hilton J 12
Hip
  fractures, thrombophylaxis 360, 362
  surgery (replacement etc.)
    mechanical thrombophylaxis 370
    pharmacological thrombophylaxis 360, 362, 633
Hippocrates 1–2
Hirudin 367
Histology, *see* Biopsy
History (of patient)
  in calf pump failure syndrome 473
  with varicose veins 169
    family 155, 169, 670
  with venous ulcers 531–2
History (of venous medicine) 1–22
  deep venous incompetence surgery 394
  thrombosis aetiology 9, 11, 15, 255
  venous repair 718
  venous ulcer treatment
    bandages/dressings 4, 4–5, 11, 15, 19, 573
    bed rest 12, 20, 580
    limb elevation 12, 580
    surgery 2, 3, 7
HIV disease/AIDS, ulcers 560
Hohenstein tester 593

Homans, J 16, 509
Homans' dorsiflexion test 293
Home E 10
Homocystinaemia 266–7
Homografts, valve, experimental 403–4
Hooks, phlebectomy 224, 225
Hormone replacement therapy, thrombosis risk 271
Hospital
  admission for varicose vein surgery, duration 231
  discharge
    thrombosis epidemiological information from 251
    varicose vein surgical patient 231
  thrombosis at-risk patient in 300
Hughes syndrome 267–9
Hunt T 575
Hunter J 9
Hunterian communicating veins, *see* Dodd's veins
Hydrocolloids 578
Hydrodynamic valve function 387
Hydrogels 578
Hydrostatic pressure 49–50
  historical observations 10
  valve function regarding 386–7
O-(-β-Hydroxyethyl)-rutoside, *see* Rutosides
Hygiene, personal, venous ulcers and 520
Hyperbaric oxygen with ulcers 591
Hypercoagulability
  axillary/subclavian vein thrombosis and 696
  deep venous thrombosis and 264, 455
Hyperfibrinolysis, postoperative 17
Hyperhomocystinaemia 266–7
Hyperlipidaemia, thrombosis risk 271
Hyperosmolar contrast media, adverse reactions 99
Hypersensitivity, *see* Allergic reactions; Sensitivity
    reactions
Hypertension
  arterial (i.e. hypertension in general)
    Martorell's ulcer and 550–1
    thrombolysis contraindicated in 323
  pulmonary, *see* Pulmonary hypertension
  venous (in calf pump failure syndrome) 492
    clinical presentation 474, 475
    microcirculation and effects of 458–67
Hypodermic needle, invention 10
Hypoplasia 666
  inferior vena cava 24, 666, 667
  superficial femoral vein 679, 681

Iatrogenic causes
  of venous injuries 715–16, 723
  of venous obstruction 414
    inferior vena cava 430
ICAM-1/2 258
Iliac artery
  internal, compressing external iliac vein 411–12
  right common, compressing left common iliac vein
    409
Iliac veins (unspecified portion/in general) 34–6
  aplasia 665, 666
  bypass operation 420–2
    damaged section 722
    history 20
    of obstruction 20, 420–2, 491–2

decompression 422
disobliteration 422
hypoplasia 667
incompetence
  calf pump function and effects of 456–7, 457–8
  combined with superficial femoral vein
    obstruction/incompetence 457–8
injuries 722
leiomyosarcoma 743
obstruction 409–12, 420–2, 456–7, 491–2
  bypass operation 20, 420–2, 491–2
  calf pump function and effects of 456–7, 457–8
  combined with superficial femoral vein
    obstruction/incompetence 457–8
  detection 114–15, 419
  external (compressive) causes 409–12, 417
  intraluminal causes 414
valves, absence 148
Iliac veins, common 34
  anatomy 34
  collateral circulation in obstruction of 415
  left
    agenesis 25
    compression 409, 416
    spurs/webs 414
  ultrasound 82, 83
Iliac veins, external 34
  anatomy 34
  obstruction
    collateral circulation 34, 35
    internal iliac artery compression causing 411–12
  ultrasound 82
Iliac veins, internal 34–6
  anatomy 34–6
  injuries 722
Iliac veins, superficial circumflex, ligation at sapheno-
    femoral junction regarding 201
Ilio-femoral thrombosis
  Palma operation 491–2
  thrombectomy 330–2, 338, 339
    phlebography following 336
Imaging *see specific methods/structures/conditions*
Immobility, prolonged, thrombosis risk 270
Immune-mediated thrombocytopenia in
    antiphospholipid syndrome 269
Impedance plethysmography 128–9
Impregnated bandages 578–80
Impregnated dressings 577
In-situ venous valve construction 402–3
Inanediones 348–51 *passim*
Incisions
  multiple oblique, for medial calf communicating vein
    approach 220
  stocking-seam 219–20
  of veins
    surgical, *see* Venotomy
    traumatic 714
Incompetence (venous/venous valve)
  calf pump outflow tract, *see* Outflow tract
  calf pump vein valve 60
  communicating veins, *see* Communicating vein
    incompetence
  deep veins (in general), *see* Deep veins

femoral veins, *see* Femoral veins, deep; Femoral
    veins, superficial
popliteal vein 390
saphenous vein, *see* Sapheno-femoral junction;
    Saphenous vein, long; Saphenous vein, short
superficial veins, *see* Superficial veins
thrombosis-related 448–9
ultrasound, *see* Ultrasound
in varicose vein aetiology 147–8
    descending 147–8, 149
in varicose vein diagnosis, determining incompetent
    vein 178
see also Insufficiency; Reflux
Indian ulcers 3
Indium-labelled platelets 307
Infection
    antibiotics with, *see* Antibiotics
    thrombus in superficial thrombophlebitis 662
    ulcers and
        in aetiology of ulcers 537, 545, 549–50, 556, 560,
          562
        in development/pathogenesis of venous ulcers 518
        in natural history of venous ulcer 524, 534, 535, 597
    varicose vein surgery and risk of 230
    venous reconstruction and risk of 724–6
    see also Micro-organisms *and specific*
        pathogens/diseases
Inflammation
    valve 388
    vein wall 658
        primary 658
        in response to thrombus 445
Informed consent, contrast media use 99
Infra-red photography 73
Infusion phlebitis 658, 661–2
Ingstron tester 593
Inherited disorder(s)
    Klippel–Trenaunay syndrome as 671
    with thrombosis risk 265, 266, 267
Inherited factors, varicose veins 155
Injection phlebitis 658, 661–2
Injection sclerotherapy, *see* Sclerotherapy
Injection ulcers 236, 561
Injury, traumatic 711–29
    concomitant to venous injury, repair 720
    to gastrocnemius/plantaris muscle 296
    local
        thrombosis secondary to 429
        ulcers caused by, *see* Ulcers (non-venous disease-
          related)
    major, thrombosis in 254
        prevention 366
    to veins 711–29, 723
        classification 714–16
        clinical presentation 717
        complications 724
        deep venous thrombosis risk 270
        incidence 711–14
        investigation 717
        phlebography 89
        superficial thrombophlebitis following 657–8
        treatment 717–26
        valvular 387

see also Fractures
Innervation of veins 52–3
Innominate vein, *see* Brachiocephalic vein
Insect bites, ulceration following 555
Inspection 69–70
    varicose veins 169–73
Inspiration, venous blood flow during 59, 122
Insufficiency
    chronic (in general) 130–2
        classification of clinical severity 70–1
        clinical application of various tests for 130–2
    deep venous
        chronic, thermography 76
        first operation for 15
    superficial venous, *see* Superficial veins
    see also Incompetence
Integrins 258
Interosseous veins, anatomy 44
Interruption, venous, *see* Vena cava, inferior
Intersex state and venous ulcers 520
Interstitial diffusion barrier, *see* 'Fibrin barrier
    hypothesis'
Interstitial space in calf pump failure syndrome 464
Intima 27
    injury causing thrombosis, historical account 11
Intra-arterial injection of sclerosant 236
Intracellular adhesion molecules 1/2 258
Intradermal venules, dilated (birch sprig/twig;
    cutaneous telangiectases; spider bursts/veins/webs;
    sunburst veins; venous stars) 164, 241, 474–5,
    536–7
    at ankle 536–7
    in calf pump failure syndrome 474–5
    treatment 241
    with varicose veins 164, 165, 241
Intramuscular angiomata 740–1
Intraosseous phlebography 94
Intravenous leiomyomatosis 745
Investigations and tests (in general) 68–144
    accuracy/sensitivity/specificity 68–70
    of venous function, *see* Function
    see also specific investigations/tests and conditions
Iron deficiency and ulceration 566, 597
Ischaemia
    arterial
        thrombosis differentiated from acute 297
        ulcers associated with 539
    in ulcer development 518–19
Isotopes, radioactive, *see* Radioisotopes

J Fast 575
Joint
    haemangioma involving 735, 741–2
    inflammation, *see* Arthritis
Jugular vein
    internal, venous repair using 719
    percutaneous access to vena cava via 645
    ultrasound 81

Kaltostat 578
Kaposi's sarcoma 560
Kasabach–Merritt syndrome in Klippel–Trenaunay
    syndrome 678

Kidney
  biopsy, thrombolytics contraindicated with 322
  carcinoma, inferior vena cava obstruction with 429,
    436
Kirstner's direct valvuloplasty (and modifications) 395–6
Klinefelter's syndrome and venous ulcers 520
Klippel–Trenaunay syndrome 671–86
  clinical presentation 673–8
    varicosities 171, 673–6
  congenital anomalies 679–81
    iliac vein hypoplasia 667
  definition 671
  differential diagnosis 681–2
  investigations 678–82
  pathophysiology 672–3
  thrombosis risk 271
  treatment 682–6
Knee (joint)
  disorders distinguished from thrombosis 299
  haemangioma affecting 735
  replacement surgery
    mechanical thrombophylaxis 370
    pharmacological thrombophylaxis 360, 366
  tourniquet below, not controlling below-knee varices
    186–7

L-selectin 258
Laboratory diagnosis of antiphospholipid syndrome 268
Lacerations, venous 714
Langer's lines in ligation/excision of tributaries 222, 223
Laser therapy, ulcers 584
Lateral communicating vein, ligation 221
Lateral limb bud veins, persistent 668
  in Klippel–Trenaunay syndrome 675, 679
Lebanese War 712
Leg
  elevation, *see* Elevation
  ulcers, *see* Ulcers
  white, historical accounts 9, 10
  see also Lower limb
Leiomyoma, *see* Leiomyosarcoma and leiomyoma
Leiomyomatosis, intravenous 745
Leiomyosarcoma and leiomyoma 742–5
  clinical presentation 742–3
  investigations 743
  pathology 742
  treatment 743–5
Leonardo da Vinci 4
Lestraflex 575
Leucocyte (white blood cells), trapping
  in calf pump failure syndrome 461–3
  ulceration and 511, 516–17
Leucocyte adhesion molecules (in thrombosis
    aetiology) 258–9
Leukaemia 551
Ligation (of vessels)
  accidental 414, 415, 715, 723
  caval 639
  communicating vein, *see* Communicating veins
  femoral veins 491
    superficial, thrombosis 'locked in' by 648–9
  first account 3
  popliteal vein, *see* Popliteal vein

at sapheno-femoral junction, *see* Sapheno-femoral
    junction
at sapheno-popliteal junction, *see* Sapheno-popliteal
    junction
superficial veins 589–90
varicose veins 195–204, 210–25
  historical account 3
  percutaneous 237
  of tributaries 195–204, 222–6
  see also specific veins
Light compression bandages 575
Light reflection rheography 115–17
Lighting for photography 72–3
Limb
  elevation, *see* Elevation
  lower, *see* Lower limb
Limb bud veins, lateral, persistent, *see* Lateral limb bud
    veins
Limb veins
  development 26–7
  lower, *see* Lower limb veins
  upper, *see* Upper limb veins
Lines of Zahn and thrombus development 273
Linton's operation, *see* Subfascial ligation
Lipodermatosclerosis 476–7, 498–500
  acute 477
  appearance 172
  biopsy 483
  in calf pump failure syndrome 465, 476–7, 483, 510
    distinguished from cellulitis 481
  chronic 477
  definition 476–7
  palpation 70
  pharmacological management 419, 494, 498–500, 582,
    595–6
  with varicose veins 169
    diagnostic pathways regarding 186–7
Lipodystrophy 168
  differentiation from thrombosis 296–7
Liquid crystal thermography 75–6
Livedo reticularis/vasculitis 557, 559
  in antiphospholipid syndrome 268–9
Liver
  biopsy, thrombolytics contraindicated with 322
  function, in congenital vena caval obstruction 670
Local and regional anaesthesia
  sapheno-femoral junction ligation 196
  thrombectomy 330
Loewenberg test 293
Lowe, Peter 6
Lower, Richard 6
Lower limb
  controlling growth in Klippel–Trenaunay syndrome
    685
  fractures, thrombosis risk 253
  microcirculation, *see* Microcirculation
  see also Leg
Lower limb veins 30–43
  anatomy 30–43
  development 26, 27
  imaging
    phlebography 88–9
    ultrasound 82–3

Lumbar sympathectomy with ulcers 591
Lumbar veins, ascending, anatomy 46, 47
Lung, *see entries under* Pulmonary
Lupus anticoagulant 268
Lupus erythematosus, systemic 547
Lupus pernio 545–6
Lusitanus, Amatus 5
Lymph, fibrinogen, venous hypertension and 460
Lymph fistula 228–9
Lymph node/gland disease
   inferior vena cava obstruction in 430
      investigations 434, 435
   ulcers and examination for 537
Lymphangioma circumscriptum 678
Lymphangiosarcoma 560, 561
Lymphangitis with ulcers 597
Lymphatic system
   in calf pump failure syndrome 464
   in Klippel–Trenaunay syndrome 678
Lymphocele 228–9
Lymphoedema
   calf pump failure distinguished from 480
   with cellulitis, differentiation from thrombosis 296
   historical account 9
   stripping of long saphenous vein contraindicated in 210
   ulcers associated with 554
Lymphography, haemangioma 735
Lyofoam 578
Lyophilized freeze dried porcine epidermis 584
Lysozymes and varicose veins 158

Macroglobulinaemia 561
Magnetic resonance imaging
   of pulmonary tree 112
   of veins (MRI phlebography/venography) 104–8
      angioma 105, 106, 107, 735
      inferior vena cava obstruction 433
      in Klippel–Trenaunay syndrome 681
      thrombosis 304, 433
Malatex 581, 582
Malformations, vascular 668
Malignant tumours 541–3, 742–5
   breast, axillary vein thrombosis associated with
      treatment for 693
   fractures associated with, thrombosis distinguished
      from 298
   iliac vein compressing 410
   inferior vena cava-obstructing
      excision 440
      thrombosis risk 429, 430, 436
   smooth muscle (of vein wall) 742–5
      clinical presentation 742–3
      investigations 743
      pathology 742
      treatment 743–5
   superior vena cava-obstructing 702, 704, 705, 707
   thrombosis risk 270–1
      inferior vena cava 429, 430, 436
   ulcers caused by/associated with 541–3, 560, 598
   see also specific histological types
Marjolin's ulcer 542, 598
Martin HA 15
Martorell's ulcer 550–1

Mass(es), causing venous compression/obstruction
   pelvic 412
   thigh 413
   see also Tumours
Massage
   calf pump failure 495
   ulcers (of surrounding area) 583
Mechanical scanners (duplex ultrasound) 79
Media, *see* Tunica media
Medial calf communicating veins, ligation 215–21
Mediastinal fibrosis 702, 703
Medical illness, thrombosis in 254, 271
   prevention
      mechanical 369, 370
      pharmacological 361, 362, 366–7
Medical services and effects of venous ulcers 572–3
Meleney's ulcer 556
Melolin 577
Membranous occlusion 665–6
Mental illness, self-induced ulceration 551–2
Mesodermal tumours, ulcerating 560
Microcirculation, lower limb 458–67, 510–18
   calf muscle pump failure affecting 458–67, 510–18
   ulceration and 510–18
Micro-organisms in venous ulcers 523–4, 564–6, 583
Mid-calf communicating vein, ligation 221
Miles clips, inferior vena cava compression by 435
Milk oedema 9
Mobilization after varicose vein surgery 231
   see also Immobility
Mobin-Uddin umbrella 640
Monoclonal antibodies, radiolabelled, in thrombosis
   diagnosis 307
Monocytes and thrombosis development 275
Morgagni GB 9
Moulds of ulcer 532, 564
Movements, passive, in calf pump failure 495
MST (Borgnis system) 593–4, 594
Munchausen's syndrome 299
Muscle
   angiomata involving 740–1
   smooth, *see* Smooth muscle
   see also specific muscles
Mycobacterium spp.
   leprae (leprosy) 561
   tuberculosis 545
   ulcerans 554–5
Myositis, differentiation from calf pump failure 480
Myositis ossificans distinguished from thrombosis 299

N-A (non-adherent) dressing 577, 580
Naevus
   haemangioma 734
   of Klippel–Trenaunay syndrome 673, 674
      management 684–5
Neck veins, occlusion 689–709
Necrobiosis lipoidica 544–5
Necrosis
   cutaneous
      sclerosant-induced 236
      secondary to warfarin or activated protein C
         resistance 562
   fat 536

Necrotizing fasciitis 556
Negative test accuracy 68, 69
Nerve(s)
  angioma involving 741
  sclerosant injected into 236
  supply to veins 52–3
Neuropathic ulcers 544–5
Neurosurgery, thrombosis after 254
NF-κB and endothelial cell activation 262
Nitric oxide (and nitric oxide synthetase) and
    thrombosis aetiology 260
'No-tourniquet' technique in phlebography of
    thrombosis 304
Northern Ireland Troubles 712
Nuclear factor-κB and endothelial cell activation 262
Nuclear magnetic resonance, *see* Magnetic resonance
    imaging
Nutrition (individual), *see* Diet
Nutritional capillaries in calf pump failure syndrome
    464–5

Obesity
  thrombosis and 271
  venous ulcers and 519, 591
Oblique incisions for medial calf communicating vein
    approach, multiple 220
Obstruction and occlusion
  blood bypassing thrombosis-related, ways 445–6
  calf pump outflow tract, *see* Outflow tract
  deep veins, *see* Deep veins
  historical observation 6
  iatrogenic causes 723
  iliac veins, *see* Iliac veins; Iliac veins, external
    membranous 665–6
  physiological tests 183
  tumours causing, thrombosis distinguished from 297
  upper arm/neck veins 689–709
  vena cava, *see* Vena cava, inferior; Vena cava,
    superior
Occlusion (pathological), *see* Obstruction and occlusion
Occlusion (technique), *see* Vena cava, inferior
Occlusive and absorbent dressings 577–8
Occupation
  thrombosis and 270
  varicose veins and 155
Oedema (and swelling)
  ankle, *see* Ankle
  in calf pump failure syndrome 474
    reducing 493, 496–8
  in deep venous obstruction 389
  in Klippel–Trenaunay syndrome 676
  lymphatic, *see* Lymphoedema
  milk 9
  thrombosis distinguished from 299
  thrombosis-related 292
  in ulcer development 518
  venous, historical account 9
Oral anticoagulants (coumarins etc.)
  pulmonary embolism therapy 621–2
    cautions 623–4
  thrombosis prophylaxis (=primary prevention of
    pulmonary embolism) 360–1, 632
    complications 361

thrombosis therapy (=secondary prevention of
    pulmonary embolism) 348–51
  complications 349, 361
  dose 349
  indications 351
  interactions with other drugs 349
  monitoring 349
  in pulmonary embolism prevention 20
  results 350–1
Oral contraceptives, thrombosis risk 271
Oriental sore 554–5
Orthopaedic surgery, thrombophylaxis
  mechanical 369, 370
  pharmacological 360, 363, 365–6, 367, 623, 633–4, 636
  new drugs 367
Osmolality of contrast media 99
Ossifying myositis 299
Osteomyelitis, ulcers over 548–9
Osteoporosis with heparin 344
Ostial valves 385–6
Outflow, venous
  in Klippel–Trenaunay syndrome 678
  strain-gauge plethysmography in assessment of 118
  in venous obstruction 418
Outflow tract (of calf pump) 58
  incompetence 60, 61, 456–8
    calf pump function and effects of 456–8
    calf vein obstruction/incompetence combined with
      458
  obstruction (in general) 60–1, 456–8
    calf pump function and effects of 456–8
    calf vein obstruction/incompetence combined with
      458
    communicating vein incompetence in 448
  superficial compartment connection with 57
  thrombosis/thrombus in
    clinical sequelae 450–3
    treatment plan 353, 450–3
  see also Popliteal veins
Overstretching of veins 715
Oxpentifylline with ulcers 583
Oxygen, hyperbaric, with ulcers 591
Oxygenation, tissue
  in calf pump failure syndrome 464–5
  ulceration and 566
Oxyrutosides, *see* Rutosides

P-selectin 258
Paediatrics, thrombosis 367
Pain
  calf pump failure syndrome 473–4
  deep venous incompetence 389
  deep venous obstruction 389
  haemangioma 734
  relief (analgesia), after varicose vein surgery 231
  superficial thrombophlebitis 659, 661
  ulcers 531
  varicose veins 164–5
Palma operation 420, 491–2
  iliac vein injuries 722
Palpation 70
  varicose veins 173–6
Pancreatitis, recurrent panniculitis secondary to 562

Panniculitis secondary to pancreatitis, recurrent 562
Paradoxical embolus 291, 623
Parietal valves 385
Parkes Weber syndrome 671
  bone overgrowth 677
Parona F 15
Paroven, *see* Rutosides
Passive movements in calf pump failure 495
Past history of varicose vein patients 169
Paste bandages for ulcers 578
  historical account 10
Patch, venous 718–19
Patency, vein
  post-thrombosis 445–8, 449
  ultrasound in assessment of 121–2
Pelvic masses (tumours etc.) 745
  causing venous obstructing/compression 412
    thrombosis distinguished from 297
Pelvic veins
  aplasia 413
  phleboliths 681, 684
Pemphigoid 557, 558
Peptic ulcers, thrombolytics contraindicated with 323
Percussion 70
  varicose veins 175
Percutaneous approach/access
  caval filter placement 645
  varicose vein ligation, out-patient 237
Perfemoral phlebography in thrombosis 304
Perfron 577
Perfusion, tissue, reduced, venous ulceration and 517
Perfusion scans (lung) 108–9, 309, 611–13
Perimeter of ulcer, tracing 532, 564
Periostitis in calf pump failure syndrome 478
Peripheral arteries, *see* Artery
Peripheral heart, calf muscle as 57
Peripheral veins, physiological measurements,
    beginnings 16
Perl L 15
Permeability, dermal capillary
  in calf pump failure 459–61, 465
  ulceration and 512–16
Peroneal veins
  anatomy 31, 32
  ultrasound 83
Perthes, Georg 15
Perthes test 72
Pharmacotherapy, *see* Drugs
Phase contrast sequences (in MRI phlebography) 105
Phased array scanners (duplex ultrasound) 79
Phlebectomy hooks 224, 225
Phlebitis, infusion/injection 658, 661–2
Phlebography/venography (non-standard)
  computed tomography (non-standard), *see* Computed
      tomography
  isotope 101–3
  MRI, *see* Magnetic resonance imaging
  in thrombosis 304
Phlebography/venography (standard/x-ray contrast)
    87–108
  anatomy 30–47
  arm (for valve transplant) 393
  artefacts 97, 98

ascending (basic aspects) 86, 88–9
  in calf pump failure 482, 483
  caval occlusion (venous interruption) preceded by
      648–9
  complications 87, 99–100
  congenital vena caval obstruction 670
  contraindications 87, 301
  descending (basic aspects) 94–7
  development 16, 18, 20
  equipment 87
  haemangioma 734–5
  incompetence/reflux
    communicating veins 92, 181, 482
    deep veins 393
    sapheno-femoral junction 97
  indications 87, 301
  indirect 94
  intraosseous, *see* Intraosseous phlebography
  in Klippel–Trenaunay syndrome 678–81
  lower limb (in general) 88–9
  obstruction of deep veins 416–17
  thrombosis 87–99, 249–51, 301–4, 311, 649–51
    accuracy 302–4, 310
    advantages/disadvantages 301–2
    axillary/subclavian vein 696
    as epidemiological evidence 249–51, 252
    in heparin therapy, post-treatment 346–8
    inferior vena cava 431
    pulmonary embolism patients 637
    in thrombectomy, postoperative 333–4, 336–7
    in thrombolysis monitoring 323
    treatment approach based on phlebography 352–3,
        649–51
  ulcers 538–9
  ultrasound compared with 86
  upper limb, *see* Arm phlebography
  varicose veins, *see* Varicography
  vena cava, *see* Venocavography
Phleboliths
  deep venous angioma containing 736
  pelvic 681, 684
Phleborheography 127–8
  venous obstruction 417
Phlebothrombosis, historical concept 15, 18, 275
Phlegmasia alba dolens (white leg)
  historical accounts 9, 10
  thrombosis causing 293
    thrombectomy 339
Phlegmasia cerulea dolens 293
Phospholipids, autoantibodies 267–9
Photography 72–3
  infra-red 73
  ulcers 532, 564
Photoplethysmography (light reflection rheography)
    115–17
  ulcers 539
Physical examination, *see* Examination
Physical treatments, ulcers 583–4
Physiological shunts in calf pump failure syndrome 465
Physiology and physiological tests, *see* Function
Pig dermis 584
Pigmentation, causes
  calf pump failure syndrome 475

Pigmentation, causes (*contd*)
  varicose veins 169
  other 480–1
PIN stripping 207–8
Pinch grafts 584
Plantar flexion, ankle (equinus deformity)
  in calf pump failure syndrome 478
  with venous ulcers 572, 597
Plantaris muscle, torn 296
Plasmin
  early description of nature 17
  in thrombosis aetiology 261
Plasmin uptake test (radioactive) 78, 306
Plasminogen 261
  deficiency 267
  radiolabelled (uptake test) 306
Plasminogen activators, *see* Streptokinase; Tissue
    plasminogen activator; Urokinase
Plaster dressings for ulcers 11
Plastic sheets 578
Platelets
  in antiphospholipid syndrome 269
  in thrombosis
    in aetiology 259–60, 269
    in diagnosis, radiolabelled 307
  see also Thrombocytopenia; Thrombocytosis
Plethysmography 115–21, 127–9, 131, 307–8
  air 118–20
  calf pump assessment by 482
  in deep venous incompetence 391–3
  foot, *see* Foot volumetry
  impedance 128–9
  isotope, *see* Radioisotope plethysmography
  in Klippel–Trenaunay syndrome 678
  strain-gauge, *see* Strain-gauge plethysmography
  thrombosis
    axillary/subclavian 696
    deep venous 307–8
  ulcers 539
Plication of valves 397
Pneumatic compression, intermittent
  in thrombophylaxis 369–70, 373
  with ulcers 576–7, 584
Poliomyelitis 546
Polycythaemia rubra vera 534
Polytetrafluoroethyelene prostheses for inferior vena
    cava bypass 439
Polyurethane dressings 578
Polyurethane sheets 578
Popliteal fossa in sapheno-popliteal junction ligation
    212, 214, 215
Popliteal veins 33
  anatomy 33
  anomalies 33, 34
  compression, masses causing 413
  entrapment 686
    in Klippel–Trenaunay syndrome 686
    thrombosis distinguished from 299
  incompetence, ultrasound 390
  ligation 491
    accidental 414, 415
  occlusion
    calf pump function and effects of 457

  by thrombosis, *see subheading below*
  as outflow tract from calf pump, *see* Popliteal veins
    thrombosis
    calf pump function and effects of 457
    imaging 85, 97
    reopening after 447
    treatment plan 353
    ultrasound
      reflux 123, 126
      thrombosis 83, 85
    valves 29
  see also Sapheno-popliteal junction
Population surveys, thrombosis epidemiological
    information from 251
Porcine dermis 584
Positive test accuracy 68
Posterior calf approach (duplex ultrasound) 83
Postero-medial approach to calf (duplex ultrasound) 83
Postero-medial superficial veins of thigh 39
  ligation at sapheno-femoral junction regarding 201
Post-mortem evidence of thrombosis/pulmonary
    embolism epidemiology 251–2
Postoperative monitoring and care
  in varicose vein surgery 230–1
    stripping of long saphenous vein 210
    subfascial ligation of medial communicating veins
      217
  with venous injury repair 723
Post-thrombotic syndrome, *see* Calf muscle pump
    failure syndrome
Posture and varicose veins, 155
  see also Erect stance
Power Doppler 80
Praxorgoras of Cos 3
Pre-aortic lymph node disease, inferior vena cava
    obstruction in 430, 434
Pregnancy
  amniotic fluid embolism in/after labour 624
  oral anticoagulants in 350
  thromboembolism in 623–4
  thrombosis in 254, 270
  varicose veins of 153, 240
Pressure, venous 49–51
  calf pump and 57–8
  fibrinolytic activity and 54, 55
  measurement 49–50, 112–15
    in deep venous incompetence 391–3
    in femoral veins 114–15, 419
    in foot during exercise 58, 112–14
    historical account 9, 19
  ulcers and 511
    historical observations 10
  see also Hydrostatic pressure
Pressure, venular capillary, measurement, historical
    account 17
Pressure ulcers 553–4
Probe, ultrasound (positioning)
  in incompetence tests 123
  in patency assessment 121–2
Procoagulant effects of endothelium 261
Propaderm 582
Prostacyclins, endothelial 54
  thrombosis aetiology and 259

Prostaglandin infusions with ulcers 583
Prostatectomy, thrombosis after 253
Prostheses
  in iliac vein disobliteration 422
  inferior vena cava bypass 439
  valve 404
  see also Stenting
Protamine sulphate with heparin-induced bleeding
    343–4
Protein C
  activated, resistance 266
  deficiency 265–6
  resistance, activated, cutaneous necrosis caused by
    562
Protein S deficiency 266
Prothrombotic changes in endothelium 259
Psoriasis 558
Psthakis' substitute valve 401
Psychological effects of venous ulcers 572
Psychological factors in venous ulcers development 520
Psychological illness, self-induced ulceration 551–2
PTFE prostheses for inferior vena cava bypass 439
Pudendal artery, external, in ligation at sapheno-
    femoral junction 201
Pudendal vein in ligation at sapheno-femoral junction
  deep external 201
  superficial external 201
Pulmonary angiography/arteriography 109–11, 613
  of acute massive embolism 620
  indications 309
  magnetic resonance 112
Pulmonary arteries, CT 111–12
Pulmonary embolism (non-thrombotic) 624–5
Pulmonary embolism (thrombotic) 105–10, 309
  acute massive 607–9, 610, 614, 618
  acute minor 607, 610, 614
  with axillary vein thrombosis 695
  calf squeezing risk 122
  clinical features (signs/symptoms) 295, 300, 309,
    606–10
  diagnosis 616
    differential (and mimicking conditions) 611, 616,
      624–5
  epidemiology 251, 251–2, 606
  investigations 300, 309, 610–15, 616
    imaging 108–10, 309, 610–11, 611–15, 616
  in Klippel–Trenaunay syndrome 675
  management 300, 309, 615, 617–22, 623–4
  natural history/prognosis 616–17
  pathology 606
  pathophysiology 606–10
  peripheral vein examination with 130
  phlebography risk 101
  predisposing/risk factors 606–7
  in pregnancy 623–4
  prevention (in general) 622–3, 631–56
  prevention, primary, *see* Thrombosis
  prevention, secondary (=secondary prophylaxis with
      thrombosis) 319, 359, 636–51
    anticoagulants in 345–6, 350–1
    historical accounts 20
    thrombectomy in 335–6, 638–9
    thrombolysis in 327–8, 638–9

repair of venous injuries and risk of 724
sources, *see* Thrombosis
subacute massive 609, 614
thrombectomy-related risk 334–5
varicose vein treatment risk
  postoperative 230
  post-sclerotherapy 230
Pulmonary function test with pulmonary embolism 611
Pulmonary hypertension, chronic thromboembolic
    609–10, 617
  clinical features/pathophysiology 609–10
  differential diagnosis 616
  investigations 611, 613, 614
  treatment 621
Pulmonary scintigraphy 108–9, 611–13
Pulmonary thromboembolism, *see* Pulmonary embolism
Pulsed Doppler 79
Pulsed-echo ultrasound 79
Pyoderma gangrenosum 553
Pyogenic granuloma 559
Pyrexia with thrombosis 294

Race
  thrombosis and 270
  varicose veins and 154
Radiography
  abdominal, in Klippel–Trenaunay syndrome 681
  chest, *see* Chest
  haemangioma 734
  veins, *see* Phlebography
Radioisotope(s)
  fibrinogen labelled with, *see* Fibrinogen uptake test
  plasmin labelled with 78, 306
  in thrombosis diagnosis 306–7
Radioisotope plethysmography 129
  in deep venous incompetence 392
  in deep venous obstruction 418
Radioisotope scans/scintigraphy
  lung 108–9, 309, 611–13, 616
  veins (phlebography) 101–3
Radiology, *see specific methods/structures/conditions*
Real time transducers 79
Recanalization in thrombosis 445
Rectal bleeding in Klippel–Trenaunay syndrome 675,
    685
Red cells, Tc-99m-labelled 306
Red-line bandages 575
Reduplication, *see* Double veins
Re-epithelialization in venous ulceration 521–2, 522–3
Refilling, venous, after exercise, strain-gauge
    plethysmography in assessment of 118
Reflection of sound waves in Duplex ultrasound 79
Reflexes
  cardiovascular 54
  venoarteriolar, *see* Venoarteriolar reflex
Reflux, venous 389, 404–5
  communicating veins, *see* Communicating veins
  deep veins, *see* Deep veins
  popliteal, ultrasound 123, 126
  prevention (in calf pump failure syndrome treatment)
    486–91
  saphenous, *see* Sapheno-femoral junction; Sapheno-
      popliteal junction; Saphenous vein

Reflux, venous (*contd*)
  strain-gauge plethysmography in assessment of 118
  see also Incompetence
Regional anaesthesia, *see* Local and regional
    anaesthesia
Release II 577
Renal problems/investigations, *see* Kidney
Renal vein
  caval filter placement and 645
  left, injury 722
  leiomyosarcoma below 743, 744–5
  leiomyosarcoma between hepatic and 745
Reopening (patency) of veins after thrombosis 445–8,
    449
Reperfusion injury to skin 517
Respiration, venous blood flow and 59, 122
Rethrombosis, *see* Thrombosis
Retroperitoneal fibrosis
  iliac vein involvement 411
  inferior vena cava obstruction in 430, 433, 435
Retrosternal goitre 702, 703
Review, patient, varicose vein surgery 231
Rheography, *see* Phleborheography;
    Photoplethysmography
Rheumatoid arthritis 543–4
  calf pump failure syndrome distinguished from 481
  ulcers in 543–4
Rib
  cervical, *see* Cervical rib
  first, resection 699
Ring, valve, dilatation 388
Rodent ulcers (basal cell carcinoma) 541, 598
Rokitansky C 11
Romans (ancient) 3
Rutosides (Paroven)
  calf pump failure 496
  ulcers 583
  varicose veins 237
Rynd, Francis 10

S1Q3T3 pattern, pulmonary embolism 610
Sacrocardinal veins, anomalies 24–5, 25
Saline administration, thrombosis risk 271
Sapheno-femoral junction 56
  anatomy 199–200
  incompetence/reflux 482
    calf pump failure syndrome and 482
    diagnostic pathways 186–7, 482
    phlebography 97
    recurrent 226–9
    ultrasound 125, 178
  ligation at (ligation of long saphenous vein and its
      tributaries; high saphenous ligation) 195–204,
      487–8
    in calf pump failure syndrome treatment 487
    incision 197–8
    preparation 196–7
    procedure 198–202
    recurrence of varicosities following 226
    technical problems 202–4
    in ulcer recurrence prevention 592
Sapheno-popliteal junction 56
  incompetence/reflux

diagnostic pathways 186–7
    recurrence 229
    ultrasound 125, 178
  ligation and division (short saphenous ligation)
      210–15
    preparation 210–12
    problems 215, 415
    technique 212–14
    in ulcer recurrence prevention 592
Saphenous nerve damage (in stripping) 210
Saphenous vein (in general)
  pressure measurement at ankle 19
  reflux
    prevention (in treatment of calf pump failure
        syndrome) 487–8
    tests 178–9
  tributaries, diagnostic pathways with
      varicosities/dilatation of 186
  varicose, examination for 171, 172
    see also Saphenous vein, long; Saphenous vein,
        short
Saphenous vein, long 37–40
  anatomy 37–40
    variations 40, 200, 201
  ascending, thrombophlebitis 661
  dilatation
    in Klippel–Trenaunay syndrome 675
    of tributaries 186
  grafts for bypass operations 420–2, 422–5, 492
  imaging
    phlebography 92–3
    ultrasound 87
  incompetence
    surgical treatment, historical account 15
    test, historical account 10
  ligation of, and its tributaries, *see* Sapheno-femoral
      junction *and* tributaries (*subheading below*)
  stripping out, *see* Strippers; Stripping
  transposition (for valve replacement) 398
  tributaries 37, 39
    dilatation 186
    ligation 222–5
    see also Sapheno-femoral junction
    varicose, historical observations 14–15
  valves 29
  varicose 172
    tributaries, historical observations 14–15
Saphenous vein, short 40–1
  anatomy 40–1
    anomalies/variations 40–1, 210, 211
  incompetence, imaging 212–13
  ligation, *see* Sapheno-popliteal junction
  stripping 212–13
  tributaries, dilatation 186
  valves 29
  varicography 91, 212–13
Sarcoma
  Kaposi's 560
  soft-tissue, distinguished from thrombosis 299
  see also Leiomyosarcoma; Lymphangiosarcoma
Scannograms in Klippel–Trenaunay syndrome 681
Scar tissue, ulcers 525
Schenck 6

Schwartz test 175
Scintigraphy, *see* Radioisotope scans
Scleroderma 547
Sclerosants 232
    adverse reactions 235–6, 560–1
Sclerosis, diathermy 237
Sclerotherapy, injection 231–6
    calf pump failure 589
    with compression bandages 231–6
        aim 232
        complications 235–6
        contraindications 233
        indications 232–3
        results 238–9
        surgery compared with 238–9
        techniques 233–4
    duplex ultrasound-guided 235
    historical accounts 12
    ulcers 589
        in preventing recurrence 593
    varicose veins 231–6
Second World War, venous injuries 711
Selectins 258
Self-induced ulceration 551–2
Sensitivity reactions, anticoagulants
    intravenous 344
    oral 349
Septicaemia with ulcers 597
Septum, congenital 689, 690
Sequential complex arrays (duplex ultrasound) 79
Sequential linear arrays (duplex ultrasound) 79
Setopress 575
Sex, *see* Gender
Sharp S 9
Shearing, communicating vein 490
Shunts, physiological, in calf pump failure syndrome 465
Sickness Surveys/Surveys of Sickness, varicose veins in
    Canada 146
    Denmark 146
    UK 146
Sigvaris stockings 594, 595
Silastic foam 578
Simon nitinol filter 641
Sinus of valves 51, 387
    properties 387
    surgery 397–8
    thrombosis starting in 52
Sinusoidal veins (of calf/soleal muscles) 28, 29, 32
Skin 557
    in antiphospholipid syndrome 268–9
    in calf pump failure syndrome, changes/damage 459, 474–7
        surgical excision of damaged areas 500
    carcinomas, ulcerating 541–3, 598
    in deep venous incompetence, changes 390
    in deep venous obstruction, changes 390
    discoloration
        sclerosant-induced 236
        thrombosis-related 293
    extravasation of contrast media into 99, 101
    flaps, *see* Flaps
    grafts, *see* Grafts

inspection for changes 69
in Klippel–Trenaunay syndrome, changes 676
necrosis, *see* Necrosis
palpation for changes 70
preparation
    for sapheno-femoral junction ligation 196
    for sapheno-popliteal junction ligation 211–12
primary diseases 557
reperfusion injury 517
substitutes, with ulcers 584
telangiectases, *see* Intradermal venules, dilated
ulceration
    sclerosant-induced 236
    with venous abnormality, *see* Ulcers (venous)
varicose vein-related changes 191–2
    diagnostic pathways regarding 186–7
    prevention 193
see also Percutaneous approach
Sliding finger control 176
Slough (with venous ulcers)
    dissolution 581–2
    surgical excision 581
Smooth muscle
    tumours of 742–5
        clinical presentation 742–3
        investigations 743
        pathology 742
        treatment 743–5
    in varicose veins
        content 151
        hypertrophy 156
    venous tone and 52–3
Smooth muscle cells in valves 386
Sodium tetradecyl sulphate (sclerosant) 232, 233
    adverse reactions 236
Soft tissue, in Klippel–Trenaunay syndrome 673
    overgrowth/hypertrophy 673, 677–8
Soft-tissue sarcoma 299
Sofwick 577
Sole, deep veins 31
Soleal muscle, sinusoidal veins 28, 29, 32
Sorbsan 578
Sore(s)
    bed 553–4
    Oriental 554–5
Spider bursts/veins/webs, *see* Intradermal venules, dilated
Spiral CT
    lungs 109, 111, 615
    veins (phlebography) 104
        thrombosis 304
Split skin grafts
    in calf pump failure syndrome 500
    for ulcer repair 584–7
Sporotrichosis 562
Spurs, left common iliac vein 414
Squamous cell carcinomas 541–3, 598
Standing and varicose veins 155
Stanozolol (Stromba)
    in lipodermatosclerosis 497, 498–500, 582, 595–6
    in superficial thrombophlebitis 662
    with ulcers 582
        in preventing recurrence 595–6

Star(s), venous, *see* Intradermal venules, dilated
Starling EH 15
Stasis
   venous, thrombosis caused by 9, 262–3
   venular and capillary, ulceration caused by 510–12
'Stasis' ('gravitational'/'varicose') ulcers, historical
   accounts 7, 13, 16, 505, 509
Stem veins of calf 31, 32
Stenting (endovascular)
   axillary/subclavian vein 699–701
   common femoral vein 424
   iliac vein 422, 423
   vena cava
      inferior 440
      superior 704, 705, 707
Steroids, anabolic, *see* Anabolic steroids
Stewart–Treves lymphangiosarcoma 561
Stocking, compression, *see* Compression stockings
Stocking-seam incision 219–20
Stones, *see* Phleboliths
Strain-gauge plethysmography 117–18
   in venous obstruction 418
Streptokinase 320–1
   analogues 321
   dose 320
   failure related to adherence 325
   historical account of use 20
   monitoring 320–1
   in prevention of recurrent thrombosis 346
   pulmonary embolus 620, 621
Streptokinase uptake test (Tc-99m) 306
Stretching of veins 715
Strippers
   long saphenous vein stripping 204–7
      failure to pass 208
      inversion of vein by 209
      perforation of vein by 209
      PIN 207–8
      recurrent varicosities after 226
   short saphenous vein stripping 212
Stripping
   long saphenous vein 204–10
      contraindications 210
      historical account 15
      postoperative care 210
      problems 208–10
      technique 204–8
      in treatment of calf pump failure syndrome 487
   short saphenous vein 212–13
Stroke patients, thrombosis prevention 367
Stromba, *see* Stanozolol
Structure of veins 27–30
   walls, *see* Walls
Subcardinal veins in development 23, 24
Subclavian vein
   thrombosis 689–702
      aetiology 689–93
      clinical features 693–4
      diagnosis/investigations 100, 695–6
      differential diagnosis 694–5
      prognosis 701–2
      treatment 696–701
Subcutaneous calcification 559

Subcutaneous veins
   of lower limb (superficial)
      acting as collateral system 448
      in calf pump failure syndrome 458
      ulcers and 537
   tone 53
Subdiaphragmatic vena caval occlusion 670
Subfascial ligation of medial communicating veins
   (Linton's operation) 215–17
   complications 221
   endoscopic 217, 218, 219
Subfascial shearing of medial communicating veins
   220–1
Sucralfate, ulcers 583
Summer ulcers 559
Sunburst veins, *see* Intradermal venules, dilated
Superficial compartment of calf pump 55–7, 57
   communications 56–7, 57
      with deep compartment 56–7, 57
Superficial thrombophlebitis 168, 443, 455–6, 657–64
   aetiology 657–9
   clinical presentation 659
   diagnosis 659–60
   idiopathic 658–9
   investigations 659–60
   in Klippel–Trenaunay syndrome 675
   pathology 657–64
   prevention 193
   thrombosis coexisting with 294, 298
   thrombosis mistakenly diagnosed in 298
   treatment 660–1
Superficial veins (in general)
   anatomy in lower limb 37–43
      ligation at sapheno-femoral junction and 201
      variations/anomalies 40
   anatomy in upper limb 44, 45
   connections between deep and, *see* Deep veins
   haemangioma 738–40
   incompetence/insufficiency 61, 62, 453–4, 455–6, 457,
      506–8
      calf pump function and failure/post-thrombotic
         syndrome and role of 453–4, 457
      clinical features 69
      deep venous incompetence and, connection
         between 11
      isolated recurrent 229
      value of various tests 131
      venous ulceration and 506–8
   in Klippel–Trenaunay syndrome, surgery 683–4
   ligation 589–90
   obstruction
      calf pump function and effects of 457
      by thrombosis, *see* Superficial thrombophlebitis
   thrombosis-related warmness/distension 293
   varicose, special investigations 178–82
   in venous ulceration
      incompetence in the genesis of ulcers 506–8
      surgery 589–90, 592
Superoxide dismutase deficiency 559
Supracardinal veins in development 23, 24
Surgery (generally/unspecified/non-vascular)
   hyperfibrinolysis after 17
   iatrogenic damage caused by, *see* Iatrogenic causes

in Klippel–Trenaunay syndrome 685
  various operations 685, 686
thrombosis/thromboembolism after 252, 252–4, 264,
    270, 622–3
  epidemiological data 252, 252–4
  mechanical prevention 369, 370
  pharmacological prevention 18, 269, 360, 361–2,
      364–6, 367, 622–3, 633–4, 635–6, 636
  recognition historically 15
  treatment 18
  with varicose vein surgery 230, 253
thrombosis/thromboembolism before, epidemiology
  252
wounds of, *see* Wounds
Surgery (vascular and in venous disease)
  in calf pump failure 486–91, 589–91
    correction of abnormality 486–91, 589–91
    palliative 500
  earliest accounts 3
  incompetent veins 394–404, 589–90
    deep 394–404, 404, 405
    long saphenous, historical account 15
  injured veins 718–26
    complications 724–6
    history 718
    postoperative monitoring 723
    results 723–4
    techniques 718–21
  insufficiency, deep venous, first operation 15
  in Klippel–Trenaunay syndrome 683–4
  leiomyosarcoma 743–5
  long saphenous vein
    for incompetence, historical account 15
    stripping out, historical account 16
  obstruction
    deep veins 419–26
    inferior vena cava 437–8, 439–40
  pulmonary embolism 621
  of thrombosis
    in axillary/subclavian vein 699–701
    thrombus removal, *see* Thrombectomy
  thrombosis after 253
    after varicose vein surgery 230, 253
  ulcers 581, 589–91, 592–3
    historical accounts 2, 3, 7
    in preventing recurrence 592–3
  varicose vein 195–231, 237–8
    complications 202–4, 208–10, 215, 230, 253
    contraindications 195, 210
    historical accounts 3, 7, 8, 17
    recurrence after 187, 194, 225–30 *passim*
    results 237–8, 238–9
    sclerotherapy compared with 238–9
  see also specific techniques
Survey of Sickness, *see* Sickness Surveys
Sutilains 582
Sutures
  in injured veins, lateral 718
  venous injury caused by 716
Swelling, *see* Oedema
Sympathectomy
  in calf pump failure 496
  with ulcers 591

Sympathetic innervation of veins 52, 53
Synergistic bacterial gangrene 556
Synthaderm 578
Syphilitic ulcers 537, 549–50
Systemic lupus erythematosus 547
Systemic sclerosis (scleroderma) 547
Systole, calf pump in 57–8

T wave inversion, pulmonary embolism 610
Tape measurement of ulcers 563–4
Tear, inferior vena cava 721
Technetium-99m
  albumin microaggregates labelled with 307
  fibrinogen labelled with 307
  lung scans 611
  phlebography 101–3
  plasmin uptake test 78, 306
  platelets labelled with 307
  red cells labelled with 306
  streptokinase uptake test 306
Telangiectases, cutaneous
  sclerotherapy-induced 236–7
  with varicose veins (birch sprig/twig; dilated
      intradermal venules; spider bursts/veins/webs;
      sunburst veins; venous stars) 164, 165, 241
    in calf pump failure syndrome 474–5
    treatment 241
Telfa 577
Tenderness
  in calf pump failure syndrome 473–4
  palpation 70
  thrombosis-related 292
Tendonitis, Achilles 299
Tension with compression stockings, measurement
    593–5
Tensopress 575, 579–80
Teratogenicity, oral anticoagulants 350
Tests, *see* Investigations *and specific tests*
Thermography 73–6
  liquid crystal 75–6
  thrombosis 74–5, 308
Thermoregulation 53
Thiersch grafts 584–7
Thigh
  colour duplex ultrasound 82
  deep veins
    anatomy 33–7
    masses compressing 413
  superficial veins of
    antero-lateral, *see* Antero-lateral superficial veins
    ligation at sapheno-femoral junction regarding 201
    postero-medial, *see* Postero-medial superficial veins
Thrombectomy/thrombus removal 319–20, 329–40,
    638–9, 697–9
  axillary/subclavian vein 697–9
  complications 334–5
  historical accounts 16, 17, 18
  indications 337–8
  inferior vena cava 339–40, 437–8
  for phlegmasia alba dolens 339
  preparation 330
  results 335–7
  technique 330–4

Thrombectomy/thrombus removal (*contd*)
  thrombolysis combined with 340
  venous injury and 720
Thrombin-antithrombin III complex assay 611
Thromboangiitis obliterans, thrombosis risk 271
Thrombocytes, *see* Platelets
Thrombocytopenia
  in antiphospholipid syndrome 269
  heparin-induced 344, 363, 605–6, 619
  thrombolysis contraindicated in 323
Thrombocytosis 269
Thromboembolic pulmonary hypertension, chronic, *see*
    Pulmonary hypertension
Thromboembolism, pulmonary, *see* Pulmonary
    embolism
Thrombolysis (natural) 84
Thrombolysis (pharmacological) 319–20, 320–9, 619–21,
    638–9
  administration techniques, new 329
  agents used 320–1
  anticoagulation compared with 328
  axillary/subclavian vein thrombosis 699
  complications and their prevention/treatment 321–2
  contraindications 322–3
  duration/termination 323–4
  historical accounts 19, 20
  indications 329
  inferior vena cava thrombus 437
  pulmonary embolus 619–21
  results 324–8
    factors affecting 324–7
    long-term 328
  thrombectomy combined with 340
Thrombomodulin (in thrombosis aetiology) 260
  defects/deficiencies 266
Thrombophilia 264–7
Thrombophlebitis 168, 271, 294, 298
  historical concept 15, 18, 275
  superficial, *see* Superficial thrombophlebitis
Thrombophlebitis migrans 659
  secondary 662
Thromboplastin time, activated partial, heparin dose
    and 341
Thrombosis
  axillary/subclavian vein, *see* Axillary vein; Subclavian
    vein
  deep venous, *see* Thrombosis, deep venous
  superficial venous, *see* Superficial thrombophlebitis
  superior vena caval, *see* Vena cava, superior
Thrombosis, deep venous (or venous thrombosis in
    general) 249–383, 444–58, 490–2
  bed rest and 20
  causes 254–72
    fibrinolytic system, *see* Fibrinolytic activity
    historical accounts 9, 11, 15, 255
    intimal injury 11
    postoperative, *see* Surgery
    predisposing/risk factors 269–72, 454–5
    sclerotherapy 236
    secondary, *see subheading below*
    stasis, *see* Stasis
  damaging/destructive effects (post-thrombotic
    damage) 17, 183–5, 444, 445

tests detecting 183–5
ulcers as 507
valvular, *see* Valves
definition 249
diagnosis 291–317
  differential 295–9, 480
  method for estimating probability 295
  missed 128
  mistaken 97, 98
epidemiology 249–54
fibrinogen uptake test, *see* Fibrinogen uptake test
function of veins affected by 444–54
imaging 81, 301–7, 615, 637
  contrast phlebography, *see* Phlebography
    (standard)
  CT phlebography 103–4
  isotope phlebography 101, 102, 103
  thermography 74–5, 308
  ultrasound, *see* Duplex ultrasound; Ultrasound
inferior vena cava, *see* Vena cava, inferior
investigations/tests 293, 301–10, 615, 637–8
  accuracy 310
  clinical application/rationale 81, 308–10
  imaging, *see subheading above*
  value 130
palpation 70
pathology 249–89, 444–58
phlegmasia alba dolens caused by 10
postoperative, *see* Surgery
previous, as risk factor for recurrence 271
prophylaxis (primary = prevention of thrombosis)
    359–83, 622–3, 632–6
  historical account 18, 19
  in Klippel–Trenaunay syndrome 686
  mechanical methods 368–71, 372, 636
  pharmacological 18, 19, 269, 360–8, 372, 622–3, 632–6
  postoperative, *see* Surgery
prophylaxis (secondary = prevention of embolism
    from thrombosis), *see* Pulmonary embolism
recurrence (rethrombosis) 301
  anticoagulants in prevention of 346–7, 351
  post-thrombectomy 334–5
  previous thrombosis as risk factor for 271
  streptokinase in prevention of 346
risk of
  hospital patients at 300
  prediction 371–2
  see also causes (*subheading above*)
secondary causes 429–30, 723
  obstruction 416
sequelae, *see* Calf muscle pump failure syndrome
signs 291–5, 299–301, 310
  discriminant value 295
  practical significance 299–301
silent, historical description 15
in sinus of valve 52
site of origin/source 275–6, 637–8
  affecting treatment success 326–7
  historical accounts 11, 12
symptom(s) 291, 295, 299–301, 310
  discriminant value 295
  inferior vena cava thrombosis (acute and chronic
    thrombosis) 430–1

practical significance 299–301
treatment/relief 319, 336
symptomatic, historical description 15
treatment 319–58, 490–2, 649–51
objectives 319
of postoperative thrombosis 18
varicose veins and, *see* Varicose veins
webs following 414
see also specific veins
Thrombus, deep vein 273–5
adherence 444, 445
thrombolysis and effects of 325
treatment plan based on 353
development of new channels through 445
formation/development/progression 255, 273–5, 444–5
in valve pockets 262
imaging 72–108, 130
phlebography 97–9
radioisotope, historical account 21
ultrasound 83–6, 130
in lung, *see* Pulmonary embolism
lysis/dissolution, *see* Thrombolysis
nature, tests determining 130
pathology, historical accounts 16
removal, historical accounts 16, 17, 18
retraction 444
squeezing of calf and risk of detachment of 122
in thrombolytic therapy (factors affecting success) 324–7
adherence 325
age 324
site 326–7
Thrombus, intracardiac 323
Thusane 575
Thyroid gland, retrosternal, enlarged 702, 703
Tibial veins
anterior
anatomy 31–2, 32, 37
ultrasound 83
posterior
anatomy 31, 32
ultrasound 83
Time of flight sequences (in MRI phlebography) 105
Tissue(s)
fluid production, principle underlying, historical explanations 15
oxygenation, *see* Oxygenation
perfusion, *see* Perfusion; Reperfusion injury
Tissue factor 260
Tissue factor pathway inhibitor 261
Tissue plasminogen activator 321
early description 19
in thromboembolic disease aetiology 261–2, 275–6
in thromboembolic disease therapy
pulmonary embolus 620, 621
thrombosis 321
Tissue plasminogen activator inhibitor in thrombosis aetiology 261–2
Tone, venous 52–4
drugs increasing, in calf pump failure 496–8
first use of term 6
Tophi, gouty 559
Topical applications, venous ulcers 581–2

Tourniquet
below-knee, below-knee varices not controlled by 186–7
phlebography of lower limb 88, 89
Tourniquet (Brodie–Trendelenburg) test 71–2
varicose veins 176–7
Towelling, *see* Drapes
Toxic reactions to sclerosant 235
Toxic substances causing venous injury/phlebitis 658, 716
Trace elements and ulceration 566
Transducers (duplex ultrasound) 79, 79–80
Transections of veins 714
Transmural pressure reduction 195, 492–5
Transplants, valve 398–401, 402–4, 490
arm phlebography for 393
in calf pump failure syndrome 490
experimental 402–4
technique 400–1
see also Grafts
Transposition, valve 398
in calf pump failure syndrome 490–11
Transverse incisions for medial calf communicating vein approach, multiple 220
'Trash foot' 550
Traumatic injury, *see* Injury
Travase 582
Trendelenburg F 15
see also Tourniquet (Brodie–Trendelenburg) test
Trental with ulcers 583
Treponema pallidum (syphilis) 537, 549–50
Treponema pertenue (yaws) 561
Tricotex 577
Tropical ulcers 554–5
Tuberculosis, ulcers associated with 545
Tubigrip 575, 579–80
Tubular bandages 575
Tularaemia 562
Tumours 541–3, 731–46
malignant, *see* Malignant tumours
mesodermal, ulcerating 560
smooth muscle, *see* Smooth muscle
venous obstruction and compression caused by
externally compressing tumours 297, 410, 412, 413, 416–17
intramural tumours 413–14
thrombosis distinguished from 297
thrombosis risk 429, 430, 436
venous spread (within lumen), historical accounts 9, 15
venous wall, *see* Wall
see also Masses *and specific histological types*
Tunica adventitia 27
Tunica intima 27
injury causing thrombosis, historical account 11
Tunica media 27, 28
venous tone and 52–3

UK Survey of Sickness (England and Wales 1950), varicose vein 146
Ulcers (non-venous disease-related)
arterial 537, 539–60
gastrointestinal, thrombolytics contraindicated with 323

Ulcers (non-venous disease-related) (*contd*)
skin, sclerosant-induced 236, 561
traumatic 518, 540–1
self-induced 551–2
Ulcers (venous) 505–603
aetiology 508–21, 532
calf pump failure 479, 508–10, 589–91
base/surface 522, 534–5
clinical features 531–7
definition 505
differential diagnosis 539–62
edge 534
effect on patient 572
epidemiology 505–8, 571
examination/assessment 532–7, 562–6
general 532
local 69, 173, 532–5, 562–6
healed/scar 525
healing 534, 535, 596
agents encouraging 582
time to, factors influencing 563, 591–2
infection and, *see* Infection
investigations 537–9, 562–6
in Klippel–Trenaunay syndrome 676
natural history/general effects 525, 571–3
pathology 521–5
post-thrombotic 507
recurrent/previous 591–8
causes 592
history of 531–2
prevention 591–8
repair 521
shape 533
site 533
size 533, 562–4
healing time and 563, 591–2
measurement 532–3, 533, 562–4
skin with
associated changes (and their causes) 520, 596–7
breakdown, causes 518–20
surrounding, *see subheading below*
surrounding skin and tissues 535–6
dermatological preparations 582
treatment 573–91
of complications and associated conditions 596–8
historical accounts, *see* History
objectives 573
with varicose veins 169, 508–9
bleeding 168
diagnostic pathways regarding ulcers 186–7
examination 173
historical accounts of connections 6, 7, 10, 13–14, 508–9
prevention 193
'varicose'/'gravitational', historical accounts 7, 13, 16, 505, 509
other historical accounts 10
Ultrasound (cardiac), pulmonary embolism 611
Ultrasound (Doppler) 78–87, 121–7
in calf pump failure 482, 483
compared with other imaging techniques 86–7, 130, 131
duplex, *see* Duplex ultrasound

haemangioma 734
incompetence, venous 123–6, 131, 390–1
communicating 124–6, 179–82, 482
deep 390–1
obstructed deep veins 417
pulsed-echo 79
thrombosis 305–6
axillary/subclavian vein 696
deficiencies 123
ulcers 538
varicose veins
deep veins 183
superficial veins 178–82, 213
Ultrasound (therapeutic), ulcers 584
Ultraviolet light treatment, ulcers 584
United Kingdom Survey of Sickness (England and Wales 1950), varicose vein 146
United States of America National Surveys (1935–36/1959–61), varicose vein 145–6
Unna boot 11
Unsightliness of varicose veins, *see* Cosmetic aspect
Upper limb veins 44
anatomy 44–7
anatomy, variations 45
in Klippel–Trenaunay syndrome 679, 683
development 26–7
imaging
phlebography, *see* Arm phlebography
ultrasound 81–2
injuries 722
occlusion (in upper arm) 689–709
physiology 62
Upstream compression 124
Urate crystals 559
Ureter, retrocaval 25, 27
Uric acid crystals 559
Urokinase
as thrombolytic 321
dose 321
monitoring 321
pulmonary embolus 620, 621
with ulcers 582
Urological surgery, thrombosis after 253
prevention
mechanical 370
pharmacological 362, 365
USA National Surveys (1935–36/1959–61), varicose vein 145–6
UV treatment, ulcers 584

Valsalva manoeuvre
ascending phlebography 89, 90
function 386–7
ultrasound assessment of valvular incompetence 123–4
Valves, venous 28–30, 51–2, 385–408
incompetence, *see* Incompetence
pathology 387–9
congenital 148, 387, 669
thrombosis-related, *see subheading below*
phlebography (lower limb) 89, 90
physical/mechanical properties 52, 386
pockets, thrombus formation in 262

spatial arrangement/distribution 51, 386
structure/anatomy 28–30, 51–2, 385–6
   historical descriptions/drawings 5, 16
surgery 394–404, 590–1
   in deep vein post-thrombotic incompetence/reflux
      490–1
     principles/aims 394–5
     reparative, *see* Valvuloplasty
     replacement 394, 398–404, 490–1
     with venous ulcers 590–1
thrombosis-related damage/effects 84–6, 388–9, 444,
    448–9
   historical account 12–13
with varicose veins
   as aetiological factors 147–8, 150, 152
   pathology 156
see also specific veins
Valvulitis 388
Valvuloplasty (valve repair) 394
   direct 395–6, 398
   indirect 397–8, 398
   with venous ulcers 590–1
Varicography (phlebography) 89–92, 179, 182–3
   defining extent and connections of varicosities 182–3
   recurrent varicosities 182, 227–8
   superficial veins 181
     short saphenous incompetence 212–13
   ulcers 539
'Varicose' ulcers, historical accounts 7, 13, 16, 505, 509
Varicose veins 145–248
   aetiology 147–55
     secondary (predisposing) factors 153–5
   anatomical distribution (of varices) 156–7, 171
     left leg greater incidence 148, 155
     recording 171
   appearance, first illustration 1
   complications, *see* symptoms (*subheading below*)
   definition 145
   diagnosis 163–89
     differential 163, 164, 167
     pathways 185–7
     of recurrence 226–9
   epidemiology 145–7
   extent and connections of varicosities, definition 182–3
   fibrinolytic activity in 454
   historical perspectives 16, 508–9
     surgery 3, 7, 8, 17
   investigations, special 178–82
     deep veins 183–5
     phlebography, *see* Varicography
     superficial veins 178–82
     thermography 76
   in Klippel–Trenaunay syndrome 171, 673–6
   natural history (of untreated/uncomplicated veins)
     191–3
   pathology 156–8
   physical signs 169–77
   in pregnancy 153, 240
   primary 178
     aetiology, *see subheading above*
     historical recognition 16
   recurrence (after treatment) 187, 193–4, 225–30
     diagnosis 226–9

     measurement 237
     postoperative 187, 194, 225–30 *passim*
   residual 225
   saphenous, *see* Saphenous vein
   secondary 178
     aetiology 155
     historical recognition 16
   symptoms and complications 158, 163–9
     determining that varicose veins are cause of 178
     prevention 193
     treatment/relief 178, 193, 194–5, 237, 241
   thrombophlebitis in 660–1
   thrombosis and 183–5, 661
     association 271
     varicose veins as result of post-thrombotic damage
      183–5
     varicosities following thrombosis 474
   treatment 178, 193–241
     decisions 192–3, 195
     objectives 193–4
     patient satisfaction 239
     results 237–9
     surgical, *see* Surgery
     of symptoms and complications 178, 193, 194–5,
      237, 241
   ulcers and, *see* Ulcers; Varicose ulcers
   vulval 240
Varidase 581
Vascular malformations 668
Vascularized free flaps 588–9
Vasculature
   endothelium, *see* Endothelium
   loss of integrity 258
   surgery, *see* Surgery (vascular)
Vasculitis 547–8, 557
   livedo, *see* Livedo reticularis
   thrombosis risk 271
   ulcers with 547–8, 557
Vasoconstriction
   local venoarteriolar, 53
   see also Venoarteriolar reflex
   thrombosis aetiology and 260
Vasodilation, thrombosis aetiology and 259–60
   see also Dilatation
Vasodilatory drugs, ulcers 583
Vasovagal attacks with sclerotherapy 235
Vena cava, inferior 36–7
   anatomy 36–7
   bypass operation 439–40, 671
   development 24
   developmental anomalies 24–5, 26
     aplasia 24, 26, 670
     double 24, 25, 666, 668
     hypoplasia 24, 666, 667
     membranous occlusion 666
   imaging
     CT phlebography (of thrombosis) 103–4
     standard phlebography, *see* Venocavography
     ultrasound 83
   injury 721–2
   leiomyosarcoma 743
     surgery 744–5
   ligation 639

Vena cava, inferior (*contd*)
  occlusion/blockade, deliberate (=venous interruption)
      438, 622, 639–49
    filters for, *see* Filters
  occlusion/obstruction (pathological) 429–41, 437–40
    aetiology/pathology 429–31, 433
    chronic 431, 438–9
    clinical presentation 430–1
    collateral circulation 36–7, 38, 415–16
    congenital 670–1
    investigations 73, 431–7
    prognosis 440–1
    treatment 437–40
  thrombosis 429–30, 437–40
    acute spontaneous/idiopathic 429, 437
    imaging 103–4
    secondary 429–30, 438–40
    symptoms (of acute and chronic thrombosis) 430–1
    treatment 339–40, 437–40
Vena cava, superior
  development 24
    anomalies 25–6
  imaging
    phlebography (superior venocavography) 88
    ultrasound 81
  occlusion and thrombosis 702–7
    aetiology 702–4
    clinical features 704–5
    investigations 705–7
Vena Tech filter 641
Venoarteriolar reflex 53
  overactivation 517
Venocavography
  inferior 88, 431–3
  superior 88
Venoconstriction of subcutaneous veins 53
Venodilation of subcutaneous veins with local heating 53
  see also Dilatation
Venography, *see* Phlebography
Venoplasty, axillary/subclavian 699–700
Venotomy (incision)
  long saphenous vein ligation 197–8
  popliteal (in short saphenous vein stripping) 197–8
  thrombectomy 331
Venotonic drugs in calf pump failure 496–8
Ventilation–perfusion scans 108–9, 309, 611, 612, 616
Venules
  in calf pump failure syndrome 459, 474–5
  dilated intradermal, *see* Intradermal venules
  see also Capillaries
Verneuil A 11, 508
Vertebral venous system 46–7
Vesalius, Andreas 5
Vietnam War 711–12
Vigilon 578
Violence, venous injury due to 711–14
Virchow R 11, 12
Viscopaste 579, 580
Vitamin K$_1$ in anticoagulant-related bleeding 349
Volume
  blood, *see* Blood volume
  calf, strain-gauge plethysmography in assessment of
      changes in 117–18
  foot, assessment, *see* Foot volumetry

Von Strauch M 15
Von Willebrand factor and thrombosis 261
V/Q scans 108–9, 309, 611, 612
Vulval varicosities 240

Wall, venous 27–8
  congenital deficiencies (aplasia etc.) 669–70
    obstruction with 413
  enzymatic changes in varicose veins (and patients'
      relatives) 157–8, 669–70
  fibrinolytic activator, *see* Fibrinolytic activator
  inferior vena cava obstruction with pathology of 430
  inflammation, *see* Inflammation
  structure 27–8, 50
    defects 148–9
  tumours 413, 731–2, 742–5
    historical account 15
    infiltrating 658
    obstructing 413
    primary 731–2, 742–5
  venous pressure and 50
  see also Transmural pressure
War, venous injury 711–13
Warfarin 320, 348–51 *passim*
  cutaneous necrosis caused by 562
  dose 349
  results 351
Warmness in superficial veins, thrombosis-related 293
Weakness, of calf (muscle) pump 59
Webs
  congenital 689, 690
  left common iliac vein 414
  post-thrombosis 414
Weible–Palade bodies 258, 261
Weight
  varicose veins and 154
  with venous ulcers, reduction 591
Welch WH 15
White C 9
White atrophy, *see* Atrophie blanche
White blood cell, *see* Leucocyte
White leg, *see* Phlegmasia alba dolens
WHO definition of varicose veins 145
Wisemann, Richard 7
Woolsorter's disease 562
World Wars, venous injuries 711
Wounds
  arterial puncture, recent, thrombolytics
      contraindicated with 322
  surgical
    fresh, thrombolytics contraindicated with 322
    infection in varicose vein surgery 230

Xenografts, valve, experimental 404
X-ray, *see* Radiography
XXY syndrome and venous ulcers 520

Yaws 562
Yellow Emperor's Classic of Internal Medicine 2

Zahn, lines of, thrombus development and 273
Zinc (and ulceration)
  deficiency 566, 582
  supplements 582